The Johns Hopkins Internal Medicine Board Review 2010–2011: Certification and Recertification

THIRD EDITION

Redonda G. Miller, MD, MBA
The Johns Hopkins University School of Medicine
Baltimore, MD

Bimal H. Ashar, MD, MBA
The Johns Hopkins University School of Medicine
Baltimore, MD

Stephen D. Sisson, MD
The Johns Hopkins University School of Medicine
Baltimore, MD

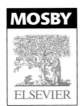

MOSBY

ELSEVIER

MOSBY
ELSEVIER

1600 John F. Kennedy Blvd.
Ste 1800
Philadelphia, PA 19103-2899

THE JOHNS HOPKINS INTERNAL
MEDICINE BOARD REVIEW 2010-2011, THIRD EDITION

ISBN: 978-0-323-06875-8

Notices

Knowledge and best practice in this field are constantly changing. As new research and experience broaden our understanding, changes in research methods, professional practices, or medical treatment may become necessary.

Practitioners and researchers must always rely on their own experience and knowledge in evaluating and using any information, methods, compounds, or experiments described herein. In using such information or methods they should be mindful of their own safety and the safety of others, including parties for whom they have a professional responsibility.

With respect to any drug or pharmaceutical products identified, readers are advised to check the most current information provided (i) on procedures featured or (ii) by the manufacturer of each product to be administered, to verify the recommended dose or formula, the method and duration of administration, and contraindications. It is the responsibility of practitioners, relying on their own experience and knowledge of their patients, to make diagnoses, to determine dosages and the best treatment for each individual patient, and to take all appropriate safety precautions.

To the fullest extent of the law, neither the Publisher nor the authors, contributors, or editors, assume any liability for any injury and/or damage to persons or property as a matter of products liability, negligence or otherwise, or from any use or operation of any methods, products, instructions, or ideas contained in the material herein.

Library of Congress Cataloging-in-Publication Data

Johns Hopkins internal medicine board review 2010–2011 : certification and recertification / [edited by] Redonda G. Miller, Bimal H. Ashar, Stephen D. Sisson.—3rd ed.
    p. ; cm.
  Includes bibliographical references and index.
  ISBN 978-0-323-06875-8
  1. Internal medicine. 2. Internal medicine—Examinations, questions, etc. 3. Physicians—Certification. I. Miller, Redonda G. II. Ashar, Bimal H.   III. Sisson, Stephen D. IV. Johns Hopkins University. V. Title: Internal medicine board review.
  [DNLM: 1. Internal Medicine—Examination Questions. 2. Internal Medicine—Outlines. WB 18.2 J652 2010]
  RC46.J57 2010
  616.0076—dc22

                                                    2009027369

Acquisitions Editor: Druanne Martin
Developmental Editor: Taylor Ball
Project Manager: Bryan Hayward
Marketing Manager: Helena Mutak
Design Direction: Steve Stave
Multi-Media Producer: Paul Coker

Printed in China

Last digit is the print number: 9 8 7 6 5 4 3 2 1

With the assistance of our publisher, Elsevier, we are pleased to offer the third edition of *The Johns Hopkins Internal Medicine Board Review*. The strength of any book of this type ultimately hinges on the quality of its contributors; in this regard, we are quite fortunate, as each chapter has been written by an accomplished faculty member with extensive knowledge of the topic discussed. The book is divided into sections weighted according to the level of emphasis on the American Board of Internal Medicine certifying examination, with additional coverage of the related (and also tested) fields of psychiatry, dermatology, and ophthalmology. Our format is unique in that it features comparative tables and decision algorithms, which lend themselves to ease of study and quick review. The book also includes a link to an exclusive Web site that provides practice questions and answers that are patterned after those seen on the actual board examination and that stress important "take home" points and allow self-assessment of knowledge retention.

In many ways, this book is the product of more than a century of medical teaching at Johns Hopkins. In the late 19th century, Sir William Osler developed the modern concept of an internal medicine training program during his tenure as the first Chair of Medicine at The Johns Hopkins Hospital. He became famous for his bedside teaching and instituted the practice of "rounds," which remains the principal method of clinical instruction in use today. Among Dr. Osler's many achievements during his remarkable life was the completion of his magnum opus, *The Principles and Practice of Medicine,* which was the first textbook to systematically categorize and describe disease with a measure of precision and clarity that had not previously been seen. In the words of Osler, "Books are tools, doctors are craftsmen, and so truly as one can measure the development of any particular handicraft by the variety and complexity of its tools, so we have no better means of judging the intelligence of a profession than by its general collection of books."

We hope you find the text to be a worthy addition to your preparation materials.

The Editors

Deborah K. Armstrong, MD
Associate Professor of Oncology
Johns Hopkins University School of Medicine

Bimal H. Ashar, MD, MBA
Associate Professor of Medicine
Johns Hopkins University School of Medicine

John N. Aucott, MD
Instructor of Medicine
Johns Hopkins University School of Medicine

Paul G. Auwaerter, MD
Associate Professor of Medicine
Johns Hopkins University School of Medicine

Ronald D. Berger, MD, PhD
Professor of Medicine
Johns Hopkins University School of Medicine

Gail Berkenblit, MD, PhD
Assistant Professor of Medicine
Johns Hopkins University School of Medicine

Katherine E. Black, MD
Pulmonary and Critical Care Fellow
Johns Hopkins University School of Medicine

Dionne Blackman, MD
Assistant Professor of Medicine
University of Chicago Medical Center

Roger S. Blumenthal, MD
Professor of Medicine
Director of Johns Hopkins Ciccarone Preventive Cardiology Center
Johns Hopkins University School of Medicine

L. Ebony Boulware, MD, MPH
Associate Professor of Medicine
Johns Hopkins University School of Medicine

Todd T. Brown, MD
Assistant Professor of Medicine
Johns Hopkins University School of Medicine

Marcia I. Canto, MD, MHS
Associate Professor of Oncology
Johns Hopkins University School of Medicine

Michael A. Carducci, MD, FACP
Professor of Oncology
Co-Director, Prostate Cancer/GU Oncology Program
Co-Director, Chemical Therapeutics
Johns Hopkins University School of Medicine

Amina A. Chaudhry, MD, MPH
Adjunct Assistant Professor of Medicine
Johns Hopkins University School of Medicine

Michael J. Choi, MD
Associate Professor of Medicine
Johns Hopkins University School of Medicine

Colleen Christmas, MD
Assistant Professor of Medicine
Johns Hopkins University School of Medicine

John O. Clarke, MD
Assistant Professor of Medicine
Johns Hopkins University School of Medicine

David S. Cooper, MD
Professor of Medicine
Johns Hopkins University School of Medicine

Mary Corretti, MD
Associate Professor of Medicine
Medical Director, Adult Echoardiography Laboratory
Johns Hopkins University School of Medicine

Sara E. Cosgrove, MD, MS
Assistant Professor of Medicine
Johns Hopkins University School of Medicine

Andrew DeFilippis, MD
Cardiology Fellow
Johns Hopkins University School of Medicine

Amy DeZern, MD
Instructor of Medicine
Johns Hopkins University School of Medicine

Susan E. Dorman, MD
Associate Professor of Medicine
Johns Hopkins University School of Medicine

M. Bradley Drummond, MD
Fellow, Division of Pulmonary and Critical Care Medicine
Johns Hopkins University School of Medicine

Kerry B. Dunbar, MD
Assistant Professor of Medicine
Johns Hopkins University School of Medicine

James P. Dunn, MD
Associate Professor of Ophthalmology
Johns Hopkins University School of Medicine

Michelle M. Estrella, MD
Assistant Professor of Medicine
Johns Hopkins University School of Medicine

Derek M. Fine, MD
Associate Professor of Medicine
Johns Hopkins University School of Medicine

John A. Flynn, MD, MBA, FACP, FACR
Professor of Medicine
Clinical Director, Division of General Internal Medicine
Medical Director, Spondyloarthritis Program
Co-Director, The Osler Center for Clinical Excellence at
    Johns Hopkins
Johns Hopkins University School of Medicine

Lawrence B. Gardner, MD
Assistant Professor
Departments of Medicine (Hematology) and Pharmacology
Langone Medical Center
New York University School of Medicine

Allan C. Gelber, MD, PhD
Associate Professor of Medicine
Director, Johns Hopkins Rheumatology Fellowship
    Program
Johns Hopkins University School of Medicine

Jonathan M. Gerber, MD
Instructor of Medicine
Johns Hopkins University School of Medicine

Michael Goggins, MD
Professor of Medicine
Johns Hopkins University School of Medicine

Sherita H. Golden, MD, MHS
Associate Professor of Medicine
Johns Hopkins University School of Medicine

Elizabeth A. Griffiths, MD
Hematology/Oncology Fellow
Sidney Kimmel Comprehensive Cancer Care Center
Johns Hopkins University School of Medicine

Thomas B. Habif, MD
Adjunct Professor of Medicine
Dartmouth Medical School

James P. Hamilton, MD
Assistant Professor of Medicine
Johns Hopkins University School of Medicine

Hans Hammers, MD, PhD
Assistant Professor of Oncology
Johns Hopkins University School of Medicine

Maureen R. Horton, MD
Associate Professor of Pulmonary and
    Critical Care Medicine
Johns Hopkins University School of Medicine

Carol Ann Huff, MD
Assistant Professor of Oncology
Johns Hopkins University School of Medicine

Mark T. Hughes, MD, MA
Assistant Professor of Medicine
Johns Hopkins University School of Medicine

H.A. Jinnah, MD, PhD
Acting Professor
Department of Neurology
Emory University School of Medicine

Clarissa Jonas, MD
Fellow, Department of Nephrology
Johns Hopkins University School of Medicine

Yvette L. Kasamon, MD
Assistant Professor of Oncology and Medicine
Johns Hopkins University School of Medicine

Edward K. Kasper, MD, FAHA, FACC
Professor of Medicine
Director of Clinical Cardiology, E. Cowles Andrus
    Professor in Cardiology
Johns Hopkins University School of Medicine

Rebecca A. Kazin, MD
Assistant Professor of Dermatology
Johns Hopkins University School of Medicine

Thomas W. Koenig, MD
Assistant Professor of Psychiatry and Behavioral Sciences
Associate Dean for Student Affairs
Johns Hopkins University School of Medicine

Paula Kue, MD
Instructor of Medicine
Johns Hopkins University School of Medicine

Sophie M. Lanzkron, MD
Assistant Professor of Medicine
Johns Hopkins University School of Medicine

Linda A. Lee, MD
Assistant Professor of Medicine
Director, Johns Hopkins Integrative Medicine & Digestive
    Center
Clinical Director, Division of Gastroenterology and
    Hepatology
Johns Hopkins University School of Medicine

Anne Marie Lennon, MD
Advanced Endoscopy Fellow
Johns Hopkins University School of Medicine

Mark Levis, MD, PhD
Associate Professor of Oncology
Johns Hopkins University School of Medicine

Howard Levy, MD, PhD
Assistant Professor of Medicine
Johns Hopkins University School of Medicine

Hyung M. Lim, MD
Instructor of Medicine
Johns Hopkins University School of Medicine

Rafael H. Llinás, MD
Associate Professor of Neurology
Johns Hopkins University School of Medicine

Meredith C. McCormack, MD
Assistant Professor of Medicine
Johns Hopkins University School of Medicine

Christian A. Merlo, MD, MPH
Assistant Professor of Medicine
Johns Hopkins University School of Medicine

Redonda G. Miller, MD, MBA
Associate Professor of Medicine
Vice-Chair for Clinical Operations,
    Department of Medicine
Johns Hopkins University School of Medicine

Kristi Mizelle, MD, MPH
Rheumatology Fellow Physician
Johns Hopkins School of Medicine

Kimberly S. Peairs, MD
Assistant Professor of Medicine
Johns Hopkins University School of Medicine

David B. Pearse, MD
Associate Professor of Medicine
Johns Hopkins University School of Medicine

Brent G. Petty, MD
Associate Professor of Medicine
Johns Hopkins University School of Medicine

Albert J. Polito, MD
Assistant Professor of Medicine
Johns Hopkins University School of Medicine

Gregory P. Prokopowicz, MD, MPH
Assistant Professor of Medicine
Johns Hopkins University School of Medicine

Rosanne Rouf, MD
Tufts-New England Medical Center

Sarbjit S. Saini, MD
Associate Professor of Medicine
Johns Hopkins University School of Medicine

Roberto Salvatori, MD
Associate Professor of Medicine
Johns Hopkins University School of Medicine

Joseph Savitt, MD, PhD
Assistant Professor of Neurology
Director, Johns Hopkins Movement Disorder Fellowship
    Program
Director, Johns Hopkins Ataxia Center
Johns Hopkins University School of Medicine

Paul Scheel, Jr., MD, MBA
Associate Professor of Medicine
Director, Division of Nephrology
Johns Hopkins University School of Medicine

Cynthia L. Sears, MD
Professor of Medicine
Johns Hopkins University School of Medicine

Philip Seo, MD, MHS
Assistant Professor
Johns Hopkins University School of Medicine

Jonathan Sevransky, MD
Assistant Professor of Medicine
Johns Hopkins University School of Medicine

Tariq Shafi, MBBS, MHS
Instructor of Medicine
Johns Hopkins University School of Medicine

Mary Sheu, MD
Assistant Professor of Dermatology
Johns Hopkins University School of Medicine

Stephen D. Sisson, MD
Associate Professor of Medicine
Johns Hopkins University School of Medicine

B. Douglas Smith, MD
Associate Professor of Oncology
Johns Hopkins University School of Medicine

Lisa A. Spacek, MD, PhD
Assistant Professor of Medicine
Johns Hopkins University School of Medicine

C. John Sperati, MD, MHS
Assistant Professor of Medicine
Johns Hopkins University School of Medicine

Michael B. Streiff, MD
Associate Professor of Medicine
Medical Director, The Johns Hopkins Hospital Special
    Coagulation Laboratory
Attending Physician, The Johns Hopkins Hospital
    Comprehensive Hemophilia Treatment Center
The Johns Hopkins University School of Medicine

Tariq Shafi, MBBS, MHS
Assistant Professor of Medicine
Johns Hopkins University School of Medicine

Aruna Subramanian, MD
Assistant Professor of Medicine
Johns Hopkins University School of Medicine

Peter B. Terry, MD, MA
Professor of Medicine
Associate Professor of Medicine
Johns Hopkins University School of Medicine

Christine Tompkins, MD
Johns Hopkins University School of Medicine

Thomas A. Traill, MD, FRCP
Professor of Medicine
Johns Hopkins University School of Medicine

Rainer von Coelln, MD, PhD
Johns Hopkins University School of Medicine

Erica Warlick, MD
Fellow of Hematology and Oncology
Johns Hopkins University School of Medicine

Robert A. Wise, MD
Professor of Medicine
Johns Hopkins University School of Medicine

Ilan S. Wittstein, MD
Assistant Professor of Medicine
Johns Hopkins University School of Medicine

Robert J. Wityk, MD
Associate Professor of Neurology
Johns Hopkins University School of Medicine

Tao Zheng, MD
Assistant Professor of Medicine
Johns Hopkins University School of Medicine

Carol M. Ziminski, MD
Associate Professor of Medicine
Johns Hopkins University School of Medicine

CONTENTS

SECTION ELEVEN Selected Topics in General and Internal Medicine

Maximizing Test Performance: Effective Study and Test-Taking Strategies

DIONNE BLACKMAN, MD

Research has identified a number of factors that affect test performance:
- Study skills
- Content knowledge
- Practice of questions in the same format as the test
- Test-taking skills
- Anxiety
- Fatigue and sleep deprivation

By reading this book, the exam taker will improve content knowledge and have the opportunity to test this knowledge with many case-based practice questions. This chapter, however, addresses the three topics not related to content knowledge: study skills, test-taking skills, and anxiety. The strategies provided will make studying for the Board Examination more effective and optimize test performance on the exam.

Strategies for More Effective Studying

Anticipate Test Content

- **Review the examination blueprint to understand the percentage of questions derived from each content area (available on the Web site for the American Board of Internal Medicine [ABIM] at www.abim.org)**
- **Complete the tutorial on taking the computer-based exam, which you can download from the ABIM Web site. The tutorial sample questions will familiarize you with the different types of exam questions and with the exam format. Specifically, you will preview how to**
  - Answer questions
  - Change answers
  - Make notes electronically
  - Access the table of normal laboratory values
  - Mark questions for review
- Board Examination questions are derived using the following criteria and will:
  - **Be patient-focused**
  - Address important clinical problems for which medical intervention has a significant effect on patient outcomes

  - Address commonly overlooked or mismanaged clinical problems
  - Pose a challenging management decision
  - Assess ability to make optimal clinical decisions
- Maintenance of Certification examination questions will not address clinical problems normally referred in practice or recent clinical advances before they are widely used in practice
- Clinical decision-making can be broken down into different tasks; the Board Examination is meant to test your ability to perform these tasks:
  - Identify characteristic clinical features of diseases
  - Identify characteristic pathophysiologic features of diseases
  - Choose the most appropriate diagnostic tests
  - Determine the diagnosis
  - Determine the prognosis or natural history of diseases
  - Select the best treatment or management strategy
  - Choose risk-appropriate prevention strategies
- **Board Examination questions will never address an area in which there is no consensus of opinion among experts in the field**
- Carefully review visual information, as this is frequently used in Board Examination questions regarding disorders with characteristic skin lesions or findings on blood smear, bone marrow, electrocardiogram, radiographs, and other visual diagnostic tests

Time Management

- **Use the Residency In-Training Examination or a full-length practice test (as on the Web site accompanying this book) to identify your areas of weakness**
- Complete practice tests in your weaker subjects first to identify specific gaps in content knowledge to address by a focused review of these subjects
- Use a "question drill to content review" ratio of 2:1 or greater to review subjects, as this has been shown to be more successful than traditional review using the reverse ratio (see McDowell 2008)
- After addressing your weaker subjects, conduct a focused review of other subjects as discussed earlier
- Create a realistic study schedule and stick to it!

- Using the examination blueprint, budget your study time to cover all of the examination content areas without last-minute cramming
- **Plan to complete your study several days before the examination**
- **Plan a question drill period for the last few days before the examination. Use answers to incorrectly answered practice questions for targeted content review.**

Effective Approaches to Studying

- The Survey, Question, Read, Recite, Review (SQ3R) Study Method has proven effective in improving reading efficiency, comprehension, and material retention
  - It provides a useful way to study for the Board Examination, regardless of study resource used
  - Steps in the method are outlined in Table 1-1
- Studying with a small group can enhance study effectiveness by providing social support and increased confidence as individuals assume responsibility to review and teach particular areas to the group

Strategies for More Effective Test Taking

The following strategies will only be effective if practiced, so plan to practice them in your question drill sessions; the Web site accompanying this book allows exam takers to practice answering questions in a timed test format.

Strategies for Time Use

- Know the examination schedule for the computer-based examination (see www.abim.org)
- **Return from breaks 10 minutes early. You must check in after breaks, and the examination clock restarts at the end of the break regardless of your return time.**
- Know the time allotted per exam question (i.e., exam time in minutes divided by number of exam questions). This is about 2 minutes per question based on the maximum 60 questions allowed per 2-hour board exam session.
- Budget your time; unfinished questions are lost scoring opportunities
- Keep track of your use of time by checking time targets at each quarter of the total exam time
- To fully use other test-taking strategies, use less than the allotted time per question (we suggest 15–30 seconds less per question)

- **To focus on pertinent data, read the question and answer options before reading the question stem (the stem is the part of the test item that precedes the question and answer options and is usually case-based)**
- Answer questions you know first and quickly guess on those you don't know

Strategies for Guessing and Reasoning

- Identify key words or phrases that affect the question's intent (e.g., at this time, now, initially, most, always, never, except, usually, least)
- Determine whether the following factors limit your thinking to certain disease categories:
  - Patient factors
    - Age, sex, race, or ethnicity
    - Habits (e.g., smoking, alcohol or illicit drug use)
    - Exposures due to occupation, travel, or residence
    - Immune status
  - Factors related to illness presentation
    - Time course of illness (i.e., acute, subacute, or chronic)
    - Symptoms or findings present or stated to be absent
    - Pattern of diagnostic data (e.g., presence of a known symptom triad, pathognomic finding)
- Eliminate answer options likely to be incorrect. Remember that incorrect options are usually written to be plausible or even partially correct.
- Examine similarities and differences between answer options (e.g., mutually exclusive options)
- Answer questions based on established standards of care, not anecdotal experiences (many current guidelines are available at National Guideline Clearinghouse at www.guideline.gov)
- Do not be afraid to use partial knowledge to eliminate answers
- When unsure of an answer, enter your best guess (research shows it is often correct) and flag the question on the computer for later review
- **Answer all questions—there is no penalty for wrong answers**

Strategies for Changing Answers

- Spending less than the allotted time per exam question allows you to finish exams early. This extra time allows you to benefit from answer changing.
- **Despite "conventional wisdom," research shows most test-takers benefit from answer changing**
- You are more likely to change from a wrong to a right answer if you:
  - Reread and better understand the test item
  - Rethink and conceptualize a better answer
  - Gain information from another test item
  - Remember more information
  - Correct a clerical error (e.g., the intended answer was not the entered answer)

Strategies for Error Avoidance

- Read each question and all answer options carefully. Be certain you understand the intent of the question before answering (e.g., questions stating "all of the following are correct except …").
- Do not "read into a question" information or interpretations that are not there

TABLE 1-1	SQ3R Study Method
Step	**Description**
Survey	Survey section headings and summaries first
Question	Convert headings, legends, and board examination tasks into "questions"
Read	Read to answer your "questions"
Recite	Recite answers and write down key phrases and cues
Review	Review notes, paraphrase major points, draw diagrams, and make flashcards for material that is difficult to recall

- Check that the answer entered is the answer you intended

Strategies for Anxiety Reduction

- Anxiety is a natural part of taking an examination, but high test anxiety will adversely affect test performance
- Consider formal counseling if you have had problems with high test anxiety in the past
- Actively manage anxiety by decreasing the effect of unknowns on your anxiety level:
  - **Test drive the travel route and time to the test site; locate parking and the site itself if it is in a building with other businesses.**
  - **Bring a sweater or dress in layers to prepare for examination room temperature variations**
  - **Bring a snack for unexpected hunger and medications for potential illness symptoms**
- Allow a minimum of 30 minutes before your test appointment for check-in procedures (see www.abim.org for details regarding check-in)
- Avoid overly anxious test takers; they heighten your anxiety level, which can hurt your test performance.

- Use relaxation techniques:
  - Deep muscle relaxation is an effective relaxation technique; it involves tensing and relaxing each muscle group until all muscles are relaxed.
  - To reduce anxiety further, engage in exercise during the period when you are preparing for the examination
- Being well-rested is imperative

SUGGESTED READINGS

Frierson HT, Hoband D: Effect of test anxiety on performance on the NBME Part I Examination, *J Med Educ* 62:431–433, 1987.

Frierson HT, Malone B, Shelton P: Enhancing NCLEX-RN performance: assessing a three-pronged intervention approach, *J Nurs Educ* 32:222–224, 1993.

Harvill LM, Davis III G: Test-taking behaviors and their impact on performance: medical students' reasons for changing answers on multiple choice tests, *Acad Med* 72:S97–S99, 1997.

Hembree R: Correlates, causes, effects, and treatment of test anxiety, *Rev Educ Res* 58:47–77, 1988.

McDowell BM: KATTS: a framework for maximizing NCLEX-RN performance, *J Nurs Educ* 47:183–186, 2008.

Robinson FP: *Effective study*, rev. ed. New York, Harper & Row, 1961.

Seipp B: Anxiety and academic performance: a meta-analysis of findings, *Anxiety Research* 4:27–41, 1991.

Waddell DL, Blankenship JC: Answer changing: a meta-analysis of the prevalence and patterns, *J Cont Educ Nurs* 25:155–158, 1994.

SECTION ONE

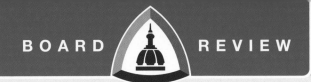

Cardiology

Hypertension

GREGORY PROKOPOWICZ, MD, MPH

Hypertension is present in more than 25% of the general population, and with the aging of the population and the increase in obesity, its prevalence is expected to increase. Hypertension is an important risk factor for many common diseases including stroke, end-stage renal disease, congestive heart failure, and myocardial infarction, and it is the most common modifiable cardiac risk factor. Aggressive control of blood pressure (BP) results in a significant decline in morbidity and mortality.

Basic Information

- Definition of hypertension
  - **Hypertension is defined as a BP of 140/90 mm Hg or higher (i.e., a systolic BP of ≥140 mm Hg, a diastolic BP of ≥90 mm Hg, or both; Table 2-1)**
    - The classification of BP applies to patients not taking antihypertensives and without acute illness (which may raise or lower BP); patients taking antihypertensive medication are considered to have hypertension.
  - BP of 140–159/90–99 mm Hg is designated as stage 1 hypertension, and BP greater than or equal to 160/100 mm Hg as stage 2 hypertension
    - If the systolic and diastolic BPs fall in different stages, the higher stage is used (e.g., a BP of 182/95 mm Hg is categorized as stage 2)
  - **BP of 120–139/80–89 mm Hg is designated as prehypertension**
    - Prehypertension is a risk category, not a disease— patients in this category are at high risk of progressing to actual hypertension and should be targeted for lifestyle modification
  - **Hypertensive urgency refers to severe hypertension requiring prompt initiation of treatment, but without acute end-organ dysfunction**
    - There is no agreed-upon BP that defines hypertensive urgency
    - Patients with hypertensive urgency may present with headache, anxiety, or medication nonadherence
  - **Hypertensive emergency implies elevated BP with acute end-organ dysfunction (Table 2-2)**
    - Although hypertensive emergency is not defined by any specific level of BP, most patients have BPs greater than or equal to 160/120 mm Hg
- Epidemiology
  - **Hypertension affects more than 60 million Americans and is the most common modifiable cardiac risk factor**
  - Hypertension is more prevalent among African Americans, who also suffer more end-organ damage

TABLE 2-1	*Classification of Blood Pressure (BP)*		
Category	Systolic BP (mm Hg)		Diastolic BP (mm Hg)
Normal	<120	and	<80
Prehypertension	120–139	or	80–89
Hypertension			
Stage 1	140–159	or	90–99
Stage 2	≥160	or	≥100

Adapted from The Seventh Report of the Joint National Committee on Prevention, Detection, Evaluation, and Treatment of High Blood Pressure. *JAMA* 289:2560–2572, 2003.

- There is a graded relationship between the level of BP and the incidence of stroke, end-stage renal disease, congestive heart failure, and ischemic heart disease
  - Below age 50, diastolic BP is the most important predictor of cardiovascular outcomes; **above age 50, systolic BP is the most important predictor**
- BP and the prevalence of hypertension rise with age (Fig. 2-1)
  - Systolic BP rises continuously; diastolic BP rises until approximately age 50 years and then declines
  - Isolated systolic hypertension (i.e., systolic > 140 mm Hg and diastolic < 90 mm Hg) is common among the elderly and is an important cardiovascular risk factor
  - Patients with prehypertension have an increased risk of progression to hypertension with aging
- Pathophysiology
  - **Most patients (>90%) do not have an identifiable cause of hypertension; this is commonly referred to as essential hypertension**
  - BP is the product of cardiac output and peripheral vascular resistance; although increased cardiac output may play a role in the initiation of hypertension, most patients with long-standing hypertension have increased peripheral resistance with normal or diminished cardiac output.
  - Certain persons respond more strongly to changes in sodium intake and extracellular fluid status and are described as salt-sensitive; salt-sensitivity occurs more commonly among African Americans and the elderly
  - End-organ damage from hypertension affects the kidneys, heart, vasculature, brain, and eyes (Table 2-3)

TABLE 2-2	*Manifestations of Acute End-Organ Damage in Hypertensive Emergency*
Hypertensive encephalopathy	Headache Altered mental status Seizures Nausea, vomiting Papilledema (see Fig. 2-2) Abnormalities on brain MRI
Intracranial hemorrhage	Headache Altered mental status Focal neurologic abnormalities Hemorrhage on brain CT
Unstable angina	Chest pain ECG abnormalities
Acute myocardial infarction	Chest pain ECG abnormalities Cardiac enzyme elevation
LV failure with pulmonary edema	Dyspnea Hypoxia Pulmonary congestion on chest radiograph
Acute aortic dissection	Chest pain Syncope End-organ ischemia
Eclampsia	Proteinuria Seizures

CT, computed tomography; ECG, electrocardiograph; LV, Left ventricular; MRI, magnetic resonance imaging.

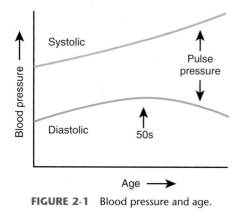

FIGURE 2-1 Blood pressure and age.

Clinical Presentation

- Most patients are asymptomatic
- Some may already have evidence of target organ damage at first presentation (see Table 2-3)
- Occasionally, patients may present with hypertensive urgencies or emergencies (see Table 2-2)

Diagnosis and Evaluation

- Measurement of BP
  - Use appropriate cuff size: The bladder of the cuff should encircle 80% or more of the arm without overlapping; use of a cuff that is too small may cause falsely elevated readings.
  - The patient should refrain from smoking or consuming caffeine for 30 minutes and sit quietly for 5 minutes before measurement
  - The arm in which BP is being measured should be supported and relaxed at the level of the heart
  - At each clinical visit, the BP should be taken at least twice, or until successive readings are within 5 mm Hg of each other
  - BP should be measured in both arms, and the higher of the two readings used
  - Systolic BP is measured at the first appearance of Korotkoff sounds and diastolic pressure at the disappearance of sounds
  - Two or more readings on each of two separate clinical visits should be obtained before classifying a patient as hypertensive
  - In elderly patients, or when orthostatic hypotension is suggested, standing BP measurements should be taken
  - For home BP monitoring, BPs above 135/85 mm Hg are considered hypertensive. For 24-hour ambulatory BP monitoring, an average BP above 130/80 mm Hg is considered hypertensive
- Goals in initial evaluation of the hypertensive patient
  - Assessment of **target organ damage** (Fig. 2-2; see also Table 2-3)
  - Identification of comorbidities
    - Diabetes mellitus (DM)
    - Chronic kidney disease (CKD)
    - Ischemic heart disease and cardiomyopathy

TABLE 2-3	*Clinical Manifestations of Chronic Target Organ Damage in Hypertension*
Heart	Left ventricular hypertrophy
	Enlarged PMI or S$_4$ gallop
	Evidence of LVH on ECG or echo
	Left ventricular dysfunction
	Signs/symptoms of CHF
	Enlarged PMI or S$_4$ gallop
	Systolic or diastolic dysfunction on echo
	Coronary artery disease
	Angina
	History of MI, PTCA, or CABG
Brain	Cerebrovascular disease
	History of stroke
	Carotid bruit
Eyes	Retinovascular disease
	Arteriolar narrowing
	Arteriovenous nicking
	Hemorrhage
	Exudates
Vasculature	Atherosclerosis
	Claudication
	Diminished or absent pulses
	Renal or femoral bruits
Kidneys	Hypertensive nephrosclerosis, ESRD
	Proteinuria or microalbuminuria
	Elevated serum creatinine

CABG, coronary artery bypass graft; CHG, congestive heart failure; ECG, electrocardiograph; echo, echocardiography; ESRD, end-stage renal disease; LVH, left ventricular hypertrophy; MI, myocardial infarction; PMI, point of maximum impulse; PTCA, percutaneous transluminal coronary angioplasty.

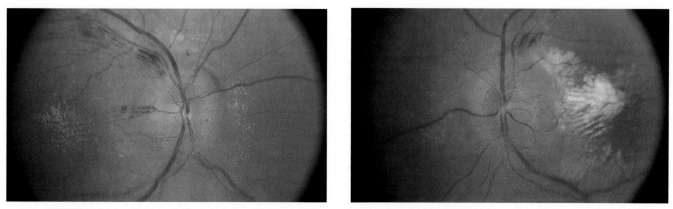

FIGURE 2-2   Papilledema in hypertension. (From Yanoff M: *Ophthalmology,* ed 2, Philadelphia, Mosby, 2004, figure 113-7.)

- Other cardiac risk factors: cigarette smoking, dyslipidemia, older age, obesity, physical inactivity, family history
- Identification of identifiable (secondary) causes of hypertension (see following discussion)
- Recommended laboratory tests for initial evaluation
  - Serum creatinine, sodium, potassium, fasting glucose
  - Urinalysis with microscopic examination
  - Electrocardiogram (or echocardiogram)
  - Fasting lipid profile
  - Optional: Serum calcium, thyroid-stimulating hormone

- Identifiable (secondary) causes of hypertension (Table 2-4)
  - When to consider secondary hypertension
    - **Sudden onset of hypertension in a previously normotensive patient**
    - **Age, history, physical examination, severity of hypertension, or initial laboratory findings suggesting a specific cause (see Table 2-4)**
    - **Recurrence of hypertension in a case of well-controlled hypertension (nonadherence should also be considered)**
    - **Resistant hypertension (defined as persistent hypertension on a regimen containing three or more drugs, including a diuretic)**

TABLE 2-4	*Major Causes of Secondary Hypertension*		
Pathophysiology	**Clinical Presentation**	**Diagnosis**	**Treatment**
Renal Artery Stenosis			
Underperfused kidney produces excess renin, which increases angiotensin II (vasoconstriction) and aldosterone (sodium retention and volume expansion) Usually due to atherosclerosis, especially in older patients May also be caused by fibromuscular dysplasia (FMD), usually in younger patients	Sudden onset of significant hypertension at older (>55 yr) or younger (<30 yr) age Abdominal bruit Patient with peripheral vascular disease Unexplained deterioration in renal function Consider FMD in young females Unusually large drop in BP with ACE inhibitors or ARBs may also suggest the diagnosis	Magnetic resonance angiography—highly sensitive, no contrast required CT angiography—highly sensitive, contrast is required Doppler ultrasound—sensitivity dependent on operator skill, no contrast required Captopril radionuclide scan—less sensitive, requires discontinuation of antihyper-tensive medications prior to test Renal artery angiography—gold standard, invasive, may be performed with CO_2 to avoid use of iodinated contrast	Goal is to improve HTN control and preserve renal function; revascularized patients usually still require medication for BP control Lesions usually progress if untreated The longer stenosis has been present, the less likely intervention will help (kidney becomes atrophic) Options Angioplasty ± stent (lesions at ostia of renal arteries often not amenable to angioplasty) Surgical bypass Surgical excision of kidney if size < 8 cm Medical therapy may be best option if recovery of renal function is unlikely
Pheochromocytoma			
Tumors that originate in the adrenal medulla or sympa-thetic ganglia and release catecholamines periodically "Rule of 10": 10% are outside the adrenals, 10% are malignant, 10% are bilateral, 10% are familial, 10% recur after resection Familial forms MEN IIA and B Neurofibromatosis von Hippel-Lindau disease (with retinal angiomas, cere-bellar hemangioblastomas, and renal cell carcinoma)	Headache Sweating Palpitations Pallor Anxiety Weight loss Orthostatic hypotension Hypertension may be episodic or sustained	Screen with 24-hour urine for catecholamines, VMA, metanephrines—best done after patient experiences symptoms Certain drugs may cause false-positive or false-negative screens If screen is positive, localize with MRI (or MIBG if MRI negative)	Surgical resection Preoperatively, patients should receive phentolamine or phenoxybenzamine to prevent crisis
Hyperaldosteronism (see Chapter 42)			
Adenoma that produces aldosterone vs. bilateral hyperplasia (zona granulosae) Rarely, aldosterone-producing carcinoma	Spontaneous hypokalemia in a hypertensive patient (may cause cramps, muscle weakness) Severe hypokalemia induced by diuretics Mild metabolic alkalosis	Screen with plasma aldosterone and renin serum—ratio of aldosterone to renin > 20 suggests disease Confirm by measuring 24-hour urine aldosterone after 3 days of salt loading: >12 µg confirms disease If screen positive, localize with CT or MRI; adrenal vein sampling	Surgical resection of adenoma May try spironolactone for hyperplasia
Hypercortisolism (see Chapter 42)			
Several possible causes ACTH-secreting pituitary tumor (Cushing's disease) Adrenal adenomas Ectopic ACTH secretion Iatrogenic steroid administration	Truncal obesity Moon facies Purple striae Proximal weakness Hirsutism Hyperglycemia Osteoporosis	Screen with 24-hour urinary free cortisol, salivary cortisol, or 1 mg overnight dexamethasone suppression test If positive, perform high-dose dexamethasone suppression test and measure plasma ACTH Localize with imaging of adrenals or pituitary	Surgical resection of tumor or discontinuation of steroid therapy

ACTH, adrenocorticotropic hormone; ACE inhibitors, angiotensin-converting enzyme inhibitors; ARB, angiotensin receptor blocker; BP, blood pressure; CT, computed tomography; FMD, fibromuscular dysplasia; HTN, hypertension; MEN, multiple endocrine neoplasia; MIBG, iodine-131-meta-iodobenzylguanidine; MRI, magnetic resonance imaging; VMA, vanillylmandelic acid.

- Substances that may cause or worsen hypertension
  - Alcohol (use or withdrawal)
  - Amphetamines, cocaine
  - Over-the-counter medications (decongestants, diet pills, nonsteroidal anti-inflammatory drugs)
  - Prescription medications (nonsteroidal anti-inflammatory drugs, oral contraceptives, cyclosporine, erythropoietin)
  - Supplements (ephedra)
  - Licorice (inhibits metabolism of endogenous cortisol to cortisone)
- Other correctable causes of hypertension
  - Acute pain or stress in hospitalized or institutionalized patients
  - Obstructive sleep apnea has a graded relationship with the development of hypertension
  - Hyperthyroidism or hypothyroidism can be associated with hypertension
  - Renal disease may increase BP because of renin oversecretion and impaired sodium excretion
  - Coarctation of the aorta may (rarely) present in adulthood
    - Delayed femoral pulses, diminished BP in the legs, and rib notching on chest radiograph suggest the diagnosis

- CT, MRI, or angiography confirms the diagnosis
- Treatment is with surgery or angioplasty

Treatment

- Initial follow-up of BP
  - The timing of follow-up for elevated BP depends on the degree of elevation (Table 2-5)
  - The suggested follow-up intervals may need to be shortened if important risk factors (e.g., diabetes) or target organ damage are present
- Risk stratification, goal BP, and therapy
  - Choice of therapy depends on the stage of hypertension and the presence of risk factors or target organ damage (Table 2-6)
  - Joint National Committee on Prevention, Detection, Evaluation, and Treatment of High Blood Pressure (JNC VII) guidelines recommend initiation of two drugs for stage 2 hypertension
  - **Goal BP is 130/80 mm Hg for DM, CKD, or coronary artery disease (CAD) and 120/80 mm Hg for congestive heart failure (CHF); otherwise, the goal is 140/90 mm Hg**
  - DM, CKD, or clinical cardiovascular disease mandates drug therapy for hypertension of any stage

TABLE 2-5	*Initial Management of Blood Pressure*	
INITIAL BP (mm Hg)		
Systolic	**Diastolic**	**Recommended Follow-up**
<120	<80	Recheck in 2 yr
120–139	80–89	Recheck in 1 yr*
140–159	90–99	Confirm within 2 mo*
160–179	100–109	Evaluate or refer within 1 mo
≥180	≥110	Evaluate and treat immediately or within 1 wk, depending on clinical situation and complications

*Provide advice about lifestyle modification.
Adapted from The Seventh Report of the Joint National Committee on Prevention, Detection, Evaluation, and Treatment of High Blood Pressure: Hypertension. *JAMA* 42:1206, 2003.

TABLE 2-6	*Treatment Recommendations by Risk Group*		
		INITIAL DRUG THERAPY	
Blood Pressure Classification	**Lifestyle Modification**	**No Compelling Indication**	**Compelling Indication(s) Present**
Normal (<120/80 mm Hg)	Encourage	None	None
Prehypertension (120–139/80–89 mm Hg)	Yes	None	Appropriate drug(s) for DM, CKD, or CAD if BP > 130/80 mm Hg, for CHF if BP > 120/80 mm Hg
Stage 1 (140–159/90–99 mm Hg)	Yes	Thiazide diuretic for most; may consider other drug classes	Appropriate drug(s) for compelling indication
Stage 2 (≥160/≥100 mm Hg)	Yes	Two-drug combination for most, including thiazide diuretic	Two-drug combination for most, usually including appropriate drug(s) for compelling indication

BP, blood pressure; CAD, coronary artery disease; CHF, congestive heart failure; CKD, chronic kidney disease; DM, diabetes mellitus.
Adapted from The Seventh Report of the Joint National Committee on Prevention, Detection, Evaluation, and Treatment of High Blood Pressure. *JAMA* 289:2561, 2003.

- DM, CKD, or CAD warrants drug therapy (in addition to lifestyle modification) for BP greater than 130/80 mm Hg
- Lifestyle modification
  - **Always start with lifestyle modification even if drug therapy is also needed**
  - Weight reduction of 10 pounds or more
  - 30 minutes or more of moderately intense physical activity (e.g., brisk walking) four or more times a week
  - Moderation of alcohol intake (1 ounce or less of alcohol per day in men, ½ ounce in women)
  - Low sodium intake (100 mmol/day, i.e., 6 g NaCl or 2.4 g Na⁺, or less)
  - Adoption of diet high in fruits, vegetables, and low-fat dairy products: Dietary Approaches to Stop Hypertension (DASH) eating plan
  - Smoking, caffeine acutely raise BP, but have not been demonstrated to cause chronic hypertension; smoking cessation and lipid modification are important for decreasing overall cardiovascular risk
  - Relaxation therapy and stress management is of uncertain benefit in lowering BP
- Drug therapy: General principles
  - If lifestyle modification is insufficient, drug therapy is initiated
  - **If possible, choose agents with 24-hour duration of action and once-daily dosing**
  - **Use of two or more drugs is usually necessary to achieve goals**
- Specific agents (Table 2-7)
- Therapeutic strategy
  - **Thiazide diuretics are the agents of choice for most patients with uncomplicated hypertension**
  - **If a compelling indication (or comorbidity) exists, choose the appropriate agent (see following)**
    - β-Blockers are increasingly seen as third-line agents, to be used only after diuretics, calcium channel blockers, and angiotensin-converting enzyme (ACE) inhibitors or angiotensin receptor blockers (ARBs) have been tried
  - If there is a partial but inadequate response to the first drug, either increase the dose of the first drug or add a second agent from a different class (Fig. 2-3)
    - Low-dose combination therapy may be preferable to higher doses of a single agent
    - Dose-dependent side effects are minimized
    - Formulations combining two drugs may offer improved convenience or lower cost
      - Low-dose diuretics with ACE inhibitors, β-blockers, or ARBs
      - Thiazides with potassium-sparing diuretics
      - Calcium antagonists with ACE inhibitors or ARBs
  - If there is no response to the first drug or if the drug is not tolerated, substitute a drug from a different class
  - **A diuretic should be part of any regimen containing three or more drugs**
  - Short-acting loop diuretics (furosemide, bumetanide) should be dosed twice daily, or a long-acting diuretic (e.g., torsemide) substituted

- Compelling indications for selection of initial antihypertensive agent
  - Chronic renal disease: ACE inhibitor, ARB
  - CHF: ACE inhibitor, ARB, diuretic, β-blocker, aldosterone antagonist
  - MI: β-blocker (non-ISA), ACE inhibitor, aldosterone antagonist
  - Other possible indications
    - Migraines: β-blockers, calcium channel antagonists
    - Benign prostatic hypertrophy: α-blockers
    - Essential tremor: β-blockers
    - Hyperthyroidism: β-blockers
- Contraindications to certain antihypertensives
  - **Pregnancy: Avoid ACE inhibitors and ARBs (absolute contraindication)**
  - Peripheral vascular disease: Avoid β-blockers
  - Gout: Avoid diuretics
  - Second-degree or third-degree heart block: Avoid β-blockers or nondihydropyridine calcium antagonists
- Treatment of hypertensive urgency and emergency
  - Hypertensive urgency (severely elevated BP without acutely progressive end-organ damage):
    - Gradual control of BP using oral agents and outpatient follow-up is appropriate
    - Short-acting nifedipine or clonidine is not indicated
  - Hypertensive emergency (severely elevated BP with acutely progressive end-organ damage):
    - BP must be brought down immediately via admission to an intensive care unit and administration of intravenous medication
    - Intravenous medication is used for rapid effect and ability to titrate (Table 2-8)
    - **Initial goal is to lower mean arterial BP by approximately 25%, but not more, within 2 hours**
    - Subsequent goal is to lower BP to approximately 160/100 mm Hg over next 2 to 24 hours (reduce BP further as tolerated for aortic dissection)

Prevention

- Patients with prehypertension (BP < 140/90 mm Hg and >120/80 mm Hg) should be provided counseling for lifestyle modification to decrease their risk of progression to hypertension

SUGGESTED READINGS

Izzo JL, Black HR (eds): *Hypertension primer: the essentials of high blood pressure*, ed 3, Baltimore, Lippincott, Williams and Wilkins, 2003.

Kaplan NM: *Clinical hypertension*, ed 9, Baltimore, Lippincott, Williams and Wilkins, 2006.

Oparil S, Weber MA (eds): *Hypertension: a companion to Brenner and Rector's the kidney*, ed 2, Philadelphia, WB Saunders, 2005.

The Seventh Report of the Joint National Committee on Prevention, Detection, Evaluation, and Treatment of High Blood Pressure: Hypertension, JAMA 42:1206–1252, 2003. [The comprehensive, unabridged version of the JNC7 report.]

The Seventh Report of the Joint National Committee on Prevention, Detection, Evaluation, and Treatment of High Blood Pressure, JAMA 289:2560–2572, 2003. [The "express," or abbreviated, version of the JNC7 report.]

TABLE 2-7 *Antihypertensive Agents*

Class	Examples	Side Effects	Comments
Thiazide diuretics	Hydrochlorothiazide Chlorthalidone Indapamide Metolazone	Hypokalemia Hyponatremia Alkalosis Hyperuricemia Dehydration	Thiazides not effective if GFR < 30 mL/min Side effects rarely a problem at low doses
Loop diuretics	Furosemide Torsemide Bumetanide	As for thiazide diuretics	Furosemide has a short half-life—dose twice a day for HTN Sodium restriction should accompany diuretics
Potassium-sparing diuretics	Distal tubule sodium channel blockers: triamterene, amiloride Aldosterone antagonists: spironolactone, eplerenone	Hyperkalemia Hyponatremia Dehydration	Often given in combination with thiazides (to prevent hypokalemia) Avoid or use with caution in renal insufficiency
β-Adrenergic antagonists (β-blockers)	β_1-selective: atenolol, metoprolol Non-β_1-selective: propranolol, nadolol α_1 and β_1 Blockade: carvedilol, labetalol Intrinsic sympathomimetic activity (ISA): pindolol, acebutolol, penbutolol	Bradycardia Fatigue Insomnia Erectile dysfunction Bronchospasm in asthma and COPD patients	ISA β-blockers useful for patients with bradycardia May mask hypoglycemic symptoms in diabetics Do not use alone in cases of catecholamine excess (cocaine intoxication, pheochromocytoma) as unopposed α_1 vasoconstriction without β_2 vasodilation may increase BP precipitously
Angiotensin-converting enzyme (ACE) inhibitors	Benazepril Captopril Enalapril Fosinopril Lisinopril Moexipril Perindopril Quinapril Ramipril Trandolapril	Cough Angioedema Hyperkalemia Decrease in CKD, renovascular disease, CHF, or dehydration	Inhibit the renin-angiotensin-aldosterone system by blocking conversion of angiotensin I to angiotensin II Dilate renal efferent arterioles Also inhibit degradation of bradykinin, which may lead to cough Avoid in pregnancy; teratogenic
Angiotensin receptor blockers (ARBs)	Candesartan Eprosartan Irbesartan Losartan Olmesartan Telmisartan Valsartan	Minimal	Inhibit the renin-angiotensin-aldosterone system by blocking the angiotensin II receptor Avoid in pregnancy; teratogenic
α-Adrenergic antagonists	Doxazosin Prazosin Terazosin	Orthostatic hypotension	Block postsynaptic α_1 receptors, causing vasodilation Favorable effect on lipid profile and glucose level May increase CHD mortality if used as a single agent
Nondihydropyridine calcium antagonists	Verapamil Diltiazem	Bradycardia, heart block Decreases cardiac contractility Constipation	Verapamil may increase cyclosporine and digoxin levels
Dihydropyridine calcium antagonists	Amlodipine Felodipine Isradipine Nicardipine Nifedipine Nisoldipine	Headache Flushing Tachycardia Pedal edema	Dilate arterioles Possible increased heart rate Short-acting nifedipine causes marked reflex tachycardia and is *not* recommended for HTN Nifedipine increases cyclosporine levels

Continued

TABLE 2-7	*Antihypertensive Agents* (Continued)		
Class	**Examples**	**Side Effects**	**Comments**
Direct vasodilators	Minoxidil Hydralazine	Headache Tachycardia Fluid retention Minoxidil Hirsutism Pericardial effusion Hydralazine Drug-induced lupus	Considered third-line agents

Central adrenergic inhibitors	Clonidine
	Guanfacine
	Methyldopa
	Reserpine
		Clonidine, guanfacine
		  Sedation
		  Dry mouth
		  Withdrawal hypertension
		Methyldopas
		  Coombs' positive hemolytic
		    anemia
		  Liver toxicity
			Inhibit sympathetic outflow from
			  CNS
			Clonidine also available in patch
			Methyldopa safe in pregnancy

ACE inhibitors, angiotensin-converting enzyme inhibitors; ARBs, angiotensin receptor blockers; BP, blood pressure; CHD, coronary heart disease; CHF, congestive heart failure; CKD, chronic kidney disease; CNS, central nervous system, COPD, chronic obstructive pulmonary disease; GFR, glomerular filtration rate; HTN, hypertension; ISA, intrinsic sympathomimetic activity.

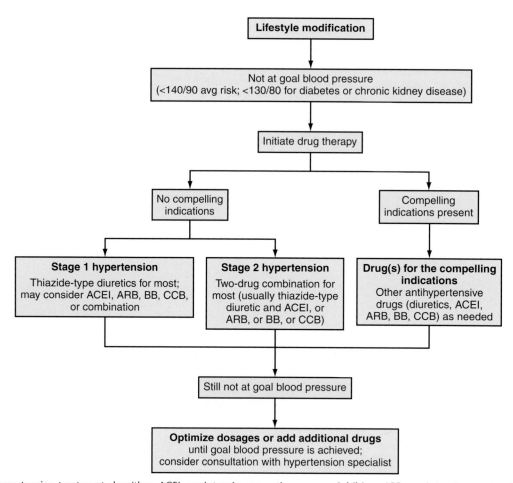

FIGURE 2-3 Hypertension treatment algorithm. ACEI, angiotensin-converting enzyme inhibitor; ARB, angiotensin receptor blocker; BB, β-blocker; CCB, calcium channel blocker.

TABLE 2-8	*Drugs Used in Treatment of Hypertensive Emergency*	
Drug	**Indication**	**Precaution**
Nitroprusside	Most emergencies	Thiocyanate toxicity
Nitroglycerin	Angina, MI	Headache, tolerance
Nicardipine	Most emergencies	Tachycardia
Labetalol	Most emergencies	CHF, bradycardia
Fenoldopam	Most emergencies	Tachycardia
Enalaprilat	CHF	Rapid, unpredictable BP drop
Esmolol	Perioperative, aortic dissection	Nausea

BP, blood pressure; CHF, congestive heart failure; MI, myocardial infarction.

2

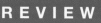
Lipid Disorders

ANDREW DeFILIPPIS, MD, and ROGER S. BLUMENTHAL, MD

Lipid disorders (dyslipidemias) are important risk factors for the development of atherosclerotic vascular disease. Many of the disorders result from both genetic and environmental factors. The Adult Treatment Panel III report and 2004 modification of the treatment algorithm summarize guidelines for cholesterol testing and management and provide a useful resource for clinicians.

Basic Information

- Cholesterol
  - Involved in vital functions such as cell membrane biogenesis, steroid synthesis, and bile acid formation
  - Liver is the primary producer of endogenous cholesterol and the main processor of dietary cholesterol
  - Cholesterol is produced when 3-hydroxy-methylglutaryl coenzyme A (HMG-CoA) is converted to mevalonic acid by HMG-CoA reductase
- Lipoproteins
  - Spherical complexes of lipid core and outer protein monolayer that transport lipids such as cholesterol and triglyceride in the circulation
  - **Most common classification divides lipoprotein particles according to increasing density;** a patient's cholesterol levels are most commonly expressed as the concentration of cholesterol in each of the individual lipoprotein particle groups as follows:
    - Chylomicrons
    - Very low-density lipoprotein (VLDL)
    - Intermediate-density lipoprotein (IDL)
    - Low-density lipoprotein (LDL)
    - High-density lipoprotein (HDL)
- Chylomicrons
  - Intestinal triglyceride-rich lipoproteins responsible for transporting dietary fat and cholesterol to the body
  - Synthesized by the intestinal epithelial cells from fatty acids
  - Increased fat consumption during meals leads to increased chylomicrons in the blood
  - Lipoprotein lipase hydrolyzes free fatty acids from chylomicrons, leaving chylomicron remnants
- VLDL
  - Synthesized in the liver from free fatty acids obtained from chylomicron catabolism (dietary fat) and from endogenously produced triglycerides (generated from excess dietary protein and carbohydrate)
  - Hydrolyzed by lipoprotein lipase and converted to smaller particles (IDL) and then into LDL
- LDL
  - **Principal cholesterol-containing lipoprotein and a major atherogenic lipoprotein**
  - Approximately 25% of LDL is cleared by the peripheral tissues
  - Approximately 75% of LDL returned to the liver, primarily via the LDL receptors
  - LDL receptor expression by hepatic cells regulates cholesterol homeostasis
    - Decreased level of cholesterol in hepatocytes leads to an increase in LDL receptor density, causing a greater clearance of LDL
    - Increased dietary saturated fatty acids decrease the production of hepatic LDL receptors, which can contribute to hypercholesterolemia
    - Dietary cholesterol inhibits the production of endogenous cholesterol, but once endogenous cholesterol production is fully suppressed, additional dietary cholesterol may result in increased serum cholesterol
- HDL
  - Small lipoprotein that participates in reverse cholesterol transport from the arteries back to the liver
  - **Levels are generally inversely associated with the risk of atherosclerotic vascular disease**
- Apolipoproteins
  - Major structural protein components of lipoproteins embedded in the surface monolayer
  - Affect the metabolism of lipoproteins by activating enzymes and aiding receptor-mediated processes
  - Are divided into five classes (Apo A–Apo E)
    - Apo A-containing lipoproteins are associated with a reduction in atherosclerosis
    - Apo B-containing lipoproteins are associated with an increased risk of atherosclerosis
- Lipoprotein(a) [Lp(a)]
  - Assembled from an LDL particle and apolipoprotein (a) [apo(a)]
  - Elevated levels of Lp(a) are associated with an increased risk of vascular disease

Clinical Presentation

- Many patients are asymptomatic until coronary heart disease (CHD) develops
- Physical signs
  - Minority of patients with lipid disorders have physical signs that suggest a diagnosis (Table 3-1 and Figs. 3-1 and 3-2)
  - Tendinous xanthomas
    - Nontender, firm nodules that appear on the extensor surfaces of various tendons including Achilles tendon, extensor tendons of the hands, patellar tendons
    - More prominent as subjects age

TABLE 3-1	*Characteristics of Various Lipid Disorders*				
Name	**Phenotype**	**Abnormal Lipid**	**Defect**	**Possible Clinical Findings**	**Risk of CHD**
Familial hypercholesterolemia	IIa	↑ LDL	Defective LDL receptor or apo-B-100; heterozygous and homozygous forms	Tendinous xanthomas Xanthelasma Planar xanthomas Corneal arcus	+++
Familial lipoprotein lipase deficiency	I, V	↑ Chylomicrons	Lipoprotein lipase deficiency	Eruptive xanthomas Lipemia retinalis Abdominal pain Hepatosplenomegaly	0
Familial hypertriglyceridemia	I, V	↑ VLDL	Genetic defect unknown	Often asymptomatic	+
Combined hyperlipidemia	IIb	↑ VLDL, LDL	Genetic defect unknown	Often asymptomatic except for CHD Yellow-orange discoloration of palmar creases	+++
Familial dysbetalipoproteinemia	III	↑VLDL, IDL	Defective or absent apo-E	Tuberoeruptive xanthomas Hyperuricemia Glucose intolerance Corneal opacities	+++
Lecithin-cholesterol acetyltransferase (LCAT) deficiency	N/A	↓ HDL	Rapid apo-A-1 catabolism	Renal insufficiency Hemolytic anemia "Fish-eye disease" in mild form	+
Tangier disease	N/A	↓ HDL	Rapid HDL catabolism	Corneal opacities Polyneuropathy Orange tonsils	0
Gain of function of proprotein convertase subtilisin-like kexin type 9 (PSCK9)	N/A	↑ LDL	Increase in LDL receptor degradation	None	+

apo, apolipoprotein; CHD, coronary heart disease; HDL, high-density lipoprotein; IDL, intermediate-density lipoprotein; LDL, low-density lipoprotein; VLDL, very low-density lipoprotein; ↑, increase; ↓, decrease.

- Xanthelasma (palpebral xanthomas)
  - Soft, off-white plaques
  - Originate near the eyelids
- Corneal arcus (arcus senilis)
  - Arcus is composed of cholesterol ester deposited in the peripheral cornea
  - Appears as a normal variant in white patients older than 40 years but a sign of hypercholesterolemia in white adults younger than 40 years
- Tuberous xanthomas
  - Raised, yellowish nodules about 0.5 to 1 cm in diameter
  - Found in areas of pressure such as elbows and knees
- Lipemia retinalis
  - Pink discoloration of the retinal vessels
  - May be seen on funduscopic examination
- Eruptive xanthomas
  - Small light yellow papules on a reddish base
  - May be present on arms, thighs, and buttocks

Diagnosis and Evaluation

- Phenotyping—describing the clinical lipid profile
  - Often classified into types I through V based on levels of LDL and VLDL

- Several familial (hereditary) forms of primary hyperlipidemia exist (see Table 3-1)
- Many patients have primary idiopathic hyperlipidemia
- Secondary dyslipidemia (caused by a concomitant disorder)
  - Sedentary lifestyle with caloric excess and excessive consumption of saturated and *trans* fatty acids and the lack of consumption of foods rich in fiber and nutrients (fruits, vegetables, whole grains), mono- and polyunsaturated fatty acids (fish, nuts, seeds, olive and canola oil) is by far the most common cause of dyslipidemia in industrialized countries, but other causes need to be considered in all patients
  - Elevated LDL differential diagnosis: Hypothyroidism, chronic liver disease, cholestasis, nephrotic syndrome
  - Hypertriglyceridemia differential diagnosis: Alcohol consumption, obesity, pregnancy, diabetes mellitus, hypothyroidism, chronic renal failure, medications (nonselective β-blockers, high-dose diuretics, oral estrogen replacement therapy, oral contraceptives)
  - Low HDL differential diagnosis: Smoking, diabetes mellitus, obesity, sedentary lifestyle, hypertriglyceridemia, medications (progestins, anabolic steroids, corticosteroids)

3

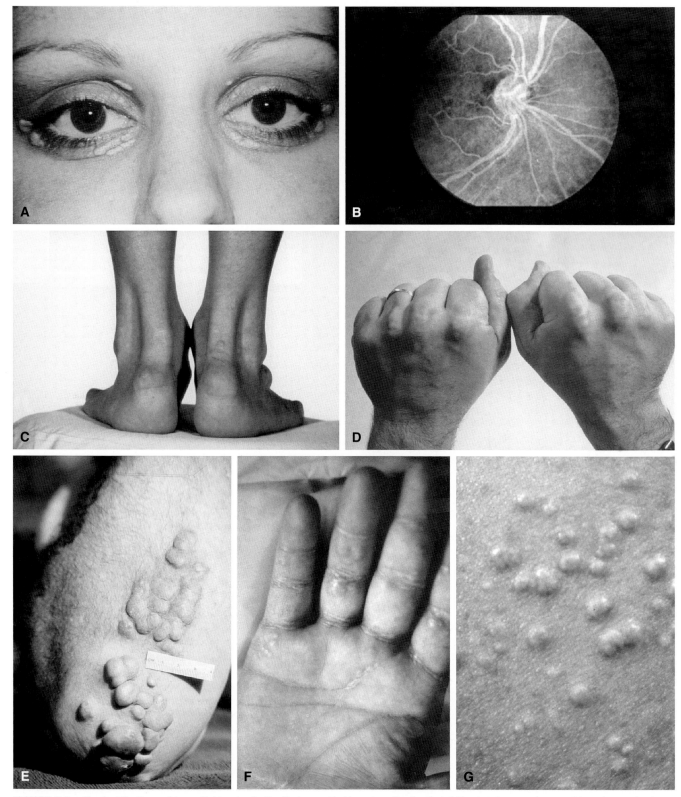

FIGURE 3-1 Physical findings of hyperlipidemia. **A,** Xanthelasma. **B,** Lipemia retinalis. **C,** Achilles tendon xanthomas. Note the marked thickening of the tendons. **D,** Tendon xanthomas. **E,** Tuberous xanthomas. **F,** Palmar xanthomas. **G,** Eruptive xanthomas. (A and B courtesy of Dr. Mark Dresner and *Hospital Practice* [May 1990, p 15]. C to F courtesy of Dr. Tom Bersot. G, Courtesy of Dr. Alan Chait. From Larsen PR, Kronenberg HM, Melmed S, et al: *Williams textbook of endocrinology*, ed 10, Philadelphia, WB Saunders, 2003, Fig. 34-26.)

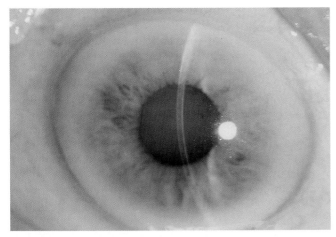

FIGURE 3-2 Corneal arcus (arcus senilis). Corneal arcus in an elderly man. (From Yanoff M, Fine BS: *Ocular pathology,* ed 5, St. Louis, Mosby, 2002, Fig. 60-4.)

- Type B pattern
  - Apolipoprotein B measurement numerically greater than the LDL, indicating the presence of small, dense atherogenic particles
  - These patients often have impaired fibrinolysis, endothelial dysfunction, and an accelerated progression of atherosclerotic vascular disease
  - This pattern is typical of the metabolic syndrome
- CHD risk assessment
  - **Adults aged 20 years or older should have fasting lipoprotein analysis (total cholesterol [TC], LDL, HDL, and triglycerides) at least once every 5 years**
  - **In nonfasting sample, only the values for TC, HDL, and non-HDL cholesterol are generally accurate**
  - Adult Treatment Panel III (ATP III) guidelines suggest the intensity of risk reduction therapy; should be adjusted to a person's absolute risk of developing CHD
  - ATP III classification (Table 3-2)
- Risk categories, Framingham Risk Score (FRS), and LDL goals

- ATP III recommends assessment of the CHD risk status of a person without CHD or other forms of atherosclerotic vascular disease
- **Assess number of risk factors for heart disease (Box 3-1)**
- **If two or more risk factors are present, estimate 10-year risk of myocardial infarction (MI) or CHD death, then determine LDL goals** (Table 3-3)
- Ten-year risk assessment uses revised FRS with risk factors of age, TC, HDL, blood pressure, and cigarette smoking (details in ATP III guidelines)
- **Zero to 1 risk factor**
  - **Minimal LDL goal of less than 160 mg/dL**
  - Patients typically have a 10-year risk of CHD less than 10%
- Two or more risk factors
  - **10-year CHD risk less than 10%**
    - LDL goal of less than 130 mg/dL
  - **10-year CHD risk 10% to 20%**
    - LDL goal of less than 130 mg/dL with optional goal of less than 100 mg/dL
    - Optional LDL goal of less than 100 mg/dL should be strongly considered for patients in this risk category with more than two risk factors, severe risk factors (e.g., significant family history of CHD), advanced age, elevated triglyceride with elevated non-HDL cholesterol and low HDL, or the metabolic syndrome
    - Emerging risk factors may also be considered (electron beam computed tomography [EBCT] or multidetector computed tomography [MDCT], showing high coronary calcium burden [>75th percentile for age and sex] or high-sensitivity (hs)-C-reactive protein > 3 mg/L)
- Known CHD (MI or >50% stenosis by angiography or ultrasound) and CHD equivalents
  - CHD equivalents refer to a risk for major coronary events equal to that of established CHD (>20% per 10 years of developing CHD death or nonfatal MI), and include
  - Other forms of atherosclerotic disease
  - Peripheral arterial disease
  - Abdominal aortic aneurysm

TABLE 3-2	*Adult Treatment Panel III Classification of LDL, Total, and HDL (mg/dL)*
LDL	
<100	Optimal
100–129	Near or above optimal
130–159	Borderline high
160–189	High
≥190	Very high
Total Cholesterol	
<200	Desirable
200–239	Borderline high
≥240	High
HDL	
<40	Low
≥60	High

HDL, high-density lipoprotein; LDL, low-density lipoprotein.

BOX 3-1	*Major Risk Factors (Exclusive of LDL) That Modify LDL Goals*

Cigarette smoking

Hypertension (BP ≥ 140/90 mm Hg or prescription of an antihypertensive medication)

Low HDL (≤40 mg/dL)

Family history of premature CHD (CHD in father, brother, or son < 55 yr of age; CHD in mother, sister, or daughter < 65 yr of age)

Age (men ≥ 45 yr; women ≥ 55 yr)

An HDL ≥ 60 mg/dL is a negative risk factor, and its presence removes one risk factor from the total count

BP, blood pressure; CHD, coronary heart disease; HDL, high-density lipoprotein; LDL, low-density lipoprotein.

3

TABLE 3-3 *LDL Goals and Cutpoints for Drug Therapy*

Risk Category	LDL Goal	LDL Level at Which to Consider Drug Therapy
CHD or CHD risk equivalents	<100 mg/dL (Optional: <70 mg/dL)	≥100 mg/dL (>70 mg/dL: consider treatment)
2 or more risk factors	<130 mg/dL (Optional: <100 mg/dL)	10-year risk 10% to 20%: ≥130 mg/dL (≥100 mg/dL: consider treatment) 10-year risk <10%: ≥160 mg/dL
0–1 risk factor	<160 mg/dL	≥190 mg/dL (160–189 mg/dL: drug therapy optional)

CHD, coronary heart disease; LDL, low-density lipoprotein.
Adapted from Grundy SM, Cleeman JL, Merz CN, et al: Implications of recent clinical trials for the National Cholesterol Education Program Adult Treatment Panel III guidelines. *Circulation* 110:227–239, 2004.

- Carotid artery disease—transient ischemic attack or stroke of carotid origin or greater than 50% obstruction of a carotid artery
- Diabetes
  - Confers a high risk of new CHD events within 10 years
  - Diabetic patients who experience an MI have a significantly worse prognosis than nondiabetics of similar age
- Multiple risk factors that confer a greater than 20% 10-year risk for CHD
- Metabolic syndrome (Table 3-4)
  - **A condition associated with a constellation of factors related to insulin resistance including**
  - **Abdominal obesity**
  - **Atherogenic/type B dyslipidemia (low HDL, elevated triglycerides, small LDL particles)**
  - **Increased blood pressure**
  - **Glucose intolerance**
  - **Prothrombotic and proinflammatory states**
  - The abnormal findings in the metabolic syndrome are secondary targets of risk-reduction therapy
  - Metabolic syndrome may be considered a "prediabetic" state, increasing CHD risk
    - Fulfillment of diagnostic criteria may warrant reevaluation of a person's ATP III risk classification
  - Lifestyle modification is initial, primary therapy for persons with metabolic syndrome
- Limitations of Framingham-based ATP III risk categorization
  - **Although clinically valuable, the FRS may underestimate a person's true atherosclerotic vascular disease risk, especially for women (this includes risk for angina requiring revascularization, stroke, and congestive heart failure)**
  - Based on published guidelines, it is difficult for women to qualify for statin and aspirin therapy (i.e., FRS = 10% over 10 years)
  - Women are less likely than men to present with an MI as the initial manifestation of cardiovascular disease
  - Several factors not considered by the FRS should be considered to reassess and refine CHD risk prediction
    - Is there a family history of premature cardiovascular disease?

TABLE 3-4 *Clinical Identification of the Metabolic Syndrome**

Risk Factor	Defining Level
Abdominal obesity (waist circumference) In men In women	>40 inches >35 inches
Triglycerides	≥150 mg/dL
HDL In men In women	<40 mg/dL <50 mg/dL
Blood pressure	≥130/85 mm Hg
Fasting glucose	≥100 mg/dL

*Three or more risk factors are required for the diagnosis.
HDL, high-density lipoprotein.

- Diagnosis of the metabolic syndrome, in particular, those with elevated triglycerides, increased waist circumference, and sedentary lifestyle
- Extent of smoking history
- Emerging risk factors
  - An elevated hsCRP above 3 mg/dL is generally associated with a doubling of predicted relative risk
  - Consider measuring hsCRP or coronary calcium burden (EBCT or MDCT) if FRS 10-year risk is 6% to 20% to refine intensity of risk-factor reduction

Treatment

- **Lifestyle modification is the cornerstone of lipid management**
  - Therapeutic lifestyle changes
    - Weight reduction if overweight
    - Increased physical activity
      - Daily energy expenditure should include at least moderately brisk physical activity, contributing at least 200 kcal/day
    - **Brisk aerobic activity should be undertaken for at least 30 minutes, three to four times per week (>10,000 steps per day)**

- Implement a diet that is rich in fruits, vegetables, whole grains, fish, lean meats; and low saturated fat or nonfat dairy products and low in simple carbohydrates, sugars, *trans* and saturated fatty acids
  - Recommended intake of saturated fat less than 7% of total calories, and recommended cholesterol intake less than 200 mg/day
  - Majority of carbohydrates should be from foods rich in complex carbohydrates such as whole grains, fruits, and vegetables
- For primary prevention: Consume fish (preferably fatty fish) a minimum of twice per week and include foods and oils rich in alpha linolenic acid in your diet
- For secondary prevention: Consume approximately 1 g of eicosapentaenoic acid (EPA) + docosahexaenoic acid (DHA) every day, preferably from fatty fish
- EPA + DHA (fish oil) supplements could be considered in consultation with a physician
- Pharmacologic options
  - Statins
    - Cholesterol is produced when 3-hydroxy-3-methylglutaryl coenzyme A (HMG-CoA) is converted into mevalonic acid by HMG-CoA reductase
    - Statins work by inhibiting this conversion and by promoting up-regulation of LDL receptors on the surface of hepatocytes
    - Options: Atorvastatin, fluvastatin, lovastatin, pravastatin, simvastatin, rosuvastatin
    - **Lower LDL by 20% to 60% (more than most other agents)**
    - Raise HDL by 5% to 15%
    - Lower triglyceride levels by 10% to 35%
    - **Statins have been shown to decrease total mortality rates, decrease CHD events, slow progression of CHD, and decrease recurrent episodes of unstable angina requiring hospitalization**
    - Side effects: Myositis and increased liver enzymes occur less than 3% of the time and often resolve without intervention or dose reduction
    - Myalgias are a more common side effect in statin- and placebo-treated patients (5–10%); the frequency depends on a person's age and the number of and type of concomitant medications
    - Rhabdomyolysis is a very rare (<0.1%) but potentially fatal side effect of statins
    - Beware of increased incidence of rhabdomyolysis, especially when used in combination with gemfibrozil and macrolide antibiotics
    - Lipid and hepatic profiles should be repeated 6 to 12 weeks after initiation or dose titration
      - Once goals achieved, lipid and hepatic profiles should generally be checked about every 12 months
  - Ezetimibe
    - Inhibits cholesterol absorption at the brush border of the small intestine
    - Decreases delivery of cholesterol to the liver, reducing hepatic stores and increasing hepatic uptake from the blood
    - Lowers LDL by 15% to 25%
    - May be given as monotherapy or in conjunction with a statin to lower LDL cholesterol

- Side effects: Abdominal and back pain, diarrhea, fatigue
- Not yet proven to reduce CVD events, and it has had variable effects on carotid intimal medial thickness trials
  - Resins (cholestyramine, colestipol, colesevelam)
    - Also known as bile acid sequestrants
    - Lower LDL by 10% to 25%, depending on the dose and agent used
    - Work synergistically with statins
    - Some types of resins decrease the absorption of other drugs
    - Resins may raise triglycerides
    - Side effects: Gastrointestinal symptoms (bloating, cramping, flatulence)
    - Small but statistically significant reduction in CVD events as monotherapy
  - Nicotinic acid (niacin)
    - Lowers LDL by 5% to 25%
    - **Raises HDL by 15% to 35% (more than most other agents)**
    - Lowers triglyceride levels by 20% to 40%
    - Extended-release niacin has been shown to slow progression of carotid intima-medial thickness, but no data yet on clinical events
    - Side effects: Flushing, hyperuricemia, hyperglycemia (in high doses), gastrointestinal distress, and hepatotoxicity
      - Flushing may be ameliorated by premedication with aspirin
    - Modest long-term decrease in mortality rates in patients following MI
  - Fibrates (gemfibrozil, fenofibrate)
    - **Lower triglycerides by 25% to 50% (more than most other agents)**
    - Raise HDL by 10% to 20%
    - Lower LDL by 5% to 20%
    - **Persons with type 2 diabetes: Reduce CHD events, but do not reduce CHD mortality rate**
      - Effects on triglycerides and HDL-C useful in managing atherogenic dyslipidemia seen in diabetes
      - Should not be used as a substitute for statins in the lowering of LDL-C (for which decreased mortality rates have been observed)
    - Side effects: Dyspepsia, myalgias, and gallstones
    - Reduces CHD events, especially in persons with above-average triglycerides

Approach to the Patient

Figure 3-3 illustrates a management algorithm for LDL.
- Measurement of lipids
  - Fasting lipid profile beginning at age 20 years
    - If nonfasting, only total cholesterol (TC) and HDL values are accurate
    - If normal, repeat measurement in 5 years
    - If abnormal, pursue appropriate therapy
  - **All patients hospitalized for a suggested coronary event should have lipid profile within 24 hours**
  - Emerging risk factors not routinely measured: Lipoprotein (a), hs-CRP, Apo B, LDL particle number, prothrombotic and proinflammatory factors
- Drug therapy to achieve LDL goals:
  - Goals and LDL levels at which to consider therapy are per updated ATP III guidelines (see Table 3-3)

3

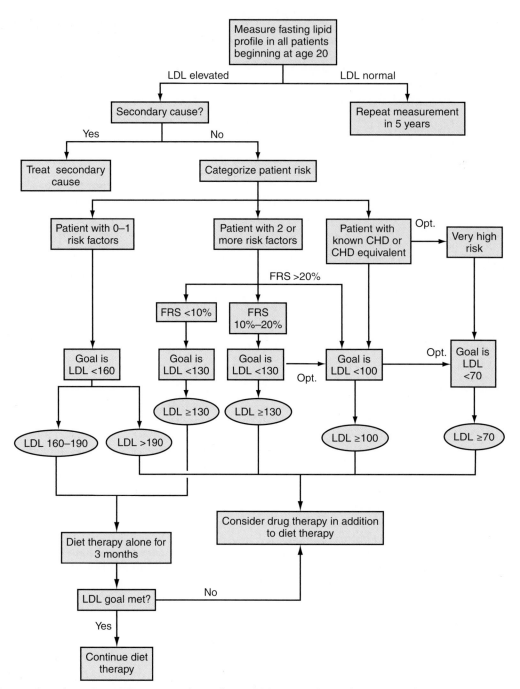

FIGURE 3-3 Approach to the patient. CHD, coronary heart disease; FRS, Framingham risk score; LDL, low-density lipoprotein; Opt., optional.

- **LDL goal of less than 100 mg/dL with optional goal of less than 70 mg/dL for CHD and CHD equivalents**
  - This optional LDL goal of less than 70 mg/dL should be considered for very high-risk patients, which includes patients with established CHD and other severe risk factors like diabetes, the metabolic syndrome, or resistant hypertension
  - Trial of diet therapy for 4 to 6 months is reasonable first-line therapy in most patients with moderately elevated LDL and no known atherosclerotic vascular disease

- If not successful, statins are often first-line choice
- If LDL goal not achieved, a higher dose of the medication or an additional type of medication should be considered
  - Ezetimibe, fibrates, niacin, and resins may be considered for combination therapy
- Management of triglyceride disorders
  - Classification
    - Normal triglycerides: Less than 150 mg/dL
    - Borderline-high: 150 to 199 mg/dL
    - High: 200 to 499 mg/dL
    - Very high: Greater than 500 mg/dL

TABLE 3-5	*Comparision of LDL and Non-HDL Goals for Three Risk Categories*	
Risk Category	**LDL Goal (mg/dL)**	**Non-HDL Goal (mg/dL)**
CHD and CHD risk equivalent	<100 (Optional: <70)	<130 (<100)
2+ risk factors and 10-year risk ≤20%	<130 (Optional: <100)	<160 (<130)
0–1 risk factor	<160	<190

CHD, coronary heart disease; HDL, high-density lipoprotein; LDL, low-density lipoprotein.

- Triglyceride levels above 150 mg/dL are associated with smaller, denser LDL particles
- Weight reduction, increased physical activity, and decreased alcohol intake (if relevant) are important lifestyle modifications
- Ingestion of omega-3 fatty acids can be beneficial
  - When triglyceride levels are greater than 500 mg/dL, a fibrate is often the preferred initial drug choice
- The sum of LDL plus VLDL cholesterol is termed non-HDL cholesterol and represents the majority of atherogenic (Apo B) lipoproteins in the serum
  - Is a secondary target of therapy in persons with high triglycerides
  - Measured as "TC minus HDL"
  - **Goal for non-HDL in person with high triglycerides is 30 mg/dL higher than for LDL, in that a VLDL less than 30 mg/dL is normal (Table 3-5)**
  - The non-HDL can be lowered by lifestyle changes, as well as through more aggressive drug therapy to lower triglycerides and/or LDL
- Management of low HDL
  - Exercise may raise HDL
  - **Nicotinic acid is the most effective drug for raising HDL**
  - Certain statins may be somewhat more effective than others in raising HDL

REVIEW QUESTIONS

For review questions, please go to www.expertconsult.com.

SUGGESTED READINGS

Ashen MD, Blumenthal RS: Clinical practice: low HDL cholesterol levels, *N Engl J Med* 353:1252–1260, 2005.

Ballantyne CM, O'Keefe JH Jr, Gotto A Jr: *Dyslipidemia essentials,* Houston, Physicians' Press, 2005.

Cui Y, Blumenthal RS, Flaws JA, et al: Non-high-density lipoprotein cholesterol level as a predictor of cardiovascular disease mortality, *Arch Intern Med* 161:1413–1419, 2001.

Expert Panel on Detection, Evaluation, and Treatment of High Blood Cholesterol in Adults: executive summary of the third report of the National Cholesterol Program (NCEP) Expert panel on Detection, Evaluation, and Treatment of High Blood Cholesterol in Adults (Adult Treatment Panel III), *JAMA* 285:2486–2497, 2001.

Gluckman TJ, Baranowski B, Ashen MD, et al: A practical and evidence-based approach to cardiovascular disease risk reduction, *Arch Intern Med* 164:1490–1500, 2004.

Lakoski SG, Greenland P, Wong ND, et al: Coronary artery calcium scores and risk for cardiovascular events in women classified as "low risk" based on Framingham risk score: the multi-ethnic study of atherosclerosis (MESA), *Arch Intern Med* 167:2437–2442, 2007.

Mora S, Musunuru K, Blumenthal RS: The clinical utility of high-sensitivity C-reactive protein in cardiovascular disease and the potential implications of JUPITER on current practice guidelines, *Clin Chem* 55:219–228, 2009.

Mudd JO, Borlaug BA, Johnston PV, et al: Beyond low-density lipoprotein cholesterol: defining the role of low-density lipoprotein heterogeneity in coronary artery disease, *J Am Coll Cardiol* 50:1735–1741, 2007.

Ridker PM, Danielson E, Fonseca FA, et al: Rosuvastatin to prevent vascular events in men and women with elevated C-reactive protein, *N Engl J Med* 359:2195–2207, 2008.

Scandinavian Simvastatin Survival Study Group: Randomized trial of cholesterol lowering in 4444 persons with coronary heart disease: the Scandinavian Simvastatin Survival Study (4S), *Lancet* 44:1383–1389, 1994.

Smith SC Jr, Allen JA, Blair SN, et al: AHA/ACC guidelines for secondary prevention for patients with coronary and other atherosclerotic vascular disease: 2006 update, *Circulation* 113:2363–2372, 2006.

Smith SC Jr, Blair SN, Bonow RO, et al: AHA/ACC Scientific Statement: AHA/ACC guidelines for preventing heart attack and death in patients with atherosclerotic cardiovascular disease: 2001 update: a statement for healthcare professionals from the American Heart Association and the American College of Cardiology, *Circulation* 104:1577–1579, 2001.

Acknowledgment

We are grateful to Dr. J. Gabriel Schneider for his help in preparing the initial draft of this chapter.

Coronary Artery Disease

ILAN S. WITTSTEIN, MD

In the United States, over 12 million people suffer from coronary artery disease (CAD), and the cost of caring for these patients is over $120 billion per year. Despite great advances in treatment, CAD remains the leading cause of death for both men and women in the United States, with approximately 1 million people dying from it each year; roughly 25% of these deaths occur suddenly.

CHRONIC CORONARY ARTERY DISEASE

Basic Information

- Atherogenesis
  - The endothelial cells lining the coronary arteries have two major roles
    - Regulation of vascular tone by vasodilatation (e.g., nitric oxide) and vasoconstriction (e.g., endothelin, angiotensin-converting enzyme [ACE])
    - Prevention of intravascular thrombosis (e.g., prostacyclin, plasminogen)
  - Numerous insults can impair normal endothelial function
    - Insults can be hemodynamic (e.g., shear stress, hypertension); chemical (e.g., low-density lipoprotein [LDL], modified LDL, homocysteine); or even biologic (e.g., viruses, bacteria, immune complexes)
    - Insults can affect both epicardial vessels and microvessels
  - Atherosclerotic plaque formation
    - Begins with interruption of endothelial cell integrity
    - Leukocytes, mostly macrophages, are attracted to the site of injury, where they collect lipids and coalesce to form the soft lipid core of a growing plaque
    - Earliest lesion of atherosclerosis is the fatty streak, made up mostly of lipid-laden macrophages containing cholesterol ester droplets
    - Chemoattractants (e.g., platelet-derived growth factor) cause smooth muscle cells to migrate to the site of the atheroma, where they produce collagen and fibrous tissue that contribute to plaque formation
    - The atherosclerotic plaque is covered by a layer of connective tissue called the fibrous cap
    - Most acute coronary syndromes (ACSs) occur when the fibrous cap ruptures, leading to thrombus formation (see the later section on Acute Coronary Syndromes)

- **It is the characteristics of a plaque, not its size, that determine its vulnerability; a large, fibrotic plaque with a thick cap is often more stable and less prone to rupture than a small plaque with a soft lipid core and a thin fibrous cap.**
- Pathophysiology of chronic CAD or chronic stable angina
  - **Fundamental problem is an imbalance between myocardial oxygen supply and demand**
  - Symptoms occur during periods of exercise or stress when increased myocardial oxygen demand (e.g., from an increase in heart rate, contractility, afterload, or wall stress) is inadequately met because of impaired coronary blood flow
  - Insufficient coronary flow can occur in one of two major ways:
    - Impaired from stenotic plaque
    - Impaired flow in the absence of severe luminal narrowing because of inadequate coronary flow reserve due to endothelial dysfunction (i.e., insufficient vasodilatory response during exercise)

Clinical Presentation

- **Risk factors for coronary atherosclerosis (Table 4-1)**
- **Special considerations**
  - **A low high-density lipoprotein (HDL) level is an independent risk factor for CAD (see Chapter 3)**
  - **Small, dense LDL has the lowest affinity for the LDL receptor and is therefore cleared to the least degree from plasma by the liver; it may be the most atherogenic type of LDL.**
    - Fenofibrate is probably best treatment
  - Homocystinuria is a rare homozygous genetic disorder of impaired homocysteine metabolism that results in severe premature atherosclerosis
    - The heterozygous form has a 1% to 2% prevalence and may account for up to 30% of cases of premature atherosclerosis
    - Though elevated homocysteine levels are associated with increased vascular events, moderate reduction in homocysteine levels by treating with folate, vitamin B_6, and vitamin B_{12} did not reduce the risk of myocardial infarction (MI) or death in a large clinical trial
  - Lipoprotein (a) [Lp(a)] is an LDL particle that contains the large glycoprotein apoprotein (a); it has a higher density than LDL and is more atherogenic.
    - Higher levels have been associated with increased CAD

TABLE 4-1	*Risk Factors for Coronary Artery Disease (CAD)*	
Strong Epidemiologic Evidence	**Moderate Epidemiologic Evidence**	**Association with CAD**
Older age Male Postmenopausal Elevated LDL Low HDL Cigarette smoking Hypertension Diabetes mellitus Obesity or sedentary lifestyle Family history of early CAD	High triglycerides Small dense LDL Elevated homocysteine Stress or depression Inflammatory markers (C-reactive protein, fibrinogen)	Lp(a) *Chlamydia pneumoniae*

HDL, high-density lipoprotein; LDL, low-density lipoprotein; Lp(a), lipoprotein(a).

- Niacin, estrogen, fenofibrate, and benzafibrate all reduce Lp(a) levels
- One should screen for Lp(a) when statin therapy does not lower LDL
- Elevated C-reactive protein (CRP) and fibrinogen levels are associated with an increased risk of MI; it is unclear whether they cause CAD or are simply markers of an associated inflammatory process.
- *Chlamydia pneumoniae* has been isolated from atheromas and may contribute to plaque inflammation. In a recent randomized clinical trial, however, patients hospitalized with an ACS who received long-term treatment with the antibiotic gatifloxacin had no reduction in cardiovascular events.
- Clinical symptoms
  - Symptoms typically occur during physical exertion and gradually resolve with cessation of the exercise
  - Symptoms can also be elicited by conditions that stress the system and increase oxygen demand (e.g., anemia, fever, sepsis, thyrotoxicosis)
  - Typical symptoms include substernal chest pressure or burning and are less commonly characterized by sharp pain
    - May radiate to the upper extremities (left arm more often than right arm), neck, jaw, or face
    - May be accompanied by dyspnea, diaphoresis
    - Symptoms may be atypical, particularly in women, diabetics, and the elderly

Diagnosis and Evaluation

- Resting electrocardiogram (ECG)
  - Approximately 50% of patients with chronic stable angina have a normal resting ECG
  - The presence of Q waves and conduction system abnormalities (e.g., left bundle branch block (LBBB), left anterior fascicular block) increases the likelihood of having underlying CAD
- Stress tests
  - Rationale
    - **Because stress tests can yield both false-negative and false-positive results (the sensitivity of an exercise treadmill test is around 70%, the specificity around 80%), the presence of CAD can never be definitively ruled in or out through stress testing alone**
    - **A better rationale for performing a stress test is to risk-stratify the patient: Use the information**

obtained from the test to determine the patient's risk for future cardiovascular events and death (see the following examples)
- Pretest probability
  - Refers to the prevalence of CAD in the population being tested (i.e., the likelihood that the patient has CAD)
  - The likelihood of a patient having CAD increases with age, with having other coronary risk factors, and with a history that is typical of exertional angina
  - The clinician should be able to determine from history and physical examination alone whether a patient has a low, medium, or high pretest probability of CAD
    - Example: A 25-year-old woman with atypical symptoms and no risk factors for CAD has a very low pretest probability
    - Example: A 75-year-old man with exertional angina and a history of hypertension (HTN), diabetes mellitus (DM), high cholesterol, and cigarette use has a high pretest probability
  - Considering pretest probability will help interpret a patient's stress test results
    - Example 1: A healthy 25-year-old woman presents with atypical symptoms of chest pain and no CAD risk factors. She exercises for 15 minutes on a Bruce protocol and has no symptoms, but her ECG shows 1- to 2-mm ST depression, and the test is read as positive. **Interpretation:** This patient has a low pretest probability, and at her age, with atypical symptoms and no risk factors, it is extremely unlikely that she has CAD. This is reinforced by her high treadmill performance without symptoms. The ECG changes almost certainly represent a false positive.
    - Example 2: For the past several months, a 75-year-old man with DM, HTN, and high cholesterol has been having substernal chest pain when he walks up a hill. His symptoms resolve quickly with rest. On a treadmill, he exercises for 6 minutes on a Bruce protocol and develops chest pain at peak exercise. The ECG shows only nonspecific changes, and the test is read as negative. **Interpretation:** This man is elderly, has a classic story for exertional angina, and has several major

risk factors. His pretest probability is very high, and it is almost a certainty that he has CAD. The stress test is likely a false negative.

- **Stress tests add little diagnostic information in patients with either high or low pretest probabilities for CAD**
- **Stress tests are most useful for diagnosing CAD in patients with intermediate pretest probability**

- Determining risk with stress testing
  - Stress test results should be categorized as
    - Inadequate
    - Negative
    - Positive—low risk
    - Positive—high risk
  - Features of a stress test that make it high risk (Box 4-1)
  - A scoring system that can be used to assess long-term risk is the Duke Treadmill Score
    - (Duration of exercise in minutes) − (5)(maximal ST deviation in mm) − (4)(treadmill angina index)
    - Treadmill angina index: 0 = no symptoms, 1 = angina that does not limit exercise, 2 = angina that limits exercise
    - Score: Less than −10: 79% 4-year survival; −10 to +4: 95% 4-year survival; +5 or greater: greater than 99% 4-year survival
  - **Patients with positive stress tests who have no high-risk features are often best treated medically**
  - **Positive tests with high-risk features suggest higher-risk coronary anatomy (e.g., left main disease, proximal left anterior descending [LAD] artery disease, three-vessel disease); the best approach here is often cardiac catheterization with the ultimate goal of revascularization.**
- Types of stress tests (Table 4-2)
  - To decide which stress test is best for a given patient, the clinician must ask two questions:

1. Can the patient exercise?

If yes, a treadmill test is the best choice. It allows you to assess your patient's functional capacity, and several studies have demonstrated a good correlation between how long a patient can exercise on the treadmill and overall long-term survival. The addition of an imaging modality such as echocardiography or thallium-201 scintigraphy can increase the sensitivity and specificity of the stress test.

If the patient cannot exercise (e.g., severe chronic obstructive pulmonary disease [COPD], peripheral vascular disease, arthritis), pharmacologic stress (e.g., persantine, dobutamine) with an accompanying imaging modality is required.

2. Does the resting ECG have ST segment abnormalities?

In patients who have baseline ST abnormalities (e.g., left ventricular hypertrophy with strain, paced rhythm, left bundle branch block (LBBB), ST depression on resting ECG), the ECG alone may not permit an accurate diagnosis of ischemia, and an imaging modality will be required

- Stress testing is very safe
  - 1 to 2 deaths per 10,000 tests

BOX 4-1	*Features of a High-Risk Stress Test*

Angina or ischemic ECG changes at low workload (<6 min or <4 METS on Bruce protocol)

ST segment depression > 2 mm

ST elevation

ST depression persisting > 6 min into recovery period

Exercise-induced hypotension

Ventricular arrhythmias

If thallium or echocardiogram used
   Reversible defects in multiple territories
   Left ventricular cavity dilatation

ECG, electrocardiogram; METS, metabolic equivalent.

- Should be avoided in patients with active symptoms of unstable angina (UA), severe aortic stenosis, possible aortic dissection
- Pharmacologic testing with dipyridamole should be avoided in patients with severe COPD
- Noninvasive imaging of coronary arteries
  - Electron beam CT (EBCT)
    - Provides a noninvasive and quantitative assessment of coronary artery calcification
    - Higher coronary artery calcium scores are associated with increased risk of MI and death
    - In asymptomatic patients, high coronary calcium scores (>75th percentile for age and sex) suggest extensive atherosclerosis and may help to identify high-risk patients who would benefit from aggressive lipid-lowering therapy
    - Has a very high negative predictive value so it can be used to reliably rule out CAD
  - Multidetector row CT (MDCT)
    - Can also measure coronary calcification
    - Improved temporal resolution of these scanners allows for direct coronary artery visualization of a beating heart with little motion artifact
- Coronary angiography
  - Considered the gold standard for the diagnosis of coronary atherosclerosis
  - Three major indications to refer for cardiac catheterization:
    - Failure of medical therapy to relieve symptoms
    - Suggested high-risk coronary anatomy (usually determined by history and stress test)
    - To confirm or exclude CAD

Treatment of Chronic Coronary Disease

- Address modifiable risk factors (e.g., lipid lowering, cigarette cessation)
- Correct illnesses that can precipitate or exacerbate angina (e.g., anemia, infection, thyroid disease)
- Medications that relieve symptoms of angina
  - β-**Blockers**
    - Reduce myocardial O_2 demand by decreasing heart rate, blood pressure (BP), and contractility
    - **Considered first-line therapy for symptoms of exertional angina**
    - Have not been shown to reduce MI or death in patients with chronic stable angina

TABLE 4-2	*Types of Stress Tests*		
	Agent	**Advantages**	**Disadvantages**
Options for Stress			
Exercise	N/A	Mimics physiologic increases in O$_2$ demand Provides useful clinical information (e.g., exercise capacity) Inexpensive	Not all patients can exercise adequately ECG alone without imaging modality has higher rates of false positives and false negatives
Pharmacologic	Dobutamine: β-agonist that ↑ heart rate and myocardial contractility (and thus O$_2$ demand) Adenosine: vasodilates coronary vascular bed and ↑ myocardial blood flow; dilation greater in normal arteries than diseased arteries resulting in steal phenomenon from diseased vascular beds Dipyridamole: coronary dilator that blocks reabsorption of adenosine	Helpful in patients who cannot exercise	More expensive Drugs can cause symptoms of chest pain, nausea, and hypotension, making test interpretation more difficult
Options for Imaging			
Nuclear isotope	Thallium-201: potassium analogue taken up by myocardial cells; hypoperf used myocardium initially shows decreased uptake; tracer redistributes overall several hours Technetium-99 m (sestamibi): also taken up by myocardial cells but binds irreversibly—no late washout makes it ideal for imaging MI and unstable angina	Helpful in distinguishing ischemia from infarcted myocardium Technetium-99 m has higher proton energy—better agent for imaging obese patients Increases sensitivity and specificity of test	More expensive More invasive Requires radiation
Echocardiography	N/A	Direct visualization of ventricular function Can quantify and localize ischemia Noninvasive Increases sensitivity and specificity of test	More expensive Imaging may be limited in obese patients Can yield false positives in patients with LBBB

ECG, electrocardiogram; LBBB, left bundle branch block; MI, myocardial infarction.

- Nitrates
  - Very good at relieving angina and improving exercise tolerance
  - Major effect comes from venodilation, which decreases preload, thereby decreasing wall stress and O$_2$ demand
  - Contraindicated in patients using sildenafil
- Calcium channel blockers
  - Considered second-line agents for chronic stable angina
  - Whereas the short-acting dihydropyridines may increase mortality rates in patients with acute ischemic syndromes (see later discussion), long-acting agents can be used safely in patients with chronic stable angina
- Medications that decrease risk of MI and death
  - Aspirin
    - Reduces risk of MI and death in patients with CAD
    - **All patients with CAD should be on aspirin unless there is a clear contraindication**

- Lipid-lowering agents
  - 3-Hydroxy-methylglutaryl coenzyme A **(HMG-CoA) reductase inhibitors (statins) reduce risk of MI and death in patients with CAD**
  - Gemfibrozil decreases MI and death risk in patients with low HDL levels and normal LDL and triglyceride levels
  - National Cholesterol Education Program (NCEP) guidelines recommend lipid-lowering therapy in patients with CAD to achieve LDL below 100 mg/dL (see Chapter 3)
- ACE inhibitors
  - Conflicting data: The largest and most recent trial showed no decrease in mortality rate in patients with coronary disease who had good left ventricular (LV) function and no heart failure
  - **Clear decrease in mortality rate in patients with CAD who have LV dysfunction and heart failure**

- Revascularization of chronic CAD
  - **Three major indications for revascularization**
    - **Relief of anginal symptoms**
    - **Prevention of nonfatal cardiac events (e.g., MI, congestive heart failure, ventricular tachycardia)**
    - **Decrease mortality**
  - Two methods of revascularization
    - Percutaneous coronary intervention (PCI)
      - PCI refers to percutaneous transluminal coronary angioplasty (PTCA) plus stent deployment
      - With PTCA, a balloon is used to split the atheromatous plaque and stretch the artery
      - Two classes of stents used:
        Bare metal stents
        Drug-eluting stents: Coated with a drug that blocks cell proliferation, thus decreasing restenosis rate
      - Because the drug also inhibits re-endothelialization of the stent, there is an increased risk of in-stent thrombosis
      - To decrease this risk, patients should be on aspirin for life and clopidogrel for at least 1 year following stent placement
      - Major benefits: Highly successful (>90%); decreases the need for bypass surgery
      - Antiplatelet agents commonly used during PCI
        Aspirin: An irreversible cyclooxygenase inhibitor
        Clopidogrel: Inhibits adenosine diphosphate (ADP)-mediated platelet activation; helps to prevent acute stent thrombosis; side effects include rash and gastrointestinal (GI) upset; can rarely cause thrombotic thrombocytopenic purpura
        Ticlopidine: Inhibits ADP-mediated platelet activation; because of associated neutropenia, it has been largely replaced by clopidogrel
        Glycoprotein IIB-IIIA inhibitors: Abciximab and eptifibatide; reduce cardiovascular complications of PCI
      - Risks and complications
        Restenosis: Renarrowing of the arterial lumen following PCI; mechanism incompletely understood but likely involves neointimal thickening because of smooth muscle cell proliferation as well as shrinkage of the dilated segment of artery; incidence of restenosis peaks between 3 and 6 months after PCI; restenosis rates have decreased significantly with the use of intracoronary stents
        1% to 2% risk of emergent bypass, 2% to 4% risk of MI, 1% risk of death; risks increase with long, tubular, eccentric, calcified lesions
      - **Although PCI is quite effective in reducing symptoms of angina in patients with stable CAD, it does not reduce the risk of death, MI, or other major cardiovascular events when compared with optimal medical therapy alone**
    - Coronary artery bypass grafting (CABG)
      - Excellent for relieving anginal symptoms
      - Need for repeated revascularization procedures is less than with PCI
      - Complications include sternal wound infection, MI, stroke, postoperative arrhythmias, and death
      - **Select groups of patients derive mortality benefit from CABG**
        Left main disease
        Three-vessel CAD and decreased LV function
        Three-vessel CAD and ischemia at low workload
        Two- or three-vessel disease with proximal LAD involvement
        Patients with DM—higher 5-year survival with CABG than with PTCA
      - Following CABG, treatment with a statin has been shown to reduce disease progression in grafts (even in patients with only mild LDL elevation)
      - How does multivessel PCI compare with CABG in patients with left main or triple-vessel CAD?
        At 1 year, rates of major adverse cardiac events are higher in the PCI group, largely due to an increased rate of repeat revascularization
        At 1 year, rates of death and MI are the same in both groups, but stroke is more likely to occur with CABG

Primary Prevention of Coronary Artery Disease and Myocardial Infarction

- Risk factor modification
  - Smoking cessation
    - Smoking cessation results in 60% reduction in coronary heart disease risk by 3 years
    - Behavior and pharmacologic intervention should be considered
  - BP control
    - A 5- to 6-mm Hg reduction in BP results in 16% reduction in cardiovascular disease
    - Approach should include lifestyle changes, weight loss, exercise, and medical management if necessary
  - Cholesterol lowering
    - Reduction in serum cholesterol by 10% reduces cardiovascular events by 18% and cardiovascular death by 10%
    - Management should include dietary modification, exercise, and lipid-lowering therapy (see NCEP III guidelines)
  - Tight glycemic control
    - DM increases risk of heart disease by two- to fourfold in men and three- to sevenfold in women
    - Data suggest that tight glycemic control reduces microvascular disease and may reduce risk of cardiovascular events
    - Patients with metabolic syndrome are at increased risk of cardiovascular disease; aggressive risk factor modification is warranted in these patients (diet, exercise, weight loss, lipid and glucose management).
  - Weight loss
    - Obesity and physical inactivity are risk factors for CAD
    - Though data are limited, trials suggest that maintaining ideal body weight and staying physically active may reduce risk of MI by 50%

- Pharmacologic therapy
  - Aspirin
    - In men, pooled data suggest a 33% reduction in first MI
    - In a recent large clinical trial, aspirin reduced the risk of stroke in women 65 years or older but had no effect on risk of MI or death from cardiovascular causes
  - Statins
    - Several large trials have shown that statins reduce the risk of first MI, even in patients with only moderately elevated cholesterol
  - Hormone therapy
    - Though cardiovascular risk increases in postmenopausal women, evidence from large trials suggests that hormone therapy may increase the risk of cardiovascular disease in the first 1 to 2 years of use; routine use for primary prevention should be avoided.
- Diet and exercise
  - Though trial data are limited, maintaining ideal body weight and a physically active lifestyle may reduce risk of MI by 50%
  - The consumption of fish and omega-3 fatty acids has been associated with reduced risk of coronary disease in both men and women
  - Moderate alcohol intake (one drink per day) decreases risk of MI by 30% to 50%; decision to recommend moderate intake should be based on risk-benefit ratio in setting of comorbidities (e.g., liver disease, peptic ulcer disease)
  - Trials with antioxidants have been disappointing; in a large study of patients with vascular disease, administration of folic acid and vitamins B_6 and B_{12} did not reduce the risk of cardiovascular death, MI, or all-cause mortality.

ACUTE CORONARY SYNDROMES

Basic Information

- Epidemiology
  - In the United States, over one million people annually suffer an MI; death results in one-third of these patients.
  - Fifty percent of the deaths from MI occur within the first hour
- Pathophysiology
  - ACSs include unstable angina (UA), non-ST segment elevation MI (NSTEMI), and ST segment elevation MI (STEMI)
  - **The common pathophysiology of all three syndromes is rupture of a vulnerable plaque that leads to platelet activation and aggregation resulting in the formation of intracoronary thrombus (Fig. 4-1)**
  - The vulnerable plaque
    - Larger, fibrotic plaques with thicker caps are less prone to rupture than are smaller plaques, which often have soft atherogenic lipid cores and thinner caps
    - Inflammation is important in plaque instability and rupture; elevated serum levels of certain inflammatory markers (e.g., CRP, fibrinogen, interleukin-6, tumor necrosis factor) correlate with an increased incidence of acute coronary events
    - Numerous factors, including inflammation, weakening of the cap from shear stress, and enzymatic degradation of the cap, can contribute to plaque vulnerability and rupture
  - Formation of thrombus
    - Following plaque rupture, the atherogenic lipid core is exposed to the bloodstream
    - Platelets adhere to the vessel wall when platelet glycoprotein binds to von Willebrand factor
    - Exposure of tissue factor activates the coagulation cascade and leads to thrombin formation, the most potent platelet activator
    - The final common pathway of platelet activation is exposure of the platelet glycoprotein IIB-IIIA receptor, which binds fibrinogen, causing platelets to stick to one another
  - Not all thrombi have the same composition
    - Red thrombi are richer in fibrinogen and red blood cells; they are seen more commonly in STEMI
    - White thrombi are more platelet-rich; they are more common in UA and NSTEMI
- Definitions
  - **Unstable angina (UA):** Defined as either rest angina (usually prolonged >20 minutes), new-onset exertional angina at least class III in severity (i.e., angina with only mild exertion), or preexisting angina that has increased in frequency or duration or that is now brought on with less exertion than before
  - **Non-ST segment elevation MI (NSTEMI):** Can be similar clinically to UA, but is distinguished by evidence of myocardial necrosis (i.e., an elevation in serum cardiac enzymes); ECG does not show ST segment elevation
  - **ST segment elevation MI (STEMI):** This type of MI is defined by the presence of elevated cardiac enzymes and ECG criteria that include greater than 1 mm ST elevation in two or more contiguous limb leads, or greater than 2 mm ST elevation in two or more contiguous precordial leads, or a new or presumed new LBBB
    - **The presence of ST segment elevation on ECG suggests total occlusion of the infarct artery by thrombus; in contrast, most patients presenting with UA or NSTEMI do not have a totally occluded infarct artery**
  - Other differences between NSTEMI and STEMI (Table 4-3)

Clinical Presentation

- Unlike chronic stable angina, in which symptoms occur with exertion, ACSs are often characterized by abrupt symptom onset while at rest
- Symptoms can include chest pain or pressure, shortness of breath, nausea, vomiting, diaphoresis, and radiation of pain to the left arm, neck, or jaw
- Symptoms can be atypical, particularly in women, diabetics, and the elderly
- Some 20% to 30% of ACSs may be clinically silent

Diagnosis and Evaluation

- ECG findings
  - UA and NSTEMI
    - A number of ECG patterns may be seen, including a normal ECG, ST segment depression, T wave inversions, or nonspecific ST and T wave changes
  - STEMI

4

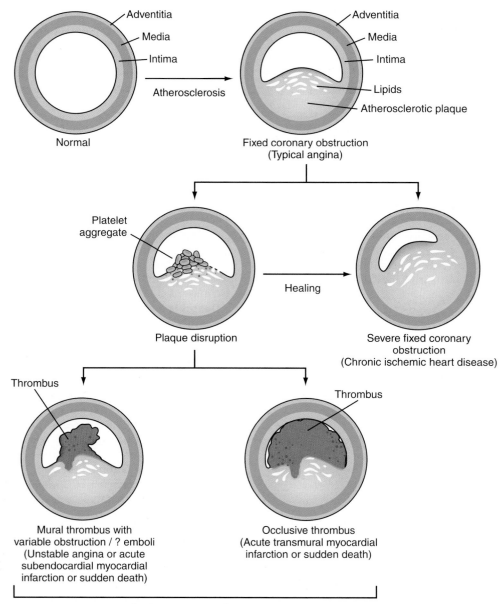

FIGURE 4-1 Schematic representation of sequential progression of coronary artery lesion morphology, beginning with stable chronic plaque responsible for typical angina and leading to the various acute coronary syndromes. (Modified and redrawn from Schoen FJ: *Interventional and surgical cardiovascular pathology: clinical correlations and basic principles,* Philadelphia, WB Saunders, 1989, p 63, and from Zipes DP, Libby P, Bonow RO, Braunwald E, editors: *Braunwald's heart disease: a textbook of cardiovascular medicine,* ed 7, Philadelphia, WB Saunders, 2005, Fig. 12-12.)

- This type of MI is defined electrocardiographically by the presence of more than 1 mm ST segment elevation in two or more contiguous limb leads, or more than 2 mm ST segment elevation in two or more contiguous precordial leads, or a new or presumed new LBBB
  - Patients who meet these ECG criteria require rapid reperfusion (either with thrombolytic therapy or PCI)
- Cardiac enzymes used to diagnose NSTEMI and STEMI (Fig. 4-2)
  - Creatine phosphokinase myocardial band (CPK-MB): First measurable in the bloodstream at 6 to 10 hours; peaks at 24 hours; baseline by 48 to 72 hours

  - Troponin T and I: Greater sensitivity than CPK-MB; appear at 4 to 6 hours; peak 24 to 48 hours and decline slowly; remain detectable for up to 7 to 10 days
  - Lactate dehydrogenase: Increases at 24 to 48 hours and remains elevated for 10 days; used less commonly now that troponins are available
- Risk stratification of UA and NSTEMI
  - Patients presenting with UA and NSTEMI should be risk stratified to determine if they are at low, intermediate, or high risk for subsequent adverse cardiac events
  - ECG and cardiac enzymes
    - The presence of ST segment depression greater than 1 mm in two or more contiguous limb leads (or >2 mm in two or more contiguous precordial leads)

TABLE 4-3	Comparison of Non-ST Segment Elevation MI and ST Segment Elevation MI	
	NSTEMI	**STEMI**
ECG findings	ST depressions; T wave inversions; nonspecific ST-T changes	ST segment elevation
Vessel at time of catheterization	Only 30–40% totally occluded	>80% totally occluded
Type of clot	Rich in platelets (white)	Rich in fibrin (red)
Extent of disease	More likely multivessel with collaterals	More commonly single vessel
Treatment	Thrombolysis not recommended; GP IIB–IIIA inhibitors indicated	Thrombolysis beneficial; GP IIB–IIIA inhibitors usually not indicated (unless PCI performed)
Hospital mortality	Lower	Higher
Reinfarction rate	Higher after hospital discharge	Lower after hospital discharge
Long-term prognosis	Higher 1-yr mortality rate after discharge	Lower 1-yr mortality rate after discharge

GP, glycoprotein; MI, myocardial infarction; NSTEMI, non-ST segment elevation myocardial infarction; PCI, percutaneous coronary intervention; STEMI, ST segment elevation myocardial infarction; ST-T, ST segment and T wave.

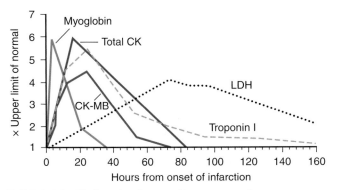

FIGURE 4-2 Timing of various cardiac enzymes after myocardial infarction. CK, creatine kinase; CK-MB, creatine kinase myocardial band; LDH, lactate dehydrogenase. (From Antman EM: General hospital management. In Julian DG, Braunwald E, editors: *Management of acute myocardial infarction*, London, WB Saunders, 1994.)

BOX 4-2	*TIMI Risk Score for Unstable Angina and Non-ST Elevation MI*

Risk Factors
1. Age > 65 yr
2. Three or more coronary artery risk factors
3. Prior coronary stenosis ≥ 50%
4. Two or more anginal events in past 24 hr
5. Aspirin use in past 7 days
6. ST segment changes
7. Positive cardiac markers

Risk of Adverse Cardiac Event by TIMI Score
0–1: 4.7%
2: 8.3%
3: 13.2%
4: 19.9%
5: 26.2%
6–7: 41%

MI, myocardial infarction; TIMI, thrombolysis in myocardial infarction.

is a predictor of an increased risk for adverse cardiac events
- An elevation of cardiac troponin I or T is a strong predictor of subsequent cardiac events
- Patients with both ST segment depression and elevated cardiac enzymes are considered to be at high risk; those with only one of the two factors are intermediate risk; patients with neither of the two factors are considered low risk.
  - The thrombolysis in myocardial infarction (TIMI) risk score for UA/NSTEMI (Box 4-2)
    - A scoring system that uses seven clinical factors to help physicians predict the risk of subsequent adverse cardiac events (defined as MI, persistent ischemia, or cardiac-related death) in patients presenting with UA or NSTEMI
    - A score of 0 to 2 is considered low risk, 3 to 4 is intermediate risk, 5 to 7 is high risk
  - **As a general rule, it is often most appropriate to treat low-risk patients conservatively (i.e., noninvasive testing, medical management); more aggressive treatment (e.g., catheterization, PCI) is**

often the best choice for intermediate-and high-risk patients
- Risk stratification of STEMI (Table 4-4)
  - The TIMI risk score for STEMI assesses risk based on history, exam, and clinical presentation; there is an increased risk in 30-day mortality rates, ranging from 1.1% to 30% for scores ranging from 0 to >8, respectively
- Differential diagnosis (diagnoses that can mimic an ACS)
  - **Always consider other conditions presenting with chest pain and ECG changes that mimic an acute MI, as the management of these conditions is often very different**
  - Aortic dissection
    - Clinical clues include "tearing" pain that radiates to the back, unequal pulses or BP in the upper extremities, new murmur of aortic regurgitation
    - ECG can reveal ST elevations if the dissection involves one or more of the coronary arteries

TABLE 4-4	*TIMI Risk Score for ST Elevation MI*
Clinical Risk Factors	**Points**
History	
≥75 yr old	3
65–74 yr old	2
History of diabetes, hypertension, or angina	1
Physical examination	
Systolic blood pressure < 100 mm Hg	3
Heart rate > 100 beats/min	2
Killip class II–IV	2
Weight < 67 kg	1
Presentation	
Anterior STEMI or left bundle branch block	1
Time to reperfusion therapy > 4 hr	1
Total possible points	14

MI, myocardial infarction; STEMI, ST segment elevation myocardial infarction; TIMI, thrombolysis in myocardial infarction.
Data from Morrow DA, Antman EM, Parsons L, et al: Application of the TIMI risk score for ST-elevation MI in the National Registry of Myocardial Infarction 3. *JAMA* 286:1356–1359, 2001.

- Thrombolytics are contraindicated
- Acute pericarditis
  - Clinical clues include chest pain that may be pleuritic or that is relieved by sitting up; friction rub may be present.
  - ECG may reveal diffuse ST segment elevation and PR segment depression
  - Heparin and thrombolytics contraindicated
- Pulmonary embolism (PE)
  - Clinical clues include risk factors for PE (e.g., sedentary or immobile, history of deep venous thrombosis, leg trauma, oral contraceptive use); sudden-onset chest pain and shortness of breath
  - ECG may show only sinus tachycardia, but classic findings include S wave in lead I, Q wave in lead III, and T wave inversion in III; or possibly a new right bundle branch block or right axis deviation

Treatment of Acute Coronary Syndromes

- Management of UA and NSTEMI (Fig. 4-3)
  - Medical therapy
    - Antiplatelet therapy
      - **Aspirin:** More than 50% reduction in risk of MI and death in patients with UA/NSTEMI
      - **Clopidogrel:** Has been shown in a large clinical trial to reduce adverse cardiac events in patients with UA/NSTEMI when given in addition to aspirin
      - **Glycoprotein IIB-IIIA inhibitors:** Clear benefit demonstrated in both UA and NSTEMI; the greatest benefit seen in patients who have positive troponins and who are going to the cath lab for PCI
        Abciximab: Fab fragment of a monoclonal antibody directed at the IIB-IIIA receptor;

clear benefit for patients undergoing PCI; no benefit seen in patients with UA/NSTEMI who do not require PCI
Eftifibitide: A synthetic peptide; benefit demonstrated in UA/NSTEMI as well as PCI
Tirofiban: A nonpeptide molecule; benefit demonstrated in UA/NSTEMI
- Antithrombotic therapy
  - Unfractionated heparin (UFH)
  - Low-molecular-weight heparin (LMWH): Compared to UFH, has less nonspecific binding and causes less thrombocytopenia; can be dosed by body weight without need to follow activated partial thromboplastin time (aPTT)
    Enoxaparin: Superior to UFH in reducing death, MI, and recurrent ischemic events
    Fondaparinux: Acts through antithrombin to neutralize factor Xa; can be used both with conservative strategy as well as invasive strategy in patients with UA/NSTEMI; preferable to UFH or enoxaparin in patients with increased risk of bleeding
  - Direct thrombin inhibitor
    Bivalirudin: This is an option only in patients where an early invasive approach is planned
- β-Blockers: In UA, β-blockers reduce ischemia and have been shown to reduce subsequent infarction; in NSTEMI, they decrease ischemia, reduce infarct size, help prevent re-infarction, and decrease mortality
- Nitrates: Decrease O_2 demand; quite effective in relieving anginal symptoms; have not been shown to improve survival
- Calcium blockers: Should not be considered first-line for UA or NSTEMI; the short-acting dihydropyridines have been associated with increased mortality in acute coronary syndromes; nondihydropyridine calcium blockers may be used to treat ischemia refractory to β-blockers and nitrates
- Statins: In addition to lipid-lowering ability, these agents have been shown to have antiplatelet and antioxidant properties as well; there is evidence to support their use during the acute presentation with UA/NSTEMI
- **Thrombolytics are not indicated in UA and NSTEMI**
- Cardiac catheterization in UA/NSTEMI
  - Indications for emergent cath
    - Persistent ischemia despite medical therapy
    - Hemodynamic instability
    - VT, ventricular fibrillation, sudden death
  - Indications to cath the patient with UA/NSTEMI who has been stabilized with medication
    - Early positive stress test
    - Large territory of ischemia on ECG
    - High risk as determined by ST segment depression on ECG and elevated cardiac enzymes
    - High or intermediate risk as determined by TIMI risk score
  - **Although stable patients with NSTEMI can be treated conservatively, data from large clinical trials suggest that these patients derive benefit (e.g., improved survival, fewer adverse cardiac**

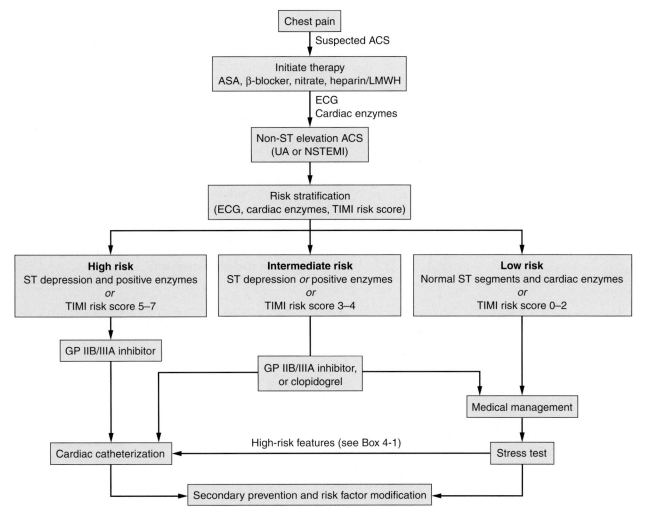

FIGURE 4-3 Approach to the patient with a non-ST segment elevation acute coronary syndrome. The thrombolysis in myocardial infarction (TIMI) risk score calculation appears in Box 4-2. ACS, acute coronary syndrome; ASA, aspirin; ECG, electrocardiogram; GP IIB/IIIA inhibitor, glycoprotein IIB/IIIA inhibitor; LMWH, low-molecular-weight heparin; NSTEMI, non-ST elevation myocardial infarction; UA, unstable angina. (Modified with permission from Yang EH, Ardehali H, Achuff SC: Acute coronary syndromes: non-ST elevation. In Cheng A, Zaas A, editors: *The Osler medical handbook,* St. Louis, Mosby, 2003, pp 95–110.)

events) if referred early for catheterization/ PCI (i.e., during first 48 to 72 hours of hospitalization)
- Management of STEMI (Fig. 4-4)
  - **Rapid recognition of an STEMI and immediate initiation of reperfusion therapy are crucial; the faster normal flow can be restored in the occluded artery, the better the prognosis.**
  - Two major reperfusion strategies
    - Thrombolytic therapy
      - About 60% success rate of opening the occluded artery
      - **Thrombolytics have the most benefit when given in the first 6 hours, but can be given up to 12 hours after onset of chest pain; after 12 hours, the benefit decreases and the risk of rupture increases.**
      - **Indications and contraindications (Table 4-5)**
      - Patients receiving thrombolytics who are at the highest risk of stroke include elderly, female,

hypertensive, and diabetic patients as well as those who have a history of prior stroke or are on warfarin
- Commonly used thrombolytics
  - Streptokinase: Derived from group C streptococcus; inexpensive; can cause allergic reactions
  - Tissue plasminogen activator (tPA): Faster and more clot-specific; more expensive; no allergic potential
  - The latest generation of lytics (e.g., r-PA, tenecteplase [TNK-tPA]): Mutants of tPA and tend to be even more clot-specific
- PCI
  - **Major advantages over thrombolytics include higher reperfusion rate (>90% success rate of opening the occluded artery) and decreased incidence of stroke**
  - More effective than thrombolytics in patients with CHF, cardiogenic shock, and prior bypass surgery

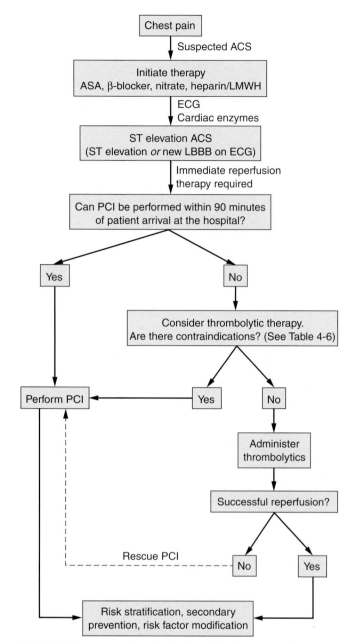

FIGURE 4-4 Approach to the patient with ST segment elevation acute coronary syndrome. ACS, acute coronary syndrome; ASA, aspirin; ECG, electrocardiogram; LBBB, left bundle branch block; LMWH, low-molecular-weight heparin; PCI, percutaneous coronary intervention.

- Major disadvantage is that it is not available in all hospitals, and it may take too much time to get the patient to the appropriate facility
- Terminology
    Primary PCI: Patient with STEMI is taken directly to the cath lab for PCI instead of receiving thrombolytics
    Rescue PCI: Urgent PCI after failure to reperfuse with thrombolytics
- Approximately 20% to 30% of patients receiving thrombolytics fail to reperfuse and have a high mortality rate; recent data show that patients

who fail to reperfuse with thrombolytics have better outcomes if they are then sent for rescue PCI
- General strategy for managing STEMI
    - Reperfusion therapy with either PCI or thrombolytics should be performed as quickly as possible
    - **PCI is usually the first choice for reperfusion if it can be performed in less than 90 minutes after patient arrival**
    - If PCI cannot be performed within 90 minutes of patient arrival, thrombolytics should be given if there are no contraindications; thrombolytics should be given **within 30 minutes of patient arrival.**
    - If a patient receives thrombolytics and fails to reperfuse, he/she should be referred for rescue PCI
- Other pharmacologic therapy for STEMI
    - **Aspirin: proven to prevent recurrent infarction and decrease mortality**
    - Clopidogrel: Improved outcomes when used in combination with aspirin
    - β-Blockers: Decrease ischemia, reduce infarct size, help prevent reinfarction, decrease mortality
    - ACE inhibitors: Proven benefit, particularly in patients with impaired LV function and heart failure; particular benefit in anterior wall MI to help prevent remodeling; angiotensin receptor blocker (ARB) should be used if there is an ACE inhibitor intolerance
    - Nitroglycerin: Good for relieving pain and ischemia; typically used for 24 to 48 hours after STEMI but can be used longer for persistent ischemia, hypertension, or heart failure
    - Heparin: Should be used unless there is a bleeding contraindication; indicated for patients going for PCI; should be given to patients receiving tPA (continued for at least 48 hours); patients receiving a nonselective thrombolytic (e.g., streptokinase) should receive heparin after coagulation factors have normalized (usually after 6 hours); typically given to keep aPTT 50 to 70 seconds for at least 48 hours
    - Statins: Have been shown to have benefit even in the acute infarct setting; can be started even before a lipid profile has been obtained
- Medications not recommended for STEMI
    - Calcium blockers: Short-acting dihydropyridines should be avoided; diltiazem should be avoided in patients with LV dysfunction
    - Empirical antiarrhythmics: Prophylactic antiarrhythmic use can actually increase mortality in the peri-MI setting
    - Glycoprotein IIB-IIIA inhibitors: Not of proven benefit to use in conjunction with thrombolytics
- Complications of acute MI (Table 4-6)

Care Following Myocardial Infarction and Secondary Prevention

- Risk factor modification (e.g., diet and weight loss, BP control, control of blood glucose, lipid lowering, smoking cessation)
- Physical rehabilitation and exercise

TABLE 4-5	**Thrombolytic Therapy in STEMI**	
Indication	**Absolute Contraindications**	**Relative Contraindications**
In a patient presenting with chest pain, the ECG criteria are ≥ 1 mm ST elevation in two contiguous leads *or* A new or presumed new left bundle branch block Duration of symptoms < 12 hr	Any history of intracranial bleed Known cerebral vascular lesion (e.g., AVM) Known malignant intracranial neoplasm Ischemic stroke within 3 mo Suspected aortic dissection Active bleeding or bleeding diathesis (excluding menses) Closed-head or facial trauma within 3 mo	Systolic BP > 180 mm Hg or diastolic BP > 110 mm Hg at presentation History of ischemic stroke > 3 mo prior Prolonged CPR (>10 min) Major surgery within <3 wk Recent internal bleeding (within 2–4 wk) Pregnancy Active peptic ulcer For streptokinase/anistreplase: Prior exposure > 5 days ago or prior allergic reaction

AVM, arteriovenous malformation; BP, blood pressure; CPR, cardiopulmonary resuscitation; ECG, electrocardiogram; STEMI, ST segment elevation myocardial infarction.

4

TABLE 4-6	**Complications of Myocardial Infarction**		
Complication	**Type of MI**	**Timing and Presentation**	**Treatment**

Bradyarrhythmias
  Mobitz type I block (Wenckebach)
 	
  Mobitz type II block
 	
  Third-degree block (complete heart block)
	Mobitz I: Usually seen with IMI; caused by ischemia or increased vagal tone; conduction block usually in AV node
	Mobitz II: Usually AMI; block typically infranodal
	Third degree: AMI or IMI
		Usually in first 24–48 hr for all types
		Asymptomatic or hypotension
			Mobitz I: Responds to atropine and usually resolves in 2–3 days
			Mobitz II: Temporary pacer because high risk for progression to complete block; many will require permanent pacer
			Third degree: Permanent pacer usually required with AMI; often resolves spontaneously with IMI

Bundle branch block	Usually AMI	First 24–48 hr	Temporary pacer indicated for alternating left and right BBB; RBBB with alternating LAFB and LPFB; LBBB or RBBB with first-degree AV block BBB associated with higher mortality
Premature ventricular contractions	Any MI	First 24–72 hr Usually asymptomatic	Treatment usually not required Avoid lidocaine (can ↑ mortality) Can use β-blockers
Ventricular tachycardia or fibrillation	Any territory, but commonly AMI	VT in first 24 hr—usually transient and benign Late VT—consider recurrent ischemia Most VF occurs in first 48 hr	Defibrillation for VF and hemodynamically significant VT For hemodynamically tolerated VT, meds can be tried before cardioversion (e.g., lidocaine, procainamide, amiodarone) β-blockers decrease incidence of lethal VF peri-infarct

Continued

TABLE 4-6	Complications of Myocardial Infarction (Continued)		
Complication	**Type of MI**	**Timing and Presentation**	**Treatment**
Papillary muscle rupture	Usually IMI	2–10 days after MI Sudden onset CHF and hypotension caused by mitral regurgitation Large V waves on Swan-Ganz tracing	IABP to help stabilize Urgent surgery required
Ventricular septal rupture	Both AMI and IMI	1–20 days after MI Pansystolic murmur and palpable thrill Hypotension Increased pulmonary artery O_2 saturation by Swan-Ganz	IABP Urgent surgery required
Ventricular free wall rupture	Both AMI and IMI	2–14 days after STEMI Sudden PEA, tamponade, or death Elderly women at greatest risk	Emergency surgery Very high mortality
Right ventricular infarct	IMI	Classic triad: ↑ JVP, clear lungs, hypotension ECG: ST ↑ in V_4 with right-sided leads	Aggressive IV fluids Avoid agents that decrease preload (e.g., nitrates, morphine) May require inotrope support (e.g., dobutamine)
Pericarditis	AMI or IMI	2–14 days after MI "Dressler's syndrome" Pericardial rub ECG may show diffuse ST elevation and PR depression	Nonsteroidal anti-inflammatory agents Avoid anticoagulation

AMI, anterior MI; AV, atrioventricular; BBB, bundle branch block; ECG, electrocardiogram; IABP, intra-aortic balloon pump; IMI, inferior MI; JVP, jugular venous pressure; LAFB, left anterior fascicular block; LBBB, left bundle branch block; LPFB, left posterior fascicular block; MI, myocardial infarction; PEA, pulseless electrical activity; RBBB, right bundle branch block; STEMI, ST segment elevation myocardial infarction; VF, ventricular fibrillation; VT, ventricular tachycardia.

- Long-term medications
  - **Aspirin: Reduces rate of second MI and improves survival; should be taken indefinitely following infarct**
  - Clopidogrel
    - In patients presenting with an acute MI, clopidogrel should be taken in combination with aspirin for at least a month, and ideally up to 12 months if patient is not at high risk for bleeding; should be used indefinitely in patients who have an intolerance or allergy to aspirin
    - In patients who undergo placement of a drug-eluting stent at the time of infarct, clopidogrel should be used in combination with aspirin for at least a year
  - β-Blockers: Improve survival; should be used indefinitely in most patients following MI
  - ACE inhibitors (or ARBs): Decrease reinfarction rate and improve survival; should clearly be used in all patients with LV dysfunction; help prevent remodeling in patients with anterior wall infarcts
  - Aldosterone blockers: Should be used long term for patients who do not have significant renal dysfunction or hyperkalemia, who are already on therapeutic doses of ACE inhibitor or ARB, have ejection fraction less than 40%, and have either symptomatic heart failure or DM
  - Statins: Reduce reinfarction rates and improve survival in patients with both high and average cholesterol levels; should be used indefinitely to keep LDL cholesterol less than 100 mg/dL
  - Warfarin: Indicated in patients who have severe LV dysfunction or evidence of apical thrombus; no proven survival benefit
- **Implantable defibrillators**
  - **Shown to improve survival in patients with ischemic cardiomyopathy and low ejection fraction (even in the absence of ventricular arrhythmias)**
  - **Indicated for patients with ejection fraction less than or equal to 30% measured at least 40 days after the acute infarction**

REVIEW QUESTIONS

For review questions, please go to www.expertconsult.com.

SUGGESTED READINGS

Antman EM, Anbe DT, Armstrong PW, et al: ACC/AHA guidelines for the management of patients with ST-elevation myocardial infarction-executive summary: a report of the American College of Cardiology/American Heart Association Task Force on Practice Guidelines (Committee to Revise the 1999 Guidelines for the Management of Patients with Acute Myocardial Infarction), *J Am Coll Cardiol* 4:E1–E211, 2004.

Antman EM, Cohen M, Bernink PJ, et al: The TIMI risk score for unstable angina/non-ST elevation MI: a method for prognostication and therapeutic decision making, *JAMA* 284:835–842, 2000.

Boden WE, O'Rourke RA, Teo KK, et al: Optimal medical therapy with or without PCI for stable coronary disease, *N Engl J Med* 356: 1503–1516, 2007.

Morrow DA, Antman EM, Parsons L, et al: Application of the TIMI risk score for ST-elevation MI in the National Registry of Myocardial Infarction 3, *JAMA* 286:1356–1359, 2001.

Morrow DA, Gersh BJ, Braunwald E: Chronic coronary artery disease. In Zipes DP, Libby P, Bonow RO, Braunwald E (eds): *Braunwald's heart disease: a textbook of cardiovascular medicine*, 7th ed. Philadelphia, 2005, WB Saunders, pp 1281–1354.

Moss AJ, Zareba W, Hall WJ, et al: Prophylactic implantation of a defibrillator in patients with myocardial infarction and reduced ejection fraction, *N Engl J Med* 346:877–883, 2002.

Mudd JO, Waters R, Keleman M: Acute coronary syndromes: ST elevation. In Cheng A, Zaas A (eds): *The Osler medical handbook*, St. Louis, 2003, Mosby, pp 111–122.

Yang EH, Ardehali H, Achuff SC: Acute coronary syndromes: non-ST elevation. In Cheng A, Zaas A (eds): *The Osler medical handbook*, St. Louis, 2003, Mosby, pp 95–110.

4

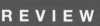
Arrhythmias

CHRISTINE TOMPKINS, MD, and RONALD D. BERGER, MD, PhD

Arrhythmias are a diverse group of disorders that account for significant morbidity and mortality affecting all age groups. They are classified as brady- or tachyarrhythmias based simply on heart rate. Bradyarrhythmias (heart rates < 60 bpm), can occur at any point along the conduction path, resulting from depressed automaticity, conduction delay, or block. Tachyarrhythmias (heart rates > 100 bpm), are typically classified as supraventricular or ventricular based on their origin. Modern-day treatment options for arrhythmias vary according to underlying cause and may encompass pharmacotherapy, electrical conversion, pacemaker or defibrillator insertion, or electrophysiologic ablation.

Bradyarrhythmias

Basic Information

Bradyarrhythmias arise from three sites: Sinoatrial node, atrioventricular node, or infranodal (Table 5-1)
- Sinoatrial node
  - Sinus node dysfunction
    - Reflected by sinus pauses
    - **Asymptomatic sinus pauses are common; treatment is only indicated in the presence of symptoms.**
- Atrioventricular (AV) node
  - First-degree AV block
  - Second-degree AV block
  - Third-degree AV block: usually associated with narrow QRS
- Infranodal
  - Third-degree AV block: usually associated with wide QRS

Clinical Presentation

- Many patients are asymptomatic
- May present with fatigue, dyspnea on exertion, presyncope, or syncope
- Often better tolerated than tachyarrhythmias due to slow progression

Diagnosis and Evaluation

- Clues often obtained from electrocardiogram (ECG) (Table 5-2)
- Event recorders allow correlation of symptoms with the bradyarrhythmia

Treatment

- Acute management of bradyarrhythmias (see Table 5-1)
- Permanent pacer placement for chronic management of bradyarrhythmias

- Indicated for
  - **Sinus node dysfunction and second-degree AV block (Mobitz I) only in the presence of symptoms that correlate with bradycardia**
  - **Second-degree AV block (Mobitz II) and third-degree AV block, even when asymptomatic**
- Dual-chamber pacemaker (senses and paces right atrium and ventricle) unless chronic atrial fibrillation is present, in which case ventricular pacing only is most appropriate

Supraventricular Tachyarrhythmias (SVT)

AV NODE RE-ENTRANT TACHYCARDIA (AVNRT)

Basic Information (Table 5-3)

- Mechanism of arrhythmia: Re-entrant pathway within AV node (Fig. 5-1)
- Dual AV nodal physiology
  - Two functionally and anatomically distinct pathways
    - Slow-conducting path with short refractory period
    - Fast-conducting path with long refractory period
- **Typical form conducts antegrade down slow pathway; retrograde up the fast**
- **Atypical form conducts antegrade down fast pathway; retrograde up the slow**

Clinical Presentation

- Age of onset can be from childhood to old age
- **Notable for abrupt onset and termination of rapid regular heart beat**
- Heart rate usually 150 to 250 bpm
- May be associated with near-syncope, but usually well tolerated; more serious symptoms occur in patients with underlying heart disease

Diagnosis and Evaluation

- Typical AVNRT findings on ECG (Table 5-4)
  - Almost always 1:1 relationship of P wave to QRS complex
  - RP interval < PR interval
  - Retrograde P wave on tail of QRS complex (pseudo-r' in V_1; pseudo-s' in II)
- Atypical AVNRT findings on ECG
  - RP interval > PR interval
- Event monitor may be useful

TABLE 5-1	*Bradyarrhythmias*			
Arrhythmia	**Location of Conduction Defect**	**Features**	**Acute Management**	
Sinus node dysfunction	Sinus node	Common with advancing age, coronary artery disease, and in association with atrial fibrillation. Nonexistent in young, healthy patients	Treat only if symptomatic Atropine Isoproterenol Rarely temporary pacer (if symptomatic)	
First-degree AV block	Slowed conduction within AV node	PR interval ≥ 0.2 sec Rarely of clinical significance	None required	
Second-degree AV block Mobitz I (Wenckebach)	AV node dysfunction	Progressive prolongation of the PR interval until a beat is dropped Can occur with high vagal tone in healthy individuals Rarely advances to complete heart block	Rarely temporary pacer (if symptomatic)	
Mobitz II	Lower conduction system (His-Purkinje) defect	Nonconducted P waves without progressive PR prolongation Almost always associated with LBBB or bifascicular block Often associated with prior anterior MI or cardiomyopathy	Rarely temporary pacer (if symptomatic)	
Third-degree (complete) AV block	Either within or below AV node conduction system defect	Complete dissociation of P waves and QRS complexes	Level of urgency depends on symptoms, QRS width, and escape rate If symptomatic with narrow QRS: atropine If symptomatic with wide QRS: temporary pacer	

AV, atrioventricular; LBBB, left bundle branch block; MI, myocardial infarction.

5

TABLE 5-2	*Electrocardiogram Examples of Common Bradyarrhythmias*

First-degree AV block

Second-degree AV block Mobitz I

Second-degree AV block Mobitz II

Third-degree AV block

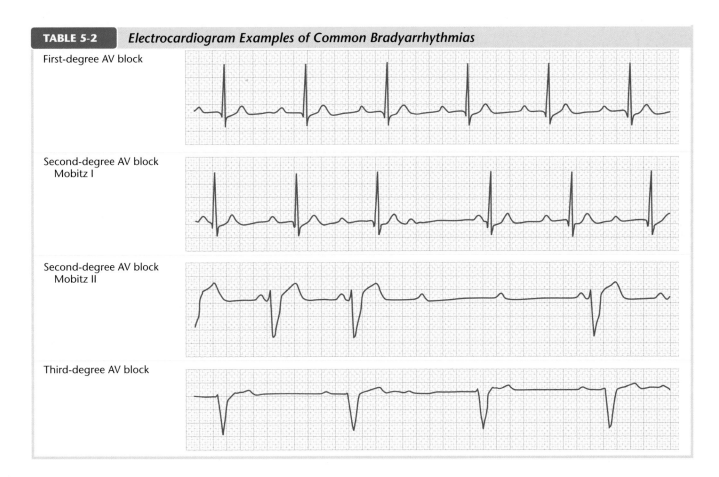

TABLE 5-3	Narrow QRS Complex Tachycardias			
Arrhythmia	**Atrial Rate (bpm)**	**Ratio of Number of Atrial Waves (A) to QRS Complexes (V)**	**P-Wave Morphology**	**Response to Carotid Sinus Massage**
Sinus tachycardia	100–200	1:1	Sinus	Slowing
AVNRT	150–250	1:1	Retrograde	Termination
ORT*	150–250	1:1	Eccentric	Termination
Atrial flutter	250–350	A > V	Sawtooth flutter waves	↑ AV block
Atrial fibrillation	350–600	A >> V	Fib (F) waves	↓ Ventricular rate
Atrial tachycardia	100–250	A ≥ V	Eccentric	↑ AV block
Junctional tachycardia	60–120	1:1	Retrograde	Slight slowing
MAT	100–180	A ≥ V	3 or more different types	Usually none

*In Wolff-Parkinson-White syndrome.
AVNRT, atrioventricular node re-entrant tachycardia; MAT, multifocal atrial tachycardia; ORT, orthodromic re-entrant tachycardia.

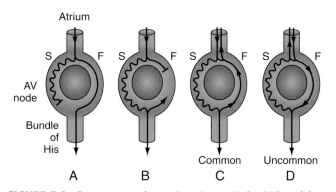

FIGURE 5-1 Re-entrant pathways in atrioventricular (AV) nodal re-entrant tachycardia (AVNRT). The AV node and perinodal tissue have dual physiology: slow-conducting pathway with a short refractory period (S) and fast-conducting pathway with a long refractory period (F). **A,** A normal sinus beat conducts through fast pathway, but conduction through slow pathway is blocked when it hits refractory period of fast pathway. **B,** A premature atrial beat cannot traverse the fast pathway because it remains refractory after prior (normal) beat. Rather, it conducts down slow pathway. **C,** In common form of AVNRT, conduction occurs down slow pathway, then retrograde up the fast pathway, with delivery of an echo beat (retrograde P wave on electrocardiogram) back up to the atrium. If slow pathway has recovered, the impulse re-enters and re-entrant tachycardia is established. **D,** In uncommon form of AVNRT, conduction occurs down the fast pathway and then retrograde up the slow pathway. The echo atrial beat appears much longer after the QRS complex because of slow retrograde conduction (RP > PR interval).

Treatment

- Acute management
  - **May respond to vagal maneuvers**
    - Carotid sinus massage
    - Valsalva maneuver
  - IV adenosine (6–12 mg rapid push) usually highly effective
- Chronic management
  - **Catheter ablation (AV node modification)**
    - **First-line treatment**
    - **Permanent cure in more than 95% of patients**
  - Medications—if not a candidate for ablation (Table 5-5)

- Suppress AV node: Verapamil, β-blocker, digoxin
- Slow conduction within the circuit: Flecainide, amiodarone

WOLFF-PARKINSON-WHITE SYNDROME (WPW)

Basic Information

- Definition: WPW syndrome is term reserved for patients with both pre-excitation on ECG and tachyarrhythmias
  - Most common tachyarrhythmia is AV re-entrant tachycardia (AVRT)
  - Not all patients with an accessory pathway have WPW syndrome
- The accessory pathway is congenital muscle fiber that connects the myocardium of atrium to ventricle across AV groove (Fig. 5-2)
- Accessory pathway may be
  - Manifest: Accessory pathway conducts in antegrade direction (usually conducts retrograde as well); baseline ECG shows pre-excitation (delta wave)
  - Concealed: Accessory pathway conducts only in retrograde direction; baseline ECG appears normal
- Age of symptom onset is childhood through middle age

Clinical Presentation

- Some patients with accessory pathways may never be symptomatic (technically do not have WPW syndrome because of lack of tachycardia)
- Patients may present with tachycardia: AVRT (70%) or atrial fibrillation (30%)
- AVRT in WPW (see Fig. 5-2)
  - Classified into orthodromic or antidromic depending on direction of conduction over the AV node
    - Orthodromic re-entrant tachycardia (ORT): Tachycardia conducts antegrade down AV node and retrograde up accessory pathway
      - Most common form of AVRT (95%)
      - Can occur with manifest pathway that conducts bidirectionally or concealed pathways

TABLE 5-4	*Echocardiogram Examples of Common Supraventricular Tachyarrhythmias*

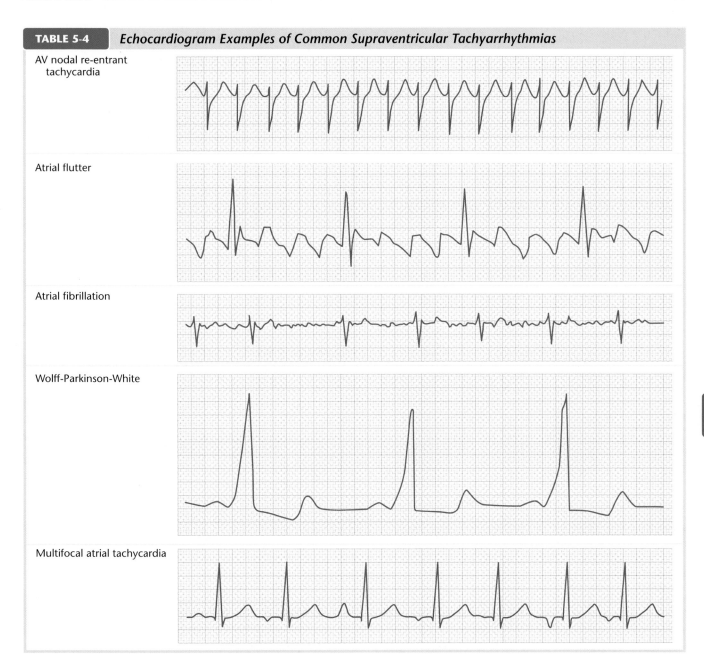

AV nodal re-entrant tachycardia	
Atrial flutter	
Atrial fibrillation	
Wolff-Parkinson-White	
Multifocal atrial tachycardia	

- Antidromic re-entrant tachycardia: Tachycardia conducts antegrade down the accessory pathway and retrograde up the AV node or a second accessory pathway
  - Less common (5%)
  - Will see wide-complex tachycardia on ECG; often confused with ventricular tachycardia (VT)
- **Atrial fibrillation in WPW**
  - **May be life-threatening**
  - **Manifest accessory pathways often conduct rapidly; may result in extremely rapid transmission of atrial fibrillation to ventricles**
  - **Will see wide, irregular QRS morphologies on ECG**
  - **Potentially leads to ventricular fibrillation and sudden death**

Diagnosis and Evaluation

- ECG findings with manifest accessory pathway (see Table 5-4)
  - **Short PR interval (<0.12 sec)**
  - **Delta wave with widened QRS**
    - Caused by ventricular activation through both the accessory pathway and the normal AV node/His-Purkinje conduction system

Treatment

- Asymptomatic patients
  - **Risk of sudden death extremely low**
  - Usually do not benefit from electrophysiologic testing, except those in high-risk occupations (e.g., pilot)

TABLE 5-5		*Common Antiarrhythmic Drugs*		
Class	**Action**		**Examples**	**Notable Side Effects**
I	Block sodium channels; varying effects on maximal velocity of depolarization and duration of action potential		Class IA: quinidine, procainamide, disopyramide Class IB: lidocaine, mexiletine Class IC: flecainide, propafenone	Class: nausea, vomiting Quinidine: hemolytic anemia, thrombocytopenia, tinnitus Procainamide: drug-induced lupus Lidocaine: dizziness, confusion, seizures, coma Mexiletine: tremor, ataxia, rash Flecainide: proarrhythmic toxicity, nausea, dizziness
II	β-Blockers; ↓ SA node automaticity and ↓ AV node conduction		Propranolol, metoprolol	Class: CHF, bronchospasm, bradycardia, hypotension
III	Prolong action potential duration		Amiodarone, sotalol bretylium	Amiodarone: hepatitis, pulmonary toxicity, hypo- and hyperthyroidism, peripheral neuropathy Sotalol: bronchospasm
IV	Calcium channel blockers; ↓ AV nodal conduction		Verapamil, diltiazem	Class: AV block, hypotension, bradycardia, constipation

AV, arteriovenous; CHF, congestive heart failure; SA, sinoatrial.

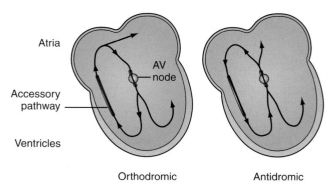

FIGURE 5-2 Re-entrant tachycardia in Wolff-Parkinson-White syndrome. In orthodromic re-entrant tachycardia, the impulse conducts down the atrioventricular (AV) node and the retrograde up the accessory pathway. In antidromic re-entrant tachycardia, the opposite occurs (down the accessory pathway and up through the AV node).

- Symptomatic patients
  - **Acute management of AVRT: IV adenosine, vagal maneuvers**
  - **Acute management of atrial fibrillation with pre-excitation**
    - **First-line therapy: Procainamide (slows accessory pathway and atrial conduction)**
    - **Avoid use of digoxin or calcium channel blockers; can cause even more rapid ventricular response by accelerating accessory pathway conduction**
    - **Emergent cardioversion if patient hypotensive or unstable**
- Chronic management
  - Catheter ablation: First-line therapy in symptomatic patients
    - Curative
    - Electrophysiology (EP) study may rarely identify a second accessory pathway
  - β-Blockers, flecainide to prevent further episodes of re-entrant tachycardia in patients with prior episodes

ATRIAL FIBRILLATION AND ATRIAL FLUTTER

Basic Information

- Atrial fibrillation and flutter often occur in the same patient
- Atrial flutter
  - Macro re-entrant circuit usually confined to the right atrium
  - Age of onset: Usually aged 30 years or older
- Atrial fibrillation
  - Most common arrhythmia
  - Multiple re-entrant wavelets within the atria
  - Increasing incidence with advancing age
  - May be paroxysmal or persistent
    - Paroxysmal form often initiated by premature atrial contraction (PAC) or burst of ectopic atrial activity (often originating in pulmonary vein); usually no structural heart disease present
    - Persistent form often associated with the following
      - Structural heart disease (mitral stenosis and other valvular disease, atrial enlargement, hypertension)
      - Alcohol ("holiday heart")
      - Hyperthyroidism

Clinical Presentation

- Atrial flutter: Palpitations; exertional dyspnea, rarely presyncope
- Atrial fibrillation: Palpitations, exertional dyspnea, presyncope
  - Patients often have underlying heart disease and are more likely to be symptomatic

Diagnosis and Evaluation (see Table 5-3)

- ECG in atrial flutter (see Table 5-4)
  - **Sawtooth P waves, especially in inferior leads**
  - **Atrial rate typically 300 bpm with 2:1 AV conduction**
  - Carotid sinus massage or adenosine will slow AV conduction and may reveal flutter waves previously hidden
- ECG in atrial fibrillation (see Table 5-4)
  - **Fibrillatory (F) waves instead of P waves; atrial rate 350 to 600 bpm**

- **Irregularly irregular and often rapid ventricular response**

Treatment

- Acute management of atrial fibrillation and flutter
  - Rate control with β-blocker, calcium channel blocker (verapamil, diltiazem)
  - Digoxin less potent but useful if heart failure present
  - The drugs themselves do not terminate fibrillation or prevent recurrence
  - Cardiovert if hemodynamically unstable
- Chronic management of atrial flutter
  - Cardioversion
  - Catheter ablation of re-entrant circuit: More than 90% successful
  - **Anticoagulation**
    - **Thromboembolic risk probably similar to that in atrial fibrillation; strong consideration should be given to warfarin therapy (same guidelines as for atrial fibrillation;** see the following)
- Chronic management of atrial fibrillation
  - Rate control as in preceding section
  - Suppression with antiarrhythmic agents
    - Class Ic antiarrhythmic agents (flecainide, propafenone) often used first-line in patients with structurally normal heart
    - Amiodarone preferable in patients with diminished left ventricular function
    - Sotalol, dofetilide are acceptable alternatives
  - Can attempt electrical cardioversion to achieve sinus rhythm
    - Before cardioversion, patients with fibrillation (or flutter) for over 48 hours should receive either
      - Anticoagulation (for at least 3 weeks before conversion and 4 weeks after conversion)
      - Transesophageal echocardiogram to exclude atrial thrombus with heparin titrated to activated partial thromboplastin ratio (rAPTT) 1.5 to 2
  - If persistent and rapid, AV node ablation to prevent conduction of rapid impulses to ventricle
    - Atria still fibrillate—therefore require chronic anticoagulation unless contraindicated
    - Requires ventricular pacemaker placement for subsequent AV block
  - If paroxysmal, may be curable by pulmonary vein isolation (catheter ablation procedure) in highly symptomatic individuals refractory or intolerant of antiarrhythmic medications
  - Chronic anticoagulation with warfarin to prevent stroke in both persistent and paroxysmal atrial fibrillation
    - Antithrombotic therapy is recommended for all patients with atrial fibrillation except lone fibrillation or contraindications.
    - Choice of antithrombotic agent is based on risk of stroke vs. bleeding
    - Indications for antithrombotic agents (Box 5-1)
    - Patients initiated on warfarin should have international normalized ratio (INR) checked weekly until achieve stable goal INR of 2 to 3

| BOX 5-1 | *Indications for Antithrombotic Agents in Atrial Fibrillation* |

Low risk: Aspirin 81–325 mg/day
Moderate risk: Warfarin for patients with more than one risk factor
  Age > 75
  Diabetes
  Hypertension
  Heart failure
  Impaired left ventricular systolic function (EF ≤ 35%)
High risk: Warfarin
  Mechanical heart valves
  Prior thromboembolism (stroke/TIA or systemic embolization)
  Rheumatic mitral stenosis

EF, ejection fraction; TIA, transient ischemic attack.

OTHER SUPRAVENTRICULAR TACHYCARDIAS

- Sinus tachycardia
  - Almost always caused by physiologic stimulus (e.g., fever, hypotension)
  - Features (see Table 5-3)
  - Treatment
    - Treat underlying cause
    - **β-Blockade helpful if caused by anxiety, thyrotoxicosis, ischemia**
    - Long-term sinus tachycardia may not be benign; may lead to high-output heart failure or rate-related cardiomyopathy
- Atrial tachycardia
  - Mechanism may be automatic (elevated sympathetic tone), triggered, or re-entrant
  - Can be associated with digitalis toxicity
  - Features (see Table 5-3)
  - Acute management: Rate control with β-blocker or verapamil
  - Chronic management: Rate control; suppression with flecainide, sotalol, or amiodarone; cure with catheter ablation
- Junctional tachycardia
  - Automatic rhythm arising in AV node
  - Occurs with enhanced automaticity (elevated sympathetic tone), after cardiac surgery, myocardial ischemia, digitalis toxicity
  - Features (see Table 5-3)
  - Acute management: Treat underlying cause
  - Chronic management: Usually none required
- Multifocal atrial tachycardia
  - Arises from multiple automatic or triggered foci
  - Occurs with elevated sympathetic tone, pulmonary disease (e.g., chronic obstructive pulmonary disease), hypoxemia
  - **ECG: Three or more P wave morphologies present (see Table 5-4)**
  - **Treatment: Treat underlying cause (e.g., hypoxemia); rate control**

5

Ventricular Tachyarrhythmias

VENTRICULAR TACHYCARDIA

Basic Information

- Characterized by wide QRS complex (Table 5-6)
- Majority (85%) of wide-complex tachycardias are ventricular; remainder are supraventricular with aberrant conduction
- Helpful clues to distinguish supraventricular vs. ventricular causes (Box 5-2)
- Several forms of VT (see Table 5-6)
  - May be sustained or nonsustained, polymorphic or monomorphic
  - General approach is dependent on presence of underlying structural heart disease or low ejection fraction (Fig. 5-3)
  - Several forms of generally benign idiopathic VT present even in healthy patients with structurally normal hearts

Clinical Presentation

- **Nonsustained VT (self-terminates within 30 seconds): May be asymptomatic or cause occasional palpitations**
- Sustained VT: More likely to cause lightheadedness, near-syncope, syncope

Diagnosis and Evaluation

- ECG findings (Table 5-7)
- Electrophysiologic study: No longer necessary before implantable cardioverter defibrillator (ICD) placement in patients with ischemic or nonischemic heart disease and ejection fraction (EF) less than 30%

Treatment

- Medications (see Table 5-6)
- If acutely hemodynamically unstable—emergent cardioversion
- Chronic treatment of most VTs based on underlying presence of ischemic heart disease
  - Patients with nonsustained VT and no underlying structural heart disease have an excellent prognosis
  - Reassurance
  - β-Blockers or amiodarone for symptoms
  - Idiopathic VT curable by catheter ablation
  - Patients with underlying heart disease and depressed left ventricular function (EF < 40%) are at increased risk of sudden death
    - ICD shown to prolong life in patients with ischemic heart disease and EF less than 30%, and in patients with ischemic or nonischemic cardiomyopathy, EF less than or equal to 35%, and New York Heart Association (NYHA) class II or III heart failure
    - EP study and catheter ablation provide useful adjunctive therapy for recurrent VT

VENTRICULAR FIBRILLATION

Basic Information

- Characterized by irregular, chaotic wide QRS (see Table 5-6)
- Causes
  - Acute myocardial infarction
  - Myocardial ischemia
  - Electrolyte abnormalities (i.e., hypokalemia)
  - Acidosis

TABLE 5-6   *Ventricular Tachyarrhythmias Examples of Common Ventricular Tachyarrhythmias*

Arrhythmia	Ventricular Rate (bpm)	QRS Morphology	Substrate	Drug Therapy	Ablatable
Sustained monomorphic VT	140–250	Any	Post-MI	Procainamide, amiodarone	Yes
Monomorphic VT associated with RVOT activity	140–220	LBBB	Normal	β-Blockers, verapamil	Yes
Ventricular fibrillation	>300	Polymorphic	Ischemia	Lidocaine, amiodarone	No
Torsades de pointes	200–300	Polymorphic	Long QT	β-Blockers	No

LBBB, left bundle branch block; MI, myocardial infarction; RVOT, right ventricular outflow tract; VT, ventricular tachyarrhythmia.

BOX 5-2   *Characteristics Suggestive of Ventricular Origin (vs. Supraventricular Origin) of Wide Complex Tachycardias*

History of structural or ischemic heart disease

Absence of an RS complex in all precordial leads

Peak of R wave to nadir of S interval > 100 ms in one precordial lead

Presence of AV dissociation (P waves unrelated to QRS complexes)

Presence of fusion (sinus QRS fuses with PVC) or captured beats (sinus QRS appears within PVCs)

If RBBB morphology present, QRS width > 0.14 sec

If LBBB morphology present, QRS width > 0.16 sec

LBBB, left bundle branch block; PVC, premature ventricular contraction; RBBB, right bundle branch block.

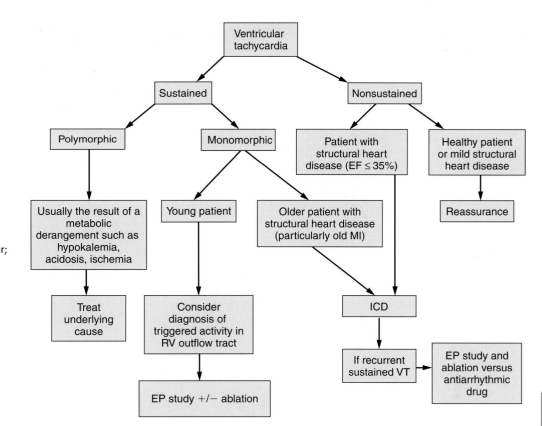

FIGURE 5-3 Approach to ventricular tachycardia. EF, ejection fraction; EP, electrophysiology; ICD, implantable cardioverter defibrillator; MI, myocardial infarction; RV, right ventricular; VT, ventricular tachycardia.

Clinical Presentation
- Sudden death

Diagnosis and Evaluation
- ECG findings (see Table 5-7)

Treatment
- Medications (see Table 5-6)
- If acutely hemodynamically unstable, emergent cardioversion
- ICD for secondary prevention

TORSADES DE POINTES

Basic Information
- Literally "twisting of the points"
- Mechanistically related to prolonged ventricular repolarization
- More common in women than men (women have longer QT intervals)
- May be seen in congenital or acquired long QT syndromes
  - Romano-Ward syndrome (family history of sudden death)
  - Jervell and Lange-Nielsen syndrome (family history of sudden death and congenital deafness)
- May be associated with certain drugs (Box 5-3)
- Tachycardia usually precipitated by a late-coupled (R on T) premature ventricular contraction

Clinical Presentation
- Syncope, presyncope, or may be asymptomatic

Diagnosis and Evaluation
- ECG: Often with prolonged QT interval (see Tables 5-6 and 5-7)

Treatment
- Acute management
  - Correct underlying metabolic abnormality or remove offending medication
  - Attempt to shorten the QT interval
  - Magnesium
  - Lidocaine, phenytoin
  - Isoproterenol
  - Temporary overdrive pacing
- Chronic management
  - If ischemia is underlying cause, consider revascularization
  - Permanent pacer/ICD
  - β-Blocker, amiodarone

Syncope

Basic Information
- Presyncope and syncope are very common presenting symptoms
- Causes vary (Box 5-4)
- In up to 25% of cases, a cause is never identified

Clinical Presentation
- In true cardiac syncope, patients do not remember "hitting the ground"

5

TABLE 5-7 *Electrocardiogram Examples of Common Ventricular Tachyarrhythmias*

Ventricular tachycardia

Ventricular fibrillation

Torsades de pointes

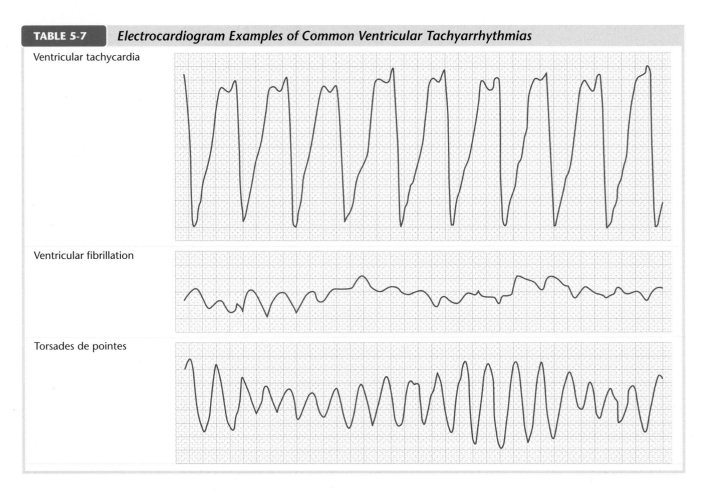

BOX 5-3 *Drugs Associated with Torsades de Pointes*

Class IA antiarrhythmics
Tricyclic antidepressants
Erythromycin
Ketoconazole
Haloperidol
Cisapride
Disopyramide
Pentamidine
Probucol
Sotalol
Dofetilide

BOX 5-4 *Causes of Syncope*

Cardiac
Anatomic: Aortic stenosis, atrial myxoma
Arrhythmic: Bradycardia, tachycardia

Vascular
Anatomic: Subclavian steal
Orthostatic: Dysautonomia, medications
Vagally mediated: Vasovagal, cough, micturition

Metabolic
Hyperventilation
Hypoglycemia

Neurologic
Seizures
Migraines

Miscellaneous
Hemorrhagic
Psychogenic

- **Usually patients arouse immediately; loss of consciousness is transient (seconds to minutes in duration).**
- History and physical examination
  - Ascertain history or symptoms of cardiac or neurologic disease
  - Characterize episode: Precipitating factors, prodromal and recovery symptoms
  - Evaluate for possible offending medications
  - Obtain orthostatic vital signs

Diagnosis and Evaluation

- History and physical examination often provide most important clues in diagnosis
- ECG

- Echocardiogram to rule out structural heart disease
  - Arrhythmia is most likely cause in presence of structural heart disease (see management in preceding sections)
    - Refer for electrophysiology study
  - Vasovagal syncope is most likely cause in absence of structural heart disease
    - Consider tilt table test to evaluate autonomic system (more useful in recurrent episodes)

Treatment

- Treat the underlying condition
- Vasovagal syncope
  - Hydration and liberalization of salt consumption
  - Educate about standing slowly from sitting position
  - Eliminate any offending medications if possible
  - Midodrine useful in refractory cases

Sudden Cardiac Death

Basic Information

- "Sudden cardiac death" describes the complete cessation of cardiac activity irrespective of whether or not the event is fatal
- Ventricular fibrillation or pulseless VT are responsible for one third of events, and the majority of events occur in patients with structural heart disease
- Often represents the first manifestation of ischemic heart disease

Diagnosis and Evaluation

- ECG for evidence of myocardial infarction or ischemia, accessory pathway (Wolff-Parkinson-White syndrome), prolonged QT interval, Brugada syndrome
- Laboratory data to rule out reversible causes, such as cardiac enzymes, electrolytes, drug levels, and urine toxicology screens
- Continuous telemetry to guard against recurrent event until definitive therapy is in place
- Echocardiogram to evaluate for structural heart disease
- Risk stratification with either coronary angiography or stress testing

Treatment

- Treat underlying causes
  - Eliminate proarrhythmic medications
  - Coronary revascularization for ischemic heart disease
- IV lidocaine and amiodarone useful in acute management of repeated arrhythmia
- ICD (Box 5-5)

REVIEW QUESTIONS

For review questions, please go to www.expertconsult.com.

SUGGESTED READINGS

A comparison of antiarrhythmic-drug therapy with implantable defibrillators in patients resuscitated from near-fatal ventricular arrhythmias. The Antiarrhythmics Versus Implantable Defibrillators (AVID) Investigators, N Engl J Med 337:1576–1583, 1997.

| BOX 5-5 | *Indications for ICD Implantation* |

1. Documented VF arrest not due to transient or reversible cause.
2. Documented sustained VT, spontaneous or induced, not associated with acute MI and not due to transient or reversible cause.
3. Documented familial or inherited conditions with high risk of life-threatening arrhythmia, such as LQTS, HCM.
4. Documented prior MI (>40 days old), LVEF < 40%, inducible sustained VT or VF at EP study (MADIT-1 criteria).
5. Documented prior MI, LVEF ≤ 30% either 40 days following MI or 3 mo following revascularization. Patients must *not* have:
   - NYHA class IV
   - Cardiogenic shock while in a stable baseline rhythm
   - CABG or PTCA within past 3 mo
   - Enzyme-positive MI within past 40 days
   - Symptoms or findings that indicate candidacy for coronary revascularization
   - Coexisting disease with expected survival < 1 yr
6. Patients with ischemic cardiomyopathy, documented prior MI, and measured LVEF < 35% and NYHA class II or III CHF
7. Patients with nonischemic dilated cardiomyopathy > 3 mo on appropriate medical therapy and measured LVEF ≤ 35% and NYHA class II or III CHF
8. Patients with NYHA class IV CHF who meet other requirements for cardiac resynchronization therapy

CABG, coronary artery bypass grafting; CHF, congestive heart failure; EP, electrophysiology; HCM, hypertrophic cardiomyopathy; LQTS, long QT syndrome; LVEF, left ventricular ejection fraction; MADIT-1, Multicenter Automatic Defibrillator Implantation Trial 1; MI, myocardial infarction; NYHA, New York Heart Association; PTCA, percutaneous transluminal coronary angioplasty; VF, ventricular fibrillation; VT, ventricular tachycardia.

Bardy GH, Lee KL, Mark DB, et al: Amiodarone or an implantable cardioverter-defibrillator for congestive heart failure, N Engl J Med 352:225–237, 2005.

Bristow MR, Saxon LA, Boehmer J, et al: Cardiac-resynchronization therapy with or without an implantable defibrillator in advanced chronic heart failure, N Engl J Med 350:2140–2150, 2004.

Buxton AE, Lee KL, Fisher JD, et al: A randomized study of the prevention of sudden death in patients with coronary artery disease. Multicenter Unsustained Tachycardia Trial Investigators, N Engl J Med 341:1882–1890, 1999.

Calkins H, Yong P, Miller JM, et al: Catheter ablation of accessory pathways, atrioventricular nodal reentrant tachycardia, and the atrioventricular junction: final results of a prospective, multicenter clinical trial. The Atakr Multicenter Investigators Group, Circulation 99:195–197, 1999.

Gregoratos G, Abrams J, Epstein AE, et al: ACC/AHA/NASPE 2002 guideline update for implantation of cardiac pacemakers and antiarrhythmia devices: summary article. A report of the American College of Cardiology/American Heart Association task force on practice guidelines (ACC/AHA/NASPE committee to update the 1998 pacemaker guidelines), Circulation 106:2145–2161, 2002.

Haissaguerre M, Jais P, Shah DC, et al: Spontaneous initiation of atrial fibrillation by ectopic beats originating in the pulmonary veins, N Engl J Med 339:659–666, 1998.

Moss AJ, Zareba W, Hall WJ, et al: Prophylactic implantation of a defibrillator in patients with myocardial infarction and reduced ejection fraction, N Engl J Med 346:877–883, 2002.

5

Heart Failure

ROSANNE ROUF, MD, and EDWARD K. KASPER, MD, FAHA, FACC

Heart failure (HF) is a common health problem that leads to significant morbidity and mortality. In the United States, approximately 5 million people have HF, and up to 550,000 cases are newly diagnosed each year. The condition exists when the heart can no longer meet the metabolic needs of the body. It can result from any disorder that impairs the ability of the ventricle to fill with or pump blood. It has been estimated that HF causes or contributes to about 290,000 deaths per year. Survival is poor, with only 50% of patients surviving longer than 5 years. Identification of the cause, followed by aggressive treatment, is crucial to improve survival.

Basic Information

- **Definition: HF is a complex clinical syndrome that occurs when the heart or circulation is unable to meet the metabolic demands of peripheral tissue at normal cardiac filling pressures; it can occur in patients with normal or depressed systolic function.**
- Commonly divided into systolic and nonsystolic heart failure (Table 6-1)
  - Systolic: Left ventricle (LV) contracts poorly and empties inadequately leading to depressed systolic function and ejection fraction
    - Often leads to right ventricular failure
    - Over time, LV dilates, increasing wall stress and oxygen demand
    - More common (60% of patients)

- Can result from pressure, volume overload, or myocardial damage
- Nonsystolic: Elevated diastolic filling pressure despite normal diastolic volumes and normal systolic function and ejection fraction
  - Poor LV filling may produce low CO state and poor perfusion
  - Occurs in 40% of patients
  - Can result from high output or diastolic function impairment
- Clinical signs and symptoms: Dyspnea, fatigue, fluid retention, effort intolerance, inadequate organ perfusion, and arrhythmias
- Caused by a variety of conditions, some unrelated to the heart
- High output: Results from a persistent need for high cardiac output, normal systolic function
  - Increased metabolic demands (thyrotoxicosis, Paget's disease, beriberi)
  - Severe anemia
  - Arteriovenous fistula
  - Persistent tachycardia
- Pressure or volume overload
  - Hypertension
  - Valvular heart disease (aortic stenosis, mitral regurgitation)
  - Intracardiac shunting (ventricular septal defect, atrial septal defect, patent ductus arteriosus)

TABLE 6-1	Comparison of Systolic versus Nonsystolic Heart Failure	
	Systolic Dysfunction	**Nonsystolic Dysfunction**
Incidence	60% of heart failure patients	40% of heart failure patients
Mechanism	Impaired ejection	Impaired filling

Physical findings	S_3 and/or S_4
	Weak carotid upstroke
	Displaced apical impulse
		S_4 more common
		Normal carotid upstroke
		Forceful apical impulse
		Hypertrophic cardiomyopathy
		    Rapid, strong carotid upstroke
		    S_4 more common
		    Outflow murmur
		    Ventricular heave

Causes	Coronary artery disease Idiopathic cardiomyopathy Valvular heart disease Hypertension Myocarditis Drug-induced Toxin-induced Systemic disease	Hypertension Fibrosis Ischemia Aging Pericardial disease Restrictive cardiomyopathy Hypertrophic cardiomyopathy Amyloidosis

- Myocyte damage or abnormality
- Myocardial infarction, ischemia
- Drugs (chemotherapeutic agents)
- Toxins (alcohol, cocaine)
- Infection/inflammation?
- Inherited/familial (dilated cardiomyopathy, muscular dystrophy, glycogen storage diseases)
- Impaired diastolic function
- Aging
- Hypertension
- Ischemia
- Constrictive pericarditis
- Infiltrative disease (amyloid, sarcoid, hemochromatosis)
- Inherited/familial (hypertrophic cardiomyopathy [HCM])
- **Most common causes are coronary artery disease, myocardial infarction, and hypertension**
- **In the elderly, 50% of cases may be caused by nonsystolic dysfunction, particularly with concurrent hypertension**
- Causes of acute HF
  - Decompensation of preexisting chronic HF from a precipitating factor (see next list)
  - Myocardial infarction or ischemia, especially if (1) the papillary muscle is involved leading to mitral regurgitation, (2) if ventricular septum rupture occurs, or (3) a right ventricular infarct results in a low cardiac output state
  - Hypertensive crisis
  - Acute arrhythmia
  - Valvular heart disease
  - Acute endocarditis (with aortic or mitral regurgitation)
  - Acute dilated cardiomyopathy (myocarditis, cocaine, toxins)
  - Cardiac tamponade
  - High-output HF (Paget's disease, thyrotoxicosis, beriberi)
- Factors precipitating decompensated HF in preexisting chronic HF
  - Natural course of disease

- Dietary indiscretion (excessive fluid or salt intake)
- Noncompliance with medications
- Infection
- New myocardial ischemia
- Metabolic stress (e.g., anemia, hyperthyroidism)
- Medications such as nonsteroidal anti-inflammatory medications (leads to sodium retention)
- **Cardiomyopathy: Primary heart muscle disease usually classified into three types**
  - **Dilated cardiomyopathy (Fig. 6-1)**
    - Ventricular dilation associated with decreased contractility (left ventricular ejection fraction [LVEF] < 45%)
    - Most common type of cardiomyopathy
    - Multiple causes (Box 6-1)
    - **Most commonly caused by coronary artery disease followed by idiopathic causes**
    - Commonly presents as decompensated HF; can also see angina, systemic emboli, syncope, and sudden death as initial presentation
    - Most forms worsen after an initial period of compensation, leading to eventual death or transplantation
    - Prognosis depends on cause; some improve spontaneously (15–20%)
      - The more symptomatic, the worse the prognosis
      - New York Heart Association (NYHA) class IV: 1-year mortality is 50%
      - For any given ejection fraction (EF), ischemic cause always has worse prognosis
      - Predictors of bad prognosis: Hyponatremia, high filling pressures, and low cardiac index
  - **Hypertrophic cardiomyopathy (see Fig. 6-1)**
    - Hypertrophy of left, right, or both ventricles
    - **Hypertrophy may be generalized or focal; if localized to septum, old term was idiopathic hypertrophic subaortic stenosis (IHSS) or asymmetrical septal hypertrophy (ASH)**
    - Most cases are caused by mutations in genes involved in contractile apparatus
      - Beta-myosin heavy chain (most common)
      - Others include troponin T and tropomyosin
      - Clinical course may depend on genotype

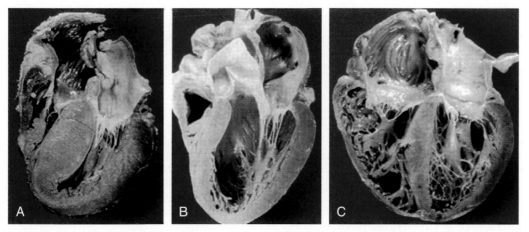

FIGURE 6-1 Gross pathology of hypertrophic and dilated cardiomyopathies. **A,** Hypertrophic cardiomyopathy showing marked hypertrophy especially of the interventricular septum. **B,** Normal heart. **C,** Dilated cardiomyopathy with increased chamber size and spherical shape of left ventricle. (From Seidman JG, Seidman C: The genetic basis for cardiomyopathy: from mutation identification to mechanistic paradigms. *Cell* 104:557, 2001.)

BOX 6-1	Selected Causes of Dilated Cardiomyopathy

Coronary artery disease
Alcohol
Peripartum
Infections (viral, Chagas' disease)
Myocarditis
Hypertension
Drugs (doxorubicin, cyclophosphamide, cocaine)
Familial
Storage disease
Thyroid disease
Vasculitis (lupus)
Pheochromocytoma
Neuromuscular diseases (Duchenne's muscular dystrophy)
Uremia
Idiopathic

- Histologically characterized by myofibril disarray
- Differential diagnosis is hypertrophy resulting from hypertension (called hypertensive HCM), renal failure, or Fabry's disease
- Pathophysiology
  - May cause left ventricular outflow tract obstruction, sometimes dynamic—made worse by increased contractility and decreased ventricular volume
  - Results in a high-pressure apical region and a low-pressure subaortic region—a gradient at the contact point between the septum and the anterior leaflet of the mitral valve during systole
  - Gradient defined as a greater than 30 mm Hg difference at rest or with stimulation (exercise, postpremature ventricular beat)
  - Ventricular volumes small and EF increased
- Presentation
  - Hypertrophy almost always presents by age 20s and symptoms by age 30s
  - **May be obstructive or nonobstructive (more common)**
  - Many never develop obstruction or symptoms
  - **Symptoms: Dyspnea, palpitations, syncope, and sudden death**
  - Outflow murmur may be augmented with maneuvers that decrease preload (Valsalva, squat-to-stand) or decrease afterload (amyl nitrite, vasodilators)
  - Carotid upstroke is rapid (in comparison with aortic stenosis)
- Variable prognosis; some patients die suddenly, often young and during organized sports (most common cause of death in a young athlete during competition); others develop HF
- A few patients will evolve into a dilated cardiomyopathy
- **Familial screening of first-degree relatives with echocardiogram and electrocardiogram (ECG) mandatory**
- **Restrictive cardiomyopathy**

- Most uncommon form of cardiomyopathy in developed world
- Characterized by restrictive filling of left or right ventricle, yet normal or near-normal ventricular function
- Hallmark is diastolic dysfunction
- Ventricular wall thickness normal or increased; biatrial enlargement
- May see "square-root sign" on cardiac catheterization (dip and plateau signifying rapid, early filling)
- Usually presents clinically as right-sided HF
- Multiple causes
  - Usually unknown (idiopathic)
  - Infiltrative diseases
  - Amyloid: Usually caused by primary (AL) form; echo often shows a hyper-refractile "ground glass" appearance of the myocardium; low voltage on ECG; frequent arrhythmias
  - Sarcoid: Many have subclinical heart involvement; conduction disturbances common
  - Hemochromatosis: 15% may present with cardiac involvement; arrhythmias may occur; rapid progression to death if untreated
  - Fabry's disease
  - Endocardial fibroelastosis
  - Löffler's syndrome
- Variable prognosis that depends on cause
  - Idiopathic variety almost always a slow, progressive decline
  - Amyloid associated with high mortality in patients with congestive HF (almost 90% mortality in 6 months)
- Pathophysiology of HF
  - Neurohormonal mechanisms
    - Neurohormonal activation often initially compensatory but detrimental long-term, leading to further ventricular dysfunction
    - Norepinephrine, renin-angiotensin-aldosterone, endothelin, atrial natriuretic peptide, vasopressin, cytokines, nitric oxide, and others (Fig. 6-2)
    - Leads to vasoconstriction and increases systemic and pulmonic vascular resistance and decreases renal blood flow
    - Enhances the vasopressin and renin-angiotensin-aldosterone system
    - Induces ventricular hypertrophy and changes in interstitium
    - Induces ischemia and possibly programmed cell death (apoptosis)
    - This process leads to further dilation termed "remodeling"; ventricular shape becomes more spherical
    - Renin-angiotensin-aldosterine-vasopressin system (RAA system)
      - Poor renal blood flow activates the RAA system increasing sodium and water retention
      - Angiotensin II enhances aldosterone production, which enhances sodium resorption and produces myocardial collagen deposition and fibrosis
      - Angiotensin II also enhances vasopressin, which decreases renal excretion of free water contributing to hyponatremia in HF

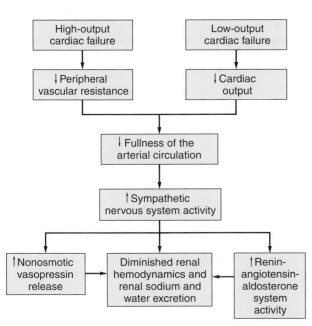

FIGURE 6-2 Pathophysiology of heart failure. Mechanism of high-output and low-output heart failure leading to activation of neurohormonal vasoconstrictor systems and renal sodium and water retention. (From Schrier RW, Abraham WT: Hormones and hemodynamics in heart failure. *N Engl J Med* 341:577, 1999.)

Clinical Presentation

- Symptoms and signs of HF—usually caused by fluid retention or poor cardiac output (or both) (Table 6-2)
- New York Heart Association Classification—a measure of severity of symptoms (Table 6-3)
- It is often difficult to differentiate dilated cardiomyopathy from HCM on history or physical examination
  - S_4 more common in HCM (because of atrial contraction against a stiff ventricle)
  - Outflow tract murmur may be present in HCM and pulse may be bisferiens (two humps)

TABLE 6-2	Symptoms and Signs of Congestive Heart Failure	
Symptoms	**Signs**	
Dyspnea	Increased jugular venous	
Cough (especially when	pressure	
recumbent)	Crackles (rales)	
Anorexia and weight loss	Hepatojugular reflux	
Orthopnea	S_3 and/or S_4	
Paroxysmal nocturnal	Pedal edema and/or ascites	
dyspnea	Hepatomegaly	
RUQ abdominal pain	Tachycardia	
(hepatic congestion)	Decreased pulse pressure	
Fatigue and poor exercise	Cachexia	
tolerance	Mitral or tricuspid	
Nocturia	regurgitation	
	Hypotension	
	Cool extremities	

RUQ, right upper quadrant.

TABLE 6-3	New York Heart Association Classification	
Class	**Severity of Symptoms**	**Description**
I	None to mild	No symptoms
II	Mild to moderate	Symptoms with moderate exertion
III	Moderate to severe	Symptoms with minimal exertion
IV	Severe	Symptoms at rest

- Outflow murmur is harsh, crescendo-decrescendo, located at lower sternal border
  - Increased by standing, postextrasystole, hypovolemia, Valsalva (during strain) (decreased preload increases the obstruction)
  - Decreased by squatting, isometric handgrip (increased afterload decreases the obstruction)
- Ventricular heave
- Restrictive cardiomyopathy and pericardial disease (tamponade, constrictive pericarditis) often present with predominately right-sided findings; findings of infiltration often present in other organs in systemic disorders (e.g., amyloid also causes enlarged tongue and liver).

Diagnosis and Evaluation

- Good history and physical examination: Severity and duration of symptoms, alcohol/cocaine use, angina, family history of HF or sudden cardiac death
  - Diagnosis of HF based on clinical history and exam
  - Strictly a clinical diagnosis
- ECG to evaluate for ischemia, evidence of old infarction, or tachyarrhythmia
- **Echocardiogram: Most cost-effective way to evaluate systolic versus nonsystolic dysfunction**
- Labs: Electrolytes, liver profile, urinalysis to evaluate possible renal or hepatic disease
- Brain natriuretic peptide (BNP) may be useful in distinguishing between cardiac and pulmonary causes of dyspnea
  - A cutoff of 100 pg/mL most commonly used; higher cutoff values improve specificity at the expense of sensitivity
  - Most patients with acutely decompensated heart failure have BNP values greater than 400 pg/mL; an important exception is patients with morbid obesity, who tend to have normal BNP levels even in HF.
- Chest radiograph: Usually shows cardiomegaly and pulmonary venous redistribution; with acute failure, chest film may also show enlarged hilar vessels and Kerley B lines (Fig. 6-3)
- Thyroid function tests if patient is in atrial fibrillation, if the patient's age is older than 60 years, or if the patient has symptoms of thyroid disease

6

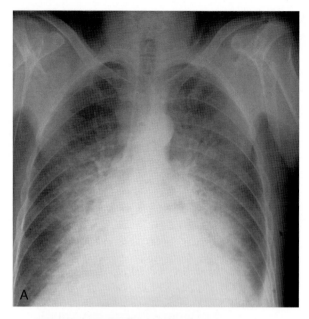

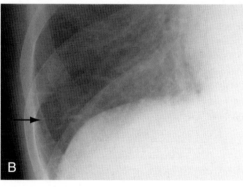

"Ground glass" appearance of alveolar edema

Prominence of upper lobe blood vessels

Enlarged hilar vessels

Septal or "Kerley B" lines

Enlarged cardiac silhouette

C

FIGURE 6-3 Radiologic features of heart failure. **A,** Chest radiograph of a patient with pulmonary edema. **B,** Enlargement of lung base showing Kerley B lines (*arrow*). **C,** Schematic highlighting the radiologic features of heart failure. (From Haslett C, Chilvers ER: *Davidson's principles and practice of medicine,* ed 19, Philadelphia, Churchill Livingstone, 2003, figures 12.22A, 12.22B, and 12.22C.)

- Stress testing is not usually done for the diagnosis of coronary artery disease; more commonly done for reasons of prognosis
- Cardiac catheterization should be done if patient has angina, shows evidence of ischemia or infarction on ECG, or has multiple risk factors

Treatment

- Treatment of acutely decompensated HF
  - Oxygen (to treat hypoxemia and promote diuresis)
  - Morphine sulfate (to decrease patient anxiety and increase arterial and venous dilation)
  - Diuretics (loop diuretics are first line)
  - Nitroglycerin (to decrease preload and pulmonary capillary wedge pressure)
  - Sodium nitroprusside (useful in hypertensive crisis)
  - Nesiritide—recombinant human BNP; works as a vasodilator
    - Questionable association with increased mortality—limit use to severe acute HF
    - Delivered as a continuous IV infusion
    - Monitor for hypotension and worsening renal function during use
  - Inotropic agents (use if peripheral signs of hypoperfusion present)
    - Dobutamine, milrinone
    - Beware of increase in ventricular arrhythmias with these agents
- **Treatment of chronic systolic HF—goal is to delay onset of symptoms if asymptomatic, ameliorate symptoms when present, and prevent sudden death**
  - **Angiotensin-converting enzyme inhibitors (ACEI)**
    - **Indicated in all patients with systolic dysfunction whether symptomatic or not**
    - Start with low dose and titrate upward, monitor potassium and creatinine
    - Titrate to highest tolerated dose or doses used in clinical trials
    - Patients with hyponatremia, hypotension, diabetes mellitus are most prone to problems with renal insufficiency
    - Side effects: Cough, angioedema, renal dysfunction are class effects
    - Contraindications to ACEI: Bilateral renal artery stenosis, previous angioedema to an ACEI. Chronic kidney disease relative contraindication depending on creatinine clearance
    - Angiotensin II receptor blocker (ARB) is an alternative, especially if patient coughs with ACEI
  - **β-Blockers**
    - Indicated in all patients with systolic dysfunction whether symptomatic or not
    - Agents of choice are carvedilol or long-acting metoprolol (succinate)
    - Do not start when patient volume-overloaded
    - Start at low dose and titrate upward to highest tolerated dose or doses used in clinical trials
  - **Both ACEI and β-blockers increase survival in patients with HF due to systolic dysfunction**
  - Diuretics for volume overload if present

- Teach patient about low-salt diet (3–4 g daily), daily weights, symptoms of HF, flexible diuretic regimen
- Loop diuretics most effective at sodium excretion
  - Thiazides used sparingly for booster effect
  - Aldosterone inhibitor (spironolactone, eplerenone) has mortality benefit in patients with severe (NYHA class IV) HF, normal renal function, and normal potassium
    - **Watch potassium carefully as risk of hyperkalemia exists!**
- Digoxin for those still symptomatic on ACEI, β-blocker, and loop diuretic
  - No effect on mortality
  - Decreases hospitalization for HF
  - Use low dose (0.125 mg/dL) and be careful in elderly, those with renal failure, and when starting amiodarone (amiodarone decreases excretion)
  - Symptoms of toxicity include heart block, atrial and ventricular tachycardia, visual disturbances (blurred or yellow vision), nausea, vomiting, dizziness
    - Toxicity exacerbated by hypokalemia
    - Treatment may require digoxin immune antibody, atropine, temporary pacer, and potassium repletion
- Hydralazine and isosorbide dinitrate
  - Recommended for African-American patients who continue to be symptomatic despite optimal therapy with ACEI and β-blocker
  - Should not be a substitute for ACEI or angiotensin receptor blocker (ARB)
  - Combination can be used as an alternative to ACEI if patient is intolerant to ACEI and ARB
- Drugs to avoid: Nonsteroidal anti-inflammatory agents, calcium channel blockers (only vaso-selective ones do not negatively affect survival), antiarrhythmic drugs (only amiodarone and dofetilide do not negatively affect survival), alcohol, cocaine, tobacco
- Warfarin: Advocated for those in atrial fibrillation, with previous embolic event, or with visible cardiac clot on echocardiography; controversial in dilated cardiomyopathy without history of embolic events
- Cardiac resynchronization therapy (CRT or biventricular pacing): To promote mechanical synchrony if LVEF less than 35%, QRS duration greater than or equal to 120 ms, in normal sinus rhythm, and NYHA class III or IV HF on maximal medical therapy
- **Internal cardioverter-defibrillator (ICD): To prevent sudden cardiac death for patients with LVEF less than or equal to 35% and NYHA class II or III HF on maximal medical therapy**
- Transplant: Associated with 90% 1-year survival and 70% 5-year survival rates
  - Strict criteria for eligibility given organ shortage
  - Major early problems are infection and rejection
  - Major late problem is transplant vasculopathy which affects coronary arteries
  - Mechanical circulatory support:
    - Can be used for short-term support, "bridge" to transplant, or "destination" (permanent) therapy for nontransplant candidates

- Treatment of chronic nonsystolic HF—less evidence-based than treatment for systolic dysfunction
  - Treat hypertension aggressively
  - Consider myocardial ischemia as potential cause
  - Diuretics to control fluid
  - Candesartan (ARB) is the only agent to be studied in a large trial of patients with nonsystolic HF; no difference in mortality but fewer hospital admissions for HF
  - Avoid digoxin and positive inotropic drugs
  - Avoid atrial fibrillation—shortens diastolic filling time
- Treatment of chronic HCM—ameliorate symptoms and prevent sudden death
  - Usually either a β-blocker or verapamil to slow heart rate, decrease inotropy, and treat hypertension
    - Verapamil may occasionally worsen gradient in patients with high resting gradient (>50 mm Hg) and severe symptoms
      - Avoid in such patients and use disopyramide instead
  - Avoid digoxin and positive inotropic drugs
  - Avoid atrial fibrillation
  - Avoid drugs that reduce preload or afterload
  - ICD for history of sudden death or syncope, family history of sudden death or syncope, sustained ventricular tachycardia, extreme hypertrophy, or a high-risk genotype
  - **Screen family for HCM with echocardiogram and ECG**
  - **Endocarditis prophylaxis is no longer recommended**
  - Treat as if patient has systolic HF if patient evolves into dilated cardiomyopathy (see previous discussion)
  - **Myectomy rarely necessary and only for obstructive HCM with severe drug-refractory symptoms and a gradient greater than 50 mm Hg**
  - Alcohol ablation of proximal septum—an alternative therapy for obstructive HCM with severe drug-refractory symptoms and a gradient greater than 50 mm Hg
- Treatment of restrictive cardiomyopathy
  - Poor options—cautious use of diuretics as noncompliant ventricle is preload dependent
  - Attempt to treat underlying cause
  - Avoid digoxin, especially in patients with amyloid (high local cardiac digoxin levels lead to increased arrhythmias)
  - Transplantation is an option
  - Avoid atrial fibrillation
  - **Make sure the patient does not have constrictive pericarditis, which is surgically correctable**

SUGGESTED READINGS

Hunt SA, Abraham WT, Chin MH, et al: Guidelines for the diagnosis and management of heart failure in adults: a report of the American College of Cardiology Foundation/American Heart Association task force on practice guidelines (Writing Committee to Update the 2005 Guidelines for the Evaluation and Management of Heart Failure), J Am Coll Cardiol 53:e1–e90, 2009.

Kushwaha SS, Fallon JT, Fuster V: Restrictive cardiomyopathy, N Engl J Med 336:267–276, 1997.

Maron BJ, McKenna WJ, Danielson GK, et al: ACC/ESC clinical expert consensus document on hypertrophic cardiomyopathy: a report of the American College of Cardiology task force on clinical expert consensus documents and the European Society of Cardiology committee for practice guidelines, J Am Coll Cardiol 43:1687–1713, 2003.

6

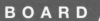
Valvular Heart Disease

THOMAS A. TRAILL, MD, FRCP

Valvular heart disease is recognized by finding a heart murmur. Here, even more than elsewhere in cardiology, the physical findings are all-important to making a diagnosis and assessing severity. Often they trump the results of special testing. Murmurs may first be detected in a symptomless patient, perhaps a young would-be athlete at a high school physical, or they may be the clue in someone with dyspnea and fluid retention that valvular disease is the reason for their cardiac failure.

Aortic Stenosis

Basic Information

- Causes and etiology
  - Congenital unicuspid valve
    - Usually severe, presents in children
  - Congenital bicuspid valve
    - Murmur present from childhood
    - Common cause of aortic regurgitation, as well as aortic stenosis (AS)
    - **AS develops in middle age with calcification**
  - Degenerative calcific disease
    - Develops usually in late middle age or later in a previously normal, trileaflet valve

- Earliest manifestation aortic sclerosis—defined as thickening of the leaflets, presence of a heart murmur, and gradient less than 25 mm Hg
- Progression of aortic sclerosis to stenosis is biologically similar to that of atherosclerosis and has been linked to the same risk factors
- Hence, interest exists in the possibility that lipid lowering will slow progression of AS (unproven)

Clinical Presentation

- Physical signs
  - Slow-rising carotid upstroke ("parvus et tardus")
  - May be difficult to detect in older patients with stiff vessels and wide pulse pressure; should be obvious in patients younger than 70 years
  - Systolic ejection murmur
    - Synonyms: crescendo-decrescendo, diamond-shaped
    - Intensity is no guide to severity
    - Murmur of severe disease sounds "late-peaking"
    - May be conducted to the apex with a musical quality ("Gallavardin murmur")
  - Reduced intensity of A_2 (aortic closure sound) in calcific disease
  - Ejection sound (close after S_1) signals bicuspid valve
  - See Table 7-1 for effects of various maneuvers

	MANEUVERS: EFFECT ON MURMUR INTENSITY*			
Valve Abnormality	**Valsalva (during Continuous Strain)**	**Amyl Nitrite**	**Handgrip**	**Squatting**
Aortic stenosis	↓	↑	↓	↑
Hypertrophic cardiomyopathy (see Chapter 6)	↑	↑	↓	↓
Chronic aortic regurgitation	↓	↓	↑	↑
Chronic mitral regurgitation	↓	↓	↑	↑
Mitral valve prolapse	Moves click and murmur onset closer to S_1	Moves click and murmur onset closer to S_1	Moves click and murmur onset closer to S_2	Moves click and murmur onset closer to S_2
Mitral stenosis	↓	↑	↑	↑

TABLE 7-1 **Effects of Maneuvers on Valvular Murmurs**

*Valsalva maneuver: During continuous strain, increases intrathoracic pressure, thereby decreasing venous return and preload. After strain, arterial pressure drops and venous return subsequently increases.
Amyl nitrite inhalation: Systemic vasodilator causing a drop in blood pressure followed by a reflex increase in heart rate and myocardial contractility.
Handgrip (isometric exercise): Increases systemic pressure and increases afterload.
Squatting: Increases peripheral resistance and thus increases venous return.

- Natural history
  - Excellent prognosis in presymptomatic patients
  - **50% 3-year mortality in patients with symptoms**
    - Classic symptoms: Angina, dyspnea, dizziness/syncope
    - Predicted by outflow tract velocity on Doppler echo
    - Greater than 4 m/sec (corresponds to gradient > 64 mm Hg); implies likely surgery or symptoms (or both) within 2 years
  - Poor prognosis in patients with left ventricular (LV) dysfunction (in whom the outflow velocity and gradient may also be misleadingly low)

Diagnosis and Evaluation

- Role of testing
  - Electrocardiogram (ECG)
    - Usually shows LV hypertrophy
    - Severe AS requiring operation is unusual with normal ECG
  - Echocardiography
    - Shows morphology of the valve
    - Allows Doppler measurement of outflow tract velocity
    - Velocity allows gradient and valve area calculations, but these have limited additional role over the raw velocity
      - More than 4 m/sec, corresponding to 64 mm Hg pressure gradient, implies disease sufficiently severe that if symptoms are not yet present they may be soon
      - Surgery for a high gradient in the absence of symptoms is not routine
    - Demonstrates aortic ectasia in certain patients with bicuspid aortic valve

Treatment

- Timing of surgery
  - Asymptomatic patients are followed, often for years
  - Symptoms of angina, dyspnea, fluid retention, syncope, or exertional dizziness require prompt surgical referral
  - Poor cardiac function requires prompt surgical referral (even if the gradient is low)
- Medical issues
  - Nitrates contraindicated (dangerous to lower preload)
  - Antibiotic prophylaxis for dental work and other potentially contaminated procedures
- Surgical options
  - Mechanical prosthetic valves require lifelong anticoagulation, but should obviate need for future surgery
  - Biologic prostheses offer 15 to 20 years' use before degenerating
    - Less time to degeneration in the young, in patients with kidney disease, and in those on corticosteroids
    - Biologic prostheses do not need anticoagulant treatment
  - Pulmonary autograft procedures are offered to a few patients, typically young people who would otherwise have a biologic xenograft (e.g., possible future pregnancy)

Chronic Aortic Regurgitation

Basic Information

- Etiology and differential diagnosis
  - Aortic regurgitation (AR) has a broad differential diagnosis, and it is critical to identify the underlying cause before determining management; AR demands a diagnosis.
  - Diseases of the valve
    - Bicuspid aortic valve
    - Following endocarditis
    - Rheumatic valve disease
  - Diseases of the aorta
    - Connective tissue disorders
      - Marfan's syndrome (Box 7-1 and Fig. 7-1)
      - Familial aortic ectasia
      - Other rare, inherited vascular disorders
    - Aortic dissection
    - Inflammatory disorders
      - Vasculitis (Takayasu's disease)
      - Giant-cell arteritis
      - Syphilis
  - Diseases affecting aorta and valve
    - Seronegative spondyloarthropathies
      - Ankylosing spondylitis
      - Reiter's syndrome
      - Psoriatic arthropathy

BOX 7-1	*Marfan's Syndrome*

Etiology: Dominant mutations in fibrillin 1, but genetic diagnosis not yet applicable to most cases
Clinical features
  Skeleton
    Height
    Wingspan > 105% of height
    Arachnodactyly
    Pectus carinatum
    Pectus excavatum
    Scoliosis
    Thumb and wrist signs
    Joint laxity
  Ocular
    Ectopia lentis
    Myopia
  Cardiovascular
    Aortic ectasia
    Mitral valve prolapse
  Other
    Dural ectasia
    Spontaneous pneumothorax
    Emphysema
Management of aortic involvement
  Periodic (every 6–12 months) evaluation of aortic dimension by echo
  β-Blocker therapy to slow progression
  Losartan may reduce aortic involvement
  Aortic root replacement for ectasia > 5 cm

7

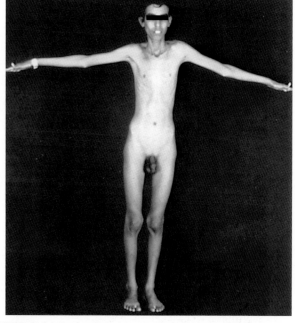

FIGURE 7-1 External phenotype of patient with Marfan's syndrome, showing long extremities and digits, tall stature, and pectus carinatum. (From Zipes DP: *Braunwald's heart disease: a textbook of cardiovascular medicine,* ed 7, Philadelphia, Saunders, 2005, figure 70-7.)

Clinical Presentation

- Physical signs and assessing severity
  - Abnormal pulses, LV enlargement, and a diastolic murmur
  - Pulses
    - Bounding pulses reflect wide pulse pressure due to runoff from the aorta
      - Differential diagnosis of such pulses includes persistent (patent) ductus arteriosus (PDA), arteriovenous fistula, and hypertrophic cardiomyopathy
        - Various eponyms attached to such pulses (Table 7-2)
    - The water hammer pulse refers to the slapping quality when the hand is held up and the arterial diastolic pressure is below approximately 25 mm Hg
  - Other peripheral findings (see Table 7-2)

TABLE 7-2	*Peripheral Pulse Findings in Chronic Aortic Regurgitation*
Sign	**Description**
Quinke's sign	Nailbed pulsation
Corrigan's pulse	Visible carotid pulsation
De Musset's sign	Head bobbing to pulse
Müller's sign	Uvula bobbing to pulse
Duroziez's sign	Diastolic bruit with compression of the femoral artery at the groin
Hill's sign	Systolic pressure in the leg >10 mm Hg higher than the measurement at the brachial artery; reflects large stroke volume
Traube's sign	Pistol shot sounds best heard over the femoral artery

- Auscultatory findings
  - Early diastolic murmur starts at the instant of aortic closure, usually medium frequency
    - Longest and loudest when AR is chronic and the patient is doing well
    - When the LV diastolic pressure rises because of failure, a torrential leak, or in the acute setting, then the murmur is less conspicuous
  - Austin Flint described a second murmur, beginning in mid- or late-diastole, caused by turbulent flow through the mitral orifice; it reflects high LV end-diastolic pressure, thus an adverse hemodynamic situation, and often indicates the need for surgical valve replacement.
  - Effects of various maneuvers on murmur intensity (see Table 7-1)

Diagnosis and Evaluation

- Role of laboratory testing
  - Echocardiography
    - Site of the problem: Valve or aortic wall
    - Morphology of valve: Bicuspid versus other
    - Vegetation, perforation
    - Associated disease of other valves
      - Mitral valve prolapse—connective tissue disorder
      - Mitral stenosis—rheumatic disease
    - Left ventricular cavity size and function

Treatment

- Natural history and timing of surgery
  - Chronic aortic regurgitation well tolerated for many years by most patients, in contrast to acute and subacute AR, but leads eventually, if uncorrected, to irreversible dilation of the LV and poor systolic function
    - The largest LVs seen are those of chronic neglected AR ("cor bovinum")
    - Small role for vasodilator treatment in chronic AR to mitigate this progression
  - Surgery recommended
    - At first hint of symptoms: Dyspnea, fatigue
      - Angina unusual in AR; may reflect coronary ostial involvement by aortitis or unrelated coronary artery atherosclerosis
    - Enlarging LV cavity
    - LV end-systolic dimension more than 5.5 cm (such a figure for dimension at end-systole implies combination of large cavity and some reduction in systolic function)
    - Aortic ectasia
    - Aortic root measurement more than 5 cm in Marfan's syndrome, more than 5.5 cm with other diagnoses

Chronic Mitral Regurgitation

Basic Information

- Differential diagnosis
  - Myxomatous (floppy) valve (i.e., mitral valve prolapse)
  - Ruptured chordae tendineae
  - Following endocarditis
  - Papillary muscle dysfunction
  - Mitral annulus calcification
  - Rheumatic
  - "Functional" (i.e., from annulus or LV dilation)
  - Rarities (e.g., Libman-Sacks endocarditis in lupus)

Clinical Presentation

- Physical signs and assessing severity
  - Hyperkinetic left ventricle
  - Pansystolic murmur
    - In acute, severe mitral regurgitation (MR), murmur may be shortened by high left atrial pressure
    - In mitral valve prolapse, late-systolic murmur implies mild regurgitation
    - **In general, loudness correlates with severity**
    - Effects of maneuvers on murmur (see Table 7-1)
  - Third heart sound

Diagnosis and Evaluation

- Role of testing
  - Chest radiography: Cardiomegaly, left atrial size, pulmonary congestion, pulmonary artery enlargement
  - ECG: May see atrial fibrillation

Treatment

- Natural history and timing of surgery
  - Chronic MR is tolerated even better than AR; hence, there has been a tendency to operate too late, at a point when the LV is irremediably damaged
  - **It is important, therefore, to follow LV size carefully and be alert to even subtle changes in effort tolerance, stamina, and energy level**
  - **Atrial fibrillation often an indication of the time to operate**
  - Enlarging LV may be reflected by end-systolic dimension of 4.5 cm
- Mitral valve repair generally preferred over replacement

Mitral Valve Prolapse

Basic Information

- Etiology
  - Mitral valve prolapse (MVP) is the bulging of the mitral leaflets past the plane of the annulus into the left atrium
    - May be accompanied by mitral regurgitation, not necessarily severe
    - Is normally the result of myxomatous change, but can occur in a normal valve under certain conditions (e.g., a hyperkinetic circulation with excessive sympathetic stimulation or an underfilled left ventricle)

Clinical Presentation

- Physical signs
  - Midsystolic click
  - Late-systolic murmur heard best at the apex
- Natural history and complications
  - Generally benign
  - Infrequent complications
    - Endocarditis; thus, a need for antibiotic prophylaxis in patients with late-systolic murmurs
    - Progressive valve degeneration leading to severe regurgitation (~10% of patients)
    - Atrial and ventricular arrhythmias
    - Sudden death—extremely rare; hence, virtually unpredictable
    - Stroke—very rare; thus, no routine antiplatelet or anticoagulant prophylaxis

Acute Valvular Regurgitation

Basic Information

- Causes
  - Endocarditis
  - Chordal rupture
  - Aortic dissection

Clinical Presentation

- Pathophysiology and presentation
  - Acute AR or MR present differently from their chronic counterparts, because the left ventricle and left atrium are of normal size
  - Thus, acute AR causes LV diastolic pressure to rise abruptly during diastole, so aortic diastolic pressure is not much reduced; pulse pressure is narrow and patients present with cardiogenic shock, small volume pulses, and an unimpressive or absent murmur
  - Acute MR causes a very abrupt tall V wave in the left atrium; hence, acute pulmonary edema, low cardiac output, and a murmur that is unimpressive and may sound like an ejection murmur

Treatment

- Natural history and management
  - Acute AR
    - Natural history is poor and early surgery is almost always advised
    - Surgery should not be delayed pending completion of antibiotic treatment
    - Antibiotic treatment should be continued after operation to finish full course
  - Acute MR
    - Natural history better than acute AR
    - Surgery advised for patients with acute pulmonary edema

Mitral Stenosis

Basic Information

- Causes
  - Acquired mitral stenosis is invariably from rheumatic fever; clinically recognized in about 50% of patients
  - Congenital mitral stenosis (MS) is recognized but rare

Clinical Presentation

- Symptoms
  - Mobile valve
    - Loud S_1
    - Opening snap (follows S_2)
    - Mid-diastolic rumble
  - Calcified valve
    - Normal or soft S_1, dull or absent snap
    - Soft but long murmur
  - Effect of various maneuvers (see Table 7-1)

Diagnosis and Evaluation

- Symptoms and management
  - Young patient, mobile valve
    - Symptoms include dyspnea, paroxysmal nocturnal dyspnea, hemoptysis, paroxysmal atrial fibrillation

7

- Balloon commissurotomy if there is pure MS (without MR) and no thrombus
- Older patient, calcified, immobile valve, or subvalve chordal disease
  - Valve replacement for symptoms or findings of fatigue, dyspnea, atrial fibrillation, pulmonary hypertension, right heart failure, edema
- Role of laboratory studies
  - Chest radiography
    - Left atrial enlargement
    - Pulmonary artery and right heart enlargement
  - Echocardiography
    - Valve morphology
    - Involvement of other valves
    - Transesophageal echocardiography (TEE) before balloon commissurotomy to examine left atrium for clot

Treatment

- Mitral stenosis and pregnancy
  - Ostensibly well young women with MS may tolerate pregnancy poorly because of combined effects of blood volume increase and high cardiac output
  - Careful preconception assessment indicated
  - In a pregnant woman with new-onset pulmonary edema, consider
    - Mitral stenosis
    - Peripartum cardiomyopathy

Antibiotic Prophylaxis

Diagnosis and Evaluation

- Goal is to prevent infective endocarditis
- Recent updated guidelines (AHA, 2007) contain major changes based on current evidence
- Patients for whom prophylaxis is indicated (only patients at highest risk):
  - Prosthetic heart valves (including bioprosthetics)
  - Personal history of infective endocarditis
  - Unrepaired congenital cyanotic heart disease
  - Incompletely repaired cyanotic heart disease or repaired using prosthetic material
  - Cardiac valvulopathy in a transplanted heart
- No longer indicated in common valvular disorders such as mitral valve prolapse, bicuspid aortic valve, acquired aortic and mitral valve disorders, hypertrophic cardiomyopathy, and others
- Procedures for which prophylaxis is indicated
  - Dental procedures that involve manipulation of gingival tissue or periapical tooth region or mucosal perforation
  - Respiratory tract procedures that involve incision or biopsy
  - Procedures in patients with GI or GU tract infections
  - Procedures on infected skin or tissue
  - Surgery to implant prosthetic valves or prosthetic intravascular or intracardiac materials

Treatment

- Standard regimen for most dental and respiratory procedures: Amoxicillin 2 g given 30 to 60 minutes before procedure
- Alternatives for penicillin-allergic patients: Cephalexin, azithromycin, clarithromycin, or clindamycin
- For other procedures, need to tailor antibiotic to likely organisms

Artificial Valves

Treatment

- Choosing a prosthesis
  - Repair preferred over replacement, but generally only available for mitral valve disease
  - **Bioprostheses last roughly 5 to 20 years—shorter lifespan than mechanical prostheses**
  - Consider biologic valves rather than the more durable mechanical prostheses when
    - Prepregnancy condition exists (and anticoagulants undesirable)
    - Anticoagulation undesirable or risky
    - Patient is in atrial fibrillation and will be on anticoagulants
    - Patients are older than 60 years (bioprosthesis should last long enough)
    - In setting of high endocarditis risk, as it is less likely to require removal in event of endocarditis
  - Bioprostheses deteriorate more rapidly in young patients, those with kidney disease, or those on corticosteroids
- Follow-up of prostheses
  - Prosthetic malfunction
    - Produces the same murmurs as in native valves (exception is paraprosthetic MR, which can be silent)
    - Consider in a patient with hemolysis
    - TEE often required for confirmation and assessing severity
  - Interrupting anticoagulants
    - Relatively safe in patients with aortic prostheses
    - Should generally use heparin (usually low-molecular-weight) for patients with mitral prostheses

SUGGESTED READINGS

Bonow RO, Carabello B, de Leon AC Jr, et al: ACC/AHA guidelines for the management of patients with valvular heart disease, *Circulation* 98:1949–1984, 1998.

Lung B, Gohlke-Barwolf C, Tornos P, et al: Working group on valvular heart disease. Recommendations on the management of the asymptomatic patient with valvular heart disease, *Eur Heart J* 23: 1252–1266, 2002.

Otto CM: Evaluation and management of chronic mitral regurgitation, *N Engl J Med* 345:740–746, 2001.

Otto CM: Valvular aortic stenosis: disease severity and timing of intervention, *J Am Coll Cardiol* 47:2141–2151, 2006.

Pericardial Disease

MARY CORRETTI, MD

Pericardial disease is a group of disorders that may manifest as an asymptomatic effusion, tamponade, acute pericarditis, or chronic constriction. Possible causes are quite varied. A thorough history and physical examination often provide clues to the underlying cause.

Acute Pericarditis

Basic Information

- Function and anatomy of normal pericardium
  - Visceral and parietal pericardial layers separated by a potential space, the pericardial cavity
  - Normally contains 15 to 50 mL of straw-colored serous pericardial fluid, an ultrafiltrate of plasma; the fluid acts as a lubricant to reduce interlayer friction during cardiac contraction
- Three main functions of pericardium
  - Suspends the heart in place—keeping the position of the heart relatively constant
  - Serves as a physical barrier to prevent spread of infection and malignancy from contiguous structures
  - Prevents acute cardiac dilatation
- Pericarditis can manifest as acute, subacute, or chronic
  - Acute pericarditis occurs when there is inflammation of the pericardium and is defined as signs or symptoms from pericardial inflammation of no more than 1 to 2 weeks' duration
  - Pericarditis is relatively common in patients presenting to emergency departments, with up to 5% of those with nonischemic chest pain and 1% with ST elevation on electrocardiogram (ECG)
- Major causes are idiopathic, infectious, neoplastic, autoimmune disorders; uremia; cardiac surgery; irradiation; traumatic events; and infarction (Table 8-1)
- **Most common cause is viral or idiopathic**

Clinical Presentation

- Clinical features
  - Chest pain can be severe
  - Sudden onset, sharp, and worse with inspiration, cough, and body movements
  - May radiate to neck, back, left shoulder, or trapezius muscle ridge
  - Is variable: May be persistent or may wax and wane
  - Pain is typically substernal or localized to left chest; left arm radiation is not typical
  - **Pain may be positional in nature: worse when patient is supine and relieved with sitting up and leaning forward**

- Patient may also complain of dyspnea
- Less common symptoms: Cough, dysphagia, and hiccups
- An antecedent history of fever and symptoms of a viral syndrome are common
- Physical examination
  - 85% of patients have an audible friction rub (high-pitched scratchy or squeaky sound best heard at the left sternal border at end expiration with the patient leaning forward)
  - Rub may be evanescent—disappearing and returning over short periods of time
  - **Rub may have three components, related to movement of the heart during the cardiac cycle: Atrial systole, ventricular systole, and ventricular diastole**
  - **In reality, the rub is triphasic in about half the patients, biphasic in a third, and monophasic in the remainder**
  - Performance of a complete, careful examination of the patient with acute pericarditis is essential to delineate specific diagnoses and to assess for the presence of coexistent myocarditis
- Special syndromes
  - Dressler's syndrome
    - Occurs weeks to months after myocardial infarction
    - Consists of fever, malaise, serositis, pulmonary infiltrates, and pleural effusion in addition to pericardial effusion
    - Due to an immunologic reaction
  - Postpericardiotomy syndrome
    - Pericarditis occurs weeks to months after cardiac surgery
    - Possibly due to hypersensitivity of injured myocardial tissue

Diagnosis and Evaluation

- Diagnosis
  - ECG findings: Classically evolves through four stages over time (Fig. 8-1)
    - Stage I: Diffuse ST segment elevation with concomitant PR segment depression in almost all leads (except aVR)
    - Stage II: Normalization of the ST and PR segments
    - Stage III: Widespread T wave inversions
    - Stage IV: Normalization of the T waves
  - Most common ECG changes of myocarditis are diffuse T-wave inversions without abnormality of the ST segment unless there is concurrent pericarditis

TABLE 8-1	*Causes of Acute Pericarditis*
Process	**Examples**
Infectious	Viral
	Bacterial
	Mycobacterial
	Fungal
	Protozoal
	HIV
Neoplastic	Primary (mesothelioma—rare, sarcomas, fibroma, lipoma)
	Secondary (breast, lung, melanoma, sarcoma, lymphoma, leukemia, ovarian)
Immune/ Inflammatory	Autoimmune and connective tissue disorders (e.g., SLE, RA, ankylosing spondylitis, scleroderma, sarcoidosis, dematomyositis, polyarteritis nodosa, Wegener's granulomatosis, Sjögren's syndrome)
	IBD
	Löffler's syndrome
	Stevens-Johns on syndrome
	Myocardial infarction
	Dressler's syndrome
	Postpericardiotomy syndrome
	Post-traumatic
	Pleural and pulmonary diseases
Metabolic	Uremia
	Dialysis-associated
	Myxedema
	Gout
Iatrogenic	Radiation injury
	Related to cardiac catheterization or placement of implantable defibrillators and pacemakers
Traumatic	Blunt trauma
	Penetrating trauma
	Chylopericardium
Drug-induced	Hydralazine, procainamide, minoxidil isoniazide, anticoagulants

IBD, inflammatory bowel disease; RA, rheumatoid arthritis; SLE, systemic lupus erythematosus.

- Chest radiography: May be normal in uncomplicated acute idiopathic pericarditis
  - Occasionally pleural effusions are present
  - Pulmonary vascular congestion may indicate severe concomitant myocarditis
- Echocardiography: Typically normal in most patients with acute idiopathic pericarditis (Fig. 8-2)
  - Most do not have effusions or they have ones that are very small and inconsequential
  - Echo is also useful to determine whether the effusion is loculated or diffuse, or contains elements of blood, fibrinous, or inflammatory material

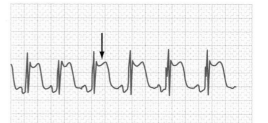

A

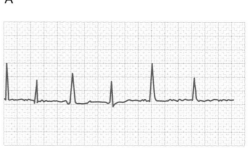

B

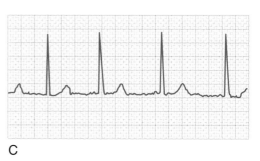

C

FIGURE 8-1 ECG changes associated with pericarditis. **A,** Acute pericarditis. Note the raised ST segment, concave upward *(arrow).* **B,** Chronic phase of pericarditis associated with a pericardial effusion. Note the T-wave flattening and inversion and the alternation of the QRS amplitude (QRS alternans). **C,** The same patient after evacuation of the pericardial fluid. Note that the QRS voltage has increased and the T waves have returned to normal. (From Kumar P, Clark M: *Clinical medicine,* ed 5, Philadelphia, Saunders, 2005, figure 13.96.)

- Can assess for tamponade or constrictive pericarditis (see later discussion) physiology
- Laboratory studies
  - Nonspecific markers of inflammation (i.e., erythrocyte sedimentation rate, C-reactive protein, and white blood cell count) usually only modestly increased
  - In the patient with concomitant myocardial inflammation, there may be a modest elevation of cardiac enzymes—creatine phosphokinase myocardial band (CPK-MB) fraction or troponin I (or both)
  - Complete blood count
    - Serum creatinine, blood urea nitrogen, antinuclear antibodies, serologic test for HIV
    - Other laboratory tests should be aimed at diagnosing the underlying cause as guided by the history and physical exam
- Evaluation
  - Guided by the history and physical exam, but usually includes
    - Electrocardiogram (frequent to detect evolutionary changes)

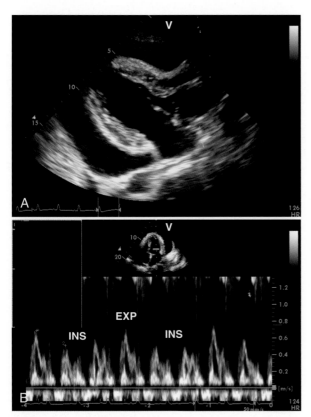

FIGURE 8-2 **A,** Echocardiogram of a large pericardial effusion with findings of tamponade physiology. Diastolic compression of the RV on 2D images. **B,** Marked variation of mitral inflow velocity by Doppler.

- Chest radiography
- Laboratory tests as previously described
- Tuberculin skin test
- Transthoracic echocardiogram
- Pericardiocentesis rarely provides diagnosis in the patient with a small or moderate effusion

Treatment

- **Acute idiopathic or viral pericarditis is usually a benign, self-limited disease that resolves within 2 to 6 weeks**
- **Treatment is primarily supportive: Bed rest and NSAIDs**
  - Aspirin (2–4 g/day), indomethacin (75–225 mg/day), and ibuprofen (1600–3200 mg/day) prescribed most often
  - Anti-inflammatory agents may be tapered after 1 to 2 weeks
  - Severe pain that does not respond to NSAIDs within 48 hours may be treated by adding colchicine (0.6 mg twice daily) or administering high doses of corticosteroids (60–80 mg of prednisone per day in divided doses)
- Other therapy is aimed at treating the underlying cause of pericarditis
- Avoid anticoagulants in the acute phase to reduce the risk of intrapericardial hemorrhage and tamponade
- Routine hospitalization usually not necessary
- Hospitalize patients with temperature greater than 38°C; subacute onset (symptoms developing over several weeks); immunosuppressed state; trauma; on oral anticoagulant therapy; myopericarditis (pericarditis with clinical or serologic evidence of myocardial involvement); large pericardial effusion (an echo-free space > 20 mm in width); cardiac tamponade; or myocardial infarction

Pericardial Effusion and Cardiac Tamponade

Basic Information

- Pericardial effusion
  - Accumulating fluid in the pericardium may be transudative or exudative
  - May occur with acute pericarditis or may accumulate in fluid-retentive states (heart failure, renal failure, or cirrhosis)
  - Features that determine whether an effusion will cause increased intrapericardial pressure and hemodynamic compromise
    - The rate of accumulation of fluid
    - The volume of the fluid
    - The physical characteristics of the pericardium itself
  - **Gradual accumulations of up to 1 to 2 L of fluid may be well tolerated, whereas the rapid addition of even 80 to 200 mL will result in markedly increased intrapericardial pressure**
- Cardiac tamponade
  - Occurs when pericardial fluid increases intrapericardial pressure, exceeding intracardiac pressures and resulting in compression of the cardiac chambers
    - Limits diastolic filling of the heart
    - Results in decreased stroke volume, cardiac output, systemic blood pressure, and elevated venous pressures
  - Any cause of acute pericarditis and pericardial effusion may lead to tamponade, but the most common causes are neoplastic, uremic, and viral/idiopathic pericarditis
  - Occurs in 15% of acute pericarditis cases

Clinical Presentation

- Symptoms of pericardial effusion
  - May be asymptomatic even if pericardial effusion is large and there is no tamponade
  - With large effusions, patients may experience dull chest pain, pressure, or a nonspecific sense of discomfort
  - Other symptoms related to mechanical compression of adjacent structures include dysphagia, cough, hoarseness (left recurrent laryngeal nerve compression), hiccups (phrenic nerve compression), nausea, or abdominal fullness
- Physical examination findings with a pericardial effusion
  - Pericardial effusions that are small or moderate may present with normal physical examination
  - Muffled heart sounds
    - Ewart's sign: Dullness to percussion and bronchial breath sounds beneath the left scapula caused by compressive atelectasis in the left lower lung field

- Symptoms of tamponade
  - Symptoms result from decreased cardiac output and elevated filling pressures
  - Fatigue, light-headedness, and dyspnea; patients may feel more comfortable sitting forward
- Physical examination findings in tamponade
  - **Classically presents with Beck's triad: (1) elevated jugular venous pressure, (2) arterial hypotension, and (3) quiet "muffled" heart sounds**
  - Other manifestations of tamponade related to reduced cardiac output include: tachypnea, diaphoresis, depressed sensorium, cool extremities, peripheral cyanosis
  - With gradual accumulation of fluid, blood pressure may be maintained and signs of right-heart failure (hepatomegaly, ascites, and lower extremity edema) may be present
  - **Pulsus paradoxus: Greater than 10-mm Hg decrease in systolic blood pressure with inspiration**
  - Kussmaul's sign: Paradoxical rise in jugular venous pressure with deep inspiration

Diagnosis and Evaluation

- Characteristic features of cardiac tamponade are shown in Table 8-2
- **ECG: Voltage may be reduced, nonspecific T-wave flattening, and electrical alternans (change in QRS voltage from beat to beat)**
- Chest radiography: Cardiac silhouette may be enlarged
- Echocardiography
  - Most useful imaging modality for demonstrating pericardial effusion and tamponade
  - Effusion is visualized as an echo-free space (black) between the pericardial layers
  - Right atrial (RA) (late diastolic) and right ventricular (RV) (early diastolic) collapse is observed when tamponade occurs
  - RV diastolic collapse is more specific (85–100%) than RA collapse for contributing evidence of tamponade physiology
  - An increase in RV volume with inspiration shifts the septum toward the left ventricle in diastole, and toward the right ventricle in systole. A decrease in RV volume occurs with expiration. This pattern of motion corresponds to the physical finding of pulsus paradoxus.

- Marked respiratory variation in echo Doppler inflow velocities across the mitral and tricuspid valves (flow velocity paradox) is seen in tamponade, as well as in constrictive pericarditis
- CT or MRI: Can detect an effusion, but less useful than echocardiogram; pericardial thickness can be measured with both CT and MRI, allowing for the severity and chronicity of inflammation and other pericardial disease entities
- Right-heart catheterization (RHC)
  - RA pressure tracings normally composed of a series of waveforms (Fig. 8-3)
    - The A wave represents atrial contraction (and follows the P wave on ECG)

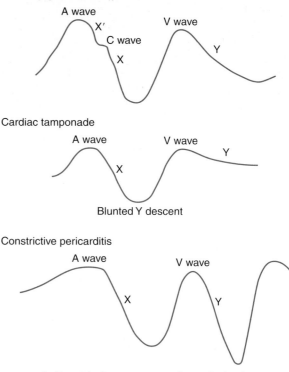

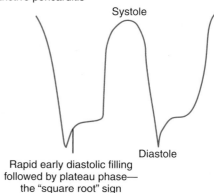

FIGURE 8-3 Typical catheterization findings in pericardial disease.

TABLE 8-2	Characteristic Features of Constrictive Pericarditis and Cardiac Tamponade	
	Constrictive Pericarditis	**Cardiac Tamponade**
Equalization of end-diastolic pressures	Yes (within 5 mm Hg)	Yes (within 5 mm Hg)
Right atrial pressure waveform	Prominent X and Y descent (X = Y or Y > X)	Blunted or absent Y descent (X > Y)
Pericardium	Thickened (>3–4 mm)	Normal
Kussmaul's sign	Present	Absent
Pulsus paradoxus	Absent	Present

- The X descent follows the A wave and represents atrial relaxation
- The V wave represents passive filling of the right atrium beginning after ventricular systole has closed the tricuspid valve
- The Y descent follows the V wave and represents the rapid flow of blood from the atrium into the ventricle in early diastole
- In tamponade, RHC findings can be diagnostic, although this modality is not usually required to make the diagnosis
  - Because increased intrapericardial pressures cause equalization of RA and RV pressures in diastole, there is a minimal pressure gradient pushing blood from the right atrium to ventricle during diastole
  - Equalization of RA, RV diastolic, and pulmonary capillary wedge pressures occur
  - **The Y descent is blunted or absent (see Fig. 8-3)**
  - The X descent, which corresponds to atrial relaxation, is preserved

Treatment

- Pericardial effusion
  - Indications for drainage of pericardial effusion by pericardiocentesis (Fig. 8-4)
    - **Evidence of hemodynamic compromise**
    - **Examination of fluid required to establish a diagnosis**
    - **Suggested purulent pericarditis**
  - Asymptomatic effusions, even large ones, may be followed indefinitely with serial echocardiograms and clinical assessments
  - As with the management of pericarditis, anticoagulation should be avoided
- Cardiac tamponade
  - Cardiac tamponade is potentially life-threatening and should be treated as a medical emergency
  - Definitive treatment for tamponade is removal of the pericardial fluid via pericardiocentesis

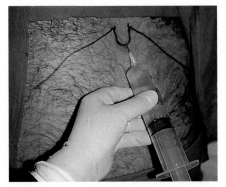

FIGURE 8-4 Aspiration of pericardial fluid. A wide-bore needle is inserted into the epigastrium below the xiphoid process and advanced in the direction of the medial third of the right clavicle. If the needle is connected to the V lead of an ECG monitor, ST elevation is usually seen if the needle touches the epicardium. This can be useful in distinguishing a bloody pericardial effusion from accidental puncture of the heart. Other complications of the procedure may include arrhythmias, vasovagal attack, and pneumothorax. (From Forbes C, Jackson W: *Color atlas and text of clinical medicine*. St. Louis, Mosby, 2003, figure 5.140.)

- Medical management
  - Temporizing until pericardiocentesis performed
  - Expansion of intravascular volume with fluids
- Recurrent episodes of pericardial effusion and tamponade may be treated with repeated pericardiocenteses, balloon pericardiotomy, surgical creation of a pericardial window, or pericardiectomy
- Another option is injection of a sclerosing agent into the pericardial space to cause adherence of the visceral and parietal pericardium

Constrictive Pericarditis

Basic Information

- Thickened (and often calcified) pericardium that may occur following any form of acute pericarditis; constrictive pericarditis is the end stage of such inflammatory process involving the pericardium
- **Most common causes are viral/idiopathic, uremic, postsurgical, tuberculous, or radiation-induced**
  - Other causes include neoplastic, autoimmune, posttrauma, sarcoid, methysergide therapy, and implantable defibrillator patches
- Typically occurs months to years after the initial episode of pericarditis
  - Pericardial effusion undergoes organization (instead of resorption) with deposition of fibrin
  - Progresses to a chronic stage with fibrous scarring and thickening of the pericardium with obliteration of the pericardial space
  - Calcium deposition may contribute to the stiffening of the pericardium
- The primary pathophysiologic feature is impaired diastolic filling caused by the presence of a rigid pericardium
  - Conceptually, constrictive pericarditis can be thought of as a normally contracting heart confined in a small box
  - Rigid pericardium impairs diastolic filling, resulting in increased and equal diastolic filling pressures in all the cardiac chambers
  - During early to mid-diastole, ventricular filling ceases abruptly when the intracardiac blood volume reaches the limit set by a stiff pericardium
  - Most ventricular filling occurs in diastole, and systemic venous congestion results
  - The myocardium may be involved in the chronic inflammatory process, leading to intrinsic contractile dysfunction as well

Clinical Presentation

- Signs and symptoms of constrictive pericarditis are the result of decreased cardiac output and increased venous pressures manifesting as right-heart failure
- Clinical features
  - Abdominal fullness (due to hepatic congestion and ascites) and peripheral edema
  - Symptoms of decreased cardiac output such as fatigue, weight loss, and muscle weakness
  - Less commonly, pulmonary congestion with orthopnea, dyspnea, and cough

8

- Physical examination
  - Elevated jugular venous pressure; signs of passive liver congestion (icterus, ascites); lower extremity edema
  - **Kussmaul's sign**
    - An increase in jugular venous pressure with inspiration (normally decreases with inspiration)
    - Occurs because the rigid pericardium insulates the heart from the decreased intrathoracic pressure that occurs with inspiration
  - **Pericardial knock:** Extra heart sound heard in early diastole (mimics an S_3), coinciding with abrupt cessation in ventricular filling due to the rigid pericardium

Diagnosis and Evaluation

- ECG: Usually nonspecific findings such as T-wave flattening or inversion
- Chest radiography: May show calcified pericardium
- Echocardiogram: 2D and M-mode may demonstrate abnormal diastolic ventricular septal motion due to interventricular interdependence, marked respiratory variation in ventricular size/filling (>25%), plethoric inferior vena cava, and at times, thickened pericardium (>4 mm)
- CT or MRI: Most useful in identifying thickened (>4 mm) and calcified pericardium
- Right-heart catheterization (RHC)
  - Important for establishing or confirming the diagnosis of constrictive pericarditis
  - Reveals elevation and equalization of RA, RV diastolic, pulmonary capillary wedge, and left ventricular diastolic pressures
  - Prominent X and Y descents result in an M or W configuration of the RA pressure tracing (see Fig. 8-3)

- The early diastolic filling of the right and left ventricles shows a characteristic "dip and plateau" pattern, or "square root" sign, caused by early rapid diastolic filling of the ventricle and then its abrupt halt (see Fig. 8-3)

Treatment

- **Total pericardiectomy (surgical removal of the pericardium) is the treatment of choice**
  - With complete pericardiectomy, 90% of patients are symptomatically improved and 50% have complete relief of symptoms
  - These results may take up to 6 months to be clinically apparent
  - Pericardiectomy is less effective when constrictive pericarditis is due to irradiation, as an underlying restrictive cardiomyopathy is often also present
  - Surgical mortality is between 5% and 19%
- Prior to pericardiectomy, calcium channel blockers and β-blockers should be avoided, because sinus tachycardia is a compensatory mechanism

REVIEW QUESTIONS

For review questions, please go to www.expertconsult.com.

SUGGESTED READINGS

Ariyarajah V, Spodicak DH: Acute pericarditis: Diagnostic cues and common electrocardiographic manifestations, Cardiol Rev 15(1): 24–30, 2007.

Lange RA, Hillis LD: Acute pericarditis, N Engl J Med 351:2195–2202, 2004.

Libby P, Bonow R, editors: Braunwald's heart disease textbook of cardiovascular medicine, ed 8, Philadelphia, 2008, WB Saunders.

Myers RB, Spodick DH: Constrictive pericarditis: Clinical and pathophysiologic characteristics, Am Heart J 138:219–232, 1999.

Electrocardiogram Review

BRENT G. PETTY, MD

The electrocardiogram (ECG) is an important tool in diagnosing a variety of cardiac conditions. A systematic approach to ECG interpretation involves evaluating heart rate, rhythm, axis, intervals, and waveforms. Putting this ECG interpretation together with the patient's clinical picture can aid in formulating a diagnosis and treatment plan.

Fundamental Features to Assess When Reading an Electrocardiogram

Rate

- Normal is 60 to 100 bpm
- **Estimate rate by dividing 300 by the R-R interval (as measured by number of large boxes from R to R)**
  - Measure R-R interval to nearest 0.01 second and divide into 60 to calculate the rate more accurately

Rhythm

See also Chapter 4 on coronary artery disease.
- Too fast or too slow?
- Regular or irregular?
- Ventricular or supraventricular?

Axis

- Normal is 0° to positive 90°
- Leftward axis, between 0° and up to negative 30°, is "borderline" but not necessarily pathologic; axis more negative than negative 30° is abnormal
- Determine axis quadrant by evaluating positive or negative deflection of the QRS complex in leads I and aVF (Table 9-1)

Intervals

Figure 9-1 illustrates intervals and waveforms of surface ECGs.
- PR interval: Normal is 0.12 to 0.2 seconds
- QRS duration: Normal is less than 0.12 seconds
- QT interval varies with heart rate
  - QT interval is inversely proportional to heart rate
  - Corrected QT ($QT_{corrected}$, or QT_c) adjusts for the heart rate
  - Calculated as: QT divided by the square root of R-R interval
  - Normal QT_c is 0.36 to 0.41 seconds

Waveform

- Pathologic Q waves (indicative of prior transmural ST-elevation myocardial infarction)

- **To be considered "pathologic," Q waves must be 1 small box wide and 1 small box deep (1 small box in width equals 0.04 seconds at correct paper speed of 25 mm per second)**
- ST segments (elevation or depression > 1 mm)
- T-wave abnormalities (inversion or pseudonormalization)

Selected Electrocardiogram Abnormalities

Low Voltage

- Definition
  - No R or S wave in limb leads greater than 5 mm
  - No R or S wave in precordial leads greater than 15 mm
- Causes
  - Obesity
  - Chronic obstructive pulmonary disease
  - Pericardial effusion
  - Hypothyroidism
  - Addison's disease
  - Infiltrative diseases (e.g., amyloidosis, hemochromatosis, sarcoidosis)

Atrioventricular Block

- **First degree**
  - **PR interval greater than 0.2 seconds**
  - By itself, of no clinical consequence
- **Second degree**
  - **Mobitz I (also called Wenckebach block)**
    - Gradually increasing PR interval until a P wave is not followed by a QRS complex
    - Usually self-limited and not clinically significant, so no treatment required
  - Mobitz II
    - Higher degree of block, where only a fraction of the P waves are followed by QRS complexes (e.g., 1:3)
    - Usually caused by disease of the His bundle system rather than the atrioventricular (AV) node itself
- **Third degree**
  - Also known as complete heart block
  - **Characterized by AV dissociation, where the P-P interval and the R-R interval are different and P waves are not responsible for the QRS complexes**
  - The QRS complexes are usually at a slow rate ("escape"), arising from intrinsic depolarization of the AV node (usually around 45–55 bpm) or the ventricle (usually around 35–45 bpm)

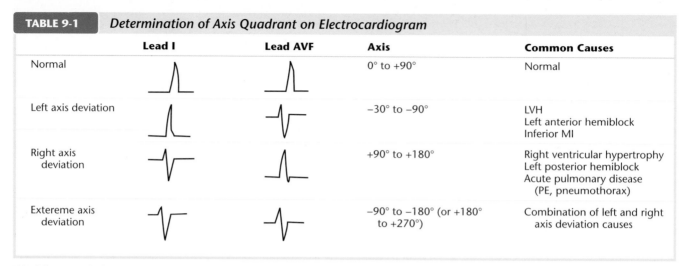

	Lead I	Lead AVF	Axis	Common Causes
Normal			0° to +90°	Normal
Left axis deviation			−30° to −90°	LVH Left anterior hemiblock Inferior MI
Right axis deviation			+90° to +180°	Right ventricular hypertrophy Left posterior hemiblock Acute pulmonary disease (PE, pneumothorax)
Extereme axis deviation			−90° to −180° (or +180° to +270°)	Combination of left and right axis deviation causes

TABLE 9-1 *Determination of Axis Quadrant on Electrocardiogram*

LVH, left ventricular hypertrophy; MI, myocardial infarction; PE, pulmonary embolism.

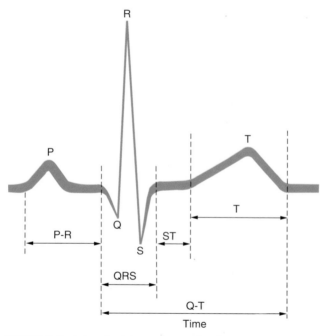

FIGURE 9-1 Intervals and waveforms of surface electrocardiogram.

Left Ventricular Hypertrophy

- The gold standard for diagnosing left ventricular hypertrophy (LVH) is echocardiogram
- ECG may be suggestive of LVH; many different ECG criteria exist
- **Common ECG standard: Increased QRS voltage plus evidence of either strain, left axis deviation, or left atrial abnormality**
  - Increased QRS voltage, as evidenced by one of the following:
    - R or S greater than 20 mm in any limb lead
    - S in V_{1-3} or R in V_{4-6} greater than 30 mm
    - (R in V_5 + S in V_1) greater than 35 mm
    - R in aVL greater than 11 mm

- "Strain": Nonspecific ST-T changes (usually mild, downward-sloping ST depression and T-wave inversion or biphasic T waves) associated with voltage criteria for LVH
  - Left axis deviation (see Table 9-1)
  - **Left atrial abnormality: Net negative P wave in V_1 and P wave in V_2 at least slightly biphasic**
- Major causes
  - Hypertension
  - Aortic valve disease, either insufficiency or stenosis
  - Mitral insufficiency
  - Hypertrophic cardiomyopathy

Wide QRS Complex

- Definition: QRS greater than or equal to 0.12 seconds
- Primary causes
  - Bundle branch block
  - Ventricular rhythm
  - Hyperkalemia
  - Wolff-Parkinson-White syndrome

Bundle Branch Block

Figure 9-2 provides a bundle branch block algorithm.
- Can determine by ECG (Table 9-2; see Fig. 9-2)
- Causes
  - Myocardial infarction
  - Infiltrative diseases (e.g., amyloidosis, hemochromatosis, sarcoidosis)
  - Degenerative diseases of the conduction system

Trifascicular Block

- Can manifest in three ways (in order of decreasing frequency):
  - Bifascicular block and prolonged PR interval
  - Complete heart block
  - Alternating right and left bundle branch block

Other Electrocardiogram Findings

- **Osborn waves**
  - **Positive deflection off declining shoulder of R wave**

TABLE 9-2	Examples of Bundle Branch Block

Type of Bundle Branch Block	Description	Example Electrocardiogram
Right bundle branch block (RBBB)	Terminal S in I and V_6 + rSR′ or tall R in V_1	
Left bundle branch block (LBBB)	Tall broad R in I and V_6 + QS or rS in V_1	
Bifascicular block	RBBB + left axis deviation beyond −30° (shown to right) *or* RBBB + right axis deviation at least +120° *or* LBBB	
Trifascicular block	Bifascicular block (at right, LBBB) + prolonged PR interval	

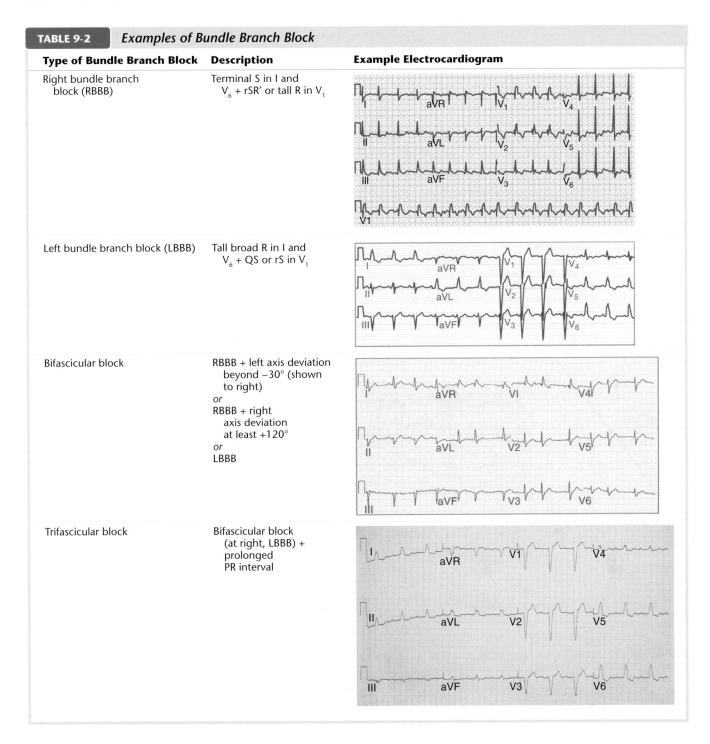

- Gives a "notched" appearance to the R wave
- **Often seen with hypothermia**
- ST elevation
  - **Consider myocardial infarction if**
    - **ST elevation in anterior (I, aVL, V_{1-4}), inferior (II, III, aVF), or lateral (V_{4-6}) pattern**
    - **ST segment elevation tends to be convex upward (sharp angle of takeoff from QRS complex) or horizontal**
    - Common sequential ECG changes in myocardial infarction (Fig. 9-3)

- Diffuse concave upward ST elevation (as may be seen in early repolarization) does not rule out infarction
- Consider ventricular aneurysm if ST elevation persists after myocardial infarction
- Consider pericarditis if
  - ST elevation is diffuse and tends to be concave upward (smooth, curved takeoff from QRS complex)
  - Rarely may have PR segment depression
- **Possible ECG findings with pulmonary embolus**
  - **Sinus tachycardia is most common ECG association**
  - T-wave inversions in inferior and precordial leads

9

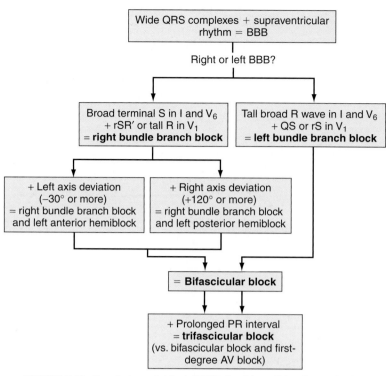

FIGURE 9-2 Bundle branch block (BBB) algorithm. AV, atrioventricular.

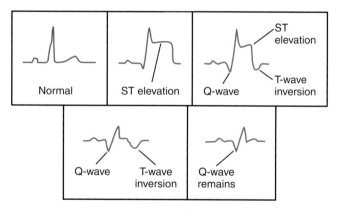

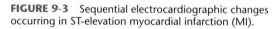
(in leads recording the area of MI)

FIGURE 9-3 Sequential electrocardiographic changes occurring in ST-elevation myocardial infarction (MI).

- Deep S wave in lead I (right axis elevation) with a Q wave and T wave inversion in lead III ($S_1Q_3T_3$)
- Electrical alternans
  - Alternating amplitude or direction of QRS complexes
  - Often seen with a pericardial effusion
- May be caused by the "to and fro" motion of the heart swinging in a pericardial sac filled with fluid
- Diffusely inverted T waves
  - Nonspecific finding, potentially related to intracranial catastrophies (hemorrhage or stroke) or evolving pericarditis
  - Also associated with "broken heart syndrome," an acute, temporary but profound cardiomyopathy frequently following sudden fear or surprise

REVIEW QUESTIONS

For review questions, please go to www.expertconsult.com.

SUGGESTED READINGS

Anguera I, Vallis V: Giant waves in hypothermia, *Circulation* 101: 1627–1628, 2000.

Sakata K, Yoshino H, Houshaku H, et al: Myocardial damage and left ventricular dysfunction in patients with and without persistent negative T waves after Q-wave anterior myocardial infarction, *Am J Cardiol* 87:510–515, 2001.

Taylor GJ, Petty BG: Electrocardiogram. In Taylor GJ, editor: *Primary care and management of heart disease*, St. Louis, 2000, Mosby, pp 54–68.

Wittstein IS, Thiemann DR, Lima JAC, et al: Neurohumoral features of myocardial stunning due to sudden emotional stress, *N Engl J Med* 352:539–548, 2005.

SECTION TWO

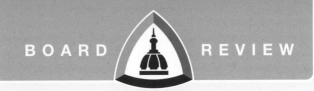

Infectious Disease

Respiratory Infections

PAUL G. AUWAERTER, MD

Infections of the respiratory tract result in more antibiotic prescriptions than any other group of medical disorders in the outpatient setting. **In many cases, respiratory tract infections do not require administration of antibiotics for cure.** The inappropriate prescription of antibiotics contributes to antibiotic resistance, particularly of concern in *Streptococcus pneumoniae*.

Bacterial Sinusitis

Basic Information

- **Acute bacterial sinusitis (ABS) is often preceded by viral upper respiratory tract infection (URTI), allergy flare, trauma, or dental manipulation**
- Symptoms often **mimicked by common cold or allergies**
- Diagnosis best made on clinical grounds, although history and physical findings are not specific
- Nasal passages also commonly involved (Fig. 10-1); thus some view this as rhinosinusitis
- **Chronic sinusitis is a poorly understood entity, diagnosed after at least 12 weeks of sinus symptoms and signs, resulting from chronic obstruction of sinus passages.** The role of bacterial pathogens in this disorder is debated.

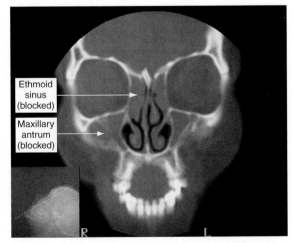

FIGURE 10-1   Coronal CT scan showing ethmoid, labyrinth, and maxillary antral opacification in a patient with sinusitis. (From Swash M: *Hutchison's clinical methods,* ed 21, Philadelphia, WB Saunders, 2002, figure 13.10.)

- **Microbiology of ABS shows that respiratory pathogens predominate (in order of decreasing frequency)**
  - *S. pneumoniae*
  - *Haemophilus influenzae*
  - *Moraxella catarrhalis*
- **Antibacterial resistance among these organisms increasingly common (>40% of *H. influenzae* and 100% of *M. catarrhalis* are now β-lactamase producers, meaning they are resistant to amoxicillin);** high-level **pneumococcal resistance to penicillin** is less frequent than previously stated as a result of revised resistance breakpoints for nonmeningeal isolates (falling from 10% to only ~1%); clinical importance of resistant bacteria in sinus conditions is debated
- Other pathogens, such as anaerobes, other streptococci, and *Staphylococcus aureus*, account for small percentages of isolates in ABS
- **In chronic sinusitis, *S. aureus, Staphylococcus epidermidis,* and anaerobes predominate. Whether antibiotic treatment helps this condition is unclear, but it is often used.**

Clinical Presentation

- **ABS most commonly follows viral URTI**
- **Change in color or character of nasal discharge is not specifically indicative of bacterial infection**
- **ABS (as opposed to viral or allergic sinusitis) is unlikely if symptoms are less than 7 days' duration**
- Historical or physical findings suggestive of ABS include
  - **Persisting or worsening of symptoms after 7 to 10 days**
  - **Unilateral sinus pain or tenderness**
  - **Purulent nasal discharge**
  - **Maxillary tooth or facial pain (particularly unilateral)**

Diagnosis

- Gold standard is culture from sinus puncture (not commonly done)
- **Best made on clinical grounds,** usually only after symptoms have lasted more than 7 days, although sensitivity and specificity of history and physical examination are poor
- **Imaging studies not recommended for uncomplicated cases** of ABS because findings are no more sensitive or specific than clinical evaluation

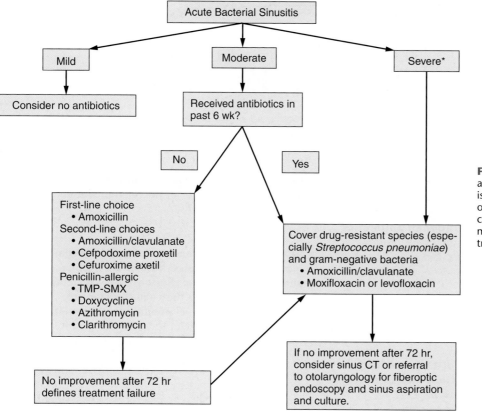

FIGURE 10-2 Management of acute bacterial sinusitis. *If patient is diabetic, immunocompromised, or in an iron-overload state and/or critically ill, consider rhinocerebral mucormycosis. TMP-SMX, trimethoprim-sulfamethoxazole.

Treatment

- Many patients, even with true ABS, will resolve **without antimicrobial therapy**; use of decongestants, analgesics, antipyretics possibly helpful but not well studied
- **Patients with moderate or severe symptoms should receive antibiotics (Fig. 10-2)**
- Goals of ABS treatment: **Avoid acute complications** (e.g., brain abscess, meningitis, or osteomyelitis—all rare; Fig. 10-3) and chronic complications (e.g., chronic sinusitis)
- Antibiotic choice dictated by local sensitivities, cost, drug allergy history. **Preferred drug: Amoxicillin**—no other antibiotic has been shown to work better for uncomplicated ABS; need to treat approximately seven patients for one to benefit.
- **True, recurrent ABS may indicate obstruction or immunodeficiency (e.g., HIV, hypogamma-globulinemia)**
- **Attempts to treat chronic sinusitis with antibiotics may result in little improvement; treatments should focus on relieving obstruction**
- Decrease mucosal swelling, exudates, and crusting with nasal saline irrigation, topical nasal corticosteroids, antihistamines, decongestants, leukotriene antagonists
- **Sinus CT scan helpful to document obstruction (e.g., polyps) in patients not responding to initial**

therapy; otolaryngology consultation is recommended
- If a patient with chronic sinusitis has an acute flare, treatment with antibiotics against *S. pneumoniae* and *H. influenzae* should be given

Otitis Media

Basic Information

- Infection of **middle ear**
- Often initiated by either **URTI or allergies** blocking the eustachian tube, resulting in pressure imbalance of inner ear with subsequent bacterial infection
- **Uncommon in adults**; less than 0.25% incidence
- Intensively studied in children; less known about infection in adults
- *S. pneumoniae* and *H. influenzae* common isolates; unclear frequency of viral and allergic inflammation

Clinical Presentation

- Commonly follows URTI or history of allergies
- **Otalgia and fever are most common symptoms**
- Severe cases complicated by meningitis, mastoiditis, or brain abscess (all rare)

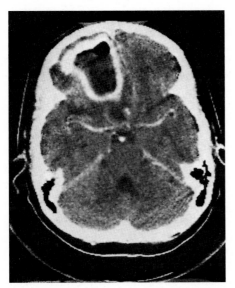

FIGURE 10-3 Cerebral abscess secondary to sinusitis. Right frontal abscess is demonstrated in a patient who had ethmoid sinusitis. An orbital abscess is also demonstrated. (From Forbes C, Jackson W: *Color atlas and text of clinical medicine,* ed 3, St. Louis, Mosby, 2003, figure 11.63.)

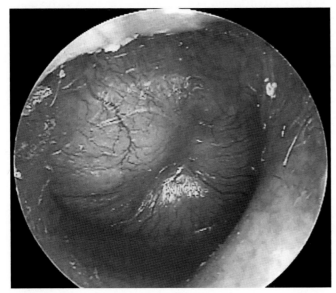

FIGURE 10-4 Acute left otitis media. (From Behrman RE: *Nelson textbook of pediatrics,* ed 16, Philadelphia, WB Saunders, 2003, figure 630-3.)

Diagnosis

- Physical examination in children imprecise, but accuracy increases with insufflation demonstrating decreased mobility of tympanic membrane
- Examination findings in adults have not been studied, but typical presentation **is bulging, red tympanic membrane** (Fig. 10-4)

Treatment

- Antimicrobial therapy not well defined; **amoxicillin/clavulanate, cefuroxime axetil, azithromycin** possible options

Pharyngitis

Basic Information

- Outpatient visits for pharyngitis account for 1% to 2% of all office visits
- Most common cause is **viral in adults**, group A streptococci in children
- Some cases may be associated with evidence of more systemic infection (Epstein-Barr virus [EBV], HIV); severe pharyngitis (*Neiserria gonorrohoeae* or group A ß-hemolytic streptococci [GABHS]); patients with a **history of rheumatic fever managed differently**, with lower threshold for prescription of antibiotics
- Viral infection causes most adult cases (~80%)
  - **Rhinovirus** (20%) is most common viral cause
  - **Coronavirus** (5–10%), **adenovirus** (5%), herpes simplex (2– 4%) less common
  - Uncommon causes include parainfluenza (2%), influenza (1%), EBV (<1%), cytomegalovirus (<1%), acute HIV type 1 (<1%), coxsackievirus (<1%)
- **Bacterial infection less common in adults** than children
- ***Streptococcus pyogenes* most common bacterial cause in adults (GABHS, 5–10%)**
  - Other streptococci less common, usually group G or C
  - Rare bacterial causes include *N. gonorrhoeae* (<1%), *Corynebacterium diphtheriae* (<1%), *Arcanobacterium haemolyticum* (<1%), *Chlamydia pneumoniae* (1%), *Mycoplasma pneumoniae* (<1%)
- Many cases unknown and presumed viral, part of the common cold

Clinical Presentation

- Typical presentations include sore throat and malaise with possible fever or cervical lymphadenopathy
- Severe sore throat with inability to swallow secretions or associated dyspnea should be evaluated in an emergency department setting; may indicate epiglottitis
- Dehydration in severe cases may require IV hydration
- **Red, beefy tonsils with exudates may be caused by either bacterial or viral causes (i.e., presence of exudate is not specific for bacterial cause; Fig. 10-5)**
- **Primary infection with EBV (infectious mononucleosis) may present with fever, sore throat, and lymphadenopathy (anterior and posterior cervical lymph nodes—may be generalized and include splenomegaly) and is easily confused with GABHS**
  - In infectious mononucleosis, laboratory abnormalities may include **predominance of lymphocytes or atypical lymphocytes**. In 90% of adult cases, the **aspartate aminotransferase, alanine aminotransferase, or lactate deyhydrogenase level is elevated** to at least two to three times normal.
  - Prescription of amoxicillin for mistakenly believed or concurrent GABHS predictably yields diffuse, pruritic, maculopapular rash in 95% to 100% of patients (rash does not mean patient is amoxicillin allergic for future dosing; Fig. 10-6)

10

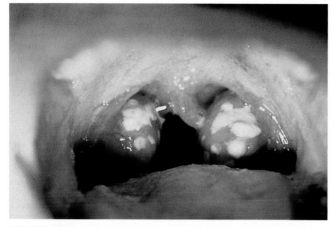

FIGURE 10-5 Acute streptococcal pharyngitis. Note purulent discharge in tonsillar crypts. A similar appearance may be seen with pharyngitis due to infectious mononucleosis. (From Forbes C, Jackson W: *Color atlas and text of clinical medicine,* ed 3, St. Louis, Mosby, 2003, figure 1.82.)

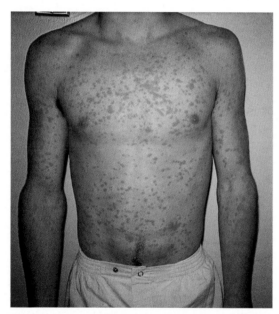

FIGURE 10-6 Generalized erythematous papular eruption of infectious mononucleosis precipitated by oral penicillin intake. (From Shah BR, Laude TA: *Atlas of pediatric clinical diagnosis,* Philadelphia, WB Saunders, 2000, figure 3-32.)

Diagnosis

Because the signs and symptoms of group A streptococcal and other viral presentations overlap, physicians are generally unable to include or exclude the diagnosis of streptococcal pharyngitis on epidemiologic and clinical grounds; therefore **laboratory testing should be done to determine whether group A streptococci are present in the pharynx** (Fig. 10-7)

- Throat culture gold standard (90% sensitive)
  - False positives may from carrier state
- Rapid strep tests
  - Throat swab detecting carbohydrate antigen

- Sensitivity 80% to 90% in adults but highly specific
- **If positive test, treat as GABHS; no further culture required**
- In children and adolescents, **negative tests should be confirmed by standard culture.** It is unclear whether this is necessary in adults.
- Sensitivity and specificity of clinical presentation 50% to 75% for GABHS (Fig. 10-8)
- The production of heterophile antibodies used to diagnose infectious mononucleosis (that are not directed against EBV but agglutinate either horse or sheep RBCs) occurs in 90% of cases and is detected by blood testing with commercial kits (e.g., Monospot, Meridian Bioscience, Cincinnati, OH)
  - **Detection of anti-EBV capsid IgM antibodies typically done if heterophilic antibodies are negative but EBV still suspected (~10% cases)**
  - Anti-EBV IgG may be present at presentation in new infection or with preexisting infection and has less clinical utility in diagnosis of acute infection

Treatment

- **Viral: Generally benign, self-limited illness remedied by rest, hydration, nonsteroidals for pain or fever, and saltwater gargles**
- **GABHS: Historically, treatment is given to avoid complications of acute rheumatic fever and may prevent suppurative complications such as tonsillar abscess. However, acute rheumatic fever is now rare in adults, and the main use of antibiotics offers shorter duration of illness (16–24 hours) if given within 72 hours of symptom onset.**
  - **All GABHS strains remain penicillin sensitive**
  - Penicillin (PCN) V standard for adults, 250 mg four times daily or 500 mg twice daily orally; long-acting intramuscular PCN given as one dose (1.2 million U benzathine ± procaine PCN G)
  - **Erythromycin 250 mg four times daily or 500 mg twice daily orally for PCN-allergic patients**

Acute Bronchitis

Basic Information

- **Most common cause of acute cough in the outpatient setting**
- Clinical challenge is to distinguish bronchitis from pneumonia
- **90% of cases are from nonbacterial cause in healthy nonsmokers**
  - Purulent sputum **may or may not** indicate bacterially induced process
  - **Viral causes predominate,** especially influenza (A or B); also coronaviruses, paramyxoviruses, rhinoviruses
- **Pertussis is uncommon cause of bronchitis but is more likely if cough is severe or persists longer than 3 weeks**

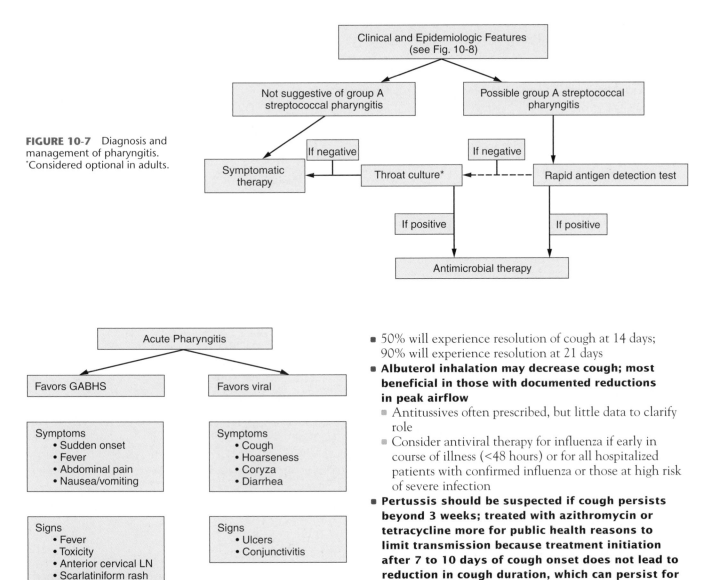

FIGURE 10-7 Diagnosis and management of pharyngitis. *Considered optional in adults.

FIGURE 10-8 Differentiation of streptococcal (group A β-hemolytic streptococci [GABHS]) pharyngitis from viral causes. LN, lymph nodes.

Clinical Presentation

- Acute respiratory infection with cough with or without phlegm for **less than 3 weeks**
- Wheezing may be present, including in those without asthma

Diagnosis

- **Diagnosis based on history and physical examination; sputum cultures are not recommended**
- **Pneumonia is uncommon if vital signs and chest examination are normal**

Treatment

- Symptomatic support; **antibiotics not recommended** regardless of cough duration, and prescription represents antibiotic abuse (Table 10-1; see notes on pertussis that follow)

- 50% will experience resolution of cough at 14 days; 90% will experience resolution at 21 days
- **Albuterol inhalation may decrease cough; most beneficial in those with documented reductions in peak airflow**
  - Antitussives often prescribed, but little data to clarify role
  - Consider antiviral therapy for influenza if early in course of illness (<48 hours) or for all hospitalized patients with confirmed influenza or those at high risk of severe infection
- **Pertussis should be suspected if cough persists beyond 3 weeks; treated with azithromycin or tetracycline more for public health reasons to limit transmission because treatment initiation after 7 to 10 days of cough onset does not lead to reduction in cough duration, which can persist for 6 to 10 weeks**
- Patient education essential: Patients not receiving an antibiotic are happier if told they have a "chest cold" rather than "bronchitis"

Acute Exacerbations of Chronic Bronchitis

Basic Information

- Part of the clinical spectrum of chronic obstructive pulmonary disease (COPD)
- **Cigarette smoking is major contributor to COPD, with less than 10% of patients with COPD having disease from occupational or environmental exposure**
- Accounts for **5% of all deaths** in United States
- **Viral or bacterial** infections may cause acute exacerbations of chronic bronchitis
- Bacterial causes
  - *H. influenzae* is most common cause (22%), particularly in smokers
  - *M. catarrhalis* (9–15%)
  - *S. pneumoniae* (10–12%)

10

TABLE 10-1	*Treatment of Bronchitis*			
Basic Clinical State	**Symptoms/Risk Factors**	**Likely Pathogens**	**First-Line Treatment**	**Alternatives/ Treatment Failure**
Acute tracheobronchitis	Cough and sputum without previous pulmonary disease	Usually viral	None	Macrolide or tetracycline if symptoms >10–14 days
Acute flare of chronic bronchitis without risk factors (group I)	Increased cough and sputum, sputum purulence, and increased dyspnea	*Haemophilus influenzae Haemophilus* spp. *Moraxella catarrhalis Streptococcus pneumoniae*	2nd-generation macrolide 2nd- or 3rd-generation cephalosporin Amoxicillin Doxycycline TMP-SMX	Fluoroquinolone or β-lactam/β-lactamase inhibitor
Acute flare of chronic bronchitis with risk factors (group II)	Symptoms as in group I *plus* at least 1 of the following: $FEV_1 < 50\%$ predicted > 4 exacerbations/yr Cardiac disease Use of home oxygen Chronic oral steroid use Antibiotic use in past 3 mo	Organisms as in group I, *plus Klebsiella* spp. Other gram-negative pathogens Increased probability of β-lactam resistance	Fluoroquinolone β lactam/β-lactamase inhibitor	May require parenteral therapy; consider referral to a specialist or hospital
Acute flare of chronic suppurative bronchitis (group III)	Symptoms as in group II, but with constant purulent sputum Some have bronchiectasis $FEV_1 < 35\%$ predicted Multiple risk factors (e.g., frequent exacerbations and $FEV_1 < 50\%$ predicted)	Organisms as in group II, *plus Pseudomonas aeruginosa* Multiresistant Enterobacteriaceae	Ambulatory patients Tailor treatment to airway pathogen (*P. aeruginosa* common; use ciprofloxacin) Hospitalized patients Parenteral therapy usually required	

FEV_1, forced expiratory volume in 1 sec; TMP-SMX, trimethoprim-sulfamethoxazole.
Adapted from Balter MS, LaForge J, Low DE, et al: Canadian guidelines for the management of acute exacerbations of chronic bronchitis. *Can Respir J* 10(suppl B):3B–32B, 2003.

BOX 10-1	*Winnipeg Criteria for Stratifying Severity of Acute Exacerbation of Chronic Bronchitis*

Symptoms
Increasing dyspnea
Increasing purulence of sputum
Increasing volume of sputum

Classification
Type 1: Severe, all three symptoms
Type 2: Moderate, two or three symptoms
Type 3: Mild, at least one symptom along with
  Upper respiratory tract infection within last 5 days
  Fever without other apparent cause
  Increased wheezing
  Increased nonproductive cough
  Increased respirations or pulse > 20% over baseline

- *Pseudomonas aeruginosa* or other gram-negative bacteria (up to 15%) seen in those with prior antibiotic use or recent hospitalization and in those with frequent flares
- Many cases without predominant bacterial species are presumed viral

Clinical Presentation

- **Patient with COPD flare has worsening dyspnea and increased sputum purulence and volume**
- Winnipeg criteria may be used to stratify severity of flares (Box 10-1)
  - Type 1 or type 2 flares **require hospitalization** and are associated with increased mortality (3–4%) that increases to 11% to 24% in-hospital mortality if care in the intensive care unit is required
- Chest radiograph (CXR) abnormalities are common
- Deep vein thrombosis and **pulmonary embolus** may be cause of exacerbation

Diagnosis

- Diagnosis made on clinical grounds
- **CXR, pulse oximetry, and arterial blood gas tests are beneficial to rule out pneumonia and gauge severity**
- May be difficult to differentiate from pneumonia if CXR is abnormal
- **Acute spirometry considered unhelpful**
- **Sputum culture not routinely recommended** but may be helpful in severe cases

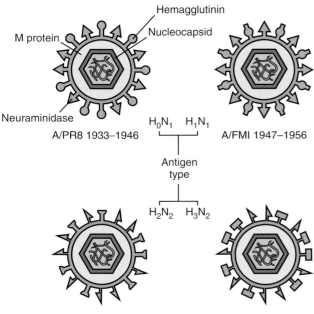

FIGURE 10-9 Schematic drawing of influenza A, demonstrating hemagglutinin and neuraminidase. Hemagglutinin is responsible for attachment to cells; neuraminidase is responsible for viral release. Figure demonstrates antigenic shifts that have caused major influenza outbreaks. (From Roitt I, Brostoff J, Male DK, editors: *Immunology,* ed 6, St Louis, Mosby, 2001, figure 14.9.)

Treatment

- Little good data to guide recommendations (see Table 10-1)
- **Bronchodilators and corticosteroids helpful**
- **Antibiotics useful for more severe flares, but data using amoxicillin and tetracycline are more than 30 years old; unclear role of emerging antimicrobial resistance and newer antibiotics**
- **Mucolytics and chest physiotherapy without clear benefit**
- **Oxygen helpful with hypoxemia** but may heighten risk of respiratory failure

Influenza

Basic Information

- Two major virus subtypes: **Influenza A and influenza B**
- Antigenic characteristics determined by surface-spike glycoproteins that have either hemagglutinin activity (HA) or neuraminidase activity (NA; Fig. 10-9)
  - **Hemagglutinin attaches to erythrocytes and is responsible for initiation of infection**
  - Neuraminidase cleaves hemagglutinin protein, **allowing viral release** from infected cells
  - **Significant antigenic variation of HA or NA bypasses prior immune memory in the host infected with influenza in the past**
    - Antigenic drift: Minor changes in HA or NA and minor changes in immunogenicity
    - Antigenic shift: Major changes in HA or NA resulting in completely new immunogenicity with risk of pandemic infection

- Avian influenza (H5N1) is a concern because of similarity to 1918 influenza severity; however, few cases to date in humans with limited human–human transmissibility
- Novel H1N1 virus arising in 2009 initially appears to behave similarly to seasonal influenza, although children and young adults more often affected; mortality seen more often in those with co-morbidities

Clinical Presentation

- Seasonal influenza outbreaks typically in epidemic pattern, peaking at 2 to 3 weeks after introduction and completed after 5 to 6 weeks in any given community
- Occurs in winter months; uncommon in other seasons
- **Symptoms for individual begin abruptly with fever, rigors, malaise, headache, myalgia, and arthralgia**
- Fever, rigors, and myalgia peak at 3 days, after which respiratory symptoms (cough) and nasal congestion predominate
- **Major complication is pneumonia**
  - **Viral pneumonia** from influenza occurs early and may be severe
  - **Postinfectious bacterial pneumonia often follows a period of recovery** from influenza and is most often caused by *S. pneumoniae, S. aureus, S. pyogenes,* or *H. influenzae*
- Other complications may include rhabdomyolysis, myocarditis, or Guillain-Barré syndrome

Diagnosis

- **Clinical presentation in individual during community outbreak is most common method and is 70% specific for influenza based on abrupt onset of cough and fever in an adult**
- Seasonal strains of influenza may be detected from sputum, nasal, or throat swab or from nasopharyngeal aspirate by rapid antigen test (70% specific) or culture (90–100% specific but slow)

Treatment

- **Optimal treatment is prevention,** with influenza vaccine recommended for all children, adults older than 50 years, and adults age 18 to 49 with comorbidities
- **Amantadine and rimantadine block ion channel function only in influenza A virus and should only be used if circulating strains are known to be susceptible;** these drugs have no role in treatment of influenza B
- **Neuraminidase inhibitors (zanamivir and oseltamivir) prevent infection of cells by inhibiting influenza neuraminidase activity for both influenza A and influenza B. Both must be administered within first 48 hours of infection to shorten the duration of influenza symptoms** in ambulatory patients, but hospitalized patients may benefit from administration during any phase of their acute illness.
  - Neuraminidase inhibitors may be the preferred treatment for influenza, although recommendations change every season based on the resistance profiles of circulating virus
  - Oseltamivir is administered orally and may result in nausea
  - Zanamivir is administered by inhalation and is well tolerated but may result in bronchospasm and should be avoided in susceptible patients, such as those with asthma or COPD

10

TABLE 10-2	Fungal Infections of the Lung		
Organism	**Presentation**	**Diagnosis**	**Treatment**
Histoplasma capsulatum	Up to 50% asymptomatic; endemic to Ohio and Mississippi River valleys Acute infection: Includes fever, infiltrates, pleurisy, hilar and mediastinal adenopathy ARDS: If inoculum sufficiently large, fulminant respiratory failure may result Progressive disseminated histoplasmosis: May result from primary infection or reactivation; more common in immunocompromised; diffuse lymphadenopathy, hepatosplenomegaly, and adrenal insufficiency may result Chronic pulmonary histoplasmosis: Usually in setting of COPD; resembles tuberculosis with cavitation	Culture is gold standard, but takes 4–6 wk *Histoplasma* antigen may be detected in serum and urine of patients with disseminated disease; may cross-react with blastomycosis and coccidioidomycosis Complement fixation of antibody to *Histoplasma capsulatum* may be used, including those with acute pulmonary infection (fourfold rise in titer consistent with acute infection)	Acute infection does not typically require treatment Chronic pulmonary infections may require treatment with itraconazole Disseminated infections treated with itraconazole or amphotericin High index of suspicion should be held for adrenal insufficiency in disseminated disease
Blastomyces dermatitidis	Endemic to region between Dakotas and Louisiana Disease may be self-limited or require treatment Pulmonary presentations include infiltrates, nodules, or cavitation Skin, bone, and genitourinary tract (prostate and epididymis) most common extrapulmonary sites of infection	Culture is gold standard Visualization of fungi in appropriate clinical setting used to initiate antimicrobial treatment Complement fixation is currently neither sensitive nor specific	Itraconazole in immunocompetent with mild to moderate disease Amphotericin in immunocompromised or with CNS involvement
Coccidioides immitis	Endemic to dry regions of southwest United States Acute pulmonary infection: Most common presentation, with fever, cough, and extensive alveolar infiltrates; may be accompanied by massive hilar and mediastinal adenopathy; cavitation may occur, with hemoptysis; erythema nodosum Dissemination may be widespread with skin, muscle, bone, and CNS involvement	Stain and culture of infected fluid or tissues Elevated complement *fixation* titers to *Coccidioides immitis*; these may be followed as markers of disease, with rising titers a poor prognostic sign	Itraconazole Fluconazole Fluconazole used if CNS involvement or refractory disease
Aspergillus fumigatus	ABPA: A hypersensitivity reaction characterized by asthma and fleeting infiltrates accompanied by eosinophilia Aspergilloma (fungal ball or mycetoma): Most common noninvasive form, occurring in old scars, cavities, or blebs Invasive aspergillosis: Usually occurs in immunocompromised, with organ transplant and hematologic malignancies common predisposers; presents as acute pneumonia with cavitation, then invades locally along with hematogenous dissemination	Diagnosis of ABPA by positive sputum culture, elevated total IgE, elevated specific antibodies to *Aspergillus*, and cutaneous reaction to *Aspergillus* immunogen Aspergilloma diagnosed by clinical presentation Invasive aspergillosis diagnosed by clinical microbiologic and radiographic presentation and CT scan; biopsy with culture usually suggested to distinguish from colonization; serum galactomannan may be elevated	ABPA: Corticosteroids; role of antifungal treatment unclear Aspergilloma may be treated with resection if hemoptysis Invasive aspergillosis: Voriconazole is treatment of choice

ABPA, allergic bronchopulmonary aspergillosis; ARDS, acute respiratory distress syndrome; COPD, chronic obstructive pulmonary disease; IgE, immunoglobulin E.

Pneumonia

Basic Information

- Remains **leading cause of infectious death** in United States; seventh overall cause of death
- Mortality highest in older patients and in those with multiple co-morbidities
- **S. pneumoniae and Legionella pneumophila are the leading bacterial causes of pneumonia death**
- Microbiology is altered by host factors (e.g., age, immunosuppression, alcohol use) and geography
  - **S. pneumoniae remains the most commonly diagnosed etiologic agent in studies of community-acquired pneumonia**
    - *S. pneumoniae* with high-level penicillin resistance is less frequent than previously stated as a result of revised resistance breakpoints for nonmeningeal isolates (declining from 10% to only ~1%)
    - Clinical significance of antibiotic-resistant organisms in pneumonia is debated
  - **Atypical agents account for 15% to 20% of community-acquired pneumonias and include infections with *L. pneumophila*, *M. pneumoniae*, and *C. pneumoniae***
  - *H. influenzae*, *S. aureus*, and gram-negative bacilli each account for 3% to 10% of community-acquired pneumonias
  - **Viral pneumonia uncommon** in adults
    - Influenza A and B most common viral causes
    - Cytomegalovirus causes pneumonia only in immunosuppressed patients
    - Adenovirus, varicella-zoster virus, and EBV are rare causes of viral pneumonia in adults
    - Hantavirus, seen mostly in the southwest United States, is a rare cause of viral pneumonia that quickly evolves to acute respiratory distress and is associated with a high mortality rate
- Fungal infections
  - More than 300 fungi capable of causing lung infection, **mostly in immunocompromised patients** with *Aspergillus* spp. and zygomycete organisms (*Rhizopus, Mucor* spp.) the leading problems
  - Endemic fungi (*Histoplasma capsulatum, Blastomyces dermatitidis, Coccidioides immitis,* and *Cryptococcus neoformans*) can infect normal hosts and cause lung disease (Table 10-2)
  - **Candida spp. are a very rare cause of pneumonia and should be considered as the causative agent only in the profoundly immunosuppressed or neutropenic patient.** Positive sputum cultures otherwise merely represent upper airway colonization.

Clinical Presentation

- Cough, fever, and new pulmonary infiltrate constitute the classic triad
- Other common symptoms include pleurisy, dyspnea, malaise, headache, nausea, vomiting, abdominal pain, and diarrhea
- Although no reliable clinical indicators have been established to differentiate "typical" pneumonia from "atypical" pneumonia, **purulent sputum without**

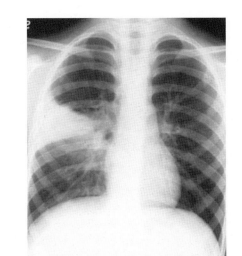

FIGURE 10-10 Right upper lobe pneumonia. On this posteroanterior chest radiograph, note that the right cardiac border is well seen. The alveolar infiltrate is seen in the right midlung. (From Mettler FA: *Essentials of radiology,* ed 2, Philadelphia, WB Saunders, 2005, figure 3-44.)

predominant organisms heightens suspicion for *Legionella, Mycoplasma,* and *Chlamydia* spp.
- Some presentations are associated with etiologic agent
  - **S. pneumoniae classically presents with sudden rigor, fever, and cough productive of rust-colored sputum (Fig. 10-10)**
  - **Legionella, which may be sporadic or cluster in an outbreak associated with aerosol spread of a contaminated water system, presents as a severe pneumonia with high-spiking fevers, classically accompanied by diarrhea and, in some cases, relative bradycardia in spite of high fevers.** Hyponatremia may be more common with *Legionella* than with other etiologic agents.
  - **The hallmark of Mycoplasma infection is a paroxysmal, nonproductive cough, often with minimal findings on CXR**; however, CXR may demonstrate pulmonary diffuse infiltrates and even effusions.
    - **Bullous myringitis, contrary to lore, is not a usual finding in Mycoplasma infection**
    - **The production of cold agglutinins (IgM produced in Mycoplasma infection that reversibly agglutinates RBCs when blood is cooled) may lead to Raynaud phenomenon and even digital necrosis (particularly in patients with sickle cell anemia)**
  - *C. pneumoniae* results in a **typically mild pneumonia** that is slowly progressive and only rarely severe; it may follow URTI symptoms (pharyngitis, sinus infection) by 1 or 2 weeks
    - There is little clinically to differentiate *C. pneumoniae* from other causes of pneumonia
  - Pneumonia is the most common initial AIDS-defining illness, with *Pneumocystis jiroveci* (Fig. 10-11) and *S. pneumoniae* the most common etiologies
  - Infiltrates with cavitation or subacute pneumonia, especially in an immunocompromised patient demands consideration of tuberculosis (1–2% of all cases of community-acquired pneumonia)

10

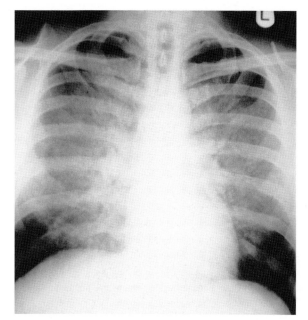

FIGURE 10-11 Chest radiograph of a patient with *Pneumocystis jiroveci* pneumonia. (From Haslett C, Chilvers ER, Boon NA, Colledge NR, editors: *Davidson's principles and practice of medicine,* ed 19, Edinburgh, Elsevier Science, 2002, figure 1.86.)

Diagnosis

- **CXR is critical to establish infiltrate** and to decrease administration of antibiotics given mistakenly for acute bronchitis
- **Chest physical examination unreliable** to include or to exclude pneumonia diagnosis
- Abnormal vital signs **heighten the likelihood** of positive CXR (see acute bronchitis section)
- **Sputum with more than 25 polymorphonuclear neutrophils and fewer than 10 epithelial cells per high-powered field considered purulent specimen that may adequately reflect pathogen of pneumonia (Fig. 10-12)**
- **Blood cultures** are considered an optional study but should be obtained in certain patients, including those with severe pneumonia, cavitary infiltrates, leukopenia, active alcohol abuse, chronic severe liver disease, asplenia, positive pneumococcal urinary antigen test, or pleural effusion
- **If significant pleural effusion is seen at presentation, thoracentesis with analysis and culture should be performed**
- **Cause of pneumonia is considered definitive only if bacteria are isolated from normally sterile space (blood, pleura)**
- Cause is probable but not definitive if only cultured from sputum unless sputum grows *Legionella*, tuberculosis, or some fungi
  - *Legionella* urinary antigen detects only type 1
  - *L. pneumophila*; sputum direct fluorescent antibody less reliable for *Legionella* spp.
- ***Chlamydia* and *Mycoplasma* infection best diagnosed by polymerase chain reaction assay of respiratory specimen; serologic tests unreliable**

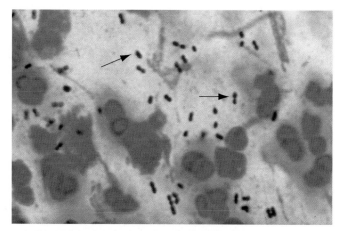

FIGURE 10-12 Purulent sputum in a patient with pneumococcal pneumonia. Gram stain shows gram-positive diplococci characteristic of *Streptococcus pneumoniae* (*arrows*). (From Haslett C, Chilvers ER, Boon NA, Colledge NR, editors: *Davidson 's principles and practice of medicine,* ed 19, Edinburgh, Elsevier Science, 2002, figure 13.30.)

Treatment

Table 10-3 summarizes the initial therapy for suspected bacterial community-acquired pneumonia.

- First decision is whether to manage as outpatient or whether hospitalization appropriate
  - Pneumonia severity index or CURB-65 score may help guide hospitalization decision (Tables 10-4 and 10-5)
  - **Usually patients who are elderly or with co-morbidities, highly abnormal vital signs, hypoxemia, or laboratory abnormalities should be treated in hospital**
- **Initial antibiotic choice typically empirical and should cover *S. pneumoniae* but should also cover atypical agents and drug-resistant *Pneumococcus* if patient is severely ill (see Table 10-3)**
- Timely antibiotic administration (within 6 hours of initial encounter) correlates with decreased mortality and now considered standard of care
- Many guidelines exist with slight variations; consider unusual factors

REVIEW QUESTIONS

For review questions, please go to www.expertconsult.com.

SUGGESTED READINGS

Bach PB, Brown C, Gelfand SE, et al: Management of acute exacerbations of chronic obstructive pulmonary disease: a summary and appraisal of published evidence, *Ann Intern Med* 134:600–620, 2001.

Balter MS, La Forge J, Low DE, et al: Canadian guidelines for the management of acute exacerbations of chronic bronchitis, *Can Respir J* 10(Suppl B):3B–32B, 2003.

Bisno AL: Acute pharyngitis, *N Engl J Med* 344:205–211, 2001.

Bisno AL, Gerber MA, Gwaltney JM Jr, et al: Practice guidelines for the diagnosis and management of group A streptococcal pharyngitis. Infectious Diseases Society of America, *Clin Infect Dis* 35:113–125, 2002.

Celin SE, Bluestone CD, Stephenson J, Yilmaz HM, Collins JJ: Bacteriology of acute otitis media in adults, *JAMA* 266:2249–2252, 1991.

Centers for Disease Control and Prevention (CDC): Effects of new penicillin susceptibility breakpoints for *Streptococcus pneumoniae*—United States, 2006–2007, *MMWR Morb Mortal Wkly Rep* 57:1353–1355, 2008.

Cooper RJ, Hoffman JR, Bartlett JG, et al: Principles of appropriate antibiotic use for acute pharyngitis in adults: background, *Ann Intern Med* 134:509–517, 2001.

Fiore AE, Shay DK, Broder K, et al: Prevention and control of seasonal influenza with vaccines: recommendations of the Advisory Committee

TABLE 10-3	*Recommended Empirical Antibiotics for Community-Acquired Pneumonia*

Outpatient Treatment

1. Previously healthy and no use of antimicrobials within previous 3 mo
   A macrolide (azithromycin, clarithromycin) (strong recommendation)
   Doxycycline (weak recommendation)
2. Presence of comorbidities such as chronic heart, lung, liver, or renal disease; diabetes mellitus; alcoholism; malignancies; asplenia; immunosuppressing conditions or use of immunosuppressing drugs; or use of antimicrobials within the previous 3 mo (in which case an alternative from a different class should be selected)
   A respiratory fluoroquinolone (moxifloxacin or levofloxacin) (strong recommendation)
   A β-lactam (amoxicillin/clavulanate, high-dose amoxicillin 1 g tid, cefpodoxime, or cefuroxime) plus a macrolide
3. In regions with a high rate (>25%) of infection with high-level (MIC ≥ 16 µg/mL) macrolide-resistant *Streptococcus pneumoniae,* consider use of alternative agents listed above in (2) for patients without co-morbidities (moderate recommendation)

Inpatients, Non-ICU Treatment

A respiratory fluoroquinolone (strong recommendation)
A β-lactam (ceftriaxone, cefotaxime, ertapenem) plus a macrolide (strong recommendation)

Inpatients, ICU Treatment

A β-lactam (cefotaxime, ceftriaxone, or ampicillin-sulbactam) plus either azithromycin or a respiratory fluoroquinolone (strong recommendation) (for penicillin-allergic patients, a respiratory fluoroquinolone and aztreonam are recommended)

Special Concerns

If *Pseudomonas* is a consideration
   An antipneumococcal, antipseudomonal β-lactam (piperacillin/tazobactam, cefepime, imipenem, or meropenem) plus either ciprofloxacin or levofloxacin (750 mg)
   or
   The above β-lactam plus an aminoglycoside and a respiratory fluoroquinolone (for penicillin-allergic patients, substitute aztreonam for above β-lactam) (moderate recommendation)
If CA-MRSA is a consideration, add vancomycin or linezolid (moderate recommendation)

CA-MRSA, community-acquired methicillin-resistant *Staphylococcus aureus*; ICU, intensive care unit; MIC, minimal inhibitory concentration.
Adapted from Mandell LA, Wunderink RG, Anzueto A, et al: Infectious Diseases Society of America/American Thoracic Society consensus guidelines on the management of community-acquired pneumonia in adults. *Clin Infect Dis* 44:S27–S73, 2007.

TABLE 10-4	*Pneumonia Severity Index*

Step 1. Is the patient at low risk (class I) based on the history and physical examination and not a resident of a nursing home?
   Age ≤ 50 yr
   and
   None of the coexisting conditions or physical examination findings listed in step 2
      No: Go to step 2
      Yes: Outpatient treatment is recommended
Step 2. Calculate risk score for classes II to V

Patient Characteristics	Points Assigned	Patient's Points
Demographic factors		
Age (yr)		
Males	Age	_____
Females	Age −10	_____
Nursing home resident	+10	_____
Coexisting conditions		
Neoplastic disease	+30	_____
Liver disease	+20	_____
Congestive heart failure	+10	_____
Cerebrovascular disease	+10	_____
Renal disease	+10	_____
Initial physical examination findings		
Altered mental status	+20	_____
Respiratory rate ≥ 30 breaths/min	+20	_____
Systolic blood pressure < 90 mm Hg	+20	_____
Temperature < 35°C (95°F) or ≥40°C (104°F)	+15	_____
Pulse ≥ 125 beats/min	+10	_____

Continued

10

TABLE 10-4	**_Pneumonia Severity Index_** _(Continued)_

Initial laboratory findings (score zero if not tested)

pH < 7.35	+30	_____
Blood urea nitrogen > 30 mg/dL (10.5 mmol/L)	+20	_____
Sodium < 130 mEq/L (130 mmol/L)	+20	_____
Glucose ≥ 250 mg/dL (13.9 mmol/L)	+10	_____
Hematocrit < 30% (0.30)	+10	_____
Arterial Po_2 < 60 mm Hg or O_2 saturation < 90%	+10	_____
Pleural effusion	+10	_____

Total score (sum of patient's points):

30-DAY MORTALITY DATA BY RISK CLASS

Total Score	Risk Class	Recommended Site of Treatment	Mortality Range Observed in Validation Cohorts (%)
None (see step 1)	I	Outpatient	0.1
≤70	II	Outpatient	0.5
71–90	III	Outpatient	0.9–2.8
91–130	IV	Inpatient	8.2–9.3
>130	V	Inpatient	27.0–29.2

O_2, oxygen; Po_2, partial oxygen pressure.

Step 1 identifies patients in risk class I on the basis of age ≤ 50 yr and the absence of all co-morbid conditions and vital sign abnormalities listed in step 2. For all patients who are not classified as risk class I, the laboratory data listed in step 2 should be collected to calculate a pneumonia severity score. Risk class and recommended site of care based on the pneumonia severity score are listed in the final table. Thirty-day mortality data are based on two independent cohorts of 40,326 patients.

From Metlay JP, Fine MJ: Testing strategies in the initial management of patients with community-acquired pneumonia. _Ann Intern Med_ 138:115, 2003.

TABLE 10-5	**_Clinical Feature Points (CURB-65) (score one point for each variable present)_**

Confusion (defined as a mental test score ≤ 8, or disorientation in person, place, or time)	1
Uremia: Blood urea ≥ 7 mmol/L (~19 mg/dL)	1
Respiratory rate: ≥ 30 breaths/min	1
Blood pressure: systolic ≤ 90 mm Hg or diastolic ≤ 60 mm Hg	1
Age > **65** yr	1
Total points	

Mortality Risks and Treatment Recommendations Based on CURB-65 Score

Score	Group
0 or 1	Mortality risk low (1.5%), consider home treatment
2	Mortality risk moderate (9.2%), consider hospital-supervised treatment
3	Mortality risk high (22%), manage in hospital
4 or 5	Consider admission to intensive care unit

From Lim WS, van der Eerden MM, Laing R, et al: Defining community acquired pneumonia severity on presentation to hospital: an international derivation and validation study. _Thorax_ 58(5):377–382, 2003.

on Immunization Practices (ACIP), 2009. *MMWR Recomm Rep* 58: 1–52, 2009; erratum in *MMWR Recomm Rep* 58:896–897, 2009.

Global strategy for the diagnosis, management, and prevention of COPD: Global Initiative for Chronic Obstructive Lung Disease (GOLD), 2008 (www.goldcopd.com/GuidelinesResources.asp, accessed 6/4/09).

Gonzales R, Bartlett JG, Besser RE, et al: Principles of appropriate antibiotic use for treatment of uncomplicated acute bronchitis: background, *Ann Intern Med* 134:521–529, 2001.

Mandell LA, Wunderink RG, Anzueto A, et al: Infectious Diseases Society of America/American Thoracic Society consensus guidelines on the management of community-acquired pneumonia in adults, *Clin Infect Dis* 44(Suppl 2):S27–S72, 2007.

Piccirillo JF: Clinical practice: acute bacterial sinusitis, *N Engl J Med* 26:902–910, 2004.

Pratter MR, Brightling CE, Boulet LP, et al: An empiric integrative approach to the management of cough: ACCP evidence-based guidelines, *Chest* 129(Suppl 1):222S–231S, 2006.

Schwartz LE, Brown RB: Purulent otitis media in adults, *Arch Intern Med* 152:2301–2304, 1992.

Stoller JK: Clinical practice: acute exacerbations of chronic obstructive pulmonary disease, *N Engl J Med* 346:988–994, 2002.

Updated interim recommendations for the use of antiviral medications in the treatment and prevention of influenza for the 2009–2010 season. Available at: www.cdc.gov/h1n1flu/recommendations.htm.

Genitourinary Infections

LISA A. SPACEK, MD, PhD

Genitourinary infections encompass a broad range of clinical manifestations and disease etiologies. Sexually transmitted diseases (STDs) are classified according to syndromes that include genital ulcer disease, urethritis, cervicitis, pelvic inflammatory disease (PID), epididymitis, vaginal discharge, genital warts, and ectoparasite infestations. **HIV testing should be considered in all patients with an STD**. Urinary tract infections (UTIs) may involve the lower genitourinary tract or both the upper and lower tract and, like STDs, are categorized according to clinical syndromes. Treatment guidelines for STDs are available at the Centers for Disease Control and Prevention (CDC) Web site: www.cdc.gov.

Genital Ulcer Disease

See Table 11-1 for a summary of the presentation and causes of urogential ulcer disease. Routine diagnostic tests include the following: Culture or antigen test for herpes simplex virus (HSV), syphilis serology, either darkfield examination or direct immunofluorescence test for *Treponema pallidum*, and culture for *Haemophilus ducreyi* (in some cases).

HERPES SIMPLEX VIRUS

Figure 11-3 shows an example of primary genital herpes.

Basic Information

- Common sites of HSV infection are **skin and mucous membranes**
- Most genital infections are HSV-2; HSV-1 predominantly causes labial lesions
- Seroprevalence of HSV-2 increases from 20% to 30% at age 15 to 19 years and to **35% to 60%** by age 60 years
- At least 50 million people have genital HSV in the United States, but most cases are **unrecognized and never diagnosed**
- Incubation period is 2 to 7 days

Clinical Presentation

- Primary genital herpes lesions are classically painful, multiple, and grouped on erythematous base, beginning as macules and papules, evolving to vesicles and ulcers
- Local symptoms may include **pain, itching, dysuria, and tender inguinal adenopathy**
- Primary lesions may be accompanied by fever, headache, malaise, and myalgias

- Recurrent disease is less severe than primary disease and occurs more commonly in immunosuppressed individuals
- Extragenital complications include aseptic meningitis and urinary retention

Diagnosis

- Clinical diagnosis can be confirmed by cell culture (low sensitivity), detection of viral antigen, polymerase chain reaction (PCR), and serology (type-specific glycoprotein G1 and G2)
- Tzanck prep may show multinucleated giant cells (low sensitivity). Asymptomatic shedding is detected in 1% to 2% of seropositive individuals by culture and up to 10% by PCR.

Treatment

- Systemic antiviral drugs (e.g., **acyclovir, famciclovir, or valacyclovir**) can be used as episodic or suppressive therapy
- Episodic treatment **does not eradicate the virus** or reduce frequency of recurrences
- Daily suppressive therapy among patients with six or more recurrences per year can reduce the frequency by up to 80% and prevents recurrences in 25% to 30% of patients; frequency of episodes may diminish over time.
- Suppressive therapy does not eliminate subclinical viral shedding

SYPHILIS

Basic Information

- Systemic illness with protean manifestations caused by *T. pallidum*
- Major routes of transmission are via **sexual intercourse** and **from mother to fetus**

Clinical Presentation

- Primary syphilis (Fig. 11-4)
  - Begins as a **chancre (a single, painless papule)** at the site of inoculation 2 to 3 weeks after initial exposure
  - Quickly erodes and becomes indurated with a clean base and raised, firm borders
  - Atypical lesions occur in 60% of cases
  - Primary lesions may be accompanied by **regional adenopathy** that is classically rubbery, painless, and bilateral
- Secondary or disseminated syphilis (Fig. 11-5)
  - Begins 2 to 8 weeks after appearance of chancre

TABLE 11-1	*Urogenital Ulcer Disease*			
Ulcerative Disease	**Causative Agent**	**Clinical Presentation**	**Diagnosis**	**Treatment**
Genital herpes	HSV-2 > HSV-1	Cluster of vesicles on erythematous base Painful and pruritic Dysuria Tender lymphadenopathy	Tzanck prep multinucleated giant cells (low sensitivity) Viral culture (gold standard)	Acyclovir or famciclovir or valacyclovir
Syphilitic chancre	*Treponema pallidum*	Single, painless papule at the site of inoculation Erodes into clean base and raised, firm borders Painless rubbery lymphadenopathy	Darkfield examination and direct fluorescent antibody tests Serology 　Nontreponemal (RPR, VDRL) 　Treponemal (FTA-ABS, TP-PA)	Penicillin
Chancroid (Fig. 11-1)	*Haemophilus ducreyi*	Painful ulcer Tender inguinal adenopathy Hallmark is suppurative adenopathy Occurs in outbreaks	Clinical diagnosis Culture available but not widely used	Azithromycin or ceftriaxone or ciprofloxacin
Donovanosis or granuloma inguinale	*Calymmatobacterium granulomatis*	Painless papule or nodule Erodes into beefy-red granulomatous ulcer with rolled edges Spread of granulomas into the groin results in edema or pseudobuboes Rare in the United States Genital ulcer disease	Donovan bodies on biopsy	Doxycycline or trimethoprim-sulfamethoxazole Treat at least 3 wk
Lymphogranuloma venereum (LGV; Fig. 11-2)	*Chlamydia trachomatis* serovars L1, L2, or L3	Induces a lymphoproliferative reaction	Clinical syndrome Serology, complement fixation titers of at least 1:64	Doxycycline Treat for 3 wk

FTA, fluorescent treponemal antibody; HSV, herpes simplex virus; RPR, rapid plasma reagin; TP-PA, *T. pallidum* particle agglutination; VDRL, Venereal Disease Research Laboratory.

- May be associated with **flulike symptoms**, generalized lymphadenopathy, and temporary patchy alopecia
- Characteristic **rash may be macular, maculopapular, papular, or pustular** and may involve the whole body or palms and soles
- **Condylomata lata** appear as raised, painless, gray-white lesions; are highly infectious; and develop in intertriginous areas and on mucous membranes
- Latent syphilis
  - Defined by a lack of clinical manifestations with positive serology
  - Latent syphilis acquired within the preceding year is **early latent syphilis**
  - **Late latent syphilis** implies acquisition more than 1 year before diagnosis
- Tertiary syphilis
  - Slowly progressive, **inflammatory** disease
  - Gummatous syphilis results in **skeletal, mucosal, ocular, and visceral lesions**
  - Average time of onset is 4 to 12 years after infection
  - Cardiovascular syphilis causes endarteritis of the aortic vasovasorum
    - Average time of onset is 15 years
    - Presents as aortic aneurysm or aortic valve insufficiency

- Neurosyphilis
  - **Can occur at any syphilis stage**
  - Clinical evidence of disease may involve **ophthalmic or auditory symptoms, cranial nerve palsies, or meningitis**
  - Ocular manifestations include **iritis, uveitis, neuroretinitis, and optic neuritis**

Diagnosis

- Darkfield examination and direct fluorescent antibody tests of lesion exudates or tissue provide definitive evidence
- Two types of serologic tests are used for presumptive diagnosis:
  - Nontreponemal tests include rapid plasma reagin (RPR) and Venereal Disease Research Laboratory (VDRL) tests
    - Used as screening tests
    - Because of low specificity, **must be confirmed by a treponemal test**
  - Treponemal tests include the fluorescent treponemal antibody absorbed (FTA-ABS) and *T. pallidum* particle agglutination tests
  - Serologic tests may be negative in primary syphilis

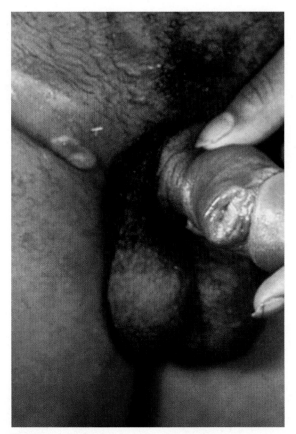

FIGURE 11-1 Chancroid presents as a painful ulcer and suppurative adenopathy. (From www.cdc.gov.)

- Neurosyphilis can occur at any stage of disease
  - Diagnosis is based on a combination of serologic tests, cerebrospinal fluid (CSF) abnormalities (>5 WBC/mm³ or abnormal protein), or a reactive CSF VDRL
    - CSF VDRL is highly specific but insensitive; negative study does not exclude the diagnosis
    - CSF FTA-ABS is less specific but very sensitive; negative study probably excludes neurosyphilis
  - CSF examination indicated if neurologic or ophthalmologic abnormalities, evidence of active tertiary syphilis (aortitis, gumma, iritis), treatment failure, or RPR greater than or equal to 1:32
  - HIV infection with CD4 ≤ 350 cells/mm³ or RPR ≥ 1:32 is associated with increased risk of neurosyphilis, and CSF examination is warranted

Treatment

- Parenteral **penicillin G** is the drug of choice (Table 11-2)
  - Only accepted therapy with documented efficacy for neurosyphilis and syphilis during pregnancy is desensitization followed by penicillin therapy
  - The **Jarisch-Herxheimer reaction**
    - Acute febrile reaction associated with headache and myalgias; thought to be activation of inflammatory cascade associated with lysis of spirochetes
    - Can occur within the first 24 hours after any therapy for syphilis
    - Treatment is supportive with use of antipyretics and anti-inflammatory agents

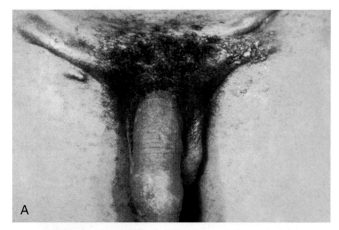

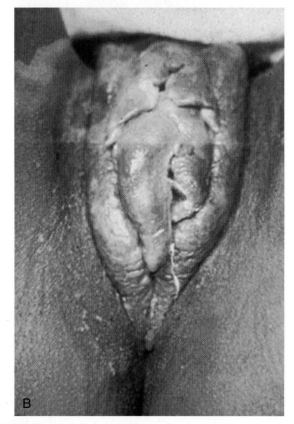

FIGURE 11-2 **A,** Early lymphogranuloma venereum (LGV) presents first as an ulcer and then as painful inguinal lymphadenopathy. **B,** Late complications of LGV include genital elephantiasis. (From www.cdc.gov.)

- Response to therapy is monitored by change in titer of a nontreponemal test (e.g., RPR) 6 months after therapy
  - A fourfold (or two-dilution) decrease in RPR or VDRL titer (e.g., from 1:64 to 1:16) indicates a cure
  - No change or increase in titer indicates failure of therapy
  - Documentation of a titer response followed by a fourfold increase indicates reinfection
  - Treponemal test (e.g., FTA-ABS) titers do not correlate with disease activity or therapy and will usually remain positive for life
- In neurosyphilis, quantitative nontreponemal serologic tests should be repeated at 6, 12, and 24 months

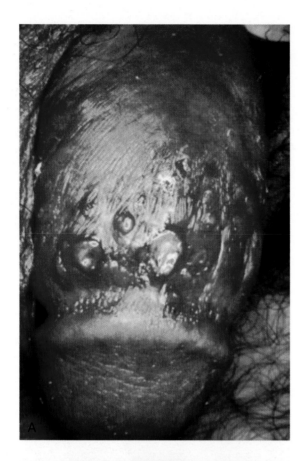

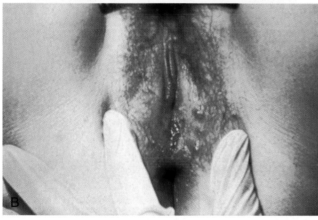

FIGURE 11-3 Primary genital herpes, along the shaft of the penis (**A**) and in the vulvar area (**B**). (From www.cdc.gov.)

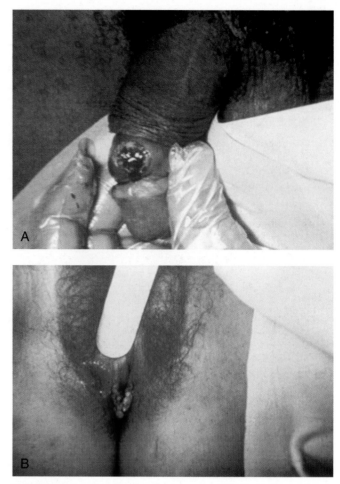

FIGURE 11-4 The chancre of primary syphilis shown in a man (**A**) and in a woman (**B**). (From www.cdc.gov.)

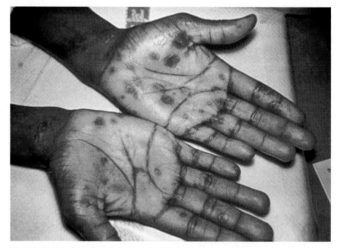

FIGURE 11-5 The characteristic rash of secondary syphilis, commonly involving the palms and soles. (From www.cdc.gov.)

Urethritis and Cervicitis

- Urethritis and cervicitis are characterized by **discharge of mucopurulent or purulent material**
- The principal etiologic agents are *Neisseria gonorrhoeae* and *Chlamydia trachomatis*

GONORRHEA

Basic Information

- Common cause of sexually transmitted infection
- Can involve the genital tract or the oropharynx, or become disseminated

- Incubation period is 3 to 7 days, and symptoms manifest within 10 to 14 days after exposure
- **Disseminated** gonococcal infection (DGI) occurs in 1% to 3%

TABLE 11-2	*Recommended Treatment Regimens for Syphilis*
Clinical Stage	**Treatment**
Primary and secondary syphilis	Benzathine penicillin G—2.4 million units IM in a single dose (If penicillin allergic—doxycycline 100 mg PO BID for 2 wk, except pregnant patients, who should be desensitized and treated with penicillin)
Early latent syphilis	Benzathine penicillin G—2.4 million units IM in a single dose
Late latent syphilis or latent syphilis of unknown duration	Benzathine penicillin G—7.2 million units, administered as 3 doses of 2.4 million units IM each at 1-week intervals
Tertiary syphilis (gummatous and cardiovascular syphilis)	Benzathine penicillin G—7.2 million units, administered as 3 doses of 2.4 million units IM each at 1-wk intervals
Neurosyphilis	Aqueous crystalline penicillin G—18–24 million units per day, administered as 3–4 million units IV every 4 hr or continuous infusion, for 10–14 days *or* Procaine penicillin— 2.4 million units IM QD, *plus* Probenecid—500 mg PO QID, both for 10–14 days

BID, twice daily; IM, intramuscularly; PO, orally; QD, daily; QID, four times daily.

Clinical Presentation

- Disease presentations are variable and differ between men and women
  - In men, symptomatic disease in 95% with **purulent urethral discharge or dysuria**
  - Women with **cervicitis** may have **vaginal discharge or bleeding**, and yet 50% may be asymptomatic
  - Other syndromes in women include **urethritis, Bartholin abscesses, or PID**
- DGI may present as triad of (1) dermatitis with petechial or pustular acral skin lesions, (2) tenosynovitis, and (3) polyarthralgias or as purulent arthritis without skin lesions
  - Perihepatitis, endocarditis, meningitis, and osteomyelitis occur less commonly

Diagnosis

- Stain of gram-negative intracellular diplococci
- Culture using modified Thayer-Martin media
- DNA amplification techniques
- Ligase chain reaction (LCR) is highly sensitive and specific
- Specimens can include cervical, urethral, oropharyngeal, and anorectal swabs; and urine

Treatment

- A third-generation cephalosporin (**cefixime** or **ceftriaxone**) is first-line therapy
- Unless ruled out, patients should receive simultaneous treatment for *Chlamydia* (see later discussion)
- Fluoroquinolones are no longer recommended because of increased prevalence of drug resistance
- **Azithromycin at 2-g dosing** is effective for both gonorrheal infections and chlamydial infections, but its use is limited by GI distress
- Pharyngeal gonorrhea is more difficult to eradicate
  - Patients require pharyngeal culture to verify response
- Sexual partners of the past 60 days or the last sexual partner should be referred for evaluation and treatment
- Patients with DGI are hospitalized and treated parenterally for 24 to 48 hours after response to therapy

CHLAMYDIA TRACHOMATIS

Basic Information

- Most common sexually transmitted bacterial infection in United States
- Risk factors include age younger than 20 years, inconsistent use of barrier contraception, and more than one sexual partner in past 3 months

Clinical Presentation

- Infection in women may present as **cervicitis or urethritis** and may involve vaginal discharge, lower abdominal pain, or dysuria
- Men develop urethritis with dysuria and mucopurulent discharge
  - **Epididymitis** manifests as unilateral testicular pain and tenderness, edema, and hydrocele

Diagnosis

- Because **asymptomatic infection is most common,** routine screening of sexually active women at risk is recommended to prevent sequelae
  - Untreated chlamydial infection in women is a major cause of PID, ectopic pregnancy, and infertility
  - In men, it may result in prostatitis
- Diagnostic methods include culture, antigen detection, gene probe hybridization, and nucleic acid amplification
- PCR and LCR of swab specimens are more than 95% sensitive and specific
  - LCR is licensed for urine and self-administered vaginal swabs

Treatment

- The CDC recommends **azithromycin or doxycycline** as first-line agents
- Alternatives include **fluoroquinolones, erythromycin, and azithromycin**
- **In pregnancy, doxycycline and fluoroquinolones are contraindicated.** Test for cure is recommended after treatment with amoxicillin or erythromycin because these regimens may not be as efficacious and side effects may discourage compliance.

- Because reinfection following treatment is common and reinfection increases the risk for PID, repeat testing is warranted
- Sexual partners of the past 60 days or the last sexual partner should be referred for evaluation and treatment
- Other causes of urethritis include *Ureaplasma*, *Trichomonas*, and HSV

Pelvic Inflammatory Disease

Basic Information

- PID encompasses inflammatory conditions that produce one or more of the following: Endometritis, salpingitis, tubo-ovarian abscess, and pelvic peritonitis
- Most commonly implicated organisms include *N. gonorrhoeae* and *C. trachomatis* as well as anaerobes, gram-negative bacilli, streptococci, and mycoplasmas

Clinical Presentation

- Fever and lower abdominal pain (usually bilateral) are the hallmarks of PID
  - Right upper quadrant tenderness from perihepatitis (Fitz-Hugh-Curtis) is seen in 10%
- Pelvic examination reveals **cervical motion tenderness, adnexal tenderness, and purulent endocervical discharge**
  - A palpable adnexal mass suggests a tubo-ovarian abscess

Diagnosis

- Minimal clinical criteria for diagnosis are **direct lower quadrant tenderness, adnexal tenderness, and cervical motion tenderness**
- Additional criteria include mucopurulent cervicitis, presence of WBCs in saline microscopy of vaginal secretions, documented *N. gonorrhoeae* or *C. trachomatis*, oral temperature above 38.3°C, and elevated erythrocyte sedimentation rate or C-reactive protein
- Definitive criteria are **histopathologic evidence of endometritis, radiologic evidence on transvaginal ultrasound, and laparoscopic evidence of PID**

TREATMENT

- CDC first-line recommended treatment for PID is either **cefotetan** *or* **cefoxitin** *plus* **doxycycline; clindamycin** *plus* **gentamicin**
- Empirical therapy is broad spectrum to cover *N. gonorrhoeae*, *C. trachomatis*, anaerobes, gram-negative bacteria, and streptococci
- Inpatient therapy is provided when surgical emergencies cannot be excluded, the patient is pregnant, there is lack of response or inability to take oral antibiotics, or the patient has a tubo-ovarian abscess

Epididymitis and Prostatitis

Basic Information

- *Epididymitis* is defined as inflammation of the epididymis caused by infection or trauma
- In men younger than 35 years, it is most often caused by *N. gonorrhoeae* or *C. trachomatis*

- In men older than 35 years, nonsexually transmitted epididymitis is more commonly caused by **gram-negative enteric organisms**
- Prostatitis, or inflammation of the prostate, is considered acute or chronic
  - Acute infection is caused by *Escherichia coli* and occasionally by *N. gonorrhoeae*
  - Chronic prostatitis is caused by gram-negative bacilli (*E. coli*) and enterococci

Clinical Presentation

- **Epididymitis** presents as unilateral testicular pain and tenderness, edema, and hydrocele
  - The major alternative diagnosis is testicular torsion, especially when onset of pain is sudden and pain is severe
  - **Pyuria** is generally seen in epididymitis, but not torsion
  - Doppler ultrasound will show decreased or absent blood flow to the affected testicle in torsion but normal or increased blood flow with epididymitis
- Acute prostatitis presents with **fever, chills, perineal pain, back pain, dysuria**
  - The prostate gland is tender on examination
- Chronic prostatitis is often indolent

Diagnosis

- For **urethritis** perform Gram stain, culture, and/or nucleic acid amplification test of urethral exudate or intraurethral swab
- Diagnosis of prostatitis is usually clinical
  - "Milking" the prostate by digital examination before voiding may induce pyuria

Treatment

- In urethritis, CDC-recommended treatment is based on suspected etiology of infection
  - For epididymitis most likely caused by gonococcal or chlamydial infection, treat with **ceftriaxone plus doxycycline**
  - For epididymitis in patients older than 35 years, treat with **ofloxacin or levofloxacin**
- Treatment for acute prostatitis includes ceftriaxone, quinolones, or trimethoprim-sulfamethoxazole (**TMP-SMX**) for 14 days
- Treatment for chronic prostatitis includes 4 to 6 weeks of **quinolone** or 6 to 12 weeks of **TMP-SMX**

Vaginitis

Table 11-3 provides a summary of the types of organisms causing vaginitis and their specific diagnoses.

Condylomata Acuminata or Anogenital Warts

Basic Information

- Caused by **human papillomavirus** (HPV) infection
- The most common viral STD in the United States; most infections asymptomatic and self-limited

		TABLE 11-3	*Vaginitis*		
Diagnosis	**Organism**	**Type of Organism**	**Discharge**	**Specific Diagnosis**
Bacterial vaginosis	Replacement of normal *Lactobacillus* spp. with high levels of anaerobes	Bacteria	White, noninflammatory coating discharge	Clue cells seen on microscopy Vaginal pH > 4.5 + whiff test (fishy odor on addition of 10% KOH)
Trichomoniasis	*Trichomonas vaginalis*	Protozoa	Foul-smelling, frothy, yellow-green discharge	Organism seen on microscopy of secretions
Vulvovaginal candidiasis	*Candida albicans*	Fungi (yeast)	White, "cottage cheese" discharge	Fungal elements seen on wet prep Vaginal pH 4–4.5

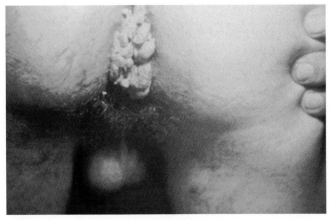

FIGURE 11-6 Anal condylomata acuminata appear as exophytic verrucous lesions. (From www.cdc.gov.)

- Types 16, 18, 31, 33, and 35 have been strongly associated with cervical neoplasia
- The same types are also associated with dysplastic and neoplastic lesions associated with anal warts
- HPV types 6 and 11 are rarely associated with neoplasia

Clinical Presentation

- Exophytic verrucous white or pigmented lesions (Fig. 11-6)
- Symptoms vary according to site and size of the lesions
- **Pain, bleeding, and pruritus** may accompany lesions
- Large exophytic masses may result in obstruction or stricture

Diagnosis

- Diagnosis is based on visual inspection
- Evaluation should include anoscopy, sigmoidoscopy, colposcopy, and/or vulvovaginal examination
  - Acetic acid 5% can be applied to facilitate identification
- **Biopsy serves to evaluate for dysplasia**
- HPV DNA detection provides a definitive diagnosis

Treatment

- Treatment of external genital warts depends on **size, location, and patient and provider preference**
- Treatments include surgical removal, cryotherapy, or topical therapy with **podophyllin, imiquimod, or trichloroacetic acid**

- Disease prevention
- HPV quadrivalent vaccine for types 6, 11, 16, 18 (Gardasil by Merck) is licensed for females aged 9 to 26 years. This does not eliminate the need for cervical cancer screening, however, because not all cancer-causing HPV types are included in the vaccine.

Ectoparasite Infestations

Basic Information

- Include **pubic lice** (pediculosis pubis) and **scabies**
- **Scabies,** caused by the mite *Sarcoptes scabiei,* is highly contagious
- **Pubic lice** and **scabies** are transmitted by intimate personal contact and are associated with **poverty, poor hygiene, and malnutrition**

Clinical Presentation

- Patients with **pubic lice** present with pruritus or notice nits or adult pubic lice attached to the base of pubic hair
  - Other affected areas may include eyelashes and coarse truncal and axillary hair
- Patients with **scabies** present with pruritic, erythematous papules and nodules and classic linear burrows, usually in web spaces between the fingers, around the nipples or periumbilical or extensor surfaces of extremities

Diagnosis

- **Pubic lice** is diagnosed by looking closely through pubic hair for nits, nymphs, or adults
- **Scabies** is confirmed by identifying the mite in **skin scrapings**

Treatment

- Treatment of **lice** includes **permethrin 1% cream or pyrethrins with piperonyl butoxide.** Malathion may be used in the setting of treatment failure due to drug resistance.
- Recommended treatment of **scabies** is **permethrin cream 5%**
  - **Lindane 1%** is an alternative regimen that cannot be used in pregnant women or young children because of systemic absorption and neurotoxicity

Urinary Tract Infections

Basic Information

- Common bacterial infections
- Represent a broad spectrum of clinical illness from **uncomplicated cystitis to pyelonephritis with bacteremia**
- Pregnancy increases the risk of UTI because of dilation of ureters, decreased ureteral peristalsis, and decreased bladder tone
  - About 20% to 40% of patients with untreated bacteriuria early in gestation progress to pyelonephritis later in pregnancy. Pyelonephritis has been associated with premature delivery.
  - Urine culture is therefore a routine part of prenatal screening
- Diabetic patients are predisposed to UTI and may progress to **perinephric abscess, papillary necrosis, or emphysematous pyelonephritis**

Clinical Presentation

- Uncomplicated acute bacterial cystitis
  - Characterized by **dysuria, frequency, and urgency**
  - Occurs in nonpregnant women with normal anatomy, no predisposing conditions, and no urologic instrumentation
  - Causative agents include primarily *E. coli* and *Staphylococcus saprophyticus*
- Complicated UTI is defined clinically by the presence of one of the following factors: **Pregnancy, diabetes, male sex, immunosuppression, catheter or urologic instrumentation, stone or abnormal structure of the genitourinary tract, or functional abnormality of the genitourinary tract**
- Acute pyelonephritis manifests with **fever, flank pain, and urinary symptoms**
- Development of perinephric abscess is suggested by an acute pyelonephritis-like illness with persistent fever and symptoms despite medical therapy

Diagnosis

- Laboratory evaluation includes microscopic examination of the urine for **pyuria** and **hematuria** or urine dipstick test for **leukocyte esterase and nitrites**
- Although a urine culture is not necessary for uncomplicated UTI, the microbiology of complicated UTI is less predictable and requires urine Gram stain and culture
- Diagnosis of pyelonephritis is supported by significant bacteriuria or greater than 10^5 colony-forming units (CFUs)/mm^3 and pyuria of more than 10 WBC/mm^3
  - Leukocyte casts are seen in 20% to 50% of cases
  - Blood cultures are positive in 20% of cases

- Diagnosis of a perinephric abscess should be confirmed by ultrasound or CT scan

Treatment

- Treatment of uncomplicated UTI is empirical
  - In areas where resistance to **TMP-SMX** is less than 20%, this drug can be used twice daily for 3 days
  - Other agents include **quinolone** therapy for 3 days or **nitrofurantoin** for 7 days
  - Antibiotic selection is based on regional surveillance
- For complicated UTI, antibiotic selection is based on culture data and duration of therapy is generally 2 weeks
- For pyelonephritis, treatment is based on severity of illness and is guided by urine or blood culture results
  - In mild cases, treatment includes **oral quinolones** or **TMP-SMX** for a 14-day course
  - Moderate to severe illness may initially require intravenous therapy with **quinolones, aminoglycosides, third-generation cephalosporins, or TMP-SMX**
  - Complicated acute pyelonephritis is treated with **imipenem or ampicillin plus aminoglycosides** to complete up to 3 weeks of therapy
- Catheter-associated bacteriuria should be treated in the setting of **symptomatic infection, suspected sepsis, renal transplant, or immunocompromise**
  - If possible, **removal** of catheter during treatment is advised
  - When chronic catheterization is required, intermittent catheterization rather than an indwelling catheter reduces the risk of infection
- For perinephric abscess, percutaneous drainage or surgery may be necessary
- Treat asymptomatic bacteriuria in the setting of pregnancy, prior to urologic procedure or renal transplant, or if neutropenia is present

REVIEW QUESTIONS

For review questions, please go to www.expertconsult.com.

SUGGESTED READINGS

Centers for Disease Control and Prevention: Sexually transmitted diseases treatment guidelines 2006, *MMWR* 55(No. RR-11):14–66, 2006.

Centers for Disease Control and Prevention: Update to CDC's Sexually Transmitted Diseases Treatment Guidelines, 2006: fluoroquinolones no longer recommended for treatment of gonococcal infections, *MMWR* 56:332–336, 2007.

Nicolle LE, Bradley S, Colgan R, et al: Infectious Diseases Society of America guidelines for the diagnosis and treatment of asymptomatic bacteriuria in adults, *CID* 40:643–654, 2005.

Warren JW, Abrutyn E, Hebel JR et al: Guidelines for antimicrobial treatment of uncomplicated acute bacterial cystitis and acute pyelonephritis in women, *CID* 29:745–758, 1999.

CHAPTER 12

Human Immunodeficiency Virus Infection

GAIL BERKENBLIT, MD, PhD

Today, more than 20 years since the first description of HIV, nearly 900,000 people are infected nationwide, with more than 55,000 new cases per year. The use of chemoprophylaxis for opportunistic infections and the advent of more effective HIV therapy have led to a decline in overall mortality. Although guidelines regarding HIV therapy are continuously changing and are usually the purview of HIV specialists, the presentation of acute HIV, common opportunistic infections, and the complications of therapy should be recognized by the general internist.

Human Immunodeficiency Virus

Basic Information

- Biology of retroviruses
    - HIV-1 and HIV-2 are RNA retroviruses that cause AIDS
    - HIV entry into T cells is mediated via binding of the CD4 receptor and associated cofactors
    - Reverse transcriptase converts the RNA genome into double-stranded DNA, which then integrates into the host genome and co-opts cellular machinery for replication
    - HIV infection selectively depletes CD4 cells, resulting in immunodeficiency
- Epidemiology
    - HIV-1 is the dominant type in the United States and worldwide
    - HIV-2 is found mainly in West Africa and has a slower clinical course
    - Both are spread via blood-borne exposure (e.g., needle sharing, transfusions), sexual intercourse, and maternal-fetal transmission

Clinical Presentation

- Acute retroviral syndrome
    - Typical onset of symptoms 1 to 6 weeks after exposure to HIV (2 to 3 weeks most commonly), but it may manifest up to 6 months later
    - Symptoms often mimic infectious mononucleosis
    - **Most common presentation: Fever, lymphadenopathy, pharyngitis, rash (Fig. 12-1), myalgias, and arthralgias**
    - Also reported: Thrombocytopenia, leukopenia, diarrhea, headache, elevated transaminases, hepatosplenomegaly, aseptic meningitis, encephalopathy

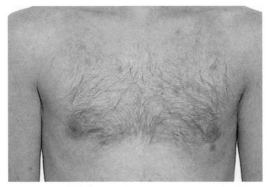

FIGURE 12-1 Typical morbilliform rash associated with acute retroviral syndrome. (From Forbes C, Jackson W: *Color atlas and text of clinical medicine,* ed 3, St. Louis, Mosby, 2003, figure 1-19.)

- Symptoms resolve without treatment within 1 to 2 weeks
- Chronic HIV infection
    - May be clinically silent for years
    - Clinical manifestations depend on CD4 count (Table 12-1)
    - Opportunistic infections and associated conditions are discussed later in this chapter

Diagnosis and Evaluation

- HIV screening
    - Routine screening now recommended for all Americans age 13 to 64 years by the Centers for Disease Control and the American College of Physicians
    - Need for repeat testing determined by risk assessment

Diagnostic Testing
- HIV antibody test (enzyme-linked immunosorbent assay [ELISA])
    - Positive 3 to 4 weeks after acute infection
    - **Test of choice in screening for chronic infection**
    - Western blot used to confirm diagnosis
- CD4 count
    - Measure of severity of immunodeficiency
    - Decline in CD4 cells confers susceptibility to opportunistic infections
    - **CD4 count lower than 200/mm³ or the presence of an indicator condition defines AIDS**
- HIV RNA viral polymerase chain reaction (PCR)
    - Positive 3 to 5 days after acute infection

TABLE 12-1	Complications and Recommended Chemoprophylaxis for Opportunistic Infections by CD4 Cell Count	
CD4 Cell Count*	**Opportunistic Infections and Other HIV-Associated Conditions**	**Recommended Chemophylaxis against Opportunistic Infections**
>500/mm³	Acute retroviral syndrome HIV-associated nephropathy	None
200–500/mm³	Oral candidiasis Community-acquired pneumonia Pulmonary TB Kaposi's sarcoma Herpes zoster CIN Lymphoma Anemia ITP	None

<200/mm³	*Pneumocystis jiroveci* pneumonia (PCP)
	Disseminated histoplasmosis
	Extrapulmonary TB
	Wasting
	HIV dementia
		PCP prophylaxis
		  Trimethoprim-sulfamethoxazole
		  or
		  Dapsone
		  or
		  Atovaquone
		  or
		  Aerosolized pentamidine

<100/mm³	CNS toxoplasmosis
	Cryptococcosis
	CNS lymphoma
		Toxoplasmosis prophylaxis (if patient is toxo IgG +)
		  Trimethoprim/sulfamethoxazole
		  or
		  Dapsone/pyrimethamine/folinic acid
		  or
		  Atovaquone

<50/mm³	Disseminated MAI
	Disseminated CMV
	Progressive multifocal leukoencephalopathy
		MAI prophylaxis
		  Azithromycin
		  or
		  Clarithromycin

*At each stage of decline in CD4 cell count, patients become at risk for further opportunistic infections and other conditions and should receive appropriate chemoprophylaxis.

CIN, Cervical intraepithelial neoplasia; CMV, cytomegalovirus; IgG, immunoglobulin G; ITP, idiopathic thrombocytopenia; MAI, *Mycobacterium avium-intracellulaire*; TB, tuberculosis.

- **Test of choice in diagnosis of acute HIV infection, although count lower than 10,000 copies/mm³ may be false positive**
- Correlates with rate of disease progression
- Used to follow response to antiretroviral therapy

Antiretroviral Therapy

- Six main classes of antiretroviral agents have different potential adverse effects (Table 12-2)
- Initiation of therapy
  - Experts agree that therapy is beneficial with CD4 count less than 350/mm³ or when AIDS indicator conditions are present
  - Current guidelines recommend initiation of antiretroviral therapy (ART) once the CD4 count declines to less than 350/mm³
  - Therapy may be considered on an individual basis in the CD4 count range greater than 350/mm³
  - **Pregnant women, patients with HIV-associated nephropathy (HIVAN), and patients undergoing treatment for hepatitis B should all be treated regardless of CD4**
  - **A combination of three antiretroviral agents from at least two different classes is recommended**

to prevent viral replication and inhibit the development of resistant HIV strains
- The best choice of initial regimen remains controversial
  - Two regimens are recommended for initial therapy: Either a non-nucleoside reverse transcriptase inhibitor (efavirenz preferred) or protease inhibitor (ritonavir-boosted darunavir, atazanavir, fosamprenavir, or lopinavir preferred) + two nucleoside reverse transcriptase inhibitors (combination of tenofovir plus emtricitabine preferred)
- Guidelines for monitoring and changing ART
  - Goal of therapy is viral suppression, which means that the viral load is undetectable or lower than 40 copies/mm³
  - CD4 count and viral load measured every 4 weeks initially and every 12 to 24 weeks once viral load suppressed
  - **ART regimen should be changed if patient fails to achieve virologic suppression in 24 to 48 weeks or has an increase in viral load (>1000 copies/mm³)**
  - Generally, do not add a single drug to a failing regimen or switch single drugs in a regimen if there is ongoing viral replication

TABLE 12-2 *Antiretroviral Medications and Commonly Associated Adverse Effects*

Class of Antiretroviral Drug	Adverse Effects
Nucleoside Reverse Transcriptase Inhibitors	

Zidovudine (AZT)	Bone marrow suppression
	Lactic acidosis
	  Presents with fatigue, nausea, myalgias
	  Labs show anion gap acidosis and elevated lactic acid
	  Can occur any time during therapy

Stavudine (d4T)	Peripheral neuropathy Lipodystrophy Lactic acidosis
Didanosine (ddI)	Peripheral neuropathy Pancreatitis Lactic acidosis
Lamivudine (3TC)	
Emtricitabine (FTC)	

Abacavir	Fatal hypersensitivity reaction
	  Presents with fever, rash, flulike symptoms
	  Usually in first 2–6 wk after starting
	  Can be fatal if drug not discontinued

Tenofovir	Renal insufficiency Fanconi's syndrome
Non-nucleoside Reverse Transcriptase Inhibitors	
Nevirapine	Rash Stevens-Johnson syndrome Hepatitis
Efavirenz	CNS side effects (confusion, nightmares) Teratogenic
Etravirine	
Protease Inhibitors	
Nelfinavir	Diarrhea
Ritonavir	Lipodystrophy
Saquinavir	Central obesity with peripheral wasting
Fosamprenavir	Hyperlipidemia
Lopinavir	Insulin resistance
Tipranavir	
Darunavir	
Atazanavir	Hyperbilirubinemia (atazanavir only)
Indinavir	Nephrolithiasis (indinavir only)
Membrane Fusion Inhibitors	
Enfuvirtide	Injection site reactions
CCR5 Antagonist	
Maraviroc	Well tolerated, but only effective against CCR5 tropic virus
Integrase Inhibitor	
Raltegravir	

BOX 12-1 *Immunization in HIV Patients*

Indicated
Hepatitis A
Hepatitis B
Pneumococcus
Influenza
Tetanus-diptheria

Contraindicated (Live Virus)
Varicella
Measles-mumps-rubella
Bacille Calmette-Guérin
Smallpox

- It is acceptable to switch single agents for side effect management if viral load is "undetectable"
- Prevention of HIV transmission: ART for postexposure prophylaxis (PEP)
  - PEP should be given for both percutaneous and mucocutaneous exposures with a combination of two drugs for lower-risk exposures and three drugs for higher-risk exposures
  - PEP should be given without delay (first dose within 1–2 hours) but is effective up to 72 hours after exposure
  - High-risk factors for percutaneous transmission include hollow needle, visible blood, needle in vessel, and high viral load
  - Recommended regimens vary, but exposed persons should be treated for 4 weeks
- Other issues in the care of HIV-infected patients
  - Prophylaxis against certain opportunistic infections should be introduced once the CD4 count has declined to below predetermined levels (see Table 12-1)
  - Immunizations are an important component of HIV care, but live-attenuated vaccines should be avoided because of risk of disseminated infection (Box 12-1)
  - **Screening purified protein derivative (PPD) should be done at diagnosis and then annually if patent is at risk; PPD greater than 5 mm is considered positive**
  - Screening and vaccination for viral hepatitis should be performed
  - Cancer screening is as per usual guidelines with the exception of cervical cancer (8- to 10-fold elevated risk in HIV patients)
    - Perform a Pap smear at the time of diagnosis and again in 6 months
    - If normal, can screen annually
  - Measures to increase adherence to medications are essential
    - Poor adherence is associated with resistance to ART
    - Factors associated with poor adherence include depression, poor social support, low self-efficacy ratings, active drug use, and complexity of regimen

12

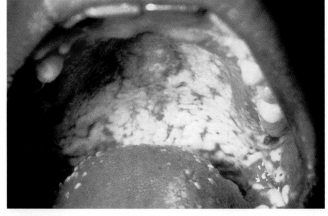

FIGURE 12-2 Oral candidiasis thrush. (From Mandell GL, Bennett JE, Dolin R, editors: *Principles and practice of infectious diseases,* ed 6, Philadelphia, Churchill Livingstone, 2005, figure 117-7.)

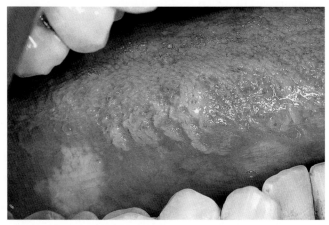

FIGURE 12-3 Oral hairy leukoplakia. Note the predilection for the lateral tongue surface and the vertical ridges. (From Cummings CW, Flint PW, Harker LA, et al, editors: *Cummings otolaryngology: Head and neck surgery,* ed 4, Philadelphia, Mosby, 2005, figure 64-8.)

Opportunistic Infections and Other HIV-Associated Conditions

CANDIDIASIS

Clinical Presentation

- At risk when CD4 count is lower than 250/mm³
- **Most commonly seen as oropharyngeal creamy white plaques (thrush) that are removable by scraping (Fig. 12-2)**
- **Differential of white oral lesions includes oral hairy leukoplakia (Fig. 12-3)**
  - Characterized by painless, white, nonremovable plaques, usually on the lateral and dorsal tongue
  - Possibly related to Epstein-Barr virus infection
- Candidal esophagitis is the most common cause of odynophagia, followed by cytomegalovirus (CMV), herpes simplex virus (HSV), and aphthous ulcers

Diagnosis

- Oral candidiasis is usually diagnosed by appearance (see Fig. 12-2).

- Swab or biopsy may be needed to differentiate from oral hairy leukoplakia
- Esophageal candidiasis is often diagnosed presumptively (odynophagia in HIV patient with low CD4 count)
  - Endoscopy is usually reserved for those for whom empirical therapy fails

Treatment

- Oral or vaginal candidal infection may be treated with topical azole therapy
- Candidal esophagitis is treated with a 2-week course of systemic fluconazole
- If azole resistance occurs, amphotericin B therapy may be necessary

PULMONARY INFECTIONS

See Figure 12-4 and Table 12-3 for common pulmonary conditions associated with HIV infections.

CNS MANIFESTATIONS

See Table 12-4 and Figure 12-5 for CNS conditions associated with HIV infections.

DISSEMINATED *MYCOBACTERIUM AVIUM-INTRACELLULARE*

Clinical Presentation

- Presents with CD4 below 50/mm³
- **Symptoms include fevers, malaise, wasting, abdominal pain, lymphadenopathy**
- Often associated with anemia and leukopenia
- **Elevated alkaline phosphatase is often a clue to this infection**

Diagnosis

- Most commonly diagnosed with mycobacterial blood cultures
  - Must hold cultures for weeks
- May suspect if acid-fast bacteria and granulomas are seen on biopsy of liver, lymph node, or bone marrow in a susceptible host

Treatment

- Treated with combination antimicrobial therapy (usually clarithromycin and ethambutol with or without rifabutin)
- **Azithromycin chemoprophylaxis is recommended when CD4 is lower than 50/mm³**

CYTOMEGALOVIRUS

Clinical Presentation

- Presents when CD4 count is lower than 50/mm³
- **Retinitis is most common end-organ complication of CMV (Fig. 12-6)**
- Symptoms include floaters and decreased visual acuity
- Retinal changes include fluffy white retinal infiltrates and hemorrhage
- Less common sites of involvement include GI tract (hemorrhagic ulcerations), lung (pneumonitis), and CNS (encephalitis)

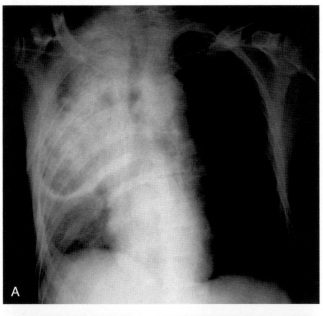

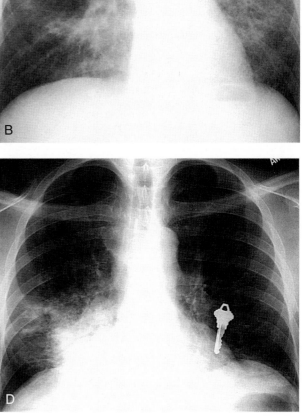

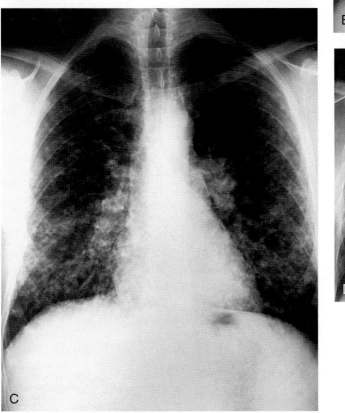

FIGURE 12-4 Chest radiographs of common pulmonary conditions associated with HIV infection. **A,** Streptococcal pneumonia, presenting with focal lobar infiltrate. **B,** *Pneumocystis* pneumonia, typical presentation with "bat wing" infiltrates (*arrows*). **C,** Diffuse bilateral infiltrates in acute pulmonary histoplasmosis. **D,** Tuberculosis pneumonia, typically presents with noncavitary, lowe-lobe infiltrates in advanced disease (key is an overlying artifact). (A, B, and D, From Mason RJ: *Murray and Nadel's textbook of respiratory medicine,* ed 4, London, Elsevier, 2005, figures 75-1, 75-5, and 75-2. C, From Mandell GL, Bennett JE, Dolin R, editors: *Principles and practice of infectious diseases,* ed 6, Philadelphia, Churchill Livingstone, 2005, figure 262-5.)

TABLE 12-3	Common Pulmonary Manifestations Associated with HIV Infection				
	CD4	**Clinical Presentation**	**Radiologic Appearance**	**Diagnostic Testing**	**Treatment**
Community-acquired pneumonia (CAP)	Any	Acute onset Fever Productive cough Pleuritic pain	Usually lobar infiltrate	Sputum Gram stain and culture	Antibiotic coverage for *Streptococcus pneumoniae* and typical CAP pathogens; cover gram-negative rods if CD4 low
Pneumocystis jiroveci pneumonia (PCP)	<200	Subacute onset Dry cough Hypoxia Fever Less likely if on prophylaxis	Usually "bat wing" perihilar infiltrate 20% have normal chest radiograph	Immunofluorescence, silver stain, or culture of induced sputum or bronchoalveolar lavage	Trimethoprim-sulfamethoxazole first-line agent Alternatives: Dapsone/trimethoprim; clindamycin/primaquine; atovaquone; or IV pentamidine Add corticosteroids if Pao$_2$ < 70 or A-a gradient > 35
Pulmonary histoplasmosis	<200	Subacute onset Dry cough Oral ulcers common Geographic risk	Diffuse interstitial infiltrates	*Histoplasma* urine antigen; bronchoalveolar lavage culture	Itraconazole or amphotericin B
Pulmonary tuberculosis	Any	Gradual onset Extrapulmonary manifestations common if CD4 < 200	Diffuse interstitial infiltrates Noncavitary in advanced HIV	AFB stain/culture PPD >5 mm considered positive in HIV-infected patients	Four-drug TB regimen for 2 mo, then two-drug maintenance for 6 mo total therapy

AFB, Acid-fast bacillus; Pao$_2$, arterial oxygen partial pressure; PPD, purified protein derivative; TB, tuberculosis.

TABLE 12-4	Common CNS Conditions Associated with HIV Infection				
Disorder	**CD4**	**Clinical Scenario**	**Appearance on MRI**	**Diagnosis**	**Treatment**
Toxoplasmosis	<100	Focal neurologic symptoms Seizures	Usually multiple ring-enhancing lesions Surrounding mass effect	Toxo IgG + in 90% Presumptive diagnosis Follow response to therapy Clinical improvement MRI in 2 wk	Sulfadiazine + pyrimethamine Suppressive therapy until CD4 > 200 for >3 mo
CNS lymphoma	<100	Focal neurologic symptoms Seizures	Usually single solid or ring-enhancing lesions Surrounding mass effect	First step is usually trial of toxoplasmosis therapy If no response, brain biopsy to diagnose lymphoma SPECT scan may be helpful if positive	Radiation therapy Begin antiretroviral therapy
Cryptococcal meningitis	<100	Severe headache High intracranial pressure Extra-CNS manifestations: Skin lesions, pneumonia	Normal in 90% of patients Mass lesion in 10%	Classically, India ink test Now, usually serum and CSF cryptococcal antigen CSF culture Low CSF WBC count is poor prognosis sign	Amphotericin B + fluconazole for suppressive therapy until CD4 > 100–200 for >6 mo
Progressive multifocal leukoencephalopathy (PML)	<50	Rapidly progressive Focal neurologic symptoms Loss of speech, vision	Focal white matter changes No mass effect Definitive diagnosis requires brain biopsy	MRI appearance CSF for JC virus PCR	No specific therapy Antiretroviral therapy may be beneficial

CSF, Cerebrospinal fluid; IgG, immunoglobulin G; PCR, polymerase chain reaction; SPECT, single-photon emission computed tomography.

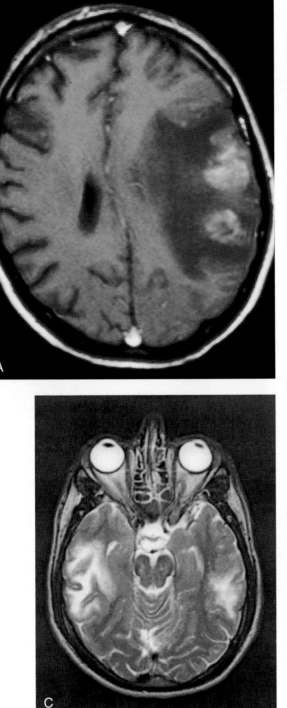

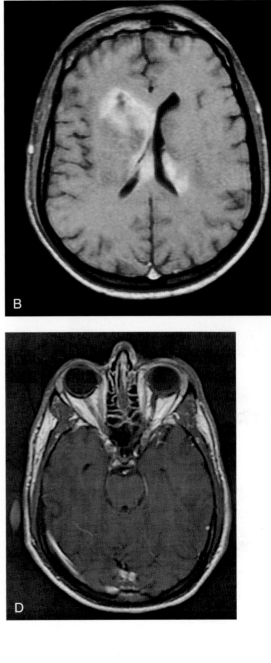

FIGURE 12-5   Imaging of common CNS conditions associated with HIV. **A,** CNS toxoplasmosis presents as multiple ring-enhancing lesions. **B,** CNS lymphoma usually presents as a solitary ring-enhancing lesion. **C,** Progressive multifocal leukoencephalopathy (PML) lesions are seen as areas of high signal intensity in the subcortical white matter (*left*) and do not enhance with gadolinium (right). (A and B, From Haslett C, Chilvers ER, Boon NA, et al, editors: *Davidson's principles and practice of medicine,* ed 19, New York, Churchill Livingstone, 2002, figures 1.88 and 1.89. C, From Mandell GL, Bennett JE, Dolin R, editors: *Principles and practice of infectious diseases,* ed 6, Philadelphia, Churchill Livingstone, 2005, figure 120-4.)

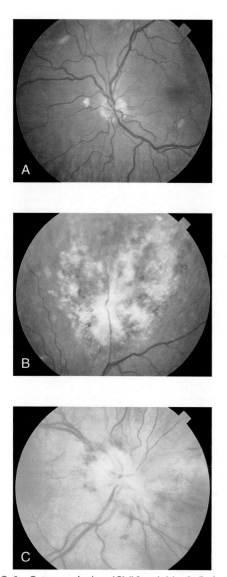

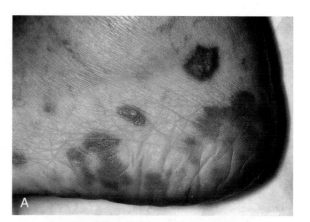

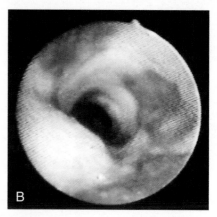

FIGURE 12-7 Kaposi's sarcoma can present cutaneously (**A**), in the oral mucosa (**B**), and internally in the lungs or GI tract (not shown). (A, From Mandell GL, Bennett JE, Dolin R: *Principles and practice of infectious diseases,* ed 6, Philadelphia, Churchill Livingstone, 2005, figure 117-12. B, From Goldman L, Ausiello D: *Cecil textbook of medicine,* ed 23, Philadelphia, WB Saunders, 2008, figure 414-12.)

FIGURE 12-6 Cytomegalovirus (CMV) retinitis. **A,** Early disease with retinal involvement along blood vessels. **B,** Extensive retinal damage and retinal hemorrhages. **C,** CMV retinitis with papillitis. (From Mandell GL, Bennett JE, Dolin R, editors: *Principles and practice of infectious diseases,* ed 6, Philadelphia, Churchill Livingstone, 2005, figure 134-2.)

Diagnosis

- **Retina reveals characteristic "ketchup and cottage cheese" lesions on fundoscopy, representing perivascular hemorrhage and exudates**
- Diagnosis at other sites is by CMV PCR, culture, or finding of viral inclusion bodies on histopathology

Treatment

- Systemic disease: Treat with either systemic ganciclovir or foscarnet
- CMV retinitis: Can use intraocular ganciclovir implants
  - Intraocular implants do not prevent nonophthalmologic manifestations of CMV

KAPOSI'S SARCOMA

Clinical Presentation

- Can be seen with a modestly depleted CD4 count (200–500/mm³ range)
- **Indurated or nodular violaceous growths on the skin or in any visceral organ (Fig. 12-7)**
- Most common malignancy in HIV/AIDS
- Predominantly among men with same-sex contact as transmission risk

Diagnosis

- Biopsy shows proliferation of abnormal vascular structures on pathology
- Human herpes virus-8 identified as causative agent but not used diagnostically

Treatment

- Cytotoxic chemotherapy
- Intralesional chemotherapy (if cutaneous)
- May regress with effective ART

NON-HODGKIN'S LYMPHOMA

Clinical Presentation

- Usually seen at CD4 less than 200/mm^3
- Heterogeneous group of malignancies
- 70% are B-cell derived
- Intermediate or high-grade B-cell lymphomas are AIDS-defining events in individual with HIV infection
- **Extranodal presentation common (GI tract, visceral, bone marrow, body cavity)**

Diagnosis

- For accessible lesions, diagnosis made by biopsy
- For CNS lesions: **Thallium single-photon emission CT (SPECT) scan is useful to differentiate lymphoma from similarly appearing lesions of toxoplasmosis; lymphoma lesions often enhance whereas toxoplasmosis does not**
- Biopsy warranted for lesions that do not respond to empirical therapy for toxoplasmosis

Treatment

- Combination chemotherapy, brain radiation if CNS involvement, and ART

HIV-ASSOCIATED NEPHROPATHY

Clinical Presentation

- Can be seen at any CD4 level, but usually CD4 is lower than 200/mm^3
- **Presents with nephrotic syndrome**
- Progressive course; if untreated, leads to renal failure over 1 to 4 months

Diagnosis

- Large echogenic kidneys seen on ultrasound
- **Diagnosis made by biopsy that shows focal segmental glomerulosclerosis**
- Differential diagnosis includes: Heroin nephropathy, drug toxicity (e.g., tenofovir, indinavir, trimethoprim-sulfamethoxazole), hepatitis-related nephropathy

Treatment

- ART
- Steroid therapy may slow progression until viral suppression is achieved

IMMUNE RECONSTITUTION SYNDROME (IRS)

Clinical Presentation

- Occurs 2 to 12 weeks after initiating ART
- Paradoxical clinical worsening owing to new ability to mount an inflammatory response against an underlying opportunistic infection or antigen (that was subclinical)
- Usually seen with low CD4 count (<100/mm^3) and rapid decline in HIV viral load

Diagnosis

- Presentations of opportunistic infections may be atypical because of brisk inflammation; high clinical suspicion needed

Treatment

- Diagnose and treat the underlying opportunistic infection
- Anti-inflammatory treatment (corticosteroids or nonsteroidal anti-inflammatory drugs) may be effective, although not proven
- Continue ART

REVIEW QUESTIONS

For review questions, please go to www.expertconsult.com.

SUGGESTED READINGS

Bartlett JG, Gallant JE: *Medical management of HIV infection*, Baltimore, 2001–2002, Johns Hopkins University Press.

Chaisson RE, Sterling TR, Gallant JE: General clinical manifestations of human immunodeficiency virus infection. In Mandell GL, Bennett JE, Dolin R, editors: *Principles and practice of infectious diseases*, ed 5, Philadelphia, 2000, Churchill Livingstone.

12

Mycobacterial Infections

SUSAN E. DORMAN, MD

Mycobacteria are aerobic bacteria that have the laboratory characteristic of retaining colorized stain when washed in an acid bath—hence they are "acid-fast" (Fig. 13-1). *Mycobacterium tuberculosis*, *Mycobacterium leprae*, and *Mycobacterium avium* complex are clinically among the most important mycobacteria. However, with the increasing prevalence of immunocompromised hosts, other mycobacterial species have become clinically relevant.

Tuberculosis

Basic Information

- Pathogenesis
  - Airborne transmission from patient with pulmonary tuberculosis (TB) disease (Fig. 13-2)
- Epidemiology
  - Global: Almost 9 million new cases and 2 million deaths per year
  - United States: 13,299 TB cases were reported in the United States in 2007 (4.4 cases per 100,000 population). African Americans and foreign-born persons are disproportionately affected.
- Impact of HIV on TB
  - **HIV increases risk of progression to active TB after *M. tuberculosis* infection**
  - **HIV increases risk of reactivation of latent *M. tuberculosis* infection**
  - HIV increases mortality from TB
  - Highly active antiretroviral therapy decreases the risk of active TB in HIV-infected persons
- Multidrug-resistant TB (MDR-TB)
  - **Defined as resistance to at least isoniazid plus rifampin**
  - Clusters in geographic areas (Russia, Latvia, Estonia, China, Iran)
  - Other risk factors: Prior TB treatment, noncompliance with TB treatment, adding one drug to a failing TB treatment regimen

Clinical Presentation

- **Primary infection: Usually asymptomatic**
  - **Minority** present with pleural effusion or pneumonia in mid- or lower-lung fields with hilar or mediastinal lymphadenopathy
  - Most (>90%) immunocompetent people control initial infection and develop clinically silent latent infection (see Fig. 13-2)
  - **HIV-infected persons have high risk of progression to active TB after initial infection**
- Reactivation TB disease
  - Typically subacute illness over weeks or months with fever, sweats, weight loss, cough
  - **Pulmonary disease typically involves upper lobe(s) or upper segments of lower lobe(s).** Cavitation is classic, but infiltrates may be lobar, nodular, or interstitial.
- Other comments
  - Nearly any organ system can be involved
  - HIV: Increased prevalence (compared with HIV-negative) of extrapulmonary TB, disseminated TB, miliary TB. **Pulmonary TB (in HIV) can present with any chest radiographic pattern, including normal chest radiograph.**
  - Miliary TB: Disease results from widespread hematogenous dissemination of bacilli. Classic chest radiographic appearance is innumerable tiny nodules (Fig. 13-3).

Diagnosis and Evaluation

- Detection of M. *tuberculosis* infection (either latent infection or active disease)
  - Tuberculin skin test (TST).
    - Intradermal inoculation of mycobacterial purified protein derivative. Readout is induration 48 to 72 hours after inoculation.

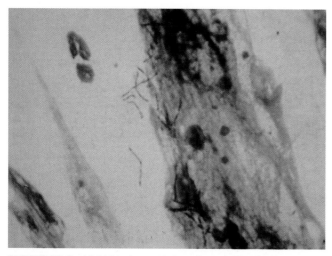

FIGURE 13-1 Ziehl-Neelsen staining of a sputum sample of a patient with pulmonary tuberculosis demonstrating acid-fast bacilli. (From Forbes C, Jackson W: *Color atlas and text of clinical medicine,* ed 3, St. Louis, Mosby, 2003, figure 4.14.)

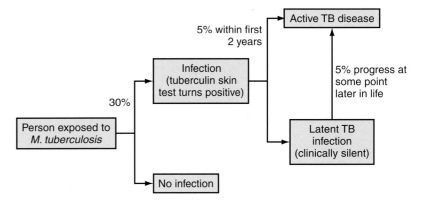

FIGURE 13-2 Pathogenesis of tuberculosis (TB) in immune-competent individuals exposed to *Mycobacterium tuberculosis*. HIV infection (not shown in this figure) substantially increases the proportion of patients who develop active TB disease after initial exposure and the proportion of patients who progress from latent infection to active TB.

13

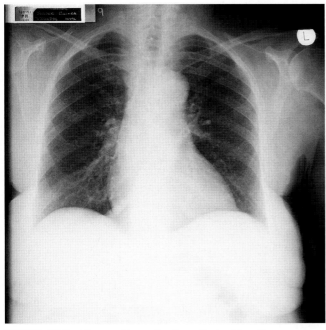

FIGURE 13-3 Chest radiograph of a patient with miliary tuberculosis. (From Swash M: *Hutchinson's clinical methods,* ed 21, Philadelphia, WB Saunders, 2002, figure 22.5.)

- **False-positive result can be due to infection with nontuberculous mycobacteria (NTM) or prior bacilli Calmette-Guérin (BCG) vaccination**
- False-negative test can result from immunosuppression
- **Positive TST does not necessarily indicate active TB disease**
- Detection of TB disease
  - Laboratory
    - Microscopic examination of sputum or other clinical specimen stained for acid-fast bacilli (AFB smear)
    - **For diagnosis of pulmonary TB, obtain three morning sputum specimens (sent for AFB smear and mycobacterial culture)**
    - AFB smear not sensitive and not specific for *M. tuberculosis* (but positive smear is highly predictive of TB in TB endemic settings)

- Culture
  - Sensitive and specific (in combination with other tests done on cultured material) for *M. tuberculosis*
  - Slow: Takes 3 to 6 weeks for *M. tuberculosis* to grow in culture
- Nucleic acid amplification (NAA) tests
  - Used to evaluate respiratory specimens from untreated patients
  - Highly specific for *M. tuberculosis*
  - Highly sensitive in AFB smear–positive patients; only 50% sensitive in AFB smear–negative patients
  - **If TB is suspected and NAA is negative, TB not excluded**
  - NAA test does not replace smear or culture

Treatment

- Treatment of latent TB infection (Fig. 13-4)
  - Decision to treat is based on individual's risk of recent *M. tuberculosis* infection and risk of progression to active TB disease if infected (Table 13-1)
  - **Exclude active TB disease before starting treatment for latent TB**
  - **Preferred regimen: Isoniazid daily for 9 months**
  - Alternative regimen: Rifampin daily for 4 months
  - **No age cutoff for treatment of latent TB infection**
- Treatment of drug-susceptible TB disease
  - Eight weeks of isoniazid plus rifampin plus pyrazinamide plus either ethambutol (commonly used) or streptomycin (not commonly used), followed by isoniazid plus rifampin "continuation phase" for an additional 4 months (total treatment duration, 6 months; Fig. 13-5)
  - Treatment extended to total of 9 months if delay (e.g., 2–3 months) in culture conversion
  - Treatment extended to 9 to 12 months for central nervous system TB
  - Streptomycin contraindicated in pregnant women; pyrazinamide not recommended for use in pregnant women
- Treatment of MDR-TB disease is 18 to 24 months, with complex regimens
- Treatment of TB disease in HIV-infected persons
  - TB treatment duration **not affected** by HIV
  - **Rifampin has drug-drug interactions with most protease inhibitors and non-nucleoside reverse transcriptase inhibitors**

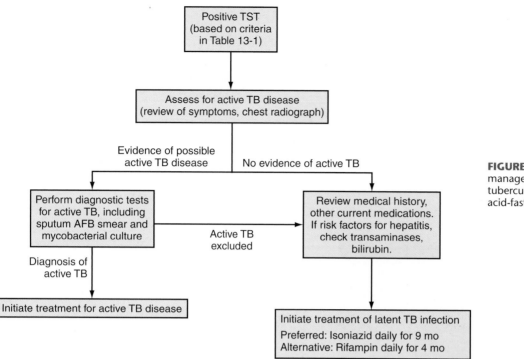

FIGURE 13-4 Clinical management of a positive tuberculin skin test (TST). AFB, acid-fast bacilli.

TABLE 13-1	Risk Groups for Targeted Tuberculin Skin Testing (TST) and Treatment of Latent Tuberculosis (TB) Infection with Tuberculin Skin Test Cut-Points
TST Induration Considered Positive	**Risk Group**
≥5 mm	HIV infection Recent contacts of active TB patients Fibrotic changes on chest radiograph Immunosuppression Use of antitumor necrosis factor α-drugs
≥10 mm	Recent immigrants Injection drug users Residents and employees of high-risk congregate settings (long-term care facilities, health care facilities, homeless shelters, prisons or jails) Mycobacteriology lab workers Persons with medical conditions that put them at risk (silicosis, diabetes mellitus, chronic renal failure, some malignancies, gastrectomy or jejunoileal bypass, underweight) Children < 4 yr old Infants, children, or adolescents exposed to adults at high risk for TB ≥10 mm increase ≥10 mm increase within 2 yr is considered evidence of recent *Mycobacterium tuberculosis* infection (a positive TST reaction)
≥15 mm	Persons without any of above risk factors (TST not recommended in this group)

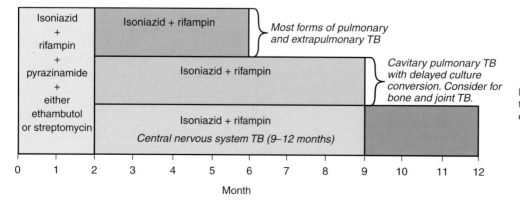

FIGURE 13-5 Recommended treatment for active tuberculosis disease, based on disease site.

TABLE 13-2	Toxicities of Commonly Used Antituberculosis Medications	
Drug	**Major Toxicities**	**Monitoring**
Isoniazid	Hepatotoxicity, peripheral neuropathy	Baseline liver chemistries. Repeat if baseline is abnormal or if other hepatitis risk factors or symptoms of hepatotoxicity are present
Rifampin	Hepatotoxicity, fever, flulike syndrome, thrombocytopenia, drug-drug interactions	Baseline liver chemistries and CBC. Repeat if baseline is abnormal or if other hepatitis risk factors or symptoms of adverse reaction are present
Pyrazinamide	Hepatotoxicity, arthralgias, rash	Baseline liver chemistries, uric acid. Repeat if baseline is abnormal or if other hepatitis risk factors or symptoms of adverse reaction are present
Ethambutol	Optic neuritis	Baseline and monthly tests of visual acuity and color vision
Streptomycin	Ototoxicity, renal toxicity, teratogenic	Monthly audiometry, renal function, electrolytes Contraindicated in pregnancy

13

- **Worsening of TB signs or symptoms can be seen in first several weeks after starting HIV and/or TB treatment (paradoxical worsening)**
- Drug toxicities and monitoring for drug toxicity (Table 13-2)
  - Rifampin stimulates the cytochrome P450 system and enhances metabolism (thereby lowering blood levels and potentially decreasing effectiveness) of many drugs, including warfarin, oral contraceptives, methadone, most HIV protease inhibitors, most HIV non-nucleoside reverse transcriptase inhibitors

Prevention of Tuberculosis Transmission

- Respiratory isolation should be initiated for all persons suspected of having pulmonary TB disease who are hospitalized or in otherwise congregate settings (e.g., prison, nursing home)
- Care providers (for persons having or suspected of having infectious pulmonary TB disease) should use personal respiratory protection (e.g., N-95 mask)

Leprosy (Hansen's Disease)

Basic Information

- Caused by M. leprae
- Prevalence highest in Africa, Asia

Clinical Presentation

- Broad spectrum of disease activity, including tuberculoid, borderline, and lepromatous forms
  - **Tuberculoid: One or few asymmetrical anesthetic skin macules;** nerve involvement (classically ulnar nerve at elbow) can be severe; biopsies of skin, nerves show few or no bacteria
  - **Lepromatous: Symmetrical skin nodules and plaques on cool areas of body;** affected tissues laden with mycobacteria; upper respiratory tract involvement common, manifest by nasal congestion, epistaxis, cartilage erosion/collapse (saddle-nose deformity; Fig. 13-6); peripheral neuropathy is common.

Diagnosis and Evaluation

- Diagnosis based on clinical presentation plus biopsy (demonstration of AFB and histology)

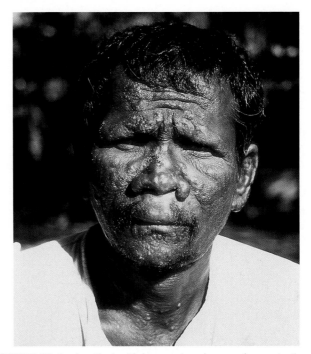

FIGURE 13-6 A patient with lepromatous leprosy demonstrating saddle-nose deformity. (From Haslett C, Chilvers ER, Boon NA, et al: *Davidson's principles and practice of medicine,* ed 19, New York, Churchill Livingstone, 2002, figure 1.69.)

Treatment

- Pauci-bacillary (skin smear negative, with five or fewer skin lesions): Dapsone daily plus rifampin monthly for 6 months
- Multibacillary (skin-smear positive, with more than five skin lesions): Dapsone daily plus rifampin monthly plus clofazimine for 1 year

Nontuberculous Mycobacteria

Basic Information

- Rapid growers (visible growth within 7 days in culture): *Mycobacterium fortuitum, Mycobacterium chelonae, Mycobacterium abscessus*

TABLE 13-3	*Clinical Features of Infections Caused by Nontuberculosis Mycobacteria*	
Species	**Reservoir**	**Common Clinical Manifestations**
Mycobacterium avium-intracellulare complex	Birds, cattle, swine, water, soil	Disseminated disease in AIDS (fevers, sweats, diarrhea, mesenteric adenopathy) Pulmonary disease (cavity, infiltrate, or bronchiectasis) in persons with underlying lung disease (COPD, cystic fibrosis) or older women
Mycobacterium kansasii	Water	Pulmonary disease resembling TB, or disseminated disease, especially in HIV-infected persons
Mycobacterium marinum	Water, marine organisms	"Fish-tank granuloma." Infection follows trauma, usually to extremities, occurring in water. Presents as enlarging nodule(s) that ulcerates, drains
Mycobacterium fortuitum *Mycobacterium abscessus* *Mycobacterium chelonae* (rapid growers)	Water	Cutaneous disease, catheter-related infections, surgical wound infections, keratitis. *M. abscessus* can cause pulmonary disease in cystic fibrosis

COPD, chronic obstructive pulmonary disease; TB, tuberculosis.

- Slow growers (visible growth requires >7 days in culture): *Mycobacterium kansasii, Mycobacterium avium-intracellulare, Mycobacterium marinum*

Clinical Presentation

- Formerly known as mycobacteria other than tuberculosis
- Isolation of NTM from clinical specimen may result from contamination (e.g., from tap water), colonization in absence of NTM disease, or NTM disease
- **Immunosuppression is a risk factor for NTM disease**
- Common clinical syndromes listed in Table 13-3

Diagnosis and Evaluation

- Diagnosis is based on clinical presentation and positive culture of clinically relevant specimen (see Table 13-3)

Treatment

- Antimicrobial agents and treatment duration vary according to organism and site of disease

REVIEW QUESTIONS

For review questions, please go to www.expertconsult.com.

SUGGESTED READINGS

American Thoracic Society: Centers for Disease Control and Prevention: Targeted tuberculin testing and treatment of latent tuberculosis infection, *Am J Respir Crit Care Med* 161:S221–S247, 2000.

American Thoracic Society: Centers for Disease Control and Prevention: Treatment of tuberculosis, *Am J Respir Crit Care Med* 167:603–662, 2003.

Blumberg HM, Leonard MK Jr, Jasmer RM: Update on the treatment of tuberculosis and latent tuberculosis infection, *JAMA* 293:2776–2784, 2005.

Griffith DE, Aksamit T, Brown-Elliott BA, et al: An official ATS/IDSA statement: diagnosis, treatment, and prevention of nontuberculous mycobacterial diseases, *Am J Respir Crit Care Med* 175:367–416, 2007.

Infectious Diarrhea

CYNTHIA L. SEARS, MD

Infectious diarrhea is the second leading cause of morbidity and mortality throughout the world, predominantly in developing countries. In the United States, between 200 and 300 million episodes of acute diarrhea occur yearly. A systematic approach to the evaluation of the patient with diarrhea is useful in identifying the cause.

Approach to a Patient with Infectious Diarrhea

Clinical Presentation

- Acute diarrhea: Three or more episodes of liquid stool in a 24-hour period; symptoms typically last less than 14 days
- Chronic diarrhea: Duration exceeds 1 month
- Clinical classification of acute diarrhea (Table 14-1)
  - **Noninflammatory: Large-volume, watery stools containing no blood or pus**
  - **Inflammatory: Frequent, small-volume stools containing blood or pus.** Fever and abdominal pain may be present.
  - Frequent overlap occurs such that common causes of inflammatory diarrhea appear to be noninflammatory diarrhea clinically

Diagnosis and Evaluation

- History should focus on duration of symptoms, features of stool (hematochezia, tenesmus), associated symptoms (fever, abdominal pain), previous antibiotic use, immune status, travel history, and risk for food-borne illness (see later discussion)
- Physical examination should include an evaluation of fever, hydration status, and abdominal tenderness

TABLE 14-1	Clinical Classification of Acute Diarrhea
Classification	**Organisms**
Noninflammatory	Noroviruses, rotavirus, enterotoxigenic *Escherichia coli*, *Clostridium* spp., *Giardia lamblia*, *Cryptosporidium*, *Vibrio cholerae*
Inflammatory	*Salmonella*, *Shigella*, *Campylobacter*, Shiga toxin–producing *E. coli* (O157 and non-O157), enteroinvasive *E. coli*, *Clostridium difficile*, *Entamoeba histolytica*, *Yersinia*, *Vibrio parahaemolyticus*

- Laboratory testing
  - Usually no laboratory assessment is needed unless inflammatory diarrhea is suspected or the patient is unstable or immunocompromised
  - Fecal leukocytes: Can help differentiate inflammatory from noninflammatory but may be able to determine whether diarrhea is inflammatory by history alone
  - Stool culture: Indicated only if patient is clinically ill, immunocompromised, and/or presence of fecal leukocytes suggests an inflammatory process
  - Occult blood cards: A positive can serve as an indicator of inflammatory diarrhea
  - **Ova and parasites: Reserve for persistent diarrhea (>14 days) or high-risk individuals (e.g., travel history or immunocompromised). Do not order routinely for acute diarrhea.**

Treatment

- Hydration: Cornerstone of therapy for all patients; oral usually sufficient
- Diet: No alteration other than avoidance of caffeine, dairy products, and sorbitol
- Antidiarrheal medications
  - **Loperamide (Imodium): Delays passage through the intestine; safe in most situations; contraindicated in inflammatory diarrheas because of concern for decreased clearance of toxin or organism (particularly for Shiga toxin–producing *Escherichia coli* (STEC) and *Clostridium difficile*)**
  - Bismuth: Moderately effective but inconvenient and leaves a bad taste; can do harm when taken in excess; will darken stools
  - Diphenoxylate (Lomotil): Has central opiate effects, so try to avoid
- Antibiotics
  - Use is controversial; data are weak that they have a true impact on course of illness in all-comers
  - Rarely indicated in noninflammatory diarrhea unless the patient is unstable or at high risk (e.g., immunocompromised, recent travel, elderly)
  - **Most guidelines recommend empirical use of quinolones in inflammatory diarrhea; azithromycin is second choice**
  - Organisms such as *Vibrio cholerae*, *Shigella* organisms, and *Giardia* spp. should always be treated with antibiotics, but invasive *E. coli* and mild to moderate nontyphoidal *Salmonella* should not be treated with antibiotics

Food-Borne Illness

Basic Information (Table 14-2)

- Can be caused by bacteria, viruses, and parasites or ingestion of bacterial toxins present in microbiologically contaminated foods
- **It is important for physicians to report cases caused by certain organisms (e.g., *Salmonella*) to their local or state health department.** Significant variations exist in state reporting guidelines.

Clinical Presentation

- Typically presents with GI symptoms (e.g., nausea, vomiting, diarrhea, abdominal pain)
- Neurologic symptoms such as paresthesias may be present in certain conditions (e.g., botulism)

Diagnosis and Evaluation

- Patients should be asked about ingestion of raw or poorly cooked food (e.g., fish, eggs, meats, shellfish); unpasteurized milk; home canned goods; or fresh produce (often imported)
- Source of food (if known) can be important in identifying a particular organism
  - Shellfish: *Vibrio cholerae, Vibrio parahaemolyticus*
  - Poultry: *Campylobacter, Salmonella* spp.
  - Meat: *Clostridium perfringens, Salmonella, E. coli*
  - Dairy: *Salmonella, Shigella, E. coli, Yersinia*
  - Prepared protein-rich foods: *Staphylococcus* (ingestion preformed toxin; Table 14-3)

TABLE 14-2	Potential Reportable Food-Borne Diseases
Category	**Illnesses or Organisms**
Bacteria	Botulism, brucellosis, cholera, *escherichia coli* O157, salmonellosis, shigellosis, typhoid fever
Viruses	Hepatitis A
Parasites	Cryptosporidiosis, cyclosporiasis, trichinosis

TABLE 14-3	Bacterial Causes of Diarrheal Illness*

Organism	Usual Incubation Period	Associated Foods	Comments
Bacillus cereus (preformed baterial enterotoxin)	1–6 hr	Fried rice, other starchy foods	Usually presents as sudden nausea and vomiting Diarrhea may not be present
Bacillus cereus (diarrhea toxin)	6–24 hr	Meats, vegetables	Diarrhea is the major manifestation
Campylobacter jejuni	1–3 days	Poultry, milk, water	Common bacterial pathogen Rarely, patients can develop Guillain-Barré syndrome or reactive arthritis after infection
Clostridium botulinum	3–30 days	Home-canned foods	Presents with vomiting, diarrhea, blurred vision, diplopia, and descending muscle weakness
Clostridium perfringens (diarrhea toxin)	6–24 hr	Meat, poultry, or gravy	Fever is rare
Escherichia coli O157:H7/other STEC	1–3 days	Beef, apple cider, water, unpasteurized milk	5–10% of infections lead to hemolytic-uremic syndrome (HUS) Antibiotics not recommended because they may increase risk of HUS If infection suspected, stool culture for specific organism must be requested
Salmonella (nontyphoidal)	1–3 days	Poultry, eggs, milk, juice, fruits, vegetables	Nontyphoidal *Salmonella* (many serotypes) are common causes of bacterial diarrhea In typhoid fever (*S. typhi*), diarrhea is uncommon; fever, fatigue, myalgias predominate
Shigella	1–3 days	Primarily person-to-person spread 20% of cases are food-borne	Variable presentation depending on infecting species Always treat with antibiotics (quinolones) for public health reasons
Staphylococcus aureus (preformed bacterial enterotoxin)	1–6 hr	Cream pastries, salads, poultry	Sudden onset of nausea and vomiting, followed later by diarrhea in some
Vibrio cholerae	1–3 days	Shellfish, contaminated water	Massive, noninflammatory diarrhea Antibiotics reduce length of illness
Vibrio parahaemolyticus	1–3 days	Raw fish, shellfish	Inflammatory diarrhea
Yersinia	1–3 days	Pork, milk	Inflammatory diarrhea Can cause right lower quadrant pain (pseudoappendicitis)

*Most causes of diarrhea can lead to postdiarrheal reactive arthritis and irritable bowel syndrome.
STEC, Shiga toxin–producing *E. coli*.

- Deli foods: *Listeria* monocytogenes
- Inquiries should be made about sick contacts, contact with daycare centers, and travel
- Etiologies can be narrowed by determining whether the diarrhea is inflammatory or noninflammatory (see Table 14-1)
- **Timing of illness (incubation period) may be helpful**
  - 1 to 6 hours: *Staphylococcus aureus*, *Bacillus cereus*
  - 8 to 16 hours: *C. perfringens*, *B. cereus*
  - 16 to 72 hours: *Campylobacter jejuni*, *Salmonella*, *Shigella*, *E. coli*, *Yersinia*, *Vibrio*

Common Pathogens

VIRAL PATHOGENS

- Account for at least 50% of all acute infectious diarrheal illnesses
- Usually the causative agent is never identified
- **Norwalk agent (norovirus) is the most commonly identified viral cause of endemic and epidemic diarrhea in adults**
  - Fecal-oral, food-borne, airborne, and fomite transmission common as a result of low inoculum required for disease
  - Incubation period is usually 24 to 48 hours
  - Noninflammatory diarrhea with or without vomiting, about 80% have both vomiting and diarrhea
- Low-grade fever in about 50%
- Treatment is supportive because symptoms usually are self-limited
- Rotavirus causes sporadic outbreaks in children; much less common in adults
  - Fecal-oral transmission usually seen
  - Vomiting, low-grade fever, transient lactase deficiency can be present
  - Episodes may last over one week
  - Treatment is supportive
- Hepatitis A (see Chapter 30)
  - Rare cause of food-borne disease
  - Long incubation period (15–50 days)
  - Transmitted by contaminated shellfish, raw produce, and foods contaminated after handling by infected people
  - Jaundice, abdominal pain, fever, elevated hepatic transaminases may be present
  - Diagnosis made by the presence of immunoglobulin M anti–hepatitis A antibodies
  - Treatment is supportive
  - Contacts should be given immune globulin

BACTERIAL PATHOGENS

See Table 14-3 for bacterial causes of diarrheal illness.

PARASITIC PATHOGENS

- *Giardia lamblia* (giardiasis)
  - Common cause of persistent or chronic diarrhea
  - Diarrhea usually watery but steatorrhea/malabsorption can arise
  - Bloating and mild nausea are common
  - **Major source is drinking water (usually well water)**
  - Usually responds to treatment with metronidazole

- *Giardia* enzyme immunoassay (EIA) available for diagnosis
- *Cryptosporidium parvum* (cryptosporidiosis)
  - Regionally variable but can be similar in incidence to *Giardia*
  - **Source is often water but can be transmitted through person-to-person, fecal-oral routes**
  - Usually self-limited in normal host but can cause persistent (>14 days) or chronic diarrhea; in HIV-infected host (particularly with CD4 count < 150 cells/mm^3), often a chronic illness
  - Symptoms are variable but can cause large-volume losses or malabsorption
  - Abdominal pain, fever, and vomiting can occur
  - Symptoms may be relapsing
  - Organisms appear on acid-fast stain as oocysts in stool (Fig. 14-1A)
  - On pathology, life-cycle forms are detected in the brush border
  - *Cryptosporidium* EIA available for diagnosis
  - Nitazoxanide available for treatment of immunocompetent children and adults
- *Cyclospora cayetanensis*
  - Also increased in HIV but can infect immunocompetent host (recent outbreak associated with imported raspberries)
  - Similar symptoms to *Cryptosporidium*
  - Responds to sulfa antibiotics
  - Organisms are also acid-fast positive in stool but twice the size of *Crytosporidium* (see Fig. 14-1B)
- *Entamoeba histolytica*
  - Spread by fecal-oral route but can contaminate food or water
  - **Presents as an inflammatory process** with bloody diarrhea and lower abdominal pain (similar to *Shigella*)
  - Often presents as chronic diarrhea
  - Diagnose by examining stool for trophozoites (Fig. 14-2), but morphologically indistinguishable from nonpathogenic *Entamoeba dispar*
  - Antigen detection methods for serum and stool to distinguish *E. histolytica* and *E. dispar* are available
  - Metronidazole is effective therapy
- *Trichinella spiralis*
  - Causes diarrhea, vomiting, abdominal pain, myalgias, fever, periorbital edema
  - Occurs days to weeks after ingestion of raw or undercooked meat (e.g., pork, bear, moose)
  - Can cause heart failure
  - Eosinophilia is usually present
  - Treatment is supportive for mild cases. Mebendazole or albendazole is used in more severe cases. Prednisone is added if inflammation is severe.

TOXINS

- *Staphylococcus aureus* and *Bacillus cereus* are the most common toxin-mediated causes of food-borne disease. Consider botulism if neurologic symptoms are present.
- Ciguatera fish poisoning
  - Illness caused by toxins concentrated in the fish
  - **Causes diarrhea, nausea, and abdominal cramps followed by tooth pain and paresthesias of the lips, tongue, and oropharynx**
  - Can lead to respiratory paralysis and bradycardia

14

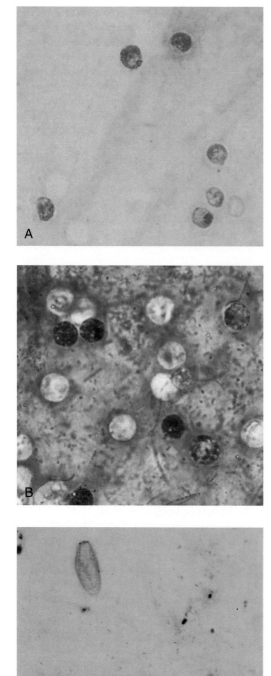

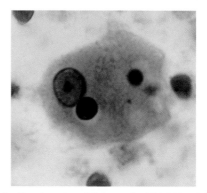

FIGURE 14-2 Trophozoite of *Entamoeba histolytica*. Note the ingested red blood cells. (From Cohen J, Powderly W: *Infectious diseases,* ed 2, St. Louis, Mosby, 2004, figure 242-1.)

- Scombroid fish poisoning
  - Ingestion of histamine present in fish results in abdominal cramps, nausea, and diarrhea and, rarely, bronchospasm
  - Incubation is less than an hour; duration is a few hours
  - Treat with antihistamines in severe cases

Special Circumstances

HIV PATIENTS

- Approximately 50% of HIV patients develop diarrhea
- Many different causes
- Common infections include the following:
  - *Cryptosporidium* (see preceding discussion): **Most common protozoal cause of diarrhea in AIDS patients**
  - Cytomegalovirus (CMV)
    - Most common cause of viral colonic disease in HIV patients
    - Typically seen with CD4 counts below 50/mm^3
    - Presentation is variable and can range from mild diarrhea to an acute abdomen
    - Biopsy is required for diagnosis
    - See characteristic "owl's-eye" nucleus with basophilic intranuclear inclusion surrounded by clear halos (Fig. 14-3)
  - *Mycobacterium avium* complex (MAC)
    - Most infections seen when CD4 counts are less than 100/mm^3
    - Can involve large or small bowel; mucosa can appear normal on colonoscopy
    - Abdominal lymph nodes may be prominent
    - Diagnose by blood culture or tissue biopsy; stool culture is not diagnostic but is predictive of risk of disease over time
    - Can treat with clarithromycin/ethambutol
  - *Isospora belli*
    - Endemic to tropical areas; rare in the United States
    - Spread by fecal-oral route
    - Can cause chronic diarrhea
    - Diagnose by ova and parasite examination or biopsy (see Fig. 14-1C)
    - Can treat with trimethoprim/sulfamethoxazole

FIGURE 14-1 Acid-fast stain of intestinal pathogens. **A,** *Cryptosporidium* spp. 4 to 6mm in diameter. **B,** *Cyclospora* spp. 8 to 10mm in diameter. **C,** Elliptical-shaped *Isospora belli.* (From Cohen J, Powderly W: *Infectious diseases,* ed 2, St. Louis, Mosby, 2004, figure 243-3.)

- Incubation is 1 to 6 hours; source is seafood; primarily seen in Florida and Hawaii
- Duration of illness can be days to months

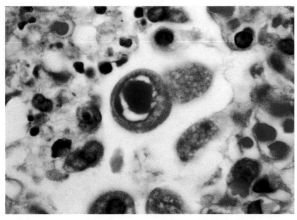

FIGURE 14-3 Cytomegalovirus colitis. Biopsy specimen reveals the typical "owl's-eye" cell. (From Kumar P, Clark M: *Clinical medicine,* ed 6, Philadelphia, WB Saunders, 2005, figure 2.16.)

- Herpes simplex virus usually causes proctitis with anorectal pain and tenesmus
- *Microsporidium*
  - Obligate intracellular pathogen seen on small bowel biopsies
  - Seen almost exclusively in AIDS with CD4 count less than 100/mm³
  - Causes chronic diarrhea and malabsorption
- Giardiasis, strongyloidiasis, and *Cyclospora* also should be considered

TRAVELER'S DIARRHEA

- **Enterotoxigenic *E. coli* most common cause, but causative agent usually not identified**
- Up to 80% of cases are bacterial in origin
- Without treatment lasts 4 to 7 days; with antibiotics lasts 24 to 48 hours
- Patients should be advised to avoid tap water, ice, raw fruits and vegetables, and undercooked meats in underdeveloped countries
- Antibiotics of choice for treatment are quinolones (although increasing resistance is being seen, particularly in southeast Asia with fluoroquinolone-resistant *C. jejuni*)
- Prophylaxis (with sulfa or quinolones) indicated for high-risk patients

Antibiotic-Associated Diarrhea

Basic Information

- **Diarrhea can occur in up to 20% of patients receiving certain antibiotics (e.g., ampicillin, amoxicillin-clavulanate, cefixime, clindamycin)**
- Only 10% to 20% of cases of antibiotic-associated diarrhea are caused by *C. difficile* infection
- *C. difficile* does, however, account for most cases of colitis caused by antibiotics

Clinical Presentation

- ***C. difficile* disease symptoms can range from mild, loose, or watery bowel movements to acute colitis**

with leukocytosis and abdominal pain. Fever occurs in only 10% to 15% of *C. difficile* patients; if present, it is a sign of severe disease.
- Symptoms of *C. difficile* can be delayed up to 4 to 8 weeks after antibiotic exposure

Diagnosis and Evaluation

- Need to rule out *C. difficile* infection in most cases of diarrhea that are not mild and self-limited after antibiotic exposure
- Diagnosis is dependent on detection of *C. difficile* toxins in stool
- Most laboratories use enzyme immunoassays for *C. difficile* that will have a false-negative rate of 10% to 30%. It may be useful to repeat the test if the index of suspicion is high.
- Most cases of *C. difficile* involve either toxin B alone or toxins A and B.

Treatment

- Antibiotic-associated diarrhea not caused by *C. difficile* is self-limited after discontinuation of the antibiotic
- *C. difficile* infection should usually be treated and the inciting antibiotics discontinued if clinically feasible. Mild cases may not need antibiotic therapy.
  - **Oral metronidazole or vancomycin can be used**
    - In severe disease (e.g., fever, low albumin, WBC >15,0000/mm³, thick colon on abdominal CT; older patients are at increased risk), vancomycin is the drug of choice. Vancomycin and metronidazole appear to be therapeutically similar in mild to moderate disease. Metronidazole is less expensive.
  - Avoid antiperistaltic agents
  - Usually treated for 10 to 14 days
- **There is a high relapse rate (20%–25%) after initial treatment for *C. difficile***
  - Initial relapses should be treated with another 10- to 14-day course of metronidazole or vancomycin
  - Method of treatment of patients with more than one relapse is controversial; prolonged, tapered treatment with vancomycin is most often used
- For severe disease: IV metronidazole, vancomycin by nasogastric tube or enema, surgical consult, and consider IV immunoglobulin

SUGGESTED READINGS

De Bruyn G, Hahn S, Borwick A: Antibiotic treatment for travellers' diarrhoea (Cochrane Review), *The Cochrane Library,* Issue 2, Oxford, 2002, Update Software.

Diagnosis and management of foodborne illnesses: a primer for physicians, MMWR 53:1–33, 2004. Available at: www.cdc.gov/mmwr/preview/mmwrhtml/rr5304a1.htm.

Dupont HL: Guidelines on acute infectious diarrhea in adults. The Practice Parameters Committee of the American College of Gastroenterology, Am J Gastroenterol 92:1962–1975, 1997.

Guerrant RL, Van Gilder T, Steiner TS, et al: IDSA practice guidelines for the management of infectious diarrhea, Clin Infect Dis 32:331–351, 2001.

Kelly CP, Lamont JT. *Clostridium difficile*—More difficult than ever, N Engl J Med 359:1932–1940, 2008.

Partnership for Food Safety Web site. Available at: www.fightbac.org.

14

Selected Topics in Infectious Disease I

ARUNA SUBRAMANIAN, MD

Patients seen by internists in both the inpatient and outpatient settings often present with a variety of infections. This chapter attempts to provide an overview of a number of infections, including meningitis, encephalitis, skin and soft tissue infections, infectious arthritis, and osteomyelitis. Additionally, an approach to the patient with fever of unknown origin (FUO) is presented.

Meningitis

Basic Information

- Defined as inflammation of the leptomeninges, the tissues surrounding the brain and spinal cord
- May be caused by bacteria, viruses, fungi, or other noninfectious etiologies

- Specific pathogens of acute bacterial meningitis (Table 15-1)
- Aseptic meningitis is strictly defined as meningeal inflammation with an absence of bacteria on cerebrospinal fluid (CSF) examination and culture
  - Mononuclear pleocytosis and normal glucose level are usually seen
  - Can result from a number of different causes (Table 15-2)
- Some pathogens may cause a subacute to chronic meningitis
  - Cryptococcal meningitis is more commonly seen in immunocompromised hosts, especially in advanced AIDS (see Chapter 12); however, it can cause a very indolent illness in healthy individuals
  - Tuberculous meningitis typically is quite protracted with a CSF profile revealing a mononuclear pleocytosis and elevated protein and lowered glucose concentrations

TABLE 15-1	*Common Etiologic Agents Causing Acute Bacterial Meningitis in Adults*	
Pathogen	**Description**	**Treatment**
Streptococcus pneumoniae	Most common etiologic agent in United States Mortality 19–26% Sometimes associated with other foci of infection (e.g., pneumonia)	Vancomycin + 3rd-generation cephalosporin until antimicrobial susceptibility is known (some experts add rifampin if dexamethasone is given)
Neisseria meningitides	Affects mostly children and young adults Patients with terminal complement deficiency are predisposed Maculopapular rash progresses to petechiae on trunk, extremities, and mucous membranes	3rd-generation cephalosporin Switch to penicillin G or ampicillin once confirmed to be highly sensitive Chemoprophylaxis Rifampin (or ciprofloxacin or ceftriaxone) recommended for household contacts, daycare center members, those directly exposed to oral secretions
Haemophilus influenzae	Mostly occurs in children Disease in adults usually associated with sinusitis, otitis media, pneumonia, sickle cell disease, splenectomy, diabetes, immune deficiency, head trauma with CSF leak, or alcoholism	3rd-generation cephalosporin
Listeria monocytogenes	Disease of neonates, the elderly, and immunocompromised Outbreaks associated with contaminated coleslaw, milk, cheese Associated with hematologic malignancy, steroid use, iron overload	Ampicillin (or penicillin G) ± aminoglycoside
Staphylococcus aureus	Usually seen after head trauma	Nafcillin or oxacillin (if methicillin susceptible) Vancomycin ± rifampin (if methicillin resistant)

CSF, cerebrospinal fluid.

TABLE 15-2	*Causes of Aseptic Meningitis*
Category	**Examples**
Viral	Mumps, echovirus, poliovirus, coxsackievirus, herpes simplex virus
Bacterial	Tuberculosis, syphilis, partially treated bacterial
Miscellaneous infections	Toxoplasmosis, coccidioidomycosis, malaria, Whipple's disease, leptospirosis
Noninfectious diseases	Brain tumors, sarcoidosis, meningeal carcinomatosis
Drugs	Trimethoprim-sulfamethoxazole, ibuprofen, carbamazepine

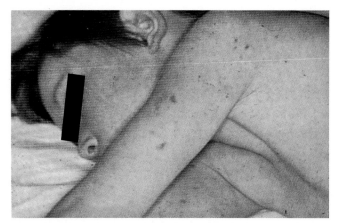

FIGURE 15-1 Typical rash of meningococcal sepsis. Fine erythematous macules and petechiae are present in some areas. (From Cohen J, Powderly W: *Infectious diseases,* ed 2, St. Louis, Mosby, 2004, figure 227.9.)

Clinical Presentation

- Fever, headache, and nuchal rigidity (neck stiffness) are seen in most cases
- Mental status change and seizures can occur
- Diffuse maculopapular rash that becomes petechial is seen with meningococcemia (Fig. 15-1)
- Physical examination may reveal signs of meningeal irritation
  - Kernig's sign—pain in the back is elicited with passive extension of the knee while the hip is flexed
  - Brudzinski's sign—passive flexion of the neck results in spontaneous flexion of the hips and knees

Diagnosis

- Blood cultures should be obtained immediately
- Diagnosis relies on examination of the CSF (Table 15-3)
- **Neuroimaging with CT or MRI is needed only in select** situations before performing a lumbar puncture (Table 15-4)
- If neuroimaging is needed, **empirical antibiotic therapy** (and dexamethasone if indicated) **must be started before scanning**

Treatment

- Bacterial meningitis
  - Empirical therapy
    - Age 1 month to 50 years: Vancomycin plus a third-generation cephalosporin (ceftriaxone or cefotaxime)
    - Older than 50 years: Ampicillin (to cover *Listeria* spp.), plus vancomycin, plus a third-generation cephalosporin
    - Penetrating head trauma, postneurosurgery, or CSF shunt: Vancomycin plus cefepime, ceftazidime, or meropenem
  - Role of adjunctive **dexamethasone**
    - Recommended in adults with suspected or proven pneumococcal meningitis
    - First dose 10 to 20 minutes before, or at least concomitant with, the first dose of antibiotics
    - Dosing: 0.15 mg/kg every 6 hours for 2 to 4 days
  - Organism-specific therapy (see Table 15-1)
- Aseptic meningitis
  - Treatment generally supportive
  - Acyclovir may be useful for herpes virus infections

15

TABLE 15-3	*Typical Cerebrospinal Fluid Abnormalities in Acute Bacterial and Aseptic Meningitis*	
	Bacterial	**Aseptic**
Opening pressure	>20 cm H$_2$O	<25 cm H$_2$O
White blood cells	10–10,000/mm^3	10–1000/mm^3
Differential	Neutrophils predominate	Lymphocytes predominate*
Glucose	<40 mg/dL	>45 mg/dL
Protein	>100 mg/dL	<200 mg/dL
Gram stain	Positive in 60–90% of cases	Negative
Culture	Positive in 70–85% of cases	Negative
Latex agglutination (for antigens of *Streptococcus pneumoniae*, *Neisseria meningitides*, *Escherichia coli*, *Haemophilus influenzae*, and group B streptococcus)	Positive in 50–90% of cases	Negative
PCR of CMV, EBV, viral nucleic acid	Negative	Positive in some cases (i.e., HSV, CMV, EBV, VZV, enteroviruses)

*Neutrophils may predominate in very early viral meningitis.
CMV, cytomegalovirus; EBV, Epstein-Barr virus; HSV, herpes simplex virus; PCR, polymerase chain reaction; VZV, varicella zoster virus.

TABLE 15-4	Indications for Head CT before Lumbar Puncture When Acute Bacterial Meningitis Is Suspected
Category	**Specific Indication**
Immunocompromised host	HIV/AIDS, transplant patient, patient on immunosuppressive medications
History of CNS disease	Mass lesion, stroke, focal infection
New-onset seizure	Onset within 1 wk of presentation
Papilledema	Especially if no venous pulsations
Abnormal level of consciousness	Inability to follow 2 consecutive commands or answer 2 consecutive questions
Focal neurologic deficit	Dilated nonreactive pupil, ocular motility abnormalities, abnormal visual fields, gaze palsy, arm or leg drift

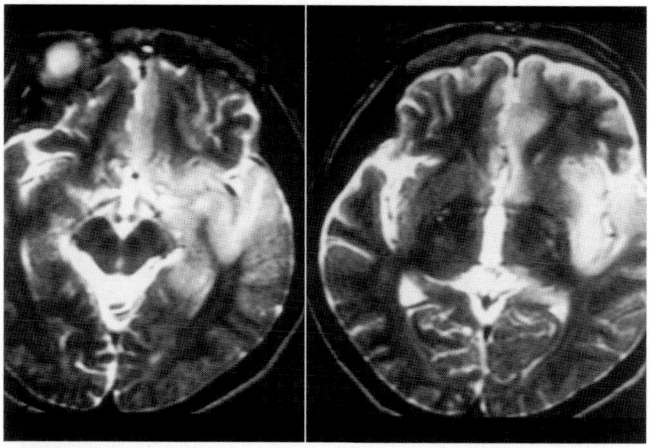

FIGURE 15-2 Herpes simplex encephalitis. T2-weighted MRI showing increased signal in left medial temporal lobe, inferior frontal lobe, and insular cortex. (From Bradley WG, Daroff RB, Fenichel GM, Jankovic J: *Neurology in clinical practice*, ed 4, Burlington, MA, Butterworth-Heinemann, 2004, figure 59B.1.)

Encephalitis

Basic Information

- Inflammation of the brain parenchyma
- Frequently concurrent with meningitis (meningoencephalitis) or inflammation of the spinal cord (encephalomyelitis)
- Can be caused by a number of different viruses (Table 15-5)

Clinical Presentation

- Headache, fever, nuchal rigidity seen as in meningitis
- Alterations in consciousness may clinically help distinguish from meningitis
  - Bizarre behavior, hallucinations, expressive aphasia can be seen with temporal lobe involvement with herpes simplex virus (HSV) infection (Fig. 15-2)
- Focal neurologic signs and seizures can also develop
- West Nile virus may be associated with flaccid weakness and reduced or absent reflexes

Diagnosis

- Basic CSF examination is similar to that seen in viral meningitis with lymphocytic pleocytosis, normal glucose level, and mildly elevated protein level
- CSF polymerase chain reaction (PCR) is useful for the detection of HSV, cytomegalovirus (CMV), Epstein-Barr virus (EBV), varicella zoster virus (VZV), West Nile virus, and enteroviruses
- Serologic testing is useful for detection of arboviruses
- Brain biopsy only needed in patients who have negative CSF PCR and serology

TABLE 15-5	Selected Viruses Causing Encephalitis			
Virus	**Transmission**	**Diagnosis**	**Treatment**	**Comments**
Arboviruses				
California encephalitis (LaCrosse)	Mosquito	Serologic testing	Supportive	Mortality is low
St. Louis encephalitis	Mosquito	Serologic testing	Supportive	Mortality seen in up to 20% of patients
West Nile	Mosquito	PCR and/or IgM in CSF or serum	Supportive; studies of higher-titer IVIG under way	Most infected patients present with febrile illness. Advanced age is greatest risk factor for severe disease
Enteroviruses	Fecal-oral	CSF PCR	Supportive	Usually occurs in summer. Rash, conjunctivitis, pleurodynia may occur
Herpes simplex virus (HSV)	Contact with mucosal surfaces	CSF PCR	Acyclovir	HSV-1 usually causes encephalitis/HSV-2 usually causes meningitis. MRI frequently reveals abnormality in the temporal lobe
Rabies virus	Bite from a rabid animal (dog, cat, bat)	Viral antigen from a nape of neck biopsy	Supportive treatment. Postexposure prophylaxis with antiserum and active immunization is important	Brainstem dysfunction causes diplopia, neuritis, excessive salivation, respiratory paralysis. Consider diagnosis in spelunkers

CSF, cerebrospinal fluid; IgM, immunoglobulin M; IVIG, intravenous immunoglobulin; PCR, polymerase chain reaction.

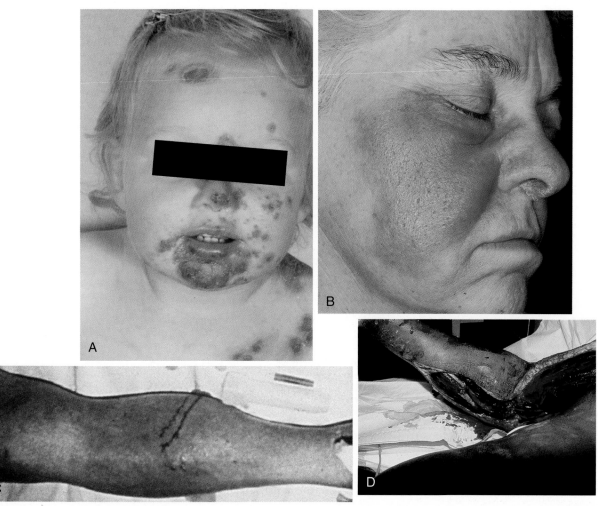

FIGURE 15-3 A, Impetigo. **B,** Erysipelas. **C,** Necrotizing fasciitis. **D,** Extensive gas gangrene of the arm. (A, C, and D, From Cohen J, Powderly W: *Infectious diseases,* ed 2, St. Louis, Mosby, 2004, figures 225.18, 225.20, and 10.19. B, From Habif TP: *Clinical dermatology,* ed 4, St. Louis, Mosby, 2004, figure 9-12.)

Treatment

- Treatment is generally supportive (see Table 15-5)
- HSV encephalitis should be treated with IV acyclovir to lower morbidity and mortality
- Postexposure prophylaxis with antiserum is given for rabies exposure

Skin and Soft Tissue Infections

See Figure 15-3 and Table 15-6 for examples and summary of skin and soft tissue infections.

Basic Information

- Community-associated methicillin-resistant *Staphylococcus aureus* (CA-MRSA)
- Frequency: Varies by location, but incidence of infection is increasing; in Atlanta in 2003, 63% of community-onset skin and soft tissue infections due to *S. aureus* were CA-MRSA

Clinical Presentation

- Most present with skin or soft tissue infection; some develop necrotizing pneumonia, necrotizing fasciitis, endocarditis, osteomyelitis, or sepsis

Treatment

- Treatment options for MRSA
  - Vancomycin is the drug of choice
  - Many CA-MRSA strains may be sensitive to trimethoprim-sulfamethoxazole (TMP-SMX)
  - Clindamycin has been used with success in children; however, resistance can be inducible
  - Newer agents such as linezolid can be considered, if needed
- When to consider empirical treatment: One should base the need for treatment on the local antimicrobial susceptibility patterns in each community. **If the local rates are high, any patient presenting with a serious community-acquired skin or soft tissue infection should be empirically treated for CA-MRSA until a cause is confirmed.**

Acute Bacterial Arthritis

Basic Information

- Usually involves one joint (*monoarticular*)
- Route of infection is usually hematogenous
- Overall, *Neisseria gonorrhoeae* is the most common pathogen in healthy young adults (Fig. 15-4)

| TABLE 15-6 | Skin and Soft Tissue Infections |

	Description	Pathogens	Treatment	Comments
Impetigo (see Fig. 15-3A)	Superficial infection Vesicular with golden crusts	Group A streptococci *Staphylococcus aureus*	Topical and oral antibiotics	Can form bullae
Furuncle (boil)	Deep infection of hair follicle Usually on buttocks, face, neck Painful and tender	*S. aureus*	Moist heat Oral antibiotics Surgical drainage may be needed	Carbuncles are infections of contiguous follicles that extend into subcutaneous fat
Erysipelas (see Fig. 15-3B)	Superficial infection Involves cutaneous lymphatics Usually involves face or extremities Raised, violaceous, painful, spreading lesions with distinct border	Group A streptococci	Oral or IV penicillin	Bullae can develop Systemic toxicity can occur
Cellulitis	Spreading infection of skin and subcutaneous tissue Localized pain, swelling, and warmth No distinct border	Most common: Group A streptococci, *S. aureus* Diabetics: Mixed gram (+) and (−) aerobic/anaerobic bacteria Lymphedema: Groups A, B, C, G streptococci	Mild: Oral PRP or erythromycin Severe: PRP ± AG Diabetic: Broad coverage (e.g., cefoxitin + AG) Lymphedema: IV PRP. Can use oral penicillin to prevent recurrences	Tinea pedis may be a portal of entry in some patients Bullae may be present. In patients with cirrhosis and saltwater exposure, consider *Vibrio vulnificus*
Necrotizing fasciitis (see Fig. 15-3C)	Severe infection of the subcutaneous soft issues Erythema and swelling progress rapidly to bullae and cutaneous gangrene Predilection for lower extremities, abdominal wall, and perineum (Fournier's gangrene)	Type I: Polymicrobial (anaerobes + streptococci + Enterobacteriaceae) Type II: Group A streptococci Recent cases now also associated with aggressive community-acquired MRSA	Surgical exploration and broad-spectrum antibiotics May need to include vancomycin if considering community-acquired MRSA	Risk factors include diabetes, peripheral vascular disease, surgery, trauma Systemic toxicity develops rapidly High mortality rate if surgical exploration not immediate
Gas gangrene (anaerobic cellulites; see Fig. 15-3D)	Begins as a localized infection in a superficial wound Rapidly spreads across fascial planes causing severe pain and swelling Crepitance may be palpable	*Clostridium perfringens* Other anaerobes	Surgical exploration Penicillin + clindamycin	Progresses from cellulitis to myositis to myonecrosis rapidly High mortality rate
Staphylococcal toxic shock syndrome	Fever, sunburn rash, hypotension progressing to multiorgan failure Desquamation occurs late	Associated with colonization of wound/vagina with toxin-producing *S. aureus* without invasive disease	IV fluid resuscitation Removal/drainage of the colonizing source Antibiotics: PRP or 1st-generation cephalosporins	Most commonly seen in the setting of menstruation Bacteremia or overt infection with *S. aureus* not usually seen
Streptococcal toxic shock syndrome	Fever and hypotension progressing to multiorgan failure Rash and desquamation usually not present	Usually associated with skin/soft tissue infection with toxin-producing group A streptococci	IV fluids Penicillin + clindamycin	Most patients are bacteremic

AG, aminoglycoside; MRSA, methicillin-resistant *S. aureus;* PRP, penicillinase-resistant penicillin.

- *S. aureus*, groups A, B, C, and G streptococci, *Streptococcus pneumoniae*, and gram-negative bacilli account for most other infections
- Specific organisms should be suspected based on the underlying host (Table 15-7)

Clinical Presentation

- Pain, decreased range of motion, effusion, and erythema are typically seen
- Fever not always present
- Knee or hip most commonly affected

Diagnosis

- Aspiration of synovial fluid is essential to proper diagnosis
  - Ultrasonography, CT scan, or MRI may be helpful for detection and aspiration with involvement of certain joints (e.g., hip, sacroiliac joint)
  - **WBC counts are usually greater than 50,000/mm³ with greater than 75% neutrophils**
  - The presence of crystals does not rule out infection because crystal-induced arthritis and septic arthritis can occasionally occur together
  - Gram stain is positive in one third of cases

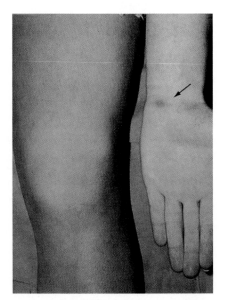

FIGURE 15-4 Gonococcal septic arthritis with an associated papular skin lesion (*arrow*). (From Forbes C, Jackson W: *Color atlas and text of clinical medicine,* ed 3, St. Louis, Mosby, 2003, figure 3.8.)

TABLE 15-7	Organisms Causing Acute Bacterial Arthritis
Organism	**Predisposing Factors and Conditions**
Neisseria gonorrhoeae	Age < 30 yr
Staphylococcus aureus	Glucocorticoid therapy Rheumatoid arthritis Diabetes Postsurgical procedure
Streptococcus pneumoniae	HIV Alcoholism Sickle cell anemia Less than half have another focus of *S. pneumoniae* infection
Mycoplasma spp.	Primary immunoglobulin deficiency
Salmonella spp.	HIV Sickle cell disease
Pasteurella multocida	Cat bites or scratches
Other gram-negative bacilli	IV drug use Immunodeficiency Neonates Elderly

- **Joint fluid cultures are positive in up to 90% of nongonococcal bacterial arthritis, but in less than 50% of gonococcal (GC) arthritis**
  - Often need genital or pharyngeal culture to confirm GC
- Blood cultures are positive in up to 60% of cases of *S. aureus* but are less helpful with other pathogens

Treatment

- Empirical antimicrobial therapy after blood cultures and joint aspiration depends on Gram stain and patient's age and sexual activity
  - If GC arthritis is suspected, ceftriaxone should be started
  - If *S. aureus* is suspected, a penicillinase-resistant penicillin (e.g., oxacillin) should be used; if hospital

BOX 15-1 *Prosthetic Joint Infection*

Early infection: Acquired at surgery, usually low-grade pathogens (e.g., coagulase-negative staphylococci, diphtheroids)

Late infection: Usually hematogenous seeding with *Staphylococcus aureus* or streptococci

Wide spectrum of severity but usually have chronic, unremitting pain and may have loosening of the joint

Definitive diagnosis made by culture of needle aspirate or surgical debridement

Most successful therapy is removal of entire prosthesis and 6 weeks of antibiotic therapy

---

acquired, consider vancomycin until sensitivity is known
  - If Gram stain is negative, a third-generation cephalosporin (e.g., ceftriaxone) is reasonable initial coverage
- Repeated aspirations may be necessary if effusions reaccumulate
- Indications for surgical drainage
  - Hip joint involvement (except in cases of GC)
  - Delay of therapy (>1 week after onset of symptoms)
  - Loculated infection or exudate too thick to aspirate
  - Poor response to therapy (e.g., failure to decrease synovial WBC)
  - Prosthetic joint infection (Box 15-1)

Chronic Monoarticular Arthritis

Basic Information

- Frequently caused by bacteria (and mycobacteria), fungi, and, rarely, parasites (Table 15-8)
- If joint culture is negative, synovial biopsy is necessary
- Treatment guided toward specific organism

Viral Arthritis

Basic Information

- Caused by direct invasion of the synovium or by an immune reaction involving certain joints
- Usually a migratory polyarthritis
- Many viruses implicated
  - Rubella
    - Can occur following infection or immunization
    - Usually seen in women
    - Self-limited disease but, rarely, can persist for years
  - Mumps
    - More common in men
    - Develops within 2 weeks of parotitis
  - Parvovirus B19
    - Hands most frequently involved
    - Infection in adults can occur without fever or rash
    - Self-limited: Usually resolves within 8 to 10 weeks
  - Hepatitis B
    - Can manifest as arthralgias or symmetrical arthritis
    - Symptoms (arthralgias or arthritis) occur before jaundice and resolve when jaundice develops
- Most are self-limited: No specific treatment for the arthritis is available

15

TABLE 15-8	Selected Pathogens Causing Chronic Monoarticular Arthritis
Borrelia burgdorferi (Lyme disease)	50% of untreated patients develop monoarthritis or oligoarthritis of large joint(s) Serology is positive in almost all patients with arthritis See Chapter 15 for further information
Mycobacterium tuberculosis	Usually involves large joints (hips, knees, or ankles) Swelling and pain worsen over months to year; systemic sign and symptoms are frequently absent; synovial fluid examination reveals about 50% neutrophils; acid-fast stain is positive in less than half of cases; culture is frequently positive; synovial biopsy culture has higher yield Treat 6–9 mo with multiple agents (see Chapter 13)
Atypical mycobacteria	Usually involves smaller joints (wrists, hands) Infection occurs from inoculation from water or soil, so may see as a result of gardening or water-related activities Synovial biopsy necessary to make the diagnosis
Brucella spp.	Can cause acute or chronic monoarthritis or asymmetrical polyarthritis Febrile illness frequently coexists Transmission is through ingestion of unpasteurized milk or cheese, ingestion of raw meat, or inhalation during contact with animals (e.g., slaughterhouse workers) Treat with doxycycline + aminoglycoside
Sporothrix schenckii	Seen in gardeners or those who work with soil
Candida spp.	Results from surgical procedures or articular injections IV drug users may have involvement of spine or sacroiliac joint Treat with drainage and antifungal therapy

Osteomyelitis

Basic Information

- Defined as an infection of bone
- Two basic types based on the route of infection
  - Hematogenous source
    - Caused by seeding of the bone during bacteremia
    - Primarily occurs in children and older adults
    - IV drug users
      - May have involvement of the vertebrae, sternoclavicular, sacroiliac, or symphysis pubis
      - S. aureus, Pseudomonas, Serratia, or Eikenella are the more common pathogens for this group
    - S. aureus is the organism most frequently isolated
    - Patients with sickle cell disease may be infected with S. aureus or Salmonella
    - Vertebral involvement caused by S. aureus, gram-negative bacilli, tuberculosis (TB; Pott's disease), or Candida

- Contiguous source
  - Accounts for most cases of osteomyelitis
  - Includes infections resulting from extension from adjacent soft tissue, injury, or surgery
  - Presentation is more indolent than with hematogenous spread
  - Diabetic foot ulcers and decubitus ulcers are common sources
  - **Most infections are polymicrobial,** although S. aureus is still frequently found
  - *Pseudomonas aeruginosa* **should be considered in the setting of a puncture wound of the foot**

Clinical Presentation

- Fever
- Bone pain over the affected site

Diagnosis

- Blood studies
  - Sedimentation rate and C-reactive protein elevated in most cases
  - Blood cultures more likely to be positive in cases of hematogenous spread
- Radiologic studies
  - Plain radiographs
    - May show periosteal elevation, soft tissue swelling, or lytic changes (Fig. 15-5)
    - Findings not present during early infection
  - Technetium bone scan
    - Detects early lesions with high sensitivity
    - Best when bone was previously normal (false positives common with previously abnormal bone)
    - Cannot distinguish infection from tumor, fracture, or infarction
  - MRI
    - As sensitive as bone scan for acute osteomyelitis
    - **Test of choice for vertebral osteomyelitis** because it better defines the surrounding soft tissue
  - Subperiosteal aspirate or bone biopsy cultures are needed to make a definitive diagnosis if blood cultures are negative
  - **Swab cultures of sinus tract or ulcer base are unreliable** for making a microbiologic diagnosis

Treatment

- Early diagnosis and treatment are important to prevent bone necrosis
- Therapy for acute osteomyelitis usually consists of 6 weeks of IV antibiotics directed by the culture results
- Chronic osteomyelitis often requires therapy for more than 3 months (until erythrocyte sedimentation rate [ESR] normalizes)
- In patients with polymicrobial (aerobic and anaerobic) infections, amoxicillin-clavulanate or clindamycin plus ciprofloxacin can be used
- Surgery may be needed to remove devitalized bone or to restore vascular supply (if there is vascular insufficiency)

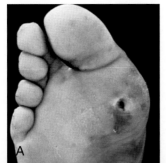

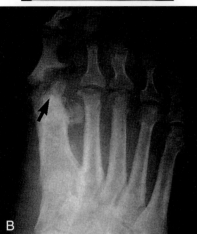

FIGURE 15-5 Diabetic abscess. **A,** Note discoloration proximal to abscess beneath first metatarsal head. **B,** Results of osteomyelitis of the first metatarsal with boney erosion (*arrow*) seen on radiograph. (A, From Canale ST: *Campbell's operative orthopaedics,* ed 10, St. Louis, Mosby, 2003, figure 82-11A. B, From Forbes C, Jackson W: *Color atlas and text of clinical medicine,* ed 3, St. Louis, Mosby, 2003, figure 3.152.)

TABLE 15-9	Classification of Fever of Unknown Origin (FUO)	
Category	**Definition**	**Common Underlying Causes**
Classic FUO	Fever ≥ 38.3°C for ≥3 wk Blood cultures negative Lack of diagnosis with 3 outpatient visits or 3 inpatient days	Infection Cancer Collagen vascular diseases Granulomatous disease
Nosocomial FUO	Hospitalized patient with no fever on admission 3 days of investigation 2 days of negative incubating cultures	*Clostridium difficile* Phlebitis Sinusitis Drug fever
Neutropenic FUO	Absolute neutrophil count < 500/μL 3 days of investigation 2 days of negative incubating cultures	Perianal infection *Aspergillus* spp. *Candida* spp.
HIV-associated FUO	HIV-positive patient Fever ≥ 3 wk in outpatients or >3 days for inpatients 3 days of investigation 2 days of negative incubating cultures	Mycobacteria Lymphoma Drug fever Cytomegalovirus *Pneumocystis jiroveci* (previously *P. carinii*) pneumonia

Fever of Unknown Origin

Basic Information
- Classified by a patient's condition and setting in which the fever manifests (Table 15-9)
- Most cases are caused by infections, noninfectious inflammatory diseases, or neoplasms
- Specific etiologies of classic FUO may be suggested by the patient's history (Table 15-10)

Diagnosis
- A thorough history, including travel, hobbies, history of TB exposure, HIV risk factors, and medications, should be obtained to guide the evaluation
- Repeated physical examinations may be necessary to detect slowly progressing diseases
- Basic testing should include the following:
  - CBC
  - Comprehensive metabolic panel
  - Urinalysis
  - ESR and C-reactive protein
  - Blood cultures (>3 sets)
  - Chest radiograph
- Purified protein derivative should be placed and HIV testing considered

TABLE 15-10	Etiologic Considerations for Classic Fever of Unknown Origin
History	**Disease**
Foreign-born individuals	Extrapulmonary tuberculosis
Age > 50 yr	Malignancy Giant cell arteritis
High fevers with arthralgias/ arthritis	Still's disease
Medical background with undocumented fevers	Factitious fever

- CT scan of abdomen plus sinuses may be helpful in the absence of other localizing signs
- Further evaluation should be based on any findings from the history, physical, and basic laboratory tests
- Administration of naproxen may help distinguish between neoplasia and infection because the fever from neoplasms is thought to be more responsive to the medication
- Try to avoid empirical antibiotics because they may suppress, but not cure, an occult infection and may interfere with the ability to make a diagnosis

15

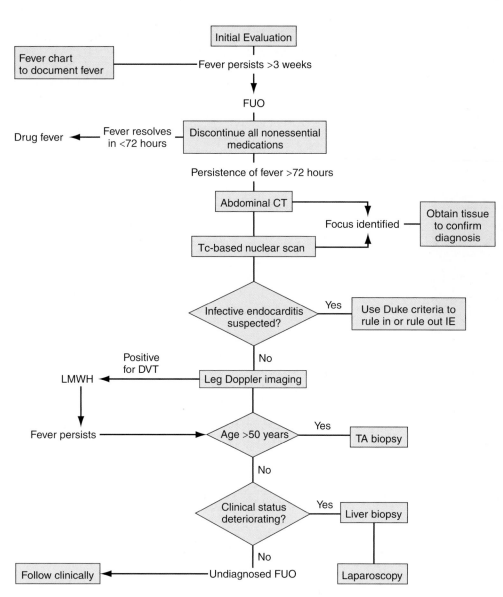

FIGURE 15-6 Diagnostic approach to fever of unknown origin (FUO). DVT, deep vein thrombosis; IE, infective endocarditis; LMWH, low-molecular-weight heparin; TA, temporal artery. (From Mourad O, Palda V, Detsky AS: A comprehensive evidence-based approach to fever of unknown origin. *Arch Intern Med 163:549, 2003, figure 2.*)

- Drug-induced fever should be considered a diagnosis of exclusion; it is confirmed by stopping the potentially offending agent
  - Usually patients do not appear as toxic as with other causes of FUO
  - **Rash and eosinophilia are sometimes present, but their absence does not rule out drug fever**
  - Some common causes are sulfonamides, β-lactam antibiotics, phenytoin, amiodarone, and nitrofurantoin
- Figure 15-6 shows an algorithm for diagnostic approach to FUO
- The cause of the FUO may not be found in approximately 30% of adults, but most of those without a diagnosis still have a good prognosis

REVIEW QUESTIONS

For review questions, please go to www.expertconsult.com.

SUGGESTED READINGS

Anaya DA, Dellinger EP: Necrotizing soft-tissue infection: diagnosis and management, *Clin Infect Dis* 44:705–710, 2007.

Cunha BA: Fever of unknown origin, *Infect Dis Clin North Am* 21:867– 915, 2007.

Durack DT, Street AC: Fever of unknown origin reexamined and redefined, *Curr Clin Top Infect Dis* 11:35–51, 1991.

Lew DP, Waldvogel FA: Osteomyelitis, *Lancet* 364:369–379, 2004, 336:999–1007, 1997.

Mandell GL, Bennett JE, Dolin R, editors: *Principles and practice of infectious diseases*, ed 6, Philadelphia, 2005, Churchill Livingstone.

Smith JW, Chalupa P, Shabaz Hasan M: Infectious arthritis: clinical features, laboratory findings and treatment, *Clin Microbiol Infect* 12:309–314, 2006.

Tunkel AR, Hartman BJ, Kaplan SL, et al: Practice guidelines for the management of bacterial meningitis, *Clin Infect Dis* 39:1267–1284, 2004.

CHAPTER 16

Selected Topics in Infectious Disease II

JOHN N. AUCOTT, MD

This chapter is divided into three sections on selected topics in infectious disease encountered by the internist: (1) endocarditis, (2) tick-borne illnesses, and (3) infections from bite and scratch wounds.

Infective Endocarditis

Basic Information

- Infective endocarditis **may present as an acute infection with devastating consequences or with a slowly progressive course and subtle clinical findings.** The diagnosis may be straightforward or may require a combination of laboratory and clinical findings. Prolonged antibiotic treatment is required, with monitoring for progression despite therapy.
  - Endocarditis most commonly refers to **infection of one of the heart valves**, but it may also occur on an atrial or ventricular septal defect or elsewhere in the endocardium
  - Bacterial and fungal organisms may cause endocarditis
  - There are noninfectious inflammatory conditions of the endocardium and valves (e.g., Libman-Sacks endocarditis associated with systemic lupus erythematosus [SLE])
  - **In subacute bacterial endocarditis, the mitral valve is the most common valve infected, followed by the aortic valve.** Much less common is tricuspid valve involvement. Infection of the pulmonic valve is rare.
    - **In acute bacterial endocarditis (usually caused by *Staphylococcus aureus*), infection of the aortic valve is most common (Fig. 16-1)**
- Acute versus subacute endocarditis
  - Classically, acute endocarditis was caused by *S. aureus* and progressed to death if not treated in 6 weeks
  - Subacute endocarditis was most commonly caused by other organisms such as the viridans group of streptococci and even if not treated could persist for up to 1 year before death
  - However, the increasing prevalence of prosthetic heart valves, along with the evolving infectious etiologies of endocarditis, have made this distinction less clinically useful

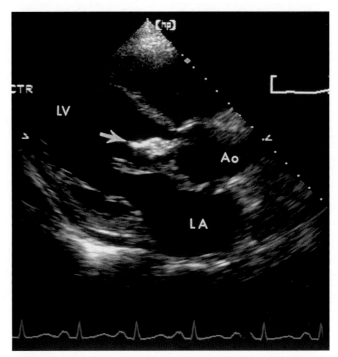

FIGURE 16-1 Infective endocarditis. Parasternal long-axis–view echocardiogram of a patient with a large aortic valve vegetation *(arrow)*. Ao, aorta; LA, left atrium; LV, left ventricle. (From Zipes DP: *Braunwald's heart disease: a textbook of cardiovascular medicine*, ed 7, Philadelphia, WB Saunders, 2005, figure 11-81.)

  - Etiologic agent, rather than acute versus subacute endocarditis, is now used to classify endocarditis because the **etiologic agent determines treatment**
- Predisposing factors
  - **Abnormal native heart valve** is the most common predisposing factor
    - Mitral valve prolapse among most common (20–30% of cases), with murmur or thickened valve associated with highest risk
    - Rheumatic heart disease less common
    - Bicuspid aortic valves usually seen as predisposing factor for endocarditis in patients older than 60 years
  - **Prosthetic valves**
  - **Congenital heart disease, including atrial and ventricular septal defects and patent ductus arteriosus**
  - **Prior endocarditis**

Clinical Presentation

- Signs and symptoms
  - **Cardiac involvement: New regurgitant murmur, vegetations on echocardiography (absence of a visible vegetation does not exclude diagnosis), conduction abnormalities (especially with endocarditis of aortic valve), myocarditis, congestive heart failure**
  - Right-sided endocarditis: Cough, chest pain, pleurisy, cavitating pulmonary infiltrates
  - Systemic inflammation: Fever, fatigue or failure to thrive, arthralgias; positive rheumatoid factor is seen in 50% of cases
  - Emboli: Seen in approximately one third of patients and may involve any organ; if CNS is involved, middle cerebral artery is most commonly affected; large emboli are more common in fungal endocarditis
  - **Mycotic aneurysms may be seen, usually in the cerebral arteries and aorta, but may also involve other major arteries**
  - Immune complex disease: Glomerulonephritis, Osler nodes (tender nodules on finger or toe pads), Janeway lesions (nodular hemorrhages on palms of hands or soles of feet), splinter hemorrhages (especially in proximal nail beds; Fig. 16-2)
  - Other: Roth spots (retinal hemorrhages; Fig. 16-3), petechiae, splenomegaly, digital clubbing
- Etiologic agents (Table 16-1)
  - Typical endocarditis organisms: **Streptococci and staphylococci account for 80% to 90% of endocarditis**
    - Streptococci cause 60% to 80% of cases, with **viridans streptococci the most common cause**
      - Pyogenic strep: Groups A, C rarely cause endocarditis
      - **Streptococcus bovis:** Associated with **GI neoplasms;** should prompt evaluation of the colon for malignancy

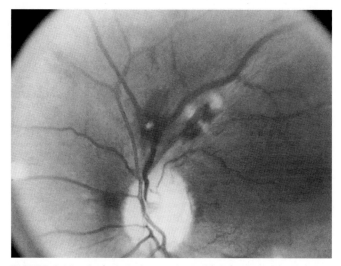

FIGURE 16-3   Roth spots in a patient with infective endocarditis. (From Zipes DP: *Braunwald's heart disease: a textbook of cardiovascular medicine*, ed 7, Philadelphia, WB Saunders, 2005, figure 58-5.)

- *Streptococcus mutans:* An oral pathogen; may cause endocarditis in the susceptible host with poor dentition
- Staphylococci cause 20% to 30% of cases, with **S. aureus the most common cause**
  - *S. aureus* infection, which **may attack normal heart valves**, results in rapid progression with valve destruction and is the most common cause of what is classically termed *acute endocarditis*
- Enterococci are an increasingly prevalent cause of endocarditis and are **common in older men following genitourinary instrumentation or in women following obstetric procedures**
- *Pseudomonas:* Typically in those with history of IV drug use; usually right-sided
- Culture-negative endocarditis: May present with endocardial vegetation or embolic events; blood culture should be held for 3 weeks if suspected
  - HACEK (*Haemophilus aphrophilus, Actinobacillus actinomycetemcomitans, Cardiobacterium hominis, Eikenella corrodens,* and *Kingella kingae*) group accounts for 3% to 5% of native valve infections (see Table 16-1)
- Unusual endocarditis organisms
  - *Coxiella burnetii* (Q fever): Diagnosed by serology; culture often negative
  - Fungi: *Candida* spp. most common, followed by *Aspergillus* spp.; susceptible hosts include those with history of injection drug use, prosthetic heart valve recipients, immunocompromised hosts
  - *Bartonella, Chlamydia, Legionella, Brucella, Mycoplasma* spp. are rare causes of endocarditis
- Prosthetic valves
  - **Early prosthetic valve endocarditis is infection of a prosthetic valve within 60 days of valve insertion**
    - **Late prosthetic valve endocarditis occurs after 60 days of valve insertion**
  - Early infection makes up one third of prosthetic valve infections, whereas **late infection makes up most** cases of prosthetic valve endocarditis

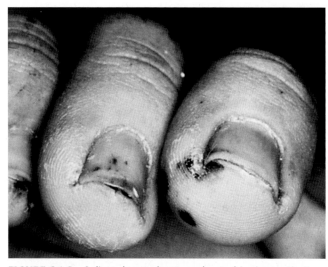

FIGURE 16-2   Splinter hemorrhages and petechiae in a patient with infective endocarditis. (From Zipes DP: *Braunwald's heart disease: a textbook of cardiovascular medicine*, ed 7, Philadelphia, WB Saunders, 2005, figure 58-4.)

TABLE 16-1	*Causes of Bacterial Endocarditis*	
Endocarditis Subtype	**Most Common Organism**	**Other Common Organisms**
"Typical"	Viridans streptococci Many species highly associated such as *Streptococcus mutans*	*Staphylococcus aureus* Other streptococcal species *Staphylococcus epidermidis* (uncommon) Enterococci (uncommon)
Culture-negative	No dominant organism	*Haemophilus aphrophilus* *Haemophilus parainfluenzae* *Actinobacillus actinomycetemcomitans* *Cardiobacterium hominis* *Eikenella corrodens* *Kingella kingii*
Injection drug use	*S. aureus*	*Pseudomonas aeruginosa* Candida Enterococci *Streptococcus viridans* *S. epidermidis* Polymicrobial
Unusual causes	No dominant organism	Fungi: *Candida, Aspergillus* *Coxiella burnetii* *Bartonella* *Chlamydia* *Legionella* *Brucella* *Mycoplasma*
Early prosthetic valve	*S. epidermidis*	*S. aureus* Gram-negative bacilli Enterococci Diphtheroids Fungi
Late prosthetic valve	*S. epidermidis*	*S. viridans* *S. aureus* Gram-negative bacilli Enterococci

16

- Whereas *Streptococcus viridans* is the most common cause of native valve endocarditis, **Staphylococcus epidermidis is the most common cause of prosthetic valve endocarditis**
- *S. viridans* is a rare cause of early prosthetic valve endocarditis but is a relatively common cause of late prosthetic valve endocarditis

Diagnosis and Evaluation

- Diagnosing endocarditis requires a high index of suspicion in the appropriate clinical setting, coupled with demonstration of microbial infection of the heart valves or endocardium
- Definite bacterial endocarditis is a pathologic diagnosis made by culture of a surgical specimen or at autopsy
  - Clinical criteria can be used to diagnose cases of definite endocarditis (Table 16-2), typically requiring **demonstration of persistent bacteremia by blood culture**, along with echocardiographic and clinical findings
    - Blood cultures: Standard initial drawing should be three separate sets of cultures drawn from three different sites over 1 hour
    - Echocardiography
      - Transthoracic echocardiography (TTE): First step with native valves; sensitivity is 44% to 63%
      - Transesophageal echocardiography (TEE): Reserve for prosthetic valves or (−) TTE with abnormal valve (+) intermediate to high probability
- Possible endocarditis, in which diagnostic criteria are not met, should be treated as endocarditis until an alternate diagnosis is confirmed

Treatment

- Treatment principles in endocarditis
  - Parenteral antibiotics preferred to ensure consistent antibiotic levels
  - Extended therapy indicated because shorter courses associated with increased risk of relapse
  - Bactericidal antibiotics are superior to bacteriostatic antibiotics in achieving cure
  - **Antimicrobial choice should be guided by culture and sensitivity results (Table 16-3)**
- Surgical considerations
  - Failure of medical therapy
    - May be manifested by prolonged fever (often indicative of aortic valve ring abscess, which may be accompanied by evidence of atrioventricular conduction abnormalities)
    - New embolic events
    - Mycotic aneurysms
    - Persistent positive blood cultures may also be evidence of failure of medical therapy

TABLE 16-2	*Diagnostic Criteria for Endocarditis*

Major Criteria	Minor Criteria

Positive blood culture
  Typical microorganism of endocarditis from two separate
    blood cultures
  Persistently positive blood cultures with a microorganism
    consistent with endocarditis, defined as blood cultures
    drawn more than 12 hr apart, or 3 of 3 positive sets of blood
    cultures drawn over the course of at least 1 hr
Evidence of endocardial involvement
  Positive echocardiogram, demonstrating oscillating
    intracardiac mass or abscess, or dehiscent prosthetic valve
New valvular regurgitation (excludes worsening of
  preexisting murmur)
	Fever 38°C or higher
	Predisposing heart condition or injection drug use
	Vascular phenomena
	  Arterial emboli
	  Septic pulmonary infarcts
	  Mycotic aneurysm
	  Intracranial hemorrhage
	  Conjunctival hemorrhage
	  Janeway lesions
	Immunologic phenomena
	  Glomerulonephritis
	  Osler nodes
	  Roth spots
	  Rheumatoid factor
	Microbiologic evidence
	  Positive blood cultures that do not meet major criteria
	Echocardiographic evidence
	  Consistent with endocarditis but not meeting major criteria

Endocarditis is diagnosed with two major criteria, one major plus three minor criteria, or five minor criteria.
Adapted from Durack DT, Lukes AS, Bright DK: New criteria for diagnosis of infective endocarditis: utilization of specific echocardiographic findings.
  Am J Med 96:200–209, 1994.

TABLE 16-3	*Synopsis of Treatment of Bacterial Endocarditis*

Organism	Standard Treatment	Comments

Streptococcus viridans, with penicillin
  MIC < 0.1
	4 wk daily penicillin or ceftriaxone	2 wk penicillin or ceftriaxone, combined
		  with gentamicin reasonable
		  alternative

S. viridans, penicillin MIC > 0.1	4 wk daily penicillin or ceftriaxone, combined with aminoglycoside for first 2 wk	

Staphylococcus aureus left-sided	4 wk daily nafcillin combined with gentamicin for
	  initial 3–5 days
		MRSA treated with 4–6 wk daily
		  vancomycin

S. aureus, right-sided	2 wk daily nafcillin combined with gentamicin	Treatment applies only to methicillin-
		  sensitive staphylococci, with no
		  embolic events

Prosthetic valve	6 wk therapy with penicillin derivative or
	  vancomycin (depending on sensitivities)
	  in combination with rifampin, plus
	  aminoglycoside for initial 2 wk
		Early surgical consultation advised
		Fungal infection of prosthetic valve
		  requires surgery in most cases

Enterococcus	6 wk daily penicillin combined with gentamicin	If aminoglycoside resistance
		  demonstrated, 8–12 wk daily
		  penicillin indicated
		Other antimicrobial resistance common
		  and should prompt consultation with
		  infectious disease team

Fungal	Early surgery usually required	

MIC, minimal infective concentration; MRSA, methicillin-resistant *Staphylococcus aureus*.

- Other indications for surgery
  - Major embolic events
  - Valvular dysfunction
  - Congestive heart failure
  - Fungal endocarditis

Prevention of Endocarditis

- Endocarditis prophylaxis
  - Endocarditis prophylaxis recommendations were recently revised because the risk of endocarditis from

dental procedures is thought to be less than previous estimates
- Prophylaxis should be done in patients with high-risk cardiac conditions, defined as:
  - Prosthetic cardiac valve or prosthetic material used for cardiac valve repair
  - Previous infective endocarditis
  - Congenital heart disease (CHD), specifically:
    - Unrepaired cyanotic CHD, including palliative shunts and conduits

TABLE 16-4	*Comparison of Tick-Borne Illnesses*			
Illness	**Etiologic Agent**	**Vector**	**Reservoir**	**Geographic Distribution**
Rocky Mountain spotted fever	*Rickettsia rickettsii*	Eastern United States: Dog tick (*Dermacentor variabilis*) Western United States: Rocky Mountain wood tick (*Dermacentor andersoni*)	Vector tick is also reservoir	South-central and mid-Atlantic states (uncommon in western United States and Rocky Mountains)
Human monocytic ehrlichiosis	*Ehrlichia chaffeensis*	Lone-star tick (*Amblyomma americanum*)	Deer	Midwest; south-central and southeastern United States
Human granulocytic anaplasmosis	*Anaplasma phagocytophilum*	Deer tick (*Ixodes scapularis*)	Unknown	Scattered east and west coast states; northern states; Florida
Babesiosis	United States: *Babesia microti* Europe: *Babesia divergens, Babesia bovis*	Ticks (*I. scapularis*)	Rodents (especially white-footed mouse); cattle	Northeast coastal states
Lyme disease	*Borrelia burgdorferi*	Deer tick (*I. scapularis*)	Mouse	Northeast; Wisconsin and Minnesota; Pacific Northwest

- Completely repaired congenital heart defect with prosthetic material or device, whether placed by surgery or by catheter intervention, during the first 6 months after the procedure
  - Repaired CHD with residual defects at the site or adjacent to the site of a prosthetic patch or prosthetic device
- Cardiac transplantation recipients who develop cardiac valvulopathy
- Dental or respiratory procedure (prophylaxis not recommended for bronchoscopy): Single-dose amoxicillin (2 g) 1 hour before procedure (clindamycin, clarithromycin, or azithromycin if penicillin allergic)
- Bowel or genitourinary procedures: Ampicillin (vancomycin if penicillin allergic) plus gentamicin 1 hour before procedure, ampicillin 6 hours later
- Low-risk patients for whom antibiotic prophylaxis is not recommended
  - Mitral valve prolapse without regurgitation or thickening
  - Pacemakers
  - Defibrillators
- Low-risk procedures for which antibiotic prophylaxis is not recommended
  - GI endoscopy (except sclerosis or dilatation/endoscopic retrograde cholangiopancreatography [ERCP])
  - Restorative dentistry
  - Gynecologic procedures: Vaginal hysterectomy, vaginal delivery, cesarean section
  - Cardiac procedures: Cardiac catheterization, balloon angioplasty

Tick-Borne Illnesses

Basic Information

- Tick-borne illnesses are best understood by understanding not only their clinical manifestations but also their vectors, reservoirs, geographic distribution, and seasonal variations (Table 16-4)
- Most people with tick-borne infections do not remember a recent tick bite, and most tick bites do not result in a tick-borne infection
- **In most cases, early manifestations of tick-borne disease are nonspecific flulike symptoms of fever, fatigue, generalized achiness with or without a rash**
- Lyme disease may present with later symptoms of arthritis or neurologic manifestions of seventh nerve palsy, symptoms of CNS infection, or peripheral neuropathy

Clinical Presentation

Table 16-5 compares the clinical features of tick-borne illnesses

- Rocky Mountain spotted fever (RMSF)
  - After incubation period of 2 to 14 days, flulike symptoms of fever, myalgias, and GI upset develop
  - Characteristic rash develops 3 to 5 days after onset of fever (Fig. 16-4)
  - **Disease may be fatal, especially if not diagnosed and treated early in illness (case fatality rate approaches 20%)**
- Ehrlichiosis and anaplasmosis (human monocytic ehrlichiosis [HME] and human granulocytic anaplasmosis [HGA])
  - After an incubation period of 1 week, flulike symptoms of high fever (>103°F), headache, myalgias, and malaise develop; often accompanied by thrombocytopenia and mild elevation of aspartate aminotransferase (AST) and alanine aminotransferase (ALT)
  - Presenting symptoms may be mild; **rash is uncommon,** and **its absence helps distinguish these disorders from RMSF and Lyme disease**
  - **HGA may occur as coinfection with Lyme disease**
  - Severe illness, with renal failure and respiratory insufficiency, is uncommon but well described
  - Most have mild illness; case fatality rate is 2%

16

TABLE 16-5	*Comparison of Clinical Features of Tick-Borne Illnesses*		
	Rash	**Laboratory**	**Diagnostic Test of Choice**
Rocky Mountain spotted fever	Begins distally (palms or soles) Spreads to involve arms, legs, then trunk Begins as maculopapular eruption, evolving to petechial or purpuric appearance Seen in 90%	Laboratory findings nonspecific WBC typically normal Renal insufficiency and acute tubular necrosis common CSF may show elevated protein if neurologic involvement	Early clinical diagnosis required to prevent death; occasionally rickettsiae may be demonstrated in biopsy of rash; diagnosis may be confirmed by acute and convalescent serology
Human monocytic ehrlichiosis (HME)	Rash seen in 1/3 Maculopapular eruption; rarely petechial	Leukopenia and thrombocytopenia neutropenia common Transaminitis and renal insufficiency common	Clinical diagnosis but fourfold increase in antibody titer to *Ehrlichia chaffeensis*; monocytic inclusions may be seen
Hemolytic granulocytic anaplasmosis (HGA)	Same as HME	Same as HME	Clinical diagnosis, but fourfold increase in antibody titer to *Anaplasma phacocytophilum* granulocytic inclusions may be seen. PCR available for acute diagnosis
Babesiosis	Rash from babesiosis unusual, but coinfection with Lyme disease is common and should be investigated in all patients with babesiosis	Hemolytic anemia (pronounced) Mild transaminitis	Thick or thin blood smear demonstrates intraerythrocytic parasites PCR of blood
Lyme disease	Erythema migrans rash 80% Not always "bull's-eye" rash	WBC typically normal without leukocytosis Mild transaminitis rarely	ELISA; negative in 70–80% in weeks 1–2; positive when repeated weeks 4–6

CSF, cerebrospinal fluid; ELISA, enzyme-linked immunosorbent assay; PCR, polymerase chain reaction.

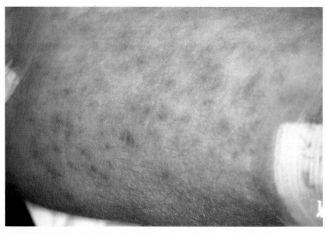

FIGURE 16-4 Florid petechial rash on the arm of a patient with Rocky Mountain spotted fever. (From Mandell GL, Bennett JE, Dolin R: *Principles and practice of infectious diseases*, ed 6, Philadelphia, Churchill Livingstone, 2005, figure 184-4.)

- Babesiosis
  - **Mild symptoms are the rule in North America, except in patients with asplenia, who may experience overwhelming infection with hypotension, acute respiratory distress syndrome**
  - After incubation of 1 to 3 weeks, flulike symptoms of fever, headache, myalgias, and arthralgias occur, often accompanied by dark urine (resulting from hemolysis)

- Coinfection with *Borrelia burgdorferi* (Lyme disease) common and should be considered in all patients with babesiosis
- Lyme disease
  - Occurs as both acute localized cutaneous rash and as disseminated early and late manifestations; as previously discussed, always consider coinfection with babesiosis or HGA when diagnosing Lyme disease
    - **Localized erythema migrans is most common acute presentation** (spreading erythematous rash minority of rashes have central clearing or classic "bull's-eye" appearance; Figs. 16-5 and 16-6)
      - The rash is noted in at least 80% of cases
  - Malaise, headache, migratory myalgias, and arthralgias are common and may occur with or without rash
  - Disseminated infection may occur within days to weeks of infection (Fig. 16-7)
    - Cutaneous dissemination with multiple areas of distant skin involvement with pleomorphic-appearing rash
    - Neurologic symptoms may include cranial neuritis (most commonly seventh nerve), meningitis, radicular pain syndromes
    - Cardiac symptoms may include atrioventricular block and myocarditis
  - Late infection results from persistent infection at systemic sites seeded during primary infection
    - Persistent infection occurs **months to years after infection**, manifested primarily with musculoskeletal disease

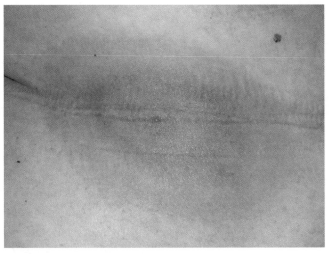

FIGURE 16-5 Erythema migrans rash of Lyme disease with classic "bull's-eye" appearance.

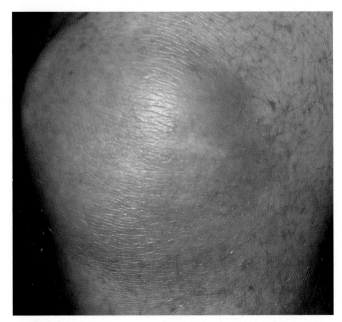

FIGURE 16-6 Erythema migrans rash of Lyme disease with uniform erythema.

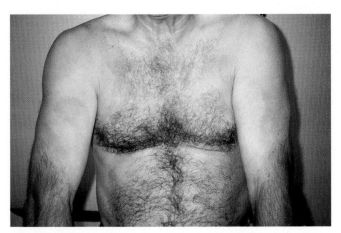

FIGURE 16-7 Cutaneous dissemination of Lyme disease presenting with pleomorphic rash.

- **Classic manifestation is monoarthritis of the knee, with effusion occurring months after infection**
  - Radiculopathy or symmetrical sensory neuropathy can occur

Diagnosis

Figure 16-8 provides an algorithm of the history of untreated Lyme disease (see also Table 16-5)
- **Early features of most tick-borne illnesses are similar;** high index of suspicion coupled with geographic distribution contribute to diagnosis
- Clinical presentation of many of these disorders should prompt initiation of treatment before definitive test results available
- Rash may assist in diagnosis of patients, particularly with RMSF and Lyme disease (see Table 16-5)
- **Other laboratory features may support diagnosis such as thrombocytopenia (which suggests anaplasmosis), but many findings, such as mild elevation of AST and ALT, are shared across disorders**

Treatment

- RMSF, ehrlichiosis, anaplasmosis, and Lyme disease all respond to **doxycycline**
  - RMSF: Doxycycline 100 mg twice daily for 1 week
  - Anaplasmosis and ehrlichiosis: Doxycycline 100 mg twice daily for 10 days
  - Lyme disease: Doxycycline 100 mg twice daily for 14 days, which will treat possibility of coinfection with HGA
    - Amoxicillin for children where doxycycline contraindicated
  - Lyme arthritis: 30 days oral doxycycline or amoxicillin; retreatment for recurrent arthritis with 28 days of oral therapy or IV ceftriaxone
    - Neuroborreliosis (i.e., meningitis or radiculopathy due to Lyme disease) or cardiac involvement: Ceftriaxone IV for 14 to 28 days
    - 200-mg single dose doxycycline effective acutely for tick bites to prevent infection
    - Vaccine for Lyme disease discontinued; long-term protection unclear, especially without availability of boosters
- Babesiosis may be asymptomatic and may not require treatment. Symptomatic patients and those with asplenia should be treated with atovaquone and azithromycin. Exchange transfusion may be necessary in cases with high-grade parasitemia greater than 10%. Relapses of symptomatic disease have been observed in patients with asplenia or underlying malignancy.

Infection from Bite and Scratch Wounds

Basic Information

- Humans, dogs, and cats harbor bacterial pathogens in the oral cavity that can cause significant infection in humans when bitten. In addition, a well-described illness may follow scratch wounds from cats.

16

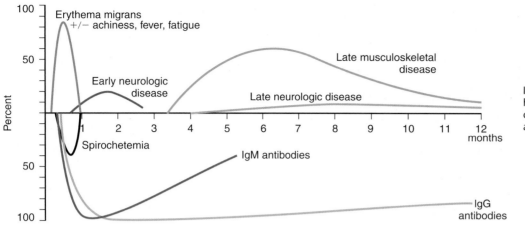

FIGURE 16-8 Natural history of untreated Lyme disease showing both acute and chronic phases of illness.

- **Treatment of infection before symptoms develop is the standard of care with bite wounds,** although dog bites become infected in a minority of cases
- **Immunization for tetanus should be current (or updated, if not),** and consideration should be given to the possibility of rabies

Clinical Presentation

- Most bite wounds occur on the upper extremities but are also commonly seen on the face and lower extremities
- **Superficial abrasions should be cleaned and otherwise need no treatment**
  - Deep bite wounds and wounds inflicted on a closed fist may need extensive debridement and surgical evaluation
- Human bites may introduce infection with *S. viridans*, *S. epidermidis*, *S. aureus*, *Eikenella*, and other species
- Dog bites may introduce infection with *Pasteurella multocida*, *S. aureus*, and, less commonly, *Bacteroides*, *Fusobacterium*, and *Capnocytophagia*
- Cat bites may introduce infection with *P. multocida* or *S. aureus*; **deep bites risk the development of osteomyelitis**
- The major risk from cat scratches (almost always from kittens) is infection with *Bartonella henselae* (i.e., cat scratch disease)
  - Regional adenopathy developing 2 weeks after a cat scratch (by which time the injury is likely to have healed) is the most common presentation and may be accompanied by malaise and fever
  - Adenopathy may progress to lymphadenitis and rarely to suppuration
  - More serious manifestations include seizures and coma and are more common in children

Diagnosis

- Bite wounds present with an obvious history and present little in the way of clinical dilemmas
  - Cat scratch disease may be missed in a patient presenting with adenopathy unless an inciting injury is specifically queried

- Antibody titers for *B. henselae* are available but unlikely to be of use in the acute setting
- *Pasteurella* infection typically becomes symptomatic in 24 hours
- Treatment for bite wounds is empirical and not based on culture results
- If the patient with a history of cat bite presents late (i.e., days or weeks after injury), consideration should be given to osteomyelitis

Treatment

- The major consideration for pathogens in animal bites, particularly in cat bites, is treatment to **cover infection with *Pasteurella multocida***
  - *P. multocida* is resistant to typical agents used to cover cellulitis (i.e., dicloxacillin, cephalexin, erythromycin)
  - Treatment is typically with **amoxicillin/clavulanate or clindamycin and a fluoroquinolone for penicillin-allergic patients**
- Dog bites may introduce *P. multocida* and rarely cause infection with *Capnocytophagia*, which in asplenic patients may result in sepsis
  - *Capnocytophagia* infection responds to amoxicillin/clavulanate or clindamycin
- If **rabies** is a consideration, **treatment should be rabies immune globulin and rabies vaccine**
- Human bites are more commonly associated with cellulitis from *Staphylococcus* or *Streptococcus* spp. and should be treated with amoxicillin/clavulanate or clindamycin
  - *Eikenella* spp. may be resistant to both and often require a fluoroquinolone for treatment
- Cat scratch disease is treated with macrolides (clarithromycin, azithromycin) or fluoroquinolones

REVIEW QUESTIONS

For review questions, please go to www.expertconsult.com.

SUGGESTED READINGS

Dajani AS, Taubert KA, Wilson W, et al: Prevention of bacterial endocarditis: recommendations by the American Heart Association, *JAMA* 2777:1794–1801, 1997.

Dumler JS, Bakken JS: Ehrlichial diseases of humans: emerging tick-borne infections, *Clin Infect Dis* 20:1102–1110, 1995.

Durack DT, Lukes AS, Bright DK: New criteria for diagnosis of infective endocarditis: utilization of specific echocardiographic findings, Duke Endocarditis Service, *Am J Med* 96:200–209, 1994.

Gilbert DN, Moellering RC, Sande MA: The Sanford guide to antimicrobial therapy 2001, Hyde Park, VT, 2001, Antimicrobial Therapy.

Roe MT, Abramson A, Li J, et al: Clinical information determines the impact of transesophageal echocardiography on the diagnosis of infective endocarditis by the Duke criteria, *Am Heart J* 139:945–951, 2000.

Wilson WR, Karchmer AW, Dajani AS, et al: Antibiotic treatment of adults with infective endocarditis caused by streptococci, enterococci, staphylococci, and HACEK microorganisms. American Heart Association, *JAMA* 274:1706–1713, 1995.

Wormser GP, Dattwyler RJ, Shapiro ED, et al: The clinical assessment, treatment, and prevention of Lyme disease, human granulocytic anaplasmosis, and babesiosis, clinical practice guidelines by the Infectious Diseases Society of America, *Clin Infect Dis* 43: 1089–1134, 2006.

16

Bioterrorism

SARA E. COSGROVE, MD, MS

The anthrax attacks of 2001, along with the increasing political instability worldwide, have reminded physicians of the importance of being familiar with the clinical features of agents that can be used in a bioterrorist attack. Here reviewed are the most likely pathogens to be used in the event of a bioterrorist attack.

Overview of Biologic Warfare

Historical Perspective

- Reports of attempts to use microbes as weapons date back to the 1700s
- After World War II, many countries, including the United States, had active programs for developing and testing biologic weapons
- These programs were officially abandoned following passage of the Biological Weapons Convention in the early 1970s, although it has recently become clear that some countries continued their programs in secret

Potential Agents of Bioterrorism

- Experts have identified several important pathogens as being the most likely agents to be used in an attack (Box 17-1)
- Characteristics of these pathogens include the following:
  - High morbidity and mortality
  - Large proportion of the population is vulnerable
  - Ease of dissemination
  - Some with person-to-person transmission (smallpox, plague, and viral hemorrhagic fevers)

BOX 17-1	*Potential Agents of Biologic Warfare*

Most Likely (Category A)
Anthrax (*Bacillus anthracis*)
Botulinum toxin
Plague (*Yersinia pestis*)
Smallpox
Tularemia (*Francisella tularensis*)
Viral hemorrhagic fevers (e.g., Ebola, Marburg)

Less Likely (Category B)
Alphaviruses (e.g., Venezuelan equine encephalitis)
Brucellosis (*Brucella* spp.)
Cholera (*Vibrio cholerae*)
Glanders
Q fever (*Coxiella burnetii*)

Role of the Primary Care Physician

- Internists, family practitioners, and emergency room physicians serve as a first line of defense against dissemination of biologic agents because they are likely to be the physicians of first contact
- Physicians should recognize the clinical presentations of infection with the more likely agents (Table 17-1)
- Physicians should know when and how to isolate patients to limit spread of disease
- Physicians should know how to activate hospital, public health, and law enforcement resources when a bioterrorism attack is suspected
- Physicians should be familiar with management strategies, which should be carried out in conjunction with infectious diseases and public health experts

Details on "Category A" Agents of Biologic Warfare

ANTHRAX (*BACILLUS ANTHRACIS*)
Basic Information

- **Infection can occur either through inhalation of (inhalational anthrax) or direct inoculation with (cutaneous anthrax) spores of *B. anthracis* that then germinate and cause disease**
- Anthrax is **not transmissible from person to person;** therefore, **patients do not require isolation**

Clinical Presentation
Diagnosis and Evaluation
- Inhalational anthrax
  - Culture of the peripheral blood is almost universally positive at presentation unless the patient has received antibiotics before the cultures are done
    - Gram stain shows a **gram-positive rod with a bamboo appearance**
  - **Mediastinal lymphadenopathy creates the characteristic appearance of a wide mediastinum on chest radiograph or CT (Fig. 17-1)**
    - Early in disease, chest CT may be more sensitive in detecting the lymphadenopathy and should be done when suspicion of anthrax is high but the chest radiograph is normal
  - **Lumbar puncture should be done if meningeal signs are present**
    - Cerebrospinal fluid (CSF) in anthrax meningitis shows elevated red and white blood cells

TABLE 17-1	*Clinical Presentation of Category A Biologic Agents*		
Agent	**Incubation**	**Route of Infection**	**Clinical Manifestations**
Inhalation anthrax	1–7 days	Inhalation	Begins with a flulike illness (e.g., malaise, fever, headache, cough, myalgias, and nausea) **No coryza (nasal discharge) seen** **Pulmonary infiltrates, severe dyspnea, and shock develop within a few days (fulminant phase)** Hemorrhagic **pleural effusions** may be present ~50% of patients with severe disease will have meningitis Death occurs rapidly after disease enters the fulminant phase
Cutaneous anthrax	1–7 days	Direct inoculation	**Pruritic macule or papule with rapid enlargement to round pustule over 24–48 hr** **Vesicles and bullae may surround the ulcer** **Erythema and nonpitting edema** develop in surrounding tissue (see Fig. 17-2) **Over 3–7 days, the pustule becomes hemorrhagic and ruptures, producing a painless eschar** **Lesions associated with painful lymphadenopathy or lymphangitis**
Smallpox	12–14 days	Person-to-person by respiratory droplet	**Initially, high fevers and malaise followed by a papular rash that starts on the oropharyngeal mucosa, face, and forearms** (see Figs. 17-3 and 17-4) Rash demonstrates **relative sparing of the trunk** Rash becomes vesicular and then pustular Lesions begin to scab by day 8 of rash Secondary bacterial skin infections can cause sepsis **Need to differentiate from chickenpox** (see Table 17-3)
Tularemia	3–5 days	Inhalation	Begins with fever, pharyngitis, bronchitis, pleuritis, and pneumonitis Untreated infections could lead to sepsis in some patients **Because signs are nonspecific, only clue to attack would come from epidemiology**

Botulism	12–72 hr	Wounds, food, inhalation*	**Initially, symmetrical cranial nerve palsies causing ptosis, diplopia, blurred vision, enlarged and less reactive pupils, dysarthria, and dysphonia**
			Neurologic symptoms progress, causing a **descending paralysis**
			   Respiratory failure can occur because of diaphragmatic weakness
			   Autonomic involvement can cause postural hypotension and urinary retention
			Patients are generally alert, afebrile, and have normal sensation

Plague	1–6 days	Natural infection from flea bites (bubonic plague), person-to-person by respiratory droplet*	Naturally occurring plague causes **swollen, tender lymph nodes** (buboes) Pneumonic symptoms can complicate bubonic plague **Biologic attack with an aerosolized strain would cause pneumonic form of plague** **Symptoms are fever, dyspnea, cough, and bloody sputum** Abdominal pain, vomiting, diarrhea can also occur Rapidly progressive and invariably fatal if not treated quickly Can resemble Hantavirus pulmonary syndrome
Viral hemorrhagic fever	5–10 days	Unclear, not thought to be aerosolized	**Begins with abrupt onset of fever, myalgia, and headache** Many patients have chest pain, cough, lymphadenopathy, conjunctival infection, and GI complaints Central nervous system involvement can cause somnolence, delirium, or coma As disease progresses, hemorrhagic manifestations present (e.g., petechiae, mucous membrane bleeding, GI bleeding)

*Most likely route of spread if used for biologic warfare.

17

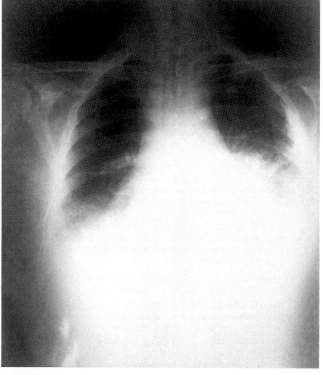

FIGURE 17-1 Chest radiograph showing a widened mediastinum in a patient with inhalational anthrax. (Courtesy of the Centers for Disease Control and Prevention and Dr. P.S. Brachman.)

- Gram stain and culture of the CSF often yield the organism
- **Nasal cultures are not helpful** in clinical decision making because they can be falsely negative. They should only be used as an epidemiologic tool.
- Cutaneous anthrax
  - **Clinical diagnosis is generally made based on the appearance of the lesion (Fig. 17-2)**
  - Swab necrotic ulcer or vesicle or bulla fluid for Gram stain and culture
  - Punch biopsy lesion for Gram stain and culture and other tests (e.g., polymerase chain reaction, immunohistochemistry done at the Centers for Disease Control and Prevention [CDC])
  - Some patients with cutaneous lesions will have disseminated disease, so blood cultures should be obtained

Treatment

Table 17-2 summarizes treatment for category A biologic agents.
- Treatment of inhalational anthrax (and cutaneous anthrax with positive blood cultures)
  - **Initially, double coverage is used in treatment of inhalational anthrax or cutaneous anthrax with positive blood cultures**
  - Acceptable regimens
    - **First agent should be either fluoroquinolone (ciprofloxacin or levofloxacin are Food and Drug Administration [FDA] approved) or doxycycline**

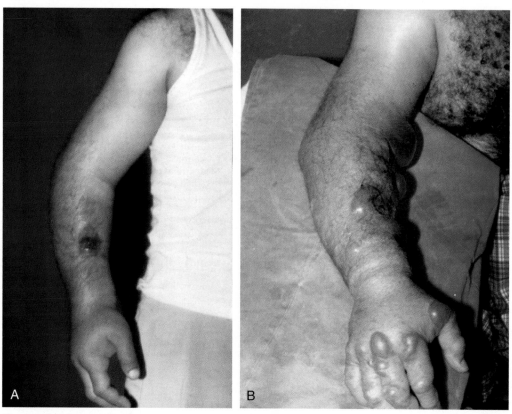

FIGURE 17-2 Characteristic lesions of anthrax at day 3. (**A**), and day 6. (**B**), with extensive tissue edema and bullae formation. (From Cohen J, Powderly W: *Infectious diseases*, ed 2, St. Louis, Mosby, 2004, figure 185-2.)

TABLE 17-2	*Treatment of Category A Biologic Agents*	
Agent	**Treatment**	**Prophylaxis**

Anthrax	Inhalation anthrax
	    Double coverage with fluoroquinolone or doxycycline
	    plus one of the following: vancomycin,
	    penicillin, clindamycin, rifampin, or clarithromycin
	Meningitis
	    Triple coverage with vancomycin, ciprofloxacin,
	    and rifampin
	Cutaneous anthrax
	    Single coverage with fluoroquinolone or
	    doxycycline
		Prophylaxis given to those potentially exposed to
		    aerosol
		Ciprofloxacin, levofloxacin, or doxycycline, all used
		    for prophylaxis

Smallpox	Supportive care	Vaccination Postexposure vaccination, if given within 4 days of exposure
Botulinum toxin	Antitoxin Supportive care, including mechanical ventilation	None

Plague	Streptomycin drug of choice
	Gentamicin, tetracycline, doxycycline,
	    ciprofloxacin, or chloramphenicol are
	    second-line agents
		Prophylaxis given to those potentially exposed
		    to aerosol and to close contacts of patients
		Doxycycline drug of choice

Tularemia	Streptomycin or gentamicin are first-line
	    agents
	Doxycycline or ciprofloxacin are second-line
	    agents
		Prophylaxis given to those potentially exposed
		    to aerosol
		Doxycycline or ciprofloxacin agent of choice

Viral hemorrhagic fevers	Supportive care	None

(avoid doxycyline if engineered resistance is suspected until susceptibilities are known)
- Acceptable second agents include **vancomycin, penicillin, clindamycin, rifampin, or clarithromycin**
- Cephalosporins are not acceptable agents because of resistance
- Duration of double coverage is unclear—consider 10 to 14 days
  - Meningitis should be treated with a combination of vancomycin, ciprofloxacin, and rifampin
    - Initial treatment should be intravenous
  - **Antibiotic courses for treatment and prophylaxis of all forms of anthrax are long because of concern for delayed spore germination**
    - There are three options for duration of treatment with fluoroquinolones or doxycycline: (1) 60 days followed by careful clinical observation, (2) 100 days, or (3) 100 days plus administration of anthrax vaccine in three doses at 2-week intervals
- Treatment of cutaneous anthrax
  - Recommendations for type and duration of treatment are the **same as for inhalational anthrax**, except a second agent is not needed
- Prophylaxis following an exposure
  - **Administration of prophylactic antibiotics is recommended for persons who have been in an air space in which anthrax spores have been aerosolized**
  - All potential exposures must be reported to public health and law enforcement officials, who should determine who should receive prophylaxis
  - **Recommended agents for prophylaxis are fluoroquinolones (ciprofloxacin or levofloxacin are FDA approved) or doxycycline**

- Ciprofloxacin is preferred for pregnant women; amoxicillin can be considered only if the strain is proven to be penicillin susceptible
- There are three options for duration of prophylaxis: (1) 60 days followed by careful clinical observation, (2) 100 days, or (3) 100 days plus administration of anthrax vaccine in three doses at 2-week intervals

SMALLPOX
Basic Information
- **Smallpox is highly infectious and spreads from person to person via respiratory droplets**
- **Smallpox is minimally contagious, if at all, before onset of the rash**
- The U.S. population is highly vulnerable to smallpox because routine vaccination was discontinued in the early 1970s and immunity has waned for those who were vaccinated before that time
- Patients with smallpox must be managed with **airborne precautions in negative-pressure rooms**, and all staff should wear N95 masks or personal air-purification respirators, along with gowns and gloves
- If smallpox is suspected, the patient area should be closed off immediately and all staff quarantined. Patients should be masked with an N95 mask, but should not be moved from the area until public health officials arrive.

Clinical Presentation
- **Need to differentiate from chickenpox (Table 17-3)**

Diagnosis and Evaluation
- **Clinical diagnosis is made based on the characteristic appearance of the rash (Figs. 17-3 and 17-4)**

17

TABLE 17-3	Distinguishing Smallpox from Chickenpox
Smallpox (Variola)	**Chickenpox (Varicella)**
Severe prodrome 1–4 days before rash (temperature ≥ 101°F, prostration, backache, abdominal pain)	No or mild prodrome
Rash (deep-seated pustules) begins in oropharynx and on face	Rash (superficial vesicles) begins on chest and back
Lesions all in the same stage of development on any one part of the body	Lesions appear in crops; on any one part of the body there are papules, vesicles, and crusts
Slow evolution over days	Rapid evolution over 24 hr

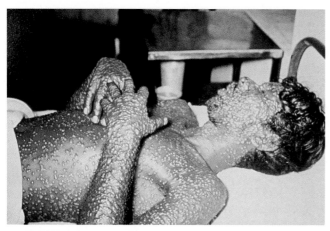

FIGURE 17-3 Patient with smallpox showing typical distribution of lesions in the same stage of development with greater involvement of the face and arms. (Courtesy of the Centers for Disease Control and Prevention and Barbara Rice.)

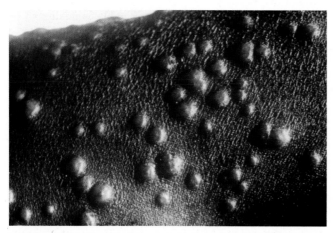

FIGURE 17-4 Characteristic pustular rash of smallpox, day 6. (Courtesy of World Health Organization Diagnosis of Smallpox Slide Series.)

- Electron microscopy and culture can be performed to confirm the diagnosis but must occur in special high-containment laboratories
- Collection of fluid from vesicles for analysis is hazardous and should only be done by someone who has been recently vaccinated

Treatment

- The mainstay of **treatment is supportive care** (fluids, antibiotics for superinfection)
- Cidofovir has in vitro activity against smallpox but unknown efficacy in clinical smallpox
- **For those who have been exposed but have not yet developed symptoms, vaccination within 4 days reduces the chance of infection twofold to threefold** and decreases morbidity and mortality if smallpox develops
  - Vaccine given 4 days after exposure also decreases mortality from smallpox

BOTULINUM TOXIN
Basic Information

- **Botulinum toxin is a potent neurotoxin produced by *Clostridium botulinum* that causes paralysis by blocking acetylcholine from binding with motor neurons, resulting in a descending flaccid paralysis**
- Intoxication with botulinum toxin can occur in one of three ways: (1) absorption of toxin produced in a wound infected with *C. botulinum*, (2) ingestion of toxin produced in food that is contaminated with *C. botulinum*, or (3) inhalation of toxin
- **Ingestion or inhalation of preformed toxin** is the most likely method of biowarfare with botulinum toxin
- Botulinum toxin is **not transmissible person to person;** therefore, **patients do not need isolation**

Clinical Presentation
See Table 17-1.

Diagnosis and Evaluation

- **Diagnosis is based on clinical findings**
- Differential diagnosis
  - Guillain-Barré syndrome (characterized by ascending paralysis, sensory involvement)
  - Myasthenia gravis (does not present with autonomic symptoms)
  - Lambert-Eaton syndrome (characterized by hip girdle weakness)
  - Tick paralysis (should have tick exposure and tick on body)
- Electrophysiologic studies can be helpful to rule out other causes of paralysis
- Specialized toxin assays are available through research laboratories and some health departments
- **Suspect botulism if more than one patient has the same symptoms**

Treatment

- If botulism is suspected, **antitoxin should be given immediately** to halt progression of disease—do not wait to confirm the diagnosis

- The antitoxin is only available from the CDC and some local health departments
- **Supportive care,** including mechanical ventilation if necessary, is the mainstay of therapy
- Because clinical features result from toxin exposure and not from infection with C. *botulinum,* there is **no role for antibiotics**

PLAGUE (*YERSINIA PESTIS*)

Basic Information

- Rodents are the primary reservoir
  - Natural infections, caused by flea bites, occur every year in the United States, mainly in the western states
- If Y. *pestis* were to be used in a biologic attack, the bacteria would probably be aerosolized to cause pneumonic plague
- **Patients with pneumonic plague are infectious and must be placed on droplet precautions for the first 48 hours of therapy**

Clinical Presentation

See Table 17-1.

Diagnosis

- Physical examination is nonspecific and includes findings consistent with **severe pneumonia**
- **Chest radiograph will usually show infiltrates that are commonly bilateral**
- **Y. pestis can be cultured from the sputum, blood, or from buboes** if cultures are obtained before antibiotics are started
- The laboratory should be notified when the diagnosis is suspected because some automated systems may misidentify the organism
- Rapid diagnostic tests are available through the CDC and some local health departments

Treatment

- **Streptomycin is the drug of choice** for treating plague but is not widely available
- **Alternatives are gentamicin (although not FDA approved for this indication), tetracycline and doxycycline, ciprofloxacin (also not FDA approved), and chloramphenicol**
- Administration of **prophylactic antibiotics is recommended for persons who have been in an air space in which Y. pestis has been aerosolized and for persons in close contact with patients** (i.e., <2 m), including family members and hospital workers
- **Doxycycline is the drug of choice for prophylaxis** and should be given for 7 days

TULAREMIA (*FRANCISELLA TULARENSIS*)

Basic Information

- Small mammals (e.g., rabbits) are the reservoir of F. *tularensis*
- Natural infections occur following exposures to infected animals or bites from infected ticks

- Although tularemia is highly infectious in the wild and in the laboratory, **person-to-person transmission does not occur, and patients do not need to be isolated**
- Inhalational disease is believed to be the most likely presentation if F. *tularensis* is used in biowarfare

Clinical Presentation

See Table 17-1.

Diagnosis and Evaluation

- **Physical findings are nonspecific and similar to those of pneumonia**
- Classic chest radiographic findings are peribronchial infiltrates with progression to multilobar involvement, effusions, and adenopathy
- Cultures of sputum and pharyngeal washings should be obtained as **growth of the organism is the definitive means of diagnosis**
- If tularemia is suspected, the laboratory must be notified because the organism **requires special media for growth and is highly infectious to laboratory personnel**
- Rapid diagnostic tests do exist but are generally only available through special laboratories
- Serologic testing is available but requires acute and convalescent samples and is not useful in making an early diagnosis

Treatment

- Infection: **Streptomycin or gentamicin**
  - Doxycycline and ciprofloxacin (not FDA approved) are alternatives for treatment
- Prophylaxis: **Doxycycline or ciprofloxacin**
  - Prophylaxis recommended for persons who have been in an air space in which F. *tularensis* has been aerosolized
  - A vaccine does exist, but it is not FDA approved and does not provide reliable protection against aerosolized F. *tularensis*

VIRAL HEMORRHAGIC FEVERS (E.G., EBOLA, MARBURG)

Basic Information

- The mode of transmission for Ebola and Marburg viruses remains unclear, although experience with outbreaks in Africa suggests that **body fluids from infected patients are highly infectious**
- Patients with viral hemorrhagic fever should be placed on **droplet precautions;** health care workers should wear gowns and gloves for all interactions and take great care to cover all mucous membranes with eye protection and masks
- Transmission by the airborne route has not been established, although airborne precautions can be considered in patients with severe pulmonary involvement

Clinical Presentation

See Table 17-1.

17

Diagnosis and Evaluation

- Early phases of the illness are relatively nonspecific and can mimic other viral infections, such as influenza
- **Hemorrhagic events, such as conjunctival hemorrhage, petechial rash, hematemesis, melena, and hematuria are the key to suspecting the diagnosis in most cases**
- The virus can be cultured but must be handled in a special, highly contained laboratory facility
- Serologic tests are also available through reference laboratories but are not useful acutely

Treatment

- Treatment of patients infected with viral hemorrhagic fevers is **supportive**
- Ribavirin is approved only for use in Lassa fever and has not been shown to be effective in Ebola or Marburg virus infections

REVIEW QUESTIONS

For review questions, please go to www.expertconsult.com.

SUGGESTED READINGS

Arnon SS, Schechter R, Inglesby TV, et al: Botulinum toxin as a biological weapon, JAMA 285:1059–1070, 2001.

Bartlett JG, Inglesby TV, Borio L: Management of anthrax, *Clin Infect Dis* 35:851–858, 2002.

Center for Biosecurity, University of Pittsburgh Medical Center. Available at www.upmc-biosecurity.org.

Centers for Disease Control and Prevention: Emergency Preparedness and Response Web site. Available at www.bt.cdc.gov.

Dennis DT, Inglesby TV, Henderson DA, et al: Tularemia as a biological weapon, JAMA 285:2763–2773, 2001.

Henderson DA, Inglesby TV, Barlett JG, et al: Smallpox as a biological weapon, JAMA 281:2127–2137, 1999.

Inglesby TV, Dennis DT, Henderson DA, et al: Plague as a biological weapon, JAMA 283:2281–2290, 2000.

Inglesby TV, Henderson DA, Bartlett JG, et al: Anthrax as a biological weapon, JAMA 281:1735–1745, 1999.

SECTION THREE

BOARD REVIEW

Pulmonary and Critical Care Medicine

Obstructive Lung Disease

ROBERT A. WISE, MD, and M. BRADLEY DRUMMOND, MD

Obstructive lung disease encompasses a wide range of processes all involving obstruction to airflow. Roughly 50% of patients die within 10 years of initial diagnosis of smoking-related chronic obstructive pulmonary disease (COPD). The most common chronic obstructive lung diseases include those that are smoking-related (chronic bronchitis and emphysema) and those that are not smoking-related (asthma, bronchiectasis, cystic fibrosis [CF], and bronchiolitis obliterans).

Asthma

Basic Information

- **Asthma is a chronic inflammatory disease of the airways that is characterized by episodes of cough, wheezing, and dyspnea**
- **It is characterized by increased sensitivity of the airways to constrict in response to nonspecific stimulation (i.e., bronchial hyper-reactivity)**
- **Approximately 80% of patients with asthma have an allergic tendency (atopy) characterized by positive immediate hypersensitivity skin tests (Fig. 18-1)**

Clinical Presentation

- Asthma may manifest with different syndromes, often overlapping
- Extrinsic asthma
  - Usual onset in **childhood**
  - Attacks **triggered by exposure to inhaled allergen**
    - Dust mites
    - Cockroaches
    - Cat antigen
    - Molds, particularly *Alternaria*
    - Pollens (e.g., ragweed, trees, grasses)
- Intrinsic asthma
  - Usual onset in **early adulthood**
  - Attacks **triggered by viral infections, nonspecific irritants**
  - May lead to chronic asthmatic bronchitis
  - Obesity is a risk factor, particularly for women
- Exercise-induced asthma
  - Characterized by **bronchospasm 10 to 20 minutes after exhausting exercise** (Fig. 18-2)
  - Occurs in nearly all asthmatics, but may occur as sole manifestation of asthma
  - **Triggered by drying or cooling (or both) of airways** with hyperventilation, particularly cold, dry air

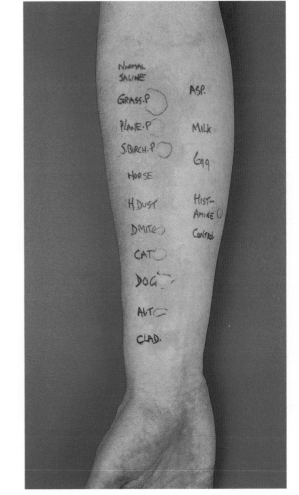

FIGURE 18-1 Multiple positive skin test results in a patient with extrinsic asthma. (From Forbes CD, Jackson WF: *Color atlas and text of clinical medicine,* ed 3, St. Louis, Mosby, 2003, figure 4.18.)

- **Can be prevented with inhaled bronchodilators (e.g., albuterol), mast-cell stabilizers (e.g., cromolyn), or leukotriene antagonists (e.g., montelukast)**
- Triad asthma (Samter's syndrome)
  - **Asthma**, often requiring systemic corticosteroids for control
  - **Nasal polyps (Fig. 18-3)**
  - **Aspirin (or other NSAID) sensitivity**
  - May require leukotriene antagonist for control of symptoms

Exercise

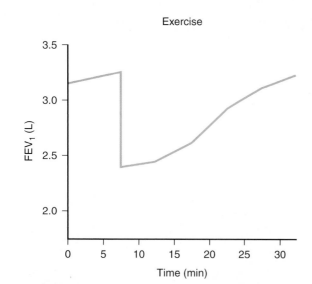

FIGURE 18-2 FEV₁ in a patient with exercise-induced asthma. Note the sudden fall of FEV₁, followed by gradual recovery. (From Haslett C, Chilvers ER, Boon NA, et al: *Davidson's principles and practice of medicine,* ed 19, New York, Churchill Livingstone, 2003, figure 13.25.)

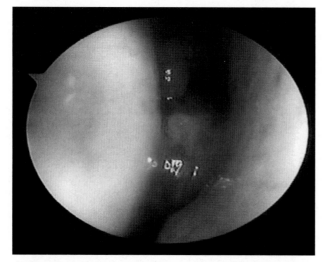

FIGURE 18-3 Endoscopic view of nasal polyps protruding from middle meatus. (From Adkinson NF Jr, Yunginger J, Busse W, et al: *Middleton's allergy: principles and practice,* ed 6, St. Louis, Mosby, 2003, figure 78-1.)

- Cough-variant asthma
  - May manifest as **cough in the absence of wheezing**
  - Responds to treatment for asthma
  - Airways hyper-reactivity present
  - One of the **three most common causes of chronic cough** (along with gastroesophageal reflux disease and chronic sinusitis/postnasal drip syndrome)
- Occupational asthma
  - Presents as **"Monday morning" symptoms** that abate during weekends
  - Symptoms usually **worse in the evening,** better in the morning
  - Prolonged exposures may lead to irreversible airflow obstruction
  - Common causes
    - Pigeons, chickens

- Epoxy resins
- Laboratory animals
- Metals (nickel, chromium)
- Plastics and rubber
- Refractory asthma
  - **Chronic unremitting wheezing** requiring long-term systemic corticosteroids
  - Often leads to chronic airway remodeling with chronic airflow obstruction
  - Possible causes for refractory asthma (Box 18-1)
- Disorders that may **mimic asthma**
  - **Congestive heart failure**
  - **Mitral stenosis**
  - **Upper airway obstructions** (e.g., laryngeal tumors, subglottic stenosis, Wegener's granulomatosis)
  - Paradoxical **vocal cord dysfunction** (more common in women and health care workers)

Evaluation and Diagnosis

- **Consider diagnosis of asthma in patients with history of wheezing or variable dyspnea with specific triggers**
- **Diagnosis confirmed by presence of obstructive lung disease on pulmonary function tests at the time of symptoms that normalize when asymptomatic**
- Diffusing capacity of the lungs for carbon monoxide (DLCO) normal between episodes
- Home monitoring with peak flow meter may be helpful for diagnosing or monitoring disease
- **Negative methacholine challenge test effectively rules out active asthma**

Treatment

Figure 18-4 shows a stepwise approach to asthma treatment.

- **The goal of asthma treatment is to avoid symptoms, minimize use of short-acting bronchodilators for relief of symptoms, prevent nocturnal awakening from asthma, and minimize systemic side effects of treatment**
- Four components of asthma treatment
  - **Monitor symptoms and pulmonary function**
  - **Control environmental exposures**
  - **Educate patient regarding avoidance of triggers and proper treatment**
  - **Drug treatment (Box 18-2)**
- Stepwise drug treatment of chronic asthma (see Fig. 18-4)
  - **For intermittent symptoms (up to two episodes per week), occasional inhaled short-acting bronchodilators**
  - **For persistent symptoms (e.g., use of short-acting bronchodilator more than twice per week), controller therapy with inhaled corticosteroids or leukotriene antagonists, supplemented by bronchodilators as needed**
  - For persistent symptoms that do not respond to moderate doses of inhaled corticosteroids, **leukotriene antagonists, theophylline, or long-acting β-agonists may be added to inhaled corticosteroids** if moderate doses do not control symptoms

Chronic exposure to an allergen (e.g., molds), irritant (e.g., air pollution), or sensitizing agent (e.g., toluene di-isocyanate)

Use of β-blockers (e.g., timolol eyedrops for glaucoma)

Use of aspirin-containing drugs

Muco-cutaneous fungal infections

Allergic bronchopulmonary aspergillosis

Churg-Strauss vasculitis

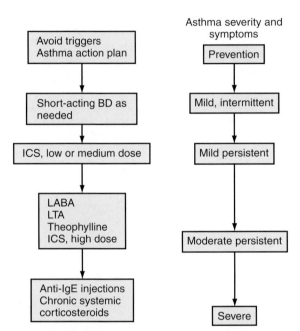

FIGURE 18-4 The stepwise approach to asthma treatment is shown. Severity of asthma is defined by the abnormality of lung function, frequency of symptomatic use of bronchodilators, and frequency of nocturnal awakenings. For patients who use their short-acting bronchodilator more than twice weekly, drugs are prescribed to control or prevent symptoms. Usually treatment is initiated with inhaled corticosteroids, and then additional controller drugs are added. Patients with recalcitrant asthma may require long-term corticosteroids or anti-IgE therapy. BD, bronchodilator; ICS, inhaled corticosteroids; LABA, long-acting β-agonist; LTA, leukotriene antagonist.

BOX 18-2 *Drug Therapy for Asthma*

β_2-Agonists
  Short-acting (albuterol)
  Long-acting (salmeterol, formoterol) (in combination with inhaled corticosteroids)
Methylxanthines
  Theophylline, Aminophylline
Corticosteroids
  Systemic
  Inhaled
Antileukotrienes
  Leukotriene receptor antagonist
  Lipoxygenase inhibitors

- For persistently low lung function, frequent exacerbations, or severe attack, **systemic corticosteroids** may be needed to gain control of disease
- Review treatment at 1- to 6-month intervals. Consider step-down of therapy if asthma has been well controlled for at least 3 months.
- Treatment of the acute asthmatic attack
  - Inhaled **short-acting bronchodilators** (e.g., albuterol) every 20 minutes for three doses
  - **Supplemental oxygen** if hypoxemia is present
  - If no relief, **systemic corticosteroids** (e.g., prednisone 60–120 mg PO or IV and repeat every 6 hours as needed)
  - **Systemic bronchodilators** (e.g., subcutaneous terbutaline or IV aminophylline) may be used in selected cases
- Indications for **hospitalization**
  - **Peak flow less than 40% baseline** after 4 to 6 hours of treatment
  - **Persistent hypoxemia**
  - **Hypercapnia**—blood gas pH may normalize if severe attack and patient is becoming fatigued
  - **Altered sensorium**
  - History of **previous near-fatal asthma** attacks

Smoking-Related Chronic Obstructive Pulmonary Disease

Basic Information

- Chronic bronchitis (chronic mucus hypersecretion syndrome)
  - Occurs in about **one out of three smokers**
  - Can occur with **occupational exposures to dust**
  - **Often remits when exposure to dust or tobacco ceases**
  - Definition
    - **Daily production of sputum for 3 or more months per year for 2 consecutive years**
    - With obstructive ventilatory defect, may be called chronic obstructive bronchitis
  - Morbid anatomy
    - **Hyperplasia of the airway mucous glands and goblet cells**
    - Mucous plugging, thickening, tortuosity, and **fibrosis** of the peripheral airways (Fig. 18-5)
  - Pathophysiology
    - Not always associated with obstructive ventilatory defect
    - Airway resistance may be increased
  - Chest radiograph
    - **Hyperinflation**
    - **Increased peribronchial markings at lung bases**
    - Thickening of **airway walls**
- Emphysema
  - **Definition** based on anatomic demonstration of **airspace enlargement**
    - **Progressive destruction of alveolar septa** and capillaries
    - **Airspace enlargement** and the development of macroscopic bullae

18

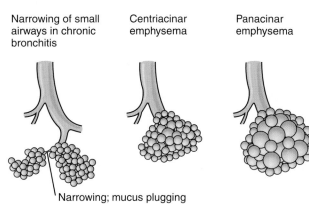

Narrowing of small airways in chronic bronchitis

Centriacinar emphysema

Panacinar emphysema

Narrowing; mucus plugging

FIGURE 18-5 Pathologic features of chronic bronchitis and emphysema. (From Kumar P, Clark M: *Clinical medicine,* ed 5, Philadelphia, Saunders, 2005, figure 14.23.)

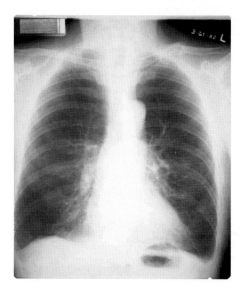

FIGURE 18-6 Chest radiograph of patient with severe COPD, showing arterial deficiency pattern of emphysema. Lungs are hyperinflated, diaphragms are low and flat, and there is paucity of vascular markings. (From Weinberger SE: *Principles of pulmonary medicine,* ed 4, Philadelphia, Saunders, 2004, figure 6-8.)

- Smoking-related disease usually involves respiratory bronchiole in the center of the pulmonary lobule (centrilobular or centriacinar emphysema; see Fig. 18-5)
- α_1-Antitrypsin deficiency usually involves the entire pulmonary lobule (panlobular or panacinar) emphysema (see later discussion)
- **Centrilobular emphysema mostly affects the upper lung zones**
- **Panacinar emphysema mostly affects the lower lung zones**
  - Pathophysiology
    - Reduced elastic recoil of the lung (increased compliance)
    - Slowing of maximum expiratory airflow (decreased forced expiratory volume in 1 second/forced vital capacity [FEV_1/FVC] ratio)
    - Hyperinflation (increased static lung volumes)
    - Decreased alveolar surface area for gas exchange (reduction in D_LCO); ventilation-perfusion mismatch (hypoxemia)
  - Chest radiograph
    - **Flattening of the diaphragm** (Fig. 18-6)
    - Attenuation of vascular markings
    - Enlargement of the central pulmonary arteries
    - **Hyperinflation**
    - Enlargement of the anterior airspace
    - Increase of the sternophrenic angle
  - CT of chest
    - **Bullae** (avascular regions)
    - Regions of decreased lung density (less than −910/−950 Hounsfield units)
  - Natural history of COPD (Fig. 18-7)
    - One in seven patients who smoke develops COPD
    - COPD develops over many years of smoking
    - Those who develop COPD have **increased rate of FEV_1 decline**
    - **Smoking cessation stops accelerated loss of lung function and prolongs survival**
    - Patients are usually **asymptomatic until FEV_1 is 30% to 50% predicted**
    - Risk factors for development of COPD in smokers (Box 18-3)

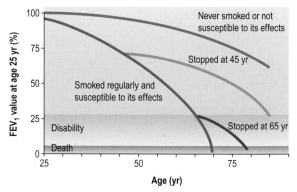

FIGURE 18-7 Natural history of COPD. Nonsmokers and smokers who are not susceptible to develop COPD lose about 25% of the early adulthood FEV_1 as a consequence of aging. Susceptible smokers lose lung function at a rate two to three times faster. By middle age, they develop symptomatic obstructive lung disease. If they continue to smoke, the disease progresses and eventually leads to disability and death. At any degree of impairment of lung function, smoking cessation leads to slowing of disease progression and extends the period of relative health.

- Survival is lower in patients with higher **BODE** index based on
  - low **b**ody mass index
  - severe **o**bstructive ventilatory defect
  - severe **d**yspnea
  - poor **e**xercise tolerance on 6-minute walk test

Clinical Presentation

- Spectrum of COPD (Table 18-1)
  - COPD includes patients with chronic obstructive bronchitis, emphysema, or both
- Physical findings in COPD (Figs. 18-8 and 18-9; Box 18-4)
  - **Physical examination not helpful in detecting mild COPD**

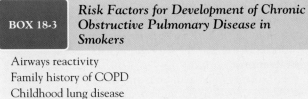

BOX 18-3 *Risk Factors for Development of Chronic Obstructive Pulmonary Disease in Smokers*

Airways reactivity
Family history of COPD
Childhood lung disease
Occupational dust exposures (e.g., silica, cotton dust, grain dust)

COPD, chronic obstructive pulmonary disease

TABLE 18-1 *Clinical Spectrum of Chronic Obstructive Pulmonary Disease*

Characteristic	Type A	Type B
Underlying lung disease	Emphysema	Chronic bronchitis disease
Lung volumes	Hyperinflated	May be normal
Physique	Slender	Obese
Dyspnea	Very dyspneic	Not dyspneic
$Paco_2$	Low until end stage	Elevated
Oxygenation with exercise	Worsens	May improve
Oxygenation at rest	Satisfactory	Low

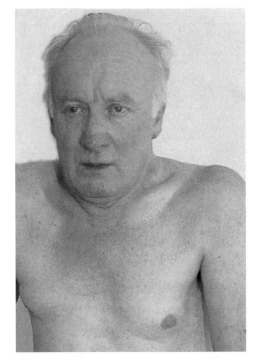

FIGURE 18-9 A "pink puffer" with emphysema. Pao_2 is maintained, but breathlessness is common, combined in the term pink puffer. (From Forbes CD, Jackson WF: *Color atlas and text of clinical medicine,* ed 3, St. Louis, Mosby, 2003, figure 4.91.)

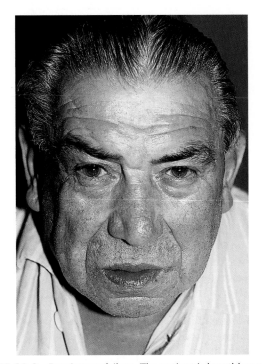

FIGURE 18-8 Respiratory failure. The patient is breathless at rest and exhibits central cyanosis with blueness of the lips and face. The lips are pursed during expiration, a characteristic feature of COPD. This facial appearance is often accompanied by heart failure with peripheral edema (cor pulmonale). The term blue bloater derives from this combination of cyanosis and edema. (From Swash M, Glynn M: *Hutchison's clinical methods,* ed 22, Philadelphia, Saunders, 2007, figure 6.1.)

BOX 18-4 *Physical Findings in Moderate Chronic Pulmonary Disorder*

Diaphragm moves <2 cm
Hyper-resonant percussion
Decreased cardiac dullness
Decreased breath sounds
Forced expiration time >10 sec
Abdominal point of maximum cardiac impulse

- **Physical examination not helpful in ruling out COPD**
- An abnormal physical examination is about 90% specific for a diagnosis of COPD

Diagnosis

- Spirometry in COPD
  - **Most sensitive measure** of disease presence and progression
  - Earliest abnormalities are decreased maximal flow at low lung volumes (seen on flow-volume loops)
  - **FEV_1/FVC less than 70%** is reasonable threshold for diagnosing obstructive lung disease
  - **FEV_1 determines the severity** (<30% predicted is very severe)

Treatment

- Treatment of stable COPD (Fig. 18-10)
  - **Smoking cessation**
    - Strong personalized message
    - Nicotine replacement (e.g., gum, patch, inhaler, lozenge, nasal spray)

18

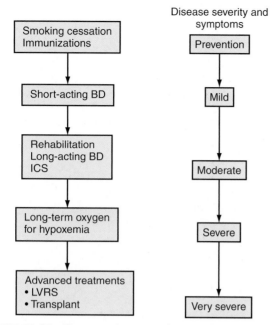

FIGURE 18-10 The step-care approach to treatment of COPD. The severity of disease is judged by the impairment of FEV_1 as a percent predicted: >80%, mild; 50–80%, moderate; 30–50%, severe; and <30%, very severe. BD, bronchodilator, either β-agonist or anticholinergic or combined; ICS, inhaled corticosteroids; LVRS, lung volume reduction surgery.

- Bupropion
- Varenicline
- Set quit date
- Group support
- Follow-up
- See Chapter 72 regarding discontinuation of addictive substances
- **Bronchodilators** for maintenance bronchodilation
  - Anticholinergic (e.g., ipratropium, tiotropium)
  - β-Agonists (e.g., salmeterol, formoterol)
- Short-acting for symptom relief (e.g., albuterol)
  - Oral theophylline
- **Inhaled corticosteroids** (ICS) to reduce exacerbation frequency
  - Not useful to prevent disease progression
  - May reduce or prevent exacerbations
  - Is associated with an increased risk of pneumonia
- **Exercise training/rehabilitation** to improve exercise tolerance
  - Improves efficiency of exercise
  - No effect on lung function or survival
- **Chronic low-flow oxygen therapy** (e.g., 2 L/min by nasal cannula)
  - **Improves survival** in patients with hypoxemia
  - Indications
    - **Partial pressure of oxygen (Pao_2) less than 55 mm Hg** in usual health
    - **Pao_2 less than 60 mm Hg with evidence of cor pulmonale or neurocognitive impairment**
- Lung transplantation candidates
  - **FEV_1 less than 20% predicted**
  - **Age under 60 years**
  - Sufficient social support

- **Lung volume reduction surgery (LVRS)**
  - Procedure removes 20% to 30% of lung volume
  - Best results in patients with upper lung zone emphysema and poor exercise capacity after rehabilitation
- **Bullectomy**
  - For single bulla occupying one third of a hemithorax
  - Best results with normal compressed lung and high $DLCO$
- Treatment of COPD exacerbation
  - **About 50% are associated with lower airway bacterial infection**
    - **Antibiotics if change in sputum volume, color, associated dyspnea**
  - **Bronchodilators** by metered dose inhaler as effective as by nebulizer in compliant patients
  - **Systemic corticosteroids** shorten duration of exacerbation
    - **No benefit of more than 2 weeks of corticosteroids**

Other Forms of Obstructive Lung Disease

α₁-ANTIPROTEASE DEFICIENCY

Basic Information
- Autosomal recessive trait
  - Also referred to as α₁-antitrypsin deficiency
- Alleles of antiprotease activity (3 most common of more than 75 identified)
  - M: Normal
  - S: Intermediate
  - Z: Marked decrease
  - Null: Absent (rare)
- Phenotypes
  - **MM, MS, MZ: No increased risk**
  - **SZ: Mild increased risk**
  - **ZZ: Increased risk for emphysema; 10% also develop chronic liver disease**
- **Panacinar emphysema** is the typical manifestation of ZZ disease
  - Affects entire respiratory lobule uniformly
  - Predominates at **lung bases**

Clinical Presentation
- Found in about **1% of patients with emphysema**
- **Premature lung disease** (age 30–40 years in smokers, age 50–60 years in nonsmokers)
- Absence of the antiprotease enzymes thought to allow proteases from inflammatory cells to damage alveolar septae
- **Bronchiectasis and chronic bronchitis may occur in deficient states along with mucous gland hyperplasia**
- **About 10% of patients have concomitant liver disease**

Diagnosis
- **Low α₁ fraction** on serum protein electrophoresis
- Plasma levels of α₁-antitrypsin reduced
- Direct **genotyping**

Treatment

- Smoking cessation
- Genetic counseling
- **Augmentation therapy with human α₁-protease inhibitor is most useful in those with moderate disease severity**

BRONCHIOLITIS OBLITERANS

Basic Information

- Causes of bronchiolitis obliterans (BO)
  - Inhalation of **toxic fumes**
    - Methane
    - Hydrochloric acid
    - Chlorine
    - Ammonia
    - Sulfuric acid
    - Nitric acid (silo-filler's disease)
  - **Viral infections** (e.g., respiratory syncytial virus, adenovirus, and influenza)
  - Connective tissue diseases—**rheumatoid arthritis**
  - **Organ transplantation**: Lung, heart, and bone marrow
  - **Neuroendocrine cell hyperplasia**
  - Idiopathic

Clinical Presentation

- Cough
- Dyspnea
- Airflow obstruction
- Air-trapping
- Physical findings
  - **Inspiratory squeaks and diffuse crackles**
  - Chest may be quiet

Diagnosis

- Chest CT
  - May appear **normal**
  - Diffuse **centriacinar nodules**
  - Diffuse **ground glass** infiltrates
  - Mosaic pattern with segmental hyperinflation on expiratory views
- Histology
  - Often requires lung biopsy for diagnosis
  - Inflammation, thickening, occlusion, and disappearance of bronchioles

Treatment

- Immunosuppressive drugs, but often there is little response
- **BO should not be confused with bronchiolitis obliterans organizing pneumonia (BOOP,** also called cryptogenic organizing pneumonia, or COP), which is a different entity involving plugging of airways with granulation tissue and postobstructive chronic pneumonia. **BOOP is often responsive to corticosteroids, whereas BO is not** (see Chapter 21).

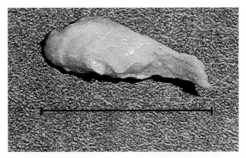

FIGURE 18-11 Typical sputum plug of allergic bronchopulmonary aspergillosis. (From Forbes CD, Jackson WF: *Color atlas and text of clinical medicine,* ed 3, St. Louis, Mosby, 2003, figure 4.12.)

ALLERGIC BRONCHOPULMONARY ASPERGILLOSIS

Basic Information

- **Hypersensitivity reaction to *Aspergillus* manifesting as worsening asthma**
- Patients with CF are also susceptible to allergic bronchopulmonary aspergillosis (ABPA), and this may be an important factor in rapid clinical deterioration

Clinical Presentation

- **Chronic steroid-dependent asthma or rapidly progressive CF**
- Recurrent **pulmonary infiltrates**
- **Brown, black, or green sputum plugs and airway casts expectorated** (Fig. 18-11)
- Culture of *Aspergillus* species from sputum
- Perihilar evanescent oval shadows on chest radiograph from mucoid impactions
- **Marked eosinophilia**
- **Elevated serum immunoglobulin E (IgE)**
- Positive *Aspergillus* skin test and serum precipitins
- Dilatation of central airways, "gloved finger" bronchiectasis

Pathophysiology

- Immune arthus-type reaction to *Aspergillus* colonizing airways

Diagnosis

- Major criteria
  - **Asthma**
  - Blood **eosinophilia**
  - Immediate skin reactivity (IgE-dependent reaction) to *Aspergillus* antigens
  - IgG antibodies (type III reaction) to *Aspergillus* antigens
  - **Transient or fixed pulmonary infiltrates**
  - Central bronchiectasis
  - **High serum IgE titer (normal level in symptomatic patient excludes ABPA)**
- Minor criteria
  - Presence of *Aspergillus* in sputum
  - Expectoration of brown mucous plugs
  - Late-phase skin test reactivity to *Aspergillus* antigen

Treatment

- **Corticosteroids** with dose adjusted by IgE levels
- Oral antifungal agents may help in some cases
- Check for CF genotype in affected patients

18

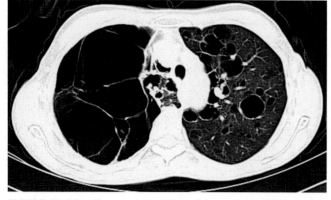

FIGURE 18-12 Characteristic CT scan from patient with lymphangioleiomyomatosis. The bullae within the left lung appear as typical punched out "Swiss-cheese" lesions. The interlobular septae are thickened giving the remaining lung parenchyma a more opaque appearance.

LYMPHANGIOLEIOMYOMATOSIS

See Figure 18-12 for a characteristic CT scan showing lymphangioleiomyomatosis.

Basic Information

- This is a rare disorder; etiology is unknown
- Affects **only fertile women**
- May be low-grade malignancy of lymphatic smooth muscle
- Associated in some cases with polymorphisms of tuberous sclerosis gene complex

Clinical Presentation

- Presents with progressive **dyspnea**
- Repeated **hemoptysis** may occur
- **Interstitial infiltrates** and airflow obstruction
- May present with pneumothorax or chylothorax

Diagnosis

- Obstructive pattern on pulmonary function tests; low DLCO
- **Characteristic "Swiss cheese" appearance on chest CT from multiple cystic spaces**
- Diffuse **proliferation of smooth muscle** within the airway walls, interstitium, and lymphatics

Treatment

- **Hormonal agents (e.g., progesterone) and induction of menopause used with no definitive success in slowing progression**
- Early referral for **lung transplantation**

CYSTIC FIBROSIS

Basic Information

- Most common lethal **autosomal recessive** disease in whites in the United States

- **Obstruction of exocrine glands** by viscous secretion
- Forty percent may not be diagnosed until adolescence
- ABPA and asthma are seen more frequently in patients with CF

Clinical Presentation

- **COPD**
- **Nasal polyps**
- **Pancreatic insufficiency**
- **Hemoptysis**
- Chronic mucoid pseudomonal infection

Diagnosis

- Abnormal sweat chloride test (**elevated** chloride)
- Genotyping

Treatment

- Management of obstructive lung disease
- Chest physiotherapy with manual percussion, flutter valves, pneumatic vest
- Long-term antibiotics including inhaled aminoglycosides
- Nutritional support and replacement of pancreatic enzymes

UNUSUAL CAUSES OF OBSTRUCTIVE LUNG DISEASE

- Immunoglobulin deficiency with bronchiectasis
  - IgA, IgG subclasses 2 and 4
- Immotile cilia syndromes
  - Kartagener's syndrome with situs inversus
  - Absence of dynein arms of cilia on electron microscopy
- Yellow nails syndrome with bronchiectasis
  - Pleural effusions, lymphedema, yellow nails
- Sarcoidosis with upper or lower airway involvement (see Chapter 21)
- Eosinophilic granuloma
- Sjögren's syndrome
- HIV with premature emphysema

REVIEW QUESTIONS

For review questions, please go to www.expertconsult.com.

SUGGESTED READINGS

Celli BR, MacNee W: ATS/ERS Task Force. Standards for the diagnosis and treatment of patients with COPD: a summary of the ATS/ERS position paper, *Eur Respir J* 23:932–946, 2004.

Global Initiative for Asthma (GINA): Global strategy for asthma management and prevention (updated 2008). Available at www.ginasthma.com.

Global strategy for the diagnosis, management, and prevention of chronic obstructive pulmonary disease (updated 2008). Available at: www.goldcopd.org.

National Asthma Education and Prevention Program Expert Panel Report III: Guidelines for the diagnosis and management of asthma: update of selected topics 2007. Available at: www.nhlbi.nih.gov/guidelines/asthma/.

Pulmonary Function Testing

ROBERT A. WISE, MD, and MEREDITH C. McCORMACK, MD

Pulmonary function tests (PFTs) are used in the evaluation of an array of lung diseases. The quality of the tests may vary depending on the patient's effort. The tests most commonly employed are spirometry, flow volume loops, bronchoprovocation testing, carbon monoxide diffusing capacity, lung volume measurements, and respiratory muscle strength. The 6-minute walk test, a simple measure of functional exercise capacity, is also performed in many pulmonary laboratories.

Pulmonary Function Tests

Spirometry

- Widely available and the most useful pulmonary function test
  - Can be performed in office and clinic as well as laboratory setting
  - Measured using flow sensors (pneumotachometers) or volume sensors (spirometers)
- **Helpful in evaluation of obstructive lung disease (i.e., COPD/asthma)**
- Performed as a forced expiration following maximum inspiration
- Recorded as volume expired per unit of time
- **Forced expiratory volume (FEV$_1$) is the volume expelled in 1 second (Fig. 19-1)**

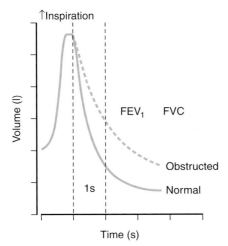

FIGURE 19-1 A spirometer tracing. The patient breathes out as fast as possible after maximum inhalation. Volume expelled is related to lung capacity. The forced expiratory volume in 1 second (FEV$_1$) is compared with the forced vital capacity (FVC). In the normal person host, this ratio is >80%; abnormal (i.e., obstructive defect) is a ratio <70%. (From Davies A, Blakeley A, Kidd C: *Human physiology,* New York, Churchill Livingstone, 2001, figure 7.1.9.)

- Correlated with maximum ventilation and with exercise
- **Reduced in both obstructive and restrictive disorders**
- **Predictive of mortality** in general population, lung cancer risk, disability
- Forced vital capacity (FVC) is the maximum volume expelled from the lung (see Fig. 19-1)
  - **May be reduced due to low total lung capacity (TLC) in restrictive ventilatory defect or due to elevated residual volume (RV) from air trapping in obstructive disease**
- **FEV$_1$/FVC is an index of the rate of emptying of the lung**
  - **Ratio less than 0.7 usually indicates obstructive ventilatory defect (Box 19-1)**
- Maximum midexpiratory flow rate (MMFR) or forced expiratory flow (FEF) 25% to 75% (forced expiratory flow at 25–75% of vital capacity) measures the mean flow during the middle 50% of expiration
  - Reportedly a measure of small airways function, but test is variable and nonspecific

Flow Volume Loops

Figure 19-2 illustrates flow volume loops.

- Displays forced expiratory and inspiratory maneuvers as flow (i.e., slope of spirogram) versus volume
- **Useful for diagnosis of upper airway obstruction**
  - Abnormality in both inspiration and expiration (fixed)
  - Abnormality in inspiration only (variable extrathoracic obstruction)
  - Abnormality in expiration only (variable intrathoracic obstruction)
- Fixed upper airway obstructions
  - Cause greater reduction in peak expiratory flow rates, but inspiratory flow rate also decreased
  - Common causes
    - **Bilateral vocal cord paralysis**
    - **Tracheal stenosis** (particularly following prolonged endotracheal intubation)

BOX 19-1 *Potential Indications for Spirometry*

Diagnosis of obstructive lung disease
Evaluation of severity of lung disease
Screen high-risk individuals (e.g., smokers)
Preoperative assessment (see Chapter 73)
Evaluation of disability/impairment
Monitoring of treatment
Assess toxic effects of exposure or drug toxicity

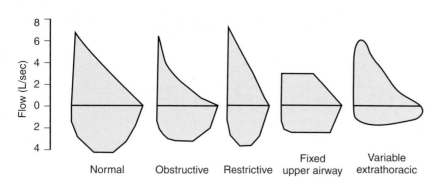

FIGURE 19-2 Flow volume loops. Curve begins at left axis and with forced expiration follows a clockwise pattern. The normal pattern appears as a triangle over a half circle. With development of chronic obstructive pulmonary disease, the expiratory limb becomes curvilinear. In restrictive lung diseases, the flows are relatively preserved and the entire curve is narrowed. With a fixed upper airway obstruction, the inspiratory and expiratory limbs are flattened.

- **Laryngeal or tracheal tumors**
- **Granulomatous diseases** (e.g., sarcoid, Wegener's granulomatosis)
- Variable extrathoracic obstruction
  - Flow during inspiration is normally greater than expiratory flow; in variable extrathoracic obstruction, **inspiratory flow is less than expiratory flow at middle lung volumes**
  - Common with **vocal cord dysfunction** or **unilateral vocal cord paralysis**
  - Found in obese individuals and those with **sleep apnea** syndrome
- Variable intrathoracic obstruction
  - **Expiratory flow is decreased,** whereas inspiratory flow is not altered
  - **Tracheal tumors, subglottic stenosis** may present this way
- Chronic obstructive pulmonary disease (COPD)
  - **Curvilinear flow volume curve caused by slowly emptying lung units**
  - Peak flow is relatively preserved, making it poor measure of COPD severity
  - Flow rates at low lung volumes are more impaired

- Asthma produces similar curve shape but with reduced flow rates at all lung volumes, including peak flow
- Vocal cord dysfunction (VCD)
  - **VCD presents as asthma, without hyperinflation on chest radiograph, and is unresponsive to steroids**
  - More common in women than men
  - Definitive diagnosis is made by visualizing vocal cord abnormalities with laryngoscopy during an attack
  - Diagnosis may be suggested by abnormal inspiratory flow patterns on flow volume loops (presents as variable extrathoracic obstruction)

Bronchoprovocation Testing

See Figure 19-3 for a methacholine challenge test.
- Performed by inhaling increasing concentrations of methacholine, followed by spirometry at each concentration
- **A positive test is defined by achieving a 20% or greater fall in FEV_1 with a dose of 16 to 25 mg/mL methacholine or less**
- The concentration required to achieve a 20% fall in FEV_1 is called the PC_{20}

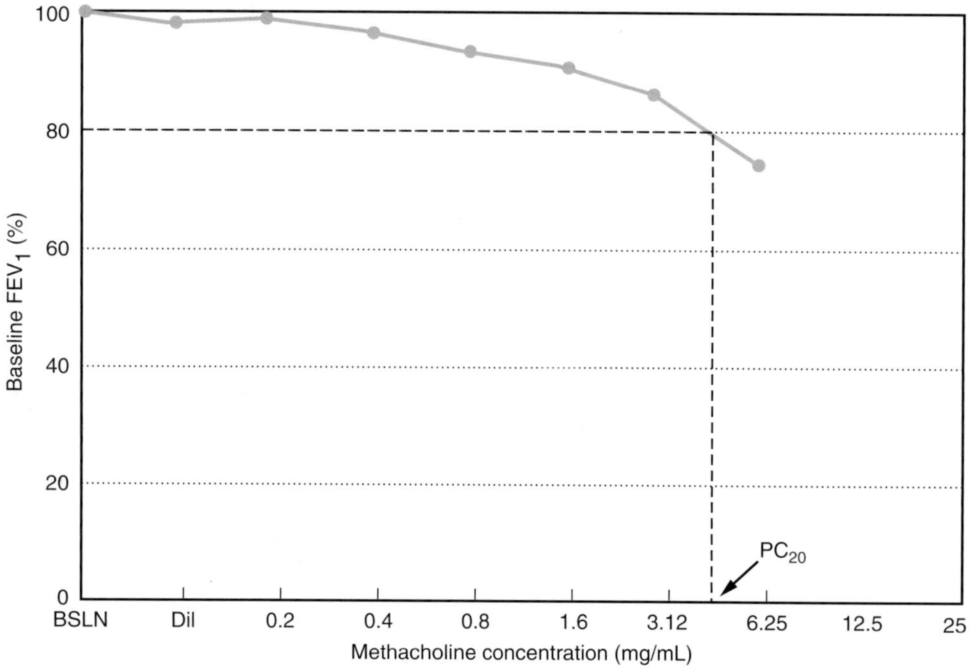

FIGURE 19-3 Methacholine challenge test. Progressively greater concentrations of inhaled methacholine are given with a nebulizer. After each concentration, spirometry is performed. In patients with airways reactivity, the forced expiratory volume in 1 second (FEV_1) will decline by more than 20% before the maximum concentration is reached (usually 25 mg/mL). The provocative concentration (PC_{20}) is determined by interpolation between concentrations. Patients with active asthma will usually show a drop in FEV_1 at <10 mg/mL. A positive test for airways reactivity is not diagnostic, however, as many normal individuals and patients with chronic obstructive pulmonary disease have a positive test.

- Half of COPD patients have positive methacholine challenge testing
- **Positive test is nonspecific**
- **Negative methacholine challenge essentially rules out active asthma**
- **Useful in the case of chronic cough to rule out cough-variant asthma**

Carbon Monoxide Diffusing Capacity

- Tests the integrity of the alveolar-capillary surface area for gas exchange
  - Carbon monoxide diffusing capacity (DLCO) less than 80% predicted is abnormal
  - DLCO less than 50% predicted predicts exercise oxygen desaturation
- DLCO is **decreased in disorders that decrease pulmonary capillary blood volume**
  - **Interstitial lung diseases**
  - **Emphysema**
  - **Pulmonary vascular disease**
- **Normal DLCO strongly rules out clinically important interstitial disease**
- DLCO changes in disease states (Table 19-1)

- Utility
  - **Distinguishing emphysema from asthma (low in emphysema, normal or high in asthma)**
  - Evaluation of dyspnea
  - Monitoring occupational/toxic exposures (e.g., bleomycin)

Lung Volume Measurements

- **Useful for distinguishing restrictive lung diseases from obstructive lung diseases (Figs. 19-4 and 19-5)**
- Resident gas methods (helium dilution and nitrogen washout) may underestimate lung volumes with obstructive defects
- Body plethysmography is more accurate in obstructive diseases
- **Restrictive ventilatory defects have a reduction in all subdivisions of lung volume, including total lung capacity (TLC), vital capacity (VC), and residual volume (RV)**
- **Obstructive ventilatory defects typically cause elevation of TLC (hyperinflation) and RV (gas trapping) and a reduction in VC**
- Obesity typically causes a disproportionate reduction in functional residual capacity (FRC) with small reductions in TLC and VC

TABLE 19-1	*DLCO Changes in Disease States*
DLCO Normal or Increased	**DLCO Decreased**
Asthma	Emphysema
Polycythemia	Anemia
Obesity	Interstitial lung disease
Left-to-right shunt	Pneumonectomy
Supine position	Pulmonary hypertension
Post exercise	Pulmonary embolism
Pulmonary hemorrhage	

DLCO, diffusing capacity of the lungs for carbon monoxide.

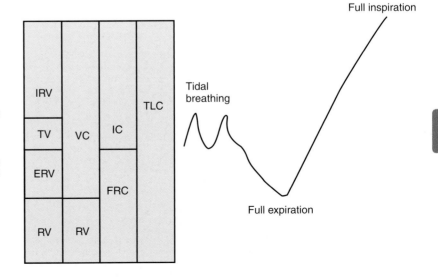

FIGURE 19-4 Lung volume subdivisions. Lung volumes are determined by measurement of FRC using a resident gas method (nitrogen washout or helium dilution) or Boyle's law method (body plethysmography). The remaining lung volumes are calculated from a period of tidal breathing followed by a slow vital capacity maneuver as shown on the right panel. ERV, expiratory reserve volume; FRC, functional residual capacity; IC, inspiratory capacity; IRV, inspiratory reserve volume; RV, residual volume; TLC, total lung capacity; TV, tidal volume; VC, vital capacity.

19

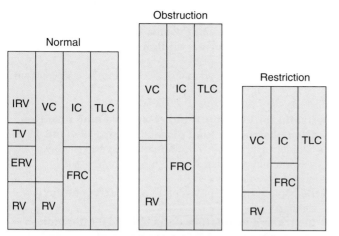

FIGURE 19-5 Abnormalities of lung volumes. Obstructive lung diseases cause elevation of TLC (hyperinflation) and RV (air trapping) with a net increase in the ratio of RV/TLC and a reduction in VC. Restrictive lung diseases cause proportionate reduction in all of the lung volumes. In obesity, however, a mild reduction in TLC is accompanied by a more marked reduction in FRC. ERV, expiratory reserve volume; FRC, functional residual capacity; IC, inspiratory capacity; IRV, inspiratory reserve volume; RV, residual volume; TLC, total lung capacity; TV, tidal volume; VC, vital capacity.

- Mnemonic for lung volumes: Four volumes that do not overlap and four capacities that do overlap

Respiratory Muscle Strength

- **Definitive test for respiratory muscle weakness is transdiaphragmatic pressure (Pdi)**
- Measured with balloon-tipped catheter to determine the pressure difference between esophagus (pleural pressure) and stomach (abdominal pressure)
- Maximum inspiratory pressure (MIP) is useful for screening for respiratory muscle weakness (i.e., diaphragmatic weakness/paralysis)
  - **Normal values between −100 and −140 cm H$_2$O**
- Bilateral diaphragm paralysis usually causes hypercapnia at moderate levels of restriction

- Clues to diaphragm paralysis
  - Orthopnea
  - Paradoxical abdominal motion with inspiration

Six-Minute Walk Test

- Simple assessment of functional exercise capacity
- Used to assess functional status (e.g., lung transplant evaluation) and response to treatment
- Predicts morbidity and mortality (COPD, pulmonary hypertension, heart failure)
- Test is performed under standard conditions
  - Patient walks as far as possible in 6 minutes
  - Patient can stop and rest during the 6 minutes as needed (clock continues)
  - Patients can use oxygen and necessary walking aids, such as canes
  - Defined course with laps of approximately 30 meters
  - Scripted language at each minute interval without coaching
  - Dyspnea and leg pain are recorded pre- and post-test (Borg scale)
- Results reported as absolute and percent predicted
- Interpretation of change in absolute value is recommended
- Clinically significant changes vary by disease

REVIEW QUESTIONS

For review questions, please go to www.expertconsult.com.

SUGGESTED READINGS

American Thoracic Society: ATS Statement: guidelines for the six-minute walk test, *Am J Respir Crit Care Med* 166:111–117, 2002.

Macintyre N, Crapo RO, Viegi G, et al: Standardisation of the single-breath determination of carbon monoxide uptake in the lung, *Eur Respir J* 26:720–735, 2005.

Miller MR, Hankinson J, Brusasco V, et al: Standardisation of spirometry, *Eur Respir J* 26:319–338, 2005.

Pellegrino R, Viegi G, Brusasco RO, et al: Interpretative strategies for lung function tests, *Eur Respir J* 26:948–968, 2005.

Wanger J, Clausen JL, Coates A, et al: Standardisation of the measurement of lung volumes, *Eur Respir J* 26:511–522, 2005.

West JB: *Respiratory physiology: the essentials,* Philadelphia, Lippincott, Williams and Wilkins, 2004.

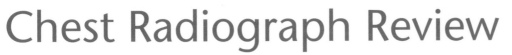

Chest Radiograph Review

CHRISTIAN A. MERLO, MD, MPH, and PETER B. TERRY, MD, MA

Pattern reading is the approach used by most radiologists to narrow the differential diagnosis when interpreting chest radiographs. This entails evaluation of both the character (e.g., nodule, mass, or infiltrate) and distribution (e.g., upper vs. lower lung field, and unilateral vs. bilateral) of pulmonary parenchymal abnormalities.

Nodules and Masses

Basic Information

- A nodule (Fig. 20-1) is defined as a lesion that measures less than 4 cm in diameter, and a mass (Figs. 20-2 to 20-5) is one that is greater than 4 cm in diameter. Lesions greater than 3 cm in diameter have a greater than 75% probability of being malignant.

Clinical Presentation

- **Smaller lesions are usually benign** because to be visible on a chest radiograph, they must be of high density, a property usually associated with calcification. Certain patterns of calcification suggest that the nodule is benign. **Eccentric calcification, although usually benign, may be associated with a malignant cause**. More benign patterns of calcification include
  - Diffuse complete calcification
  - Laminated calcification
  - Eggshell calcification
  - Central/"bull's-eye" calcification
  - Popcorn calcification
  - Onion skin calcification

Diagnosis and Evaluation

- The **differential diagnosis of nodules** includes
  - Infections
    - Bacterial (including abscesses)
    - Mycobacterial
    - Fungal
    - Parasitic (e.g., human infection with *Dirofilaria immitis* [dog heartworm])
  - Granulomata
  - Rheumatoid nodules
  - Wegener's granulomatosis
  - Vascular malformations
  - Bronchogenic cysts
  - Hamartoma
  - Primary or secondary lung neoplasms

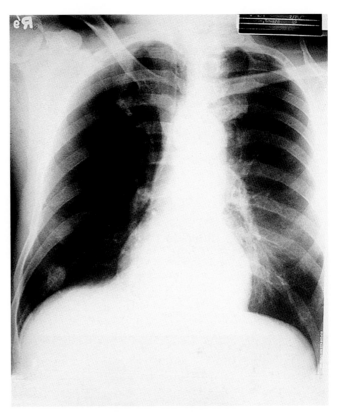

FIGURE 20-1 Nodule.

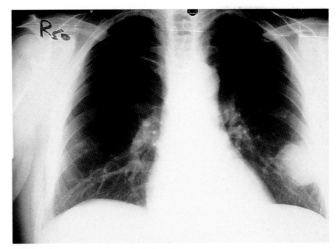

FIGURE 20-2 Mass.

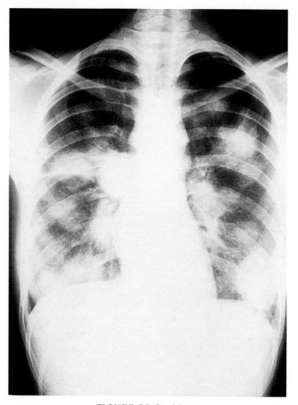

FIGURE 20-3 Mass.

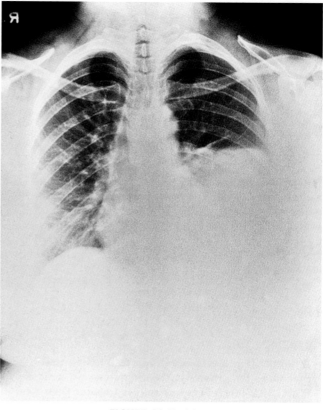

FIGURE 20-5 Mass.

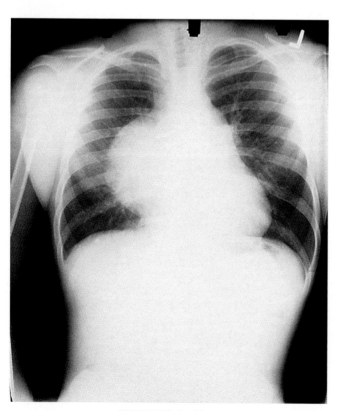

FIGURE 20-4 Mass.

- **The differential diagnosis of masses includes the preceding possibilities and is expanded to include sarcomas, fibromas, and progressive massive fibrosis (PMF)**
- **The differential diagnosis for anterior mediastinal masses ("terrible Ts") deserves particular attention and includes**
  - **T**eratoma
  - **T**hymoma
  - **T**hymolipoma
  - **T**hymic carcinoma/carcinoid
  - **T**hymic cyst
  - **T**horacic thyroid
  - **T**errible lymphoma

Infiltrates

Basic Information

- The radiographic pattern and constituents of infiltrates provide clues to their etiology

Clinical Presentation

- **Alveolar infiltrates (Figs. 20-6 to 20-8) are marked by their homogeneity, their irregular and often fluffy appearance, and the presence of air bronchograms (Fig. 20-9);** they may consist of
  - Water
    - Cardiogenic pulmonary edema
    - Noncardiogenic pulmonary edema

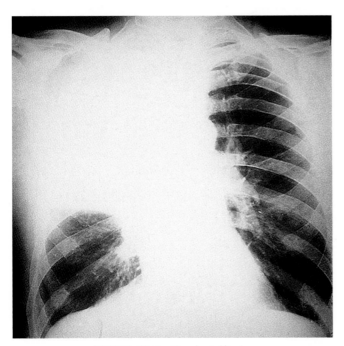

FIGURE 20-6   Alveolar infiltrate.

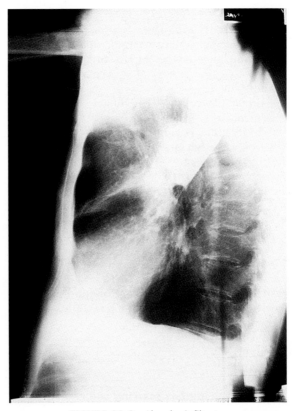

FIGURE 20-8   Alveolar infiltrate.

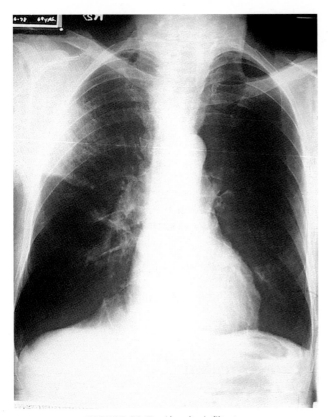

FIGURE 20-7   Alveolar infiltrate.

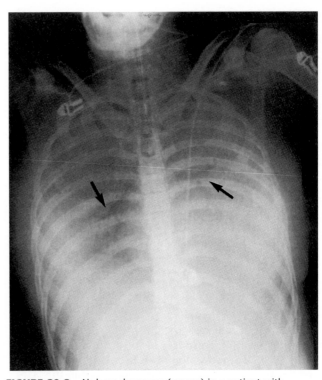

FIGURE 20-9   Air bronchograms (*arrows*) in a patient with alveolar infiltrates due to *Pneumocystis jiroveci* pneumonia. (From Souhami R: *Textbook of medicine,* New York, Churchill Livingstone, 2002, figure 13.12.)

20

- Blood
  - Goodpasture's syndrome
  - Idiopathic pulmonary hemosiderosis (IPH)
  - Systemic lupus erythematosus (SLE)
- Cells
  - Malignant
    - Bronchoalveolar cell carcinoma
  - Benign
    - Eosinophilic pneumonia
    - Desquamative interstitial pneumonitis–(DIP)
- Pus
  - Bacterial pneumonia
- Protein
  - Alveolar proteinosis
  - *Pneumocystis jiroveci* pneumonia (PCP)–associated protein in alveoli
- Calcium
  - Alveolar microlithiasis (very rare)
- **Interstitial infiltrates (Figs. 20-10 and 20-11) have a broad differential diagnosis, although the pattern helps to narrow the diagnostic possibilities:**
  - Reticular
  - Nodular
  - Combined—a very common pattern with a broad differential diagnosis
  - Linear
  - **Honeycomb—implies scarring and end-stage disease and is usually seen with IPF**
  - Ground glass
    - Bronchiolitis obliterans with organizing pneumonia (BOOP)
    - Sarcoidosis
    - Viral pneumonitis

Diagnosis and Evaluation

- **The pattern of distribution of interstitial infiltrates may provide clues to the specific diagnosis**
  - The **differential diagnosis of upper lobe infiltrates is generally small** and depends on the clinical history and whether the abnormality is unilateral or bilateral
    - Diffuse **bilateral** upper lobe infiltrates (Figs. 20-12 and 20-13)
      - Sarcoidosis
      - Eosinophilic granuloma
      - Ankylosing spondylitis
      - Cystic fibrosis
      - Hypersensitivity pneumonitis
      - Old tuberculosis or histoplasmosis
      - Pneumoconiosis (e.g., silicosis)
    - **Unilateral** upper lobe infiltrates (Figs. 20-14 to 20-16)
      - Infections
    - Tuberculosis
    - Histoplasmosis
    - Coccidioidomycosis
    - *Klebsiella* pneumonia
      - Primary lung neoplasms
- **The differential diagnosis of lower lobe infiltrates (Fig. 20-17) is generally much broader, but 80% of the time the differential is found within the following list:**
  - **Bronchiectasis (look for "tram tracks")**
  - **Aspiration (usually found in the superior or posterior basilar segments)**

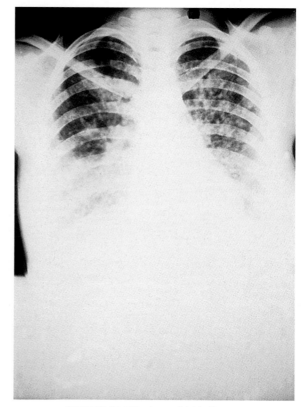

FIGURE 20-10   Interstitial infiltrate.

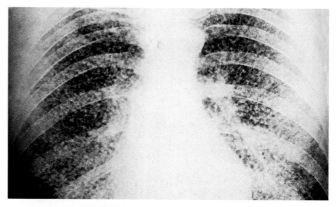

FIGURE 20-11   Interstitial infiltrate.

- Dermatomyositis/polymyositis
- **Asbestosis (always associated with rales on examination)**
- Scleroderma, SLE, Sjögren's syndrome
- Sarcoidosis (pleural thickening and effusions are seldom seen)
- Early Hamman-Rich syndrome/IPF (pleural disease is uncommon)
- Rheumatoid arthritis

Pleural Effusions

Basic Information

- **Both the size and side of a pleural effusion provide clues to its etiology**

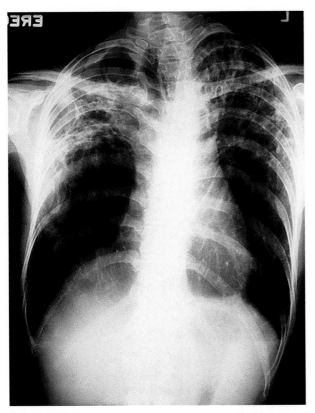

FIGURE 20-12   Bilateral upper lobe infiltrate.

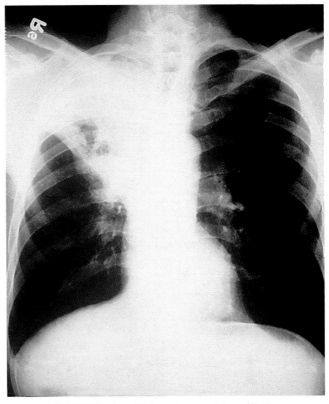

FIGURE 20-14   Unilateral upper lobe infiltrate.

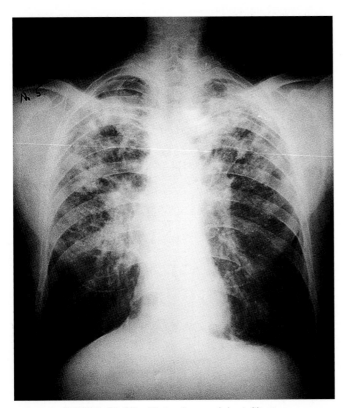

FIGURE 20-13   Bilateral upper lobe infiltrate.

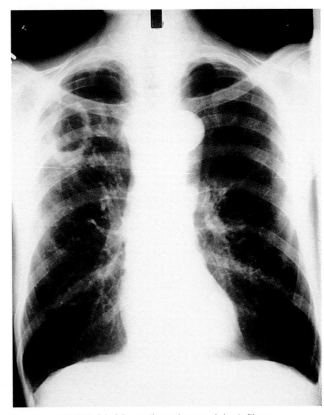

FIGURE 20-15   Unilateral upper lobe infiltrate.

20

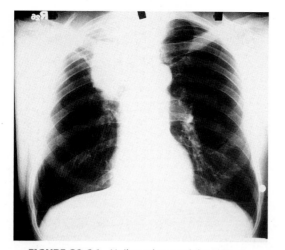

FIGURE 20-16 Unilateral upper lobe infiltrate.

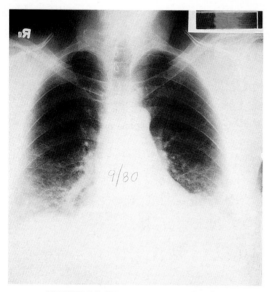

FIGURE 20-17 Lower lobe infiltrate.

- **A pleural effusion filling more than half (Fig. 20-18) of the hemithorax is likely caused by**
  - Trauma
  - Tumor
  - Tuberculosis
  - Hepatic hydrothorax (in patients with cirrhosis and ascites)
  - Chylothorax (caused by thoracic duct obstruction or disruption)

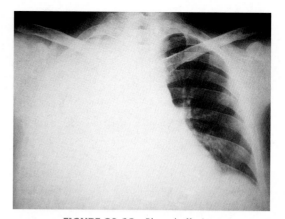

FIGURE 20-18 Pleural effusion.

- **An effusion that is bilateral and with a normal heart** is generally caused by
  - Tumor
  - Connective tissue disease
  - Viral infection
  - Congestive heart failure (less often)
- **An effusion that is bilateral and with an enlarged heart is generally caused by congestive heart failure**
- **Right-sided effusions** suggest
  - Congestive heart failure
  - Hepatic hydrothorax
  - Meigs' syndrome (in patients with benign ovarian tumors or fibroids)
- **Left-sided effusions** suggest
  - Aortic aneurysm dissection
  - Boerhaave's syndrome (esophageal rupture)
  - Pancreatitis
  - Splenic rupture or infarction

REVIEW QUESTIONS

For review questions, please go to www.expertconsult.com.

SUGGESTED READINGS

Fraser RG, Pare JAP, Pare PD, et al: *Diagnosis of diseases of the chest*, Philadelphia, WB Saunders, 1991.

Sherman CB: Inflammatory disease of the lung. In Barondess JA, Carpenter CJ (eds): *Differential diagnosis*, Philadelphia, Lea & Febiger, 1994.

Teeter JG, Terry PB: Pulmonary nodules, masses and mediastinal disease. In Barondess JA, Carpenter CJ (eds): *Differential diagnosis*, Philadelphia, Lea & Febiger, 1994.

Interstitial Lung Disease

MAUREEN R. HORTON, MD, and KATHARINE E. BLACK, MD

This chapter covers a group of diseases that all produce diffuse involvement of the lung parenchyma but are very distinct pathophysiologically. Some are primary pulmonary diseases; others are seen in association with systemic disorders. The pace of symptom onset, the presence or absence of extrapulmonary signs and symptoms, and the radiographic pattern of the process often provide clues to the etiology.

Idiopathic Pulmonary Fibrosis

Basic Information

- Two thirds of patient have onset of disease **when older than 60 years of age**
- No gender predominance
- Most common idiopathic interstitial pneumonia; over 60% of cases
- No known cause, cure, or effective treatment

Clinical Presentation

- Insidious onset over years; usually symptoms for 3 to 5 years prior to diagnosis
- Acute exacerbations portend worse prognosis
- **Exertional dyspnea; nonproductive cough; rare constitutional symptoms**
- Physical examination
  - "Dry, Velcro-like" crackles
  - Clubbing
  - Signs of elevated right-sided pressure on cardiac examination late in disease (e.g., elevated jugular venous pressure, edema, and right ventricular heave)

Diagnosis, Evaluation, and Treatment

- Imaging
  - Subpleural, peripheral reticular, and nodular infiltrates increased in the **basilar lung zones** with areas of honeycombing (Figs. 21-1 and 21-2)
  - Minimal ground glass infiltrates
  - May be asymmetrical
  - Decreasing lung volumes on serial chest radiographs
  - Honeycombing on CT scan correlates with fibrosis on biopsy
- Labs are nonspecific
- Pulmonary function tests (PFTs)
  - **Restrictive disease with decreased forced vital capacity (FVC), total lung capacity (TLC), and diffusing capacity for carbon monoxide (DLCO)**

- Diagnosis
  - Made from constellation of clinical history, radiographic findings, and the absence of other identifiable causes for fibrosis
  - Surgical lung biopsy demonstrating usual interstitial pneumonitis (UIP) is the gold standard for diagnosing idiopathic pulmonary fibrosis (IPF)
  - Not all patients require surgical lung biopsy if clinical picture is overwhelmingly suggestive
  - Table 21-1 lists diagnostic categories of alternative idiopathic interstitial pneumonias
- Therapy
  - No proven effective treatment for IPF
  - N-Acetylcysteine 600 mg tid has been demonstrated in one study to slow down the progression of IPF compared with placebo
  - Steroids have not been demonstrated to be effective; historic response rates less than 5% to 10%
  - Cytotoxic agents (azathioprine, cyclophosphamide) have been demonstrated to be ineffective
  - Lung transplantation remains the only effective treatment

Desquamative Interstitial Pneumonia

Basic Information

- Rare
- Name is misnomer, as histologic finding is not desquamated cells but macrophage infiltrate
- Ninety percent of patients are smokers
- Relation to respiratory bronchiolitis-associated interstitial lung disease (RBILD) controversial
- RBILD also smoking-related, involves infiltration of bronchioles, and is less severe

Imaging

- Linear opacities on chest radiograph, high-resolution computed tomography shows ground glass (50% basilar predominant); honeycombing not typically seen

Diagnosis

- Histology shows diffuse accumulation of intra-alveolar macrophages

Treatment

- Smoking cessation, steroids; up to 25% progress despite therapy (see Table 21-1)

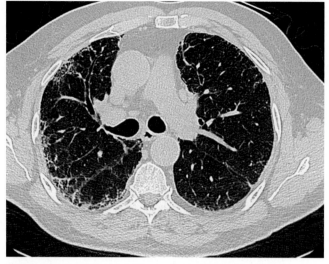

FIGURE 21-1   Reticular infiltrates in a patient with idiopathic pulmonary fibrosis. Note subpleural, peripheral distribution of infiltrates.

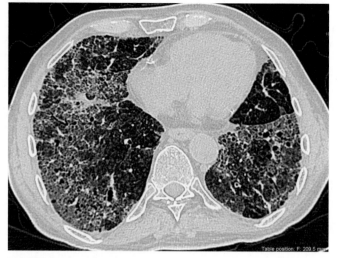

FIGURE 21-2   Lungs of a patient with end-stage idiopathic pulmonary fibrosis.

TABLE 21-1	*Idiopathic Interstitial Pneumonias*			
	UIP	**DIP**	**AIP**	**NSIP**
Onset	Insidious	Insidious	Acute	Subacute
Steroid response	Poor	Good	Poor	Good
Complete recovery?	No	Yes	Yes	Yes

AIP, acute interstitial pneumonitis; DIP, desquamative interstitial pneumonitis; NSIP, nonspecific interstitial pneumonitis; UIP, usual interstitial pneumonitis.

Connective Tissue Diseases

SYSTEMIC LUPUS ERYTHEMATOSUS

Basic Information

- Systemic lupus erythematosus (SLE) is a systemic disease that may involve the lung or pleura
- Rarely causes chronic interstitial lung disease (ILD)
- More than one manifestation may be present in a single patient

Clinical Presentation

Table 21-2 summarizes the clinical presentations of pulmonary SLE.
- Other clinical presentations may include
  - **Alveolar hemorrhage**
    - Acute fever, dyspnea, cough, with or without hemoptysis
    - **Falling hematocrit with new infiltrates suggests alveolar hemorrhage**
    - Can be diagnosed with bronchoscopy
    - May be seen in the presence or absence of the antiphospholipid antibody syndrome
  - **Diaphragm dysfunction**
    - "Shrinking lung syndrome": **Smaller lung volumes resulting from diaphragm weakness**

RHEUMATOID ARTHRITIS

Basic Information

- Although rheumatoid arthritis (RA) is more common in females, **RA lung disease is more common in males (3:1)**
- **RA lung disease precedes the disease in the joint in 20% of cases**
- Multiple pulmonary manifestations of RA

Clinical Presentation

See Table 21-2 for a summary of the clinical presentation of RA.
- Other clinical presentations may include
  - Rheumatoid (necrobiotic) nodules
    - **May be single or multiple and may cavitate**
    - Pathology of nodules reveals histiocytic palisades, specific for RA
    - Caplan's syndrome: Rheumatoid nodules in coal miners
  - Bronchiolitis obliterans
    - **Dyspnea, dry cough; chest radiograph clear or hyperinflated**
    - Obstruction on PFTs
    - Pathology reveals lymphoplasmacytic infiltration of airway wall
    - Poor response to therapy
  - Cricoarytenoid arthritis
    - **Pain, hoarseness, dyspnea, stridor, obstruction**
    - Symptoms in 25% of patients with RA

SCLERODERMA

Basic Information

- **60% to 100% of patients with scleroderma have ILD at autopsy**
- There are several manifestations of lung disease in scleroderma

Clinical Presentation

See Table 21-2.

TABLE 21-2 *Pulmonary Manifestations of Connective Tissue Diseases*

	SLE	RA	Scleroderma	PM
Acute pneumonitis	May be initial manifestation of SLE Acute onset fever, pneumonic symptoms Diffuse or patchy infiltrates in chest film Pleuritis, pericarditis are common	None	Aspiration pneumonia is common consequence of esophageal dysmotility	None
Interstitial disease	Progression from acute pneumonitis gradual; dyspnea, ± pleuritis, ± productive cough Lower lobe infiltrates on chest film, with increasing restriction of PFTs	Similar to IPF Dyspnea and cough are common Clubbing is common Lower lobe infiltrates, with or without honeycombing Variable response to corticosteroids	Can be seen in patients with CREST or diffuse disease Usually after skin disease Infiltrates are predominantly lower lobe Clubbing is rare Recurrent aspiration may present as interstitial disease	Progressive DOE ± Muscle symptoms Lower lobe infiltrates
Pleural disease	Pain, dyspnea, fever, and effusion are common Pleural fluid is exudative, with normal glucose and normal PH Pleural fluid ANA may be increased LE cells diagnostic	Symptoms related to pleural disease are present in 20% of patients Pleural fluid: Low pH, glucose <30 mg/dL in 70–80% of patients Pleural fluid RF may be increased and greater than serum RF	Thickening or effusions in 10–25%, but rarely symptomatic	None
Pulmonary hypertension	Rare without parenchymal disease May be primary arteriolar disease or secondary to interstitial lung disease	Secondary to hypoxia with severe ILD Idiopathic secondary to RA	Seen in 10% of patients with CREST Pulmonary hypertension in patients with scleroderma is a primary vascular disease, and occurs independent of parenchymal disease	Usually secondary to parenchymal disease

ANA, antinuclear antibody; CREST, calcinosis, Raynaud's syndrome, esophageal dysmotility, sclerodactyly, telangiectasia; DOE, dyspnea on exertion; ILD, interstitial lung disease; IPF, idiopathic pulmonary fibrosis; LE, lupus erythematosus; PFTs, pulmonary function tests; PM, polymyositis; RA, rheumatoid arthritis; RF, rheumatoid factor; SLE, systemic lupus erythematosus.

POLYMYOSITIS/DERMATOMYOSITIS

Basic Information

- More common in females
- 10% present with ILD prior to myositis
- Associated with anti-Jo or other antisynthetase antibodies
- Antisynthetase syndrome is ILD with minimal or subclinical muscle symptoms

Clinical Presentation

- Dyspnea on exertion (DOE), proximal muscle weakness, skin rash, "heliotrope" rash around eyes in polymyositis, "mechanic's hands"

Pulmonary/Renal Syndromes

WEGENER'S GRANULOMATOSIS

Basic Information

- Also known as "antineutrophil cytoplasmic antibody (ANCA)-positive granulomatous vasculitis"
- Two forms described

  - **Classic disease: Involving the upper and lower respiratory tracts and kidney**
  - **Limited disease: Isolated respiratory tract involvement**
- Characteristic pathology reveals necrotizing granulomatous inflammation and small-vessel vasculitis of the upper and lower respiratory tracts and necrotizing glomerulonephritis in the kidney

Clinical Presentation

See Table 21-3.

GOODPASTURE'S SYNDROME

Basic Information

- Disease affecting the lung and kidney associated with **circulating antiglomerular basement membrane antibodies** that may be the cause of the process (Fig. 21-3)
- The **lung and kidney are both involved in 60% to 80% of cases;** in the remainder the kidney is involved alone

Clinical Presentation

See Table 21-3.

TABLE 21-3	*Comparison of Pulmonary–Renal Disorders*	
	Wegener's Syndrome	**Goodpasture's Syndrome**
Presentation	Ears, nose, and throat are involved in 85% of patients Kidney is ultimately involved in 85% of cases Cough and dyspnea Pleural effusion, subglottic/bronchial stenoses or endobronchial lesions seen Wegener's granulomatosis can involve skin, joints, eyes, and neurologic system	Hemoptysis, dyspnea, cough, and fatigue are the primary symptoms Fever, chills, and weight loss occur in <25% of patients
Radiographic findings	Infiltrates, nodules, or cavitation may be seen Infiltrates or nodules may be unilateral or bilateral	Bilateral infiltrates are the most common chest radiographic finding
Diagnostic studies	ESR commonly increased Abnormal urinalysis 80% c-ANCA most strongly correlated with Wegener's granulomatosis, but sensitivity and specificity variable	Anemia is common Hematuria and proteinuria are seen in 90% of patients Anti-GBM antibodies are seen in 90% of patients Bilateral infiltrates are the most common chest radiograph finding Suspect when patient has the constellation of alveolar infiltrates, anemia, and renal disease Linear IgG in biopsy, or anti-GBM antibodies are diagnostic
Treatment	Limited disease: Methotrexate plus prednisone Life- or organ-threatening disease: Oral daily cytoxan plus prednisone If patient is severely ill, give solumedrol 1 g/d for 3 days followed by oral prednisone Cyclophosphamide for 3–6 mo; taper steroids over 6 mo 75–90% complete remission	Corticosteroids, cyclophosphamide, plasmapheresis

cANCA, antineutrophil cytoplasmic antibody; ESR, erythrocyte sedimentation rate; GBM, glomerular basement membrane; IgG, immunoglobulin.

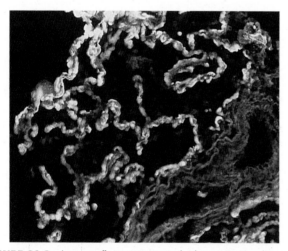

FIGURE 21-3 Immunofluorescence study demonstrating linear staining (immunoglobulin G) of alveolar walls in a patient with Goodpasture's syndrome. (Original magnification ×10.) (From Mason RJ: *Murray and Nadel's textbook of respiratory medicine,* ed 4, London, Elsevier, 2005, figure 56.8.)

Eosinophilic Lung Diseases

Basic Information

- Diverse group of diseases, all of which exhibit blood or tissue eosinophilia

Clinical Presentation and Treatment

- Acute eosinophilic pneumonia
  - Acute presentation with infiltrates and hypoxemia with or without peripheral eosinophilia
  - **Diagnosis requires eosinophilia in bronchoalveolar lavage (BAL) fluid or lung tissue**
  - Very steroid-responsive
- Chronic eosinophilic pneumonia
  - Subacute presentation with constitutional symptoms, cough, dyspnea, and **peripheral eosinophilia**
  - Chest radiograph with peripheral infiltrates ("**reverse pulmonary edema**"; Fig. 21-4)
  - Diagnosis requires BAL eosinophilia (>40% diagnostic) or lung tissue eosinophilia
  - Very steroid-responsive
  - May develop severe asthma and require chronic steroid use
- Hypereosinophilic syndrome
  - Defined as more than **1500 eosinophils/mm³ in peripheral blood for 6 months**
  - Primary targets include the **heart, central nervous system, peripheral nervous system, and skin; the lung is less commonly involved**
  - Therapy with corticosteroids or cytotoxic agents (or both)
- Allergic bronchopulmonary aspergillosis (ABPA)
  - Clinical constellation of **asthma, eosinophilia, infiltrates, and mucous plugs**

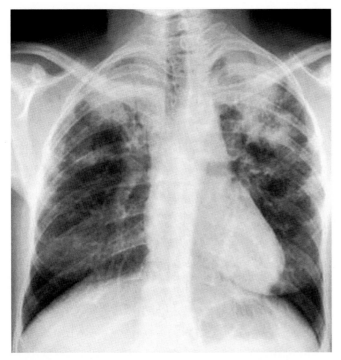

FIGURE 21-4 Chest radiograph of a patient with idiopathic chronic eosinophilic pneumonia showing bilateral alveolar opacities predominating in the upper lobes ("reverse pulmonary edema"). (From Mason RJ: *Murray and Nadel's textbook of respiratory medicine,* ed 4, London, Elsevier, 2005, figure 57-3.)

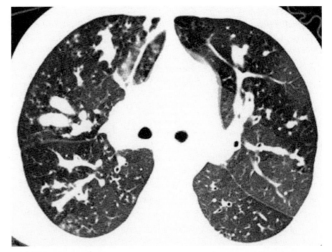

FIGURE 21-5 Axial computed tomography scan of a patient with allergic bronchopulmonary aspergillosis showing central bronchiectasis with mucoid impaction. Diffuse bilateral inhomogeneous lung opacity is present, with areas of low attenuation throughout the pulmonary parenchyma representing mosaic perfusion resulting from a combination of large and small airway inflammation. (From Mason RJ: *Murray and Nadel's textbook of respiratory medicine,* ed 4, London, Elsevier, 2005, figure 57-7.)

- Bronchiectasis may result (Fig. 21-5)
- Diagnosis is made by demonstrating eosinophilia, a positive skin test or antibodies to *Aspergillus,* an increased total and specific IgE, and recurrent infiltrates on chest film
  - Very responsive to corticosteroids and itraconazole
- Allergic angiitis and granulomatosis (i.e., Churg-Strauss syndrome)
  - Clinical constellation of **asthma, eosinophilia, and systemic vasculitis**
  - Lung biopsies reveal eosinophilia and extravascular granulomas
  - **Asthma is present in more than 80% of patients** and radiographic infiltrates are present in more than 90% of patients; 30% have pleural effusions
  - Disease may be unmasked after tapering systemic steroids in an asthmatic
  - **This is a systemic illness, with skin (75% of patients) and peripheral nervous system (mononeuritis multiplex in 60% of cases) involvement**
    - **The heart and GI tract may also be involved**
    - The kidney is rarely involved
  - Usually responsive to corticosteroids
- Eosinophilic granuloma (pulmonary Langerhans cell histiocytosis)
  - Pulmonary Langerhans cell histiocytosis—non-neoplastic collection of Langerhans cells
  - Despite name, not actually eosinophilic lung disease but rather a variant of histiocytosis X seen in smoking adults (Box 21-1)

BOX 21-1	*Eosinophilic Granuloma*

Pulmonary Langerhans cell histiocytosis

Cough and dyspnea in two thirds of patients

Smoking history in 90% of patients

Radiographic manifestations: Progression from diffuse nodules to reticulonodular pattern to diffuse cystic changes in severe disease

Spares costophrenic angles

Pneumothorax common

May have associated central diabetes insipidus and bone cysts

Biopsies reveal CD1a(+), s100+ Langerhans cells on light microscopy with Birbeck granules on electron microscopy

Prognosis usually good with smoking cessation

Bronchiolitis Obliterans Organizing Pneumonia/Cryptogenic Organizing Pneumonia

Basic Information

- **Pathologic diagnosis** of fibroblast and inflammatory cell plugs filling bronchioles, alveolar ducts, and alveoli
- This is a nonspecific histologic reaction that can be **seen in response to infections, connective tissue diseases, or drugs, or may be idiopathic**
- A diagnosis of bronchiolitis obliterans organizing pneumonia (BOOP) typically means the idiopathic form
- This is a different entity from bronchiolitis obliterans (Box 21-2)

Basic Information

A variety of associations, including postinfection (viral primarily); post-transplant; toxin/fumes exposure; drugs (e.g., penicillamine, gold); and connective tissue diseases

There is also an idiopathic form

Clinical Presentation

The primary clinical manifestation is dyspnea

Evaluation and Diagnosis

Pulmonary function tests reveal obstruction or air-trapping with high residual volumes

Chest radiographs may reveal hyperinflation or may be normal

Lung biopsies demonstrate a constrictive bronchiolitis

Treatment

The response to corticosteroid therapy is generally poor

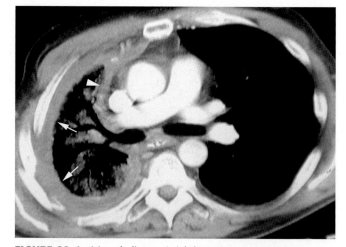

FIGURE 21-6   Mesothelioma. Axial thoracic computed tomography scan shows diffuse right pleural thickening (*arrows*) associated with marked volume loss in the right thorax. Note the presence of mediastinal pleural involvement (*arrowhead*). (From Mason RJ: *Murray and Nadel's textbook of respiratory medicine,* ed 4, London, Elsevier, 2005, figure 70.2.)

Clinical Presentation

- Idiopathic BOOP commonly presents as a subacute illness with an infectious-like onset
  - Cough, dyspnea, and fever are the most common symptoms
  - Crackles or squeaks are present on lung examination in 75% of patients

Evaluation and Diagnosis

- **Patchy infiltrates,** which may migrate, are the most common radiographic finding
- **Pulmonary function tests reveal restriction and hypoxemia, in contrast to bronchiolitis obliterans, which is characterized by an obstructive PFT pattern**
- Obstruction is seen in only 20% of patients with BOOP; nearly all are smokers

Treatment

- Idiopathic **BOOP is steroid-responsive,** with typical doses 0.75 to 1.5 mg/kg prednisone/day
- Relapse is common if the duration of therapy is less than six months
- The response to therapy in drug- and connective tissue disease-associated BOOP is much less predictable

Asbestos-Related Lung Disease

Basic Information

- Disease results from chronic exposure over prolonged periods, usually years
- Sources of exposure include the auto industry (brakes), construction, demolition, shipbuilding and renovation, cement industry, and mining

Clinical Presentation

- Asbestosis
  - Manifests as progressive dyspnea, usually 10+ years after exposure

- Intensity of asbestos exposure affects expression and latency
- Interstitial fibrosis, primarily in the lower lobe infiltrates similar to IPF
- Pleural disease
  - Benign pleural disease typically first manifestation; includes pleural plaques, thickening, and benign effusions
    - **Mesothelioma is a malignant tumor of the pleura,** presenting with chest pain that may be pleuritic, dyspnea, weight loss, and cough, after a latency of 20 to 40 years (Fig. 21-6)
    - **Mesothelioma is not affected by smoking**
    - There is no effective therapy
- Lung cancer and asbestos
  - The risk of lung cancer in an asbestos-exposed individual is increased four- to fivefold in a nonsmoker and by 50-fold in smokers, compared with nonasbestos-exposed nonsmokers

Sarcoidosis

Basic Information

- Sarcoidosis is a systemic disease of unknown origin
- Pathologic **hallmark is the noncaseating granuloma**
- Presentation
  - Most instances (70–80%) occur between the ages of 20 and 50 years
  - More common in blacks, females in the United States
  - 30% to 60% of cases are asymptomatic

Clinical Presentation

- Constitutional symptoms including weight loss, fatigue, fever, and malaise may occur
- Respiratory tract
  - The lung is involved in more than 90% of cases
  - Cough, dyspnea, sputum production, and hemoptysis can be seen

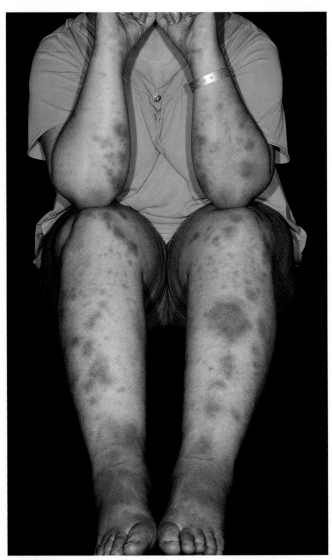

FIGURE 21-7 Erythema nodosum. (From Habif TP: *Clinical dermatology: a color guide to diagnostic therapy,* ed 4, St. Louis, Mosby, 2004, figure 18-9.)

- Endobronchial disease may produce obstructive symptoms
- The upper respiratory tract can be involved, producing nasal and upper airway obstruction or hoarseness
- Mycetomas often seen in fibrocystic sarcoid lesions
- Eye
  - Uveitis and keratoconjunctivitis
  - Sicca syndrome (dry eyes and mouth)
  - Uveoparotid fever in sarcoidosis (Heerfordt-Waldenström syndrome) is the constellation of bilateral lacrimal and parotid gland enlargement, fever, and anterior uveitis
- Heart
  - Myocardial granulomatous inflammation can produce conduction abnormalities, tachyarrhythmias, cardiomyopathy, and sudden death
  - Cor pulmonale can be seen in patients with chronic severe pulmonary disease
- Neurologic
  - Up to 5% of patients with sarcoidosis have neurologic manifestations

- Central nervous system findings may precede other findings but peripheral nerves are typically involved late
- Cranial nerves (VII, II, IX, X, VIII), meninges, and pituitary most involved
- Lumbar puncture may reveal increased cells (typically monocyte predominant), protein, or opening pressure or decreased glucose, but CSF is normal in up to 30% of patients with neurosarcoid
- Skin
  - Erythema nodosum most common skin finding (Fig. 21-7)
    - **Löfgren's syndrome: Erythema nodosum with hilar adenopathy, arthralgias, and fever; spontaneous resolution common**
  - Lupus pernio: Purplish nodules or plaques on cheeks, nose, and ears
  - Treatment of skin disease may be with chloroquine or pentoxifylline rather than corticosteroids
- Liver
  - Granulomas in liver in 75% of patients
  - Only 35% have elevated liver function tests, alkaline phosphatase best predictor
  - Symptomatic liver disease uncommon

Evaluation and Diagnosis

- Chest radiographs in patients with sarcoidosis have been typed (or staged) based on the pattern of abnormalities (Table 21-4 and Fig. 21-8)

TABLE 21-4	*Chest Radiographic Staging in Sarcoidosis*	
Type	**Distribution**	**Frequency (%)**
0	Normal	10
I	Hilar nodes	40
II	Hilar nodes + infiltrates	35
III	Infiltrates ± fibrosis/ honeycomb	15

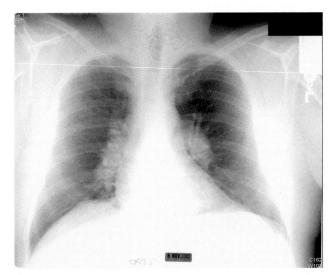

FIGURE 21-8 Posteroanterior chest radiograph of stage I sarcoidosis. Important features include prominent hilar lymphade-nopathy and normal lungs. (From Mason RJ: *Murray and Nadel's textbook of respiratory medicine,* ed 4, London, Elsevier, 2005, figure 55-1.)

- Disease progression not necessarily from one stage to next
- **Tissue biopsy revealing noncaseating granulomas is required for the diagnosis**
- Serum angiotensin-converting enzyme level may be elevated in patients with sarcoidosis and may track with disease activity but is nonspecific and nondiagnostic, so its role in management is undefined

Treatment

- Treatment should be limited to symptomatic or progressive pulmonary disease or any involvement of heart, eye, or nervous system
- Corticosteroids (usually low to moderate doses) are mainstay of therapy; alternative regimens are under investigation

REVIEW QUESTIONS

For review questions, please go to www.expertconsult.com.

SUGGESTED READINGS

Browne K: Asbestos-related disorders. In Parkes WR (ed): *Occupational lung disorders,* Boston, Butterworth Heinemann, 1994.

Delaney P: Neurologic manifestations of sarcoidosis, *Ann Intern Med* 87: 336–345, 1977.

Epler GR (ed): *Diseases of the bronchioles,* New York, Raven Press, 1994.

Johns CJ, Scott PP, Schonfeld SA: Sarcoidosis, *Ann Rev Med* 40: 353–371, 1989.

Katzenstein A-L: *Katzenstein and Askin's surgical pathology of non-neoplastic lung disease,* Philadelphia, WB Saunders, 1997.

Katzenstein A-L, Myers JL: Idiopathic pulmonary fibrosis, *Am J Respir Crit Care Med* 157:1301–1315, 1998.

Nothe I, Martinez F: Recent advances in idiopathic pulmonary fibrosis, *Chest* 132(2):637–650, 2007.

Schwarz MI, King TE, Cherniak RM: Principles of and approach to the patient with interstitial lung disease. In Murray JF, Nadel JA, editors: *Textbook of respiratory medicine,* ed 3, Philadelphia, WB Saunders, 2000.

Venous Thromboembolic Disease

DAVID B. PEARSE, MD

Venous thromboembolism, which includes deep venous thrombosis (DVT) and pulmonary thromboembolism (PE), occurs for the first time in approximately 100 persons per 100,000 in the United States each year. **More than 80% of clinically significant pulmonary emboli occur from DVTs in the lower extremities;** the remaining emboli originate from pelvic and upper extremity veins. The estimated short-term mortality rate from untreated PE (30%) is markedly reduced (<5%) by successful diagnosis and appropriate therapy. Unfortunately, the diagnoses of DVT and PE are frequently missed, and effective prophylactic treatment is underused.

Deep Venous Thrombosis

Basic Information

- Virchow's triad
  - Venous stasis
    - Immobility
    - Elevated venous pressure
    - Elevated blood viscosity
  - **Vessel wall damage**
  - **Increased blood coagulability**
    - Activation of clotting
    - Inhibition of fibrinolytic system
    - Deficiencies of coagulation factors
- Mechanisms
  - **Most important clinical risk is venous stasis from immobility**

Clinical Risk Factors

- Lower extremity DVT
  - Recent surgery
  - Major trauma **(>50% develop DVT if prophylaxis not implemented)**
  - Previous DVT **(30% recurrence over 8 years after first DVT)**
  - Increasing age (exponential increase after age 50 years)
  - Pregnancy/puerperium (PE is second leading cause of death; 75% occur postpartum)
  - Oral contraception
  - Medical conditions with immobility/hypercoagulability
    - Common: Cancer, heart failure, myocardial infarction, obesity, myeloproliferative disorder, nephrotic syndrome

- Uncommon: Systemic lupus erythematosus, antiphospholipid antibody, sickle cell anemia, homocystinuria, Behçet's syndrome
- Upper extremity DVT
  - Central venous catheter
  - Cancer

Familial Thrombophilic Disorders

- Common
  - Activated protein C resistance (factor V Leiden)
    - Autosomal dominant defect of factor V: Prevents inactivation by protein C
    - 5% normal white population; rare in those of African or Asian descent
    - 20% unselected DVT patients; 60% idiopathic, recurrent DVT
  - Prothrombin 20210A
    - Gene defect causing increased prothrombin and thrombin
    - 2% normal white population; rare in those of African or Asian descent
    - 5% unselected DVT, problematic when coexisting with other defects
- Rare
  - Deficiencies of antithrombin III, protein C, protein S
    - Autosomal dominant
    - **Protein C or S deficiency associated with warfarin-induced skin necrosis**

Clinical Presentation

- Symptoms and signs neither sensitive nor specific
  - Only 35% of symptomatic patients have leg DVT
  - Leg pain or swelling may be present
  - Homans' sign (pain and tenderness with dorsiflexion of ankle) present in less than 40%
- Starts in calf (except leg trauma, orthopedic surgery); most self-limited
- 25% of calf DVT extend to thigh
- **Thigh DVT strongly associated with PE**
  - Untreated symptomatic proximal DVT: 20% mortality from acute PE
  - 40% to 50% of patients with symptomatic thigh DVT have silent PE
- DVT recurs in 30% by 8 years; 50% of recurrences in contralateral leg

Diagnosis and Evaluation

- Noninvasive
  - B-mode compression ultrasonography (US)
    - Visualizes noncompressable clot in proximal veins; **poor for calf DVT**
    - 97% sensitive and specific for symptomatic proximal leg DVT
    - 30% to 60% sensitive, 98% specific for asymptomatic proximal leg DVT
    - **Initial test of choice for upper extremity DVT evaluation** but sensitivity and specificity 80%
    - Addition of Doppler flow or color adds little to sensitivity
  - CT venography
    - Performed with spiral chest CT; able to visualize clot in thigh, pelvic veins, inferior vena cava (IVC)
    - **Performed with injured or casted leg** as US cannot be performed in this scenario
    - Contrast dye load
    - **Sensitivity and specificity comparable to compression US**
  - MRI
    - Able to visualize clot in calf, thigh, pelvic veins, IVC, upper extremities
    - Performed with injured or casted leg as US cannot be performed in this scenario
    - No contrast dye load
    - **Sensitivity and specificity greater than 90%**
- D-Dimer
  - Degradation product of cross-linked fibrin
  - Elevated in DVT/PE but also in
    - Surgery, trauma, malignancy, disseminated intravascular coagulopathy, pregnancy, infection
  - Assay
    - Enzyme-linked immunosorbent assay (ELISA) more sensitive than latex agglutination
    - Positive D-dimer not helpful; negative (i.e., normal) D-dimer more clinically useful as follows
      - Normal D-dimer with low pretest probability for DVT or PE excludes thromboembolism
      - Normal highly sensitive D-dimer with nondiagnostic $\dot{V}/\dot{Q}$ scan excludes PE
  - Usefulness limited in inpatients
- Invasive: Venography
  - **Gold standard,** detects thigh, calf, and upper extremity DVT regardless of symptoms
  - **Can distinguish between acute and recurrent clot**
  - Requires risks of contrast dye
  - Painful, can cause thrombosis
  - Decreasing availability
- DVT diagnosis in the **symptomatic** lower extremity
  - Determine pretest clinical risk using Well's prediction rule (Table 22-1)
  - Low clinical suspicion and normal D-dimer
    - Further testing unnecessary, low incidence of DVT/PE if no therapy given
  - Low clinical suspicion and negative US (if D-dimer not available)
    - Further testing unnecessary, low incidence of DVT/PE if no therapy given
  - Moderate or high clinical suspicion: US necessary

TABLE 22-1	*Assessment of Pretest Probability of Deep-Vein Thrombosis (DVT)*
Variables	**Points**
Active cancer	1
Paralysis, paresis, or recent plaster immobilization of lower extremities	1
Bedridden > 3 days or major surgery within 12 wk	1
Localized tenderness along deep veins	1
Swelling of entire leg	1
Calf swelling > 3 cm larger than other side	1
Pitting edema of symptomatic leg	1
Collateral superficial veins	1
Alternative diagnosis at least as likely as DVT	−2

Clinical pretest probability for PE: Low, <1; intermediate, 1–2; high, >2. Data from Wells PS, Hirsh J, Anderson DR, et al: Accuracy of clinical assessment of deep-vein thrombosis. *Lancet* 345:1326–1330, 1995.

- **Negative initial US:** 15% of these patients have calf DVT; 20% to 30% of which will extend to thigh
  - US should be repeated at 1 week
- Negative serial US: Acceptable 1% to 2% risk of thromboembolism if untreated
- Immediate venogram is alternative to serial US

DVT Treatment/Prophylaxis

- Treatment of DVT—see PE treatment
- Prophylaxis choice depends on the risk of thrombosis for an individual (Table 22-2)

Pulmonary Embolism

Basic Information

- Effects of pulmonary emboli on gas exchange
  - Dead space increased but **arterial partial pressure of carbon dioxide ($Paco_2$) normal or low** (from hyperventilation)
  - **Hypoxemia variable** because it is epiphenomenon of clot (atelectasis, interatrial shunt)
- Effects of pulmonary emboli on pulmonary and systemic hemodynamics
  - In previously healthy patients
    - Peripheral vascular resistance (PVR) increase proportional to obstruction
    - Pulmonary artery pressure (Ppa) increases after 30% to 50% bed occluded
    - Normal right ventricle (RV): Maximal mean Ppa of 40 mm Hg
  - In patients with preexisting heart/lung disease
    - No correlation of clot burden with PVR or Ppa
  - Shock
    - Increased right atrial pressure decreases venous return
    - RV distension leads to shift interventricular septum, causing impaired left ventricular function

TABLE 22-2	*DVT Prophylaxis*	
	Clinical Risks	**Prophylaxis**
Low risk (<10% DVT*)	Minor surgery in mobile patients Medical patients who are fully mobile	Early ambulation Compression stockings
Moderate risk (10–40% DVT)	Most general, open gynecologic or urogenital surgery Medical patients, bed rest or sick Moderate risk plus high bleeding risk	LMWH (e.g., enoxaparin 40 mg SQ qd) LDUH (5000 U SQ bid or tid), fondaparinux Mechanical thromboprophylaxis†
High risk (40–80% DVT)	Hip or knee arthroplasty Hip fracture surgery Extensive trauma Stroke, spinal cord injury Major cancer surgery or major surgery with history of DVT	LMWH (e.g., enoxaparin 40 mg qd or 30 mg bid) fondaparinux (hip surgery or fracture), or moderate-dose warfarin (INR 2–3) Continue LMWH after hospital discharge for up to 28 days

*Rates based on objective diagnostic screening for DVT in patients not receiving thromboprophylaxis.
†Mechanical thromboprophylaxis includes intermittent pneumatic compression and/or graduated compression stockings.
DVT, deep-vein thromboembolism; INR, international normalized rate; LDUH, low-dose unfractionated heparin; LMWH, low-molecular-weight heparin.
From Geerts WH, Bergqvist D, Pineo GH, et al: Prevention of venous thromboembolism. *Chest* 133:381S–453S, 2008.

Clinical Presentation

- **PE presents as**
  - **Infarction-like syndrome: Chest pain, cough, hemoptysis (65%)**
  - **Dyspnea syndrome (22%)**
  - **Circulatory collapse (8%)**
- **Major symptoms: Dyspnea, chest pain, cough**
- **Major signs: Tachypnea, crackles, tachycardia**
  - Dyspnea, tachypnea, or pleuritic chest pain present in 97% PE

Diagnosis and Evaluation

See Figures 22-1 and 22-2.
- Chest radiograph and electrocardiogram (ECG)
  - Abnormal 70% to 90%, but nonspecific
    - Atelectasis, consolidation, diaphragm elevation on chest film
    - Nonspecific ST changes on ECG
- Arterial blood gases
  - **Wide alveolar-to-arterial O₂ gradient**
  - **Respiratory alkalosis**
  - Hypoxemia with the following caveats
    - 12% to 25% of patients have an arterial oxygen partial pressure (Pao_2) greater than 80 mm Hg
    - 20% have normal age-defined alveolar-to-arterial O_2 gradient
- PE diagnosis in the symptomatic patient
  - Determine pretest clinical risk using Well's prediction rule (Table 22-3)
  - Low or intermediate clinical risk and normal D-dimer
    - Further testing unnecessary, low incidence of DVT/PE if no therapy given
  - Low clinical risk and elevated D-dimer or high clinical risk
- Lung imaging with ventilation/perfusion ($\dot{V}/\dot{Q}$) scan (Fig. 22-3 and Table 22-4) or spiral CT scan
  - Normal $\dot{V}/\dot{Q}$ scan rules out PE regardless of clinical suspicion or ventilation scan findings
    - High probability $\dot{V}/\dot{Q}$ and moderate/high clinical probability: 88% to 96% positive predictive value

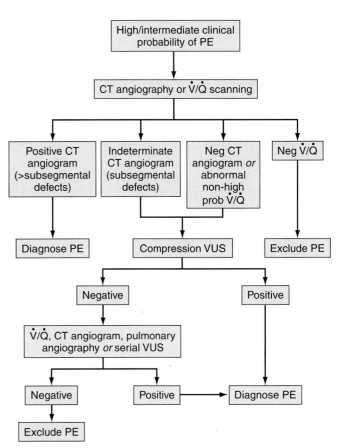

FIGURE 22-1 Proposed diagnostic algorithm for pulmonary embolism (PE) in patients with high or intermediate pretest probability using either $\dot{V}/\dot{Q}$ scan or CT angiography as initial test. $\dot{V}/\dot{Q}$, ventilation perfusion scan; VUS, venous ultrasound. (Modified from Fedullo PF, Tapson VF: Clinical practice: the evaluation of suspected pulmonary embolism, *N Engl J Med* 349:1247, 2003.)

- High probability $\dot{V}/\dot{Q}$ and low clinical probability: 50% positive predictive value
- All other abnormal scan/clinical probability combinations: PE risk unpredictable but substantial (20–40%)

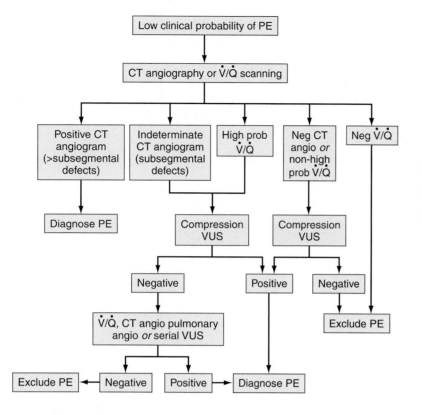

FIGURE 22-2 Proposed diagnostic algorithm for pulmonary embolism (PE) in patients with low pretest probability using either V̇/Q̇ scan or CT angiography as initial test. V̇/Q̇, ventilation perfusion scan; VUS, venous ultrasound. (Modified from Fedullo PF, Tapson VF: Clinical practice: the evaluation of suspected pulmonary embolism, *N Engl J Med* 349:1247, 2003.)

TABLE 22-3	*Assessment of Pretest Probability of Pulmonary Embolism*
Variables	**Points**
Clinical signs and symptoms of DVT	3.0
Alternative diagnosis less likely than PE	3.0
Heart rate > 100/min	1.5
Immobilization or surgery in preceding 4 weeks	1.5
Previous DVT or PE	1.5
Hemoptysis	1.0
Cancer	1.0

Clinical pretest probability for PE: Low, <2; intermediate, 2–6; high, >6. DVT, deep-vein thromboembolism; PE, pulmonary thromboembolism. From Wells PS, Ginsberg JS, Anderson DR, et al: Use of a clinical model for safe management of patients with suspected pulmonary embolism, *Ann Intern Med* 129:997–1005, 1998.

- Specificity of high probability V̇/Q̇ not altered by underlying lung disease such as COPD
- Proximal filling defects on spiral CT scan diagnostic (Fig. 22-4); single distal filling defects can be false positive, so further testing generally necessary
- Negative multidetector spiral CT adequate stopping point only if low or intermediate pretest risk
- If additional testing needed, can perform V̇/Q̇, spiral CT, pulmonary angiography or lower extremity US as secondary test depending on initial test choice

- Role for serial leg studies
  - Low/intermediate clinical probability, intermediate or low probability V̇/Q̇, negative leg US, and good cardiopulmonary reserve
    - Two additional leg studies at 7 and 14 days off anticoagulant; if negative, no treatment
  - Poor cardiopulmonary reserve (shock, syncope, RV dysfunction, respiratory failure) or severe symptoms
- Lung imaging with spiral CT or angiography
  - This strategy results in
    - Less than 10% overall need for pulmonary angiography in PE workup
    - Less than 3% subsequent thromboembolism at 3 months if anticoagulant withheld

Treatment

- Acceptable forms of therapy
  - Unfractionated heparin (UH) 80 U/kg IV bolus, 18 U/kg/hour, activated partial thromboplastin time (aPTT) 1.5 to 2.5 continuous *or*
  - UH 17,500 U SQ every 12 hours, aPTT 1.5 to 2.5 continuous, *or*
  - Low-molecular-weight heparin (LMWH) 100 U/kg every 12 hours or 200 U/kg once per day (no monitoring, contraindicated if renal failure), *then*
  - Warfarin 5 mg/day started day 1, overlapped with heparin 2 days, target international normalized ration (INR) 2 to 3
    - Protein C and S decline when warfarin is started during an active thrombotic state. This decline causes an increase in thrombogenic potential. Heparin can counteract this temporary procoagulant effect.

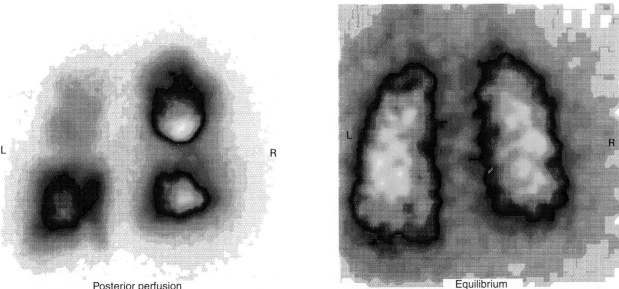

22

Posterior perfusion

Equilibrium

FIGURE 22-3 Lung ventilation and perfusion scintigraphy. **A,** Multiple perfusion defects in left upper lobe and right midzone on perfusion scan. **B,** Normal ventilation scan. This combination is consistent with high probability of pulmonary embolism. (From Haslett C, Chilvers ER, Boon NA, et al: *Davidson's principles and practice of medicine*, ed 19, New York, Churchill Livingstone, 2002, figure 13.6.)

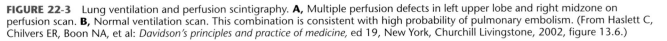

TABLE 22-4	*Ventilation/Perfusion Lung Scanning: The PIOPED Study Criteria*	
Scan Pattern (Prevalence)	**Original Definition**	**Revised Definition**
High probability (13%)	Segmental mismatches ≥ 2 large 1 large + 2 moderate ≥4 moderate	≥2 moderate/large segmental mismatch
Intermediate (39%)	Not high or low	1 moderate/large segmental mismatch or match Not high or low
Low (34%)	1 moderate/large segmental mismatch ≤4 moderate/large segmental match	>3 small subsegmental defects Nonsegmental perfusion defects
Very low/normal (14%)	Normal perfusion ≤3 small subsegmental perfusion defects	Normal perfusion ≤3 small subsegmental perfusion defects

PIOPED, Prospective Investigation of Pulmonary Embolism Diagnosis.

- PE/DVT: Duration of therapy
  - **Three months with reversible major risk factors**
  - **Six months with reversible minor risk factors** (estrogen therapy, partial immobilization)
  - **Six months to indefinite for idiopathic DVT/PE**
    - Indefinite if low bleeding risk and patient agrees
    - Six months if significant bleeding risk or patient refuses indefinite treatment
  - **Twelve months to indefinite for**
    - First DVT/PE with cancer, antiphospholipid antibody, deficiency of antithrombin III (ATIII), or
    - Second DVT/PE, which is idiopathic or associated with thrombophilic disorder
    - Indefinite if low bleeding risk and patient agrees
    - Twelve months if significant bleeding risk or patient refuses indefinite treatment
- Thrombolytic therapy (TT)
  - TT indicated for

- **PE with severe hemodynamic/oxygenation compromise**
  - In PE, TT accelerates resolution of physiologic abnormalities and scan defects
  - However, no difference at 7 days compared with heparin
- **Extensive iliofemoral DVT**
  - Decreases postphlebitic syndrome
  - Use of TT in submassive PE (normal blood pressure but RV dysfunction) controversial
    - Submassive PE associated with increased mortality on heparin therapy
- TT not shown to decrease mortality in this subgroup
- Risk of TT
  - Serious bleeding 6% to 45% (threefold > heparin)
  - Fatal bleeding 2% (10-fold > heparin)
- Approved drugs
  - Streptokinase infusion over 24 hours

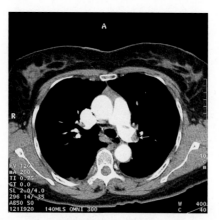

FIGURE 22-4 CT scan demonstrating filling defect in proximal left pulmonary artery (*arrow*) from thrombus. Distal branches of artery are occluded. (From Souhami R: *Textbook of medicine,* New York, Churchill Livingstone, 2002, figure 13.6.2A.)

- Urokinase infusion over 12 to 24 hours
- Recombinant tissue-type plasminogen activator (rt-PA) infusion over 2 hours
- Contraindications of TT
  - Absolute
    - **Intracranial or intraspinal disorders, surgery, trauma in preceding 2 months**
    - **Active bleeding**
  - Relative
    - Surgery, organ biopsy, large vessel puncture, CPR, within 10 days postpartum
- Inferior vena caval filters
  - Indications
    - Contraindication to anticoagulation
    - Recurrence of DVT/PE on therapeutic anticoagulation
  - Effects
    - Decrease early recurrent PE after anticoagulation without mortality effect
    - Increase incidence of later DVT

REVIEW QUESTIONS

For review questions, please go to www.expertconsult.com.

SUGGESTED READINGS

Baarslag HJ, van Beek EJ, Koopman MM, et al: Prospective study of color duplex ultrasonography compared with contrast venography in patients suspected of having deep venous thrombosis of the upper extremities, *Ann Intern Med* 136:865–872, 2002.

Decousus H, Leizorovicz A, Parent F, et al: A clinical trial of vena caval filters in the prevention of pulmonary embolism in patients with proximal deep-vein thrombosis, *N Engl J Med* 338:409–415, 1998.

Geerts WH, Bergqvist D, Pineo GH, Heit JA, et al: Prevention of venous thromboembolism, *Chest* 133:381S–453S, 2008.

Haas S: Venous thromboembolism in medical patients: the scope of the problem, *Semin Thromb Hemost* 29:17–21, 2003.

Hargett WC, Tapson VF: Clinical probability and D-dimer testing: how should we use them in clinical practice? *Semin Respir Crit Care Med* 29:15–24, 2008.

Kearon C, Crowther M, Hirsh J, et al: Management of patients with hereditary hypercoagulable disorders, *Annu Rev Med* 51:169–185, 2000.

Kearon C: Duration of therapy for acute venous thromboembolism, *Clin Chest Med* 24:63–72, 2003.

Musset D, Parent F, Meyer G, et al: Diagnostic strategy for patients with suspected pulmonary embolism: a prospective multicentre outcome study, *Lancet* 360:1914–1920, 2002.

Qaseem A, Snow V, Barry P, et al: Current diagnosis of venous thromboembolism in primary care: a clinical practice guideline from AAFP and ACP, *Ann Family Med* 5:57–62, 2007.

Scarvelis D, Wells PS: Diagnosis and treatment of deep-vein thrombosis, *CMAJ* 175:1087–1092, 2006.

Stein PD, Fowler SE, Goodman LR, et al: For PIOPED II. Multidetector computed tomography for acute pulmonary embolism, *N Engl J Med* 354:2317–2327, 2006.

Stein PD, Hull RD, Patel KC, et al: D-Dimer for the exclusion of acute venous thrombosis and pulmonary embolism: a systematic review, *Ann Intern Med* 140:589–602, 2004.

Stein PD, Terrin ML, Hales CA, et al: Clinical, laboratory, x-ray, and EKG findings in patients with acute PE and no preexisting cardiac or pulmonary disease, *Chest* 100:598–603, 1991.

Tapson VF: Acute pulmonary embolism, *N Engl J Med* 358:1037–1052, 2008.

Todd JL, Tapson VF: Thrombolytic therapy for acute pulmonary embolism, *Chest* 135:1321–1329, 2009.

Wells PS, Ginsberg JS, Anderson DR, et al: Use of a clinical model for safe management of patients with suspected pulmonary embolism, *Ann Intern Med* 129:997–1005, 1998.

Wells PS, Hirsh J, Anderson DR, et al: Accuracy of clinical assessment of deep-vein thrombosis, *Lancet* 345:1326–1330, 1995.

Selected Topics in Pulmonary Medicine

ALBERT J. POLITO, MD

Pulmonary medicine encompasses a variety of disorders that fall outside such traditionally broad topics as chronic obstructive pulmonary disease (COPD), asthma, interstitial lung disease, and thromboembolic disease. This chapter addresses four important smaller topics: (1) sleep disorders, (2) the solitary pulmonary nodule, (3) hemoptysis, and (4) pulmonary hypertension.

Sleep Disorders and Obstructive Sleep Apnea

Basic Information

- Apnea: Cessation of airflow for more than 10 seconds
- Respiratory disturbance index (RDI), also known as the apnea-hypopnea index (AHI): Number of apneas and hypopneas per hour of sleep; normal is five or fewer events per hour
- **Obstructive apnea: Patient continues to make respiratory efforts against an obstruction (typically a narrowing or closure in the upper airway)**
  - Occurs in 2% to 4% of middle-aged adults (Box 23-1 lists risk factors)
  - Recurrent decrements in airflow (i.e., apneas or hypopneas) most commonly occur during sleep (obstructive sleep apnea, OSA)

BOX 23-1	*Risk Factors for Obstructive Sleep Apnea*

Gender
   Male:female ratio, 2:1
   Risk increases for postmenopausal women
Age
   Predominantly 40–70 years old
Body habitus
   Obese (BMI ≥ 30 kg/m²)
Alcohol use
Medications
   Sedatives
   Hypnotics
Endocrine disease
   Acromegaly
   Hypothyroidism

- Events usually more prominent during rapid eye movement sleep, caused by associated hypotonia of upper airway musculature
- **Central apnea: Patient makes no respiratory effort during the apnea** (Box 23-2 lists diseases associated with central apnea)
  - Occurs most commonly during sleep (central sleep apnea, CSA)
  - During sleep, transient abnormalities of central drive to the respiratory muscles occur in affected individuals
  - Much less common than OSA
- Mixed apnea: Apnea with features of both OSA and CSA
- Hypopnea: A 50% or greater decrease in airflow or a less than 50% decrease in airflow associated with at least a 4% drop in oxygen saturation or an arousal
- Upper airway resistance syndrome (UARS)
  - Repeated arousals secondary to increased upper airway resistance ("crescendo snoring")
  - RDI is normal
  - No significant oxygen desaturation episodes
- Obesity-hypoventilation syndrome (OHS; "Pickwickian syndrome")
  - Syndrome of morbid obesity and chronic hypoventilation with daytime hypercapnia (arterial partial pressure of carbon dioxide [$Paco_2$] > 45 mm Hg)
  - OSA present in majority of patients
- Cheyne-Stokes respirations
  - Cyclic rise and fall in respiratory pattern with recurrent periods of apnea
  - Apneas are typically central
  - Most commonly seen with congestive heart failure, central neurologic disease, or administration of sedative agents, but may occur in normal patients

BOX 23-2	*Diseases Associated with Central Sleep Apnea*

Multiple system atrophy (Shy-Drager syndrome)
Autonomic dysfunction
Myasthenia gravis
Neuromuscular disease
Bulbar poliomyelitis
Brainstem infarction
Encephalitis

Clinical Presentation

- OSA
  - History obtained from the patient alone may be unreliable
    - Input of bed partner or housemate often helpful
    - Symptoms of OSA include loud, disruptive snoring (patient "wakes the dead"); daytime sleepiness; witnessed apneas (most sensitive medical history question: "Have you ever been told that you stop breathing while you are sleeping?")
    - Patients also describe sleep as nonrefreshing, complain of morning headaches, irritability/personality change/depression, cognitive impairment, and decreased libido
    - Nocturia/enuresis may also be seen
  - **Physical examination findings in OSA include obesity, increased neck circumference, large tonsils and adenoids, large uvula, low soft palate, systemic hypertension, and lower extremity edema**
    - Retrognathia, micrognathia, and other craniofacial abnormalities also described
  - Medical consequences of OSA are listed in Table 23-1
- CSA
  - Historical findings include daytime sleepiness and witnessed apneas
    - Snoring not a prominent finding
  - Physical examination findings in CSA
    - Patients may have any body habitus
    - Underlying neurologic disease, if present, determines many of the physical findings

Diagnosis and Evaluation

- Diagnosis of a suggested apnea syndrome is obtained with an overnight polysomnogram ("sleep study"; Fig. 23-1)
- Physiologic parameters measured include airflow, chest/abdominal wall effort, oxygen saturation, electroencephalogram (EEG), electrocardiogram (ECG), electro-oculogram (EOG), and body position
- Recording time should be 6 to 8 hours
- **If RDI more than five events per hour, sleep study is positive for sleep apnea**
  - **OSA versus CSA is determined by presence versus absence of chest/abdominal wall efforts, respectively**
  - Mild: 6 to 20 events per hour
  - Moderate: 21 to 50 events per hour
  - Severe: More than 50 events per hour

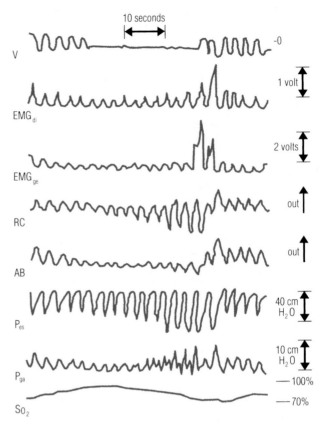

FIGURE 23-1 Polysomnogram in obstructive sleep apnea. The study shows a period when ventilation is obstructed and there is no airflow (V). At this time, the diaphragm continues to contract (EMG_{di}), esophageal (P_{es}) and gastric (P_{ga}) pressure swings occur, and there is ribcage and abdominal movement (RC and AB). As obstruction continues, arterial oxygen saturation (SO_2) falls. Eventually the activity of the upper airway muscles, including the genioglossus muscle (EMG_{ge}), increases, the upper airway becomes patent, and airflow is restored. Patients can have hundreds of similar episodes during the night. (From Onal E, Lopata M, O'Connor T: Pathogenesis of apneas in hypersomnia–sleep syndrome, *Am Rev Respir Dis* 125:167, 1982; and Souhami R: *Textbook of medicine*, New York, Churchill Livingstone, 2002, figure 13.42.)

Treatment

- OSA
  - Three components to treatment: Behavioral, medical, and surgical (Table 23-2 and Fig. 23-2)
  - **Behavioral treatment is commonly the only intervention recommended for patients with mild OSA**
  - Compliance a major problem with nasal CPAP; discomfort of apparatus, claustrophobia, aerophagia, and difficulty with exhalation are common side effects
- CSA
  - Nasal CPAP usually not effective
  - Treatment of choice: Nocturnal nasal noninvasive ventilation with a backup respiratory rate and bilevel (inspiratory and expiratory) pressure settings (BiPAP)
  - Ventilatory stimulants (e.g., acetazolamide) have not proven useful

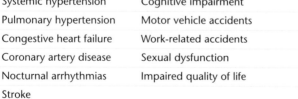

TABLE 23-1	**Medical Consequences of Obstructive Sleep Apnea**	
Cardiovascular Effects	**Noncardiovascular Effects**	
Systemic hypertension	Cognitive impairment	
Pulmonary hypertension	Motor vehicle accidents	
Congestive heart failure	Work-related accidents	
Coronary artery disease	Sexual dysfunction	
Nocturnal arrhythmias	Impaired quality of life	
Stroke		

TABLE 23-2	*Treatment of Obstructive Sleep Apnea (OSA)*	
Modality	**Options**	**Comments**
Behavioral	Weight loss Avoidance of alcohol, sedatives, and hypnotics Position therapy	Small amounts of weight loss can significantly improve symptoms Lateral decubitus sleeping position helps alleviate symptoms in many
Medical	Nasal continuous positive airway pressure (CPAP) Oral appliances Protriptyline Medroxyprogesterone acetate Oxygen	Nasal CPAP is treatment of choice for moderate to severe OSA; apnea, snoring, daytime somnolence, and hypertension all may improve Oral appliances most useful in retrognathia and micrognathia; not effective in severe OSA No medication has been shown to be successful in treating OSA Medroxyprogesterone increases respiratory drive and improves daytime arterial blood gases but has no effect on OSA
Surgical	Nasal surgery (e.g., septoplasty, sinus surgery) Tonsillectomy/adenoidectomy Uvulopalatopharyngoplasty (UPPP) Laser-assisted uvuloplasty Maxillofacial surgery Tracheostomy	Nasal surgery rarely effective in directly treating OSA Tonsillectomy/adenoidectomy most effective in children with OSA UPPP most common surgical procedure for OSA; at least 50% will not improve despite surgery Tracheostomy 100% effective but should be reserved for patients with severe/incapacitating disease that has failed standard aggressive therapy

Untreated obstructive sleep apnea

Obstructive sleep apnea treated with continuous positive airway pressure

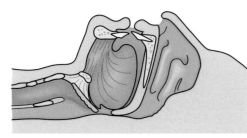
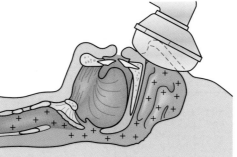

FIGURE 23-2 Effect of continuous positive airway pressure (CPAP) on obstructive sleep apnea (OSA). The chief mechanism of CPAP in the treatment of OSA is airway splinting and dilatation of obstructed pharyngeal segments. (From Albert RK, Spiro SG, Jett JR: *Clinical respiratory medicine,* ed 2, St. Louis, Mosby, 2004, figure 71-9.)

Solitary Pulmonary Nodule

Basic Information

- Pulmonary nodule: A single, well-defined lesion, usually rounded or slightly ovoid, surrounded by normal lung tissue
  - **Diameter must be 3 cm or less**
    - **If diameter greater than 3 cm, process is called a mass, of which 90% are malignant**
- Solitary pulmonary nodules are found in 1 out of every 500 chest radiographs
  - Nodular mimics: Nipple shadows, skin moles, prominent costochondral junction
- Etiologies (Table 23-3)
  - **60% benign (most common: Healed granulomas secondary to tuberculosis or fungal infection)**
  - **40% malignant (most common: Bronchogenic carcinoma)**

Clinical Presentation

- The solitary pulmonary nodule is usually an unexpected finding on routine chest film
  - Most patients are asymptomatic; some have cough

Diagnosis and Evaluation

- Key features of the history include
  - Age (malignancy uncommon in patients younger than 35 years)
  - Smoking (increases likelihood of malignancy)
  - Occupational exposure (asbestos, silica)
  - Prior history of cancer
  - Travel or history of living in endemic area
    - **Mississippi and Ohio River valleys: Suggests histoplasmosis (most common); blastomycosis**
    - **Southwestern United States: Suggests coccidioidomycosis**
- Physical examination
  - Most patients have normal lung examinations
  - Occasionally, with a proximally located nodule, a localized wheeze (from airway impingement) may be present
  - Clubbing may be present with a malignant pulmonary nodule
- Further imaging (Fig. 23-3)
  - The initial step is always to locate older chest radiographs to evaluate stability or change in size of the nodule; allows approximate calculation of doubling time

23

TABLE 23-3	Causes of the Solitary Pulmonary Nodule

Benign Causes	Malignant Causes
Infectious granuloma (tuberculosis, histoplasmosis, coccidioidomycosis) Hamartoma "Round" pneumonia Bronchogenic cyst Pulmonary infarction Arteriovenous malformation Rheumatoid nodule Wegener's granulomatosis Amyloidosis Parasitic infection (*Ascaris, Echinococcus*)	Bronchogenic carcinoma Bronchial carcinoid Pulmonary lymphoma Pulmonary sarcoma Solitary metastasis from extrapulmonary site

TABLE 23-4	Characteristics of Benign and Malignant Pulmonary Nodules

Characteristic	Benign	Malignant
Size	<2 cm	>2 cm
Edge	Smooth, sharp	Spiculated, ragged
Cavitation	No	Yes
Satellite lesions	Yes	No
Doubling time	<25 days or >450 days	25–450 days

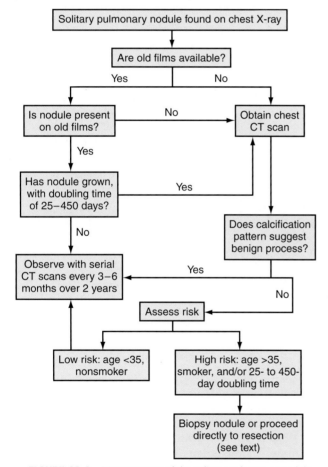

FIGURE 23-3 Management of the solitary pulmonary nodule.

Central ("target")   Diffuse   Popcorn   Laminar (concentric)

4 patterns seen only in benign lesions

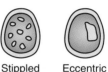

Stippled   Eccentric

2 patterns seen with either benign or malignant lesions

FIGURE 23-4 Calcification patterns in solitary pulmonary nodules. (Adapted from Lillington GA: Management of solitary pulmonary nodules, *Dis Mon 37:271, 1991.*)

- The pattern of calcification may be useful in diagnosis (Figs. 23-4 and 23-5)
  - Hamartomas show a "popcorn" calcification pattern or areas of low-attenuation fat deposits (or both) (Fig. 23-6)
  - Pulmonary arteriovenous malformations (AVMs) fill with contrast material
- Positron emission tomography (PET): Used to define metabolic activity of pulmonary nodule
  - In general, malignant lesions have an increased rate of label uptake compared with benign lesions or normal tissue; however, active infections, granulomatous diseases, and other inflammatory conditions also can have increased uptake (false positives)
  - False negatives can occur with small tumors (<1 cm), tumors with low metabolic activity (e.g., bronchial carcinoid), and hyperglycemia
  - For diagnosis of malignant solitary pulmonary nodules, sensitivity is 97% and specificity is 82%
  - Role in evaluating solitary pulmonary nodules is still being determined; some suggest use in borderline cases, with biopsy recommended if PET scan positive

Treatment

- General principles
  - If a nodule has grown with a doubling time of 25 to 450 days and the patient's cardiopulmonary status permits surgery, thoracotomy with resection is indicated
  - If no previous films are available, the patient's risk of cancer must be assessed to determine whether the approach should be observation or biopsy (see Fig. 23-3)

- **Doubling time of 25 to 450 days suggests a malignant process**
- **Doubling time of less than 25 days or more than 450 days suggests a benign process**
- Doubling time refers to the volume of the nodule (i.e., an increase of 28% in nodule diameter indicates doubling)
- Chest CT: Important for defining the characteristics of the nodule (Table 23-4)

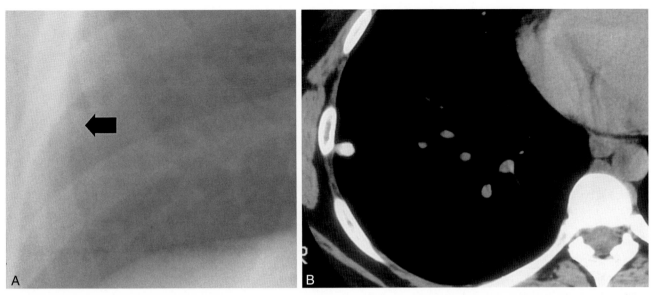

FIGURE 23-5 The use of CT to characterize a solitary pulmonary nodule. **A,** Chest radiograph shows a peripheral nodule (*arrow*) that does not appear to be calcified. **B,** CT scan through the nodule demonstrates dense, diffuse calcification, consistent with a benign lesion. The other gray densities on the scan are pulmonary vessels rather than nodules. (From Mason RJ: *Murray and Nadel's textbook of respiratory medicine,* ed 4, London, Elsevier, 2005, figure 20-36.)

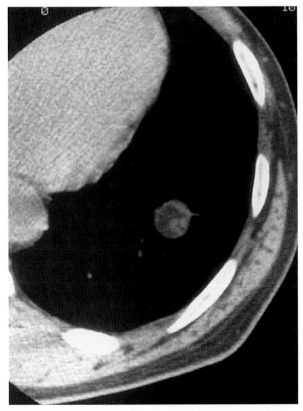

FIGURE 23-6 Hamartoma. CT scan shows low attenuation within the solitary pulmonary nodule, consistent with fat. (From Mason RJ: *Murray and Nadel's textbook of respiratory medicine,* ed 4, London, Elsevier, 2005, figure 20-37.)

- Patient preferences must always be taken into account; some patients fear the uncertainty of observation and want to "do something" right away to make a diagnosis (this may not be possible or appropriate)

- Biopsy techniques
  - Fiberoptic bronchoscopy: Limited usefulness in evaluation of the solitary pulmonary nodule
    - Most useful if the nodule is greater than 2 cm in diameter, is located proximally, or has a bronchus leading into it on chest CT
    - Diagnostic yield: 10% to 20% if less than 2 cm, 55% if greater than 2 cm
  - Percutaneous transthoracic needle aspiration: Usually performed with CT guidance
    - Most useful for peripheral lesions in the outer one third of the lung
    - **Higher diagnostic yield than bronchoscopic biopsy: 80% to 95% (even in lesions < 2 cm)**
    - Major limitation: 10% to 30% rate of pneumothorax
  - Once diagnosis is confirmed, treat the underlying disease

Hemoptysis

Basic Information

- Hemoptysis: Expectoration of blood from the airways
- Pathophysiology: **In the majority of cases, hemoptysis originates from bronchial arterial circulation**
  - Bronchial arteries increase in size and number in the setting of chronic inflammation (e.g., bronchiectasis) or malignancy and are susceptible to rupture
  - Bleeding may be profuse because of the high pressure of the systemic circulation
  - **Clinically significant bleeding from pulmonary arterial circulation is rare because it is a low-pressure system and hypoxic pulmonary vasoconstriction diverts blood flow away from diseased portions of the lung**
- Causes are listed in Box 23-3
  - Bronchitis and bronchogenic carcinoma, the two most common causes, account for 40% and 25% of cases, respectively

23

BOX 23-3	*Causes of Hemoptysis*

Infectious
Bronchitis
Bronchiectasis
Pneumonia
Tuberculosis

Neoplastic
Bronchogenic carcinoma
Bronchial carcinoid
Pulmonary metastasis from other site

Cardiovascular
Congestive heart failure
Mitral stenosis
Pulmonary embolism/infarction
Pulmonary arteriovenous malformation

Miscellaneous
Idiopathic (as much as 20–30% of cases)
Lung contusion
Goodpasture's syndrome
Wegener's granulomatosis
Pseudohemoptysis (from *Serratia marcescens* pneumonia)

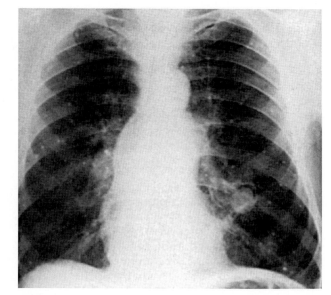

FIGURE 23-7   Chest radiograph showing an aspergilloma in the left lower lung zone of an asymptomatic patient. A dark rim of air is readily seen around the upper edge of the fungus ball ("air crescent sign"). (From Mason RJ: *Murray and Nadel's textbook of respiratory medicine,* ed 4, London, Elsevier, 2005, figure 34-15.)

Clinical Presentation

- Amount of blood may be small or large; massive hemoptysis is defined most commonly as loss of more than 600 mL of blood in 24 hours
- Hemoptysis may be accompanied by mucopurulent sputum and fever (bacterial pneumonia), hematuria (pulmonary-renal syndromes, including Goodpasture's), or prominent sinusitis (Wegener's granulomatosis), the presence of which may offer clues to etiology

Diagnosis and Evaluation

- Key features of the history start with a careful questioning of the patient's symptoms to help determine source of blood; many patients confuse hemoptysis with hematemesis or epistaxis
  - Other features include estimation of the quantity of blood and the duration of bleeding
- Physical examination
  - Crackles or rhonchi may be present in the area of the bleeding and can help localize site of bleeding
- Radiographic studies
  - Chest radiograph should be obtained in every patient and may suggest the diagnosis
    - Nodule or mass suggests neoplasm
    - Lobar atelectasis suggests obstructing endobronchial lesion
    - **Mass within a cavity ("air crescent sign") suggests aspergilloma** (fungus ball; Fig. 23-7)
    - Thickened bronchial walls ("tram tracking") suggest bronchiectasis
  - 30% of patients have normal or nonlocalizing chest films
  - Chest CT is generally not an important tool for evaluation of hemoptysis, except in those patients with normal or nonlocalizing chest radiographs

- Fiberoptic bronchoscopy: The invasive procedure of choice for nonmassive hemoptysis
  - Helpful for localizing the bleeding side or the specific site of bleeding
  - Not useful for massive hemoptysis (field of vision through bronchoscope is obscured by large amounts of blood)

Treatment

- Therapy should be directed at the underlying cause of the hemoptysis (e.g., antibiotics for bronchitis or pneumonia; diuresis for congestive heart failure; resection and chemotherapy/radiotherapy for bronchogenic carcinoma)
- Massive hemoptysis requires special attention
  - **Airway protection: Position patient with the bleeding lung in the dependent position (prevents spillage of blood into the nonbleeding lung)**
    - Intubation may be needed to isolate the lungs from each other, using a double-lumen endotracheal tube
  - Fluid resuscitation to support volume
  - Gentle cough suppression to prevent the airway trauma of vigorous coughing
    - Avoid excessive cough suppression because airway compromise can result
  - Correction of coagulopathy, if present
  - Bronchial artery embolization is effective at immediately halting bleeding in 80% to 95% of patients
    - 30% will rebleed within 3 months
  - Surgery: Indicated for massive, unilateral hemoptysis unresponsive to other measures, provided that the patient has adequate pulmonary reserve
    - High mortality rate (35%) for patients actively bleeding at the time of surgery

Pulmonary Hypertension

Basic Information

- Normal pulmonary artery (PA) pressures are 18 to 30 mm Hg systolic and 4 to 12 mm Hg diastolic
- **Pulmonary hypertension is defined as mean PA pressure greater than 25 mm Hg at rest or greater than 30 mm Hg with exercise**
  - Severe pulmonary hypertension is defined as mean PA pressure greater than or equal to 40 mm Hg at rest
- Classified as either primary or secondary (Box 23-4 lists causes of secondary pulmonary hypertension)

Clinical Presentation

- Demographics
  - **Primary pulmonary hypertension (PPH) is three times more common in women than in men and generally occurs in younger patients (typical age of onset is 20–40 years)**
- Symptoms
  - Similar for both primary and secondary etiologies, though for the latter, other symptoms of the underlying disorder may be present (e.g., snoring and hypersomnolence in OSA, skin changes in scleroderma)
  - Patients with mild pulmonary hypertension are usually asymptomatic
  - Exertional dyspnea is most common presenting complaint
  - May also have chest pain or dizziness; syncope portends a poor prognosis

BOX 23-4	*Causes of Secondary Pulmonary Hypertension*

Cardiac Disease
Congenital
Eisenmenger's syndrome
Left-sided heart failure

Parenchymal Lung Disease
Chronic obstructive pulmonary disease
Interstitial lung disease

Vascular Impairment
Chronic thromboembolic disease
Pulmonary veno-occlusive disease
Sickle cell disease

Infections
HIV
Schistosomiasis

Drugs/Toxins
Anorexigens

Miscellaneous
Obstructive sleep apnea
Collagen vascular diseases (through either direct vascular effect or interstitial changes in the parenchyma)

Diagnosis and Evaluation

- Physical examination
  - **Prominent pulmonic component (P_2) of the second heart sound is a reliable indicator of elevated PA pressure**
  - May also see elevated jugular venous pressure with large a wave, left parasternal heave (from right ventricular hypertrophy), right-sided S_3, or tricuspid regurgitation murmur
  - Pedal edema common
- Chest radiography
  - Shows enlarged pulmonary arteries with rapid tapering of vessels toward the periphery of the lungs (a "pruned tree" appearance; Fig. 23-8)
  - May also see right-heart enlargement
  - For secondary pulmonary hypertension caused by parenchymal lung disease, look for hyperinflation and bullous disease (suggestive of COPD) or increased interstitial markings (suggestive of interstitial lung disease)
- Other studies
  - Echocardiography: Permits noninvasive estimation of PA pressure, as well as size of right heart
  - Pulmonary function tests: Typically show decreased diffusing capacity
  - Ventilation-perfusion scan: Helps identify patients with secondary pulmonary hypertension because of chronic thromboembolic disease, but PPH can also produce abnormal scans
  - Right-heart catheterization: Permits direct measurement of PA pressure and, with angiography, definitive diagnosis of chronic thromboembolic disease

Treatment

- PPH
  - Right-heart catheterization should be performed in all patients to determine if there is a positive response to acute administration of a vasodilator (typically nitric oxide)
    - **5% to 10% of patients are "responders" (PA pressure declines by at least 10 mm Hg to a value < 40 mm Hg) and should be treated with oral calcium channel-blockers**
    - **"Nonresponders" have an increased risk of death with calcium channel-blockers and should receive other therapy (prostacyclins, bosentan, or sildenafil)**
  - Continuous infusion of epoprostenol (prostacyclin), a direct pulmonary vasodilator, is indicated in patients with New York Heart Association class III or IV symptoms
    - Adverse effects of epoprostenol include flushing and diarrhea
    - Prostacyclin analogues: Trepostinil, iloprost
  - Other treatment options
    - Bosentan—oral endothelin receptor antagonist
    - Sildenafil—phosphodiesterase inhibitor (enhances nitric oxide-mediated vasodilation)
  - **Chronic anticoagulation is indicated in all patients to prevent intravascular thrombosis in the pulmonary circulation as well as deep venous thrombosis**

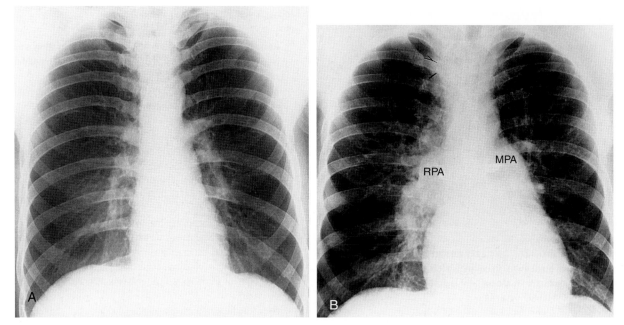

FIGURE 23-8   Progressive pulmonary arterial hypertension. **A,** The patient initially had a normal chest radiograph. **B,** Several years later, however, increasing heart size and marked dilatation of the main pulmonary artery (MPA) and right pulmonary artery (RPA) are noted. Pulmonary artery enlargement can be recognized by a bulging along the left cardiac border just below the aortic arch. (From Mettler FA: *Essentials of radiology,* ed 2, Philadelphia, WB Saunders, 2005, figure 5-12.)

- ▪ Many patients require chronic diuretic therapy
- ▪ Supplemental oxygen
- Secondary pulmonary hypertension
  - ▪ Treat underlying disease
  - ▪ Epoprostenol and bosentan are used frequently for secondary pulmonary hypertension caused by scleroderma
  - ▪ Sildenafil is used increasingly in a variety of secondary settings
  - ▪ Chronic anticoagulation should be instituted for all patients with severe pulmonary hypertension, provided there is no contraindication
  - ▪ Supplemental oxygen helps reduce hypoxic pulmonary vasoconstriction
  - ▪ For severe chronic thromboembolic pulmonary hypertension, consider pulmonary thromboendarterectomy

REVIEW QUESTIONS

For review questions, please go to www.expertconsult.com.

SUGGESTED READINGS

Cahill BC, Ingbar DH: Massive hemoptysis: assessment and management, *Clin Chest Med* 15:147–167, 1994.

Farber HW, Loscalzo J: Pulmonary arterial hypertension, *N Engl J Med* 351:1655–1665, 2004.

Lillington GA: Management of solitary pulmonary nodules, *Dis Mon* 37:271–318, 1991.

Malhotra A, White DP: Obstructive sleep apnoea, *Lancet* 360:237–245, 2002.

McGoon MD: The assessment of pulmonary hypertension, *Clin Chest Med* 22:493–508, 2001.

Midthun DE, Swensen SJ, Jett JR: Clinical strategies for solitary pulmonary nodule, *Annu Rev Med* 43:195–208, 1992.

Ost D, Fein A: Evaluation and management of the solitary pulmonary nodule, *Am J Respir Crit Care Med* 162:782–787, 2000.

Runo JR, Loyd JE: Primary pulmonary hypertension, *Lancet* 361: 1533–1544, 2003.

Strollo PJ, Rogers RM: Obstructive sleep apnea, *N Engl J Med* 334:99–104, 1996.

Critical Care Medicine

JONATHAN SEVRANSKY, MD

Critical care medicine focuses on the management of acute organ failure and other life-threatening illnesses. Treatment of acute respiratory failure and its common causes, including pneumonia, chronic obstructive pulmonary disease (COPD), and the acute respiratory distress syndrome (ARDS), is an important component of critical care management. The timely diagnosis and rapid treatment of septic, cardiogenic, and hypovolemic shock are crucial to the survival of patients with these life-threatening conditions. Recent emphasis on minimizing and preventing the complications of critical care therapies is also highlighted here. Because toxin exposures often require acute management in a critical care setting, a review of the major types of toxin exposures is included.

Acute Respiratory Failure

Basic Information

- Two pathophysiologic causes of acute respiratory failure
  - **Failure of oxygenation**
    - Defined as an **inadequate arterial oxygen partial pressure (Pao$_2$)** despite high levels of supplemental inspired O$_2$
    - Five major etiologic classes
      - Right-to-left shunt via pathologic vascular communications (e.g., pulmonary ateriovenous malformations [AVMs], intracardiac right-to-left shunts), or space-filling pulmonary parenchymal lesions (e.g., atelectasis or pneumonia)
      - Ventilation/perfusion ($\dot{V}/\dot{Q}$) mismatch: Regional imbalances between blood flow and ventilation (e.g., pulmonary embolism or lung parenchymal disease)
      - Reduced diffusion capacity (e.g., interstitial lung disease, emphysema); may be minimal at rest; more pronounced with exercise
      - Alveolar hypoventilation (e.g., from CNS depression, neuromuscular disease, or chest wall abnormality)
      - Low fraction of inspired oxygen (Fio$_2$, e.g., high altitude)
  - **Failure of ventilation**
    - Defined as **elevated partial pressure of carbon dioxide (PaCo$_2$) with decreased pH**
    - Caused by either
      - Increased CO$_2$ production (e.g., sepsis, overfeeding, thyrotoxicosis)
      - Decreased CO$_2$ elimination (caused by obstructive lung disease, pneumonia, increased dead space)

  - Decreased minute ventilation (e.g., CNS depression)
  - Decreased alveolar ventilation (e.g., COPD, increased dead space)

Clinical Presentation

- Depends on underlying cause
- Agitation or altered mental status commonly seen in hypoxia and hypercarbia
- **Cyanosis occurs only once deoxyhemoglobin level is greater than 5 g/dL, which corresponds to an arterial oxygen saturation (Sao$_2$) around 67%**

Diagnosis and Evaluation

- **Pulse oximeter may be unreliable in the following situations:**
  - On the steep portion of the oxyhemoglobin dissociation curve (i.e., at saturation levels < 90%; Fig. 24-1)
  - In patients with carboxyhemoglobin or methemoglobin
  - In patients with decreased peripheral perfusion (e.g., shock)
  - In patients with pigmented skin or nail polish
- Arterial blood gas measurement is the gold standard
  - Most oxygen is delivered to tissues bound to hemoglobin, which is reflected in measured saturation obtained with arterial blood gas rather than dissolved in the plasma (i.e., measured by Pao$_2$)
  - **Consider mechanical ventilation when Pao$_2$ is less than 60 to 70 mm Hg with Fio$_2$ greater than 0.8 to 1 mm Hg or PaCo$_2$ greater than 45 mm Hg with decreased pH**
  - **Work of breathing (high respiratory rate with use of accessory muscles) and ability to protect airway are additional important considerations**

Treatment

- Supplemental oxygen to **maintain O$_2$ saturation greater than 88% or Pao$_2$ greater than 55% to 60%**
  - Do not deliver inadequate amounts of oxygen out of concern about suppressing central respiratory drive
- Mechanical ventilation (Box 24-1)
  - Consider whether noninvasive ventilation candidate (Table 24-1)
    - Noninvasive ventilation decreases complications, such as ventilator-associated pneumonia and decreased length of ICU stay, and improves mortality rates for selected patients with hypercarbic respiratory failure in setting of COPD and immunosuppressed patients with bilateral infiltrates and hypoxemic respiratory failure

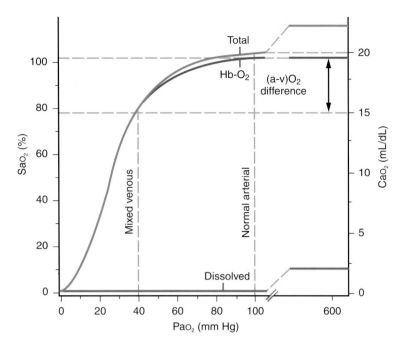

FIGURE 24-1 Oxyhemoglobin dissociation curve. (From Goldman L, Bennett JC, Ausiello D: *Cecil textbook of medicine,* ed 22, Philadelphia, Saunders, 2004, figure 100.5.)

- Treat underlying cause (e.g., antibiotics for pneumonia, bronchodilators and corticosteroids for status asthmaticus)
- Protocol-driven weaning strategies for ventilators and methods to limit doses of sedative analgesic infusions (e.g., daily interruption of sedation) will decrease the length of time that patients require mechanical ventilation

Acute Respiratory Distress Syndrome

Basic Information

- Divided into pulmonary and nonpulmonary causes (although no clear difference in outcomes)
  - **Sepsis and pneumonia are most common causes**
  - Other: Aspiration, irritant gases and smoke inhalation, medications, blood transfusions, burns, pancreatitis, and trauma
- Incidence increases with increasing age
  - Estimated 15 to 78 cases per 100,000 population
  - At-risk patients who develop ARDS generally do so within 48 to 72 hours of acquiring risk factor, although some may take as long as a week to meet criteria
  - Some suggestion that African Americans may have higher risk than whites
- **Overall mortality related to number of organ system failures**
  - Single-organ system failure mortality rate 25% to 40%
  - Three-organ system failure has up to 90% mortality rate
  - Mortality rates increase with age
- **Sepsis and multiorgan system failure most common causes of death**
  - Rare for patients to die solely from intractable hypoxemia
  - May be difficult to diagnosis ventilator-associated pneumonia in patients with ARDS
- Survivors of acute illness may have long-term sequelae
  - Two thirds of survivors have minimal to moderate respiratory impairment 1 year after event

- Recent studies have reported muscle wasting, weakness, and post-traumatic stress disorder as late as 1 year after illness in survivors of ARDS. Only half of the patients return to work 1 year after discharge.

Clinical Presentation, Diagnosis, and Epidemiology

- Syndrome definition from the European-American Consensus Statement requires
  - **Acute onset of symptoms**
  - **Diffuse bilateral infiltrates on chest radiograph (Fig. 24-2)**
  - **Pao_2/Fio_2 ratio less than 200** (Pao_2/Fio_2 ratio < 300 defines acute lung injury [ALI])
  - **No evidence of left heart failure (pulmonary capillary wedge pressure < 18 mm Hg)**

Treatment

- **Use lung-protective ventilatory strategy**
  - **Small tidal volumes (6 mL/kg) coupled with low plateau pressures (<30 cm H_2O) to minimize ventilator-induced lung injury**
  - This approach decreased mortality from ARDS, reduced incidence of multiorgan system failure, and decreased measures of local and systemic inflammation
  - Higher levels of PEEP coupled with lung protective ventilation do not change mortality rates, but may decrease duration of ventilation
- Supportive care: Mechanical ventilation, treatment of underlying cause, hemodynamic renal support, and nutritional support if necessary
- **Routine modulation of proinflammatory mediators is of no proven value**
- **Corticosteroids' role uncertain** in treatment of late-phase ARDS, with conflicting results from studies
- Prone positioning and inhaled nitric oxide improve oxygenation in many patients but have no effect on length of ventilation or survival

BOX 24-1	*Mechanical Ventilation*

Volume cycled: Ventilator delivers a set volume, using whatever pressure is required to overcome airway resistance and lung compliance. Examples include assist control and synchronized intermittent mandatory ventilation

Assist control: Patient receives a set tidal volume for every initiated breath. A preset number of breaths per minute prevents hypoventilation

Synchronized intermittent mandatory ventilation (SIMV): Patient receives a set tidal volume for only a designated number of breaths per minute. Additional patient-initiated breaths have no support

Pressure-regulated volume control (PRVC): Patient receives set tidal volume for every initiated breath as long as the pressure required to deliver remains below a preset value

Pressure cycled: Ventilator maintains a set pressure; tidal volume delivered depends on lung mechanics. Examples include pressure control and pressure support

Pressure support: Ventilator provides a constant preset pressure for each patient-initiated breath; primarily used in awake patients or as a weaning mode. Should not be used in patients without intacted respiratory drive

Complications

Auto-positive end-expiratory pressure (PEEP) (dynamic hyperinflation): Caused by air trapping because of inadequate emptying during expiration in patient with airflow obstruction (e.g., asthma or chronic obstructive pulmonary disease)

The increased intrathoracic pressure causes increased work of breathing and may decrease venous return to the heart, producing hypotension

Treatment includes disconnecting the patient from the ventilator as a temporary measure if decompensating; changing the ventilator parameters to allow increased expiratory time by increasing inspiratory flow rate; decreasing tidal volume and respiratory rate; and increasing sedation

Volutrauma or barotrauma: Can cause pneumothorax, pneumomediastinum, and diffuse alveolar damage

Increased infection rate: Ventilator-associated pneumonia

Endotracheal tube complications: Subglottal stenosis, vocal cord dysfunction, tracheoesophageal fistula, sinusitis

Noninvasive Ventilation

Definition: Mechanical ventilation without endotracheal intubation

Does not protect airway; avoid using in patients with depressed level of consciousness

Continuous positive airway pressure (CPAP): Constant pressure provided throughout respiratory cycle

Bilevel positive airway pressure (BiPAP): Different pressures provided upon inspiration and expiration

TABLE 24-1	*Criteria for Use of Noninvasive Ventilation*	
Disease	**Patient Characteristics**	**Contraindications**
COPD exacerbation	Hypercapneic respiratory failure (pH 7.25–7.35, RR, 20–25) Able to manage secretions	Shock Not able to tolerate mask GCS <8
Respiratory failure in immuno-suppressed patients with bilateral infiltrates	Immunosuppression (e.g., s/p bone marrow transplant, HIV, or post-chemotherapy neutropenia)	Shock Not able to tolerate mask GCS < 8

COPD, chronic obstructive pulmonary disease; GCS, Glasgow Coma Scale; RR, respiration rate.

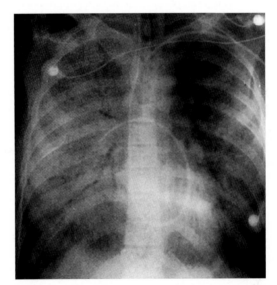

FIGURE 24-2 Chest radiograph of a patient with acute respiratory distress syndrome. Note diffuse bilateral infiltrates. (From Mason RJ: *Murray and Nadel's textbook of respiratory medicine*, ed 4, Philadelphia, Saunders, 2005, figure 51.2.)

Sepsis

Basic Information

- Etiology
  - Bacterial products (e.g., endotoxin, peptidoglycans, teichoic acid) stimulate host defense cells (monocyte or macrophage)
  - Host defense cells respond by **producing proinflammatory mediators** (e.g., tumor necrosis

factor α [TNF-α], interleukin-1 [IL-1], arachidonic acid metabolites, platelet-activating factor, complement components, and nitric oxide)
  - Proinflammatory mediators cause **dysregulation of the coagulation cascade**
- Epidemiology
  - Incidence 80 cases per 100,000 population
    - More common at the extremes of age (i.e., very young or very old)
    - Incidence may be increased in African Americans
  - May occur in the setting of a wide number of infections (i.e., gram-positive, gram-negative, viral, or fungal organisms)
  - Infections may occur in community, facility, or hospitalized person; both immunocompetent and immunosuppresed patients may develop sepsis

24

- The lungs, central venous catheters, and bladder catheters are the most common sites of nosocomial infections in ICU patients
- **Gram-positive organisms now most common cause of sepsis, followed closely by gram-negative organisms**
- Mortality related to number of organs that fail (may also be affected by underlying disease)

Clinical Presentation and Diagnosis

- Bacteremia is defined as the **presence of bacteria in the bloodstream**
- Sepsis syndrome is defined as the presence of the following four components:
  - Temperature (>38°C or <36°C)
  - Pulse (>90 bpm)
  - Respiration rate (>24/min, $PaCo_2$ < 32 mm Hg), or need for mechanical ventilation
  - WBC (>12,000/mm^3 or <4000/mm^3)
    - Evidence of infection (i.e., positive blood, urine, or sputum cultures, positive Gram stain, or presence of pus)
      - Microbiologic proof not required since patients sometimes are on antibiotics when sepsis develops
  - Note definition of syndrome is not specific, as there are many causes of elevated pulse, temperature, respiration rate in hospitalized patients
- **Severe sepsis defined as sepsis plus organ failure (e.g., renal, hematologic, respiratory, cardiovascular, neurologic)**
- **Septic shock is defined by hypotension unresponsive to fluid resuscitation and the presence of end-organ damage**
  - Mortality rates 15% to 20% for sepsis; 50% to 60% for septic shock

Treatment

- Timely antibiotics, fluids, and hemodynamic support, renal Support if necessary
  - Appropriate antibiotics should be infused within 1 hour in patients with hypotension due to sepsis (door-to-infusion time < 1 hour); selection of antibiotics should be driven by patient characteristics and place that patient developed infection (i.e., home versus hospital)
- No benefit seen with attempts to modulate proinflammatory cytokines (e.g., anti-TNF monoclonal antibody, soluble TNF receptor, IL-1 receptor antagonist)
- **Recombinant activated protein C may be beneficial** by modulating coagulation system in patients with severe sepsis and high predicted mortality rates (APACHE II score > 25)
  - No beneficial effect seen in patients at low risk of dying (APACHE II scores < 25)
- **No value with physiologic corticosteroids for patients with septic shock for patients on vasopressors. May be role for physiologic corticosteroids in patients with shock who are hypotensive while on vasopressors**
  - No role for high-dose (pulsed) corticosteroids
- Routine use of **dopamine to prevent renal failure is of no proven value**
- Goal-directed therapy early in presentation (e.g., protocol-based strategy using fluids, vasopressors, and, if necessary, packed red blood cell transfusions, inotropes, and endotracheal intubation/mechanical ventilation to reach a target mean arterial pressure > 65 mm Hg and venous O_2 saturation > 70% for 6 hours) improves outcomes in patients with severe sepsis
  - Goal-directed therapy late in management (i.e., after 24 hours) does not improve outcomes

Shock

Basic Information

- Shock is defined as **inadequate end-organ perfusion** (not synonymous with hypotension)
- Results from any combination of malfunction of
  - Arterial perfusion
  - Cardiac performance
  - Vascular performance
  - Cellular function

Clinical Presentation

- Decreased urine output
- Decreased peripheral perfusion (e.g., cool extremities, cyanosis)
- Altered mental status
- Tissue hypoxia (elevated lactic acid)

Diagnosis

See Figure 24-3 for a diagnostic algorithm for treating shock.
- Four types of shock are distinguished (Table 24-2)
- Pulmonary artery (Swan-Ganz) catheter
  - May be useful as diagnostic tool to measure cardiac output and filling pressures (noninvasive methods less accurate)
  - Limitations on usefulness
    - Varied levels of interpretation skills
    - Pulmonary artery occlusion pressure is not always a good surrogate for left ventricular end-diastolic volume
  - Routine use is controversial because no studies have demonstrated improved outcomes with its use

Treatment for Septic Shock

- Volume resuscitation
  - Crystalloids (e.g., saline, lactated Ringer's) are the initial fluid of choice
    - Inexpensive, easily available
    - No proven benefit to use of colloids (e.g., albumin) in critically ill patients requiring fluid resuscitation in randomized trials
- In patients with critical illness **without coronary artery disease or active bleeding,** a transfusion threshold of hemoglobin of 7 g/dL was as effective, and possibly superior to, using a transfusion threshold of hemoglobin of 10 g/dL
- Vasopressor support to maintain organ perfusion
  - Benefit of norepinephrine compared with dopamine as first-line vasopressor agent unclear; no randomized trials done to support use of either one
  - Dopamine recommended by expert opinions, but patient may be more likely to develop tachyarrythmias
  - Norepinephrine is more potent vasopressor
    - The addition of vasopressin to patients requiring norepinephrine is reasonable but does not alter mortality rates

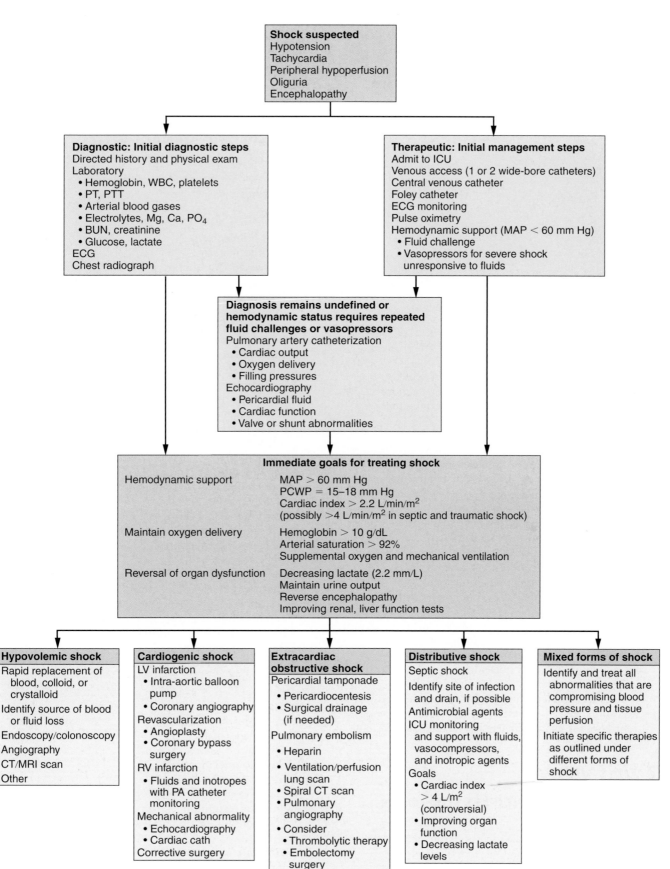

Shock suspected
Hypotension
Tachycardia
Peripheral hypoperfusion
Oliguria
Encephalopathy

Diagnostic: Initial diagnostic steps
Directed history and physical exam
Laboratory
• Hemoglobin, WBC, platelets
• PT, PTT
• Arterial blood gases
• Electrolytes, Mg, Ca, PO_4
• BUN, creatinine
• Glucose, lactate
ECG
Chest radiograph

Therapeutic: Initial management steps
Admit to ICU
Venous access (1 or 2 wide-bore catheters)
Central venous catheter
Foley catheter
ECG monitoring
Pulse oximetry
Hemodynamic support (MAP < 60 mm Hg)
• Fluid challenge
• Vasopressors for severe shock
unresponsive to fluids

Diagnosis remains undefined or hemodynamic status requires repeated fluid challenges or vasopressors
Pulmonary artery catheterization
• Cardiac output
• Oxygen delivery
• Filling pressures
Echocardiography
• Pericardial fluid
• Cardiac function
• Valve or shunt abnormalities

Immediate goals for treating shock

Hemodynamic support	MAP > 60 mm Hg PCWP = 15–18 mm Hg Cardiac index > 2.2 L/min/m² (possibly >4 L/min/m² in septic and traumatic shock)
Maintain oxygen delivery	Hemoglobin > 10 g/dL Arterial saturation > 92% Supplemental oxygen and mechanical ventilation
Reversal of organ dysfunction	Decreasing lactate (2.2 mm/L) Maintain urine output Reverse encephalopathy Improving renal, liver function tests

Hypovolemic shock
Rapid replacement of
blood, colloid, or
crystalloid
Identify source of blood
or fluid loss
Endoscopy/colonoscopy
Angiography
CT/MRI scan
Other

Cardiogenic shock
LV infarction
• Intra-aortic balloon
pump
• Coronary angiography
Revascularization
• Angioplasty
• Coronary bypass
surgery
RV infarction
• Fluids and inotropes
with PA catheter
monitoring
Mechanical abnormality
• Echocardiography
• Cardiac cath
Corrective surgery

Extracardiac obstructive shock
Pericardial tamponade
• Pericardiocentesis
• Surgical drainage
(if needed)
Pulmonary embolism
• Heparin
• Ventilation/perfusion
lung scan
• Spiral CT scan
• Pulmonary
angiography
• Consider
• Thrombolytic therapy
• Embolectomy
surgery

Distributive shock
Septic shock
Identify site of infection
and drain, if possible
Antimicrobial agents
ICU monitoring
and support with fluids,
vasocompressors,
and inotropic agents
Goals
• Cardiac index
> 4 L/m²
(controversial)
• Improving organ
function
• Decreasing lactate
levels

Mixed forms of shock
Identify and treat all
abnormalities that are
compromising blood
pressure and tissue
perfusion
Initiate specific therapies
as outlined under
different forms of
shock

FIGURE 24-3 Diagnosis of shock. BUN, blood urea nitrogen; ECG, electrocardiogram; ICU, intensive care unit; MAP, mean arterial pressure; PA, pulmonary artery; PCWP, pulmonary capillary wedge pressure; PT, prothrombin time; PTT, partial thromboplastin time; RV, right ventricular. (From Goldman L, Bennett JC, Ausiello D: *Cecil textbook of medicine,* ed 22, Philadelphia, 2004, Saunders, figure 102.3.)

24

TABLE 24-2	Differentiation of the Four Different Types of Shock*		
Type of Shock	Cardiac Output	Filling Pressure	SVR
Distributive	↑	↓ or normal	↓
Septic			
Anaphylactic			
Neurogenic			
Hypovolemic	↓	↓	↑
Cardiogenic (pump failure)	↓	↓	↑
Extracardiac obstructive	↓	↓ or ↑	↑
Pericardial tamponade			
Acute PE			
Air embolus			

*Can be made based on PA catheter parameters.
PE, pulmonary embolism; SVR, systemic vascular resistance.

- Supplemental oxygen to increase oxygen delivery
- Antibiotics directed at likely pathogens (site of infection and location of infection important determinants)

Preventing Complications

- Most life-sustaining therapies used in the ICU have potential mechanical or infectious complications (e.g., ventilator-induced lung injury, ventilator-associated pneumonia)
- Important to use these therapies only when necessary and to discontinue when risk-benefit ratio no longer favors use
  - Use ventilator protocols to wean patients off ventilators
  - Use sterile technique to place catheters
    - Subclavian site less likely to have mechanical or infectious complications than femoral site
    - Remove catheters when no longer essential
  - Use deep vein thromboembolism prophylaxis for at-risk patients
  - Stress ulcer prophylaxis for at-risk patients (mechanical ventilation > 48 hours or coagulopathy)
  - Sedation protocols to minimize dose of sedatives
    - Daily interruption or nurse-driven protocols both are acceptable
    - Both decrease length of intubation and ICU stay
  - Elevation of head of bed 30° to 45° to reduce risk of ventilator-associated pneumonia in intubated patients

Toxin Exposures

MANAGEMENT PRINCIPLES FOR TOXIN EXPOSURES

- Obtain history: Time since ingestion, number and type of pills taken, formulation (e.g., extended release), concomitant ingestions (alcohol, illicit drugs)
- Obtain IV access, nasogastric intubation
- Activated charcoal blocks absorption of most drugs
  - **Exceptions include alkalis, lithium, iron, and insecticides**

- **Ipecac is no longer routinely recommended to induce emesis**
  - May be used in the alert, awake patient
- **Gastric lavage is of unproven efficacy but often used and may be useful if recent ingestion (<1 hour)**
- **Endotracheal intubation should be considered in patients who are obtunded or have a poor gag reflex**

TOXIN-SPECIFIC MANAGEMENT

Analgesics and Sedatives

See Table 24-3 for a summary of analgesic and sedative toxin exposures.

Cardioactive Medications

- Tricyclic antidepressants
  - Basic information
    - Possess anticholinergic, α-adrenergic blocking, and adrenergic uptake-inhibiting properties
    - Ingestion of 10 to 20 mg/kg may cause moderate to severe toxicity, and 30 to 40 mg/kg may be life-threatening
    - Best predictor of toxicity is **QRS interval greater than 100 ms**
  - Clinical presentation
    - Arrhythmias, hypotension, and anticholinergic effects (e.g., hyperthermia, flushing, dilated pupils, intestinal ileus, urinary retention, and sinus tachycardia; Fig. 24-4)
    - CNS effects are common with initial agitation followed by seizures and depressed consciousness
  - Treatment
    - **Alkalinization** to serum pH of 7.4 to 7.5 with IV sodium bicarbonate is indicated to reduce occurrence of arrhythmias
    - If patient is on a ventilator, may also hyperventilate
    - Carefully monitor pH during therapy (pH > 7.55 increases risk of seizures)
- β-Blockers
  - Basic information
    - Negative inotropic and chronotropic effects
    - Non-$β_1$-selective agents may have respiratory effects, and lipophilic agents (e.g., propranolol) can cross blood-brain barrier, causing CNS depression
  - Clinical presentation
    - Hypotension, bradycardia, and varying degrees of heart block
  - Treatment
    - **Glucagon**
    - IV fluids if hypotensive
    - If needed, pacing and vasopressor or inotrope with $β_1$ activity
- Calcium channel blockers
  - Basic information
    - Negative inotropic and chronotropic effects
  - Clinical presentation
    - Hypotension, bradycardia, and low cardiac output
  - Treatment
    - **10% calcium chloride**
    - If needed, pacing and vasopressor with β and α activity
- Digitalis
  - Basic information
    - Therapeutic inotropic agent/antiarrhythmic with a narrow therapeutic window

TABLE 24-3	*Toxin Exposures: Analgesics and Sedatives*			
Toxin Exposure	**Basic Information**	**Clinical Picture**	**Diagnosis**	**Treatment**
Acetaminophen	Toxicity caused by reactive metabolite Metabolite detoxified by glutathione	Hepatotoxicity If ingestion >7.5 g Less in alcoholics	Acetaminophen level Nomogram helpful in determining potential for toxicity over time	N-Acetyl cysteine Best results within 8 hr of exposure May be beneficial up to 24 hr
Salicylate	Uncouples oxidative phosphorylation	Acute toxicity Respiratory alkalosis Anion gap acidosis Hyperthermia Coagulopathy Pulmonary edema Hyper- or hypoglycemia Seizures	Salicylate level >40 mg/dL in acute ingestion >30 mg/dL in chronic ingestion Potential toxicity by dose <150 mg/kg low risk >300 mg/kg severe toxicity >500 mg/kg may be lethal	Hydration Alkalinization of urine Gastric lavage, activated charcoal Hemodialysis (for seizures, refractory acidosis, or levels >90–100 mg/dL)
Opiates	Bind opiate receptors	Hypotension Respiratory depression CNS depression	Urine testing for opiate metabolites	Naloxone Opiate antagonist Short acting
Benzodiazepines	Bind the GABA receptor	Hypotension Respiratory depression CNS depression Synergistic effect with opiates	Urine testing for metabolites	Flumazenil Benzodiazepine receptor antagonist Short acting. Use with caution. May precipitate seizures in patients with chronic benzodiazepine use or concomitant TCA overdose.

GABA, γ-aminobutyric acid; TCA, tricyclic antidepressant.

- Clinical presentation
  - Nausea, malaise, weakness, bradycardia, heart block, hyperkalemia, visual complaints of seeing yellow halos around lights
- Treatment
  - **Digoxin-specific antibody**
    - Indicated for **hemodynamically compromising conduction disturbances or for hyperkalemia**
  - Calcium is relatively contraindicated in this setting because hypercalcemia may potentiate digitalis toxicity
  - Cardiac monitor for at least 6 hours after ingestion
- Theophylline
  - Basic information
    - Methylxanthine bronchodilator with a narrow therapeutic window
  - Clinical presentation
    - Nausea and vomiting, agitation, seizures and arrhythmias, especially supraventricular
  - Treatment
    - **Hemodialysis or charcoal hemoperfusion may be initiated for markedly elevated levels (>60–100 mg/mL), seizures, or persistently unstable hemodynamics**
    - Supraventricular arrhythmias may be treated with β-blockers

Toxins That Alter Hemoglobin/Oxygen-Binding Properties

- Carbon monoxide poisoning
  - Basic information

- Colorless odorless gas emitted by faulty heaters
- Seen primarily in winter months
- Clinical presentation
  - Dizziness, headache, weakness, confusion, dyspnea, chest pain
  - In severe cases: Loss of consciousness, focal CNS symptoms, cardiac ischemia
  - Lips and skin may appear cherry red, but this is an insensitive sign
  - Diagnosis is made by measurement of carboxyhemoglobin
- Treatment
  - Remove patient from the source
  - **Deliver 100% Fio$_2$ by nonrebreathing mask**
  - **Hyperbaric oxygen** appears to prevent delayed neurologic sequelae in high-risk patients (loss of consciousness, confusion, lactic acidosis)
- Methemoglobinemia
  - Basic information
    - Occurs when the ferrous ions (Fe^{2+}) of heme are oxidized to the ferric (Fe^{3+}) state that has a lower affinity for oxygen
    - Methemoglobin formation may be caused by exogenous agents, including sulfonamides, nitrates, topical anesthetics, antimalarials, and occupational exposures
    - Higher levels of methemoglobin occur in individuals with deficiency of the cytochrome b_5 reductase enzyme, which reduces Fe^{3+} to the Fe^{2+} state
  - Clinical presentation
    - Hypoxia, cyanosis, and chocolate color of arterial blood

24

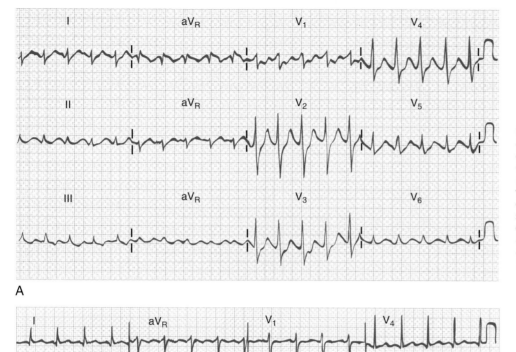

FIGURE 24-4 Electrocardiogram (ECG) in tricyclic antidepressant overdose. **A,** Sinus tachycardia, QRS widening, and QT prolongation in a patient with tricyclic antidepressant overdose. **B,** Normal ECG in the same individual four days later. (From Goldberger AL: *Clinical electrocardiography: a simplified approach,* ed 6, St. Louis, Mosby, 1999, figure 10-4.)

TABLE 24-4	*Alcohol-Induced Toxicity*				
Alcohol	**Example**	**Clinical Presentation**	**Anion Gap***	**Osmolar Gap†**	**Treatment**
Methanol	Antifreeze Bootleg whiskey	Abdominal pain Nausea/vomiting Loss of vision	+	+	Fomepizole (alcohol dehydrogenase inhibitor)
Ethylene glycol	Antifreeze Windshield deicer	Ataxia Seizures Abdominal pain Nausea/vomiting	+	+	Fomepizole
Isopropanol	Rubbing alcohol	Abdominal pain Nausea/vomiting Headache Ataxia Coma	−	+	Fomepizole

*Anion gap, $[Na^+] - ([Cl^-] + [HCO3^-])$.
†Osmolar gap, measured osmolality $- \{2[Na^+] + (BUN/2.8) + ([glucose]/18)\}$.

- Suggested in a patient with **a low pulse oximeter reading, but a normal arterial blood gas Pao_2**
- Diagnosis
- Measurement of methemoglobin level
- Treatment
- Discontinuation of the offending agent
- Administration of **methylene blue** to reduce the methemoglobin to hemoglobin

Alcohols

See Table 24-4 for a summary of alcohol-induced toxicity.

SUGGESTED READINGS

The Acute Respiratory Distress Syndrome Network: Ventilation with lower tidal volumes as compared with traditional tidal volumes for acute lung injury and the acute respiratory distress syndrome, *N Engl J Med* 342:1301–1308, 2000.

Connors AF Jr, Speroff T, Dawson NV, Thomas C, et al: The effectiveness of right heart catheterization in the initial care of critically ill patients. SUPPORT Investigators, *JAMA* 276:889–897, 1996.

Finfer S, Bellamo R, Boyce N, et al: A comparison of albumin and saline for fluid resuscitation in the intensive care unit, *N Engl J Med* 350:2247–2256, 2004.

Hebert PC, Wells G, Blajchman MA, et al: A multicenter, randomized, controlled clinical trial of transfusion requirements in critical care. Transfusion Requirements in Critical Care Investigators, Canadian Critical Care Trials Group, *N Engl J Med* 340:409–417, 1999.

Knaus WA, Zimmerman JE, Wagner DP, et al: APACHE—acute physiology and chronic health evaluation: physiologically based classification system, *Crit Care Med* 9:591–597, 1981.

Sandham JD, Hull RD, Brant RF, et al: A randomized, controlled trial of the use of pulmonary-artery catheters in high-risk surgical patients, *N Engl J Med* 348:5–14, 2003.

Tobin MJ: Advances in mechanical ventilation, *N Engl J Med* 344:1986–1996, 2001.

Wheeler AP, Bernard GR: Treating patients with severe sepsis, *N Engl J Med* 340:207–214, 1999.

Pleural Disease

ALBERT J. POLITO, MD

Pleural diseases are among the most frequently encountered problems in chest medicine. Two of the most common such diseases are pleural effusions and pneumothoraces. The former reflect an excessive accumulation of fluid in the pleural space, whereas the latter occur when air enters the pleural space.

Pleural Effusions

Basic Information

- The most common causes of pleural effusion in the United States are congestive heart failure, pneumonia, malignancy, and pulmonary embolism
- Pathophysiology of pleural effusions
  - Pleural fluid originates from capillaries in parietal pleura and is drained by lymphatics in parietal pleura
  - Pleural effusion forms when more fluid is formed than can be reabsorbed
  - Effusion can also originate from interstitial spaces of lung, intrathoracic lymphatics, or the peritoneal cavity
    - Mechanisms of pleural fluid accumulation are shown in Table 25-1
  - Subpulmonic effusions develop when fluid becomes loculated between the lower aspect of the lung and the diaphragm
  - Parapneumonic effusions and empyema are pleural effusions associated with bacterial pneumonia or lung

abscess; they are associated with a higher mortality rate than pneumonia and abscess without effusions

Clinical Presentation

- Symptoms of pleural effusion differ markedly according to cause and rapidity of onset
  - Pleural effusions are often asymptomatic, but small to moderate effusions may be symptomatic if they develop rapidly
  - Dyspnea; pleuritic chest pain (although pain may be dull and aching); and dry, nonproductive cough are typical symptoms of pleural effusion
    - Patients with infectious causes (e.g., pneumonia, tuberculosis) present with acute febrile illness and chest pain
    - **Patients with malignant pleural effusions typically present with dyspnea**
      - **Malignancy is the most common cause of massive pleural effusions that cause complete opacification of one hemithorax**
  - Patients with a pulmonary embolus present with pleuritic chest pain and dyspnea
    - Effusions (seen in 30–50% of cases) are usually small to moderate in size and unilateral
  - Rheumatoid pleurisy may be asymptomatic and occur in the absence of joint disease activity
    - Classic presentation is an elderly man with subcutaneous rheumatoid nodules and a unilateral pleural effusion
    - **Frequently mimics a complicated parapneumonic effusion, with high lactate dehydrogenase (>1000 U/L), low glucose (<40 mg/dL), and low pH (<7.2)**
  - Lupus pleuritis is typically painful and occurs in 15% to 40% of patients with lupus at some point in the disease
    - Small, bilateral effusions commonly seen
    - It is the presenting feature of lupus in 5% of cases
    - **Lupus pleuritis may be seen in drug-induced lupus because of procainamide, hydralazine, or isoniazid, among others**
  - Chylothorax manifests with (typically) unilateral pleural effusion (Fig. 25-1)
    - Thoracic duct course (Fig. 25-2): Originates in abdomen as cisterna chyli, enters the thorax with the aorta, runs along the right anterolateral surface of the vertebrae, crosses the midline at the fourth thoracic vertebra, continues up along the left antero-lateral vertebral surface, and empties into the junction of the left internal jugular and subclavian veins

TABLE 25-1	*Mechanisms of Pleural Fluid Accumulation*
Mechanism	**Representative Disease State**
Increased hydrostatic pressure of vasculature	Congestive heart failure
Decreased oncotic pressure of vasculature	Nephrotic syndrome
Decreased pleural pressure	Atelectasis
Obstruction of lymphatic drainage	Malignancy
Increased capillary permeability	Parapneumonic effusion
Rupture of thoracic duct	Chylothorax
Increased fluid in peritoneal cavity	Hepatic hydrothorax
Iatrogenic	Placement of central line into pleural space

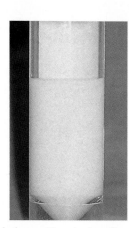

FIGURE 25-1 Chylothorax. The classic milky-appearing pleural fluid of a chylothorax. (From Forbes CD, Jackson WF: *Color atlas and text of clinical medicine*, ed 3, St. Louis, Mosby, 2003, figure 4.53.)

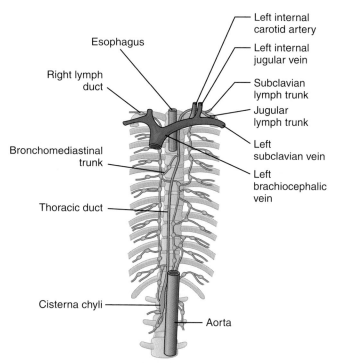

FIGURE 25-2 Lymphatics of the thorax. (From Jacob S: *Atlas of human anatomy*, New York, Churchill Livingstone, 2002, figure 3.4h.)

- **Site of interruption of thoracic duct determines side of pleural effusion (right-sided if below the fourth thoracic vertebra; left-sided if above it)**
- **Lymphoma is cause in 75% of cases**
- Thoracic duct trauma from injury or surgery makes up the majority of the remainder of cases
- Occasionally idiopathic; rarely seen with tuberculosis or sarcoid
- Patients with asbestos exposure may present with benign asbestos pleural effusion (BAPE) 5 to 15 years after exposure to asbestos
  - Effusions are typically unilateral, persist for a mean of 4 months, and resolve spontaneously
  - Patients may go on to develop pleural plaques (20 years after exposure) or mesothelioma (20–30 years after exposure)

- **Physical examination findings over the site of the effusion include dullness to percussion, with decreased or absent breath sounds and the absence of tactile fremitus**
  - Pleural rub (creaky, leathery sound) not common; suggests pleural inflammation alone or with small effusion
  - Other physical findings vary depending on cause of effusion

Diagnosis and Evaluation

- Evaluation of pleural effusions is done by imaging of the effusion and sampling of the effusion with thoracentesis
- Imaging
  - As pleural effusion develops, small amounts of fluid obscure posterior costophrenic angle on lateral imaging, followed by blunting of lateral costophrenic angle on posteroanterior imaging (Fig. 25-3)
    - Sensitivity of posteroanterior and lateral films is 200 mL
    - Lateral decubitus film extremely helpful in detecting effusion; can detect as little as 15 mL of fluid
    - **If lateral decubitus film shows fluid is free-flowing and depth of pleural fluid is greater than 10 mm, diagnostic thoracentesis can be performed**
  - Consider subpulmonic effusion if one hemidiaphragm appears elevated and apex of diaphragm is laterally displaced
    - On left side, consider if top of hemidiaphragm is separated from gastric air bubble
  - Ultrasound is useful for identifying loculated areas of pleural fluid or for localizing placement of thoracentesis needle and distinguishing pleural fluid from pleural thickening
  - CT scanning helps distinguish between pleural and parenchymal disease and can differentiate between empyema and lung abscess

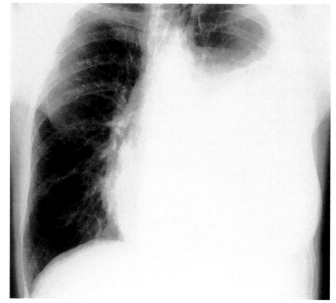

FIGURE 25-3 Large, left pleural effusion. This patient had a previous mastectomy on the right and the pleural effusion is malignant. The mediastinal shift to the right results from the space-occupying effects of the fluid. (From Albert RK, Spiro SG, Jett JR: *Clinical respiratory medicine*, ed 2, St. Louis, Mosby, 2004, figure 1.83.)

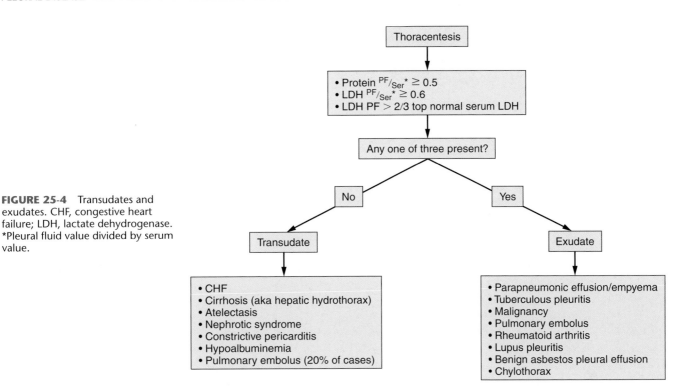

FIGURE 25-4 Transudates and exudates. CHF, congestive heart failure; LDH, lactate dehydrogenase. *Pleural fluid value divided by serum value.

Flowchart content:

Thoracentesis
↓
- Protein $^{PF}/_{Ser}* \geq 0.5$
- LDH $^{PF}/_{Ser}* \geq 0.6$
- LDH PF $> 2/3$ top normal serum LDH
↓
Any one of three present?

No → Transudate
- CHF
- Cirrhosis (aka hepatic hydrothorax)
- Atelectasis
- Nephrotic syndrome
- Constrictive pericarditis
- Hypoalbuminemia
- Pulmonary embolus (20% of cases)

Yes → Exudate
- Parapneumonic effusion/empyema
- Tuberculous pleuritis
- Malignancy
- Pulmonary embolus
- Rheumatoid arthritis
- Lupus pleuritis
- Benign asbestos pleural effusion
- Chylothorax

25

- Thoracentesis
  - For undiagnosed pleural effusions, thoracentesis is indicated
  - Differential diagnosis of pleural effusion is narrowed by determining whether pleural fluid is transudate or exudate (Fig. 25-4)
    - Note that pulmonary embolus usually (80%) results in an exudative effusion but manifests with a transudate in 20% of cases
  - **If any one of the three criteria shown in Figure 25-4 (known as Light's criteria) is met, the effusion is classified as an exudate**
    - **Application of Light's criteria occasionally leads to misclassification of a transudate as an exudate, but does not lead to misclassifying exudates**
  - Cytopathology: Important for diagnosing malignant effusions
    - Most common causes of malignant pleural effusions include lung cancer (33%, usually adenocarcinoma), breast cancer (25%), and lymphoma/leukemia (15%)
    - **Sensitivity of single thoracentesis sample for diagnosing malignancy is 60%; three sequential thoracenteses increase sensitivity to 80%**
    - Cytology more likely to be positive with pleural metastases or with mediastinal lymph node involvement
  - Culture
    - Most common organisms in parapneumonic effusion are *Staphylococcus aureus*, anaerobes such as *Bacteroides* and *Peptostreptococcus*, *Streptococcus pneumoniae*, and gram-negative organisms such as *Escherichia coli* and *Klebsiella*

- **Yield for mycobacterial cultures is only 35%; pleural biopsy typically performed if tuberculosis suggested**
  - **With pleural biopsy, granulomas seen in 80% of cases; acid-fast bacterial (AFB) stain positive in 25% of cases; and AFB culture positive in 55% of cases**
  - **Tuberculin skin test (purified protein derivative [PPD]) positive in only two thirds of patients with a tuberculous pleural effusion**
- Other tests used in evaluation of pleural fluid are shown in Table 25-2
- In patients with pneumonia, characteristics used to distinguish parapneumonic effusion from empyema are shown in Table 25-3

Treatment

- Treatment of pleural effusions determined by size of effusion, presence of symptoms, and cause of effusion
- Treatment options include therapeutic thoracentesis, chest tube drainage, thoracotomy with decortication, and pleurodesis (fusion of visceral and parietal pleura to prevent recurrence of symptomatic effusion)
  - **Chemical pleurodesis: Done with doxycycline (agent of choice)** or bleomycin (less effective and more expensive) introduced through chest tube after fluid is drained and lung has reexpanded
    - **Talc no longer used because of risk of acute respiratory distress syndrome**
  - Surgical pleurodesis performed with mechanical abrasion of pleura via thoracotomy
- Specific treatment
  - Parapneumonic effusion (see Table 25-3)

TABLE 25-2	Tests Used in the Evaluation of Pleural Fluid
Test	**Result**

Cell counts	RBC count > 100,000/μL suggests
	  Trauma
	  Malignancy
	  Pulmonary embolism with infarction
	WBC count
	  <1000/μL suggests transudate
	  >1000/μL suggests exudate
	WBC differential
	  >10,000 neutrophils/μL suggests parapneumonic effusion or empyema; occasionally seen with pulmonary embolus, pancreatitis, or early tuberculosis
	  >50% lymphocytes suggests tuberculosis or malignancy; also seen after coronary artery bypass graft surgery
	  Eosinophilia nonspecific, but may suggest parasitic infection, drug reaction, malignant effusion, or Churg-Strauss syndrome

pH	pH < 7.2 suggests
	  Complicated parapneumonic effusion
	  Empyema
	  Esophageal rupture
	  Rheumatoid pleurisy
	  Malignant effusion
	pH > 7.8 suggests *Proteus* infection

Glucose	Glucose < 60 mg/dL suggests
	  Parapneumonic effusion
	  Empyema
	  Rheumatoid pleurisy
	  Malignant effusion
	  Tuberculous pleuritis

Amylase	If elevated, suggests
	  Pancreatic disease
	  Esophageal rupture (salivary isoenzymes elevated); typically results in left-sided effusion
	  Malignant effusion (salivary isoenzymes not elevated)

Triglycerides (TG)	TG > 110 mg/dL indicates chylothorax If TG 50–110 mg/dL, send fluid for chylomicrons Presence of chylomicrons indicates chylothorax TG < 50 mg/dL indicates no chylothorax

Cholesterol	Causes a "pseudochylothorax" (milky fluid but not a true chylothorax)
	Usually seen in long-standing effusions
	  Old tuberculous effusion
	  Rheumatoid pleurisy
	  Nephrotic syndrome

Antinuclear antibody (ANA)	Pleural fluid ANA titer commonly elevated to >1:160 in lupus, but is not specific for the disease

- **Chylothorax: Treatment includes chest tube, bed rest, enteral feeding with medium-chain triglycerides (absorbed to circulation via portal vein, avoiding thoracic duct)**
  - Occasionally thoracic duct ligation or placement of pleuroperitoneal shunt needed
  - Lack of treatment results in loss of protein, fat, and lymphocytes, risking malnutrition and infection

Pneumothorax

Basic Information

- Pneumothorax results from the introduction of air into the pleural space
  - May occur spontaneously or result from trauma or iatrogenic causes (e.g., surgery, central venous access placement, thoracentesis)
- Primary spontaneous pneumothorax occurs when no clinically apparent lung disease is present

- **Incidence in men compared with women is 6 to 1**
- **Typical patient is a tall, thin male younger than age 40 years who smokes**
  - Most patients have radiographically inapparent subpleural bullae
- Secondary spontaneous pneumothorax occurs as a result of underlying lung disease
  - Obstructive lung diseases associated with secondary spontaneous pneumothorax include asthma, chronic obstructive pulmonary disease, and cystic fibrosis
  - Associated interstitial lung diseases include idiopathic pulmonary fibrosis, eosinophilic granuloma, and lymphangioleiomyomatosis
  - *Pneumocystis jiroveci* (formerly *carinii*) pneumonia and Marfan's syndrome also are associated with secondary spontaneous pneumothorax

Clinical Presentation

- Typical symptoms include ipsilateral pleuritic chest pain and dyspnea

TABLE 25-3 *Parapneumonic Effusions and Empyema*

Effusion Type	Definition	Treatment*
Simple parapneumonic effusion	pH > 7.2 Glucose > 40 mg/dL LDH < 3 times top normal serum LDH	Antibiotics alone often sufficient
Complicated parapneumonic effusion	Gross appearance does not resemble pus pH < 7.0 Glucose < 40 mg/dL "Borderline" complicated pH 7.0–7.2, with glucose > 40 mg/dL and/or LDH < 3 times normal	Antibiotics Chest tube Serial thoracentesis acceptable in borderline cases
Empyema	Appearance of frank pus pH < 7.0 Glucose < 40 mg/dL WBC typically > 15,000/μL Bacterial culture commonly positive	Antibiotics Chest tube Decortication may be required Fibrinolytics or thoracoscopy occasionally used if loculations present

*Treatment of each disorder will be determined in part by volume of fluid and presence of loculations.
LDH, lactate dehydrogenase.

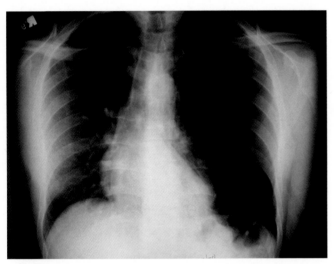

FIGURE 25-5 Anteroposterior chest radiograph of simple pneumothorax. Note absence of lung marking on the affected side and deviation of the trachea contralaterally. (From Roberts JR: *Clinical procedures in emergency medicine,* ed 4, Philadelphia, Saunders, 2004, figure 10-1.)

- Physical findings normal with small pneumothorax (<15%)
  - **Tachycardia is the most common finding in pneumothorax**
  - **Hyper-resonance to percussion, decreased chest wall movement, decreased fremitus, and decreased or absent breath sounds common with large pneumothorax**
  - Hypotension, cyanosis, and shift of the trachea to the contralateral side seen with tension pneumothorax

Diagnosis and Evaluation

- Radiographic imaging used to confirm diagnosis
  - Visceral pleural edge separated from chest wall on chest radiograph (Fig. 25-5)
  - May be difficult to diagnose with underlying lung disease (e.g., bullous emphysema)
  - Chest CT may be needed if suggested but not apparent on chest film

Treatment

- Treatment is similar for primary and secondary spontaneous pneumothorax, although the threshold for placing a chest tube is lower (i.e., done sooner) for secondary spontaneous pneumothorax
  - **Administer 100% oxygen and observe patient if pneumothorax is small (<15%)**
    - **Increases rate of reabsorption of air from pleural space fourfold**
  - Larger (>15%) pneumothoraces require removal of air, either with catheter (works best with young patients) or with chest tube (required for most patients)
- Recurrence rate
  - Similar for primary and secondary forms
  - **30% after first episode; more than 50% after second episode**
  - Usually occurs within 2 years after initial pneumothorax
  - Advise patients to avoid scuba diving
  - **After second pneumothorax, recommend intervention to prevent recurrence**
    - Chemical pleurodesis through chest tube
    - If present, blebs/bullae should be surgically resected, with concomitant mechanical abrasion of pleura (surgical pleurodesis)

REVIEW QUESTIONS

For review questions, please go to www.expertconsult.com.

SUGGESTED READINGS

Light RW: *Pleural diseases,* ed 4, Philadelphia, Lippincott, Williams & Wilkins, 2001.
Light RW: Pleural effusion, N Engl J Med 346:1971–1977, 2002.
Sahn SA, Heffner JE: Spontaneous pneumothorax, N Engl J Med 342:868–874, 2000.
Schiza S, Siafakas SM: Clinical presentation and management of empyema, lung abscess, and pleural effusion, Curr Opin Pulm Med 12:205–211, 2006.

25

SECTION FOUR

Gastroenterology

Peptic Ulcer Disease and Gastrointestinal Bleeding

JOHN O. CLARKE, MD, and LINDA A. LEE, MD

Causes of GI blood loss have been divided into two basic categories based on the anatomic location of the bleeding source in relation to the ligament of Treitz. *Upper GI bleeding* refers to blood loss originating above this area, whereas *lower GI bleeding* stems from sources below. This chapter focuses on the approach to patients with suspected upper or lower GI bleeding and describes the most common specific causes within each category.

Background

Stomach Anatomy

Figure 26-1 illustrates the anatomy of the stomach.
- Antrum
  - Pyloric glands
    - G cells: Secrete gastrin, which stimulates acid production
    - D cells: Secrete somatostatin, which inhibits gastrin secretion
    - Goblet cells: Secrete mucus to coat and protect the stomach from corrosive injury
- Fundus/body
  - Oxyntic glands
    - Parietal cells: Secrete acid (HCl)
    - Chief cells: Secrete pepsinogen, which is converted to pepsin by HCl. Pepsin can damage the gastric epithelium.

Gastric Acid Secretion

- Three pathways by which acid production/secretion occurs
  - Vagus innervation leads to release of acetylcholine, which leads to stimulation of H+/K+ adenosine triphosphatase (ATPase) and acid production/secretion
  - Gastrin release leads to direct stimulation of H+/K+ ATPase, which leads to acid production/secretion
  - Histamine release leads to stimulation of adenylate cyclase, which leads to cyclic adenosine monophosphate (cAMP), which leads to stimulation of H+/K+ ATPase and leads to acid production/secretion
- Regulation of acid secretion
  - Basal acid secretion: Mediated by vagal tone; highest levels at nighttime
  - Food-stimulated secretion
    - Cephalic phase: Sight, smell, and taste stimulate the vagus nerve
    - Gastric phase: Triggered by gastric distention and protein digestion caused by food entering the stomach; gastrin is then released
    - Intestinal phase: Triggered by protein in small bowel

Peptic Ulcer Disease

Causes

- Direct mucosal injury (e.g., toxins, ethanol, NSAIDs, *Helicobacter pylori*, bile)
- Inhibition of prostaglandin synthesis (NSAIDs)
- Disruption of the protective mucus layer (NSAIDs, *H. pylori*)
- Increased gastric acid secretion (*H. pylori*, gastrinoma, hypercalcemia, sepsis, central nervous system, burns)
- Mucosal ischemia (anastomotic ulcers)

Epidemiology

- **Most patients have normal acid secretion**
- Gastric ulcers may represent an underlying malignancy (~3%)
- Duodenal ulcers rarely represent an underlying malignancy
- Lifetime prevalence of peptic ulcer disease (PUD) is 5% to 10%

Clinical Presentation

- Epigastric abdominal pain is the most common symptom
- Nausea and vomiting may occur
- Gastrointestinal bleeding (see later discussion): 20% of patients will bleed and can present with hematemesis, coffee-ground emesis, hematochezia, or melena

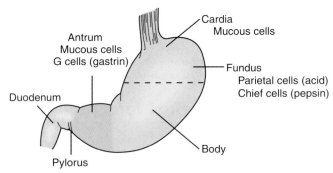

FIGURE 26-1 Anatomy of the stomach. (From Kumar V, Fausto N, Abbas A: *Robbins & Cotran's pathologic basis of disease*, ed 7, Philadelphia, WB Saunders, 2004, figure 17-12A.)

- Perforation
  - Seen in 5% of patients
  - Abdominal examination reveals rigid abdomen with rebound tenderness
  - Duodenal ulcers may penetrate posterior to the pancreas, resulting in elevations in amylase and lipase
- Gastric outlet obstruction
  - Usually caused by peripyloric scar formation
  - Presents with abdominal bloating, nausea, vomiting, weight loss

Diagnosis

- Endoscopy versus barium study
  - Four studies show that endoscopy is far superior to barium study for detecting gastric and duodenal ulcers
  - American College of Physicians 1985 guidelines recommend endoscopy

Therapy

- Antacids
  - Neutralize acid
  - Magnesium and aluminum compounds can be toxic in patients with renal failure
  - Calcium carbonate antacids can cause milk-alkali syndrome (hypercalcemia, hyperphosphatemia) with prolonged use
- Histamine 2 (H_2) blockers (e.g., cimetidine, ranitidine, famotidine, nizatidine)
  - Block H_2 receptor on parietal cells
  - Effective for both duodenal and gastric ulcers
  - Inhibit cytochrome P-450 drug metabolism (more common with cimetidine); need to monitor levels of some drugs (e.g., warfarin, phenytoin, theophylline)
- Proton-pump (H+/K+ ATPase) inhibitors (e.g., omeprazole, lansoprazole, rabeprazole, pantoprazole, esomeprazole)
  - Irreversibly block H+/K+ ATPase; take 3 days to block 90% of pumps
  - Effective for both duodenal and gastric ulcers
  - Can interfere with the absorption of other drugs (e.g., ketoconazole, ampicillin, iron, digoxin)
  - Emerging data suggest long-term use may be associated with decreased bone mineral density and increased community-acquired infection
  - Emerging data to suggest it may interfere with clopidogrel
- Sucralfate
  - Stimulates endogenous prostaglandins and enhances mucosal defenses and repair
  - Effective for duodenal ulcer
  - Avoid in patients with renal insufficiency because of the potential for aluminum toxicity

Duration of Therapy

- Duodenal ulcers: 4 to 6 weeks
- **Gastric ulcers: 6 to 8 weeks; repeat endoscopy with biopsies to rule out gastric cancer in 8 weeks**

NSAID-Associated GI Toxicity

Epidemiology

- Dyspepsia occurs in 10% to 20% of patients taking NSAIDs
- 1.3% of those taking it for arthritis have a serious GI complication

- Mortality rate for those hospitalized with NSAID-related bleeding is 5% to 10%
- **An increased risk of GI bleeding is associated with even low-dose aspirin use (<75 mg per day)**
- Enteric-coated aspirin has a similar rate of complication to nonenteric-coated preparations

Risk Factors

- Prior history of ulcer
- Concomitant use of corticosteroids
- Concomitant use of other anticoagulants
- High doses of NSAIDs
- Advanced age (>70 years)
- *H. pylori*–controversial

Mechanisms

- Topical: NSAIDs are acidic and can migrate through the protective layer of mucus to the gastric epithelium, where they dissociate into the ionized form. The disruption in the layer of mucus also permits further injury by gastric acid and pepsin.
- Inhibition of prostaglandin synthesis: Most important cause of gastroduodenal NSAID injury

Therapy

- Withdraw NSAIDs
- Treat *H. pylori* (see later discussion) if ulcer is present
- Proton-pump inhibitor

Prophylaxis

- Not indicated in the absence of prior PUD or symptoms
- Misoprostol
  - Prostaglandin E derivative shown to decrease the incidence of NSAID-induced ulceration
  - Diarrhea is a common side effect
  - Contraindicated in pregnancy
- Proton-pump inhibitor is also effective
- H_2 blockers found to be inferior to proton-pump inhibitors and misoprostol
- **Eradicate *H. pylori* before initiating NSAID therapy if patient is *H. pylori* positive and has a history of PUD**

Alternative to Prophylaxis

- Cyclooxygenase-2 (COX-2)-selective inhibitors
- Based on the fact that COX-1 is constitutively expressed and maintains GI mucosal integrity and COX-2 expression is induced by inflammation
- Studies show that COX-2-selective inhibitors are less likely to cause PUD than are nonselective NSAIDs
- Lack cardiovascular protective effects (COX-1 participates in platelet aggregation)
  - **Protective effect of COX-2-selective inhibitor is lost if the patient uses regular or baby acetylsalicylic acid concomitantly**

Helicobacter pylori *Infection*

Features

- Gram-negative, spiral-shaped, flagellated rod
- Accounts for most cases of PUD in the United States
- Found in mucous layer; produces a urease that splits urea into ammonia and bicarbonate

- Humans are the principal reservoir
- Mode of transmission thought to be fecal-oral and/or oral-oral routes
- Infection thought to occur in childhood
- In the United States, 40% to 50% of those older than 60 years are infected
- More prevalent in developing countries
- Risk factors for infection include low socioeconomic status, domestic crowding, exposure to unclean food or water

Diagnosis

- Noninvasive tests
  - Serum immunoglobulin G (IgG): About 90% sensitivity
    - Serum qualitative antibody test
    - Whole-blood qualitative antibody test
    - Quantitative antibody test: A 30% decrease in titer can be used to document post-treatment eradication (rarely done). A qualitative test is not useful to document post-treatment eradication because IgG remains positive after treatment.
  - Urea breath test (95% sensitivity, >95% specificity)
    - Urea labeled with C-13 or C-14 cleaved by urease into ammonia and CO_2
    - Stop proton-pump inhibitor 1 week and antibiotics 4 weeks before test; should also stop bismuth and high doses of H_2-receptor antagonists
  - Stool *H. pylori* antigen test
    - Sensitivity 93.2%, specificity 93.2%
    - Useful for initial diagnosis and also documentation of post-therapy eradication
    - More widely available than breath test
- Invasive tests
  - Rapid urease test (~90% sensitivity, >95% specificity)
    - Biopsy is placed on a card that is spotted with urea; when urease is present, it cleaves the urea, inducing a pH and color change on the card
  - Histology
  - Presence of active chronic gastritis suggests the presence of *H. pylori* even in the absence of visible organisms
  - Organisms can be detected by Giemsa, hematoxylin and eosin, and silver stains
  - Culture
    - Useful only for detecting antibiotic resistance and not often obtained in clinical practice
- Use of *H. pylori* testing
  - Antibody tests are useful in those who have not been previously treated
  - **Stool antigen test or urea breath test is useful to detect active infections or monitor response to therapy**
  - Endoscopy is useful to detect *H. pylori*–associated ulcers or cancers

Therapy

- Overview
  - **Triple-drug therapy far superior to dual-drug therapy**
  - Reinfection is rare
  - Metronidazole resistance is 43%
  - Clarithromycin resistance is 8%

- Food and Drug Administration–approved regimens
  - 14 days: Bismuth subsalicylate two tablets four times a day, metronidazole 250 mg four times a day, tetracycline 500 mg four times a day, H_2 blocker (BMT)
  - 14 days: Lansoprazole 30 mg twice a day, amoxicillin 1 g twice a day, clarithromycin 500 mg twice a day (LAC)
  - 10 days: Omeprazole 20 mg twice a day, amoxicillin 1 g twice a day, clarithromycin 500 mg twice a day (OAC)

Diseases Associated with *H. pylori*

- Peptic ulcer disease
  - **_H. pylori_ is present in 70% of patients with gastric ulcers and in nearly 100% of patients with duodenal ulcers**
- Active chronic gastritis
- Gastric adenocarcinoma
- **Gastric mucosa–associated lymphoid tissue lymphoma: Treatment of infection causes tumor regression in most patients with this disease**

Zollinger-Ellison Syndrome

- Hypersecretion of gastrin from tumors arising from the pancreas or wall of the duodenum (*gastrinoma*)
- Presents with peptic ulceration, which may be refractory to treatment
- Ulceration may be single or multiple and involve the stomach, duodenum, or jejunum (classic location is post-bulbar duodenum)
- Diarrhea results from the high volumes of gastric acid produced. Steatorrhea may result from inactivation of pancreatic enzymes as a result of the high volume of gastric acid in the duodenum.
- Two thirds of gastrinomas are malignant and may metastasize to the lymph nodes or liver
- About one third of gastrinomas are associated with multiple endocrine neoplasia type 1, so adenomas of the parathyroid (causing hypercalcemia) and pituitary may also be seen
- Diagnosis
  - Elevated basal acid output levels (not sensitive)
  - **Increased serum gastrin levels (value > 1000 pg/mL) with a gastric pH less than 2 mEq is virtually diagnostic**
  - Patients with gastrin levels less than 1000 pg/mL and with a pH less than 2 mEq/mL need provocative testing
    - Secretin test: IV infusion of secretin results in a paradoxical rise in serum gastrin in patients with Zollinger-Ellison syndrome but not in other conditions. A secretin stimulation test has a sensitivity of approximately 85%.
      - Calcium infusion test has a much lower sensitivity and specificity and should be used only if the secretin test does not confirm the diagnosis and suspicion is high
  - Tumor localization
    - Radiologic imaging: Abdominal CT—**90% of gastrinomas are located within the "gastrinoma triangle,"** bordered by the head of the pancreas, the second portion of the duodenum, and the cystic and common bile duct

26

- Octreotide scintigraphy scan: ^{111}In-DTPA-D-Phe1 octreotide binds to the somatostatin type 2 receptors on gastrinomas. Using whole-body scintigraphy, gastrinomas can be localized with a sensitivity of 71% to 75% and a specificity of 86% to 100%.

Dyspepsia

- Definition: Chronic or recurrent epigastric pain in the absence of reflux symptoms, acute severe pain, abdominal wall pain, or dysphagia
- Differential diagnosis of dyspepsia
  - Functional dyspepsia: 60% of cases
  - Disordered motility
    - Hypersensitive visceral sensation
    - Altered intestinogastric reflexes
    - Psychological stress
  - Peptic ulcer disease: 15% to 25% of cases
  - Gastroesophageal reflux disease: 5% to 15% of cases
  - Malignancy: Less than 2% of cases
- Clinical evaluation and therapy
  - 2001 American Gastroenterology Association Guidelines: If age younger than 45 years and no warning symptoms (e.g., weight loss, dysphagia, anemia), check *H. pylori* serology (or stool antigen test), and treat if positive; trial of antisecretory therapy if serology negative; if no response, then endoscopy; if age older than 45 years or warning symptoms are present, proceed directly to endoscopy

Gastrointestinal Bleeding

Approach to the Patient with Gastrointestinal Bleeding

- Evaluation
  - Determine heart rate, blood pressure, the presence of orthostatic hypotension

- Check hematocrit—may initially be misleadingly normal in patients with severe bleeding
- **Volume resuscitation with IV fluids or blood**
- Differentiate between upper (UGIB) and lower GI bleeding (LGIB)
  - Hematemesis: Indicates an upper source (above the ligament of Treitz)
  - Melena: Indicates that blood has been present in the GI tract for a number of hours; can be seen in upper GI as well as proximal lower (i.e., right colon) GI bleeding
  - Hematochezia: Usually suggests a lower GI source but can be from a massive upper GI bleed
  - Nasogastric aspirate: Look for fresh blood or coffee grounds; can occasionally see a nonbloody aspirate in patients with UGIB
- Diagnosis (Fig. 26-2)
  - Suspected UGIB: Proceed with upper endoscopy
  - Suspected LGIB: Controversial; many sources recommend performing sigmoidoscopy or colonoscopy first and then proceeding with angiography or technetium-99m (^{99m}Tc)-labeled red cell scan if bleeding persists; however, because of issues of preparation and timing, if the bleed is significant, in practice the order is often reversed and a tagged RBC scan or angiography is obtained first to evaluate for bleeding activity and offer potential therapy
  - Hematochezia with hemodynamic instability: **Initially perform upper endoscopy to rule out an upper GI source**
  - Occult GI bleed: Refers to hemoccult-positive stool without a clear source; workup usually consists of an upper endoscopy and lower endoscopy (yield, ~50%); if negative, the small bowel should be evaluated (push enteroscopy, video capsule endoscopy, single/double balloon enteroscopy or small bowel series)
- Treatment: Based on the cause of the bleed; H_2 blockers and proton-pump inhibitors do not reduce the risk of

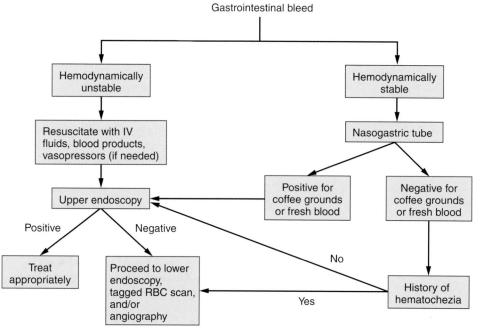

FIGURE 26-2 Evaluation of patient with gastrointestinal bleeding.

TABLE 26-1	Causes of Gastrointestinal (GI) Bleeding	
	Upper GI	**Lower GI**
Acute GI bleeding	Peptic ulcer disease Gastric erosions Esophagitis Mallory-Weiss tear (5–15%) Portal hypertension– related Dieulafoy's lesion	Diverticulosis Vascular ectasia Colitis Neoplasms
Chronic GI bleeding	Esophagitis Gastric ulcer Gastritis Duodenal ulcer Vascular ectasia	Adenomas > 1 cm Carcinoma Colitis Vascular ectasia

rebleeding in the absence of endoscopic stigmata of recent bleeding; if UGIB is suspected, may wish to start IV proton-pump inhibitor empirically because it might reduce the risk of rebleeding in patients with ulcers with visible vessels injected with epinephrine

Etiology

See Table 26-1 for a summary of the causes of GI bleeding.
- Upper GI source
  - Consider in a patient who presents with melena, hematemesis, or brisk hematochezia associated with orthostatic hypotension
- Lower GI source
  - Accounts for only 20% of all episodes of acute GI bleeding
  - Consider in a patient who presents with hematochezia, occasionally with melena
  - In more than half the cases of acute LGIB, diverticular bleed is the cause

Specific Etiologies

- Gastric/duodenal ulcers
  - Bleeding ulcers tend to be located on the lesser curve or in the posterior duodenal bulb, where erosion into large vessels may occur
  - *H. pylori* does not appear to be a risk factor for ulcer bleeding, unlike age and NSAID use
  - Endoscopic therapy is warranted in patients with a visible vessel observed in an ulcer crater, even if there is no active bleeding; chance of rebleeding is 50% to 70% without therapy, 20% with therapy
  - IV omeprazole administered after endoscopic therapy decreased the rate of recurrent bleeding from 22.5% to 6.7%
  - Refer patients for surgery if endoscopic therapy is unsuccessful
  - Consider long-term prophylactic therapy in those who have bled; 33% PUD recurrence rate in 3 years without prophylaxis
- Mallory-Weiss tear
  - Laceration of the mucosa at the gastroesophageal junction

- Often associated with a history of vomiting or dry heaves before the bleeding episode
  - May also be associated with heavy alcohol use
  - Bleeding usually stops spontaneously, although rebleeding may occur in 5% of patients
  - Angiography with embolization can be performed. Surgery is rarely required.
  - **Distinguished from Boerhaave's syndrome, which is esophageal perforation caused by retching**
- Vascular malformations
  - Angiodysplasia
    - Flat, red lesions; can be found anywhere in the small intestine and colon
    - Diagnosed by endoscopy
    - Associated with chronic renal failure, valvular heart disease
    - Treat with iron supplements or with estrogens
    - Brisk bleeds can be evaluated by bleeding scan or arteriography and treated by embolization, surgical resection
  - Watermelon stomach (Fig. 26-3)
    - Vascular ectasia of the gastric antrum
    - Seen predominantly in elderly women
    - **Possible association with chronic liver disease and scleroderma**
    - Usually manifests as iron deficiency anemia
    - Treat with iron supplementation, but sometimes cautery or surgery is necessary
- Dieulafoy's lesion
  - Ectatic artery that erodes into the stomach, causing brisk bleeding
  - Endoscopy may fail to identify the lesion if the bleeding has ceased
  - Treat endoscopically with cautery; embolization or surgery may be necessary

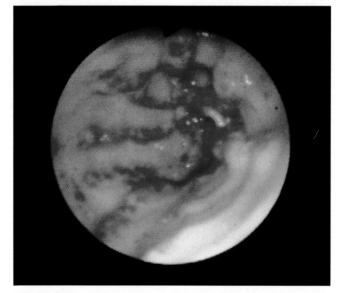

FIGURE 26-3   Endoscopic view of watermelon stomach. (From Feldman M: *Sleisenger and Fordtran's gastrointestinal and liver disease,* ed 7, Philadelphia, WB Saunders, 2002, figure 120-9.)

26

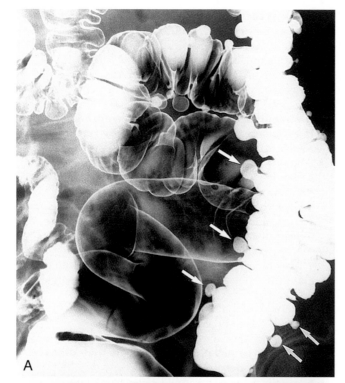

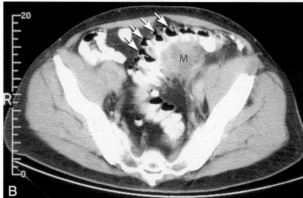

FIGURE 26-4 Diverticulosis of the colon. **A,** Double-contrast barium enema showing outpouchings *(arrows)* that represent diverticula. **B,** CT showing outpouchings *(arrows)* and a focal mass (M), a developing abscess. (From Mettler FA: *Essentials of radiology,* ed 2, Philadelphia, WB Saunders, 2005, figure 6-73.)

- Diverticulosis—"outpouchings" of colonic mucosa and submucosa (Fig. 26-4)
  - Most common cause of acute LGIB
  - Usually affects the left colon, but bleeding is often from the right colon
  - Low recurrence rate of bleeding
  - In only 20% of cases will the bleeding diverticulum be identified
  - **Most patients do well, and bleeding stops spontaneously**
  - Resection in those with refractory bleeding or recurrent bleeding
  - Diverticulitis
    - Inflammation around the diverticular sac
    - Usually occurs in the left colon
    - Typically presents with abdominal pain, fever, and leukocytosis
    - Microscopic bleeding can occur commonly, but gross bleeding is rare
    - **CT scan can aid in the diagnosis, but barium enema and colonoscopy should be avoided with acute infection**
    - Complications include perforation, peritonitis, abscess, and fistula formation
    - Treat with broad-spectrum antibiotics (e.g., ciprofloxacin plus metronidazole) to cover gram-negative aerobes and anaerobes
- Bleeding associated with portal hypertension
  - Bleeding can occur if portal pressure is greater than 12 mm Hg
  - Prevent bleeding with β-blockers, which also reduce mortality associated with bleeding
  - Esophageal/gastric varices
    - Likelihood of varices in cirrhotic patients is 35% to 80%, with 30% experiencing bleeding
    - Mortality rate for each bleeding episode is 35% to 50%
    - **Poor prognostic indicator: Only one third of patients with a history of variceal bleeding are alive at 1 year**
    - Acute therapy
      - Volume replacement/blood products
      - Sengstaken-Blakemore tube is only a temporizing measure for another therapy
      - Octreotide (minimal impact on systemic hemodynamics, in contrast to vasopressin)
      - Endoscopic sclerotherapy or band ligation
      - Transjugular intrahepatic portosystemic shunt (TIPS)
      - No mortality advantage over endoscopic therapy
      - High incidence of hepatic encephalopathy
      - Useful as a bridge to transplantation
      - Surgical shunting
      - Orthotopic liver transplantation
  - Portal hypertensive gastropathy
    - Vascular congestion of the gastric mucosa, imparts a "mosaic appearance" endoscopically
    - Treat with somatostatin to lower splanchnic blood flow
    - Consider TIPS
  - Secondary prevention of recurrent bleeding associated with portal hypertension
    - Nonselective β-adrenergic blocker drugs (e.g., propranolol)
    - Variceal banding: Useful for esophageal varices only; not gastropathy or gastric varices
    - TIPS
- Colitis
  - Infectious (see Chapter 14)
  - Inflammatory: Crohn's disease, ulcerative colitis (see Chapter 29)
  - Ischemic
    - Patients usually over age 60 years
    - Arises from low flow rate, not occlusion
    - **Watershed areas affected—right colon, splenic flexure, and rectum**
    - Symptoms include mild abdominal pain, cramping, bloody diarrhea
    - Diagnose by clinical presentation, colonoscopy

- Can be associated with estrogen use, hypercoagulable states, vasculitis
- Chronic GI bleeding
  - Can present as iron deficiency anemia from causes such as PUD, colon cancer, vascular malformations
  - Can also present with heme-positive stool in the absence of iron deficiency
    - UGIB causes include esophagitis, gastritis, PUD
    - LGIB causes include colon cancer, colonic adenomas larger than 1 cm, colitis, vascular ectasia
    - Presence of upper GI symptoms is usually associated with detection of an upper GI lesion
    - In patients with or without symptoms, upper GI lesion is more common than lower GI lesion
      - Workup: Upper endoscopy, colonoscopy, push enteroscopy, capsule enteroscopy, single/double balloon enteroscopy, dedicated small bowel series; bleeding scan and angiography are only useful if there is acute bleeding at a fairly brisk rate (0.1 mL/min for scan, 0.5 mL/min for angiography); diagnostic yield of capsule enteroscopy is greater than for push enteroscopy; single/double balloon enteroscopy allows both diagnosis and treatment, but it is time-consuming and not widely available

REVIEW QUESTIONS

For review questions, please go to www.expertconsult.com.

SUGGESTED READINGS

Gralnek IM, Barkun AN, Bardou M: Management of acute bleeding from a peptic ulcer, *N Engl J Med* 359:928–937; 2008.

Green BT, Rockey DC: Lower gastrointestinal bleeding—management, *Gastroenterol Clin North Am* 34:665–78; 2005.

Lanza FL, Chan FK, Quigley EM: Guidelines for prevention of NSAID related ulcer complications, *Am J Gastroenterol* 104:728–738; 2009.

Rockey DC, Cello JP: Evaluation of the gastrointestinal tract in patients with iron-deficiency anemia, *N Engl J Med* 329:1691–1695, 1993.

Rockey DC, Koch J, Cello JP, et al: Relative frequency of upper gastrointestinal and colonic lesions in patients with positive fecal occult-blood tests, *N Engl J Med* 339:153–159, 1998.

Wolfe MM, Lichtenstein DR, Singh G: Gastrointestinal toxicity of nonsteroidal anti-inflammatory drugs, N Engl J Med 340:888–1899, 1999.

26

Esophageal Disease

JOHN O. CLARKE, MD, and LINDA A. LEE, MD

Diseases of the esophagus include a number of conditions caused by abnormalities in anatomic structure or function. This chapter reviews many of those conditions, including gastroesophageal reflux disease (GERD) and esophagitis, esophageal cancer, and dysmotility syndromes. Before describing specific disease processes, basic esophageal anatomy is reviewed.

Normal Esophageal Structure and Function

Figure 27-1 shows the anatomy of the esophagus.
- Upper esophageal sphincter
  - Striated muscle
  - Relaxes in response to a swallow
  - Functions to prevent aspiration
- Esophageal body
  - Upper one third striated muscle, lower two thirds smooth muscle

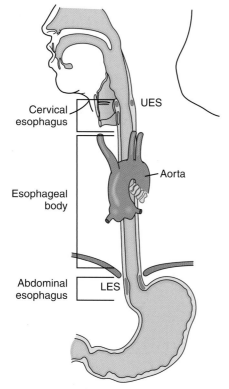

- Innervated by the vagus nerve
- Swallowing initiates contractions in the upper esophagus, and enteric nervous system perpetuates it through the body
- Lower esophageal sphincter (LES)
  - High-pressure zone in distal esophagus
  - Relaxes in response to a swallow (vagally mediated)
  - Prevents GERD
  - Relaxation regulated by a variety of neuropeptides and hormones

Gastroesophageal Reflux Disease

Basic Information
- Protective mechanisms against reflux include the LES, peristalsis, saliva, and gravity
- **Caused by increased frequency of transient relaxations of the LES and decreased LES tone**
- There are numerous potential complications of GERD (Box 27-1)

Clinical Presentation
- Heartburn, indigestion
- Acid regurgitation

BOX 27-1	*Potential Complications of GERD*

Esophagitis
Esophageal ulceration
Esophageal stricture
Pulmonary aspiration
Barrett's esophagus
   Occurs in up to 14% of patients with reflux symptoms undergoing endoscopy
   Replacement of the squamous epithelium with columnar epithelium
   Increased cancer risk associated only with specialized columnar epithelium (i.e., goblet cells present)
   Increased rate of adenocarcinoma estimated to be 10%
   Surveillance endoscopy every 3 years with biopsies from multiple levels is recommended but has not yet been shown to reduce mortality
   Treatment is antireflux therapy, although this may not cause regression of Barrett's or reduce the risk of progression to high-grade dysplasia or cancer
   Presence of high-grade dysplasia is an indication for esophagectomy or endoscopic ablative therapy, particularly for those patients who are not good surgical candidates

FIGURE 27-1 Anatomy of the esophagus showing the upper esophageal sphincter (UES), lower esophageal sphincter (LES), and esophageal body.

- Water brash: Vagal-mediated saliva production that occurs in response to esophagitis; distinguished from regurgitation
- Dyspnea: Vagal-mediated bronchoconstriction, microaspiration
- Dysphagia: Triggered by esophageal spasm
- Chronic cough
- Hoarseness
- Chest pain

Diagnosis and Evaluation

- In patients who present "typically" (heartburn and/or acid regurgitation), testing might not be necessary; a therapeutic trial (see following) may be sufficient
- Testing is indicated when atypical presentations, refractory symptoms, weight loss, or dysphagia is present
- Endoscopy with biopsies is often the first-line diagnostic study and is very specific for reflux (>95%) if esophagitis or Barrett's esophagus is identified; however, it is relatively insensitive (~20% in most studies)
- A 24-hour catheter–based pH probe has been the traditional "gold standard" (79–95% sensitivity, 86%–100% specificity) when symptoms are persistent and endoscopy is unrevealing. However, two new modalities have now entered the clinical arena: (1) the wireless pH capsule that can be attached temporarily to the esophageal wall and records the pH telemetrically; and (2) combined 24-hour pH/impedance, which combines standard pH monitoring with impedance flow, thereby allowing detection of flow (allowing detection of non–acid reflux).
- Barium swallow: Used primarily to evaluate dysphagia; insensitive for nonerosive esophagitis
- Bernstein test (acid infusion): A provocative test to evaluate atypical chest pain; symptoms are reproduced with the infusion of 0.1 N HCl but not with the infusion of saline; not used clinically in most centers and of limited diagnostic utility

Treatment

- Greater amount of acid suppression is needed to control GERD than to control peptic ulcer disease
- Lifestyle changes
  - Smoking cessation
  - Avoidance of alcohol
  - Low-fat diet
  - Elevate the head of the bed (6 inches)
  - Eat several hours before going to bed
  - Avoid medications that lower LES tone (e.g., anticholinergics, sedatives, nitrates, calcium blockers, theophylline)
  - Avoid foods known to lower LES tone (e.g., tomatoes, citrus, garlic, onions, peppermint, chocolate)
- Antacids: Treat symptoms, not esophagitis
- Histamine 2 (H_2) blockers (cimetidine, ranitidine, famotidine, nizatidine) are useful for cases of moderate severity
- Proton-pump inhibitors (omeprazole, pantoprazole, rabeprazole, lansoprazole, esomeprazole)
  - **Superior to H$_2$ blocker in controlling symptoms and healing esophagitis**
  - Duration of therapy should be at least 6 weeks
  - Prolonged use is necessary for severe cases

- No increased risk of tumors (carcinoid or gastrinoma) with long-term use
- Emerging data to suggest long-term use may be associated with decreased bone mineral density and increase in community-acquired infections
- May interfere with the anti-platelet activity of clopidogrel
- Prokinetic agents (e.g., metoclopramide) increase LES pressure and/or gastric emptying
- γ-Aminobutyric acid (GABA)-agonists (e.g., baclofen) decrease the frequency of transient LES relaxation and subsequently the number of reflux episodes; limited utility because of dose-related side effects
- Endoscopic antireflux devices: Available for those patients who cannot or will not take proton-pump inhibitors (PPIs) to control their symptoms; currently consists of two methods: Endoscopic suturing or delivery of thermal energy to the distal esophagus (Stretta); both methods are associated with a reduction in PPI use but have failed to show any significant reduction in reflux episodes by pH-metry; the long-term consequences of these therapies are not yet known, and they are not recommended in routine cases at present
- Antireflux surgery (fundoplication) is indicated in patients with refractory symptoms. Laparoscopic Nissen fundoplication is a proven effective alternative to PPI use and may be effective in up to 90% of cases.
- **In cases of refractory GERD, consider alternative diagnoses, such as gastroparesis, gastrinoma (rare), gallbladder dysfunction,** or cardiac etiology

Esophagitis: Causes

- GERD (see preceding)
- Pill-induced
  - Common offenders include KCl, NSAIDs, tetracycline, alendronate, quinidine, FeSO$_4$, and ascorbic acid
- Occurs more often in elderly patients
- Caustic ingestion
  - **Ingestion of alkali worse than acid**
    - Induction of vomiting is not recommended for lye ingestion
    - Increased risk of squamous cell carcinoma with lye strictures
  - Stricture formation is common
  - Can also cause perforation, bleeding, and death
- Eosinophilic esophagitis
  - Deposition of eosinophils in esophagus leads to a ringed esophagus
  - Results in solid food dysphagia
  - Believed to be related to either food or airborne allergies but mechanism uncertain
  - Clusters with asthma and atopic disorders
  - Diagnosed with endoscopic biopsy
  - Increasing in incidence and prevalence
  - Treated in most cases with dietary modification or topical steroids
- Infectious
  - Presence or absence of oral lesions does not correlate with esophagitis
    - Diagnosis best made by endoscopy

27

- Viral esophagitis
  - Cytomegalovirus (CMV)
    - Only in immunocompromised patients
    - Endoscopy shows serpiginous ulcers within normal mucosa
    - Histology shows intranuclear and intracytoplasmic inclusions
    - Treat with ganciclovir or foscarnet (if resistance occurs)
  - Herpes virus
    - Type 1 rarely causes esophagitis in immunocompetent patients
    - Type 1 or 2 can cause esophagitis in immunosuppressed patients
    - Endoscopy shows vesicles and small ulcers
    - Histology can show eosinophilic intranuclear inclusions and giant cell formation
    - Treat with acyclovir or foscarnet (if acyclovir resistance occurs)
  - Varicella-zoster virus (VZV)
    - Can cause esophagitis in immunocompetent and immunosuppressed patients
    - Similar presentation to herpes simplex virus (HSV)
    - Acyclovir can reduce symptom duration
  - HIV (see Chapter 12)
    - Self-limited ulceration can accompany seroconversion
    - Persistent ulceration can exist in patients with more advanced disease; glucocorticoids or thalidomide may be used to treat
- Candidal esophagitis
  - Endoscopy shows whitish-yellow plaques (Fig. 27-2)
  - Diagnose by demonstrating yeast or hyphal forms on KOH preparation
  - Fluconazole is the preferred treatment

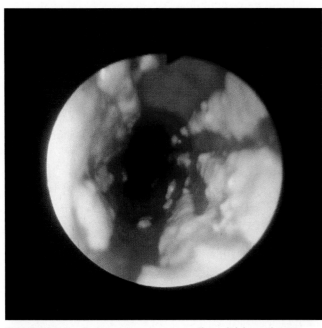

FIGURE 27-2 Endoscopic appearance of candidal esophagitis. (From Cohen J, Powderly W: *Infectious diseases,* ed 2, St. Louis, Mosby, 2004, figure 237-2.)

- Ketoconazole and amphotericin are acceptable alternatives
- Bacterial esophagitis (rare): In immunocompromised hosts, *Lactobacillus* and β-hemolytic streptococci can be the cause

Structural Disorders

- Zenker's diverticulum
  - Outpouching of the wall above the upper esophageal sphincter
  - Symptoms include halitosis and regurgitation of saliva and food
  - Commonly associated with underlying dysmotility
  - Treatment with surgery (cricopharyngeal myotomy/ diverticulectomy), if needed
- Esophageal webs and rings
  - Schatzki's ring
    - Causes intermittent dysphagia to solids **("steakhouse syndrome")**
    - Congenital ring at distal esophagus just above or at the LES
    - Endoscopic dilatation usually effective in treating
  - Plummer-Vinson syndrome
    - Web in cervical esophagus
    - Presents as intermittent dysphagia
    - Associated with iron deficiency anemia
    - Associated with squamous cell esophageal cancer
- Hiatal hernia: Movement of part of the stomach into the thoracic cavity
  - Sliding type
    - Very common with increasing age
    - Gastroesophageal junction (GEJ) and fundus slide upward
    - Can contribute to reflux esophagitis
  - Paraesophageal type
    - GEJ remains fixed
    - Pouch of stomach herniates through the esophageal hiatus next to the GEJ
    - Can cause bleeding and strangulation
    - **Surgery is necessary for symptomatic or large hernias of this type**

Esophageal Dysmotility Syndromes

- Oropharyngeal dysmotility
  - Diminished ability to move food to esophagus
  - Characterized by dysphagia, nasal regurgitation, coughing, and aspiration
  - Most often caused by neurologic disorders (e.g., myasthenia gravis, multiple sclerosis, amyotrophic lateral sclerosis)
  - Collagen-vascular diseases that affect striated muscle (polymyositis, dermatomyositis) can also cause oropharyngeal dysmotility
- Achalasia
  - Most cases in the United States are idiopathic
  - Presentation: Dysphagia, regurgitation, chest pain, weight loss

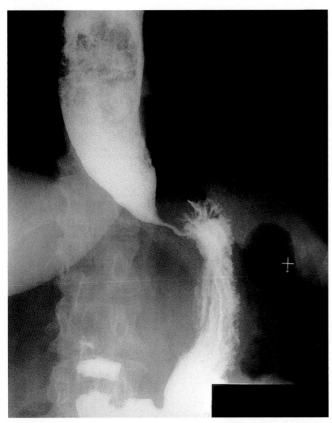

FIGURE 27-3 Barium swallow showing an air-fluid level in the esophagus and a "bird's-beak" deformity consistent with achalasia.

- Diagnosis: Barium swallow can be highly suggestive, but manometry is the most sensitive study
- Radiologic studies: Barium swallow—dilated esophagus that tapers to a "bird's beak" and air/fluid level in the esophagus (Fig. 27-3); chest radiograph—absent gastric bubble; esophageal manometry—absence of peristalsis and failure of the LES to relax in response to a swallow
- Esophagogastroduodenoscopy (EGD) is necessary to rule out pseudoachalasia/secondary cause
- Therapy
  - Medications (smooth-muscle relaxants)—rarely effective
  - Endoscopic dilatation of LES (success rates of 60–70%)
  - Myotomy—surgical or laparoscopic; reflux esophagitis and stricture may be a complication of surgery (success rates of up to 90%)
  - Botulinum toxin produces short-term results but can be diagnostically helpful in atypical presentations
- Secondary causes
  - Gastric cancer involving the GEJ (pseudoachalasia)
  - Neurologic disorders (e.g., myasthenia gravis, amyotrophic lateral sclerosis)
  - Chagas' disease (American trypanosomiasis)
    - Transmission: Through reduviid bugs carrying the parasite *Trypanosoma cruzi*; transmission also occurs through blood transfusions
    - Epidemiology: Found mainly in Central and South America, although cases have been reported in the southern United States

- Presentation
  Acute disease (usually self-limited): Skin induration (chagoma), fever, lymphadenopathy; myocarditis and heart failure can occur
  Chronic disease (years or decades after primary infection): Cardiomyopathy, arrhythmias, megaesophagus, megacolon, aspiration pneumonia
  Diagnosis: Examination of blood smear for parasites in acute disease; serologic tests for antibodies to *T. cruzi* for chronic disease
  Treatment: Nifurtimox or benznidazole recommended; referral for cardiac transplantation may be needed for severe cardiomyopathy
- Scleroderma (see Chapter 46)
  - Presentation: Severe GERD, dysphagia
  - More than 90% have esophageal involvement
  - More than 90% have Raynaud's phenomenon
  - Peptic stricture in distal esophagus may occur
  - Diagnosis: Esophageal manometry shows absent peristalsis and low LES tone; barium swallow shows dilation and loss of peristaltic contractions
  - Therapy
    - PPIs
    - Esophageal dilatation for peptic stricture
- Diffuse esophageal spasm
  - Presentation: Dysphagia, chest pain that can be aggravated by stress
  - Commonly associated with GERD (70%)
  - Diagnosis
    - Esophageal manometry test may be normal if patient is asymptomatic at the time
    - Barium swallow can show "corkscrew" esophagus, uncoordinated contractions along the esophageal wall (Fig. 27-4)
  - Treatment
    - Treat GERD
    - Smooth-muscle relaxants (isosorbide dinitrate, dicyclomine, calcium channel blockers) if GERD is not present
    - Antidepressants (selective serotonin reuptake inhibitors, trazodone)
    - Benzodiazepines
    - Antipsychotics

Esophageal Cancer

- Can present with solid-food dysphagia, odynophagia, weight loss, and/or pneumonia from tracheoesophageal fistulas
- Squamous cell carcinoma
  - Incidence decreasing
  - More common in men and African Americans
  - Usually occurs in mid-to-lower esophagus
  - Risk factors include alcohol, smoking, achalasia, nitrate consumption, lye ingestion, Plummer-Vinson syndrome
- Adenocarcinoma
  - Incidence increasing

27

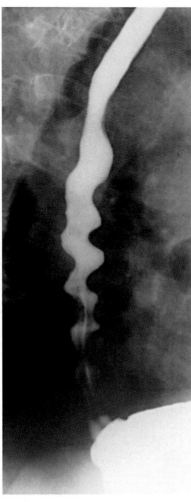

FIGURE 27-4 Diffuse esophageal spasm leading to "corkscrew" esophagus. (From Feldman M: *Sleisenger and Fordtran's gastrointestinal and liver disease,* ed 7, Philadelphia, WB Saunders, 2002, figure 32-14.)

- More common in men and in whites
- Usually occurs in the distal esophagus
- Major risk factor is GERD and Barrett's esophagus (see Box 27-1)
- Diagnosis: Endoscopic biopsy and tumor brushings; CT scan and endoscopic ultrasound to assess regional spread
- Therapy
  - Prognosis is generally poor (5-year survival is 5%)
  - Surgical resection appropriate for less than half of all patients; 5-year survival rate after esophagectomy is about 20%
  - Palliative measures include radiation, chemotherapy, photodynamic therapy, stenting, and endsoscopic fulguration with lasers

Approach to the Patient with Dysphagia/Odynophagia

- Age, gender, immunosuppression, duration of symptoms, and associated symptoms (e.g., weight loss, chest pain) may suggest a particular cause
- Barium swallow is almost always the first test to obtain
- Symptom-based evaluation is often helpful (Fig. 27-5)

SUGGESTED READINGS

American Gastroenterological Association Institute technical review on the management of gastroesophageal reflux disease, *Gastroenterology* 135:1392–1413, 2008.

American Gastroenterological Association Medical Position Statement on Treatment of Patients with Dysphagia Caused by Benign Disorders of the Distal Esophagus, *Gastroenterology* 117:229–233, 1999.

DeVault KR, Castell DO: Updated guidelines for the diagnosis and treatment of gastroesophageal reflux disease, *Am J Gastroenterol* 100:190–200, 2005.

Kahrilas PJ: Clinical practice: gastroesophageal reflux disease, *N Engl J Med* 359: 1700–1707, 2008.

Shaheen NJ, Richter JE: Barrett's oesophagus, *Lancet* 373:850–861, 2009.

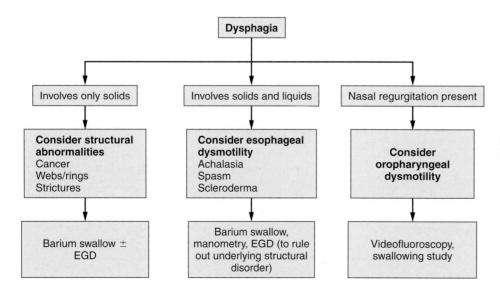

FIGURE 27-5 Evaluation of dysphagia. EGD, esophagogastroduodenoscopy.

Pancreatic and Biliary Disease

KERRY B. DUNBAR, MD, and MARCIA I. CANTO, MD, MHS

The pancreas is a lobular structure responsible for secretion of digestive enzymes, bicarbonate, and certain hormones. The gallbladder and biliary tree serve to excrete cholesterol, assist in the absorption of fats, and influence water and electrolyte transport. Diseases of the pancreas and biliary system include a number of acute and chronic conditions responsible for a large percentage of intra-abdominal pathology.

Pancreatic Disease

OVERVIEW OF PANCREATIC STRUCTURE AND FUNCTION

- Anatomy and physiology (Fig. 28-1A)
  - Pancreas: Soft, elongated gland that lies behind the peritoneum of the posterior abdominal wall
  - Anatomic parts of the pancreas are the head with the uncinate process, the neck, the body, and the tail

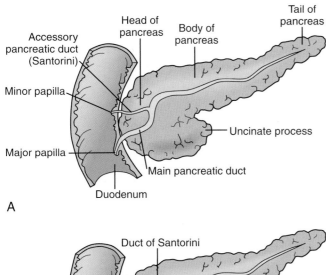

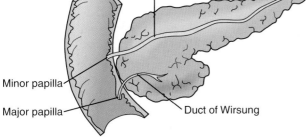

FIGURE 28-1 **A,** Normal anatomy of the pancreatic ductal system. **B,** Pancreas divisum.

- Main pancreatic duct (duct of Wirsung) opens in the major duodenal papilla
- The accessory pancreatic duct (duct of Santorini) drains via the minor duodenal papilla
- The pancreas has a lobular structure and consists of an exocrine portion, which secretes digestive enzymes and bicarbonate, and an endocrine portion, which secretes hormones into the blood
- The exocrine portion is composed of ductal, acinar, and centroacinar cells
- **More than 95% of pancreatic masses arise from acinar cells**
- The endocrine pancreas consists of islet cells (1–2%) that produce insulin, glucagon, somatostatin, and pancreatic polypeptide
- Exocrine pancreatic secretion occurs via acinar cell secretion into pancreatic ductules; islet cells secrete hormones directly into the blood
- Developmental abnormalities
  - Pancreas divisum (see Fig. 28-1B)
    - Incomplete fusion of the ducts results in the duct of Wirsung draining only the ventral pancreas and the duct of Santorini draining the entire dorsal pancreas
    - Present in 5% to 10% of the general population
  - A long common channel between the bile duct and pancreatic duct may facilitate bile reflux into the pancreatic duct and predispose to development of acute pancreatitis
  - Annular pancreas
    - Congenital anomaly, in which a concentric band of pancreatic tissue forms around the duodenum
    - It usually presents in infancy as duodenal obstruction but can also present in adulthood
    - Can be associated with many other congenital abnormalities (e.g., intestinal malrotation, Meckel's diverticulum, Down's syndrome, and tracheoesophageal fistulas)

ACUTE PANCREATITIS

Basic Information

- Epidemiology
  - Acute pancreatitis is a common disorder that results in thousands of hospitalizations
  - The incidence of acute pancreatitis ranges from 1 to 5 per 10,000 per year
- Etiology (Table 28-1)
  - **Ethanol and gallstones are the two most common causes of acute pancreatitis**

TABLE 28-1	Etiologic Association of Acute Pancreatitis
Category	**Examples**
Obstruction	Choledocholithiasis, biliary microlithiasis, ampullary or pancreatic tumor, pancreas divisum, mucinous ductal ectasia or intraductal papillary mucinous neoplasm, choledochocele, parasites, periampullary duodenal diverticula, hypertensive sphincter of Oddi, duodenal loop obstruction
Toxins	Ethanol, methanol, scorpion venom, organophosphorus insecticides
Drugs	Definite: Azathioprine, 6-MP, valproic acid, estrogens, tetracycline, metronidazole, pentamidine, furosemide, sulfonamides, methyldopa, cimetidine, ranitidine, sulindac, dideoxyinosine, nitrofurantoin
Metabolic	Hypertriglyceridemia (types I, IV, V), hypercalcemia
Trauma	Blunt trauma to abdomen, postoperative, post-ERCP/endoscopic sphincterotomy/sphincter of Oddi manometry
Infections	Parasites (ascariasis, chlonorchiasis), viral (mumps, rubella, hepatitis A, B, non-A non-B, coxsackievirus, echovirus, adenovirus, cytomegalovirus, varicella, Epstein-Barr virus, HIV)
Vascular	Ischemia (postcardiac surgery), atherosclerotic emboli, vasculitis (SLE, PAN, malignant hypertension)
Miscellaneous	Penetrating peptic ulcer, Crohn's disease of the duodenum, autoimmune pancreatitis, pregnancy-associated, cystic fibrosis, Reye's syndrome, idiopathic
Inherited	Autosomal dominant disorder; can develop into chronic pancreatitis

ERCP, endoscopic retrograde cholangiopancreatography; PAN, polyarteritis nodosa; SLE, systemic lupus erythematosus.

- Drug-induced pancreatitis usually occurs within the first month of drug administration
- The incidence of post-endoscopic retrograde cholangiopancreatography (ERCP) pancreatitis is 1% to 10%, and the risk is higher following sphincter of Oddi manometry
- About 10% to 30% of acute pancreatitis is idiopathic
- Autoimmune pancreatitis causes recurrent episodes of acute pancreatitis and chronic pancreatitis
  - Characterized by pancreatic and biliary strictures
  - CT shows diffuse enlargement of the pancreas or a focal inflammatory mass
  - Serum immunoglobulin G4 (IgG4) is often elevated
  - Responds to corticosteroids
- Examination of bile for crystals, sludge, and microlithiasis can help diagnose biliary sludge, a treatable cause of acute recurrent pancreatitis
- Pathophysiology
  - Poorly understood, but the triggering event is thought to vary according to the cause

- The initiating event is the intra-acinar activation of trypsinogen to trypsin with damage to the microcirculation of the pancreas
- Activation and release of phospholipase A2, elastase, kallikrein, complement, and coagulation factors can result in systemic toxicity seen in severe cases of pancreatitis

Clinical Presentation

- Symptoms
  - Epigastric abdominal pain radiating to the back
  - Nausea, vomiting, abdominal distention
- Physical examination
  - Low-grade fever, tachycardia, hypotension
  - Abdominal tenderness
  - Diminished bowel sounds
  - **Discoloration around umbilicus (Cullen's sign) or flanks (Grey-Turner sign) suggests hemoperitoneum and hemorrhagic pancreatitis**
- Clinical course and complications
  - Most patients with acute pancreatitis have mild, self-limited disease
  - In those with recurrent attacks, the first attack is usually the most severe and has the highest associated risk of death
  - Early complications are those that develop less than 14 days from admission (Box 28-1)
  - Late complications are those that develop after 14 days
    - Pseudocyst formation with or without infection (Fig. 28-2)
      - **Most pseudocysts resolve spontaneously within 6 weeks**
      - Those that persist, enlarge, or become symptomatic need drainage
    - Infected pancreatic necrosis leading to phlegmon
  - Pancreatic sepsis is the most common cause of death in patients with severe acute pancreatitis

Diagnosis and Evaluation

- Blood tests
  - Serum amylase and lipase: Most often used to diagnose pancreatitis
    - Amylase is the most commonly used test, but it is less sensitive and specific than serum lipase
    - **If the amylase is elevated but lipase is not, consider a nonpancreatic process**

BOX 28-1	Early Complications of Pancreatitis

Vascular instability and shock
Pulmonary complications (ARDS, effusions, atelectasis)
Renal (acute renal failure, acute tubular necrosis)
Endocrine and metabolic derangements (hyperglycemia, acidosis, hypocalcemia)
Infected pancreatic necrosis
Pancreatic or retroperitoneal hemorrhage
Massive GI bleeding caused by pseudoaneurysm of the splenic artery (hemosuccus pancreaticus)
Disseminated intravascular coagulation

ARDS, acute respiratory distress syndrome.

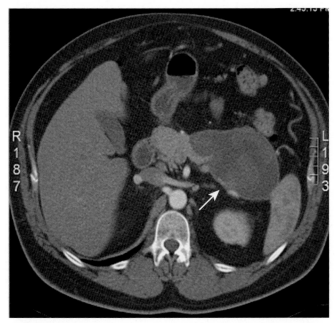

FIGURE 28-2 CT scan: Pancreatic pseudocyst in the tail of the pancreas (*arrow*).

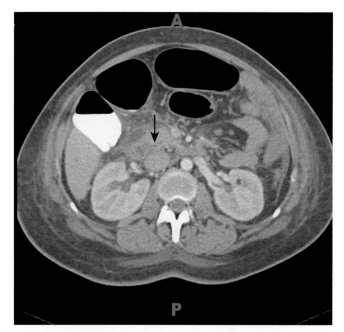

FIGURE 28-3 CT scan: Acute pancreatitis (*arrow*).

- Both amylase and lipase can be elevated in other intra-abdominal processes (e.g., bowel infarction, perforation, or obstruction) that may also present with an acute abdomen
- **The levels of pancreatic enzymes do not correlate with the severity of disease**
- Renal failure alone (without pancreatitis) may be associated with elevated amylase and lipase up to five to six times normal
- Serum liver function tests
  - Serum alanine aminotransferase (ALT) is a useful predictor of biliary origin of pancreatitis (more than threefold rise has a positive predictive value of 95% in acute gallstone pancreatitis)
  - Elevations of serum bilirubin and alkaline phosphatase are not specific for the diagnosis of gallstone pancreatitis
- Radiologic tests
  - Plain radiographs
    - Useful for detecting free air, which suggests bowel perforation
    - Abnormal gas signs in pancreatitis include local "sentinel loop" and general small bowel ileus
    - Chest radiograph may show pleural effusions (left greater than right), atelectasis, or acute respiratory distress syndrome–like pattern
  - Transabdominal ultrasonography
    - Useful for diagnosis of gallstone disease and bile duct dilation in gallstone pancreatitis
    - Not usually helpful in visualizing the pancreas because of overlying bowel gas
  - **CT is the most informative radiologic test**
    - Mild pancreatitis may be associated with a normal CT scan
    - Severe pancreatitis can result in pancreatic enlargement, peripancreatic fluid or debris, abdominal fluid collections, hemorrhage, and

necrosis. IV contrast can help identify pancreatic necrosis (Fig. 28-3).
- Serial CT scans are helpful (1/week) in detecting pancreatic abscesses; gas in fluid collections may suggest a pancreatic abscess caused by gas-forming organisms
- Magnetic resonance cholangiopancreatography (MRCP) can be used to identify the cause of acute pancreatitis and stage severity
  - Provides a better view of pancreatic and bile ducts than CT
  - Can detect choledocholithiasis, fluid collections, necrosis, and pseudocysts
- ERCP helps to diagnose the cause of acute recurrent pancreatitis, such as choledocholithiasis (gallstone pancreatitis), papillary stenosis, complete or incomplete pancreas divisum, tumor, stones, and sphincter of Oddi dysfunction
- Endoscopic ultrasonography (EUS) may be helpful for diagnosing tumors not evident by CT scan that may present with acute pancreatitis
- Clinical measurements of severity
  - Ranson's criteria (Table 28-2)
    - Reliable for predicting mortality

28

TABLE 28-2	Ranson's Criteria for Acute Pancreatitis	
On Admission		**Within 48 Hours**
Age > 55 yr		Hematocrit decrease = 10%
WBC > 16,000/mm^3		BUN increase = 5 mg/dL
Glucose > 200 mg/dL		Calcium < 8 mg/dL
Lactate dehydrogenase > 350 U/L		Po$_2$ < 60 mm Hg Base deficit > 4 mEq/L
Aspartate aminotransferase > 250 U/L		Fluid deficit > 6 L

- Fulfillment of three or more criteria indicates severe disease and poor prognosis. **Those with three or four risk factors have a 15% mortality rate; those with six or seven risk factors have a 100% mortality rate.**
- CT scan: The presence of pancreatic necrosis, abscess, or pseudocyst usually predicts severe disease

Treatment

- Supportive care: Bowel rest, IV fluids, analgesic medications
- Enteral nutrition: Jejunal feeding in acute pancreatitis reduces the incidence of infection and shortens length of stay in the hospital
- Parenteral nutrition: May be required for moderate and severe pancreatitis
- Antibiotics: Imipenem and third-generation cephalosporins achieve high pancreatic tissue levels and may be effective for reducing the incidence of pancreatic sepsis in patients with severe necrotizing pancreatitis; **empirical antibiotic therapy is currently recommended only for such severe cases**
- A CT scan should be obtained if there is no clinical improvement within 72 hours. If necrosis is found and infection is suspected, fine-needle aspiration (FNA) should be considered.
- Surgery is indicated for drainage of pancreatic abscess and debridement of infected pancreatic phlegmon
- Urgent ERCP
  - Indicated for gallstone pancreatitis, especially with coexisting cholangitis, jaundice, dilated common bile duct (CBD), or in patients with clinical deterioration (Fig. 28-4)
  - ERCP with sphincterotomy and stenting of the minor papilla is also useful for treatment of acute recurrent pancreatitis in patients with pancreas divisum

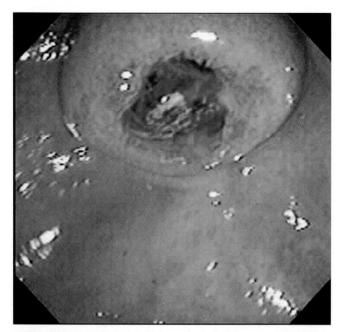

FIGURE 28-4 Endoscopic retrograde cholangiopancreatography: Gallstone pancreatitis caused by stone impacted in major duodenal papilla.

- Nasogastric tube suction, histamine 2 (H₂) receptor antagonists, fresh-frozen plasma, and peritoneal lavage have no proven efficacy. Pancreatic duct stents have been shown to reduce the risk of post-ERCP pancreatitis.

CHRONIC PANCREATITIS

Basic Information

- Definition and cause
  - Chronic pancreatitis is manifested by abdominal pain and abnormal secretory function of the exocrine pancreas associated with histologic findings of atrophy and fibrosis of exocrine parenchyma
  - If alcoholism is excluded, most patients in the United States with chronic pancreatitis have no identifiable cause
  - Idiopathic chronic pancreatitis presents at any age but is most commonly seen in middle-aged women
  - Autosomal dominant familial pancreatitis can present as acute or chronic pancreatitis with prominent pancreatolithiasis
    - Mutation is present in the *PRSS1* gene
    - Familial pancreatitis can also be caused by mutations in the serine protease inhibitor SPINK1 and in the cystic fibrosis transmembrane conductance regulator gene (*CFTR*)
  - Autoimmune pancreatitis can also cause chronic pancreatitis
- Pathophysiology
  - Pancreatic duct obstruction occurs from hypersecretion of pancreatic fluid, rich in protein and calcium carbonate, which can precipitate in branches of the pancreatic duct
  - Mononuclear cell parenchymal infiltration, atrophy, and fibrosis of the exocrine tissue may be seen on pathology

Clinical Presentation

- Signs and symptoms
  - Abdominal pain: Recurrent bouts or continuous
  - Pancreatic insufficiency: Diarrhea (steatorrhea) and weight loss caused by malabsorption
  - Diabetes: Occurs in advanced chronic pancreatitis
- Occasionally, patients may have no pain but may have malabsorption with or without diabetes
  - Painful attacks tend to diminish over time (5–10 years) as the exocrine and endocrine insufficiency progresses
  - Cessation of alcohol intake may decrease the frequency of painful attacks, but pancreatic insufficiency may still develop despite abstinence
- Complications include pseudocysts, ascites, and biliary obstruction (Fig. 28-5)

Diagnosis and Evaluation

- Blood tests
  - **Amylase and lipase levels may be normal**
  - Low serum trypsinogen or immunolipase may suggest pancreatic cancer or chronic pancreatitis (specificity > 98%)
- Pancreatic function tests
  - Bentiromide test

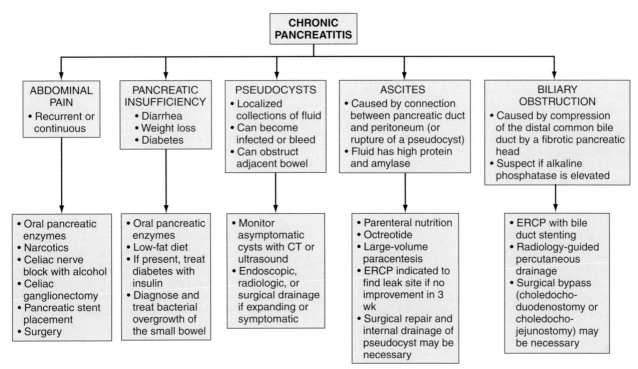

FIGURE 28-5 Sequelae and treatment of chronic pancreatitis. ERCP, endoscopic retrograde cholangiopancreatography.

- Bentiromide is *N*-benzoyl-L-tyrosyl-para-aminobenzoic acid (NBT-PABA), which is cleaved by pancreatic chymotrypsin in the duodenum
- PABA is absorbed by the small intestine, conjugated by the liver, and excreted in the urine if pancreatic exocrine function is normal
- Decreased urinary excretion or serum levels suggests pancreatic exocrine insufficiency (assuming small bowel function is normal)
- Pancreatic intubation function tests: Bicarbonate and enzyme concentrations measured from direct samples obtained from an ERCP
- Stool tests
  - 72-hour fecal fat collection: Still the most definitive test for diagnosing steatorrhea, which may be pancreatic or nonpancreatic
    - Greater than 7 g/24 hours of fecal fat while consuming a high-fat diet is considered abnormal
    - Pancreatic steatorrhea does not occur until the pancreatic lipase output decreases to less than 5% to 10% of normal
    - Fecal chymotrypsin and fecal elastase are simpler tests of pancreatic exocrine function. Low fecal levels of chymotrypsin or fecal elastase suggest pancreatic dysfunction.
- Radiology
  - Plain radiographs: Useful for detecting pancreatic calcifications, which are suggestive of chronic pancreatitis
  - CT scan: More sensitive for pancreatic calcification; can also diagnose pseudocysts, tumors, focal fibrotic masses, and associated bile duct and/or pancreatic duct dilatation
  - MRCP: Useful for visualizing the pancreatic duct and cysts and in diagnosing pancreas divisum
  - ERCP: Useful for evaluating pancreatic ductal changes; less helpful in differentiating chronic pancreatitis from pancreatic cancer

- EUS
  - The high-resolution images of the pancreas can help in diagnosing early chronic pancreatitis, even when ERCP is normal
  - Complements ERCP in evaluation of chronic pancreatitis
  - Secretin-stimulated pancreatic ductal dilation can be detected, which can diagnose SOD dysfunction or obstruction of the pancreatic duct
  - Currently it is the best test for early diagnosis and staging of pancreatic cancer

Treatment
See Figure 28-5 for treatment options.

PANCREATIC CANCER
Basic Information
- Epidemiology
  - Pancreatic cancer is the second most common GI malignancy (after colorectal cancer) in the United States
  - Types of pancreatic cancer
    - **Adenocarcinoma is the most common type of malignancy and has the worst prognosis; usually located in the pancreatic head**
    - Cystadenocarcinoma, papillary cystic carcinoma, ampullary carcinoma, endocrine tumors, and lymphoma are rarely seen
- Etiology
  - Risk factors for pancreatic cancer include cigarette smoking, obesity, age, male sex, African-American race
  - Most cases of pancreatic cancer are sporadic
  - Cases of familial pancreatic cancer suggest a genetic linkage
  - Gene mutations in hereditary chronic pancreatitis, Peutz-Jeghers syndrome, and hereditary breast

28

cancer (*BRCA2*) are associated with pancreatic cancer

Clinical Presentation

- Most common presenting symptoms are abdominal pain (frequently radiating to the back) and weight loss
- Jaundice caused by biliary obstruction commonly found in patients with tumors of the pancreatic head
- On examination, a palpable gallbladder (Courvoisier's sign) may be present but is not sensitive or specific
- Glucose intolerance, venous thrombosis (Trousseau's syndrome), and GI variceal bleeding (from compression of the portal system) may occur
- **Most patients present with advanced disease**

Diagnosis and Evaluation

- CT scan (Fig. 28-6)
  - A specific diagnosis of a pancreatic mass can be made with up to 95% accuracy
  - Pancreatic protocol (high-resolution CT with IV contrast and water contrast in the stomach) improves sensitivity
  - Necessary for staging and to rule out metastatic disease
- Serum CA 19-9
  - Has a sensitivity of 80% to 90% and specificity of 85% to 95% in patients with signs and symptoms of pancreatic cancer
  - In patients with pancreatic masses on CT scan, high levels may be suggestive of malignancy
  - Can be elevated in colon, gastric, and bile duct cancers
  - **Not considered an appropriate screening test at this time**
- EUS: Can diagnose potentially curable small tumors (<1–2 cm) not evident by CT scan
  - Provides staging information as well as histology (via EUS-guided FNA) at the same procedure

- EUS is also useful in diagnosing and localizing pancreatic endocrine tumors, including gastrinomas (associated with Zollinger-Ellison syndrome) and insulinomas (associated with hypoglycemia)
- ERCP
  - Cytologic sampling at the time of ERCP is possible but not as informative as EUS plus FNA, particularly in nonjaundiced patients
  - ERCP is most useful in the setting of biliary obstruction because endoscopic sphincterotomy and biliary stent placement can be done with the same procedure

Treatment

- Surgery: Results vary from 0% to 35% 5-year survival in curative resections, with better outcome in ampullary carcinomas (up to 50% survival)
  - Patients who have the best chance for curative resection are those who present with painless obstructive jaundice
  - **Patients with tumors in the body or tail are rarely eligible for resection for cure (because of late presentation)**
- Palliation
  - Endoscopic or percutaneous stenting or biliary bypass at the time of surgery may relieve obstruction and jaundice
  - Pain can be palliated with celiac axis nerve block during surgery or under CT or EUS guidance
  - Chemotherapy with gemcitabine and 5-fluorouracil (5-FU)-based chemoradiotherapy are also used for treatment

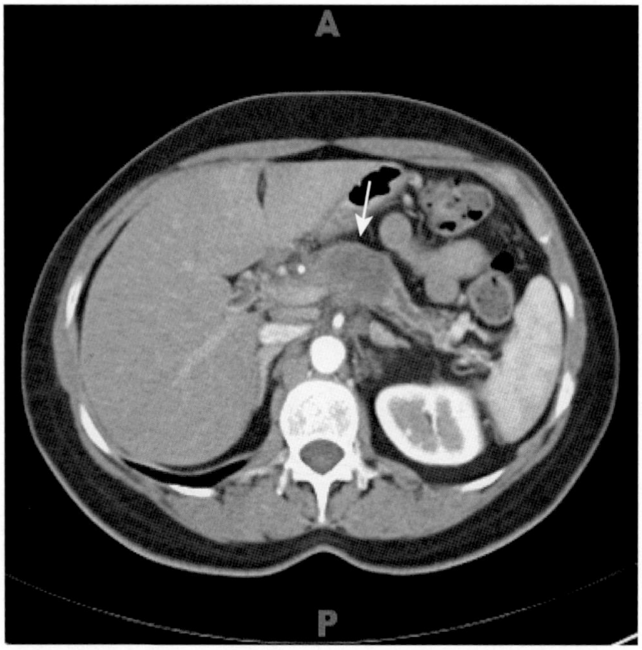

Biliary Diseases

OVERVIEW OF ANATOMY AND PHYSIOLOGY

- Gallbladder (Fig. 28-7)
  - The anatomic parts of the gallbladder are the fundus, body, infundibulum, and neck

FIGURE 28-6 CT scan: Mass in the body of the pancreas.

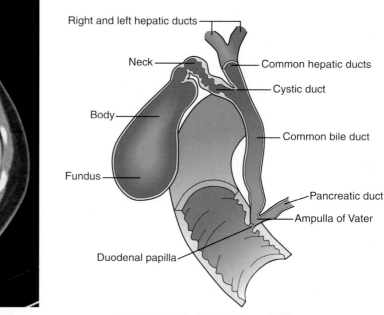

Right and left hepatic ducts

Neck

Common hepatic ducts

Cystic duct

Body

Common bile duct

Fundus

Pancreatic duct

Ampulla of Vater

Duodenal papilla

FIGURE 28-7 Gallbladder and biliary tree.

- Accumulates and concentrates bile and stores concentrated bile between meals
- Filling and emptying of the gallbladder are controlled by neural and hormonal factors, including cholecystokinin (CCK), cholinergic vagal stimulation, motilin, and pancreatic polypeptide
- In response to hormonal stimulation after meals, the gallbladder releases concentrated bile into the duodenum for activation of digestive enzymes and digestion of dietary lipids
- Extrahepatic biliary tree
  - Main right and left hepatic ducts join to form the common hepatic duct, which joins with the cystic duct to form the CBD; in most patients, the CBD joins with the pancreatic duct to open into the major duodenal papilla
  - Bile flow from liver to duodenum is controlled by gallbladder contraction and sphincter of Oddi activity

GALLSTONE DISEASE

Basic Information

- Definition and epidemiology
  - Cholelithiasis describes presence of microscopic crystals or large stones in the gallbladder
  - Choledocholithiasis refers to presence of gallstones in extrahepatic bile ducts
  - **Women are diagnosed with gallstones two to three times more often than men of the same age**
  - Most gallstones are cholesterol stones (contain >50% cholesterol) that have centers with calcium, pigment, and glycoprotein
  - A minority of gallstones are pigment stones (have <20% cholesterol content) that contain calcium salts of carbonate, phosphate, and bilirubin distributed evenly throughout the stone; these usually form in the setting of hemolysis (e.g., sickle cell anemia), cirrhosis, or chronic biliary infection
- Pathogenesis and risk factors
  - The healthy gallbladder prevents gallstone formation by acidifying bile, absorbing cholesterol, concentrating bile (which in turn promotes micelle formation), and expelling crystals and sludge
  - Risk factors for development of cholelithiasis (Box 28-2)

BOX 28-2	*Risk Factors for the Development of Cholelithiasis*

Genetic predisposition (Pima Indians, Native Americans, Mexican Americans, Scandinavians)

Older age (>50 yr)

Obesity

Pregnancy

Medications (e.g., oral contraceptives, octreotide, ceftriaxone)

Prolonged total parenteral nutrition

Rapid weight loss

Diseases of the terminal ileum causing decreased reabsorption of bile acids

Clinical Presentation

- Biliary colic (chronic cholecystitis): Transient episodes of pain caused by intermittent obstruction of the cystic duct or CBD by passing stone
  - The pain typically occurs in the right upper quadrant or epigastrium and can radiate to the shoulder or back
  - **The pain can be sharp and intense, often related to meals (particularly fatty food)**
- Acute cholecystitis: Results from lasting obstruction of the cystic duct by a gallstone
  - Abdominal pain is more intense and prolonged than that of biliary colic
  - Fevers, chills, nausea, and vomiting commonly accompany the pain
  - Obstructive jaundice may occur when migration and obstruction of the gallstone into the extrahepatic bile duct occurs; it may also occur when a cystic duct stone erodes into or compresses the adjacent common bile duct (Mirizzi's syndrome)
  - Acalculous cholecystitis may be seen in up to 10% of patients with cholecystitis symptoms
    - Usually associated with other underlying illness (e.g., patients in the intensive care unit, those with diabetes)
    - Has a higher complication rate than that for calculous cholecystitis
  - Complications of cholecystitis
    - Empyema: Carries a high incidence of perforation and sepsis
    - Gangrene: From ischemia of the gallbladder wall; advanced age and diabetes are commonly present
    - Emphysematous cholecystitis may occur with gangrene and infection of the gallbladder with gas-forming bacteria
    - Gallstone ileus: Bowel obstruction caused by large stones that erode into the duodenum from an inflamed gallbladder (Bouvaret's syndrome) or pass into the small bowel from the bile duct
- Cholangitis: Patients present with spiking fever, right upper quadrant abdominal pain, and jaundice (Charcot's triad) caused by complete obstruction of the CBD
  - Charcot's triad with hypotension and confusion indicate Reynold's pentad
  - May have cholangitis without all the symptoms listed
- Gallstone pancreatitis
  - Caused by acute impaction of gallstones in the major duodenal papilla
  - Urgent ERCP with sphincterotomy is necessary to remove the impacted stone and to restore adequate drainage from biliary and pancreatic ducts

Diagnosis and Evaluation

- Physical examination (for acute cholecystitis)
  - Right upper quadrant tenderness with or without peritoneal signs
  - Inspiratory arrest with right upper quadrant palpation (Murphy's sign) may also be seen
  - The gallbladder is palpable in less than half of cases
- Leukocytosis and elevated liver function tests commonly noted in cases of acute cholecystitis or cholangitis

28

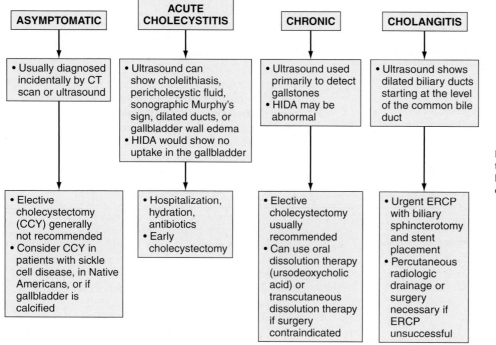

FIGURE 28-8 Diagnosis and treatment of gallstone disease. ERCP, endoscopic retrograde cholangiopancreatography.

- Most common organisms cultured are *Escherichia coli*, *Klebsiella* spp., group D *Streptococcus*, *Staphylococcus* spp., and *Clostridium* spp.
- Radiologic tests can be helpful (Fig. 28-8)

Treatment

See Figure 28-8 for treatment options.

POSTCHOLECYSTECTOMY SYNDROME

Basic Information

- Postcholecystectomy syndrome: A complex of symptoms (abdominal discomfort or pain, nausea) persisting or presenting after cholecystectomy with or without abnormal liver function tests, and possibly with an abnormal amylase and lipase
- Most common causes of the postcholecystectomy syndrome:
  - Papillary stenosis: Fixed narrowing of the distal CBD and/or pancreatic duct as a result of fibrosis
  - Retained bile duct stone
  - Consequences of the intraoperative bile duct injury (strictures, bile leak)
  - Biliary dyskinesia (also called *sphincter of Oddi dysfunction*): Primary motility disorder of the sphincter of Oddi leading to elevated intraductal pressure

Clinical Presentation

- **Persistent or recurrent pain in the right upper quadrant and/or epigastric area that can be accompanied by nausea and vomiting and that resembles symptoms that occurred before cholecystectomy**
- Patients with postoperative bile duct strictures can present with pruritus, jaundice, or cholangitis

Diagnosis and Evaluation

- A biliary cause for postcholecystectomy pain should be suspected in the presence of bile duct dilation and abnormalities in liver function tests during painful attacks
- If ductal dilation and laboratory abnormalities are absent, patients may require ERCP with sphincter of Oddi manometry to document an elevated intraductal pressure. There is a high risk of post-ERCP pancreatitis after sphincter of Oddi manometry.
- The less-invasive CCK-HIDA scan has been reported to correlate well with sphincter of Oddi manometry.

Treatment

- Most causes of postcholecystectomy syndrome can be corrected endoscopically during ERCP

CHOLANGIOCARCINOMA

Basic Information

- Rare tumor of the biliary tree that is challenging to diagnose
- Defined as a primary malignant tumor originating from cells resembling biliary epithelium and distinguished from gallbladder cancer. These tumors may arise from
  - Small peripheral intrahepatic bile ducts
  - Larger intrahepatic bile ducts at or near the hilar confluence of the right and left hepatic ducts (Klatskin's tumor)
  - Extrahepatic bile ducts (distal bile duct carcinoma)
- Associated risk factors include the following:
  - Primary sclerosing cholangitis (PSC) (lifetime risk of 30%); more than 50% of PSC patients have inflammatory bowel disease (ulcerative colitis)
  - Chronic parasitic infection of the biliary tree with *Clonorchis sinensis*, *Opisthorchis* spp., *Ascaris*, and other parasites (Asia)

- Cystic dilatations of any segment of the biliary system (intrahepatic and/or extrahepatic)
- Can present with abdominal pain, jaundice, and right upper quadrant mass
- Bile duct obstruction and pancreatitis can occur
- Surgical excision usually indicated to prevent malignant transformation
- Types of choledochal cysts
  Type I—cystic dilation of the common bile duct (most common)
  Type III—choledochocele. Intraduodenal choledochal cyst
  Type V—Caroli's syndrome
    Autosomal-recessive condition
    Patients have widespread saccular dilatations of the bile ducts
    Bile collections may become infected
    Associated with polycystic kidney disease

- Exposure to thorium dioxide (Thorotrast, a radiocontrast medium used in the 1930s and 1940s)
- Choledochal cysts (Box 28-3)
- Oriental cholangiohepatitis—brown pigment intrahepatic biliary stones develop as a result of chronic inflammation from chronic bacterial infection
- Multiple biliary papillomatosis
- Hereditary nonpolyposis colorectal cancer
- It is more common in older patients, particularly men

Clinical Presentation

- Patients typically present with jaundice, weight loss, abdominal pain, and pruritus; may also have dark urine and acholic stools
- The gallbladder may be palpable (Courvoisier's sign)

Diagnosis and Evaluation

- Transabdominal ultrasonography, CT scanning, or MRCP may show biliary dilation, a level of obstruction, and possibly a ductal mass
- Cholangiography (percutaneous or endoscopic via ERCP) will show irregular, tight strictures with proximal dilation and allow for histologic sampling; however, brushings and biopsies may be falsely negative
- EUS can be used to identify small tumors and lymph nodes. Histologic sampling can be performed by FNA.
- Ca 19-9 may be elevated but is nonspecific for cholangiocarcinoma

Treatment

- The overall prognosis is poor with a 5% 5-year survival rate
- **The diagnosis is typically made late and most tumors are unresectable for cure**
- Surgical resection may be possible in up to 20% of patients

- Chemotherapy and radiation therapy have little effect on outcome

GALLBLADDER CANCER

Basic Information

- Rare GI cancer that presents late in life and is usually unresectable when symptomatic
- It is potentially curable when incidentally found or removed by cholecystectomy (2% of all gallbladders removed for symptomatic gallstones or cholecystitis)
- Predisposing risk factors include
  - Older age
  - Female gender
  - Obesity
  - Gallbladder adenomas/polyps (particularly those > 1 cm in diameter)
  - Chronic cholecystitis (e.g., large gallstones)
  - Chronic *Salmonella typhi* infection
  - Calcified or (porcelain) gallbladder

Clinical Presentation

- Weight loss, abdominal pain, biliary obstruction, nausea, or right upper quadrant mass

Diagnosis and Evaluation

- Ultrasound may show a mass, thickening of the gallbladder wall, or extraluminal extension of the tumor
- CT and MRCP can also be used to identify gallbladder masses and polyps
- Laboratory studies are less helpful

Treatment

- The prognosis is very poor because these cancers are very aggressive and patients usually present with advanced form of disease
- Treatment options are limited for tumors that extend beyond the gallbladder and include aggressive surgery, chemotherapy, and radiation
- Surgery for very limited disease may be curative. Overall survival rates for more advanced disease are poor

REVIEW QUESTIONS

For review questions, please go to www.expertconsult.com.

SUGGESTED READINGS

Ahmed A, Cheung RC, Keeffe EB: Management of gallstones and their complications, *Am Fam Physician* 61:1673–1680, 2000.
Feldman M, Friedman LS, Brandt LJ, et al: *Sleisenger and Fordtran's gastrointestinal and liver disease: pathophyisiology/diagnosis/management*, ed 8, Philadelphia, Saunders Elsevier, 2006.
Godil A, Chen YK: Endoscopic management of benign pancreatic disease, *Pancreas* 20:1–13, 2000.
Kalloo AN, Kantsevoy SV: Gallstones and biliary disease, *Primary Care* 28:591–606, 2001.
Ranson JH: Etiological and prognostic factors in human acute pancreatitis: a review, *Am J Gastroenterol* 77:633–638, 1982.

28

Disorders of the Small and Large Intestine

ANNE MARIE LENNON, MD, and MICHAEL GOGGINS, MD

The small and large bowels are primarily responsible for the absorption of nutrients and fluid and excretion of waste. Diseases that affect the intestinal system are likely to interfere with at least one of these two functions and lead to problems with motility or malabsorption. Diseases that disrupt the mucosal integrity can also cause bleeding, as discussed in Chapter 26.

Diarrhea: General Principles

Basic Information

- Defined as an increase in the fluidity, frequency, or volume of stool output; usually results in increased daily stool weight (**>200 g/day** in the United States)
- Mechanisms of diarrhea (Table 29-1)
  - Osmotic diarrhea
    - Results from osmotically active solutes that are not absorbed from the gut lumen
    - Higher osmolality in the lumen causes passive water loss across the mucosa of the duodenum and jejunum, overwhelming the absorptive capacities of the ileum and colon
    - **Diarrhea stops when oral intake stops**
    - Volume is usually less than 1 L/day
  - Secretory diarrhea
    - Increased fluid secretion and impaired electrolyte absorption across the intestinal mucosa
    - **Diarrhea continues even when oral intake stops**
    - Stool volume usually large (>1 L/day), watery, without pus or blood
  - Altered motility
    - Increased motility
      - Causes decreased contact time between the gut and digesting food (*chyme*)
      - Leads to less absorption and large amounts of fluid delivered to the colon

TABLE 29-1	*Mechanisms of Diarrheal Disease*	
Category	**Example Conditions**	**Comments**
Osmotic	Maldigestion of carbohydrates (e.g., lactase deficiency, sucrase deficiency) Ingestion of nonabsorbed solutes (e.g., mannitol, sorbitol) Ingestion of poorly absorbed salts (magnesium hydroxide)	Small stool volume Osmolar gap present Stops with fasting Stool pH < 6
Secretory	Bacterial toxins (e.g., cholera, *Escherichia coli*) Hormonal secretagogues (e.g., vasoactive intestinal peptides, serotonin) Gastric hypersecretion (e.g., Zollinger-Ellison syndrome) Laxatives (e.g., senna, phenolphthalein) Bile salt malabsorption	Large volume of stool No osmolar gap Persistent diarrhea with fasting
Abnormal motility	Increased motility—hyperthyroidism, carcinoid, postgastrectomy dumping syndrome Decreased motility—diabetes, hypothyroidism, scleroderma, amyloidosis, postvagotomy syndromes	Bacterial overgrowth motility usually secondary to decreased motility
Exudative	Inflammatory bowel disease Bacterial pathogens (e.g., *Salmonella, Shigella*) Vasculitis Radiation enteritis Severe diverticulitis Ischemic injury	Volume can be small or large
Anorectal dysfunction	Neurologic disease Postsurgical complication Inflammatory bowel disease	Small volume of stools

- Decreased motility
  - Causes bacterial overgrowth
  - Leads to impaired bile salt function
- Exudative diarrhea
  - Inflamed or ulcerated mucosa permits mucus, blood, and pus to leak into lumen
  - Diarrhea can result directly from the increased osmotic load, increased motility (stimulation of the enteric nervous system), or secretion of the products of inflammation
  - Stool volume can be large or small, depending on the part of the bowel affected
  - Anorectal dysfunction or injury
    - Leads to the inability to retain feces
    - Characterized by fecal incontinence and small-volume stools
- Many diseases have more than one mechanism (e.g., diseases of malabsorption)

Clinical Presentation

- Acute diarrhea
  - Most cases are infectious (see Chapter 14)
  - Consider medications (e.g., laxatives, magnesium-containing antacids, proton-pump inhibitors, colchicine, furosemide)
  - Usually self-limited (<4 weeks' duration)
  - If abdominal pain and bloody diarrhea occur together in a patient older than 50 years, consider ischemic colitis
- Chronic diarrhea
  - Lasts longer than 4 weeks
  - Stools can be watery, bloody, contain grease, and be foul-smelling
  - Steatorrhea is defined as more than 7 g of fat per day by 72-hour fecal fat while on a high-fat diet

- Abdominal pain or cramping is often present
- Associated signs and symptoms that suggest an organic rather than a functional (e.g., irritable bowel syndrome [IBS]) cause are
  - Fever
  - Weight loss
  - Arthritis
  - Signs and symptoms of malabsorption (Table 29-2)
- Can result from a number of different etiologies (Table 29-3)

Diagnosis and Evaluation

- History and physical examination
  - Should focus on stool character, associated symptoms, and predisposing conditions (e.g., travel, HIV, family history of inflammatory bowel disease [IBD], antibiotic use)

TABLE 29-2	Nutrient Malabsorption	
Location of Normal Absorption	**Nutrient**	**Consequences of Malabsorption**
Proximal small bowel	Iron	Glossitis, pallor Anemia, pica
	Calcium	Bone pain, tetany Osteoporosis
	Folate	Glossitis, pallor Anemia, depression
Distal small bowel	Vitamin A	Night blindness Hyperkeratosis Corneal ulcers
	Vitamin D	Bone pain Muscle weakness Osteomalacia
	Vitamin E	Peripheral neuropathy Retinopathy
	Vitamin K	Bleeding Bruising
	Vitamin B_{12}	Peripheral neuropathy, subacute combined degeneration of the spinal cord Dementia, neuropsychiatric effects Anemia

TABLE 29-3	Selected Causes of Chronic Diarrhea
Category	**Examples**
Infections	Amebiasis Giardiasis *Clostridium difficile* HIV enteropathy *Yersinia, Campylobacter Cryptosporidium, Cyclospora* Intestinal schistosomiasis
Inflammatory	Ulcerative colitis Crohn's disease Microscopic colitis Eosinophilic gastroenteritis
Hormonal abnormalities/tumors	Diabetes Hyperthyroidism Adrenal insufficiency Vasoactive intestinal peptide tumors (VIPomas) Carcinoid syndrome Medullary thyroid cancer Gastrinoma Mastocytosis
Nonendocrine neoplasms	Villous adenoma secreting bicarbonate Obstructive colon cancer causing impaction and overflow diarrhea of liquid feces
Steatorrheal causes—maldigestion	Pancreatic exocrine insufficiency Bacterial overgrowth Liver disease
Steatorrheal causes—mucosal malabsorption	Celiac sprue Tropical sprue Whipple's disease Ischemia
Structural	Bile salt diarrhea after ileal resection Vagotomy Short gut syndrome
Osmotic	Laxatives (magnesium) Carbohydrate enzyme deficiencies (e.g., lactase) Sorbitol, lactulose ingestion
Functional	Irritable bowel syndrome
Anorectal dysfunction	Neurologic disease

29

- Acute diarrhea in a nonimmunocompromised patient does not require evaluation unless dehydration, bloody stools, fever, or severe abdominal pain is present (see Chapter 14)
- Diagnostic tests for chronic diarrhea
  - General blood studies: CBC with differential, chemistry panel that includes renal and liver function should initially be obtained
  - Use of further testing needs to be guided by history, physical findings, and results of general blood studies
  - Stool studies
    - Fecal leukocytes: Suggest inflammatory or infectious process
    - Bacterial culture: Most useful for acute diarrhea
    - Ova and parasites
    - *Clostridium difficile* toxin assay: Particularly useful if antibiotics recently administered
    - 72-hour quantitative stool collection for volume
    - Stool electrolyte concentration to calculate osmolar gap
      - Measure stool Na+ and K+ concentrations
      - **Osmolar gap = 290 − ([Na+] + [K+]) × 2**
      - **Osmolar gap greater than 40 suggests osmotic diarrhea**
      - **Osmolar gap less than 40 suggests secretory diarrhea**
    - Qualitative and quantitative fecal fat on a high-fat diet (e.g., 72 hour/100 g fat/day)
    - Stool phenolphthalein (if laxative abuse is suspected)
  - Tests for malabsorption
    - D-Xylose test
      - Measures the absorptive capacity of the proximal small bowel
      - Urine and blood are collected after 25 g oral xylose is administered
      - Abnormal test suggests small bowel mucosal disease or bacterial overgrowth
      - It is normal in pancreatic enzyme deficiency
    - Hydrogen breath test
      - Tests for lactose intolerance
      - After ingestion of lactose, the amount of hydrogen in expired air is measured

- If substantial levels are recorded, lactose intolerance is suggested
- This test is generally unnecessary since a therapeutic trial of lactose restriction is more cost-effective
- Endoscopy
  - Not routinely indicated
  - Colonoscopy and sigmoidoscopy are useful in cases where bloody diarrhea is present
    - Colonic biopsies are needed to diagnose microscopic colitis
  - Upper endoscopy with small bowel biopsy helpful in suspected cases of malabsorption, such as celiac disease
- Radiologic studies may also be useful in certain cases
- Capsule endoscopy may be helpful to evaluate the cause of suspected small intestinal diarrhea if radiology and endoscopy are nondiagnostic
- Specific blood and urine studies assist in searching for specific etiologies

Treatment

- Directed at the specific cause
- Treat dehydration
- Avoid caffeine and other secretagogues
- Antimotility agents (e.g., loperamide) can be useful if infection has been ruled out

Diarrheal Diseases

CELIAC SPRUE (GLUTEN-SENSITIVE ENTEROPATHY)

Basic Information

- Predominantly seen in white population
- Causes flattened villi of the proximal small bowel (Fig. 29-1)
- Most patients express human leukocyte antigen (HLA) DQ2 or DQ8, reflecting their genetic predisposition
- **Serology studies suggest celiac disease has a prevalence of approximately 1 in 200 individuals in the United States**
- Recent studies have shown that type 1 diabetes mellitus and celiac disease share common alleles, suggesting that they share biologic mechanisms

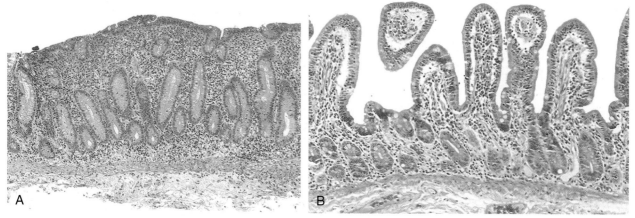

FIGURE 29-1   Celiac disease (gluten-sensitive enteropathy). **A,** A peroral jejunal biopsy specimen of diseased mucosa shows diffuse severe atrophy and blunting of villi, with a chronic inflammatory infiltrate of the lamina propria. **B,** A normal mucosal biopsy. (From Kumar V, Fausto N, Abbas A: *Robbins and Cotran: Pathologic basis of disease,* ed 7, Philadelphia, WB Saunders, 2005, figure 17-38.)

Clinical Presentation

- Diarrhea is common but might not be present
- Iron-deficiency anemia seen in 50% of adults with celiac disease
- Osteomalacia and osteoporosis can develop from vitamin D and calcium malabsorption
- Most adult patients do not present with classic features of malabsorption (e.g., steatorrhea)
- 42% of patients with celiac disease have elevation of aminotransferases
- **Diagnosis is often delayed for many years after the onset of symptoms**
- **Patients often have been given a diagnosis of IBS**
- Associated with a number of diseases:
  - Dermatitis herpetiformis (papulovesicular rash usually on the elbows, knees, buttocks, or scalp; Fig. 29-2)
  - Type 1 diabetes mellitus and other autoimmune disorders
  - IgA deficiency; occurs in 2% to 5% of patients with celiac disease compared with less than 5% of the general population
  - Autoimmune hepatitis
  - Autoimmune thyroid disease
  - It is also more common in people with Down's, Turner's, or Williams' syndrome
  - Increased incidence of small bowel lymphoma

Diagnosis and Evaluation

- Initial screening is usually performed with antibodies
  - Anti–endomysial antibody is an IgA antibody that is 85% to 98% sensitive and 97% to 100% specific
  - Tissue transglutaminase antibody (tTG) is an IgA antibody that is 90% to 98% sensitive and 95% to 97% specific
  - Anti-gliadin antibody (immunoglobulin G [IgG] and IgA) has lower sensitivity and specificity
  - **If there is a high suspicion of disease but negative antibodies, the total serum IgA concentration should be checked to rule out IgA deficiency.** In these cases, an IgG-based assay (serum IgG tTG) can be used or an upper endoscopy with biopsies performed.
- The diagnosis of celiac disease requires a small bowel biopsy, which demonstrates flattened or blunted villi and increased lymphocytes (see Fig. 29-1B). A minimum of four biopsies should be taken from the second and third parts of the duodenum, as histologic changes can be patchy.
- The gold standard for the diagnosis of celiac disease includes a repeat endoscopy with biopsies once the patient is on a gluten-free diet. These biopsies should demonstrate resolution of the histologic changes. This is rarely performed nowadays, with the diagnosis made on positive antibodies, histology consistent with celiac disease, and a response to treatment on a gluten-free diet.

Treatment

- Lifelong complete gluten-free diet—highly effective in resolving symptoms and reversing pathologic abnormalities
- Most relapses are caused by dietary noncompliance or hidden sources of gluten
- Refractory cases can be treated with corticosteroids or other immunosuppressives
- The possibility of early-onset small bowel lymphoma should be considered in refractory cases
- Response to treatment can be monitored using either IgA tTG or IgA anti–gliadin antibody with a return to normal baseline expected within 3 to 12 months after initiation of gluten-free diet
- Nutritional deficiencies (iron, calcium, phosphorus, folate, B_{12}, fat-soluble vitamins) should be identified and treated
- Patients should be screened for osteoporosis

TROPICAL SPRUE

- Suspect in patients with chronic diarrhea and malabsorption after residing or traveling to a tropical area
- **Most patients have evidence of folate deficiency**
- Infectious agents (e.g., *Klebsiella*) have been implicated
- Pathology from a small bowel biopsy can be similar to celiac sprue, but the patient is unresponsive to a gluten-free diet
- Treatment is with tetracycline and folate

WHIPPLE'S DISEASE

- Usually seen in middle-aged men
- **Caused by gram-positive bacilli (*Tropheryma whippelii*)**
- Presents with diarrhea, steatorrhea, abdominal pain, weight loss, migratory arthritis, and fever
- Neurologic (dementia, ocular disturbances, meningoencephalitis, cerebellar symptoms), cardiac (congestive heart failure, pericarditis, valvular heart disease), and ophthalmologic features may be present
- The diagnosis is made by showing periodic acid-Schiff (PAS)-positive macrophages containing the small bacillus in any affected tissue (usually small bowel). Antibodies to the protein and polymerase chain reaction (PCR) to the DNA of *Tropheryma whippelii* can also help to establish the diagnosis.
- Treatment is with trimethoprim-sulfamethoxazole for 1 year

BACTERIAL OVERGROWTH SYNDROME

Basic Information

- Caused by
  - Small bowel stasis
    - Anatomic abnormalities (postsurgical, diverticulae)
    - Abnormal small bowel motility (scleroderma, diabetes mellitus)

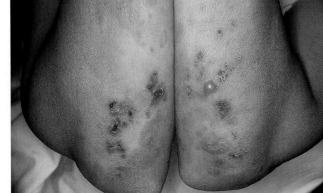

FIGURE 29-2 Dermatitis herpetiformis of the elbows. (From Callen JP: *Color atlas of dermatology,* ed 2, Philadelphia, WB Saunders, 2000.)

29

- Abnormal communication (Crohn's fistula, resection of the ileocecal valve) between the small bowel and colon
  - Multifactorial (chronic pancreatitis, cirrhosis, achlorhydria, immunodeficiency)
  - 90% associated with intestinal dysmotility syndrome and chronic pancreatitis

Clinical Presentation

- Bloating, flatulence, abdominal pain
- Diarrhea
- Weight loss
- Steatorrhea is caused by impaired micelle formation because of bacterial deconjugation of bile acids in the proximal small bowel
- Dermatitis, arthritis
- Vitamin deficiencies:
  - Vitamin B_{12} deficiency is common
  - Vitamin A deficiency with night blindness
  - Hypocalcemia secondary to vitamin D deficiency
  - Folate may be elevated because it is produced by enteric bacteria

Diagnosis and Evaluation

- The gold standard is small bowel aspirate demonstrating bacterial overgrowth (>10^5 colony-forming units/mL)
- Breath tests:
  - Lactose: Hydrogen breath test
    - Lactose is normally broken down in the colon. In bacterial overgrowth, an early hydrogen peak is seen.
    - Low sensitivity and specificity
  - ^{14}C-glycocholate breath test and ^{14}C-D-xylose breath test:
    - Detect the release of radiolabeled carbon dioxide resulting from bacterial deconjugation of bile acid and metabolism of xylose
    - D-Xylose sensitivity and specificity approach 90%
- Normalization of the Schilling test after antibiotics is highly suggestive of bacterial overgrowth (see Chapter 47)

Treatment

- Treat any anatomic abnormality with surgery, if possible
- Treat any underlying disease
  - Broad-spectrum antibiotics (ciprofloxacin, tetracycline, metronidazole, and rifamixin) can be administered for 2 to 3 weeks
  - Bacterial overgrowth often recurs in nonfunctional cases, and repeated cycles of antibiotics or alternating antibiotics are often required
  - Dietary supplements if required to treat nutritional deficiencies

BILE ACID MALABSORPTION

- Bile acids are absorbed in the ileum. Diseases that affect the ileum (i.e., Crohn's disease) or where the ileum has been resected will cause bile acid diarrhea.
- Two basic forms of the disease:
  - Bile acid diarrhea
    - Associated with limited ileal abnormality or resection
    - Impaired bile acid absorption in the ileum leads to chloride and water secretion in the colon
    - Steatorrhea does not develop because the liver is able to compensate for the loss of bile acids in the stool

- Responds to cholestyramine
- Fatty acid diarrhea
  - Associated with extensive ileal abnormality/resection
  - Liver is unable to compensate for the loss of bile acids in the stool, so steatorrhea develops
  - Does not respond to cholestyramine
  - May respond to low-fat diet

MICROSCOPIC COLITIS

Basic Information

- Usually occurs in patients in their 50s and 60s
- **Accounts for up to 10% of cases of chronic diarrhea**
- There are two types of microscopic colitis based on histology: collagenous colitis and lymphocytic colitis
  - Lymphocytic colitis is more common
  - Collagenous colitis occurs more frequently in women
- Microscopic colitis is associated with certain drugs, especially NSAIDs
- Associated with other diseases, especially celiac disease
- Consider it in the differential diagnosis of patient with celiac disease who is maintaining a strict diet but continues to have diarrhea

Clinical Presentation

- Microcytic anemia
- Diarrhea
- Weight loss
- Abdominal discomfort
- Fatigue

Diagnosis and Evaluation

- Colonoscopy
  - Will be grossly normal endoscopically, but biopsies should be taken from both the right and left colon
  - Diagnosis is made by histologic examination
- Histologic criteria for diagnosing microscopic colitis are
  - Increased chronic inflammatory infiltrate in the lamina propria
  - Increased number of intraepithelial lymphocytes (>15–20 lymphocytes per 1000 epithelial cells)
  - Damage of the surface epithelium with flattening of the epithelial cells
  - The presence of subepithelial collagenous band distinguishes collegenous colitis from lymphocytic colitis

Treatment

- Microscopic colitis can resolve spontaneously
- Stop NSAIDs or other associated drugs
- **First-line treatment is budesonide**
- A 5-aminosalicylic acid (5-ASA; mesalamine, sulfasalazine) compound can be tried if budesonide is ineffective
- Other alternatives include bismuth and oral steroids other than budesonide
- Symptoms of diarrhea will often respond to cholestyramine

OTHER DISEASES

See Table 29-4 for selected diseases that cause chronic diarrhea.

TABLE 29-4	Selected Diseases Causing Chronic Diarrhea			
Category/Disease	**Extradiarrheal Manifestations**	**Diagnosis**	**Treatment**	**Comments**
Infections				
Giardia lamblia	Bloating Nausea	Stool examination for ova and parasites of Giardia antigen	Metronidazole	Suspect in those with exposure to surface water (e.g., campers)
Secretory				
Vasoactive intestinal peptide tumors (VIPomas)	Hypokalemia Achlorhydria Non–anion gap metabolic acidosis	Elevated plasma VIP	Somatostatin analogues Surgery	Causes massive diarrhea WDHA syndrome (watery diarrhea, hypokalemia, achlorhydria)
Carcinoid syndrome	Flushing Abdominal pain Wheezing Right-sided valvular disease	Elevated urinary 5-hydroxyindoleacetic acid	Somatostatin analogues	Syndrome generally present when hepatic metastases present
Mastocytosis	Pruritus Flushing Abdominal pain Headache Urticaria pigmentosa—macular lesions that urticate when stroked (Darier's sign)	Elevated 24-hr urine for histamine and metabolites Elevated serum tryptase levels Skin biopsy	Histamine receptor blockers Glucocorticoids	Symptoms can be episodic
Osmotic				
Lactase deficiency	Abdominal cramps Flatulence	Empirical trial of lactose-free diet Hydrogen breath test	Lactose-free diet	Common disorder Symptoms typically occur after ingestion of dairy products
Inflammatory				
Microscopic/collagenous colitis	None	Colonoscopy shows grossly normal colon Increased collagen or in basement membrane or lymphocytic infiltrate microscopically	Corticosteroids Aminosalicylic acid	More commonly seen in women over age 50 yr

WDHA, watery diarrhea–hypokalemia–achlorhydria.

Constipation

Basic Information

- Subjectively defined as difficult-to-pass or hard feces or bowel movements occurring less frequently than usual
- Objective definition is less than three bowel movements per week
- Increases with age
- Women have a greater incidence than men
- Can result from a number of different conditions (Table 29-5)

Clinical Presentation

- Can be acute or chronic
- New-onset, persistent constipation can be a symptom of underlying organic disease
- Abdominal discomfort may also be present but is less prominent than in patients with constipation-predominant IBS

Diagnosis and Evaluation

- History and physical examination should look for secondary causes of constipation. Rectal examination may point to anorectal dysfunction.
- Blood work should include CBC, electrolytes, Ca2+, thyroid-stimulating hormone (TSH)
- In problematic cases, consider abdominal radiograph, colonic transit studies, colonoscopy (especially in elderly patients), anorectal motility (if anorectal dysfunction is suspected)
- Constipation is often due to slow transit. Occasionally it is due to pelvic floor dysfunction. With pelvic floor dysfunction, straining is a dominant symptom and soft stool and even enemas may be difficult to pass.

Treatment

- Functional constipation
  - Hydration
  - Exercise
  - Dietary fiber (15–25 g/day)
  - Psychological counseling
  - Consider osmotic laxatives (e.g., polyethylene glycol, lactulose, sorbitol)
  - Tegaserod (a serotonin type 4 agonist) is often helpful if other approaches fail
  - Reserve stimulant laxatives (e.g., bisacodyl, senna) for acute constipation
  - Pelvic floor dysfunction requires enemas and biofeedback
- Secondary causes
  - Remove offending drugs
  - Treat specific condition

29

TABLE 29-5	*Causes of Constipation*
Functional (most common)	Psychogenic Irritable bowel syndrome Mental illness (e.g., depression, eating disorders) Inactivity Low dietary fiber
Drugs	Side effects from anticholinergics, calcium channel blockers, diuretics, calcium/aluminum antacids, opiates Laxative abuse leading to diminished neurologic function of the colon Metal toxicity (e.g., arsenic, lead, mercury, phosphates)
Endocrine/ metabolic	Hypothyroidism Diabetes Hypokalemia Hypercalcemia Uremia Amyloid neuropathy Porphyria
Neurogenic	Colonic pseudo-obstruction Occurs postoperatively, with infections, narcotic use, or electrolyte disorders Risk of perforation when cecum > 13 cm Peripheral nerve injury—cauda equina syndrome Hirschsprung's disease Can present in adults as chronic constipation Rectal biopsy shows aganglionosis Autonomic neuropathy CNS disorders (e.g., MS, Parkinson's disease, stroke)
Diseases of the large bowel and rectum	Tumors Volvulus, hernia Colitis, proctitis Infection Scleroderma
Anorectal diseases	Fissure Rectal prolapse, rectocele, pelvic floor injury

Irritable Bowel Syndrome

Basic Information

- Characterized by chronic recurrent abdominal pain and altered bowel habits in absence of structural disorder
- Patients may have predominant diarrhea (never nocturnal), constipation, or intermittent episodes of the two. Pain is often relieved with defecation.
- Affects 20% of Western adults
- Women more often affected than men
- Second leading cause of work absenteeism (next to the common cold)
- Patient characteristics
  - Diet may be unhealthy: Fast foods, low-fiber diet
  - Emotional or psychological factors: Stress is associated with increase in symptoms; sexual abuse is more common in these patients; an increase in anxiety and depression but possibly only in those who seek medical attention
  - Innate sensitivity or susceptibility: Positive family history of irritable bowel, increased occurrence of other disorders with somatization features (e.g., fibromyalgia)

- Motility disturbance (slower myoelectric rhythm in colon) and abnormal sensitivity to rectal distention have been demonstrated
- Postinfectious: Infectious gastroenteritis predisposes to the development of IBS
- Small bowel bacterial overgrowth may cause IBS symptoms and is found in a minority of patients diagnosed with IBS
- Celiac disease may cause IBS symptoms

Clinical Presentation

- Pain most commonly in left iliac fossa or hypogastrium
- Knotting, burning, cramping sensation
- Distention, bloating, fullness, especially postprandially
- Small-volume stools whether diarrhea or constipation
- Constipation stools often scybalous (pebble-like); diarrhea often in morning, following normal bowel movements; **mucus is common**
- **Relief of pain often with bowel movement**
- Dyspepsia, heartburn, nausea, headaches, urinary frequency, dysmenorrhea can also be seen
- No history of weight loss, awakening from sleep, rectal bleeding, fever, rigidity on examination (if present, think of other disorders)
- No specific findings on examination except for mild abdominal tenderness—more often over sigmoid colon

Diagnosis and Evaluation

- Diagnostic criteria (Rome III criteria) are based on history (Box 29-1). Extensive investigation is usually not necessary.
- CBC, erythrocyte sedimentation rate, stool studies, occult blood examination are normal
- With diarrhea-predominant IBS, need to rule out lactose intolerance, celiac disease, IBD
- In more severe or unresponsive cases, stool volume (should be normal) can be examined and sigmoidoscopy performed
- If constipation is severe, rule out hypothyroidism, hyperparathyroidism, diverticulosis, anorectal dysfunction, and malignancy
- Occasionally, pelvic pain and altered bowel habit with gynecologic conditions, such as endometriosis, can mimic IBS

Treatment

- Educate patient about condition
- High-fiber diet or supplementation, reduce or remove offending foods (e.g., high-fat, high-carbohydrate diet)
- Antispasmodics (e.g., dicyclomine, hyoscyamine) and low-dose tricyclics may be helpful for abdominal pain

BOX 29-1	*Diagnostic Criteria for Irritable Bowel Syndrome (Rome III)*

At least 3 months, with onset at least 6 months previously, of recurrent abdominal pain or discomfort associated with two or more of the following:
1. Improvement with defecation
2. Onset associated with change in frequency of stool
3. Onset associated with change in form (appearance) of stool

- Antimotility agents (e.g., loperamide) may be helpful for diarrhea
- Probiotics may be useful, particularly for postinfectious IBS. Further studies are required to determine the type and dose of probiotics required.
- Gas symptoms may respond to diet changes, simethicone, or bismuth
- Treat depression and anxiety (avoid narcotics and benzodiazepines)
- Drugs
  - Tegaserod, a 5-hydroxytryptamine-4 partial agonist, may be useful for women with constipation-predominant symptoms
  - Alosetron, a 5-hydroxytryptamine-3 agonist, modulates visceral afferent activity from the GI tract and was found to be helpful in IBS in women with diarrhea-predominant symptoms. This drug was withdrawn following its release because of an apparent increased incidence of ischemic colitis; however, it has now been reintroduced.

Inflammatory Bowel Disease

Basic Information

- Defined as an idiopathic chronic inflammation of the GI tract: Primarily Crohn's disease (CD) and ulcerative colitis (UC)
- **Bimodal peak age distribution: Initial 15 to 25 years, second peak 50 to 80 years**
- Significantly greater incidence in Western developed countries
- Smoking as a risk factor
  - Increased risk in CD
  - Decreased risk of current smokers and increased risk of ex-smokers in UC
- Genetics
  - 10% to 20% of patients with IBD have additional relatives with IBD
  - First-degree relatives of patients with IBD are 3 to 20 times more likely to develop the disease than the general population
  - Increased risk of IBD in patients with other autoimmune diseases
  - *NOD2/CARD15* mutation is a risk factor for CD but not UC (mutation carriers often do not have disease)
- Crohn's disease can affect any part of the bowel from the mouth to the anus. It can have "skip lesions" with a normal section of bowel between diseased sections.
  - 80% of patients have small bowel involvement, usually in the distal ileum
  - 50% have involvement of both the ileum and the colon
  - A small number of patients have involvement of the upper GI tract (esophagus, stomach, proximal small bowel)
  - 30% have perianal disease
- UC affects the large bowel and is continuous from the rectum to the proximal extent of the disease
  - Proctitis: Ulcerative colitis limited to the rectum
  - Distal colitis: Affects the rectum and sigmoid colon
  - Left-sided colitis: Affects area from the rectum to the splenic flexure
  - Extensive colitis: Extends from the rectum past the spenic flexure but does not involve the cecum
  - Pancolitis: Extends from the rectum to the cecum

Clinical Presentation

- Typically characterized by recurrence of a number of symptoms
  - Diarrhea
  - Abdominal pain
  - Weight loss
  - Rectal bleeding
  - Fever
- Causes of exacerbations
  - Usually not identifiable
  - NSAID use, tobacco use (in CD), infections, and medication noncompliance may predispose to attacks
- Extraintestinal manifestations may present without symptoms of abdominal disease (Box 29-2)

BOX 29-2	***Extraintestinal Manifestations and Complications of Inflammatory Bowel Disease***

Arthritis
  Peripheral arthritis involving large joints
  Spondyloarthropathy/ankylosing
    spondylitis
Uveitis/iritis
Skin manifestations
Pyoderma gangrenosum
Erythema nodosum
Hepatobiliary manifestations
Primary sclerosing cholangitis (PSC)
  70% of PSC patients have inflammatory bowel
    disease (IBD)
  All PSC patients should be screened for IBD with
    colonoscopy
Cholelithiasis
Fistulas (Crohn's disease [CD])
  Often involves perianal area, but any area of bowel may
    be involved, can lead to abscess formation
  Usually extends to skin, bowel, or vagina
Hemorrhage
Bowel obstruction/perforation
  Stricturing can lead to obstruction
  Spontaneous perforation more common in CD
  Toxic megacolon (abdominal distention, diarrhea, colonic
    dilation on radiograph)
    More commonly seen in ulcerative colitis
    Fever, tachycardia, leukocytosis, anemia
    50% of patients will require surgery
    15% mortality rate
Nutritional manifestations/malabsorption
Malnutrition
Dehydration
Anemia (iron deficiency, vitamin B_{12} deficiency)
Osteoporosis
  Can occur even without corticosteroid use
  Bone density scans should be checked routinely
Thromboembolism
Spontaneous abortion/premature delivery
Protein-losing enteropathy
Nephrolithiasis (calcium oxalate and uric acid stones)
Amyloid
Colorectal carcinoma

29

- Cancer
  - Colorectal cancer
    - The risk is related to the duration and extent of the disease
    - **Overall risk in UC and extensive colitis from CD is 2% to 5%**
    - **Screen for dysplasia and cancer 8 to 10 years after diagnosis of IBD is made, then every 1 to 2 years**
  - Small bowel cancer increased in CD

Diagnosis and Evaluation

- Laboratory tests
  - Increased C-reactive protein and sedimentation rate; leukocytosis, anemia, and thrombocytosis are commonly seen
  - Stool studies for ova and parasites, culture, and *C. difficile* should be obtained to rule out infection
  - Peripheral antineutrophil cytoplasmic antibody (p-ANCA) is elevated in 60% of patients with CD or UC. Anti-*Saccharomyces cerevisiae* antibody is elevated in 80% of CD patients. Neither is adequate for diagnosis.
- Radiographic features
  - Barium enema can show mucosal granularity or ulceration (in UC; Fig. 29-3)
  - Small bowel series may show ulcerations in between normal mucosa, fistulas ("cobblestoning"), or strictures (in CD)
  - MRI is also helpful in evaluating Crohn's disease, particularly of the small intestine
- Sigmoidoscopy or colonoscopy is most often used to make the diagnosis and to distinguish between UC and colonic CD (Table 29-6)
- Capsule endoscopy is useful for staging small bowel Crohn's disease
- Complications of IBD and therapies, such as malnutrition, osteoporosis, and gallstones, should be sought and treated (e.g., nutritional supplementation, bone densitometry; see Box 29-2)

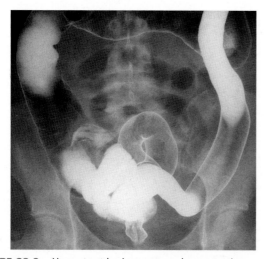

FIGURE 29-3   Air contrast barium enema demonstrating luminal narrowing and loss of haustral markings in the sigmoid and descending colon in a patient with ulcerative colitis. (From Goldman L, Bennett JC, Ausiello D: *Cecil textbook of medicine,* ed 22, Philadelphia, WB Saunders, 2004, figure 142-1.)

TABLE 29-6	*Differentiating Ulcerative Colitis from Crohn's Disease**	
	UC	**CD**
Perianal disease	–	+
Fistula formation	–	+
Small bowel involvement	–	+
Granuloma formation on biopsy	–	+
Transmural inflammation	–	+
Inflammation limited to mucosa	+	–
Continuous colonic inflammation	+	–

*In 10% of patients ulcerative colitis (UC) and Crohn's disease (CD) will be indistinguishable.

- Assessment of severity of a disease flare
  - Mild to moderate: Able to tolerate oral diet; no dehydration, toxicity, abdominal tenderness, mass or obstruction
  - Moderate to severe: Failed treatment for mild to moderate disease or symptoms of fever, weight loss, abdominal pain and tenderness, intermittent nausea, vomiting, or anemia
  - Severe: Fulminant—persisting symptoms despite treatment with steroids or high temperature, persistent vomiting, intestinal obstruction, rebound tenderness, cachexia, or abscess

Treatment

- Medical (Table 29-7)
  - 5-ASA medications (sulfasalazine, mesalamine, olsalazine)
    - Mainstay of therapy for mild to moderate cases of UC and CD
    - Inhibits lipoxygenase pathway, prostaglandin cytokine synthesis, free radical scavenger
  - Corticosteroids
    - Initial therapy for most moderate cases and all severe cases
    - Can be used intravenously, orally, or as an enema (for isolated rectal involvement or proctitis)
    - Oral budesonide undergoes extensive first-pass metabolism and has fewer side effects
  - Antibiotics (metronidazole, ciprofloxacin)
    - No clear role in treatment of UC
    - Most effective in fistulous and perianal disease of CD
  - Immunosuppressants
    - Usually indicated in steroid-resistant or steroid-dependent patients
    - Specific agents
      - Azathioprine/6-mercaptopurine: Most frequently used; these agents are used both to induce and maintain remission
      - Cyclosporine: Used for UC, not CD; given over 2 to 4 months to induce remission
      - Methotrexate: Mainly used for CD
      - Anti–tumor necrosis factor (TNF) therapies
        Infliximab: Chimeric mouse/human monoclonal antibody against TNF-α; given as IV infusion; licensed for CD and UC both to induce and maintain remission; also used to treat fistulizing Crohn's disease

TABLE 29-7	*Medications Used for the Treatment of Inflammatory Bowel Disease*
Medication	**Side Effects**
Sulfasalazine	GI distress Allergy (fever and rash, similar to other sulfa drugs) Folic acid deficiency Hemolysis, neutropenia Male infertility
Other aminosalicylates (mesalamine, olsalazine, balsalazide)	Fewer than sulfasalazine; no hemolysis or infertility; rarely nephritis
Corticosteroids (including budesonide)	Hyperglycemia Cataracts Mood disorders Avascular necrosis Osteoporosis
Metronidazole	Metallic taste Peripheral neuropathy
Ciprofloxacin	GI distress Photosensitivity Elevated transaminases
Azathioprine/ 6-mercaptopurine	Pancreatitis Leukopenia Elevated transaminases
Cyclosporine	Hypertension Renal failure Tremors Paresthesias Seizures Infections
Methotrexate	Leukopenia Hepatic fibrosis Pneumonitis
Infliximab	Infusion reaction Tuberculosis and other infections related to immunosuppression Lupus-like syndrome

Adalimumab: Recombinant human IgG$_1$ monoclonal antibody against TNF-α; subcutaneous administration every 2 weeks; can be used in patients who have lost response to infliximab

Certolizumab: Humanized monoclonal antibody Fab fragment linked to polyethylene glycol, which neutralizes TNF; subcutaneous administration every 4 weeks

Patients need to be screened for tuberculosis (TB; tuberculin skin test and chest radiograph) before starting anti-TNF therapy because patients are at increased risk of developing TB and other serious infections

Lymphoma risk is also slightly increased, as is risk for demyelinating disease, hematologic disease, and liver toxicity

- Miscellaneous agents
  - Fibrin sealant for fistulas
  - Fish oil (in UC)
- Surgical
  - UC
    - Because UC is limited to the colon, total proctocolectomy cures UC. An ileal pouch can be

formed, replacing the rectum. This can be affected by pouchitis.

- Indications for surgery:
  - Fulminant disease (toxic megacolon)
  - Colitis refractory to medical therapy
  - Dysplasia or concern for colorectal cancer
  - Stricture
  - Massive bleeding
- Crohn's disease (Fig. 29-4)
  - Indications for surgery include obstructive symptoms, refractory severe inflammation, and repair of fistulas
  - More than 40% of patients require surgery within first 10 years of diagnosis
  - Up to 80% of patients will have evidence of recurrence endoscopically, and 10% to 15% will have clinical recurrence
  - There is an increased risk of recurrence in patients who smoke or have perforating disease
  - The aim of surgery is to preserve as much small bowel as possible
  - A stricturoplasty can be performed to treat strictures, avoiding removing large sections of bowel
  - Bile salt diarrhea and fat malabsorption may occur following ileal resection
- Nutritional (enteral therapy)
  - Effective therapy in patients with active CD for treating flare and decreasing fistula output
  - Useful in children, but adults can find enteral therapy unpalatable
  - Not effective as lone therapy in UC

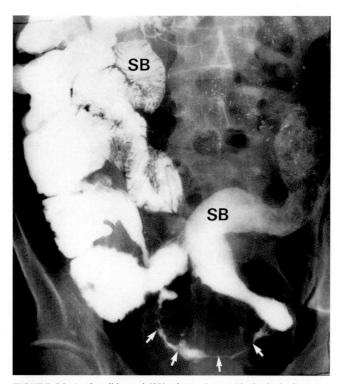

FIGURE 29-4 Small bowel (SB) of a patient with Crohn's disease. Note the stricture in the terminal ileum (*arrows*). (From Burkitt GH, Quick CRG: *Essential surgery,* ed 3, New York, Churchill Livingstone, 2002, figure 21.8.)

29

REVIEW QUESTIONS

For review questions, please go to www.expertconsult.com.

SUGGESTED READINGS

AGA Institute medical position statement on the diagnosis and management of celiac disease, *Gastroenterology* 131:1977–1980, 2006.

American Gastroenterological Association medical position statement: guidelines on constipation, *Gastroenterology* 119:1761–1778, 2000.

Donowitz M, Kokke FT, Saidi R: Evaluation of patients with chronic diarrhea, *N Engl J Med* 332:725–729, 1995.

Drossman DA, Camilleri M, Mayer EA, Whitehead WE: AGA technical review on irritable bowel syndrome, *Gastroenterology* 123:2108–2131, 2002.

Green PHR, Cellier C: Celiac disease, *N Engl J Med* 357:1731–1743, 2007.

Longstreth GL, Thompson WG, Chey WD, et al: Functional bowel disorders, *Gastroenterology* 130:1480–1491, 2006.

Mayer EA: Irritable bowel syndrome, *N Engl J Med* 358:1692–1699, 2008.

Podolsky DK: Inflammatory bowel disease, *N Engl J Med* 347:417–429, 2002.

CHAPTER 30

Acute and Chronic Liver Disease

JAMES P. HAMILTON, MD

The widespread use of serum liver chemistries has led to an increase in the identification of diseases of the liver. Diseases such as hepatitis C, hemochromatosis, and nonalcoholic fatty liver disease have been found to be quite prevalent in the general population. A systematic approach designed to assess liver function and disease severity via laboratory testing and imaging can direct the need for more invasive evaluation and defined treatment.

Evaluation of Elevated Liver Tests

Basic Information

- Biochemical liver tests lack sensitivity and specificity, but both the pattern and degree of elevation may sometimes give clues to disease processes
- **Persistently or markedly (>10× normal) elevated liver tests should always be fully evaluated**

Clinical Presentation

- Elevated aminotransferases (aspartate aminotransferase [AST] and alanine aminotransferase [ALT]) are usually indicative of hepatic inflammation and hepatocyte necrosis
  - Alcoholic hepatitis, viral hepatitis, drug-induced injury, autoimmune hepatitis, toxic injury, and non-alcoholic fatty liver disease are common causes
  - **The pattern of enzyme elevation, i.e., hepatic *versus* cholestatic, is a critical first step in the interpretation of liver chemistries**
  - **An AST/ALT ratio of greater than 2 is suggestive of alcoholic liver disease in the appropriate clinical scenario**
  - AST and ALT values greater than 1000 IU/mL are usually indicative of acute viral, toxic, or ischemic hepatitis. Alcoholic hepatitis almost never raises the enzymes above 400 IU/mL.
- Alkaline phosphatase (AP) is elevated in diseases associated with impaired flow of bile, such as cholestatic diseases, infiltrative diseases, biliary tract obstruction, and drug-induced toxic injury
- γ-Glutamyl transpeptidase (GGT) and 5′-nucleotidase are tests that can be used to confirm that the elevation in AP is from the liver and not from another source (e.g., bone)
- Liver function tests (bilirubin, prothrombin time [PT], and albumin) reflect synthetic capacity of the liver

- Bilirubin is elevated in a variety of hepatocellular and biliary diseases in addition to some nonhepatic causes (e.g., hemolysis)
- PT is prolonged when vitamin K–dependent coagulation factors I, II, V, VII, and X are insufficiently synthesized by the liver. Vitamin K malabsorption in cholestatic liver disease is common.
- Albumin is produced by the liver, has a half-life of 3 weeks, and decreases as synthetic function of the liver fails

Diagnosis: Investigating Elevated Liver Enzymes

- The pattern of elevation dictates the evaluation process and diseases to be considered (Table 30-1)
- A careful history and review of patient's medications, both prescribed and over-the-counter, are critical
- Elevated aminotransferases should first be evaluated by serologic and biochemical tests (Fig. 30-1)
- Elevated bilirubin or AP should be evaluated by an ultrasound of the biliary tree and an antimitochondrial antibody (see Fig. 30-1)
- If ascites is present, Doppler studies of hepatic veins can be used to rule out outflow obstruction of the liver (e.g., hepatic vein thrombosis [Budd-Chiari syndrome])
- **Liver biopsy should be considered when diagnostic confirmation is required or if serologic and biochemical tests have not revealed the cause of liver enzyme abnormality**
- Endoscopic retrograde cholangiopancreatography (ERCP) or magnetic resonance cholangiopancreatography (MRCP) can be used to evaluate biliary tract disease
- CT and MRI scans can be used in place of or to complement ultrasound

Acute Liver Failure

Basic Information

- *Acute liver failure* (ALF) is defined as hepatocellular dysfunction as evidenced by jaundice with encephalopathy in the setting of no prior liver disease
- Most commonly caused by medications, toxins (mushrooms), or viruses (hepatitis B, herpes)
- **Most commonly implicated drug is acetaminophen,** and acetaminophen toxicity is the most common cause of ALF in the United States

TABLE 30-1	*Summary of Common Liver Disorders*		
Disease	**Liver Test Abnormalities**	**Diagnostic Testing**	**Treatment**
Autoimmune hepatitis	AST, ALT	ANA, anti–smooth muscle Ab	Prednisone plus azathioprine, transplant
Primary biliary cirrhosis	AP	Antimitochondrial Ab	UDCA, transplant
Primary sclerosing cholangitis	AP	ERCP, pANCA	UDCA, transplant
Alcoholic liver disease	AST/ALT ratio > 2:1	History suggestive; improvement with abstention from alcohol	Pentoxifylline, corticosteroids, transplant
Hemochromatosis	AST, ALT	Iron saturation, ferritin, genetic analysis	Transplant
Wilson's disease	AST, ALT	AP low, ceruloplasmin low, high 24-hr urine Cu, hepatic Cu high	Chelation, transplant
Hepatitis A	AST, ALT	Anti-HAV-IgM	Supportive
Hepatitis B	AST, ALT	HBSAg, anti-HB$_c$-IgM, HepBeAg, HBVDNA	PEG-interferon-α, nucleoside analogues, transplant
Hepatitis C	AST, ALT	Anti-HCV, HCV RNA	Interferon plus ribavarin, transplant

Ab, antibody; ALT, alanine aminotransferase; ANA, antinuclear antibodies; AP, alkaline phosphatase; AST, aspartate aminotransferase; ERCP, endoscopic retrograde cholangiopancreatography; HAV, hepatitis A virus; HB$_c$, hepatitis B core; HBSAg, hepatitis B serum antigen; HBV, hepatis B virus; HCV, hepatitis C virus; HepBeAg, hepatitis B antigen; IgG, immunoglobulin G; pANCA, perinuclear antineutrophil cytoplasmic antibody; PEG, percutaneous endoscopic gastronomy; UDCA, ursodeoxycholic acid.

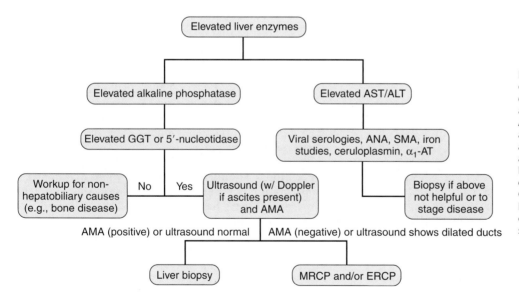

FIGURE 30-1 Evaluation of elevated liver enzymes. α_1-AT, α_1-antitrypsin; ALT, alanine aminotransferase; AMA, antimitochondrial antibody; ANA, antinuclear antibody; AST, aspartate aminotransferase; AT, antitrypsin; ERCP, endoscopic retrograde cholangiopancreatography; GGT, γ-glutamyl transpeptidase; MRCP, magnetic resonance cholangiopancreatography; SMA, smooth muscle antibody.

- Other causes of ALF are Wilson's disease, Budd-Chiari syndrome, acute fatty liver of pregnancy, autoimmune hepatitis, Reye's syndrome, and other idiosyncratic drug reactions (e.g., isoniazid, phenytoin, sulfonamides, propylthiouracil, azoles)

Clinical Presentation

- Patients present with encephalopathy, which can lead to coma and cerebral edema. Cerebral edema can result in brainstem herniation, which is the leading cause of death in ALF.

- Presentation is often complicated by sepsis, multisystem organ failure (including renal failure and pancreatitis), gastrointestinal bleeding, and coagulopathy
- With progressive coagulopathy, hemorrhage is commonly seen
- With collapse of hepatocytes, loss of glycogen stores and impaired gluconeogenesis lead to hypoglycemia

Diagnosis

- Careful history from family and friends, history of toxin exposure, drug use, medications

TABLE 30-2	Indicators of Poor Prognosis in Acute Liver Failure (King's College Criteria)

Acetaminophen Overdose

Arterial pH < 7.3 or all of the following

    PT > 100 sec (INR > 7.7)

    Cr > 3.4 mg/dL

    Grade 3–4 encephalopathy (HE)

Other Causes of ALF

PT > 100 sec (INR > 7.7) or any three of the following

    Non-A or B hepatitis or drug reaction

    Jaundice > 7 days before HE

    Age < 10 yr or >40 yr

    PT > 50 sec (INR > 3.85)

    Bilirubin > 17.4 mg/dL

ALF, acute liver failure; Cr, creatinine; HE, hepatic encephalopathy; INR, international normalized ratio; PT, prothrombin time.

- Toxicology screen, including acetaminophen level, should be sent immediately
- Viral serologies, Doppler study of hepatic veins, CT imaging, ceruloplasmin, and 24-hour urinary copper excretion may be helpful in establishing the underlying diagnosis
- Prognosis can be made using King's College criteria (Table 30-2) or the Clichy criteria

Treatment

- Monitor PT, pH, glucose level, liver enzymes, cultures, fluid balance, central venous pressure
- Enteral feeding, dextrose infusion, thiamine
- Prophylactic antibiotics, antifungals
- Proton-pump inhibitor or H$_2$ receptor antagonist
- **N-Acetylcysteine for acetaminophen toxicity**
- Mechanical ventilation to protect airway in patients with delirium
- Elevate head of bed, hyperventilate initially, mannitol if serum osmolality is less than 320 mOsm to keep intracranial pressure (ICP) low
- ICP monitor, when available, should be used to monitor perfusion pressures and ICP
- Continuous venovenous hemofiltration for renal failure
- **Transfuse clotting factors (including recombinant factor VII) only for bleeding or before invasive procedures**
- Disease-specific treatments such as penicillin for mushroom poisoning and acyclovir for herpes hepatitis
- Transfer to transplant center as soon as possible

Drug-Induced Hepatitis

Basic Information

- 5% of all adverse drug reactions involve the liver
- Approximately 20% to 30% of acute liver failures are drug induced
- Reactions can be dose dependent or idiosyncratic

TABLE 30-3	Hepatic Injury Caused by Various Medications
Injury Pattern	**Drug**
Nonspecific or viral-like hepatitis	Aspirin, amiodarone, diclofenac, isoniazid, methyldopa, nitrofurantoin, phenytoin, propylthiouracil, sulfonamides
Cholestasis	Carbamazepine, chlorpromazine, co-trimoxazole, haloperidol, tricyclics, estrogens, 17-alpha substituted steroids
Steatosis	Alcohol, prednisone, tetracycline, valproic acid, amiodarone, zidovudine
Granulomatous hepatitis	Allopurinol, quinidine, sulfonamides, sulfonylurea agents
Veno-occlusive disease	Anti-neoplastics, azathioprine, pyrrolizidine alkaloids
Adenomas and hepatocellular carcinoma	Estrogens and anabolic steroids

Clinical Presentation

- Usually asymptomatic
- Can follow several patterns of injury: hepatitis, cholestasis, cholestatic hepatitis, and progressive bile duct injury known as "vanishing bile duct syndrome"
- Most biochemical parameters return to normal after eliminating the offending drug
- Injury pattern can give clue to offending agent (Table 30-3)
- Several medications require regular monitoring (Table 30-4)

TABLE 30-4	Liver Monitoring Schedule for Hepatotoxic Medications		
Medication	**Every Month**	**Every Month for 3 Months, Then Every 3 Months**	**Every 3 Months**
Amiodarone			X
Antiepileptics			X
Azathioprine	X		
Diclofenac			X
HMG-CoA reductase inhibitors			X
Herbal remedies			X
All conazoles (e.g., fluconazole)	X		
Nicotinic acid	X		
NSAIDs (other)			X (3–6 mo)
Tacrine		X	
Protease inhibitors	X		

HMG-CoA, 3-hydroxy-3-methylglutaryl-coenzyme A.

30

TABLE 30-5	Herbs and Associated Hepatic Injuries	
Remedy	**Toxic Component**	**Injury**
Gordolobo yerba tea, comfrey	Pyrrolizidine alkaloids	Veno-occlusive disease
Chinese herbal tea	Compositae	Veno-occlusive disease
Jin Bu Huan	*Lycopodium serratum*	Acute hepatitis, steatosis
Germander	Teucrin A	Hepatitis
Chaparral leaf	*Larrea tridentata*	Necrosis, chronic hepatitis
Mistletoe, skullcap, valerian	Unknown	Hepatitis
Natural laxatives	Senna, podophyllin	Elevated aminotransferases
Dai-saiko-to and Sho-saiko-to	*Scutellaria* and others	Hepatitis, fibrosis, steatosis
Kava kava	Kavalactones	Hepatitis

TABLE 30-6	Serologic Features of Autoimmune Hepatitis Variants	
Serologic Features	**Type 1**	**Type 2**
Smooth-muscle antibodies	+/–	–
Antinuclear antibodies	+/–	–
Liver kidney microsomal Ab	–	+
Anti-actin	+/–	–
Anti-liver cytosol-1	–	+/–
Soluble liver antigen/liver pancrea	+/–	–

Diagnosis

- Thorough history is critical to diagnosis
- Temporal relationship to medication use is critical to the diagnosis

Treatment

- Discontinue medication and do not rechallenge
- Biopsy liver if enzymes do not normalize within several weeks or if diagnosis is in question
- Transfer to transplant center if liver failure ensues

Herbal Remedies and Natural Products

Basic Information

- Increased use of herbal remedies has led to recognition of potential hepatotoxicity
- Few over-the-counter agents have been put through any rigorous scientific testing
- **Most reactions are idiosyncratic, although some are dose dependent**

Clinical Presentation

- Elevated aminotransferases are the most common presentation
- Can also present with ascites and/or hepatomegaly
- Cirrhosis or liver failure can occur with ongoing use of offending agent
- Table 30-5 lists herbs and associated hepatic injuries

Diagnosis

- Thorough history (patients do not think of herbs as medicines)
- Exclude other forms of liver disease

Treatment

- Discontinue herbal medication and do not rechallenge
- Monitor liver enzymes and biopsy liver if they do not normalize within several weeks

Autoimmune Hepatitis

Basic Information

- Autoimmune hepatitis (AIH) is a diagnosis of exclusion when nonviral, immune-mediated hepatocellular injury is present
- **Should be considered when liver enzymes are elevated and patient has negative viral serologies and no drug injury is implicated**
- Cause of AIH is not known, but pathogenesis likely involves genetic susceptibility with etiologic trigger such as viral infection or medication
- Variant, overlapping, or mixed forms of AIH exist that share features with other autoimmune diseases, such as primary biliary cirrhosis and primary sclerosing cholangitis

Clinical Presentation

- Two established forms of AIH with different autoantibodies (Table 30-6)
  - Both are more common in women, with age of onset in third to fourth decades of life
- Range of presentation varies from mild enzyme elevations to liver failure
- Nonspecific fatigue, lethargy, abdominal pain, and arthralgias may be present
- Concomitant autoimmune diseases (thyroiditis, type 1 diabetes, systemic lupus erythematosus, Sjögren's syndrome) are common
- Liver enzyme elevations tend to wax and wane

Diagnosis

- Elevated liver enzymes with negative hepatitis serologies, elevated gamma globulin (especially immunoglobulin G [IgG])
- Supported by histologic pattern of interface hepatitis, plasma cell infiltrate, and portal tract inflammation
- Autoantibodies usually but not invariably present (see Table 30-6)

Treatment

- Treatment indicated in patients with ALT 10 times or more than normal; ALT 5 or more times normal and gamma globulin 2 or more times normal; or necrosis on liver biopsy
- **Prednisone with or without azathioprine for at least 18 to 36 months (many patients require lifelong therapy)**
- 30% of patients not responsive to this regimen and require more potent immunosuppressives
- Treatment progress is followed by monitoring transaminases, gamma globulin, and liver biopsies
- Consider liver transplantation for decompensated cirrhosis
- 30% recurrence rate after transplantation

Primary Biliary Cirrhosis

Basic Information

- Immune-mediated destruction of small bile ducts
- Genetic predisposition plus triggering event such as viral infection or medication underlie many cases
- Prevalence in North America is 2 per 100,000
- 6% prevalence in first-degree relatives

Clinical Presentation

- Mean age at diagnosis is 55 years
- **90% of patients are women**
- **Intermittent pruritus,** fatigue, and abdominal pain; jaundice late in disease
- Progresses over 5 to 15 years from diagnosis
- Impaired fat-soluble vitamin (A, D, E, K) absorption leading to osteomalacia, night blindness
- Elevated total cholesterol without increased cardiac risk
- Can lead to cirrhosis, portal hypertension, and hepatocellular carcinoma

Diagnosis

- Alkaline phosphatase almost always elevated
- Aminotransferases typically mildly elevated
- Antimitochondrial antibody (AMA) is present in 97% of cases
- Antinuclear antibody (ANA) is also positive in most cases
- Liver biopsy reveals portal tract infiltrates and bile duct injury (Fig. 30-2)

Treatment

- Ursodeoxycholic acid (UDCA, 12–15 mg/kg/day) improves transplant-free survival, improves liver chemistries, and slows histologic progression
- UDCA works by increasing canalicular excretion of toxic bile acids, inhibiting intestinal bile acid reabsorption, and scavenging reactive oxygen species
- Corticosteroids, colchicine, and other immunosuppressants may improve liver chemistries but do not alter disease progression and should not be recommended
- Liver transplantation should be considered once cirrhosis and jaundice develop. The five-year post-transplant survival rate is 80% (among the highest for all liver diseases).

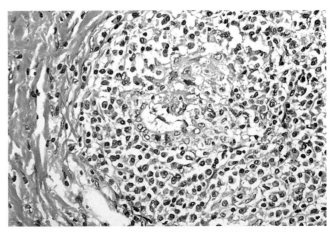

FIGURE 30-2 Primary biliary cirrhosis. Note the portal tract inflammation and injury to the bile duct. (From Kumar V, Fausto N, Abbas A: *Robbins and Cotran's pathologic basis of disease,* ed 7, Philadelphia, WB Saunders, 2005, figure18-31.)

Primary Sclerosing Cholangitis

Basic Information

- Autoimmune disease typically seen in young men
- Progressive inflammatory destruction of medium and large bile ducts
- **Most (80%) cases are associated with inflammatory bowel disease, typically ulcerative colitis (UC)**
  - 10% of patients with UC have primary sclerosing cholangitis (PSC)
  - Increased risk of colon cancer in patients with UC and PSC (more than UC alone)
- Increased risk of cholangiocarcinoma
- Prevalence is 1 to 6 of 100,000 in the United States

Clinical Presentation

- Generally asymptomatic but can present with abdominal pain, jaundice, cholangitis, or pruritus
- Mean age at presentation is 30 to 40 years
- Progresses over a mean of 12 years from diagnosis

Diagnosis

- AP is usually elevated, with mild elevation of aminotransferases
- Bilirubin is typically normal, except when common hepatic duct or common bile duct is involved and in late stages of disease
- Diagnosis made by ERCP or MRCP, which demonstrates strictures or beading of the intrahepatic or extrahepatic bile ducts (Fig. 30-3)
- Liver biopsy typically shows pericholangitis and periductular fibrosis but is often not diagnostic in early disease
- Perinuclear antineutrophil cytoplasmic antibody (pANCA) positive in two thirds of cases

Treatment

- High-dose (25–28 mg/kg/day) UDCA may improve liver chemistries but does not slow disease progression and may actually hasten development of portal hypertension

30

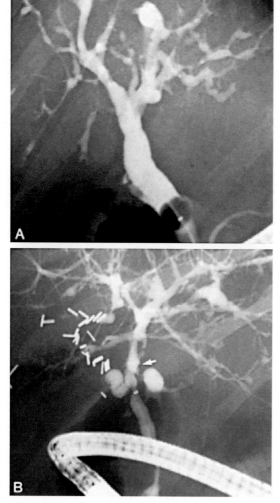

FIGURE 30-3 **A,** Primary sclerosing cholangitis. **B,** Endoscopic retrograde cholangiopancreatography showing beading and strictures of the intrahepatic ducts *(arrow).* (From Feldman M: *Sleisenger and Fordtran's gastrointestinal and liver disease,* ed 8, Philadelphia, WB Saunders, 2006, figure 65-1.)

- Periodic dilation of strictures via ERCP or percutaneous approach may be necessary
- Annual screening for colon cancer in patients with concomitant UC
- Liver transplantation should be offered to those with advanced liver disease or repeated bouts of cholangitis
- Disease can recur after transplantation

Alcoholic Liver Disease (Alcoholic Hepatitis)

Basic Information

- Chronic liver disease occurs in 15% to 20% of alcoholics
- Variables leading to higher likelihood of alcoholic liver disease include malnutrition and obesity, female gender, concomitant drug toxicity, and coexisting viral hepatitis

- Pathophysiology related to increased reactive oxygen species and inflammatory cytokines (tumor necrosis factor [TNF]-α)—this is the rationale for anti-inflammatory therapy (see later discussion)

Clinical Presentation

- Physical examination in acute alcoholic hepatitis can reveal fever, malnutrition, jaundice, encephalopathy, tremor, parotid gland enlargement, hepatomegaly, right upper quadrant pain, ascites, spider nevi, and leukocytosis
- Tender hepatomegaly can occur secondary to fatty infiltration
- Can present with portal hypertension and ascites as disease progresses; hepatorenal syndrome is a frequent cause of death in severe acute alcoholic liver disease

Diagnosis

- History of alcohol use (at least 20–40 g/day for 10 years or longer)
- **Patients present with elevated aminotransferases, often with AST-ALT ratio greater than 2:1**
- Bilirubin and PT may be elevated
- GGT and red blood cell mean cell volume are often elevated
- Liver biopsy can be used to stage fibrosis and exclude other forms of liver disease
- Histopathology reveals acute (neutrophilic) and chronic (lymphocytic) inflammatory infiltrate, steatosis, steatonecrosis, or cirrhosis
- Mallory bodies are a classic finding on biopsy but are not specific for alcoholic liver disease

Treatment

- Abstinence is the most crucial component of therapy
- Adequate nutrition is important, although survival benefits using enteral nutrition or parenteral nutrition have not been shown
- Corticosteroids may be of modest benefit in improving short-term survival (see later discussion)
  - The discriminant function (DF) = 4.6 × [PT – control (in seconds)] + serum bilirubin (in mg/dL), determines the need for corticosteroid therapy
  - Score of greater than 32 predicts a greater than 50% 30-day mortality rate and is used to indicate the need for corticosteroid therapy
  - **Long-term survival benefits of corticosteroids have not been shown**
  - Steroids are not recommended for patients with concomitant infection or poorly controlled diabetes
- Pentoxifylline 400 mg thrice daily improves short-term survival by decreasing the risk of hepatorenal syndrome and should be considered as a surrogate for prednisone in patients with severe alcoholic hepatitis (DF > 32) in addition to volume repletion, nutritional support, thiamine, and a proton-pump inhibitor. Pentoxifylline is not approved by the Food and Drug Administration (FDA) for this indication.
- Nephrotoxins should be carefully avoided (including contrast dye)

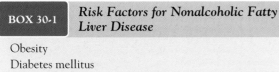

BOX 30-1 *Risk Factors for Nonalcoholic Fatty Liver Disease*

Obesity
Diabetes mellitus
Hyperlipidemia
Jejunoileal bypass and rapid weight loss
Prolonged total parenteral nutrition
Small bowel bacterial overgrowth
Advanced HIV/AIDS with lipodystrophy
Medications
    Amiodarone
    Corticosteroids
    Tamoxifen
    Perihexiline maleate
    Tetracycline
    Calcium channel blockers
Methotrexate

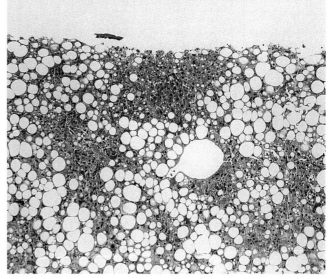

FIGURE 30-4 Nonalcoholic fatty liver disease. Liver biopsy specimen showing diffuse steatosis and focal inflammation and necrosis. (From Feldman M: *Sleisenger and Fordtran's gastrointestinal and liver disease,* ed 8, Philadelphia, WB Saunders, 2006, figure 82-3.)

- Liver transplantation may be considered if a patient has abstained from alcohol use for the period of time required by the local transplant program (usually at least 6 months)
- Reversal of portal hypertension and remarkable clinical improvement can be seen after prolonged abstinence

Nonalcoholic Fatty Liver Disease

Basic Information

- Nonalcoholic fatty liver disease (NAFLD) was previously known as nonalcoholic steatohepatitis
- **Most common liver disorder causing elevated liver enzymes**
- Histologically similar to alcoholic liver disease
- Occurs in up to 25% of the U.S. population
- Spectrum of disease ranging from benign hepatic steatosis, which may progress to steatohepatitis and can progress to fibrosis and cirrhosis
- **Up to one third of patients with NAFLD can progress to cirrhosis by the fifth or sixth decade of life**

Clinical Presentation

- The main risk factor is coexisting features of the metabolic syndrome, most notably obesity and diabetes mellitus, but several other risk factors exist (Box 30-1). Insulin resistance is the hallmark of the disease.
- Aminotransferases can be elevated severalfold
- Hepatomegaly typically presents with signs of portal hypertension in more advanced disease

Diagnosis

- Alcohol use should be ruled out by history
- Imaging with ultrasound, CT scan, or MRI often reveals hepatomegaly and suggests fatty infiltration. Ultrasound may miss subtle steatosis but is less expensive.
- Liver chemistry elevation pattern not typically helpful in diagnosis

- Histology is the key to diagnosis, revealing either steatosis or steatonecrosis with or without fibrosis (Fig. 30-4)

Treatment

- Weight loss, strict glucose control, treatment of hypertension, and lipid control are recommended (cardiac disease is the leading cause of death in patients with NAFLD)
- Antioxidants, insulin sensitizers, and cholesterol-lowering medications have been studied, but no clear benefit has been found
- Potentially offending medications should be discontinued
- Liver transplantation can be an effective option, although risk of recurrence is significant if risk factors remain

Hereditary Hemochromatosis

Basic Information

- Most common autosomal recessive disease of whites with 1/10 carrier rate
- Mutant *HFE* gene identified on chromosome 6
- **Disease may be present in homozygotes with the *C282Y* mutation**
- Pathogenesis involves increased intestinal iron absorption, possibly due to decreased production of the hepatic hormone hepcidin, resulting in hepatic accumulation of iron

Clinical Presentation

- Typically presents in men in the fourth to sixth decade of life and in postmenopausal women
- Nonspecific elevation of liver enzymes
- **In addition to the liver, the joints (caused by calcium pyrophosphate deposition), pituitary gland, testes, pancreas, and heart can be affected**

- Symptoms typically include weakness, fatigue, myalgias, arthralgias, loss of libido
- Hepatomegaly may be present, especially early in disease
- As disease advances, patients can develop skin pigmentation, diabetes, cardiomyopathy, or conduction abnormalities
- Hepatocellular carcinoma risk is significant, especially once cirrhosis develops

Diagnosis

- Elevated transferrin saturation greater than 50% and ferritin greater than 300 mg/L are present in more than 95% of cases
- *HFE* mutational analysis to detect *C282Y* or *H63D* mutations
- Liver biopsy for quantification of iron per gram of dry liver weight remains the gold standard; values greater than 71 mmol/g are highly suggestive
- First-degree family members need screening, either through serum transferrin saturation and ferritin or by genetic testing

Treatment

- Phlebotomy of 1 unit of blood weekly until ferritin level falls from more than 200 mg/L to 10 to 20 mg/L, followed by maintenance phlebotomy every several weeks as needed to keep the ferritin below 50 mg/L
- Iron chelation with deferoxamine is an alternative when phlebotomy is restricted by anemia
- Liver transplantation can be considered once cirrhosis has developed

α_1-Antitrypsin Deficiency

Basic Information

- 1 in 600 births
- Common in Northern Europe
- Mutation in α_1-antitrypsin (AAT), a protein that prevents protease enzymes such as elastin from degrading normal host tissue; mutated protein is abnormally folded and cannot exit hepatocytes
- Absolute deficiency of AAT leads to lung disease, and relative deficiency leads to liver and or lung disease

Clinical Presentation

- Can present with elevated liver enzymes, hepatomegaly, or cirrhosis in children and adults
- Panacinar emphysema may be present alone or in addition to cirrhosis
- May also be associated with panniculitis and Wegener's granulomatosis
- Patients are at high risk for the development of hepatocellular carcinoma

Diagnosis

- Reduced serum levels of α_1-antitrypsin
- Phenotype analysis and liver biopsy are key to diagnosis if levels are found to be low
- Phenotype ZZ most typically seen with advanced liver disease

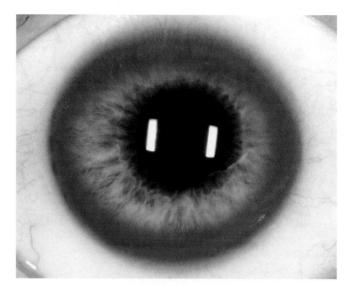

FIGURE 30-5 Kayser-Fleischer ring in a patient with Wilson's disease. Note the brown-green pigment around the cornea. (From Goldman, L, Bennett JC, Aussiello D: *Cecil textbook of medicine,* ed 22, Philadelphia, WB Saunders, 2004, figure 224-1.)

- Liver biopsy positive for periodic acid-Schiff (PAS), diastase-resistant globules

Treatment

- IV infusions of α_1-antitrypsin derived from pooled plasma or obtained by recombinant DNA methods are under investigation for treatment of pulmonary disease but have not been successfully used for liver disease
- **Liver transplantation is the only viable therapy for the liver disease component and is curative**

Wilson's Disease

Basic Information

- Autosomal recessive disorder of copper metabolism
- Defective mobilization of copper from liver resulting in accumulation in the liver, brain, and eyes
- 1 in 30,000 live births

Clinical Presentation

- Typically presents before the age of 40 years
- Can present with Coombs' negative hemolytic anemia, elevated liver chemistries, cholestatic jaundice, or acute liver failure
- AP inappropriately low
- Some cases present with neurologic abnormalities, including psychosis, coma, or movement disorders

Diagnosis

- Consider in any young patient with acute hepatitis, jaundice, or hemolysis
- **Kayser-Fleischer rings are nearly 100% sensitive if neurologic abnormalities are present (Fig. 30-5)**
- Serum ceruloplasmin is typically low but may be normal because it is an acute phase reactant
- 24-hour urine copper level greater than 100 μg
- Liver biopsy for quantification of copper revealing greater than 200 μg/g of dry liver weight is the gold standard

Treatment

- Oral chelation with D-penicillamine or trientine is generally used as primary therapy
- Oral zinc may be used to inhibit copper absorption and prevent reaccumulation after treatment with penicillamine or trientine
- Transplantation is curative and should be offered to patients with advanced or acute fulminant disease

Pregnancy-Related Liver Disease

Basic Information

- Complicates less than 0.1% of pregnancies
- Several different disease processes but no clearly defined causes
- All tend to be recurrent in subsequent pregnancies except acute fatty liver of pregnancy
- **Children of mothers who had preeclampsia, HELLP (hemolysis, elevated liver enzymes, low platelets) syndrome, or acute fatty liver of pregnancy should be screened for long-chain 3-hydroxyacyl-CoA dehydrogenase (LCHAD) deficiency because this may be the underlying etiology**

Clinical Presentation

See Table 30-7 for a summary of liver diseases in pregnancy.

Diagnosis

See Table 30-7.

Treatment

See Table 30-7.

Viral Hepatitis

Overview

- Several human hepatatropic viruses exist, the most significant being hepatitis A, B, and C
- Hepatitis A commonly found in developing countries with occasional outbreaks in the United States
- Hepatitis B is the most common chronic viral hepatitis worldwide
- Hepatitis C is the most common in the United States

HEPATITIS A

Basic Information

- 38% of the U.S. population has positive antibodies for past infection
- **Incubation period of 2 to 6 weeks**

Clinical Presentation

- Fecal-oral spread
- Nausea, vomiting, diarrhea
- Children usually are asymptomatic, but adults are often jaundiced
- **Fatal disease can occur in older patients and in those with chronic liver disease, but most cases are self-limited**
- Never becomes chronic but cases of relapsing and cholestatic disease can occur

TABLE 30-7	Liver Diseases of Pregnancy				
Disease	**Symptoms/Signs**	**Lab(s)**	**Treatment**	**Mortality Risk: Mother/Fetus**
Hyperemesis gravidarum	Nausea/vomiting (N/V), dehydration in 1st trimester	Bilirubin up to 5 × normal AST/ALT 2–3 × normal	Antiemetics, hydration	–/– (Resolves spontaneously)
Intrahepatic cholestasis of pregnancy	Pruritus, jaundice in 2nd or 3rd trimester	Bilirubin up to 10 × normal AST/ALT up to 1000	Cholestyramine, UDCA; deliver if fetal distress	–/Low
Preeclampsia/ eclampsia	N/V, hypertension (HTN), edema, seizures/coma in late 2nd or 3rd trimester	Bilirubin normal AST/ALT can be >1000	Treat HTN and edema; magnesium sulfate; deliver in severe cases	+/Low
HELLP syndrome	RUQ pain, N/V, HTN, edema in late 2nd or 3rd trimester	Bilirubin up to 20 × normal AST/ALT can be >1000 Low haptoglobin Platelets <100 K	Delivery	+/+
Acute fatty liver of pregnancy	RUQ pain, N/V, fatigue, jaundice, hepatomegaly in 3rd trimester	Bilirubin up to 20 × normal AST/ALT up to >1000 Hyperammonemia Azotemia Disseminated intravascular coagulation can develop	Delivery	+/+
Hepatic rupture	Severe abdominal pain, shock in 3rd trimester	Variable	Immediate surgery	+/+

ALT, alanine aminotransferase; AST, aspartate aminotransferase; RUQ, right upper guadrant; UDCA, ursodeoxycholic acid.

30

Diagnosis

- Acute disease is diagnosed by serum anti-hepatitis A virus (HAV) IgM
- Immunity conferred by presence of anti-HAV IgG

Treatment

- Supportive care
- **Vaccinate those at risk of exposure, including close contacts of index case**
- Vaccinate travelers to endemic areas, military workers, IV drug users, those with chronic liver disease
- **Immune globulin can be given for passive protection before or within 2 weeks of exposure**

HEPATITIS B

Basic Information

- 5% of U.S. population has serologic markers of past infection, with chronic infection in 0.7%
- More than 400 million people infected worldwide
- **Incubation period of 6 weeks to 6 months**
- Transmitted parenterally and by sexual contact
- **High risk for vertical transmission**
- Likelihood of chronic infection inversely related to age at time of infection

Clinical Presentation

- Symptomatic disease (e.g., abdominal pain, nausea, jaundice) occurs in only 25% of adults
- Many are chronic "carriers" with normal liver chemistries and no evidence of or low levels of viral replication
- The vast majority of adults infected will clear virus spontaneously, whereas 5% develop chronic hepatitis and 1% fulminant hepatitis
- Death caused by hepatocellular carcinoma (HCC) and cirrhosis particularly high in those infected as neonates; HCC risk high even in those without cirrhosis
- Reactivation in the setting of immunosuppression (i.e., chemotherapy) may occur in patients who have had prior exposure to hepatitis B (hep B core IgG positive)
- Extrahepatic manifestations
  - Polyarteritis nodosa that may improve with antiviral therapy
  - Membranous nephropathy or mebranoproliferative glomerulonephritis

Diagnosis

- Based on serologic patterns (Table 30-8)
- **Hepatitis B serum antigen (HBsAg) is the first positive marker of acute infection (Fig. 30-6). It usually disappears within 6 months but persists in chronic disease.**
- Screening for chronic infection should utilize HbsAg
- Anti-HBc-IgM positive with acute infection, whereas anti-HBc-IgG indicates past infection
- HBe antigen positivity indicates active replication, although this is negative in some strains
- HBV DNA positivity indicates active replication
- **Presence of anti-HBsAb denotes immunity**
- To determine presence of viral replication in chronic infection, check HBe antigen and HBV DNA

TABLE 30-8	Serologic Diagnosis of Hepatitis B			
HBsAg	HBsAb	HBcAb–IgM	HBcAb–IgG	Disease Pattern
+	−	+	−	Acute infection
+	−	−	+	Chronic or late acute infection
−	−	+	−	Acute infection or window before HBcAb seroconversion (or HBsAb conversion)
−	+	−	+	Past infection
−	+	−	−	Immunized against hepatitis B or remote infection

HBcAb, hepatitis B core antibody; HBsAb, hepatitis B surface antibody; HBsAg, hepatitis B surface antigen.

Treatment

- Percutaneous endoscopic gastrostomy (PEG)-interferon-α, lamivudine, adefovir, entecavir, tenofovir, and telbirudine are all FDA approved for treatment of chronic hepatitis B
- Interferon-α may provide a more durable response but is quite expensive and is associated with more side effects than the others (e.g., flulike symptoms, cytopenias, elevated liver tests, mood changes)

HEPATITIS C

Basic Information

- Hepatitis D is partial RNA virus and requires the presence of HBV for replication
- Up to 40% of IV drug users are coinfected but less than 2% of others with HBV

Clinical Presentation

- Can coinfect or superinfect with HBV
- In superinfection, disease is more severe with higher rates of cirrhosis and liver failure
- More common in Mediterranean countries and the Far East

Diagnosis

- Can be diagnosed by presence of hepatitis D virus antigen (HDV-Ag) or anti-HDV
- Polymerase chain reaction (PCR) test available only through research laboratories

Treatment

- No clearly proven benefit for treatment with interferon; however, it is currently recommended because of lack of other effective therapies

HEPATITIS D

Basic Information

- RNA virus with incubation from 2 to 26 weeks
- Chronic infections occur in 75% to 85% of cases

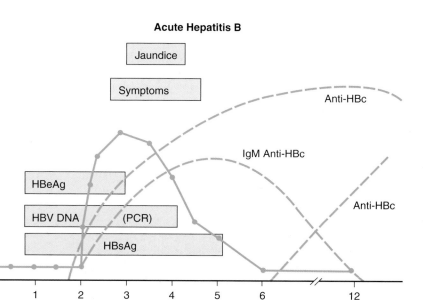

FIGURE 30-6 Serologic response to acute hepatitis B infection. HBc, hepatitis B core protein; HBsAg, hepatitis B serum antigen; HBV, hepatitis B virus; IgM, immunoglobulin M; PCR, polymerase chain reaction.

- Leads to cirrhosis in 20% to 50% of those infected, usually after about 20 years
- Heavy alcohol use accelerates fibrosis
- Most common hepatotropic viral infection in America, with 4 million anti-HCV positive
- Risk factors for hepatitis C include IV drug use, transfusions before 1990, high-risk sexual behavior, dialysis, and hemophilia

Clinical Presentation

- Acute disease is often asymptomatic, although profound hepatitis occurs rarely
- Common symptoms of chronic infection include fatigue and periodic right upper quadrant discomfort
- May be complicated by HCC once cirrhosis develops (2–5% risk per year)
- Extrahepatic manifestations include cryoglobulinemia, vasculitis, glomerulonephritis, porphyria cutanea tarda, cardiomyopathy, and lymphoma

Diagnosis

- Hepatitis C antibody develops within 6 months of infection
- Diagnosis of persistent or past infection indicated by anti-hepatitis C virus (HCV) positivity
- Aminotransferases may be normal, periodically elevated, or persistently elevated to any degree
- Aminotransferase levels should not be used as an indication of presence or absence of disease (one third of infected patients will have normal liver enzymes)
- Active viral replication determined by presence of serum RNA
- Most commonly used test to detect RNA is PCR and less commonly used test is branched-chain DNA assay
- Liver biopsy is a useful tool to stage disease and render prognosis
- Strain or genotype of the virus and the viral load should be determined if therapy is considered
  - Genotype 1 is associated with reduced responsiveness to therapy and is the most common

Treatment

- Standard of care is pegylated interferon and ribavirin for 6 to 12 months, depending on genotype
- If serum RNA persists after 6 months of therapy, there is nearly no likelihood of cure
- Multiple side effects exist with therapy, including flulike symptoms, depression, anemia, thrombocytopenia, leukopenia, and teratogenicity

HEPATITIS E

Basic Information

- RNA virus transmitted by contaminated water supply
- Endemic in India and parts of Asia
- Two to eight weeks incubation

Clinical Presentation

- Generally mild acute disease and often subclinical
- Rarely fatal except in pregnancy, when mortality can reach 20%
- Disease is never chronic

Diagnosis

- Anti-hepatitis E virus (HEV) IgM and IgG
- Suspect disease in patient presenting with acute hepatitis and recent travel to endemic areas

Treatment

- Supportive
- Vaccine is in development
- Liver transplantation should be considered for fulminant disease

Liver Lesions

Overview

- Focal lesions of the liver are found frequently, and often incidentally, during abdominal imaging studies for other disorders

30

- It is important to diagnose these lesions accurately, if possible
- In addition to hepatic malignancy, there are two broad categories of liver lesions: cysts or abscesses and other benign conditions

Cysts and Abscesses

- Simple cysts (solitary or a few cysts) are found in about 1% of the adult population and are usually congenital and benign
  - Tend to have a uniform fluid density and a thin, regular wall without mass effect or complexity
  - Hydatid cysts are diagnosed by the presence of daughter cysts and the presence of echinococcal serologies
  - Aspiration of simple cysts usually results in recurrence of the fluid, and needle aspiration of hydatid cyst is contraindicated due to the risk of tracking or rupture
- Hepatic abscesses are usually associated with fever, right upper quadrant pain, or other systemic signs of infection
- May be pyogenic or amebic
- Sonogram-guided needle aspiration of pyogenic abscesses can help guide antibiotic treatment and allow placement of a percutaneous catheter for large abscesses
- Surgery rarely needed
- Amebic abscesses are usually difficult to diagnose with aspiration and frequently respond to metronidazole treatment

Other Benign Lesions

- Hemangioma
  - Most frequent benign lesion of the liver; occurs in about 4% of the population
  - Complications and need for intervention are rare unless they achieve a large size (>5 cm) with replacement of a significant part of the hepatic parenchyma. In such cases, resection may be indicated.
  - Diagnosis requires sonogram, triphasic CT, or MRI, with occasional use of tagged technetium-99 RBC SPECT (single-photon emission CT) studies
- Focal nodular hyperplasia
  - Occurs in 0.4% of the population
  - Lesions have a characteristic central stellate scar that may be seen on sonogram, CT, or MRI
  - Liver biopsies tend to be nondiagnostic, but occasional use of sulfur-colloid hepatic scans is helpful because

these lesions contain nonparenchymal cells that take up the sulfur-colloid particles leading to a contrast pattern equivalent to the hepatic parenchyma (i.e., a disappearing mass lesion)
  - Treatment or surgical intervention is not required, except in rare cases of diagnostic uncertainty; no risk of malignancy
  - Not associated with oral contraceptives
- Hepatic adenoma
  - A rare benign tumor, most often seen in the setting of oral contraceptive use in women of childbearing age; has the ability to transform to HCC
  - Can occasionally be associated with diabetes mellitus, glycogen storage disease, or pregnancy
  - Large lesions can cause pain, intraperitoneal bleeding, and occasionally a "mass-effect" with replacement of an entire lobe
  - Surgical resection or liver transplantation in extreme cases has been used effectively. Discontinuation of any offending agents (e.g., oral contraceptives, anabolic steroids, etc.) is a cornerstone of treatment. Regular follow-up with imaging studies is recommended to monitor any changes, including malignant degeneration.

REVIEW QUESTIONS

For review questions, please go to www.expertconsult.com.

SUGGESTED READINGS

de Alwis NM, Day CP: Non-alcoholic fatty liver disease: the mist gradually clears, *J Hepatol* 48(Suppl 1):S104–S112, 2008.
Dienstag JL, McHutchison JG: American Gastroenterological Association medical position statement on the management of hepatitis C, *Gastroenterology* 130:225–230, 2006.
Krawitt E: Autoimmune hepatitis, *N Engl J Med* 354:54–66, 2006.
Lok ASF, McMahon BJ: Chronic hepatitis B, *Hepatology* 45(2):507–539, 2007.
Maddrey WC: Drug-induced hepatoxicity, *J Clin Gastroenterol* 39 (4 Suppl 2):S83–S89, 2005.
Seeff LB: Herbal hepatotoxicity, *Clin Liver Dis* 11:577–596, 2007.
Su GL: Pregnancy and liver disease, *Curr Gastroenterol Rep* 10(1):15–21, 2008.

Acknowledgment

This chapter is adapted from a chapter written by F. Fred Poordad for the first edition and Rudra Rai from the second edition of the Johns Hopkins Internal Medicine Board Review.

Complications of Liver Disease

JAMES P. HAMILTON, MD

In the previous chapter, a number of causes of liver disease were described. This chapter focuses on the consequences that can result from those disease entities. Morbidity and mortality from cirrhosis can result from numerous different processes, including infection (spontaneous bacterial peritonitis), encephalopathy, renal failure (hepatorenal syndrome), pulmonary disease, and hepatocellular carcinoma. Liver transplantation offers the only cure.

Overview of Cirrhotic Liver Disease

- Definitions
  - Hepatic fibrosis is a reversible wound healing response characterized by accumulation of extracellular matrix (ECM)
  - **Cirrhosis is marked by progression to an irreversible state with worsening fibrosis and organ damage**
- Pathophysiology
  - Chronic inflammation leads to activation of hepatic stellate cells and is the critical event in the pathogenesis of hepatic fibrosis. These perisinusoidal cells lead to deposition of scar tissue with subsequent vascular and organ contraction.
- Causes (Table 31-1)
- Clinical consequences of cirrhosis (Table 31-2)

Portal Hypertension

Basic Information

- Definition
  - The most common and morbid consequence of liver disease and cirrhosis

- Complications of portal hypertension begin to develop when portal pressure reaches values equal to or greater than 12 mm Hg (normal, up to 10 mm Hg)
- Direct measurement of portal pressure is difficult, but indirect measurement of the hepatic vein pressure gradient (HVPG) is possible by catheterizing the hepatic vein
- Classification of portal hypertension (Fig. 31-1)
  - Presinusoidal: Obstruction proximal to hepatic sinusoids
    - Prehepatic (e.g., splanchnic arteriovenous fistula, splenic vein thrombosis, portal vein thrombosis [idiopathic or associated with hypercoagulable states])
    - Hepatic (e.g., schistosomiasis, sarcoidosis, myeloproliferative disorders)
  - Sinusoidal: Results from cirrhotic liver disease
  - Postsinusoidal: Obstruction distal to the hepatic sinusoids
    - Posthepatic (e.g., inferior vena cava obstruction, Budd-Chiari syndrome [hepatic vein thrombosis often associated with hypercoagulable states], cardiac disease)
    - Hepatic (e.g., veno-occlusive disease, perivenular sclerosis)

Clinical Presentation

- The major complication of portal hypertension is development of portosystemic collaterals, the most clinically significant of which are gastroesophageal varices (Fig. 31-2) and hemorrhoids
- For other clinical consequences of portal hypertension, see Table 31-2

TABLE 31-1	Causes of Chronic or Cirrhotic Liver Disease
Infections	Viral hepatitis (hepatitis B, C), *Echinococcus* infections, brucellosis, congenital tertiary syphilis, schistosomiasis
Drugs and toxins	Alcohol, methotrexate, isoniazid, vitamin A, amiodarone, perhexilene maleate, α-methyldopa
Metabolic or genetic diseases	Wilson's disease, hereditary disorders, hemochromatosis, α_1-antitrypsin deficiency, carbohydrate metabolism disorders, lipid metabolism disorders, amino acid disorders, metabolism disorders, porphyria
Biliary obstruction	Chronic biliary obstruction, primary biliary cirrhosis, secondary biliary cirrhosis, cystic fibrosis, congenital biliary cysts
Vascular abnormalities	Veno-occlusive disease, Budd-Chiari syndrome, inferior vena cava obstruction, cardiac disease, hereditary hemorrhagic telangiectasias
Miscellaneous	Autoimmune chronic hepatitis, nonalcoholic steatohepatitis, granulomatous liver disease, sarcoidosis, polycystic liver disease

TABLE 31-2	*Clinical Consequences of Cirrhosis*
Synthetic defects	Decreased production of procoagulants, albumin, and fibrinogen
Renal	Sodium retention Hepatorenal syndrome Acute tubular necrosis Renal tubular acidosis
Endocrine	Impotence Anovulation Euthyroid-sick syndrome Hepatic osteodystrophy
Cardiopulmonary	Hypotension Portal-pulmonary hypertension Hepatopulmonary syndrome
Oncologic	Hepatocellular carcinoma Cholangiocarcinoma
Portal hypertension	Portosystemic encephalopathy Variceal hemorrhage Ascites Spontaneous bacterial peritonitis Splenomegaly

Diagnosis

- Laboratory studies should focus on evaluation of hepatic synthetic function, renal function, and hematologic values. Thrombocytopenia may develop from splenic sequestration.
- Radiographic studies may aid in the diagnosis and treatment of various conditions

Treatment

- Usually directed at the specific complication of portal hypertension
- Attempts to decrease the portal pressure can be made through several different modalities
  - Non-cardioselective β-blockers (propranolol or nadolol) are beneficial for the primary prophylaxis of bleeding in patients with medium and large varices
  - Transjugular intrahepatic portosystemic shunt (TIPS) can offer an alternative to surgery (Fig. 31-3)
  - Surgical decompression (portal systemic shunt) has not been shown to improve survival in patients with cirrhosis
- Treatment of acute variceal hemorrhage consists of somatostatin analogues to induce splanchnic vasoconstriction, variceal band ligation, balloon tamponade, and TIPS

Ascites

Basic Information

- Ascites is the presence of excess fluid in the peritoneal cavity
- Fluid is formed because of a number of contributing factors, including elevated hydrostatic pressure caused by portal hypertension, increased sympathetic outflow, reduced oncotic pressure caused by hypoalbuminemia, and increased renal sodium reabsorption (Fig. 31-4)

Clinical Presentation

- Patients may be asymptomatic or may complain of early satiety, increased abdominal girth, or respiratory distress

- Physical examination can reveal abdominal distention, bulging flanks, shifting dullness, or a fluid wave if there is greater than 500 mL of fluid present

Diagnosis

- Clinical symptoms and examination may be suggestive
- Laboratory studies
- Blood tests may show evidence of underlying liver disease
- Ultrasound and Doppler examinations are indicated to detect small amounts of fluid and to evaluate for portal vein thrombosis or Budd-Chiari syndrome
- Ascitic fluid analysis
  - Indicated for every patient with new-onset ascites
  - Tests ordered include WBC count with differential, total protein, albumin, Gram stain, culture and sensitivity, cytology (if malignancy suspected), amylase (if pancreatic cause suspected), and triglycerides (if chylous ascites suspected)
  - Serum ascites albumin gradient (SAAG)
    - Calculated by subtracting the albumin level of the ascitic fluid from the albumin level in the serum
    - Levels greater than 1.1 g/dL are more than 90% sensitive for portal hypertension
    - Levels less than 1.1 g/dL usually exclude cirrhosis and portal hypertension
    - Total protein levels greater than 4 and ascitic albumin levels greater than 2.5 suggest a cardiac cause

Treatment

- Sodium restriction to less than 2 g/day
- Free water restriction only needed if hyponatremia is present
- Diuretic therapy to reduce sodium retention by the kidneys is generally required
  - Spironolactone: Works by inhibition of distal tubular and collecting duct sodium reabsorption and by abrogation of the renin-angiotensin system
  - Loop diuretics function at the ascending limb of the loop of Henle

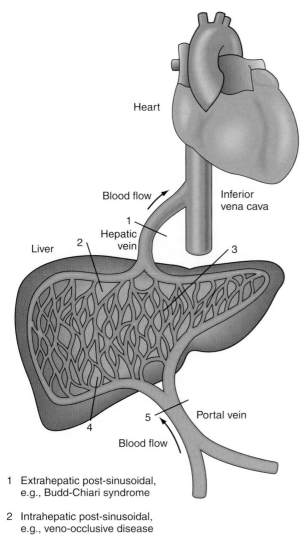

1 Extrahepatic post-sinusoidal,
  e.g., Budd-Chiari syndrome

2 Intrahepatic post-sinusoidal,
  e.g., veno-occlusive disease

3 Sinusoidal,
  e.g., cirrhosis

4 Intrahepatic pre-sinusoidal,
  e.g., sarcoidosis, schistosomiasis

5 Extrahepatic pre-sinusoidal,
  e.g., portal vein thrombosis

FIGURE 31-1 Classification of portal hypertension. (From Boon NA, Colledge NR, Walker BR: *Davidson's principles and practice of medicine,* ed 20, New York, Churchill Livingstone, 2006, figure 23.19.)

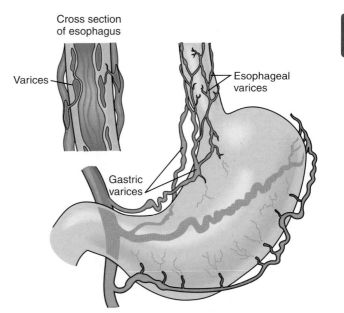

FIGURE 31-2 Esophageal and gastric varices. (From http://hopkins-gi.nts.jhu.edu/pages/latin/templates/index.cfm?pg=disease4& organ = 2&disease=25&lang_id=1.)

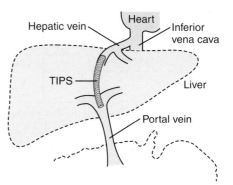

FIGURE 31-3 Transjugular intrahepatic portosystemic shunt (TIPS). A stent is placed from the portal vein to the right hepatic vein, allowing for decompression of the portal system. (From Boon NA, Colledge NR, Walker BR: *Davidson's principles and practice of medicine,* ed 19, New York, Churchill Livingstone, 2006, figure 23.24B.)

Spontaneous Bacterial Peritonitis

Basic Information

- The most important sequela of ascites is the risk for development of spontaneous bacterial peritonitis (SBP)
- Because of the low protein content (including bacterial opsonins) and oncotic pressure of portal hypertensive ascitic fluid, the risk of infection is very high
- Risk factors for developing SBP in cirrhosis include GI hemorrhage, ascitic fluid protein content less than 1 g/dL, and a previous episode of SBP
- **Most infections are caused by transmigration of bacteria through the bowel wall, so enteric gram-negative bacilli are common pathogens (70% of cases)**
- Streptococci and staphylococci make up most of other cases
- Polymicrobial infection may suggest bowel perforation

- Generally a combination of spironolactone or other potassium-sparing diuretic, along with a loop diuretic, is required for complete diuresis
  - Need to monitor for side effects that may include electrolyte disorders, dehydration, hypotension, and azotemia
- Large-volume paracentesis is still required at times in patients with difficult-to-control ascites or in patients who do not tolerate diuretic therapy. IV albumin (8 g/dL of ascites removed) may be beneficial to prevent post-paracentesis circulatory collapse.
- Liver transplantation should also be considered in patients with refractory ascites

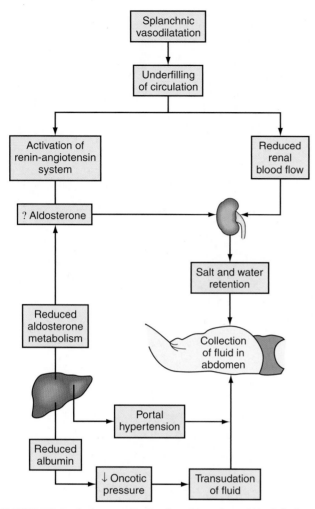

FIGURE 31-4 Pathogenesis of ascites. (From Boon NA, Colledge NR, Walker BR: *Davidson's principles and practice of medicine,* ed 20, New York, Churchill Livingstone, 2006, figure 23.12.)

Clinical Presentation

- Fevers, chills, and generalized abdominal pain can be seen; 33% of patients with cirrhosis and SBP will not have a fever or leukocytosis
- Often a clinical diagnosis is difficult to make because of inconsistent signs and symptoms. Pain is often absent, and the only reliable way to diagnose this condition is by paracentesis.
- Need to suspect SBP in patients with worsening jaundice, encephalopathy, or renal failure

Diagnosis

- The diagnosis of SBP is made based on an ascitic fluid polymorphonuclear (PMN) cell count greater than 250/mL. A very high ascitic PMN count (>1000/mL) suggests bowel perforation.
- Cultures of ascitic fluid taken at the time of paracentesis are often positive if done properly. The preferred method is to inoculate two blood culture bottles with 10 to 20 mL of ascitic fluid.
- Gram stain is commonly negative
- Basic classification of ascitic fluid infection
  - Spontaneous bacterial peritonitis

- Culture positive
- Greater than 250 neutrophils
- Culture-negative neutrocytic ascites
  - Culture negative
  - Greater than 250 neutrophils
- Monomicrobial non-neutrocytic bacterascites
  - Culture positive
  - Less than 250 neutrophils

Treatment

- The treatment of choice for documented SBP is cefotaxime (1 g IV every 8 hours for a minimum of 5 days)
- Repeat paracentesis at 48 to 72 hours should be done to check response to therapy
- Recurrent episodes of SBP are common, with about 70% of patients experiencing a second infection within 1 year
- Prophylactic therapy using ciprofloxacin, norfloxacin, or trimethoprim-sulfamethoxazole should be initiated in patients with recurrent episodes of SBP
- Primary prevention indicated in high-risk patients (ascitic fluid protein < 1 g/dL) and in patients with acute variceal hemorrhage

Hepatorenal Syndrome

Basic Information

- Hepatorenal syndrome is a functional renal failure that occurs in the setting of advanced liver disease. It is exhibited by decreased urine production, azotemia, and reduced urinary sodium excretion.
- It is seen in up to 10% of patients hospitalized with liver failure
- The exact pathogenesis is not fully understood, but evidence suggests that splanchnic vasodilation leads to reduction in effective circulatory volume. The kidneys compensate by increasing renin, constricting efferent arterioles, increasing sodium resorption, and decreasing urine output. The kidney structure remains essentially normal, and the kidneys will often return to normal function if the liver disease is corrected (e.g., by liver transplantation).
- Risk factors include cirrhosis, alcoholic hepatitis, acute liver failure, recent large-volume paracentesis, infection, GI bleeding, use of diuretics, nephrotoxic agents (i.e., NSAIDs and contrast dye), and the presence of orthostatic hypotension

Clinical Presentation

- Hypotension, azotemia, hyponatremia, and progressive oliguria are typically seen
- Hepatorenal syndrome was recently classified into two types:
  - Type 1: Severe, with rapid lowering of creatinine clearance below 20 mL/minute; has virtually 100% mortality; patients will usually have massive ascites
  - Type 2: More insidious, less severe

Diagnosis

- It is typically diagnosed when other causes of kidney failure are excluded

BOX 31-1	*Diagnostic Criteria for Hepatorenal Syndrome*

Low glomerular filtration rate (creatinine > 1.5 g/dL or 24-hr urine creatinine clearance < 40 mL/min) that progresses over days to weeks
Absence of any apparent cause for renal disease
Urine sodium concentration < 10 mEq/L and a urine osmolality greater than plasma osmolality
No improvement in renal function with volume expansion or withdrawal of diuretics

- A number of diagnostic criteria have been developed (Box 31-1)

Treatment

- **No established effective medical therapies are available.** Combinations of mitodrine, albumin, and octreotide are commonly used with modest benefit.
- Liver transplantation can be curative

Hepatic Encephalopathy

Basic Information

- Defined as disturbances in behavior and consciousness associated with liver disease and/or portal-systemic shunting
- Can be associated with acute liver failure, chronic liver disease/cirrhosis, or portosystemic bypass without intrinsic liver disease
- The pathogenesis of hepatic encephalopathy is unknown, but the accumulation of toxins (e.g., ammonia, mercaptans, short-chain fatty acids, phenol) in the systemic circulation because of bypass of the liver (from hepatocellular disease or shunting) is thought to be a major contributing factor
- Precipitating factors for hepatic encephalopathy (Box 31-2)

Clinical Presentation

- Disturbances in behavior and mentation that can progress to coma
- Asterixis, hyperreflexia, abnormal Babinski reflexes can be seen
- Fetor hepaticus: Musty odor emanating from the urine or breath

BOX 31-2	*Precipitating Factors for the Development of Hepatic Encephalopathy*

Acute hepatitis, progression of liver disease, portal systemic shunts
Azotemia
Constipation
Dehydration
Drugs (benzodiazepines, narcotics, sedatives, diuretics)

Electrolyte disorders (hypokalemia, hyponatremia)
GI bleeding
Sepsis

TABLE 31-3	*Stages of Hepatic Encephalopathy*
Stage	**Clinical Description**
0	No alteration in consciousness, intellectual function, personality, or behavior
1	Hypersomnia, insomnia, euphoria or anxiety, short attention span, irritability
2	Lethargy, disorientation, impaired cognition, inappropriate behavior, slurred speech, and ataxia
3	Somnolence, gross confusion, response to noxious stimuli
4	Coma, no response to noxious stimuli

Diagnosis

- Based primarily on clinical presentation in a patient with acute or chronic liver disease and/or portosystemic shunting
- Electroencephalography can show symmetrical, high-voltage, triphasic slow-waves
- **Many patients will have elevated ammonia levels, but this is not sensitive or specific for diagnosis**
- Grading of hepatic encephalopathy based on change in mental status (Table 31-3)

Treatment

- Supportive measures: Nutrition (reduced-protein diet), fluid and electrolyte maintenance, pressure-sore prevention, aspiration precautions
- Eliminate or treat precipitating factors
  - Treat GI bleeding and SBP or other infections
  - Discontinue sedatives or narcotics (treat with naloxone or flumazenil, if appropriate)
  - Avoid nephrotoxic agents
- Eliminate toxins from the systemic circulation
  - Administer lactulose, nonabsorbable disaccharide that fosters the removal of ammonia in the stool and helps convert ammonia to ammonium ion (which is poorly absorbed); dose is titrated to maintain two to four loose bowel movements per day
  - Neomycin, metronidazole, and rifaximin are antibiotics that diminish GI tract bacterial production of ammonia (not Food and Drug Administration approved for this indication)
  - Gut clearance with cathartics or enemas may be necessary in the setting of GI bleeding
  - Branched-chain amino acid infusion may be beneficial
- Hepatic support
  - Artificial liver systems have not been successfully developed
  - Liver transplantation

Pulmonary Manifestations of Cirrhosis and Portal Hypertension

Basic Information

- One third of patients with chronic liver disease develop some form of hypoxemia
- Lung disease can take many forms:

- Parenchymal lung disease
  - Primary biliary cirrhosis—lymphocytic or fibrosing alveolitis and organizing pneumonitis
  - α_1-Antitrypsin deficiency—emphysematous lung disease
  - Pleural space disease
    - Hepatic hydrothorax associated with cirrhosis
    - Elevated hemidiaphragms because of ascites or hepatomegaly
- Infected pleural fluid associated with ascites
  - Diseases of the pulmonary circulation
    - Impaired gas exchange
    - Hypoxic vasoconstriction
    - Hepatopulmonary syndrome
      - Hypoxemia related to vasodilation of pulmonary capillary bed resulting in right-to-left shunt
      - **Clinical presentation includes hypoxemia, platypnea (difficulty breathing upon sitting up), and orthodeoxia (decreased oxygen saturation when changing from the lying to sitting position)**
      - Can be diagnosed with contrast-enhanced echocardiography or albumin lung perfusion scan
      - Condition is reversed by liver transplantation
    - Portopulmonary hypertension
      - Pulmonary hypertension is related to cirrhosis by unclear mechanisms
      - Moderate to severe elevations of right ventricular systolic pressures are a contraindication to transplantation
      - Pulmonary varices

Treatment

- Liver transplantation may result in complete resolution of severe pulmonary manifestation of liver disease, hepatic hydrothorax, and hypoxemia associated with hepatopulmonary syndrome. Pulmonary hypertension may resolve in carefully selected patients following liver transplantation.

Hepatocellular Carcinoma

Basic Information

- One of the most common malignancies worldwide, predominantly because of the prevalence of chronic viral hepatitis (hepatitis B and C); incidence is rising in the United States
- Chronic liver disease of any etiology is a risk factor for development of hepatocellular carcinoma (HCC)
- Aflatoxins, alcohol, hemochromatosis, and anabolic steroids are other potential etiologic factors
- Fibrolamellar hepatocellular carcinoma is a distinct form of HCC with a characteristic histopathologic and clinical appearance. It typically occurs in younger adults without cirrhosis.
- **Hepatitis C is now associated with HCC in nearly 80% of cases diagnosed in the United States and is almost always found in the setting of established cirrhosis**
- **Hepatitis B may be frequently associated with HCC in the absence of cirrhosis**
  - Caused by the presence of a proto-oncogene

- Careful radiographic surveillance of chronic hepatitis B carriers should be performed, especially in young adults who may have acquired it vertically at birth or through household contact in early childhood

Clinical Presentation

- Findings may be nonspecific and are often confused with progression of cirrhotic liver disease
- Abdominal pain is the most common symptom
- Examination may reveal a right upper quadrant abdominal mass and/or a bruit over the liver
- **Paraneoplastic syndromes are occasionally seen:**
  - Erythrocytosis—caused by erythropoietin-like activity emanating from tumor cells
  - Hypercalcemia—caused by parathyroid hormone (PTH)–like hormone secretion
  - Acquired porphyria cutanea tarda
  - Carcinoid syndrome
  - Vitiligo

Diagnosis

- Ultrasound, CT, and MRI are commonly used to image the liver
- α-Fetoprotein (AFP) levels greater than 500 mg/L are about 80% sensitive for HCC
- Liver biopsy is not required when the lesion meets radiologic requirements and the patient has chronic liver disease
- Measurement of serum α-fetoprotein and ultrasound examination may be used to screen for early HCC in cirrhotic patients
  - Many hepatologists recommend every 6 months
  - A clear benefit to this type of screening has yet to be proven

Treatment

- Surgical resection is indicated in patients without or with well-compensated cirrhosis (Child's class A)
- Liver transplantation is indicated in patients with advanced cirrhosis and small tumors (one tumor 2–5 cm or up to 3 tumors all less than 3 cm). The 5-year survival rates are around 75%. Metastases are a contraindication to transplant (including portal vein invasion).
- Patients with advanced cancers are candidates for locoregional therapy, such as hepatic artery embolization with chemotherapy, cryoablation, radiofrequency ablation, or alcohol ablation. Sorafaneb, an oral chemotherapeutic agent, was recently approved for the treatment of advanced HCC.

Liver Transplantation

Basic Information

- Acceptable indications for liver transplantation may include the following:
  - Acute liver failure
  - Advanced or chronic liver disease
  - Inherited metabolic liver disease
  - HCC using strict selection guidelines (Milan criteria)
- Contraindications to transplantation to be considered (Table 31-4)

TABLE 31-4	*Contraindications to Liver Transplant*
Absolute Contraindications	**Relative Contraindications**
Metastatic cancer of the liver or other organs	Alcoholism
Irreversible cardiac or pulmonary disease	Drug abuse
Acute infection outside the liver	HIV positivity
AIDS syndrome	HBV DNA positivity
	Advanced renal disease

HBV, hepatitis B virus.

- There are different sources of donor livers:
  - Cadaveric—Most common type of transplantation performed; long waiting times because of liver shortages
  - Living-related donor—Portion of the liver from a friend or relative is transplanted
- After an evaluation is completed, the patient is placed on the liver transplant waiting list with United Network for Organ Sharing (UNOS). In February 2002, UNOS changed its criteria for prioritizing patients for liver transplantation to the following:
  - Status 1: Acute liver failure with stage 3 or 4 encephalopathy and retransplantation or failed liver transplant resulting from primary graft nonfunction or hepatic artery thrombosis
  - Status 2: Model for End-Stage Liver Disease (MELD) score ranging from 6 to 40 points
  - Status 7: Inactive
- The waiting time depends on the severity of liver disease as assessed by the MELD score in all patients with chronic liver disease, but there are variations based on blood type, body size, and geographic regions. The MELD score provides a reliable estimate of short-term survival for patients with a wide range of liver

BOX 31-3	*MELD Score*

Based on the values of serum creatinine, total bilirubin, and INR

Formula

$$MELD\ Score = 10\ \{0.957\ Ln(Scr) + 0.378\ Ln(Tbil) + 1.12\ Ln(INR) + 0.643\}$$

General Rules

- Minimum value for any variable is 1
- Maximum value for creatinine is 4
- Maximum MELD score is 40
  An online calculator is available at: www.unos.org/resources/MeldPeldCalculator.asp? index=98

INR, international normalized ratio; MELD, model for end-stage liver disease.

diseases and is based on easily obtainable and objective laboratory parameters (Box 31-3).

- The 5-year survival rate is now close to 85% at well-established liver transplant centers, and the 1-year survival rate exceeds 90%

REVIEW QUESTIONS

For review questions, please go to www.expertconsult.com.

SUGGESTED READINGS

Dib N, Oberti F, Calès P: Current management of the complications of cirrhosis and portal hypertension: variceal bleeding and ascites, *CMAJ* 174:1433–1443, 2006.

El-Serag HB, Marrero JA, Rudolph L, Reddy KR: Diagnosis and treatment of hepatocellular carcinoma, *Gastroenterology* 134:1752–1763, 2008.

Munoz SJ: Hepatic encephalopathy, *Med Clin North Am* 92(4):795–812, 2008.

Munoz SJ: The hepatorenal syndrome, *Med Clin North Am* 92(4):813–837, 2008.

Runyan BA: Management of adult patients with ascites due to cirrhosis, *Hepatology* 39:841–856, 2004.

31

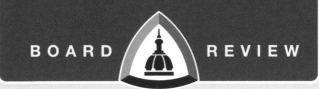
Nephrology

Acid-Base Disorders and Renal Tubular Acidosis

STEPHEN D. SISSON, MD

Acid-base disorders are extremely common in clinical medicine and can be seen in numerous disease states. The lungs and kidneys help maintain acid-base equilibrium (in the lungs via CO_2, in the kidneys via bicarbonate [HCO_3^-]; Fig. 32-1). **The body never overcorrects for a single acid-base disorder. When evaluating acid-base status, begin by looking at the serum pH to decide if acidosis or alkalosis is present** (pH < 7.4 indicates acidosis; pH > 7.4 indicates alkalosis). Then look at the partial pressure of carbon dioxide (Pco_2) and serum HCO_3^- to see which one (or both) is consistent with the pH, to determine if the primary disorder is respiratory or metabolic. **Note that a normal pH does not exclude an acid-base disorder; for instance, with a coexisting metabolic acidosis and metabolic alkalosis, the pH may be normal.**

Metabolic Acidosis

Basic Information

- Primary defect in metabolic acidosis is decreased serum HCO_3^-
- Calculation of the anion gap is used to help narrow differential diagnosis
  - Anion gap calculated as $Na^+ - (Cl^- + HCO_3^-)$
  - **The normal anion gap is 12±2** and is made of phosphates, sulfates, organic acids, and negatively charged plasma proteins
- When metabolic acidosis develops, determining whether anion gap increases, remains unchanged, or decreases will indicate a group of potential causes

Metabolic Acidosis with Increased Anion Gap

- **The differential diagnosis of the most common causes of an anion gap acidosis is remembered by the mnemonic MUDPILES (Box 32-1)**
- Besides a thorough history and physical examination, **evaluation of serum ketones, serum lactate, toxicology screen, and salicylate level should be considered**

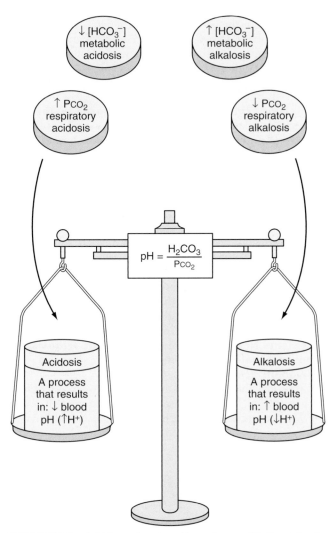

BOX 32-1	*Differential Diagnosis of Metabolic Acidosis with Increased Anion Gap*

M: Methanol
U: Uremia
D: Diabetic ketoacidosis (Fig. 32-2) or alcoholic ketoacidosis; drugs[*]
P: Phosphate or paraldehyde
I: Ischemia or isoniazid (rare) or iron toxicity (rare)
L: Lactate
E: Ethylene glycol
S: Starvation or salicylates

FIGURE 32-1 Acid-base disorders. (From Baynes JW, Dominiczak MH: *Medical biochemistry*, ed 2, St. Louis, Mosby, 2004, figure 22-5.)

*For example, metformin, nucleoside reverse transcriptase inhibitors.

In the figure:

$\downarrow$ [HCO_3^-] metabolic acidosis

$\uparrow$ [HCO_3^-] metabolic alkalosis

$\uparrow$ Pco_2 respiratory acidosis

$\downarrow$ Pco_2 respiratory alkalosis

$$pH = \frac{H_2CO_3}{Pco_2}$$

Acidosis: A process that results in: $\downarrow$ blood pH ($\uparrow H^+$)

Alkalosis: A process that results in: $\uparrow$ blood pH ($\downarrow H^+$)

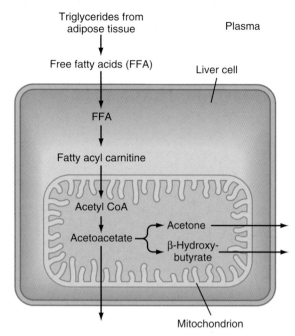

FIGURE 32-2 Pathogenesis of metabolic acidosis in ketogenesis. Acetoacetate, acetone, and β-hydroxybutyrate pass into the bloodstream, producing acidosis. (From Kumar P, Clark M: *Clinical medicine,* ed 5, Philadelphia, WB Saunders, 2005, figure 19-12.)

BOX 32-2	*Differential Diagnosis of Metabolic Acidosis with Normal Anion Gap*

D: Diarrhea

U: Ureteral diversion

R: Renal tubular acidosis

H: Hyperalimentation

A: Addison's disease, acetazolamide, ammonium chloride

M: Miscellaneous (chloridorrhea, amphotericin B, toluene,* others)

*Toluene initially results in an anion gap metabolic acidosis, but as it is cleared, a hyperchloremic normal anion gap acidosis develops.

Metabolic Acidosis with Normal Anion Gap

- Also referred to as a non–anion gap acidosis, although an anion gap is present but normal
- In this group, the increased anion is chloride (Cl^-), and the anion gap does not change
- **The mnemonic for the most common causes of a normal-anion gap acidosis is DURHAM (Box 32-2)**
- **Calculation of the urine anion gap may be helpful in evaluating normal-anion gap metabolic acidosis** to differentiate renal tubular acidoses (RTAs) from other causes of normal-anion gap metabolic acidosis
  - Normal kidney response to acidosis is to excrete acid, in the form of NH_4^+, which is balanced by increases in urine chloride. In type 1 or type 4 RTA, NH_4^+ excretion does not occur
  - **Formula for urine anion gap: Urine (Na + K – Cl)**
    - In normal patient (without RTA) with metabolic acidosis, the sum of this equation is less than 0

- If normal-anion gap metabolic acidosis exists, and urine anion gap is greater than 0, type 1 or type 4 RTA likely

Metabolic Acidosis with Decreased Anion Gap

- Low-anion gap acidoses are less commonly seen
  - **May be caused by hypoalbuminemia, multiple myeloma, ingestion of bromide**
  - The acid-base disorders in these diseases are of little clinical consequence

Investigation of Coexistent Anion Gap and Normal-Anion Gap Metabolic Acidoses

- **An anion gap acidosis and a normal-anion gap acidosis may coexist**
- To determine if the metabolic acidosis is caused by more than one process, compare the increase in the anion gap with the decrease in HCO_3^-
  - In pure anion gap metabolic acidosis, the decrease in HCO_3^- equals the increase in the anion gap
  - **If the HCO_3^- decreases significantly more than the anion gap increases, then a coexisting normal-anion gap metabolic acidosis is present**
  - Expressed as the "delta-delta equation": Change (Δ) in anion gap = change (Δ) in HCO_3^-
    - Note that the actual values of the HCO_3^- and anion gap are not compared, but rather the change in each of these values from their baseline (baseline HCO_3^- is 24 mEq/dL; baseline anion gap is 12)

Osmolar Gap

- **Metabolic acidosis is occasionally caused by the ingestion of toxic compounds that are osmotically active (e.g., methanol, ethylene glycol, toluene)**
- May be investigated in the clinically appropriate setting by calculating the difference between the measured osmolality and the calculated osmolality; in normal host, difference between measured and calculated osmolality is less than 10
- If this difference is greater than 10 (i.e., measured osmolality > 10 units higher than estimated osmolality), there are extra osmotically active compounds in the blood; **compare clinical picture with signs and symptoms of suggested toxin, including methanol (associated with papilledema and retinal hemorrhages), ethylene glycol (associated with calcium oxalate crystals in the urine), toluene (presents first with anion gap metabolic acidosis, then metabolized resulting in normal anion gap metabolic acidosis)**
  - Isopropyl alcohol ingestion also results in an osmolar gap, although no acid-base disorder is associated
  - Written mathematically, the osmolar gap is calculated as

$$\text{Osmolality(measured)} - \text{Osmolality(calculated)}$$

where

$$\text{Osm}_{calc} = [2 \times Na] + [\text{Blood urea nitrogen}/2.8] + [\text{Glucose}/18]$$

(normal < 10)

Clinical Presentation

- Respiratory compensation in patients presenting with metabolic acidosis
  - The body compensates for metabolic acidosis by creating respiratory alkalosis
  - Pco_2 may be predicted by the following equation (Winter's formula):

$$[1.5 (HCO_3^-) + 8] \pm 2 = Pco_2$$

  - Equation only valid when primary disorder is metabolic acidosis; do not use this equation when the primary disorder is not a metabolic acidosis
  - If the measured Pco_2 is not close to what we predict, a second disorder coexists
    - If the Pco_2 is less than predicted, second disorder is respiratory alkalosis
    - If the Pco_2 is higher than predicted, second disorder is respiratory acidosis

Metabolic Alkalosis

Basic Information

- **The primary defect in a metabolic alkalosis is an increase in the serum HCO_3^-, implying either a gain of HCO_3^- or a loss of acid**
  - **Examples of HCO_3^- gain**
    - Administration of sodium bicarbonate ($NaHCO_3$), baking soda, or medication formulations that include citrate or lactate
  - **Examples of acid loss**
    - Gastric losses, such as vomiting or nasogastric suction

- Renal causes (e.g., side effects from diuretics), as well as administration of nonresorbable anions (e.g., IV penicillin or carbenicillin)
- Hypermineralocorticoid states

Clinical Presentation

- The presence of a metabolic alkalosis always implies that two events have occurred: (1) initiation of the alkalosis and (2) maintenance of the alkalosis
  - The initiating factors are the gain of HCO_3^- or loss of acid described previously
  - The kidneys always are responsible for the maintenance of alkalosis; two states favor maintenance of alkalosis by the kidney
    - **Volume depletion:** The kidney responds to volume depletion by becoming Na^+ avid, and Na^+ is resorbed along with an anion (HCO_3^-, because Cl^- is depleted in volume depletion)
    - **Hypermineralocorticoid states:** Mineralocorticoids stimulate renal hydrogen ion (H^+) excretion; examples include hyperaldosteronism (Conn's syndrome; Fig. 32-3) and Cushing's disease

Diagnosis and Evaluation

- **Measurement of a spot urine Cl^- is helpful in evaluating the cause of the metabolic alkalosis (Box 32-3)**
- Respiratory compensation in primary metabolic alkalosis
  - **Response to metabolic alkalosis requires respiratory acidosis; response therefore limited**
  - In general, the Pco_2 rises 0.5 to 1 mm Hg for every 1 unit increase in serum HCO_3^- from a baseline of 24 mmol/L
  - The maximum Pco_2 in compensation is 55 to 60 mm Hg

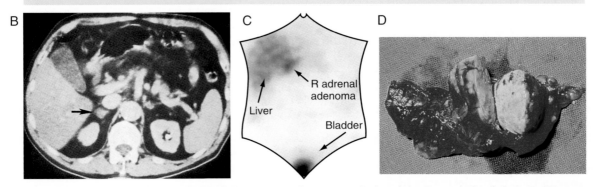

A 35-year-old male

- Mild polyuria
- Blood pressure 188/104 mm Hg

Plasma biochemistry
- Na 144 mmol/L (132–144)
- K 3.1 mmol/L (3.3–4.7)
- HCO_3^- 29 mmol/L (21–27)

Lying at 0900 hr
- Renin activity <0.5 (0.4–1.5)
- Aldosterone 850 pmol/L (30–440)

Standing at 1200 hr
- Renin activity <0.5 (1–2.5)
- Aldosterone 750 pmol/L (110–860)

FIGURE 32-3 Conn's adenoma causing metabolic alkalosis. **A,** Note hypernatremic, hypokalemic metabolic alkalosis. **B,** CT appearance of right adrenal adenoma. **C,** Unilateral uptake of radiolabeled cholesterol in right adrenal gland. **D,** Pathologic specimen following surgical excision. (From Haslett C, Chilvers ER, Boon NA, et al: *Davidson's principles and practice of medicine,* ed 19, New York, Churchill Livingstone, 2002, figure 16.19.)

BOX 32-3 *Differential Diagnosis of Metabolic Alkalosis*

Causes of a saline-responsive alkalosis (urine chloride < 10 mEq/L)
1. NG suction
2. Vomiting
3. Diuretics
4. Posthypercapnia

Causes of a saline-resistant alkalosis (urine chloride >10 mEq/L) are further divided according to BP:
1. With elevated BP: Primary aldosteronism, Cushing's, renal artery stenosis, renal failure plus alkali administration
2. With normal BP: Hypomagnesemia, severe hypokalemia, Bartter's syndrome, $NaHCO_3$ administration, licorice ingestion (enzymatically inhibits degradation of cortisol)

BP, blood pressure; NG, nasogastric.

Respiratory Acidosis

Basic Information

- **The primary defect in respiratory acidosis is an increase in P_{CO_2}**
- Whereas the lungs can respond rapidly to a metabolic challenge, the kidneys cannot respond immediately to a challenge from the lungs
  - **Respiratory processes (both acidosis and alkalosis) have an acute compensatory phase, in which plasma buffers help maintain pH; and a chronic phase, in which the kidney participates**
  - The acute response takes minutes to hours, whereas the chronic response takes 3 to 5 days
- Prediction of pH and HCO_3^- in respiratory acidosis
  - **Acute respiratory acidosis: For every 10-mm Hg that P_{CO_2} increases, pH decreases by 0.08, and serum HCO_3^- increases by 1**
  - **Chronic respiratory acidosis: For every 10-mm Hg increase in P_{CO_2}, pH decreases by 0.03, and serum HCO_3^- increases by 3 to 4**

Differential Diagnosis

- Differential diagnosis of respiratory acidosis is shown in Box 32-4

Respiratory Alkalosis

Basic Information

- **The primary defect in respiratory alkalosis is a decrease in P_{CO_2}**
- As with respiratory acidosis, there are acute and chronic phases to respiratory alkalosis
  - **Acute respiratory alkalosis: For every 10-mm Hg decrease in P_{CO_2}, HCO_3^- decreases by 2.5**
  - **Chronic respiratory alkalosis: For every 10-mm Hg decrease in P_{CO_2}, HCO_3^- decreases by 5; maximum compensation of HCO_3^- is 15**

BOX 32-4 *Differential Diagnosis of Respiratory Acidosis*

Chest Cavity
Neurologic disorders (e.g., amyotrophic lateral sclerosis)
Muscular disorders
Kyphoscoliosis (severe)
Pleural effusion
Pneumothorax

Central
Sedation or narcotics
Respiratory center hypofunction (infection, ischemia, infarction)
Obstructive sleep apnea

Lung/Airways
Pneumonia
Pulmonary edema
Bronchospasm or laryngospasm
Chronic obstructive pulmonary disease
Mechanical obstruction (foreign body/tumor)

BOX 32-5 *Differential Diagnosis of Respiratory Alkalosis*

Systemic
Sepsis
Salicylates
Liver failure
Hyperthyroidism
Pregnancy
High-altitude residence
Hypotension

Central
Ischemia or cerebrovascular accident
Tumor
Infection
Progesterone
Anxiety
Fever

Pulmonary
Pulmonary embolus
Restrictive lung disease
Hypoxemia (e.g., pneumonia, pulmonary edema)

- Although many use the same estimates of pH change seen in respiratory acidosis (i.e., acutely for each 10-mm Hg decrease in P_{CO_2}, pH increases 0.08), the pH changes in respiratory alkalosis are less predictable
- In respiratory alkalosis the body can return the pH to normal

Differential Diagnosis

- Differential diagnosis of respiratory alkalosis is shown in Box 32-5

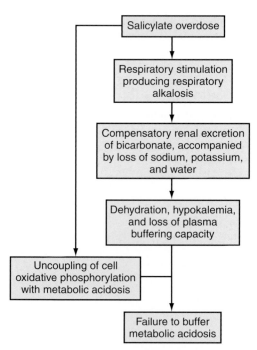

FIGURE 32-4 Salicylate overdose results in metabolic acidosis and respiratory alkalosis. (From Waller D, Renwick A: *Medical pharmacology and therapeutics,* ed 2, Philadelphia, WB Saunders, 2005, figure 53-9.)

- **Note that sepsis and salicylate toxicity result in both a metabolic acidosis and respiratory alkalosis (Fig. 32-4)**

Renal Tubular Acidosis

See Table 32-1 for the characteristics of renal tubular acidosis.

Basic Information

- The kidney contributes to maintaining the acid-base equilibrium of the serum by either resorbing or excreting acid (in the form of NH_4^+) and HCO_3^- as needed
- If the kidney does not appropriately excrete acid (NH_4^+) or resorb HCO_3^-, acidosis will develop
- Because a renal tubular defect is responsible when this acidosis occurs, these disorders are termed the renal tubular acidoses

TYPE 1 RTA

Basic Information

- **Distal renal tubular defect in NH_4^+ excretion, resulting in severe acidosis and an inability to acidify urine below a pH of 5.5, even with an acid challenge**
- Potassium conservation in most patients with type 1 RTA is typically impaired, and **hypokalemia often accompanies this disorder**
- Causes may include
  - Congenital autosomal dominant disorder (most common cause of type 1 RTA)
  - Other genetic disorders (Marfan's syndrome, Ehlers-Danlos syndrome)

TABLE 32-1	Characteristics of Renal Tubular Acidoses		
	Type 1	**Type 2**	**Type 4**
Basic defect	Distal renal tubular defect in NH_4^+ excretion	Proximal tubular defect in HCO_3^- resorption	Hyporeninemic hypoaldosteronism
Serum potassium	Low	Low	High
Able to acidify urine to pH < 5.5	No	Yes	Yes
Responds to $NaHCO_3$	Yes	No	N/A

- Autoimmune diseases (systemic lupus erythematosus, rheumatoid arthritis, Sjögren's syndrome)
- Medications such as amphotericin, lithium, and high doses of salicylates
- Urinary tract obstruction and the renal defects seen in sickle cell anemia (usually associated with hyperkalemia)

Clinical Presentation

- **Clinical manifestations include hypercalciuria and calcium oxalate stones**
  - Hyperparathyroidism and low vitamin D levels may develop, leading to rickets in children and osteomalacia in adults
  - Other clinical manifestations are related to associated diseases

Diagnosis

- **Diagnosis is made on clinical grounds and confirmed by ammonium chloride (NH_4Cl) administration, which will result in worsening systemic acidosis without drop in urine pH below 5.5**
  - Urine anion gap is also greater than 0

Treatment

- **Treatment consists of $NaHCO_3$,** which is titrated until the serum HCO_3^- and urine calcium excretion normalize

TYPE 2 RTA

Basic Information

- **A proximal renal tubular defect in HCO_3^- resorption leading to a mild acidosis**
- **Able to acidify urine below a pH of 5.5 with an acid challenge**
- Low levels of proximal tubular resorption do occur, which prevent severe acidosis
  - There is no defect in renal H^+ excretion
  - Because potassium often complexes with HCO_3^-, **hypokalemia is common with type 2 RTA**
  - Calcium resorption is also typically impaired, but not as severely as in type 1

32

- Commonly seen in conjunction with defective resorption of other molecules, such as glucose and amino acids (as seen in Fanconi's syndrome)
- Other causes: Carbonic anhydrase inhibitors, outdated tetracycline, lead and mercury toxicity

Diagnosis and Evaluation

- Diagnosis is suggested on clinical grounds
  - Administration of NH_4Cl results in normal acidification of urine because acid excretion is normal in type 2 RTA
  - **Administration of $NaHCO_3$ results in alkaline urine despite systemic acidosis because renal HCO_3^- resorption does not occur**
  - Urine anion gap is not useful in evaluation, since defect is HCO_3^- resorption, not acid excretion

Treatment

- Treatment is usually not indicated
- If necessary, can try very high doses of HCO_3^-

TYPE 4 RTA

Basic Information

- **Type 4 RTA is an acquired diffuse renal defect in NH_4^+ excretion, resulting in mild non–anion gap acidosis**
- **Able to acidify urine below a pH of 5.5 with an acid challenge**
- Mechanism in type 4 RTA is not completely understood; the majority of patients with type 4 RTA have low levels of renin and aldosterone (referred to as "hyporeninemic, hypoaldosterone" states)
- **A distinguishing feature is the coexisting inability of the kidney to excrete potassium, leading to high serum potassium (types 1 and 2 RTAs usually hypokalemic)**

- **Causes include diabetes (the most common cause),** mineralocorticoid deficiency (including Addison's disease), therapy with NSAIDs, heparin, or angiotensin-converting enzyme inhibitors

Diagnosis and Evaluation

- **Diagnosis usually made on clinical grounds**
  - Administration of NH_4Cl results in some acidification of urine because some renal acid excretion occurs; urine pH declines below 5.5
- Urine anion gap is greater than 0

Treatment

- If treatment is desired, a mineralocorticoid may be administered (e.g., fludrocortisone)
- Another option is treatment with furosemide, as long as sodium intake is adequate

REVIEW QUESTIONS

For review questions, please go to www.expertconsult.com.

SUGGESTED READINGS

Androgue HJ, Madias NE: Management of life-threatening acid-base disorders (Part 1), N Engl J Med 338:26–34, 1998.

Androgue HJ, Madias NE: Management of life-threatening acid-base disorders (Part 2), N Engl J Med 338:107–111, 1998.

Battle DC, Hizon M, Cohen E, et al: The use of the urinary anion gap in the diagnosis of hyperchloremic metabolic acidosis, N Engl J Med 318:594–599, 1988.

Narins RG, Emmett M: Simple and mixed acid-base disorders: a practical approach, Medicine 59:161–187, 1980.

Rose BD: Renal tubular acidosis. In Rose BD, editor: Clinical physiology of acid-base and electrolyte disorders, ed 3, New York, McGraw Hill, 1989.

Stewart PA: Modern quantitative acid-base chemistry, Can J Physiol Pharmacol 61:1444–1461, 1983.

Electrolyte Disorders

C. JOHN SPERATI, MD, MHS, and STEPHEN D. SISSON, MD

The maintenance of proper electrolyte concentrations is crucial to normal organ function and regulation of body volume. Alterations in the balance between electrolyte and water content may change electrolyte concentrations, osmolality, body volume status, and cellular function.

Osmolality

- Number of particles (osmoles, Osm) dissolved in solution
- Water moves between body compartments along osmolal gradients from an area of lower osmolality to an area of higher osmolality
- Only *effective* osmoles (substances that do not freely cross cell membranes) induce a water shift
  - Predominant effective osmole: Sodium
  - Ineffective osmole (does not induce fluid shift): Urea
- The body attempts to regulate osmolality *primarily* via retention or excretion of water, not osmoles (i.e., sodium, Na^+)

Sodium and Water Balance

Sodium

- As the major extracellular cation, Na^+ is the predominant solute contributing to osmolality
  - Na^+ is actively pumped from the intracellular to the extracellular space
  - Na^+ leaves the body primarily through urinary excretion, which is tightly regulated
- Serum osmolality may be estimated using the following equation:
  Serum osmolality = [2 × serum Na^+ (mEq/L)] + [BUN (mg/dL)/2.8] + [glucose (mg/dL)/18]

Aldosterone

- Mineralocorticoid produced in the zona glomerulosa of the adrenal glands
- **Major actions are to reabsorb Na^+ and to secrete potassium (K^+) and hydrogen (H^+) in the collecting duct of the kidney**
- **Aldosterone release is stimulated by:**
  - **Hyperkalemia**
  - Angiotensin-II
- The renin-angiotensin-aldosterone axis modulates Na^+ retention and excretion to regulate total body volume (and hence blood pressure)

Water

- Total body water (TBW) represents 60% of body weight in men and 50% in women
  - TBW is distributed:
    - Intracellular $^2/_3$
    - Extracellular $^1/_3$
      - Interstitial $^3/_4$ of extracellular
      - Intravascular ¼ of extracellular
- Water losses occur via the kidney, GI tract, skin, and respiratory tract
  - Renal water excretion is tightly regulated via concentration or dilution of urine
  - 500 to 1000 mL per day lost through skin and respiratory tract ("insensible losses")
- Thirst is an essential mechanism for preventing and correcting a water deficit
  - Stimulated by hypovolemia and an elevated serum osmolality

Antidiuretic Hormone (ADH, vasopressin)

- ADH is the principal hormone regulating osmolality
  - ADH increases water reabsorption from the collecting duct lumen back into the circulation
    - ADH present: concentrated urine; smaller urine volume
    - ADH absent: dilute urine; larger urine volume
- ADH release from the posterior pituitary is stimulated by:
  - Increases in plasma osmolality as small as 1%
  - Pain, nausea, multiple medications
  - Greater than or equal to 10% decrease in effective circulating volume
- See Fig. 33-1

HYPONATREMIA

Basic Information

- Serum Na^+ concentration less than 135 mEq/L
- Most common electrolyte disturbance in hospitalized patients
- **Can occur with low, normal, or high total body Na^+; hyponatremia requires the presence of too much water relative to the quantity of total body Na^+**

Clinical Presentation

- Not all hyponatremia is symptomatic (see later information on iso-osmolar hyponatremia)
- Signs and symptoms are due to swelling of the central nervous system (CNS)

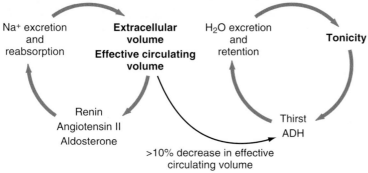

FIGURE 33-1 Regulation of body fluid compartments and osmolality. The renin-angiotensin-aldosterone pathway regulates body volume, while antidiuretic hormone (ADH) regulates osmolality via excretion/retention of water. A greater than 10% decrease in effective circulating volume will stimulate a nonosmotic release of ADH.

- As serum osmolality falls, water shifts intracellularly to an area of higher osmolality until an osmolal gradient no longer exists
- Signs and symptoms: See Table 33-1

Diagnosis and Evaluation

- Figure 33-2 shows an algorithm for the differential diagnosis of hyponatremia
- Determine osmolality
  - Normal
    - Pseudohyponatremia: Hyperlipidemia and hyperproteinemia can cause an artifactual decrease in serum Na^+
      - Asymptomatic; exclude before pursuing evaluation of hyponatremia
  - High
    - Osmotically active particles may pull water into the extracellular space, creating a dilutional hyponatremia
      - Examples: Glucose, mannitol, maltose
      - For every 100 mg/dL increase in glucose above 100, serum Na^+ decreases around 1.6 to 2.4 mEq/L
- Determine volume status
  - Findings suggestive of hypovolemia
    - Hypotension, tachycardia, dry mucous membranes, skin tenting, absence of edema
  - Findings suggestive of hypervolemia
    - Edema, elevated jugular venous pressure, rales, S_3, pulmonary edema
  - Evaluate urine indices
    - Can be seen in hypovolemia or hypervolemia (congestive heart failure, cirrhosis)
      - Urine Na^+ less than 10 mEq/L
      - Fractional excretion of sodium (Fe_{Na}) less than 1%: [(Urine Na^+ × serum creatinine)/(Serum Na^+ × urine creatinine)] × 100
      - Urine osmolality greater than serum osmolality
    - Suggestive of euvolemia or recent diuretic use
      - Urine Na^+ greater than 20 mEq/L
- Special consideration: Syndrome of inappropriate antidiuresis (SIAD)
  - Must exclude known stimuli of ADH release before labeling *idiopathic*
  - Must be clinically euvolemic
  - Urine sodium greater than 20 mEq/L
  - Urine osmolality greater than serum osmolality
  - Causes of SIAD are listed in Box 33-1 (medications, pulmonary disease, and CNS disease are major causes)

TABLE 33-1	*Signs and Symptoms of Hyponatremia*	
Mild	**Moderate**	**Severe**
[Na⁺] = 125–135 mEq/L	[Na⁺] = 120–125 mEq/L	[Na⁺] < 120 mEq/L
Anorexia	Agitation	Seizures
Apathy	Disorientation	Coma
Restlessness	Headache	Areflexia
Nausea		Cheyne-Stokes respirations
Lethargy		Incontinence
Muscle cramps		Death

Treatment

- Treat underlying cause
  - Hypovolemic hypo-osmolar: Isotonic saline
  - Hypervolemic hypo-osmolar: Fluid restriction, diuresis, dialysis
  - Euvolemic hypo-osmolar: Fluid restriction, consider use of V_2 receptor antagonists
- V_2 receptor antagonists ("vaptans")
  - Block the V_2 ADH receptor in collecting duct
  - Example: Conivaptan (delivered intravenously)
  - Only for use in euvolemic (SIAD) and potentially hypervolemic disorders
  - Results in aquaresis without significant natriuresis
  - Hyponatremia will reoccur with discontinuation of drug if underlying cause not addressed
  - Demeclocycline is an older therapy to antagonize ADH action that is rarely used
- Severe CNS symptoms (e.g., seizure, obtundation)
  - Raise Na^+ concentration 1 to 2 mEq/L/hour with 3% saline until symptoms abate
- Rate of correction is usually proportional to rate at which hyponatremia developed
  - Chronic hyponatremia (>24–48 hours): Raise Na^+ concentration 0.5 to 1 mEq/L/hour and no more than 8 to 10 mEq/L in 24 hours
  - Acute hyponatremia (<24–36 hours): Can raise 1 to 2 mEq/L/hour usually without the need for 3% saline unless severe CNS symptoms are present
  - Rapid correction can result in prompt cerebral dehydration and irreversible osmotic demyelination of the CNS (i.e., central pontine myelinolysis, Fig. 33-3)

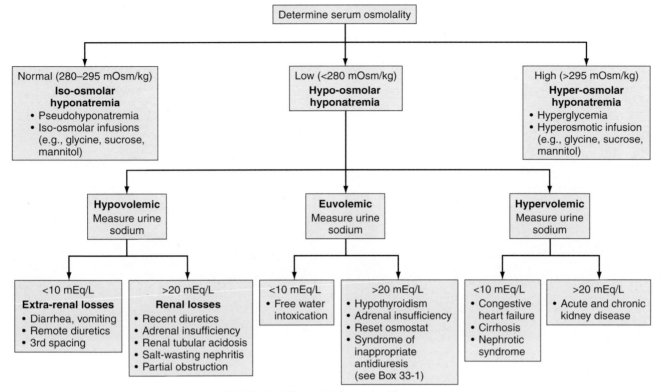

FIGURE 33-2 Differential diagnosis of hyponatremia.

BOX 33-1	*Causes of Syndrome of Inappropriate Antidiuresis*

Idiopathic

Pulmonary disease

Ectopic ADH production (e.g., small-cell carcinoma of lung)

Infections: Meningitis, encephalitis, abscess, VZV

Vascular: Subarachnoid hemorrhage, CVA, temporal arteritis

Severe nausea/vomiting

Drugs: SSRI, narcotics, cyclophosphamide, chlorpropamide

Ecstasy ingestion (aggravated by copious fluid intake)

HIV

Prolactinoma

Waldenström's macroglobulinemia

Shy-Drager syndrome

Delirium tremens

Oxytocin

Marathon runner

ADH, antidiuretic hormone; CVA, cerebrovascular accident; SSRI, selective serotonin reuptake inhibitor; VZV, varicella-zoster virus.

HYPERNATREMIA

Overview

- Serum Na^+ concentration greater than 145 mEq/L
- **Thirst is the major defense against the development of hypernatremia**
  - Usually requires impaired access to water
  - If free access to water is present, consider impaired thirst mechanism
- Most cases occur in hospitalized patients
  - Classic outpatient presentation: Elderly female nursing home resident with underlying infection

Clinical Presentation

- Signs and symptoms are due to dehydration of the CNS
  - As serum osmolality rises, water flows from inside cells of the CNS into the extracellular space along the osmolal gradient
- **Patients may experience restlessness, irritability, lethargy, muscle twitching, hyper-reflexia, spasticity, and in severe cases, intracranial hemorrhage**

Diagnosis and Evaluation

- Differential diagnosis of hypernatremia shown in Figure 33-4
- Special consideration: Diabetes insipidus (DI)
  - Insufficient ADH action leads to polyuria and free water loss
    - Central: Lack of pituitary ADH production
    - Nephrogenic: Renal resistance to ADH action
  - High normal to high serum Na^+ concentration with low urine osmolality (<300 mOsm/kg)
  - Differential diagnosis—Rule out polyuria due to:
    - Primary polydipsia
    - Diuretics
    - Osmotic diuresis (e.g., hyperglycemia)
  - Major causes of DI include pituitary tumor or apoplexy, lithium, hypercalcemia, hyperkalemia, and pregnancy

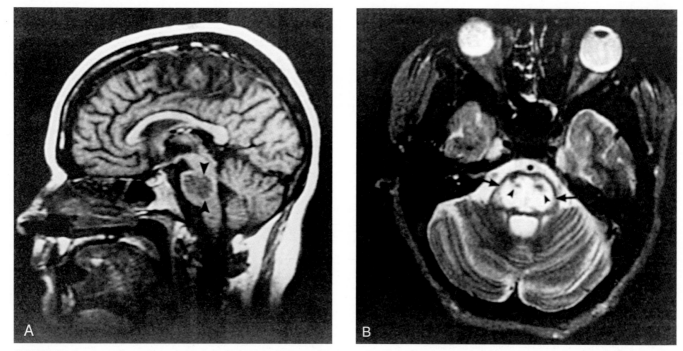

FIGURE 33-3 Central pontine myelinolysis (*arrowheads*, **A**; *arrows*, **B**) in a patient who presents with serum sodium of 99 mmol/L corrected to 125 mmol/L in 24 hours. (From Goetz CG: *Textbook of clinical neurology*, ed 2, Philadelphia, WB Saunders 2003. In Hart BL, Eaton RP: Images in clinical medicine—osmotic myelinolysis, *N Engl J Med* 333:1259, 1995.)

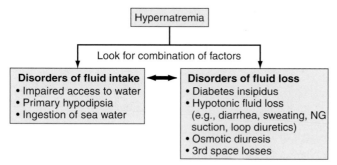

FIGURE 33-4 Differential diagnosis of hypernatremia. NG, nasogastric.

Treatment

- Address underlying cause
- **Overly rapid correction can result in cerebral edema**
- If evidence of circulatory collapse, first correct hypovolemia with isotonic saline
- To calculate free water deficit:

$$\text{Free water deficit} = \text{TBW} \times [(\text{Serum sodium concentration}/140) - 1]$$

- Decrease serum Na⁺ concentration approximately 0.5 mEq/L/hour and no more than 8 to 10 mEq/L in 24 hours

Potassium Disorders

POTASSIUM BALANCE

- K⁺ is the major intracellular cation
  - Intracellular K⁺ is maintained at a high concentration by the 3Na-2K-ATPase pump
- 95% to 98% of total body K⁺ is stored intracellularly
- 80% of K⁺ excretion occurs via the kidney, with the remainder in the stool and sweat
  - Renal K⁺ excretion increased by aldosterone
  - Increased Na⁺ delivery to the distal nephron increases K⁺ excretion
- Disorders of K⁺ concentration occur via:
  - Gain or loss in total body K⁺ stores
  - Shifts between intracellular and extracellular compartments
- Changes in the electrical potential of cellular membranes lead to the major signs and symptoms

HYPOKALEMIA

Basic Information

- Serum K⁺ concentration less than 3.5 mEq/L
- In the absence of intracellular shifting, **hypokalemia implies low total body K⁺**
- Most commonly results when K⁺ losses exceed intake
  - More rarely may result simply from inadequate daily intake

Clinical Presentation

- May result in fatigue progressing to muscle weakness and arrhythmia, followed by tetany or rhabdomyolysis at K⁺ less than 2.5 mEq/L and then paralysis when less than 2 mEq/L
- Cardiac conduction is affected, resulting in T wave flattening, the development of U waves, and arrhythmias (e.g., atrial tachycardia, atrioventricular dissociation, ventricular tachycardia, and ventricular fibrillation; Fig. 33-5)
  - Risk of arrhythmia is increased in the presence of high concentrations of digoxin

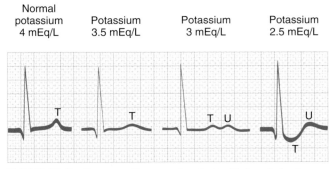

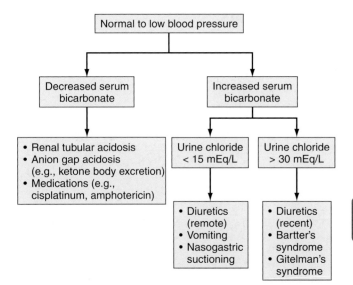

FIGURE 33-5 Electrocardiogram of patient with hypokalemia. Note flattening of T waves and prominent U waves. (From Goldberger AL: *Clinical electrocardiography: a simplified approach,* ed 6, St. Louis, Mosby, 1998.)

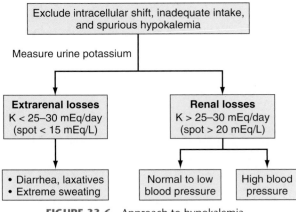

FIGURE 33-6 Approach to hypokalemia.

- Hypokalemia may increase the risk of osmotic demyelination when correcting hyponatremia
  - If neurologically stable, correct hypokalemia before correcting hyponatremia

Diagnosis and Evaluation

- Differential diagnosis of hypokalemia is shown in Figures 33-6 to 33-8
- Evaluate for spurious hypokalemia, intracellular shift, and inadequate intake
  - Spurious hypokalemia due to increased uptake after venipuncture when leukocytosis greater than 100,000 cells/mm³ is present
  - Intracellular shift due to insulin, β₂-receptor stimulation, or alkalosis
- Renal K⁺ wasting
  - Urine K⁺ concentration greater than 25 to 30 mEq/day or spot greater than 20 mEq/L
- Extra-renal K⁺ wasting
  - Urine K⁺ concentration less than 25 to 30 mEq/day or spot less than 15 mEq/L

Treatment

- Investigate and treat underlying cause
- Nature of treatment determined by degree of hypokalemia and presence or absence of symptoms

FIGURE 33-7 Renal potassium loss with normal to low blood pressure.

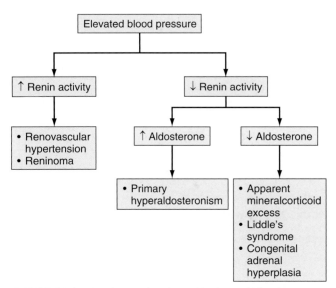

FIGURE 33-8 Renal potassium loss with elevated blood pressure.

- Patients at increased risk of arrhythmia (e.g., digoxin therapy, coronary artery disease) merit more aggressive treatment
- In patients with total body depletion, serum K⁺ concentration of 3 mEq/L represents loss of approximately 200 to 300 mEq of K⁺
  - K⁺ concentration 3 to 3.5 mEq/L: Prevent further K⁺ loss and consider oral repletion
  - K⁺ concentration less than 3 mEq/L: Intravenous K⁺ repletion with cardiac monitoring should be considered
- Hypomagnesemia and hypocalcemia may render correction of hypokalemia more difficult
- In patients with impaired renal function, intravenous K⁺ repletion can lead to unpredictable serum concentrations and should be employed with caution

HYPERKALEMIA

Basic Information

- Serum K^+ concentration greater than 5.5 mEq/L
- Rarely caused by excess intake alone, as normally functioning kidneys have a substantial excretory capacity

Clinical Presentation

- Mild elevations (5.5–6 mEq/L): Usually asymptomatic
- Greater than 6.5 mEq/L: Progressive weakness, muscle aches, areflexia, paresthesias, electrocardiogram (ECG) changes
- Greater than 7 mEq/L: Paralysis, respiratory failure, life-threatening arrhythmias
- ECG changes are not a sensitive marker for presence or severity of hyperkalemia (Fig. 33-9)
  - 6 to 7 mEq/L: Peaked T waves (height > 5 mm)
  - 7 to 8 mEq/L: Widening of QRS complex, prolonged PR interval with flattening of P wave
- Greater than 8 mEq/L: Atrial standstill, progressive QRS widening and fusion with T wave to form sine wave pattern, ventricular tachycardia and fibrillation

Diagnosis and Evaluation

- Differential diagnosis of hyperkalemia is shown in Figure 33-10
- Evaluate for extracellular shift and pseudohyperkalemia
  - Pseudohyperkalemia may occur with:
    - Hemolysis during venipuncture
    - Leukocytosis greater than 100,000 cells/mm³ or thrombocytosis greater than 500,000 cells/mm³. Plasma K^+ should be normal
    - Familial pseudohyperkalemia (autosomal dominant)
- Evaluate for mechanisms of impaired renal excretion
  - Calculate transtubular potassium gradient (TTKG)
    - TTKG = (Urine K/Plasma K)/(Urine Osm/ Plasma Osm)

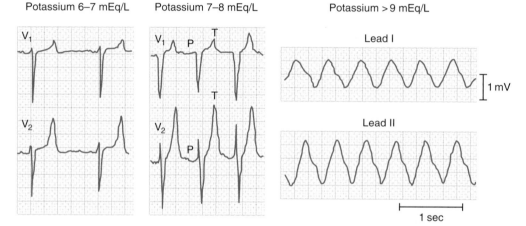

FIGURE 33-9 Electrocardiogram changes in hyperkalemia. The first panel demonstrates peaked T waves, which worsen as the P waves begin to disappear in the second panel. A sine wave configuration is shown in panel 3, as seen in a patient with severe hyperkalemia. (From Goldberger AL: *Clinical electrocardiography: a simplified approach,* ed 6, St. Louis, Mosby, 1998.)

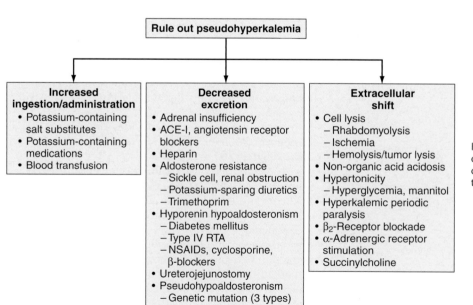

FIGURE 33-10 Differential diagnosis of hyperkalemia. ACE-I, angiotensin-converting enzyme inhibitor; RTA, renal tubular acidosis.

- Value less than 5 suggests hypoaldosteronism or K⁺ secretory defect

Treatment

- For K⁺ greater than 6.5 mEq/L or in the presence of ECG changes, administer IV calcium to decrease myocardial excitability
- **Decrease the intake of K⁺**
  - Examine medications and dietary factors high in K⁺
  - Avoid medications that inhibit K⁺ excretion
- Shift K⁺ intracellularly
  - Correct hyperglycemia, if present
  - 10 units of regular insulin administered intravenously with an ampule of 50% dextrose in water ($D_{50}W$) to prevent hypoglycemia
  - Consider IV bicarbonate, although effectiveness is marginal
- Increase K⁺ elimination from the body

- Oral or rectal administration of a K⁺ exchange resin, sodium polystyrene sulfonate (SPS); SPS is ineffective in patients with prior colectomy
- Loop diuretics may be of utility in a stable patient with mild hyperkalemia
- Dialysis if severe and life-threatening

REVIEW QUESTIONS

For review questions, please go to www.expertconsult.com.

SUGGESTED READINGS

Androgue HJ, Madias NE: Hypernatremia, *N Engl J Med* 342:1493–1499 and 1581–1589, 2000.

Ellison DH, Berl T: The syndrome of inappropriate antidiuresis, *N Engl J Med* 356:2064–2072, 2007.

Fried LF, Palevsky PM: Hyponatremia and hypernatremia, *Med Clin North Am* 81:585–609, 1997.

Mandal AK: Hypokalemia and hyperkalemia, *Med Clin North Am* 81: 611–639, 1997.

Soupart A, Decaux G: Therapeutic recommendations for management of severe hyponatremia: current concepts on pathogenesis and prevention of neurologic complications, *Clin Nephrol* 46:149–169, 1996.

Sumit K, Thomas B: Sodium, *Lancet* 352:220–228, 1998.

33

Acute Renal Failure

HYUNG M. LIM, MD

Acute renal failure (ARF), or acute kidney injury (AKI), may result from a wide array of renal insults in both hospitalized patients and outpatients. A systematic approach that includes a detailed history, focused physical examination, and supporting laboratory or radiologic evaluation is needed to determine the diagnosis. Supportive care, specifically dialysis, may be needed until renal function returns.

Basic Information

- Definition: AKI is deterioration in renal function manifested by an acute rise in serum creatinine (Cr) and blood urea nitrogen (BUN) caused by the inability to clear water, electrolytes, and nitrogenous wastes, occurring over hours to days
    - **Doubling of serum Cr indicates approximately 50% reduction in renal function**
    - ARF results in altered urine output, classified as either **oliguric (<400 mL/day) or nonoliguric (>400 mL/day)**
- RIFLE (risk, injury, failure, loss, and ESRD [end-stage renal disease]) criteria
    - Risk: 1.5× increase in the serum Cr or glomerular filtration rate (GFR) decrease by 25% or urine output less than 0.5 mL/kg/hour for 6 hours
- Injury: 2× increase in the serum Cr or GFR decrease by 50% or urine output less than 0.5 mL/kg/hour for 12 hours
- Failure: 3× increase in the serum Cr or GFR decrease by 75% or urine output less than 0.3 mL/kg/hour for 24 hours, or anuria for 12 hours
- Loss: Persistent ARF = complete loss of renal function for more than 4 weeks
- ESRD: ARF more than 3 months
- AKIN (Acute Kidney Injury Network)—modified RIFLE criteria
    - Abrupt absolute increase in serum Cr of 0.3 mg/dL from baseline
    - Serum Cr concentration increase of 50%
    - Oliguria of less than 0.5 mL/kg/hour for more than 6 hours
- Categories of ARF (Fig. 34-1)
    - **Prerenal:** Reduction in effective circulating volume and renal perfusion or bilateral renal artery occlusion
    - **Intrarenal:** Vascular, glomerular, or tubular injuries
    - **Postrenal:** Obstruction of urinary tract or bilateral renal veins
- General approach to the evaluation of the patient with ARF (Fig. 34-2)
- General principles for treatment of ARF

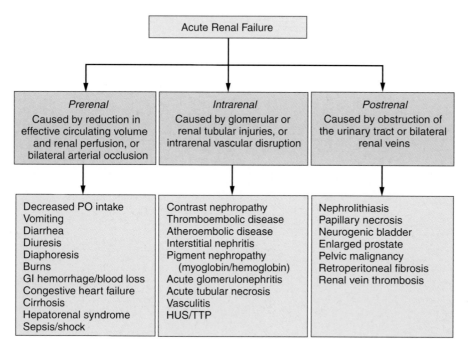

FIGURE 34-1 Differential diagnosis of acute renal failure. HUS/TTP, hemolytic uremic syndrome/thrombotic thrombocytopenic purpura.

History	Ask about existing and new medications, toxin exposure, volume depletion, invasive tests, and hypotensive episodes

↓

Physical exam	Check BP/pulse (with orthostatics), look for skin tenting or edema, palpate for full bladder, check skin for palpable purpura or rash, check fundi and skin for evidence of thromboemboli

↓

Urinalysis	Presence of protein and RBC casts suggests glomerulonephritis; WBCs or WBC casts suggest infection or interstitial nephritis; hyaline casts suggest acute tubular necrosis; granular casts suggest ATN, ischemia, or nephrotoxin

↓

Other labs	Serum: electrolytes, uric acid, LFTs, CPK, CBC, toxicology screen Urine: sodium, FE_{Na}* (eosinophils)

↓

Imaging studies	Renal ultrasound, CT scan, IVP, MRI/MRA,† furosemide renogram

↓

When to biopsy	H&P, labs, and imaging have ruled out prerenal and postrenal causes. Intrarenal cause due to primary renal disease felt to be likely. Biopsy also if glomerulonephritis is suspected.

FIGURE 34-2 Initial evaluation of the patient with acute renal failure. *$FE_{Na} = U_{Na}/P_{Na} \times P_{Cr}/U_{Cr} \times 100\%$. †Gadolinium contraindicated in moderate to severe renal failure due to risk of nephrogenic systemic fibrosis. ATN, acute tubular necrosis; CPK, creatine phosphokinase; FE_{Na}, fractional excretion of sodium; H&P, history and physical examination; IVP, intravenous pyelogram; LFTs, liver function tests; MRI/MRA, magnetic resonance imaging/ magnetic resonance angiography; P_{Cr}, plasma creatinine; P_{Na}, plasma sodium; U_{Cr}, urine creatinine; U_{Na}, urine sodium.

TABLE 34-1	*Indications for Dialysis*

Indication	Findings
Volume overload	Congestive heart failure Uncontrolled hypertension Massive edema
Severe metabolic acidosis	Hyperventilation Hyperkalemia
Hyperkalemia	Cardiac arrhythmias
Uremia	Pericarditis; stupor; seizures; asterixis; platelet dysfunction
Drug toxicity (e.g., lithium, digoxin)	Specific to drug

- **Correct any reversible causes**
- Assess potassium, acid-base status, fluid status, toxin accumulation, and need for dialysis (Table 34-1)
- **Adjust dosage of renally cleared medications**
- Fluid challenge if appropriate
- Discontinue all nephrotoxic drugs
- Avoid angiotensin-converting enzyme inhibitors, angiotensin receptor blockers, and NSAIDs

Prerenal Causes of Acute Renal Failure

Basic Information

- ARF that is caused by reduction of effective circulating volume or decreased renal blood flow
- **Prerenal causes are the second most common general cause of ARF in the hospital setting (most common is acute tubular necrosis)**
- Patients can present with severe oliguric renal failure
- Once the effective circulating volume has been restored, renal recovery is the general rule

Clinical Presentation

- **True volume depletion**
  - Lack of oral intake or vomiting
  - GI loss: Bleeding or diarrhea
  - Renal loss: Diuretics, hyperglycemia, salt-wasting nephropathy, diabetes insipidus
  - Skin loss: Sweats or burns
- **Reduction in effective circulating volume**
  - Congestive heart failure
  - Cirrhosis
  - Sepsis and shock
  - **Hepatorenal syndrome: A poorly understood, relentless worsening of renal function in the patient with advanced liver disease, with no other apparent cause (a diagnosis of exclusion)**
    - Pathophysiology includes dilation of the splanchnic bed vasculature, which pools blood and results in a fall in the systemic vascular resistance and blood pressure, with reduced renal perfusion
    - The renin-angiotensin and sympathetic nervous systems are activated, and vasopressin is released, resulting in renal artery vasoconstriction

Diagnosis

- **BUN/Cr ratio greater than 20:1** because of increased water and urea reabsorption
- Low urine sodium concentration (**usually <20mEq/L**)
- **Low urine fractional excretion of sodium (FE_{Na} < 1%; Table 34-2)**
- Urine osmolality greater than 500 mOsm/kg
- Urine Cr/Plasma Cr ratio greater than 40

TABLE 34-2	*Use of Fractional Excretion of Sodium (FE_{Na}) in ARF*

Causes of ARF	FE_{Na}* (%)
Prerenal causes of ARF because of hypovolemia	<1
Prerenal causes of ARF because of decreased effective circulating volume	<1
Acute tubular necrosis, from any cause	>2
Hepatorenal syndrome	<1

*$FE_{Na} = U_{Na}/P_{Na} \times P_{Cr}/U_{Cr} \times 100\%$.
ARF, acute renal failure; P_{Cr}, plasma creatinine; P_{Na}, plasma sodium; U_{Cr}, urine creatinine; U_{Na}, urine sodium.

34

Treatment

- Volume depletion: **Vigorous IV fluid resuscitation typically improves renal function and urine output within 24 to 48 hours**
- Reduced effective volume: Treatment of the underlying disease process; **maximize cardiac output**
- **Hepatorenal syndrome is best treated by liver transplantation.** Dialysis may be needed in the interim.
  - Peritoneovenous shunt or transjugular intrahepatic portosystemic shunt (TIPS) may prolong renal function but can cause worsening of encephalopathy of liver disease
  - **Omnipressin (an antidiuretic hormone analogue that constricts the splanchnic bed) may be administered with IV albumin, which may improve renal function but can cause ischemia**
  - Midodrine (systemic vasoconstrictor) and octreotide (blocks vasodilator release) may be of some benefit

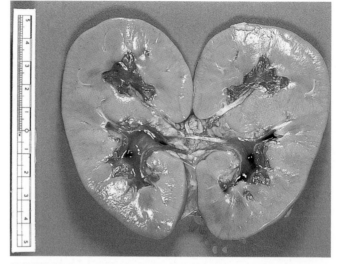

FIGURE 34-3 Acute tubular necrosis. In acute tubular necrosis, kidneys are swollen and pale, particularly in the renal cortex. (From Stevens A, Lowe J: *Pathology*, ed 2, St. Louis, Mosby, 2000, figure 17.23.)

Intrarenal Causes of Acute Renal Failure

Table 34-3 lists the intrarenal causes of ARF. Acute glomerulonephritis and vasculitis are covered in Chapter 35.

Acute Tubular Necrosis

See Figure 34-3 for an illustration of acute tubular necrosis.

Basic Information

- **The most common cause of ARF in the hospital setting**
  - Results from ischemic (i.e., prerenal) or nephrotoxic (i.e., intrarenal) injury to renal tubules
  - Damaged tubular cells accumulate in tubular lumen, resulting in occlusion
    - Injury commonly most severe in early proximal tubule and medullary segment

Clinical Presentation

- Appropriate clinical setting, such as ischemic event or exposure to nephrotoxin, precedes deterioration in renal function
- **Clinical course typically progresses, then resolves over 1 to 3 weeks**

Diagnosis

- **BUN/Cr ratio is normal,** usually less than 20:1
- Urinalysis shows **muddy brown granular casts and epithelial cell casts**
- **High urine sodium concentration (usually >40 mEq/L)** is caused by tubular injury and decreased sodium reabsorption
- High urine fractional excretion of sodium **(FE_{Na} > 2%; see Table 34-2)**
- Urine osmolality less than 450 mOsm/kg

TABLE 34-3	*Intrarenal Causes of ARF*	
Disorder	**Suggestive Features**	**Treatment**
Contrast nephropathy	Appropriate clinical setting, such as recent (<72 hr) contrast radiography	Prevention; supportive measures until recovery of renal function
Interstitial nephritis	Fever; skin rash; WBC casts in urine; eosinophilia and eosinophiluria	Discontinue offending drug; prednisone
Acute glomerulonephritis	Hypertension; fluid retention; hematuria; proteinuria	Differs based on underlying cause of glomerulonephritis
Acute tubular necrosis	Recent hypotensive event; recent exposure to nephrotoxin	Supportive care until renal function returns
Pigment nephropathy	High serum CPK (typically >10,000 IU/L); pigmented casts, hemoglobinuria, but no RBCs in urine	IV hydration; alkalinize urine to pH > 6.5
Renal artery atheroembolic disease	Low serum complement; eosinophilia; eosinophiluria; cholesterol crystals on renal or skin biopsy	Supportive measures, but prognosis poor
Renal artery thromboembolic disease	Flank pain, hematuria, elevated LDH	Supportive measures, anticoagulation

ARF, acute renal failure; CPK, creatine phosphokinase; LDH, lactate dehydrogenase.

- **Urine Cr/Plasma Cr ratio less than 20:1** (measure of tubular water reabsorption)

Treatment

- **Supportive care** until renal function returns
- Avoid nephrotoxins

Interstitial Nephritis

Basic Information

- Results from the infiltration of the interstitial space by inflammatory cells (mostly T cells and monocytes; Fig. 34-4)
- Process **initiated by reaction to medication**
  - **β-Lactam antibiotics and cephalosporins** are the most common
  - **NSAIDs** are associated with
    - Either pure interstitial disease or additional glomerular disease **(minimal change disease or membranous glomerulonephritis)**
    - NSAIDs can also cause **acute ischemic renal injury (hemodynamic change), analgesic nephropathy, or papillary necrosis**
    - **Urine sediment may not contain significant eosinophils**
  - **Rifampin** is associated with acute tubulointerstitial disease even with intermittent dosing or after discontinuation of the drug
  - **Sulfonamides** can cause vasculitis

Clinical Presentation

- Acute worsening of renal function after starting a new medication
- **Fever and skin rash are also common**

Diagnosis

- Diagnosis is made based on clinical presentation or renal biopsy and is supported by
  - **Hematuria, pyuria, and WBC casts in urine**
  - **Eosinophilia and eosinophiluria are seen in more than 75% of cases**
  - Mild proteinuria also seen

Treatment

- Discontinuation of offending agent(s)
- **Corticosteroids: Prednisone 1 mg/kg/day**

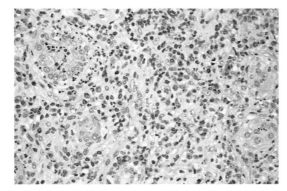

FIGURE 34-4 Drug-induced interstitial nephritis, with prominent eosinophilic and mononuclear cell infiltrate. (From Kumar V, Fausto N, Abbas A: *Robbins and Cotran: pathologic basis of disease,* ed 7, Philadelphia, Saunders, 2005, figure 20-44.)

Contrast-Induced Nephropathy

Basic Information

- **Caused by renal vasoconstriction** from the release of endothelin and adenosine as well as from the high osmolality of the contrast material
- **Also caused by direct tubular injury** by the contrast agent
- Those at greatest risk include those with
  - Underlying renal insufficiency with **plasma Cr greater than 1.5 mg/dL**
  - **Diabetic nephropathy** with renal insufficiency
  - Poor renal perfusion: **Heart failure, dehydration, or liver failure**
  - **Multiple myeloma**
  - High doses of contrast agent
- **Magnetic resonance gadolinium contrast media may also be associated with nephrotoxicity in high concentrations**
  - Use of gadolinium in the setting of advanced renal failure has been associated with nephrogenic systemic fibrosis

Clinical Presentation

- Acute rise of serum BUN/Cr occurs within 24 to 48 hours of IV contrast exposure
- **Cr peaks within 7 days and usually returns to baseline within 10 days**
- Renal failure is usually reversible

Diagnosis

- Clinical diagnosis based on **history of exposure in appropriate time period**
- Imaging of the kidneys, ureter, and bladder reveals enhanced outline of kidneys secondary to retained IV contrast

Treatment

- No specific therapy; supportive measures only
- Maintain renal perfusion with IV hydration, but with risk of volume overload
- Avoid repeated contrast exposure
- **Best treatment is prevention**
  - **IV hydration with normal saline** 1 mL/kg/hour, 12 hours before and after administration of IV contrast agent
  - **Sodium bicarbonate** hydration may also be of benefit before IV contrast
  - N-Acetyl cysteine (Mucomyst) 600 to 1200 mg PO twice a day for 2 days, starting 1 day before IV contrast exposure
  - **Minimize** IV contrast volume
  - Use **nonionic contrast or dilute contrast media**
  - Prophylactic dialysis to remove contrast has no proven benefit

Renal Artery Embolic Disease

Basic Information

- ARF results from cholesterol emboli, which lodge in medium or small renal arteries
- Inflammatory reaction causes **intimal proliferation, fibrosis, and irreversible blockages**

34

Clinical Presentation

- Two common presentations, caused by either thromboembolic or atheroembolic event
  - **Thromboembolic: Occurs after myocardial infarction or with atrial arrhythmias,** resulting in complete arterial obstruction and renal infarction
    - Individual notes flank pain, hematuria
    - Lactate dehydrogenase is elevated
  - **Atheroembolic: Occurs spontaneously or following a catheter manipulation in aorta or surgery;** produces incomplete obstruction and renal atrophy; renal function worsens acutely and continues to progress over several weeks
    - Other physical findings include cyanosis, gangrene of toes or feet, livedo reticularis (Fig. 34-5)
    - If pancreatic or mesenteric emboli also occur, abdominal pain may result

Diagnosis

- Clinical suggestion in appropriate setting
- Laboratory findings include **eosinophilia, eosinophiluria, and hypocomplementemia**
- Cholesterol crystals may be present on renal or **skin biopsy,** or elsewhere in body (Fig. 34-6)

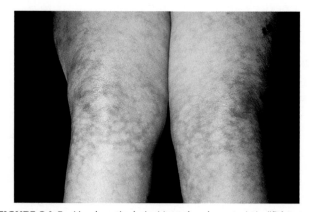

FIGURE 34-5 Livedo reticularis. Note the characteristic "fishnet stocking" pattern of the rash. (From Haslett C, Chilvers ER, Boon NA, et al: *Davidson's principles and practice of medicine,* ed 19, New York, Churchill Livingstone, 2002, figure 20.48.)

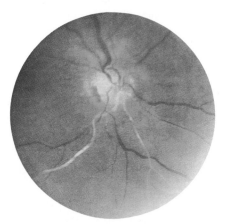

FIGURE 34-6 Cholesterol emboli noted in the funduscopic exam. (From Swash M: *Hutchinson's clinical methods,* ed 21, Philadelphia, WB Saunders, 2002, figure 12.14.)

Treatment

- Supportive care only; prognosis is poor
- Consider anticoagulation with thromboembolic disease

Pigment Nephropathy

Basic Information

- Acute renal tubular injury from **myoglobin or hemoglobin**
- Pathogenesis is **tubular cell injury from free chelatable iron** (ferrihemate), which results in intrarenal vasoconstriction
- **Obstruction of tubules** with pigment casts, which results in renal failure

Clinical Presentation

- Patient often notes dark urine ("Coca-Cola urine") because of presence of myoglobin/hemoglobin pigments in urine
- Usually **associated with traumatic muscle injuries** (extreme exercises, trauma, seizures, ischemia), **muscle** toxins (drugs, including cocaine and 3-hydroxy-methylglutaryl coenzyme A reductase inhibitors), or others (infections, electrolyte abnormalities, endocrine, inflammatory myopathies)
  - Release of intracellular electrolytes results in **hyperkalemia, hyperphosphatemia, and hyperuricemia**
  - Sequestration of fluid and calcium into injured muscles leading to **volume depletion and hypocalcemia**

Diagnosis

- ARF in appropriate clinical setting
- Associated with high serum creatine phosphokinase (CPK); **renal injury often associated with CPK greater than 10,000 IU/L**
- Hyperkalemia, hyperphosphatemia, and hypocalcemia also common and support the diagnosis
- Urinalysis reveals pigmented casts (**but no RBCs**) with myoglobin or hemoglobin in the urine

Treatment

- **Aggressive IV hydration**
- **Alkalinize urine to pH above 6.5** (2–3 ampules of bicarbonate mixed in 1 L of 5% dextrose in water) to prevent formation of ferrihemate from myoglobin or hemoglobin
- Recovery is the general rule, but dialysis may be needed until renal function returns

Postrenal Causes of Acute Renal Failure

Basic Information

- **Group of disorders resulting from the physical obstruction of the ureters (e.g., obstructing nephrolithiasis, malignancy, retroperitonal fibrosis), bladder (e.g., prostatic hypertrophy, clots, tumors), or renal veins (e.g., renal vein thrombosis, see Chapter 35; Fig. 34-7)**

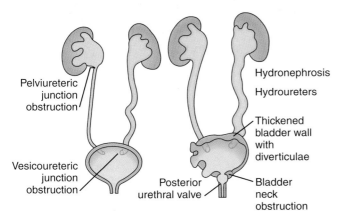

FIGURE 34-7 Postrenal causes of acute renal failure include any obstruction along the urinary outflow tract. (From Lissauer T, Clayden G: *Illustrated textbook of paediatrics,* ed 2, St. Louis, Mosby, 2001, figure 16-6a.)

Clinical Presentation

- If onset sudden, patient will note flank pain
  - **If obstruction complete, anuria results**
- **Partial obstruction may result in polyuria or oliguria**
- Physical examination may note abdominal mass from hydronephrosis, or pelvic mass from distended bladder

Diagnosis

- **Ultrasound is the test of choice to determine the presence of obstruction** because of high sensitivity (90%) and specificity (90%), low cost, and safety
- **IV pyelography is the test of choice to define the location of obstruction** and anatomy of the ureters; however, one must consider the potential toxicity of IV contrast medium and poor visualization of the kidneys with low GFR (Fig. 34-8)
- **CT is able to diagnose hydronephrosis without IV contrast** and is useful in determining extrinsic mass, hematoma, or stones
- **Nuclear medicine furosemide renogram can provide functional status of the kidneys** and avoid risk of IV contrast; however, anatomic visualization is poor

Treatment

- The most effective treatment is determined by the location of the obstruction. **Emergency relief of the obstruction is indicated if ARF or urosepsis has resulted.**
  - Obstruction distal to the bladder can be relieved by a Foley catheter or a suprapubic catheter
  - Upper urinary tract obstruction can be relieved by either a percutaneous nephrostomy tube or ureteral stent placement
- Recovery of renal function depends on the duration of the obstruction

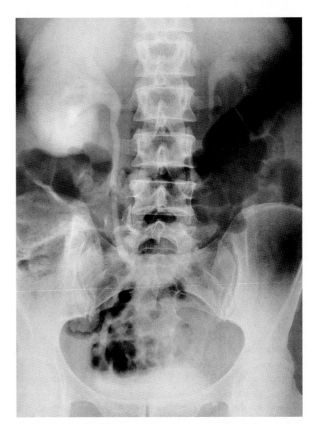

FIGURE 34-8 Unilateral urinary outflow tract obstruction. This patient has an obstructing kidney stone at the lower end of the right ureter. This image, taken 2 hours after contrast injection, demonstrates persistent contrast in the right kidney and collecting system as compared with that on the left. (From Haslett C, Chilvers ER, Boon NA, et al: *Davidson's principles and practice of medicine,* ed 19, New York, Churchill Livingstone, 2002, figure 14.38.)

- **Postobstructive diuresis: Marked polyuria with loss of water, sodium, potassium, and other electrolytes**
  - Replacement fluid should be half normal saline initially and readjusted according to serum electrolyte changes
  - Etiology of massive diuresis is volume expansion, urea accumulation, tubular damage, and accumulation of natriuretic factors
    - Prolonged fluid replacement should be avoided, as it will perpetuate postobstructive diuresis by continued replacement of sodium and water

REVIEW QUESTIONS

For review questions, please go to www.expertconsult.com.

SUGGESTED READINGS

Brenner BM, Rector FC: *The kidney,* ed 8, Philadelphia, WB Saunders, 2007.
Jacobson HR, Striker GE, Klahr S: *The principles and practices of nephrology,* Philadelphia, BC Decker, 1994.
Rose BD: Up-To-Date Online, Nephrology and Hypertension 2009.

34

CHAPTER 35

BOARD REVIEW

Glomerular Disease

Ur. loss of Ig → Immunosuppression
" loss of albumin → edema
" loss of anti-coag → thrombosis, esp in renal V.

TARIQ SHAFI, MBBS, MHS, and DEREK M. FINE, MD

Glomerular diseases include a group of disorders in which the glomerular filtration barrier is altered. The resultant change in filtration may be accompanied by proteinuria (in nephrotic disorders) or hematuria (in nephritic disorders), or both. Familiarity with the causes of nephrotic and nephritic disorders will guide the history, physical, and laboratory examination of patients presenting with abnormal urinary sediment.

Basic Information

- **Glomerular disease refers to disorders of the glomerular filtration barrier that occur either as a primary disorder or as a result of other diseases, toxins, or infections**
- **The glomerular filtration barrier may be affected so that proteinuria results; if the proteinuria is greater than 3.5 g/24 hours (nephrotic range proteinuria), a nephrotic syndrome may result**
- **If glomerular filtration barrier is affected so that hematuria results (often accompanied by proteinuria), the disorder is classified as nephritic (glomerulonephritis [GN])**
- Additional clinical features typically accompany nephrotic and nephritic disorders (see following)
- Significant overlap may exist among disorders that result in nephrotic syndrome and GN

Nephrotic Syndrome

Basic Information

- General features of nephrotic syndrome
  - **Nephrotic syndrome is defined by the presence of**
    - **Proteinuria (>3.5 g/24 hours)**
    - **Hypoalbuminemia**
    - **Hyperlipidemia**
  - Edema results from hypoalbuminemia
  - Blood pressure is variable depending on the underlying disease
    - Usually normal in minimal change disease and membranous nephropathy
    - Frequently elevated in focal segmental glomerulosclerosis (FSGS)
  - **Urinary loss of anticoagulant proteins (e.g., protein C, protein S, antithrombin III) may result in hypercoagulable state**
    - Renal vein thrombosis may occur with any cause of nephrotic syndrome but is most common with membranous GN
    - **Renal vein thrombosis often presents as sudden-onset worsening of renal insufficiency, worsening proteinuria, hematuria, or flank pain**
  - Loss of immunoglobulins may result in a relative immune-deficient state

Clinical Presentation

- Features of specific causes of nephrotic syndrome—all may be idiopathic or related to secondary causes (Table 35-1)
  - **Minimal change disease**
    - **Rapid onset; patient is normal one day and has edema the next**
    - **Glomerular filtration rate (GFR) remains normal**
      - **Massive proteinuria common (>4 g/24 hr)**
      - **Pathologic hallmark is normal-appearing glomeruli on microscopy and generalized loss of foot processes of podocytes on electron microscopy** (Fig. 35-1)
  - Focal segmental glomerulosclerosis (FSGS)
    - "Classic" FSGS common in African Americans
    - Slow onset with progressive decrease in GFR if untreated
    - Creatinine (Cr) normal, but may be elevated at presentation (elevated Cr indicates poorer prognosis)
    - Proteinuria not massive (2–4 g/24 hours)
    - Includes findings seen with hyperfiltration injury (secondary FSGS)
    - HIV-associated nephropathy (HIVAN) presents with a collapsing FSGS (vs. classic FSGS)
      - Characterized by a very rapid onset of renal failure (over months) with massive proteinuria
      - Collapsing FSGS may occasionally be seen in non-HIV-infected patients
  - **Membranous GN**
    - **The most common cause of nephrotic syndrome in adults**
    - **Slow onset with loss of GFR, usually over years**
    - Cr often normal; if Cr deteriorates rapidly, consider renal vein thrombosis
    - Proteinuria varies from subnephrotic range to massive (>20 g/24 hours)
- Secondary causes of nephrotic syndrome
  - Diabetes
    - Diabetic nephropathy is the most common cause of nephrotic proteinuria
    - Earliest evidence of diabetic nephropathy is microalbuminuria (30–300 mg albumin/24 hours), which then progresses to overt proteinuria (>300 mg/24 hours) and may progress to nephrotic-range proteinuria

TABLE 35-1	*Diagnosis of Causes of Nephrotic Syndrome*		
Cause	**Typical Age of Onset**	**Associated Diseases**	**Pathologic Findings**
Minimal change disease	<12 years or mid-60s	NSAIDs Lymphoma Bee sting	Light microscopy: Normal Immunofluorescence: Normal Electron microscopy: Diffuse podocyte foot process effacement
Focal segmental glomerulosclerosis (FSGS)	Early teens to mid-30s	Hyperfiltration (seen in morbid obesity; may result from nephron loss due to other causes) HIV (collapsing variant) Heroin nephropathy	Light microscopy: Focal and segmental glomerulosclerosis Immunofluorescence: May show nonspecific IgM deposition Electron microscopy: Foot process effacement Collapsing variant seen on light microscopy in those with HIV
Membranous glomerulonephritis	Mid-30s to mid-60s	Adenocarcinoma (breast, bowel, lung) Hepatitis B Systemic lupus erythematosus Drug reaction (NSAID)	Light microscopy: Thickened capillary loops Immunofluorescence: Deposition of immunoglobulin and complement Electron microscopy: Subepithelial immune complex deposition
Membranoproliferative glomerulonephritis	Idiopathic: 8–16 years Secondary: More common in adults	Type I: Hepatitis C Chronic hepatitis B Endocarditis Idiopathic Type II: Lipodystrophy Type III: Can be inherited	Light microscopy: Glomerular lobulation, capillary wall thickening and mesangial expansion Immunofluorescence Type I: C3, early complement components, IgG deposits Type II: ±C3, IgM Electron microscopy Type I: Subendothelial electron-dense deposits Type II: Dense "ribbon-like" deposits along basement membrane; dense-deposit disease Type III: Large lucent areas in basement membrane

IgM, immunoglobulin M.

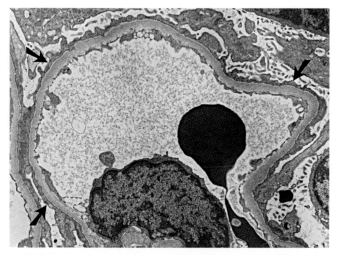

FIGURE 35-1 Electron micrograph of a glomerular capillary wall from a patient with minimal change glomerulopathy, showing extensive foot process effacement (*arrows*) and microvillous transformation (magnification ×5000). (From Brenner BM: *Brenner and Rector's the kidney,* ed 7, Philadelphia, WB Saunders, 2004, figure 28-4.)

- Once overt proteinuria has set in, renal function inevitably declines
  - Average time to end-stage renal disease after onset of proteinuria is 10 years
  - May be attenuated by angiotensin-converting enzyme (ACE) inhibitors or angiotensin receptor blockers

- Diabetic nephropathy rarely develops before 10 years' duration of diabetes
- Type 1 diabetics with nephropathy
  - 95% also have retinopathy
  - In a patient with type 1 diabetes and nephropathy, the absence of retinopathy should prompt consideration of nondiabetic etiology of proteinuria/nephropathy
- Type 2 diabetics with nephropathy
  - 50% to 75% have retinopathy
  - Nephropathy in the absence of retinopathy in a patient with type 2 diabetes is therefore more common than with type 1 diabetes, but should still prompt consideration of other causes of nephropathy
  - If retinopathy is present in patients with type 2, almost 100% have nephropathy
- **All diabetic patients with proteinuria should be evaluated for other systemic diseases (e.g., hepatitis B and C, systemic lupus erythematosus [SLE], and monoclonal gammopathy) because up to 20% have either primary or superimposed nondiabetic cause of proteinuria**
- Clinical scenarios in which to consider renal biopsy in diabetics
  - Presence of proteinuria with less than 10 years' duration of diabetes
  - Presence of significant hematuria or RBC casts on urinalysis

TABLE 35-2	*Treatment of Idiopathic Nephrotic and Nephritic Disorders*	
Disorder	**Treatment**	**Response**
Minimal change disease	Corticosteroids Cyclosporin or cyclophosphamide or mycophenolate mofetil for relapse	Children respond within 2 wk Adults respond in 4–8 wk, but often relapse
Focal segmental glomerulonephritis	Corticosteroids + ACE-I Cyclosporin or mycophenolate mofetil may be added to steroids	40–60% Response takes 4–13 mo
Membranous glomerulonephritis	ACE-I for all patients Corticosteroids added if hypertension, nephrotic-range proteinuria (>4 g/day over a period of 6 mo), or renal insufficiency (creatinine clearance < 80 mL/min) present Cytotoxic agents added if poor response	Variable, dependent on prognostic indicators One-third remit spontaneously without treatment
Membranoproliferative glomerulonephritis	Corticosteroids ± cytotoxic agents Antiplatelet agents (aspirin; dipyridamole) may slow disease progression	Spontaneous remission in <10% Prolonged course of slowly deteriorating renal function seen in many

ACE-I, angiotensin-converting enzyme inhibitor.

- Absence of retinopathy in type 1 diabetics and possibly type 2 diabetics
- Any clinical or laboratory evidence of other systemic disease
- Amyloidosis
  - Systemic disease with extracellular deposition of amyloid in various organs (see Chapter 57)
  - Most common is AL-amyloid (primary amyloidosis) with deposits of light-chain immunoglobulin
  - Secondary (AA-amyloid) associated with chronic inflammatory or infectious states
  - AL-amyloid is caused by plasma cell dyscrasia with overt multiple myeloma in 20% of cases
  - 90% have monoclonal light chains (Bence Jones proteins) in urine or blood
  - Proteinuria is the consistent feature with associated renal insufficiency
  - Nephrotic syndrome in patient older than 50 years—should have a high index of suspicion for AL-amyloid
  - Generally poor prognosis, but may respond to chemotherapy (AL amyloid: Melphalan, dexamethasone ± stem cell transplant; AA amyloid: Eprodisate)

Diagnosis

- **Serologic evaluation: Antinuclear antibody, hepatitis B surface antigen, anti-hepatitis C antibody, serum and urine protein electrophoreses, HIV antibody, complement levels**
- **Kidney biopsy needed in most patients**
  - All patients with rapidly rising Cr, biopsy is urgent
  - Diabetics with consistent time course (>10 years disease), no other systemic disease or serologic abnormalities, and presence of retinopathy may not require biopsy for diagnosis
  - Nephrotic patients with amyloid diagnosed by biopsy of other organ (e.g., heart, skin, or bone marrow) may not need kidney biopsy

Treatment

- When nephrotic syndrome is secondary to a systemic disease, treat the underlying disorder
- Additional renoprotective measures including
  - Strict blood pressure control (<130/80 mm Hg)
  - Use of ACE-inhibitors
  - Aggressive control of cardiovascular risk factors
  - Diabetes control essential in the diabetic patient
- Treatment of idiopathic causes of nephrotic syndrome is described in Table 35-2

Nephritic Disorders

Basic Information

- General features of nephritic disorders (GN)
  - **Nephritic disorders are commonly associated with systemic diseases**
  - **Patients typically present with deteriorating renal function, mild to moderate proteinuria, and an active urine sediment (RBCs and RBC casts in the urine; Fig. 35-2)**
  - Patients may report dark urine
  - Blood pressure is typically elevated; peripheral edema may be seen (which may progress to include ascites or pleural effusions)
  - Urine output may be normal or oliguric

Clinical Presentation

- Features of specific causes of GN
  - When evaluating the patient with a diagnosis of nephritis, consideration should be given to a search for a systemic, infectious, or postinfectious cause because GN is often secondary to another disorder
- Systemic diseases associated with GN
  - Frequently present with rapid-onset renal insufficiency in the setting of immune dysregulation
  - The role of complement in evaluation of GN is shown in Figure 35-3

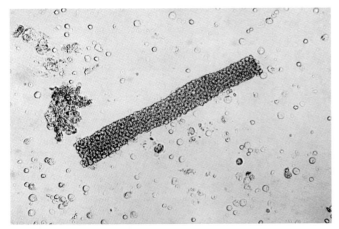

FIGURE 35-2 Red cell casts typically seen in acute glomerulonephritis. (From Noble J, Greene HL, Levinson W, et al: *Textbook of primary care medicine,* ed 3, St. Louis, Mosby, 2000, figure 144-6.)

- The role of immune serologies is shown in Figure 35-4
- Immunofluorescence (IF) of the pathologic sample is essential in defining the underlying process:
  - Immune complex GN (immune complexes seen on IF)
  - Pauci-immune GN (no immune staining, hence the term *pauci*-immune)
  - Antiglomerular basement membrane (anti-GBM) disease (linear GBM staining)
- SLE: A secondary cause of proliferative or membranous GN (see Chapter 46)
- **Henoch-Schönlein purpura (HSP)**
  - **Manifestation often includes purpuric rash (Fig. 35-5), arthralgias, abdominal pain, and renal involvement**
  - Commonly follows upper respiratory infection

- Immunoglobulin A (IgA) deposition seen in renal mesangial cells (looks exactly like IgA nephropathy)
- Uncommon in adults—more common in children; predominates in males
- Vasculitis (includes Wegener's granulomatosis, microscopic polyangiitis, and Churg-Strauss syndrome; see Chapter 45)
- **Goodpasture's syndrome**
  - Results from production of anti-GBM antibodies
  - The presence of both lung and kidney involvement with linear anti-GBM staining on immunofluorescence defines the syndrome
  - Pathology reveals "crescent formation" in glomeruli; number of crescents relates to severity and prognosis
  - If pulmonary disease is absent in the presence of anti-GBM antibodies, diagnosis of the kidney-specific anti-GBM disease is made
- Infectious diseases associated with GN
  - Endocarditis
  - Hepatitis B and C
  - Less common: Syphilis, malaria
- Postinfectious etiologies associated with GN
  - Includes poststreptococcal GN, endocarditis-related GN, various viral infections
  - With poststreptococcal GN, patients present with hypertension, oliguria, and elevated antistreptolysin O (ASO) antibody titers 7 to 14 days after throat or skin infection with group A *Streptococcus*
    - Certain streptococcal strains more likely to cause GN (types 12 and 49)
    - Presentation can be highly variable—from asymptomatic microscopic hematuria to florid nephritic syndrome
  - GN may also occur after staphylococcal and other bacterial infections

FIGURE 35-3 Role of complement levels in diagnosis of the patient with glomerulonephritis. *Refers to infection of a ventriculoatrial shunt. HUS/TTP, hemolytic uremic syndrome/thrombotic thrombocytopenic purpura. (Adapted from Madaio MP, Harrington JT: The diagnosis of acute glomerulonephritis, *N Engl J Med* 309:1299–1302, 1983.)

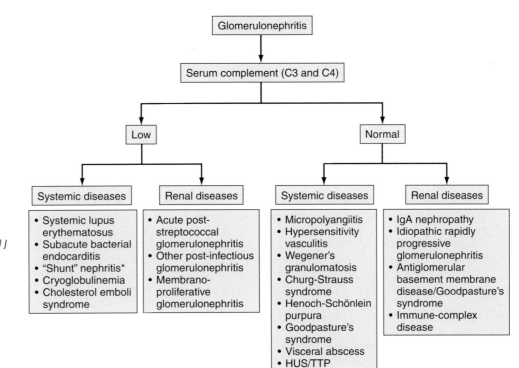

35

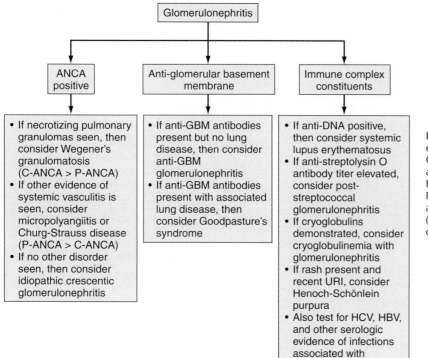

Glomerulonephritis

ANCA positive
- If necrotizing pulmonary granulomas seen, then consider Wegener's granulomatosis (C-ANCA > P-ANCA)
- If other evidence of systemic vasculitis is seen, consider micropolyangiitis or Churg-Strauss disease (P-ANCA > C-ANCA)
- If no other disorder seen, then consider idiopathic crescentic glomerulonephritis

Anti-glomerular basement membrane
- If anti-GBM antibodies present but no lung disease, then consider anti-GBM glomerulonephritis
- If anti-GBM antibodies present with associated lung disease, then consider Goodpasture's syndrome

Immune complex constituents
- If anti-DNA positive, then consider systemic lupus erythematosus
- If anti-streptolysin O antibody titer elevated, consider post-streptococcal glomerulonephritis
- If cryoglobulins demonstrated, consider cryoglobulinemia with glomerulonephritis
- If rash present and recent URI, consider Henoch-Schönlein purpura
- Also test for HCV, HBV, and other serologic evidence of infections associated with glomerulonephritis

FIGURE 35-4 Role of immune serologies in evaluation of the patient with glomerulonephritis. C-ANCA; cytoplasmic antineutrophil cytoplasmic antibody; GBM, glomerular basement membrane; HBV, hepatitis B virus; HCV, hepatitis C virus; P-ANCA, perinuclear antineutrophil cytoplasmic antibody; URI, upper respiratory infection. (Adapted from Falk RJ: ANCA-associated renal disease, *Kidney Int* 38:998–1010, 1990.)

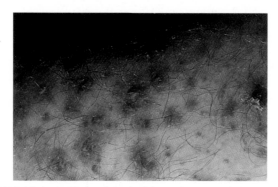

FIGURE 35-5 Typical rash (palpable purpura) on the lower extremities seen in Henoch-Schönlein purpura. (From Goldman L, Bennett JC, Ausiello D: *Cecil textbook of medicine,* ed 22, Philadelphia, WB Saunders, 2004, figure 475.4.)

- **IgA nephropathy (Berger's disease)**
  - **Most common cause of GN in adults (although rare in African Americans)**
  - **Classic presentation is gross hematuria following upper respiratory infection (majority of patients)**
  - Others present with persistent, microscopic hematuria long after viral upper respiratory infection has been forgotten; less than 10% have a nephrotic presentation
  - Mesangial IgA deposition is seen on biopsy (establishes the diagnosis)
  - In contrast to HSP, rash is not seen and course is less aggressive
- Membranoproliferative glomerulonephritis (MPGN)
  - Clinical presentation may be nephrotic, nephritic, or mixed

- **Most often secondary to hepatitis C infection (type I MPGN)**
  - Idiopathic forms of type I and type II
  - Course varies depending on presentation—from slowly progressive nephrotic syndrome similar to membranous GN to a rapidly progressive GN as is seen with the necrotizing vasculitides
  - Associated with cryoglobulins when related to hepatitis C (essential mixed cryoglobulinemia—type II cryoglobulins)

Diagnosis

- Clinical presentation and testing for specific diseases (e.g., ASO titers, hepatitis serologies) may be sufficient to diagnose likely, underlying cause of nephritic syndrome
- The evaluation and testing performed differs based on the clinical suggestion
- Immunologic testing may also help narrow differential diagnosis (see Figs. 35-1 and 35-2)
- Some diseases manifest with rapidly progressive renal failure and may mimic GN (Box 35-1)
- Renal biopsy should be performed when the following occur
  - Diagnosis/prognosis remains unclear
  - Rapidly progressive GN
  - Nephrotic-range proteinuria
  - Subnephrotic-range proteinuria (>2 g/day); use same approach as nephrotic patient
  - Presence of a systemic disease if accompanied by proteinuria or hematuria
  - Progressive renal insufficiency
  - Suspected acute tubular necrosis not improving after 3 to 4 weeks
  - Course atypical for diabetic nephropathy in diabetic patient

BOX 35-1	*Diseases That May Present with Rapidly Progressive Renal Failure and Mimic Glomerulonephritis*

Cholesterol emboli syndrome (transient hypocomplementemia may be seen in 25%)

Thrombotic microangiopathies—include HUS, TTP, and antiphospholipid antibody syndrome

Scleroderma renal crisis

Myeloma cast nephropathy

Collapsing FSGS (usually associated with HIVAN)

FSGS, focal segmental glomerulosclerosis; HIVAN, HIV-associated nephropathy; HUS, hemolytic uremic syndrome; TTP, thrombotic thrombocytopenic purpura.

Treatment

- When GN is secondary to a systemic disease or infection, treatment is aimed at the underlying disorder
- Table 35-3 outlines therapy for selected nephritic disorders
- Some patients may require dialysis therapy temporarily or indefinitely

REVIEW QUESTIONS

For review questions, please go to www.expertconsult.com.

SUGGESTED READINGS

Falk RJ: ANCA-associated renal disease, *Kidney Int* 38:998–1010, 1990.

Madaio MP, Harrington JT: The diagnosis of acute glomerulonephritis, *N Engl J Med* 309:1299–1302, 1983.

Orth S, Ritz E: The nephrotic syndrome, *N Engl J Med* 338:1202–1211, 1998.

TABLE 35-3	*Treatment of Selected Nephritic Disorders*

Disorder	Treatment	Response

Henoch-Schönlein purpura	Supportive care
	  Rest
	  Fluids
	  Pain relief
	Hospitalize for
	  Inadequate oral intake
	  GI bleeding
	  Renal failure
	Glucocorticoids for severe disease (unproven efficacy, but reasonable)
		Excellent prognosis
		Roughly one-third relapse within 4 mo
		Acute morbidity: Due to GI bleeding
		Chronic morbidity: Renal involvement; 10% develop ESRD

Goodpasture's syndrome	Plasmapheresis (to remove anti-GBM antibodies) + corticosteroids + cyclophosphamide Among those with higher creatinine requiring dialysis: Therapy less likely to be beneficial; most would still use above regimen	Prognosis (patient and kidney survival) correlates with number of crescents on biopsy and level of renal insufficiency on presentation Relapses are uncommon unless patient is also ANCA-positive
Postinfectious GN	Immunosuppressive therapy generally not helpful Rapidly progressive GN with crescents: Consider pulse steroids (though unproven efficacy)	Prognosis generally quite good Spontaneous resolution usually occurs over 3–4 wk

IgA nephropathy	Treat progessive disease (not all disease is progressive)
	ACE inhibitors or ARBs to treat hypertension and reduce intraglomerular pressure
	Corticosteroids may be of use in some patients
	Fish oil (omega-3 fatty acid) use is controversial, but frequently used
	Combined therapy with prednisone and other immunosuppressives may be needed in patients who continue to progress and in those with rapidly progressive disease
		Not all patients progress; some have stable course, some experience remission
		In patients who progress, deterioration is usually gradual
		Predictors of progression
		  Elevated creatinine at diagnosis
		  Increase in blood pressure
		  Protein excretion above 500–1000 mg/24 hr
		ESRD eventually develops in 15% at 10 yr and 20% in 20 yr

ACE, angiotensin-converting enzyme; ANCA, antineutrophil cytoplasmic antibody; ARB, angiotensin receptor blocker; ESRD, end-stage renal disease; GBM, glomerular basement membrane; GI, gastrointestinal; GN, glomerulonephritis.

35

Chronic Kidney Disease and End-Stage Renal Disease

TARIQ SHAFI, MBBS, MHS, PAUL J. SCHEEL JR., MD, MBA, and DEREK M. FINE, MD

Chronic kidney disease (CKD) is a rising public health problem in the United States, predominantly because of the increasing prevalence of diabetes and hypertension with resultant renal disease. CKD often leads to end-stage renal disease (ESRD) and the need for renal replacement therapy.

Basic Information

- Definition: Defined by structural or functional abnormalities of the kidney for 3 months or longer, with or without decreased glomerular filtration rate (GFR)
- **The National Kidney Foundation has established the following stages of CKD:**
  - **Stage I: Kidney damage (proteinuria, cyst formation, etc.) with normal or increased GFR**
  - **Stage II: Kidney damage with mild decrease in GFR (GFR 60–89 mL/min/1.73 m²)**
  - **Stage III: Moderate decrease in GFR (GFR 30–59 mL/min/1.73 m²)**
  - **Stage IV: Severe decrease in GFR (GFR 15–29 mL/min/1.73 m²)**
  - **Stage V: Kidney failure (GFR 15 mL/min/1.73 m² or dialysis)**
- Epidemiology
  - Many patients with CKD progress to ESRD
  - Prevalence increases with age
  - Estimated ESRD prevalence in the United States in 2007 was over 500,000 with an annual incidence of greater than 110,000
- Etiology
  - Diabetes (~40%)
  - Hypertension (~25%)
  - Glomerulonephritis (~10%)
  - Genetic or congenital (i.e., polycystic kidney disease, ~3%)
  - Urologic (~2%)

Clinical Presentation

- Usually asymptomatic until the late stages of renal failure
- **Onset of symptoms is usual indication for initiation of dialysis**
- **Early symptoms: Anorexia, nausea, lethargy, fatigue**
- **Late symptoms: Pruritis, mental status changes due to encephalopathy, volume overload, chest pain from pericarditis, neuropathy**
- Metabolic abnormalities often seen (Table 36-1)
  - Anemia

- Secondary and tertiary hyperparathyroidism (associated with hypocalcemia, hyperphosphatemia, and metabolic bone disease)
  - Acidosis
  - Hyperkalemia
- Physical examination findings
  - Asterixis (indicative of encephalopathy)
  - Pericardial friction rub
  - Signs of volume overload
  - Uremic fetor: Foul-smelling breath similar to urine or fish
  - Pallor
  - Calciphylaxis: Calcification of arterioles (Fig. 36-1) seen in patients with ESRD (not just CKD)
    - Usually in the setting of a high calcium × phosphorus product
    - Violaceous, indurated skin lesions that may ulcerate
    - Predilection for the lower extremities and trunk

Diagnosis

- Diagnose by estimated or actual GFR, not serum creatinine (Cr) levels
  - Normal GFR is usually greater than 90 mL/min in women and greater than 100 mL/min in men
  - **CKD is underdiagnosed if serum Cr is used as sole measure**
  - **Need to use GFR estimation equations**
    - Modification of Diet in Renal Disease (MDRD) formula is preferred for estimating GFR. It is used for GFR estimation by clinical laboratories and in most clinical trials (available at www.kidney.org).
  - **Cockcroft-Gault equation is an alternative:**

$$\frac{(140 - \text{age}) \times \text{lean body weight (kg)}}{\text{Serum Cr (mg/dL)} \times 72}$$

- For GFR in women, multiply equation by 0.85
- Other features that indicate CKD
  - Evidence that compromised GFR is long-standing (more than one measure over longer than 3 months)
  - Small kidneys on renal ultrasound (normal kidney size is 10 to 12 cm; kidneys are smaller in women)
  - Presence of manifestations of CKD: Anemia, secondary hyperparathyroidism, acidosis
- Should rule out reversible causes in any patient with renal insufficiency
  - Obstruction and prerenal causes (see Chapter 34)

TABLE 36-1	*Manifestations of Chronic Renal Insufficiency*			
Manifestation	**Mechanism**	**Clinical Features**	**Diagnosis**	**Treatment**
Anemia	Erythropoietin (EPO) deficiency	Onset: GFR 25–50 mL/min Early: Asymptomatic Late: Decrease in functional capacity and quality of life, left ventricular hypertrophy	Rule out other causes of anemia Reticulocyte count Smear iron studies Hemoccult stool EPO levels *not* useful	**Goal hemoglobin:** 10–12 g/dL **Erythropoietin:** Start dose: 50–70 U/kg SC weekly **Darbepoetin:** Start dose: 0.45 µg/kg SC weekly **Iron replacement** (all patients) Monitor hemoglobin weekly until "in range," then monthly Avoid hemoglobin > 13 g/dL Follow ferritin and TSAT at least quarterly in CKD, monthly in ESRD—inadequate iron stores if ferritin < 100, TSAT < 20% IV iron if stores inadequate with oral iron
Metabolic bone disease	**Low 1,25-dihydroxyvitamin D** (poor conversion from 25-hydroxyvitamin D) **High phosphate** (low excretion) **Low calcium** (due to low vitamin D) ↓ All lead to high intact PTH (iPTH) secondary hyperparathyroidism ↓ Renal osteodystrophy	Onset: GFR 25–40 mL/min Usually asymptomatic Bone pain—late manifestation Risk of fractures	High iPTH High phosphate Low calcium	**Goal iPTH:** 1.5–2 times upper limit of normal for the lab K/DOQI goals: CKD 3: 35–70 pg/mL CKD 4: 70–110 pg/mL CKD 5 or ESRD: 150–300 pg/mL **Goal serum phosphorus** 2.7–4.6 mg/dL (CKD 3, 4) 3.5–5.5 mg/dL (CKD 5 or ESRD) **Restrict dietary phosphorus** < 800–1000 mg/day **Phosphate binders** Calcium-based Calcium carbonate Calcium acetate Non–calcium-based (if high calcium × phosphorus product [> 72]) Sevelamer Lanthanum carbonate **Check vitamin D-25 levels if iPTH is above goal (CKD 3–5):** If <30 ng/mL: Supplement with ergocalciferol (caution if serum phosphorus ≥ 4.6 mg/dL or serum calcium ≥ 10.2 mg/dL) **Goal serum calcium:** 8.4–10.2 mg/dL **Vitamin D analogues** Calcitriol Paricalcitol Doxercalciferol
Acidosis	Inability of kidney to excrete acid load Usually a distal RTA	Chronic acidosis can result in hypercatabolism with poor nutritional status Calcium mobilization from the bone—exacerbation of osteoporosis	Low serum bicarbonate	**Goal serum bicarbonate** > 22 mEq/L Start therapy if serum bicarbonate < 18 mEg/L **Sodium citrate** 10 mL 3 times daily *or* **Sodium bicarbonate** 650 mg 3 times daily Monitor bicarbonate to avoid alkalosis
Volume overload	Inability of kidney to excrete water and salt	CHF Lower extremity edema	Physical exam Chest radiograph	**Sodium restriction** < 2 g/day (<100 mEq on a 24-hr urine collection) **Fluid restriction** < 1500 mL/day **Diuretics** Loop—increase dose until maximum; bid dosing Thiazide—add to regimen if patient unresponsive to loop diuretic to overcome distal sodium retention
Hyperkalemia	Inability of kidney to excrete potassium load	Usually asymptomatic May cause paralysis or respiratory failure Cardiac arrhythmias	High serum potassium ECG changes Peaked T waves Flat or absent P wave Wide QRS Sine waves ECG changes	**Acute** Calcium gluconate, insulin/glucose, β-agonist, diuretic, sodium polystyrene, dialysis **Long-term** Dietary restriction (high-potassium foods include orange, potato, tomato, banana, cantaloupe, and many others) Loop or thiazide diuretic Correct concurrent acidosis (see above) Consider discontinuation of β-blockers Sodium polystyrene resin

CHF, congestive heart failure; CKD, chronic kidney disease; ECG, electrocardiogam; ESRD, end-stage renal disease; GFR, glomerular filtration rate; K/DOQI, National Kidney Foundation Kidney Disease Outcomes Quality Initiative; PTH, parathyroid hormone; RTA, renal tubular acidosis; TSAT, transferrin saturation.

36

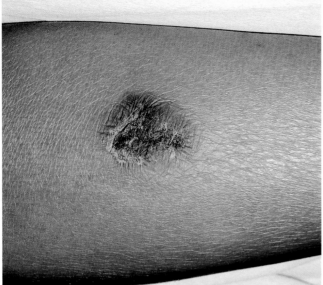

FIGURE 36-1 Typical skin lesion of calciphylaxis. (From Dharmadhikari A, Sukkar A, Mani S: Cases from the Osler Medical Service at Johns Hopkins University. *Am J Med* 114:765–767, 2003, figure 1.)

- Treatable glomerular disease (see Chapter 35)
- Atherosclerotic renal vascular disease (Box 36-1)

Management

- Early recognition of CKD
  - **Early referral to nephrologist shown to improve outcomes (at least by the time GFR is 30 mL/min)**
  - Allows for early intervention (Fig. 36-2)
- Delay progression of CKD
  - **Angiotensin-converting enzyme (ACE) inhibitors and angiotensin receptor blockers (ARBs)**
    - Mechanism: Decrease intraglomerular pressure and hyperfiltration
    - Problem: May lead to elevation of serum Cr and potassium
      - Cr rise is 20% or less: Can continue therapy as there is long-term benefit in preservation of GFR
    - If potassium is elevated (goal to maintain ACE-I or ARB therapy)
      - Exclude renal artery stenosis
      - Dietary potassium restriction (major culprits include bananas, cantaloupe, oranges, potatoes, tomatoes)
      - Use of potassium-wasting diuretic (thiazide-type or loop diuretic)
      - Elimination of potassium-sparing diuretics (triamterene, spironolactone, or eplerenone)
      - Consider β-blocker dose reduction (though usually would try to maintain dose because of other benefits)
      - Use of sodium polystyrene
  - Management of hypertension
    - Hypertension is a very important risk factor for acceleration in decline in GFR
    - Lowering of blood pressure reduces rate of decline in GFR

BOX 36-1 *Atherosclerotic Renal Vascular Disease*

Common in patients with evidence of atherosclerotic disease in other vascular beds (20% of these patients)
45% to 50% of renal artery stenosis patients will have bilateral disease
Consider if any of the following are present
  New-onset hypertension after age 50 years
  Newly difficult to control hypertension (requiring >2 medications) in known hypertensive patient
  Unexplained increase in creatinine in patient with suspected vascular disease (CAD, PVD, smoker, diabetic)
  Hypotension or worsening creatinine after initiation of ACE-inhibitor
  Flash pulmonary edema without evidence of cardiac cause
Diagnosis
  Renal angiography (gold standard)
  Magnetic resonance angiography (less invasive, >90% sensitivity and specificity)
  CT angiogram (best in those who can tolerate IV contrast)
  Doppler ultrasound (accuracy is very user dependent)
Treatment
  Angioplasty and endovascular stenting
  Stenting associated with better outcomes, except in fibromuscular dysplasia
  Stenting especially important with ostial lesions, which have highest restenosis rates
Outcomes
  Improvement in GFR
  Improved blood pressure control requiring fewer antihypertensives (occasional cure of hypertension)

ACE, angiotensin-converting enzyme; CAD, coronary artery disease; GFR, glomerular filtration rate; PVD, peripheral vascular disease.

  - **Further reduction in blood pressure below 130/80 mm Hg (<125/75 mm Hg) may have added benefit in patients, especially those with proteinuria** (Joint National Committee-VII guidelines)
  - ACE-inhibitors or ARBs should be first line, given their independent benefits on halting progression of renal disease
  - Atenolol is cleared by the kidney; therefore, use with caution or consider switch to hepatically cleared β-blocker such as metoprolol
  - **Dietary protein restriction**
    - Mechanism: In theory, reduced protein intake decreases intraglomerular pressure and metabolic demands on kidney
    - Conflicting efficacy data from trials
    - Recommendation (largely opinion-based): Maximum dietary restriction for a patient with CKD would be 0.7 g of protein/kg of body weight/day; many would suggest that 1 g of protein/kg of body weight/day would be more appropriate
    - If patient is placed on protein-restricted diet, must have close follow-up of nutritional status to avoid malnutrition
  - Management of glucose in patients with diabetes mellitus and CKD
    - Tight control of patient's blood glucose slows progression of diabetic nephropathy

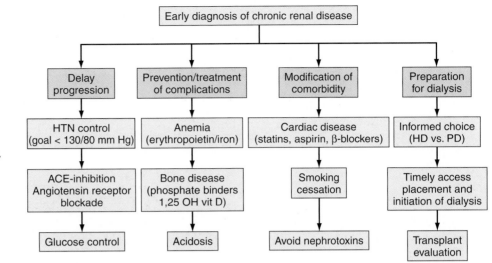

FIGURE 36-2 Management of chronic renal disease. ACE, angiotensin-converting enzyme; HD, hemodialysis; HTN, hypertension; PD, peritoneal dialysis; 1,25 OH vit D, 1,25-dihydroxyvitamin D.

- Goal HgbA$_{1c}$ is 6%
- Modify other cardiovascular risk factors (e.g., tobacco use, hypercholesterolemia)
- Avoid nephrotoxins and use renally cleared drugs with caution (Table 36-2)
- Prevent and treat complications of CKD
  - Anemia, metabolic bone disease, acidosis, and volume overload (see Table 36-1)
    - Recent studies suggest increased risk of cardiovascular events with normalization of hemoglobin (>13 g/dL)
    - Maintenance of hemoglobin in the 11- to 12-g/dL range is therefore important
  - Other endocrine complications
    - **Decreased GFR leads to prolonged half-life of insulin**
    - **Patients with progressive renal failure need a downward titration of insulin and sulphonylurea dosing to avoid hypoglycemia**
- Avoid additional insults
  - Radiocontrast
    - Risk of acute renal failure 20% to 90%
    - Patients with diabetes at highest risk
    - Choose alternative imaging modality if possible
      - Gadolinium-based contrast agent contraindicated in those with estimated GFR less than 30 due to risk of nephrogenic systemic fibrosis (NSF)—if its use is essential in this high-risk group use a low dose of a macrocyclic agent (gadoteridol)
    - If radiocontrast use unavoidable:
      - **Ensure adequate hydration with isotonic saline or sodium bicarbonate**
      - **Minimize contrast volume**
      - **Utilize nonionic contrast**
      - **N-Acetylcysteine 600 mg twice a day for 24 hours before procedure and 48 hours following procedure may reduce incidence of acute renal failure in high-risk groups**
  - Avoid volume depletion
    - Tolerated poorly in this patient population
    - May lead to worsening of CKD secondary to acute tubular necrosis

- Low threshold for IV fluids for hydration
- Avoid iatrogenic complications from medications
  - Adjust dose and interval of all renally metabolized medications
  - See Table 36-2 for specific drugs
- **Renal transplantation**
- **Preferred treatment of ESRD**
- Every patient with ESRD should be considered a candidate for transplantation until proven otherwise
- **Contraindications to transplantation**
  - **Anticipated life span less than 4 years**
  - **HIV infection (currently under study)**
  - **Recent malignancy (time varies according to cancer type)**
  - **Active infection**
- Sources of organs
  - **Living related (best option: Better antigen matches with recipient)**
  - Living unrelated (second best option: But less well matched than related)
  - Deceased donor (less optimal because of cold ischemic times in transport to recipient—may result in cell death and antigen release)
- **Refer to transplant center for evaluation when GFR 30 mL/min or less**
- Patients can be listed for cadaveric transplant when GFR less than 20 mL/min
- **Treatment goal, for suitable candidate, is to receive a transplant before need for dialysis**
- Prognosis: The 5-year survival is 80% for deceased donor, 85% for living unrelated donor, and 90% for living related donor
- Dialysis
  - 90% of patients are candidates for either hemodialysis (HD) or peritoneal dialysis (PD)
  - **If therapy prescribed and monitored correctly, HD equals PD in effectiveness**
  - Initiation of therapy
    - Diabetics: Estimated GFR less than 15 mL/min/1.73 m^2
    - Nondiabetics: Estimated GFR less than 10 mL/min/1.73 m^2

36

TABLE 36-2 *Drugs to Use with Caution in Renal Insufficiency*

Drug Name	Side Effect	Mechanism
Gadolinium-based contrast agents	Nephrogenic systemic fibrosis	Poor clearance with extended half-life and deposition of free gadolinium in tissues. Avoid in GFR < 30 and ESRD. Macrocyclic agent (gadoteridol) safer than linear agents (gadodiamide = Omniscan or gadopentetate = Magnevist) if exposure is essential
Phosphate-containing bowel preps or enemas	Phosphate deposition in kidneys (phosphate nephropathy) or high anion gap acidosis	Poor clearance with renal failure
Aminoglycosides	ARF	Tubular toxicity
Atenolol	Bradycardia	Decreased renal clearance
NSAIDs and COX-2 inhibitors	ARF	Prostacyclin-induced afferent vasoconstriction
Sulfonylureas	Hypoglycemia (glyburide worse than glipizide)	Decreased renal clearance
Metformin	Lactic acidosis (should really avoid in most CKD patients; hold before contrast studies)	Mitochondrial toxicity
Magnesium-containing medications	Hypermagnesemia	Decreased clearance of magnesium
Meperidine	Seizure	Low clearance of toxic metabolite normeperidine
Sucralfate	Aluminum toxicity	High aluminum content with decreased clearance in renal failure, especially ESRD
Potassium supplements or potassium-sparing diuretics	Hyperkalemia	Absorption or retention of potassium

ARF, acute renal failure; COX-2, cyclooxygenase-2; ESRD, end-stage renal disease; GFR, glomerular filtration rate.

- **Absolute dialysis indications (ideal goal is to avoid these manifestations and initiate dialysis at the onset of early symptoms)**
  - **Uremic encephalopathy or pericarditis**
  - **Volume overload not responsive to diuretics**
  - **Hyperkalemia despite medical management**
  - **Acidosis despite medical management**
- Prognosis for dialysis patients is poor in general
  - Median 5-year survival: 33% (1 in 3 dialysis patients will survive for 5 years after starting dialysis)
  - Most common cause of death: Heart disease, followed by infection
- Peritoneal dialysis
  - Can be continuous ambulatory peritoneal dialysis (CAPD) or automated peritoneal dialysis (APD) done over only 12 to 13 hours
  - **Major risk is peritonitis; occurs at a rate of 0.5 episodes per patient per year**
  - Preparing patient for PD
    - Electively repair ventral and inguinal hernias
    - PD catheter placement 4 to 6 weeks before initiation of therapy
- Hemodialysis
  - Procedure: Dialyze three times per week for 3 to 5 hours each treatment
  - Requires access to bloodstream (following options in order of preference)
    - Arteriovenous fistula (AVF)
    - Prosthetic bridge graft
    - Dual-lumen catheter

- AVF preferred access given decreased risk of infection, superior longevity, and high blood-flow rates
- AVF may take 2 to 8 months to mature, and multiple attempts may be necessary to achieve desired result
- Once a patient decides on HD as modality of renal replacement therapy
  - Patient should be referred to vascular surgeon 6 to 12 months before need for dialysis; need to place AVF early to mature
  - Phlebotomy and blood pressure measurement should be performed on dominant arm, reserving nondominant arm for dialysis access; preferably use hand veins

REVIEW QUESTIONS

For review questions, please go to www.expertconsult.com.

SUGGESTED READINGS

Kimmel PL: Management of the patient with chronic renal disease. In Greenberg A, editor: *Primer on kidney diseases*, ed 2, San Diego, Academic Press, 1998.

National Kidney Foundation: K/DOQI clinical practice guidelines on chronic kidney disease: evaluation, classification and stratification, Available at: www.kidney.org/professionals/ doqi/kdoqi/toc.htm.

Perazella MA: Current status of gadolinium toxicity in patients with kidney disease, *Clin J Am Soc Nephrol* 4:461–469, 2009.

Post TW, Rose BD: Overview of the management of chronic renal failure, Available at: Up-to-Date online.

Winearls CG: Clinical evaluation and manifestations of chronic renal failure. In Johnson RJ, Feehally J, editors: *Comprehensive clinical nephrology*, London, Harcourt, 2000.

Selected Topics in Nephrology

CLARISSA JONAS, MD, MICHELLE M. ESTRELLA, MD, and MICHAEL J. CHOI, MD

Hematuria and nephrolithiasis are among the most common clinical problems in nephrology. The differential diagnosis and associated conditions for both hematuria and nephrolithiasis can be narrowed by a stepwise approach to the clinical presentation.

Hematuria

Basic Information

- Microscopic hematuria
  - Typically discovered on urinalysis in the **asymptomatic** adult
  - Incidence **increases with increasing age;** some series show 2% to 18% of those older than 50 years have microscopic hematuria
  - Definition is variable, but most suggest **more than 3 RBCs/hpf** as criterion for microscopic hematuria
  - Urine dipstick testing is highly sensitive for microscopic hematuria but is not specific. **It may indicate the presence of heme despite the absence of RBCs. This may occur with myoglobinuria, intravascular hemolysis, povidone-iodine administration, or the presence of oxidizing agents.**
- Gross hematuria
  - Less common than microscopic hematuria
  - **The presenting symptom in up to 85% of patients diagnosed with bladder cancer and 40% in those with renal cell carcinoma**
  - **Pseudohematuria is the presence of red urine without blood; may be seen after ingestion of certain foods (e.g., beets, rhubarb) or medications (e.g., pyridium, phenothiazines) or may result from other medical diseases (e.g., porphyria)**
- General approach to the evaluation of the patient with hematuria
  - History: Important details include timing, associated symptoms, social and family history (Table 37-1)
  - Laboratory evaluation: Important details include associated abnormalities in urine (e.g., protein, WBCs) and appearance of RBCs (Table 37-2)
  - The differential diagnosis of hematuria may be divided between glomerular and nonglomerular causes (Fig. 37-1). Depending on the clinical picture, several radiologic studies may be of diagnostic use (Table 37-3). The general approach to the workup of hematuria is summarized in Figure 37-2.

TABLE 37-1	Historical Details in the Evaluation of the Patient with Hematuria
Historical Details	
Timing	Transient
	Can be caused by fever, exercise, CHF
	Rule out contamination by menstrual blood
	Initial
	Often implies urethral source
	Terminal
	Often implies bladder source
Associated symptoms	Dysuria
	Suggests urinary tract infection
	Flank pain
	Suggests nephrolithiasis or papillary necrosis
	Weight loss, fatigue
	Suggests vasculitis or cancer
Medications	
Analgesics	Suggests papillary necrosis
Antibiotics, other	Consider acute interstitial nephritis, especially if other evidence of hypersensitivity
Family/Social History	
FH of renal failure	Suggests autosomal dominant polycystic kidney disease (ADPKD)
FH of hematuria in men only	Suggests Alport's syndrome (especially if associated with deafness)
SH of tobacco use or dye exposure	Suggests bladder cancer

CHF, congestive heart failure; FH, family history; SH, social history.

- **Anticoagulation alone does not induce hematuria.** Patients on anticoagulation who have hematuria should undergo evaluation unless there is massive bleeding from overanticoagulation

Nonglomerular Causes of Hematuria

- Extrarenal disorders
  - **The most common cause of hematuria, with infections and nephrolithiasis the most common disorders**
  - Neoplasms of the bladder, prostate, and ureters may manifest with either microscopic or gross hematuria
- Nonglomerular renal disorders
  - **Autosomal dominant polycystic kidney disease (ADPKD)**
    - Seen in 1 in 500 to 1 in 1000 people

TABLE 37-2	*Laboratory Evaluation of the Patient with Hematuria*

Urinalysis
Clots
  Rules out glomerular source
Proteinuria, dysmorphic RBCs, RBC casts
  Indicates glomerular source; consider serologic evaluation with ANA, complement levels, cryoglobulins, ANCA, anti-GBM, ASO, hepatitis serologies, and rheumatoid factor
Pyuria
  Suggests infection or interstitial nephritis; consider urine culture and Hansel's stain for eosinophils

Urine Cytopathology
Obtain if bladder cancer suspected
May detect bladder carcinoma in situ missed by cytoscopy

ANA, antinuclear antibody; ANCA, antineutrophil cytoplasmic antibody; ASO, antistreptolysin O; GBM, glomerular basement membrane.

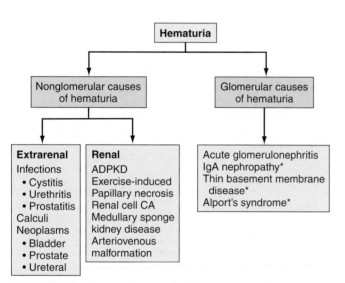

FIGURE 37-1 Causes of hematuria. *Can present with <500 mg/day of proteinuria. ADPKD, autosomal dominant polycystic kidney disease; CA, cancer; IgA, immunoglobulin A.

- Two subtypes: 85% to 95% of cases are ADPKD1 located on chromosome 16; the remaining 5% to 15% are ADPKD2 located on chromosome 14
- **Clinical presentation includes gross or microscopic hematuria in 50% of patients; hypertension is common. Many have episodes of flank pain and a palpable abdominal mass on examination (Fig. 37-3).**
- **Renal cysts are evident on CT or ultrasound by age 30 years**
- **Intracranial aneurysms seen in less than 10%; screen individual with ADPKD for aneurysm if positive family history or symptoms**
- **Other extrarenal manifestations include hepatic involvement and ovarian cysts, mitral valve prolapse, diverticulosis, and hernias**

TABLE 37-3	*Imaging Modalities for Evaluation of Hematuria*

IVP	Use when nonglomerular cause suggested Definitive test for medullary sponge kidney disease and papillary necrosis Superior to ultrasound for detection of stones or cancer in the ureters Cannot distinguish between solid and cystic renal masses
Ultrasound	Use when glomerular cause suspected Use when dye allergy or renal insufficiency present Superior to IVP for ADPKD, renal cell CA, small bladder CA Limited in detection of small solid lesions (< 3 cm)
CT scan	Superior to IVP for nephrolithiasis Better defines mass that may have been observed with ultrasound More expensive than IVP or ultrasound
CT urogram	Most sensitive test for hematuria Noncontrast CT performed first to look for stones If negative, contrast CT is performed with visualization of kidneys, ureters, and bladder

ADPKD, autosomal dominant polycystic kidney disease; CA, cancer; IVP, intravenous pyelogram.

- **Exercise-induced hematuria**
  - Usually **microscopic;** may rarely be associated with **RBC casts**
  - Mechanism unclear, but some suggest bladder trauma or glomerular ischemia cause
  - Seen in both contact and noncontact sports
  - Typically resolves with 1 to 3 days of rest
- **Papillary necrosis**
  - Results from **ischemic damage** to renal papilla
  - **May be precipitated by sickle cell disease, diabetes mellitus, nonsteroidal anti-inflammatory analgesics (by decreasing vasodilator prostaglandins), urinary tract obstruction, and tuberculosis**
  - Diagnosis is by intravenous pyelogram (IVP) or CT urogram, which reveals characteristic changes (Fig. 37-4). Occasionally, necrotic papillary debris can be identified in the urine.

Glomerular Causes of Hematuria

- **The urinalysis serves as an important diagnostic tool in determining a glomerular cause of hematuria by indicating the presence of proteinuria or demonstrating the presence of either dysmorphic RBCs or RBC casts**
- **Dysmorphic RBCs are thought to form when RBCs passing through the glomerular basement membrane lyse and damage other RBCs, resulting in dysmorphic, crenated, misshapen RBCs (>80% dysmorphic RBCs on examination slide is diagnostic of glomerular hematuria; Fig. 37-5)**

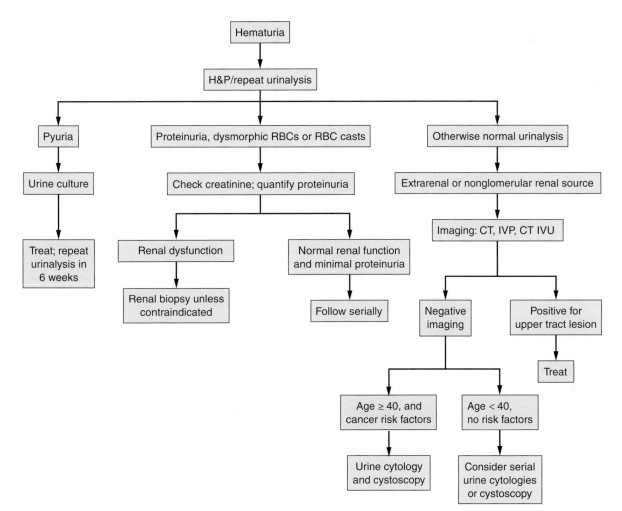

FIGURE 37-2 Algorithm for workup of microscopic hematuria. CT, computed tomography; H&P, history and physical; IVP, intravenous pyelogram; IVU, intravenous urogram.

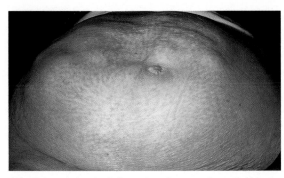

FIGURE 37-3 Abdominal distention due to polycystic kidney disease. An enlarged, cystic liver is also present. (From Haslett C, Chilvers ER, Boon NA, et al: *Davidson's principles and practice of medicine,* ed 19, New York, Churchill Livingstone, 2002, figure 11.8.)

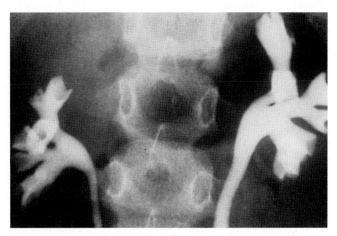

FIGURE 37-4 Grades II and III reflux in a voiding cystourethrographic study from a young boy who presented with recurrent urinary tract infection. Note early clubbing of the calyces and dilatation of the ureter on the left side. (From Mandell GL, Bennett JE, Dolin R: *Principles and practice of infectious diseases,* ed 6, Philadelphia, Churchill Livingstone, 2005, figure 66-19.)

- **RBC casts** result from RBCs adhering to one another in the presence of Tamm-Horsfall protein, forming a "cast" of the tubule (Fig. 37-6)
- **Immunoglobulin A (IgA) nephropathy, thin basement membrane disease, and Alport's syndrome are the three most common glomerular causes of isolated hematuria without significant proteinuria (<500**

mg/day). Causes of acute glomerulonephritis cause glomerular hematuria with proteinuria (Table 37-4; see also Fig. 37-1 and Chapter 35)

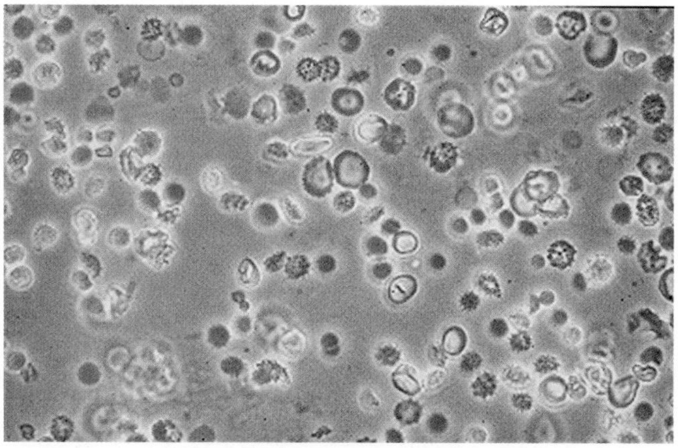

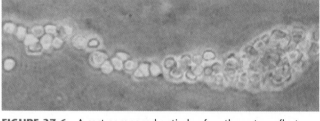

FIGURE 37-5 Dysmorphic erythrocytes. These dysmorphic erythrocytes vary in size, shape, and hemoglobin content and reflect glomerular bleeding. (From Johnson RJ, Feehally J: *Comprehensive clinical nephrology*, London, Mosby, 2000, figure 4.4.)

FIGURE 37-6 A cast composed entirely of erythrocytes reflects heavy hematuria and active glomerular disease. Crescentic nephritis is likely to be present if erythrocyte casts are greater than 100/mL. (From Johnson RJ, Feehally J: *Comprehensive clinical nephrology*, London, Mosby, 2000, figure 4.8B.)

- Evidence of systemic illness (e.g., fatigue, athralgias, hemoptysis, and sore throat) should prompt consideration for collagen-vascular disease, other autoimmune disease, postinfectious glomerulonephritis, or viral hepatitis

Nephrolithiasis

Basic Information

- Incidence: 1% in middle-aged white men
- Stone types
  - Calcium-based (oxalate and phosphate): 75% (pure calcium phosphate: 5%)
  - Uric acid: 10% to 12%
  - Struvite: 10% to 20%
  - Cystine: Less than 1%
  - Other (triamterene, indinavir): Rare

Clinical Presentation

- Patients typically present with **severe flank pain radiating to the groin,** often described as worst pain for men, and worst (other than childbirth) for women
- Some patients have no symptoms of pain, with the stone discovered during the evaluation of microscopic or gross hematuria

Diagnosis

- Initial step is to image stone and rule out obstruction with IVP (Fig. 37-7), ultrasound, or CT

TABLE 37-4	**Glomerular Causes of Hematuria Without Proteinuria**		
Disorder	**Diagnosis**	**Associated Findings**	**Treatment**
IgA nephropathy (Berger's disease)	Renal biopsy; IgA immune complex deposits along glomerular mesangium Usually seen in young men (M:F 3:1)	Idiopathic form presents as microscopic hematuria or gross hematuria 1–3 days after URI May be associated with cirrhosis, inflammatory bowel disease Increased serum creatinine at diagnosis, >1 g/day proteinuria, hypertension and scarring on biopsy portend worse prognosis ESRD in 20% after 20 years	ACE-I if proteinuria present Immunosuppressive agents if creatinine rising rapidly Fish oil (controversial) if >1 g/day proteinuria
Thin basement membrane disease (benign familial hematuria)	Familial; autosomal dominant; glomerular basement membrane is half normal thickness	90% present with microscopic hematuria; gross hematuria uncommon Proteinuria may be present, usually < 1.5 g/day	No treatment needed
Alport's syndrome (hereditary nephritis)	Familial, 80% are X-linked due to mutations in genes for type IV collagen	Microscopic or gross hematuria Proteinuria (late) High-tone sensorineural deafness Lenticonus or cataracts ESRD in majority by age 35	Supportive measures

ACE-I, angiotensin-converting enzyme inhibitor; ESRD, end-stage renal disease; IgA, immunoglobulin A; URI, upper respiratory infection.

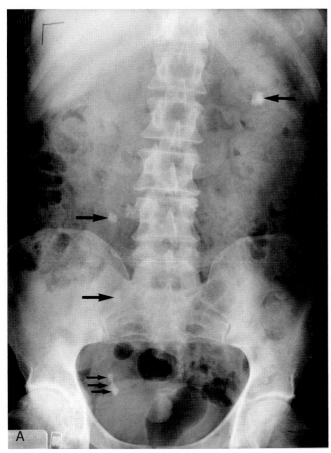

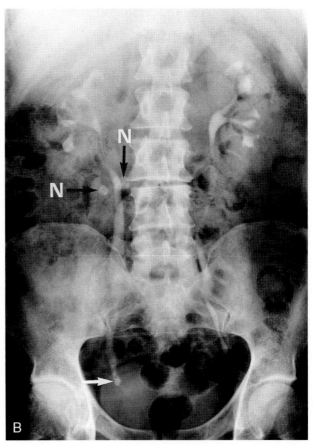

FIGURE 37-7 Intravenous pyelogram of a patient with nephrolithiasis, before and after administration of contrast agent. **A** and **B,** Multiple kidney stones are noted throughout the urinary collecting system (*black arrows*), with evidence of obstruction (*white arrow*). Calcified lymph nodes (N) are noted outside the collecting system. (From Burkitt GH, Quick CRG: *Essential surgery,* ed 3, New York, Churchill Livingstone, 2003, figure 31.3.)

- In the past, IVP was the gold-standard imaging study, but it has been largely replaced by **noncontrast stone protocol CT**
- IVP and CT urogram remain the best for diagnosing medullary sponge kidney disease (anatomic abnormality with outpouching of collecting ducts leading to urinary stasis)
- Urinalysis and culture should be obtained. **The presence of WBCs may indicate inflammation without infection.** Infected kidney stones need antibiotic treatment and removal.
- Strain urine to capture stone for laboratory analysis of its composition
- **Standard initial studies include serum electrolytes, calcium, phosphorus, and uric acid levels**
- Obtain 24-hour urine collection for stone risk profile if patient has risk factors for stone recurrence
  - Risk factors: **Positive family history in middle-aged white men, malabsorption, chronic diarrhea, gout, and procedure required to remove stone**
  - The 24-hour urine should be sent for volume, creatinine, calcium, sodium, sulfate or urea nitrogen, oxalate, uric acid, citrate, phosphate, cystine (if suggested), and pH

Treatment

- See Table 37-5 for risk factors and treatment of nephrolithiasis.
- There is debate about treatment of the first episode of calcium nephrolithiasis
- **Risk of recurrence after single episode is approximately 50% over the next 10 years**

REVIEW QUESTIONS

For review questions, please go to www.expertconsult.com.

SUGGESTED READINGS

Coe FL, Parks JH, Asplin JR: The pathogenesis and treatment of kidney stones, *N Engl J Med* 327:1141–1152, 1992.
Reynolds TM: Chemical pathology clinical investigation and management of nephrolithaisis, *J Clin Pathol* 58:134–140, 2005.
Yun EJ, Meng MV, Carroll PR: Evaluation of the patient with hematuria, *Med Clin North Am* 88:329–343, 2004.

37

TABLE 37-5	*Nephrolithiasis: Risk Factors and Treatment*		
Stone Type	**Risk Factors**	**Treatment**	**Comments**
Calcium oxalate	*Hypercalciuria* (urine calcium > 300 mg/day in men; 250 mg/day in women); most common risk factor (e.g., hyperparathyroidism, sarcoidosis)	Low-sodium diet (urine sodium excretion parallels urine calcium excretion) Thiazide diuretics	Envelope-shaped crystals "Idiopathic" most common cause of hypercalciuria
	Hyperoxaluria (urine oxalate > 40 mg/day), e.g., malabsorption (increased colonic absorption of oxalate)	Avoid calcium limitation as it increases stone risk by leading to increased urine oxalate excretion	Strawberries, okra, spinach, brewed tea, nuts, and chocolate high in oxalate
	Hypocitraturia (urine citrate < 300 mg/day), e.g., distal RTA, diarrhea	Potassium citrate	
	Hyperuricosuria	Decrease purine intake Allopurinol	
Calcium phosphate	Distal (type 1) RTA Primary hyperparathyroidism Alkaline urine	See hypercalciuria treatment	Pure calcium phosphate stones are rare
Uric acid	High urine uric acid, e.g., gout, myeloproliferative disorder Acidic urine	Restrict purine intake; allopurinol Potassium citrate	Radiolucent crystals
Struvite	Urinary tract infection with urease-producing bacteria (e.g., *Proteus*)	Antibiotics Urologic procedure to remove stone	Crystals resemble coffin lids Form staghorn calculi
Cystine	Genetic defect resulting in decreased tubular reabsorption of cystine (urine cystine excretion > 400 mg/day)	High fluid intake to decrease urine cystine concentration Alkalinize urine Use medications with sulfhydryl groups to increase cystine solubility (e.g., captopril, penicillamine)	Hexagonal greenish/yellow crystals pathognomonic Respond poorly to lithotripsy

RTA, renal tubular acidosis.

SECTION SIX

BOARD REVIEW

Endocrinology

Diabetes Mellitus

SHERITA H. GOLDEN, MD, MHS

Diabetes is a major health problem. Approximately 8% of the U.S. population, or 17.9 million individuals, have been diagnosed with diabetes and it is estimated that 5.4 million individuals have undiagnosed diabetes. Type 2 diabetes accounts for 90% to 95% of cases. Significant complications of diabetes include retinopathy, nephropathy, neuropathy, and cardiovascular disease. Approximately 182,000 deaths per year are related to diabetes and its complications, making it the third largest killer in this country. Whereas death from cardiovascular disease has declined over the past two decades, death from diabetes continues to increase.

Diabetes Mellitus

Basic Information

- Diabetes mellitus encompasses several syndromes of altered insulin secretion and/or peripheral resistance that result in hyperglycemia
- Classification of diabetes
  - Type 1 diabetes
  - Type 2 diabetes
  - Gestational diabetes
  - Other specific types
- Genetic defects: β-Cell function, insulin action
- Disease of exocrine pancreas
- Endocrinopathies
- Drug- or chemical-induced
- Infection-related
- Other genetic syndromes associated with diabetes
- Pathogenesis of type 1 diabetes mellitus
  - Pancreatic β-cell destruction with resulting complete insulinopenia
- Immune-mediated: Anti-islet cell antibodies and anti-insulin antibodies are humoral markers of islet cell inflammation
- Idiopathic
  - Patients require insulin to prevent hyperglycemia and ketosis
- Pathogenesis of type 2 diabetes mellitus
  - Impaired insulin secretion because of β-cell dysfunction
  - Insulin resistance leads to increased hepatic glucose production and decreased peripheral glucose uptake
- Distinguishing between type 1 and type 2 (Table 38-1)

TABLE 38-1	*Distinguishing Between Types 1 and 2 Diabetes Mellitus*	
	Type 1	**Type 2**
Body weight	Lean or normal History of weight loss before presentation	Overweight or obese History of weight gain before diagnosis
Family history	<20% first-degree relatives with diabetes	Strong family history of first-degree relatives with diabetes
Other autoimmune disorders	May be present: Hashimoto's thyroiditis, Graves' disease, vitiligo, adrenal insufficiency, pernicious anemia	Absent
Glycemic patterns	Greater daily variability Exaggerated hyperglycemic response to stressors and meals	Blood sugars more stable throughout day
Response to oral agents	Nonresponse	Responsive
Insulin sensitivity	Normal	Very reduced
Islet cell antibodies	~80% have detectable titers at onset	Not present
C-peptide	Very low or undetectable	Detectable or elevated

Clinical Presentation

- Main symptoms include polyphagia, polydipsia, and polyuria
  - Type 1 diabetes typically presents in the first two decades of life; however, type 1 diabetes can present in adulthood and is then referred to as latent autoimmune diabetes of adulthood (LADA)
  - Type 2 diabetes typically presents after age 40 years
- Acute complications include diabetic ketoacidosis and nonketotic hypertonicity (Table 38-2)
- Chronic complications
  - Nephropathy (see section on diabetic nephropathy)
  - Retinopathy (see section on diabetic retinopathy)
  - Neuropathy (see section on diabetic neuropathy)
  - Cardiovascular disease (see section on cardiovascular disease)
  - Skin manifestations
    - Acanthosis nigricans (Fig. 38-1)

TABLE 38-2	*Management of Diabetic Ketoacidosis (DKA) and Nonketotic Hypertonicity (NKH)*	
	Diabetic Ketoacidosis	**Nonketotic Hypertonicity**
Occurrence	Occurs in both type 1 and 2 diabetes	Occurs mainly in type 2 diabetes, but can occur in type 1
Definition	1. Blood glucose (>250 mg/dL) 2. Low bicarbonate (<15 mEq/L) 3. Low pH (<7.3)	1. Effective osmolarity $\geq$ 320 mOsm/L [calculated as $2 \times (Na + K) + (glucose/18) + (BUN/2.8)$] 2. Blood glucose $\geq$ 600 mg/dL 3. pH $\geq$ 7.3
Presentation	1. Fatigue, blurred vision, polydipsia, polyuria, weight loss 2. Nausea, vomiting, and vague abdominal pain are common 3. Obtundation, shock, and coma may ensue 4. Kussmaul respirations and fruity breath suggest ketoacidosis	1. Fatigue, blurred vision, polydipsia, polyuria, weight loss 2. Severe dehydration 3. Obtundation, shock, and coma may ensue
Precipitants	Infection, omission or inadequate use of insulin, new-onset diabetes	Infection, new-onset diabetes, stroke, myocardial infarction, pancreatitis, uremia, burns, subdural hematoma, acromegaly, ectopic ACTH
Treatment	1. Hydration Usually a total of 4–5 L needed 1 L isotonic saline in first hour; add colloid if hypovolemic shock present Switch to hypotonic saline at 200–1000 mL/hr once initial fluid resuscitation complete Add dextrose when glucose < 200 mg/dL 2. Insulin therapy Initial priming dose: 0.3–0.4 units/kg regular insulin IV followed by infusion at ~7 units/hr Titrate as needed Continue until pH and serum bicarbonate normal Do not follow serum ketones; as DKA resolves, β-hydroxybutyrate is converted to acetoacetate and acetone, so ketones appear to be increasing In obtunded, hyperosmolar patient, lower glucose to 300 and maintain until patient is alert 3. Electrolyte replacement Hyperkalemia may be seen initially because of insulin deficiency and acidosis, but total body potassium is low After initial liter of normal saline, add 20–30 mEq potassium (2/3 as KCl and 1/3 as KPO_4) to each liter of fluid to correct hypokalemia and hypophosphatemia	1. Hydration 1–2 L fluid in first 2 hours then 7–9 L over next 2–3 days; give normal saline until blood pressure and urine flow restored, then switch to hypotonic saline Replace half the free water deficit in the first 12 hr and the remainder in the next 24 hr Add dextrose when glucose < 250 mg/dL 2. Electrolyte replacement Replace potassium with 20–40 mEq/L once urine flow is normal and serum potassium begins to fall 3. Insulin therapy Additive to fluid therapy but not a primary therapy here; hydration alone can correct hyperglycemia 10-unit bolus of regular insulin IV, then infuse 0.1–0.15 units/kg/hr
Follow-up	Check glucose once every hour for first several hours then every 4 hr while on IV fluids Check electrolytes every 2 hr until normal then every 4–6 hr while on IV fluids Check venous pH to follow resolution of acidosis	Check glucose once every hour for first several hours then every 4 hr while on IV fluids Check electrolytes every 2 hr until normal then every 4–6 hr while on IV fluids
Complications	Cerebral edema ARDS Hyperchloremic acidosis Vascular thromboembolism	Vascular thromboembolism Rhabdomyolysis ARDS

ACTH, adrenocorticotropic hormone; ARDS, acute respiratory distress syndrome; BUN, blood urea nitrogen.

- Frequently associated with insulin resistance and obesity; can also be related to underlying malignancy (especially GI and lung)
    - Dark, velvety, thickened plaques occurring in flexural areas (axilla, inguinal crease, back and sides of neck)
- Treatment
    - Weight reduction, treatment of the diabetes or underlying disorder
    - For severe, odorous lesions: Antibacterial soaps, topical antibiotics
- Necrobiosis lipoidica (Fig. 38-2)
    - Inflammatory skin condition of unknown etiology; frequently associated with diabetes or impaired glucose tolerance

- Often asymptomatic lesions; usually occur on the shin
- Indurated, oval plaques with central atrophy and yellow pigmentation; red-brown margins
- Treatment is often suboptimal
    - First-line: Topical or intralesional steroids
    - For ulcers: Cyclosporine, hyperbaric oxygen, infliximab, and others can be tried

Diagnosis and Evaluation

- Three main criteria are used for diagnosis of diabetes (only one of three is required for diagnosis)
    - Symptoms of diabetes (e.g., polyuria, polydipsia, weight loss, ketoacidosis, hyperosmolarity) plus random plasma glucose greater than 200 mg/dL

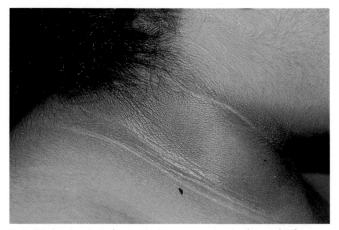

FIGURE 38-1 Acanthosis nigricans occurring in the neck of a patient with severe insulin resistance associated with obesity. (From Besser GM, Thorner M: *Comprehensive clinical endocrinology,* ed 3, St. Louis, Mosby, 2002, figure 36.7.)

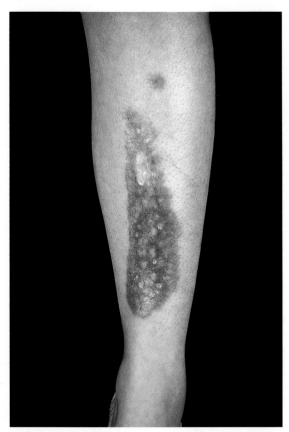

FIGURE 38-2 Necrobiosis lipoidica. (From Swash M: *Hutchinson's clinical methods,* ed 21, Philadelphia, WB Saunders, 2002, figure 8.8.)

- Fasting plasma glucose of 126 mg/dL or greater or random plasma glucose greater than 200 mg/dL on two separate occasions
- Two-hour plasma glucose of 200 mg/dL or greater after ingestion of a 75-g glucose load (oral glucose tolerance test, OGTT) on two occasions
- Other related conditions
  - Impaired glucose tolerance: Two-hour plasma glucose 140 to 199 mg/dL during OGTT

TABLE 38-3	*American Diabetes Association Recommended Glycemic Targets for Nonpregnant Adults*
	Glycemic Goals
Preprandial capillary plasma glucose	70–130 mg/dL
Postprandial capillary plasma glucose	<180 mg/dL
HbA$_{1c}$	<7%

HbA$_{1c}$, glycosylated hemoglobin.

TABLE 38-4	*Types of Insulin*		
	Onset of Action	**Peak of Action**	**Duration of Action**
Rapid-acting			
Lispro, Aspart	5–15 min	1–2 hr	3–5 hr
Regular	30–60 min	2–4 hr	6–8 hr
Intermediate-acting			
Neutral protamine Hagedorn	1–3 hr	5–7 hr	13–18 hr
Long-acting			
Ultralente	2–4 hr	8–14 hr	18–30 hr
Glargine	Within 4 hr	Peakless	>24 hr
Detemir	Within 4 hr	Peakless	18–24 hr

- Impaired fasting glucose: Fasting plasma glucose 100 to 125 mg/dL

Treatment

- Treatment objective is glycemic control
  - Glycemic control reduces long-term microvascular complications (e.g., nephropathy, neuropathy, and retinopathy) in both type 1 and type 2 diabetic patients
  - **Goals for glycemic control (Table 38-3)**
  - **Insulin therapy is necessary for type 1 diabetics**
  - Oral agents and/or insulin therapy may be used in type 2 diabetics
- Insulin therapy
  - Different forms of insulin are characterized by their duration of action (Table 38-4)
  - **Total daily dosage (TDD) of insulin depends on the type of diabetes, diet, exercise, and degree of insulin resistance**
    - Type 1 diabetes: 0.5 units/kg/day
    - Type 2 diabetes: 1 to 2 units/kg/day for patient on only insulin therapy and not on oral agents; daily insulin requirements may be less in patients on insulin-sensitizing agents
  - For both type 1 and type 2 diabetic patients, the insulin regimen should be divided as follows:
    - Determine TDD by multiplying body weight in kilograms by
      - 0.5 to 0.7 units if patient has type 1 diabetes
      - 0.4 to 1 unit (or more) if patient has type 2 diabetes
    - Determine the basal insulin requirement
      - 40% to 50% of TDD
      - Options for administration

38

Continuous subcutaneous insulin infusion (CSII)

Long-acting insulin analogue (glargine or detemir) once daily in the morning or at bedtime

Intermediate (neutral protamine Hagedorn [NPH]) twice a day

- Determine prandial insulin requirement
  - TDD minus basal insulin dose
  - Split to cover meals
    Lispro or aspart: Divide into three injections (prior to breakfast, lunch, and dinner)
    Regular: Divide into two injections (before breakfast and dinner)
    May also give rapid-acting analogues after meals based on carbohydrate amount consumed
- Correction or supplemental insulin
  - Treats hyperglycemia before meals or between meals
  - Corrects hyperglycemia in NPO patient or in patient receiving scheduled nutritional or basal insulin but not eating discrete meals
  - Sliding scale correction dose based on preprandial blood sugar
    1 unit per 50 mg/dL increment over 180 mg/dL (type 1)
    1 unit per 30 mg/dL increment over 180 mg/dL (type 2)
- Insulin is the preferable first-line therapy in certain clinical situations
  - Pregnancy: Only insulin is approved for use in pregnancy
  - Polyuria/polydipsia: Indicates severe hyperglycemia that should be rapidly reversed with insulin therapy
  - Ketosis: Indicates insulinopenia
  - LADA
    - Suspect in lean individuals presenting in middle age who do not respond to oral agents
    - These individuals are really type 1 diabetics presenting later in life and require insulin therapy
    - Insulin antibodies (antiglutamic acid decarboxylase and anti-islet cell) may be positive within the first year of diagnosis
- Oral antihyperglycemic agents
  - Classes of oral agents (Table 38-5)
  - Multiple factors should be considered in selecting initial oral hypoglycemic agents for patients with type 2 diabetes (Fig. 38-3 gives suggested algorithm)
  - Degree of reduction needed in glycosylated hemoglobin A$_{1c}$ (HbA$_{1c}$) and/or fasting blood glucose
    - Sulfonlyureas, biguanides (metformin), and thiazolidinediones all lower HbA$_{1c}$ 1 to 2 percentage points on average when used as monotherapy
    - Agents targeted at reducing postprandial hyperglycemia, meglitinides, α-glucosidase inhibitors, and dipeptidyl peptidase-4 (DPP-4) inhibitors are less potent, lowering HbA$_{1c}$ 0.5 to 1 percentage point when used as monotherapy
  - Body habitus and estimated degree of insulin resistance
    - In obese individuals, insulin resistance is very likely. Thus, an insulin sensitizer (metformin or

thiazolidinediones) would be the preferable therapy. Because thiazolidinediones can be associated with weight gain and edema, they are not generally recommended as the agent of first choice.
- Lean individuals are less likely to be insulin resistant and are more likely to have some β-cell reserve, so a sulfonylurea is a preferable first-line agent
- Contraindications to agents (see Table 38-5)
  - Metformin is contraindicated in renal insufficiency (creatinine $\geq$1.4 mg/dL in women and $\geq$1.5 mg/dL in men), treated congestive heart failure, hypoxemia, hypotension, and binge alcohol use, as these conditions increase the risk of lactic acidosis
- Potential for adverse health risks of hypoglycemia in patients with cerebrovascular or cardiovascular disease
  - Metformin, the thiazolidinediones, acarbose, and sitagliptin do not cause hypoglycemia when used as monotherapy
- Possibility of postprandial hyperglycemia (should be suspected when there is a poor correlation between fasting glucose readings and the HbA$_{1c}$)
  - Agents that target postprandial hyperglycemia are the meglitinides, acarbose, and sitagliptin
- Presence of a coexisting lipid disorder
  - Metformin lowers low-density lipoprotein (LDL) and triglycerides and has no effect on high-density lipoprotein (HDL)
  - Compared with rosiglitazone, pioglitazone resulted in a significant reduction in triglycerides, a greater increase in HDL-cholesterol, a smaller rise in LDL-cholesterol, and a greater increase in LDL particle size
- Subcutaneous noninsulin glucoregulatory hormone replacement
  - The incretins, glucagon-like peptide and glucose-dependent insulinotropic polypeptide, are gut-derived hormones released in response to meals
  - Amylin is a β-cell hormone co-secreted with insulin in response to meals
  - **The incretin mimetic, exenatide, a glucagon-like peptide-1 analogue, and the amylin agonist, pramlintide, both stimulate glucose-dependent insulin release in response to meals, inhibit glucagon release, and slow gastric emptying in patients with type 2 diabetes when administered by subcutaneous injection**
  - Dosages and indications
    - Exenatide
      - Exenatide lowers HbA$_{1c}$ by 0.4% to 1% when added to sulfonylurea, metformin, or combination therapy
      - Indicated for patients with type 2 diabetes who have not attained adequate glycemic control on maximal sulfonylurea, metformin, and combination sulfonylurea and metformin therapy
      - 5 μg subcutaneously twice daily for 1 month and then increase to 10 μg twice daily
    - Pramlintide
      - Pramlintide lowers HbA$_{1c}$ by 0.43% when added to insulin alone or insulin in combination with metformin and sulfonylureas

TABLE 38-5	*Oral Agents for Diabetes Mellitus*		
Therapy	**Mechanism**	**Benefits**	**Precautions**
Metformin	Suppresses hepatic glucose output	No weight gain No hypoglycemia when used as monotherapy	GI side effects: nausea, diarrhea (titrate dose upward slowly to minimize) Contraindicated in renal compromise (Cr ≥ 1.4 in women; Cr ≥ 1.5 in men; Cr clearance ≤ 60) Contraindicated in CHF requiring treatment Discontinuation required before contrast dye studies (may re-start in 48 hr if normal renal function) Increased risk of lactic acidosis Older age: Use over age 80 yr only if Cr clearance normal Avoid excessive alcohol consumption
Thiazolidinediones Rosiglitazone Pioglitazone	Enhance peripheral muscle sensitivity to insulin	↓ C-peptide and insulin levels No hypoglycemia when used as monotherapy	Monitor LFTs at baseline and every 2 mo for first year Contraindicated in active liver disease and/or LFTs > 2.5× upper limit of normal Weight gain (~1–3 kg) Contraindicated in class III/IV CHF Plasma volume expansion (↓ Hct 3–4%) Edema Possible increased MI risk with rosiglitazone
Sulfonylureas Glimepiride Glyburide Glipizide	Increase pancreatic secretion of insulin	Ease of use and familiarity	Weight gain Hypoglycemia Sulfa sensitivity
Metglitinides Repaglinide Nateglinide	Increase pancreatic secretion of insulin	Reduces postprandial hyperglycemia	↓ Compliance due to multiple daily doses with meals Mild hypoglycemia Use cautiously with liver impairment
Acarbose	Delays glucose absorption by inhibition of pancreatic α-amylase and intestinal α-glucoside	No hypoglycemia as monotherapy Reduces postprandial hyperglycemia	GI: Flatulence, cramps, diarrhea Requires multiple dosing with meals Cannot treat hypoglycemia with sucrose
Dipeptidyl peptidase-4 inhibitor Sitagliptin	Inhibits breakdown of endogenous incretins resulting in inhibition of postprandial glucagon release, increased satiety, slowed gastric emptying, and stimulation of glucose-dependent insulin release	No hypoglycemia as monotherapy Reduces postprandial hyperglycemia Weight neutral	Pharyngitis, urinary tract infections, possible pancreatitis; long-term safety not established

CHF, congestive heart failure; Cr, creatinine; Hct, hematocrit; LFTs, liver function tests; MI, myocardial infarction.
Adapted from Ratner R: *Clinical endocrinology update 1999 syllabus.* Chevy Chase, Md., Endocrine Society, 1999.

38

- Indicated for use in patients with type 1 or type 2 diabetes who have not achieved adequate glycemic control on insulin therapy
- Dosage for type 1 diabetes: 2.5 units (15 μg) to initiate, then increase dose by 2.5 units every 3 days to a maximum dose of 10 units (60 μg); given subcutaneously twice a day before meals
- Dosage for type 2 diabetes: 10 units (60 μg) to initiate, then increase dose by 2.5 units every 3 days to a maximum dose of 20 units (120 μg); given subcutaneously twice a day before meals
- Mealtime insulin should be decreased by 50% to prevent severe hypoglycemia
- Both therapies are associated with nausea and vomiting and are contraindicated in patients with gastroparesis; exenatide may be associated with pancreatitis
- Combination therapy (see Fig. 38-3)
  - Combination therapy (using multiple modalities) is often required even at an early stage to achieve near normoglycemia
    - Combination oral agents
      - Metformin + sulfonylurea
      - Metformin + thiazolidinedione
        Metformin + sitagliptin
        Sitagliptin + sulfonylurea
        Sitagliptin + thiazolidinedione

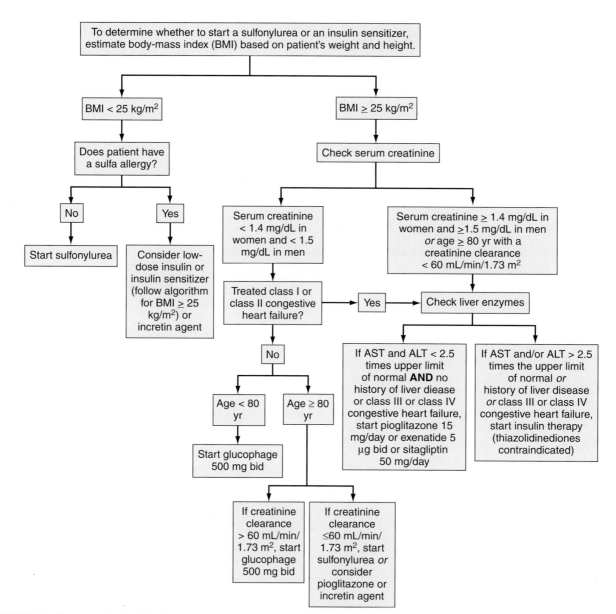

FIGURE 38-3 A suggested algorithm for initiating oral therapy in type 2 diabetes. ALT, alanine transaminase; AST, aspartate transaminase; bid, twice daily; BMI, body-mass index. (From Golden SH: Treatment of the metabolic syndrome. In *Clinical endocrinology update,* 2004 Syllabus, October 3–6, Baltimore, Md., p. 42. Chevy Chase, MD, Endocrine Society Press, 2004, adapted with permission from the Endocrine Society.)

- Monotherapy fails because of multiple factors
  - Decreasing β-cell function
  - Obesity
  - Noncompliance with treatment
  - Lack of exercise
  - Intercurrent illness
- Oral agents can be combined and/or used with insulin therapy to improve glycemic control
  - Methods of adding insulin to an established oral regimen
    - NPH or lantus insulin at bedtime
    - 70/30 or 75/25 insulin at evening meal
    - Dose based on weight and blood glucose, but most patients start with 8 to 10 units/day

- Method of adding oral agents to an established insulin therapy
  - Continue current insulin dosage initially, then decrease the dose by 15% to 25% if hypoglycemia develops or the fasting blood glucose levels are less than 100 mg/dL
- Exenatide can be added to oral therapy with metformin and/or sulfonylureas in type 2 diabetes
- Pramlintide can be added to insulin therapy in type 1 diabetes and to insulin therapy alone or insulin therapy in combination with sulfonylureas and/or metformin in type 2 diabetes
- Treatment of diabetic ketoacidosis and nonketotic hypertonicity (see Table 38-2)

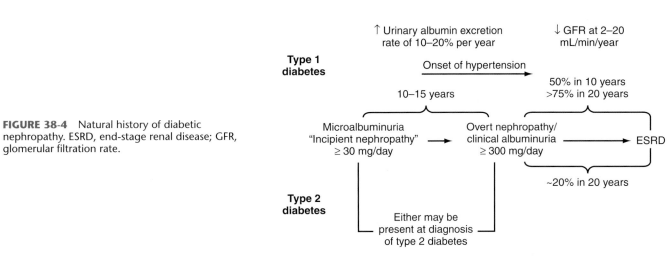

FIGURE 38-4 Natural history of diabetic nephropathy. ESRD, end-stage renal disease; GFR, glomerular filtration rate.

Diabetic Nephropathy

Basic Information

- 20% to 30% of patients with type 1 or type 2 diabetes develop evidence of nephropathy but a smaller fraction progress to end-stage renal disease (ESRD) in type 2 diabetes
- Native Americans, Mexican Americans, and African Americans have higher risk of developing ESRD than do white individuals
- Natural history is summarized in Figure 38-4

Clinical Presentation

- Patients usually asymptomatic until late in course
- Characterized by proteinuria and rising creatinine

Diagnosis and Evaluation

- Urine microalbumin measurement should be performed annually to screen for diabetic nephropathy after 5 years of disease duration in patients with type 1 diabetes and at diagnosis in patients with type 2 diabetes
  - See Table 38-6 for a definition of microalbuminuria; two of three specimens collected within a 3- to 6-month period should be abnormal before confirming the diagnosis
  - **Factors that may increase urinary albumin excretion over baseline values: Exercise within 24 hours, fever, infection, congestive heart failure, marked hyperglycemia, marked hypertension, pyuria, hematuria**
  - If initial screening tests are negative, patients should undergo annual screen; whether to continue annual screening after microalbuminuria has been diagnosed and appropriately treated is less clear

Treatment

- Pharmacologic therapy
  - Use of angiotensin-converting enzyme (ACE) inhibitors is recommended for all hypertensive and nonhypertensive patients with type 1 diabetes and microalbuminuria or clinical albuminuria
  - Angiotensin II receptor blockers (ARBs) are the agents of first choice in hypertensive type 2 diabetic patients with microalbuminuria or clinical albuminuria

TABLE 38-6	Definition of Microalbuminuria
Category	**Spot Collection (μg/mg creatinine)**
Normal	<30
Microalbuminuria	30–299
Clinical albuminuria	≥300

  - Aggressive treatment of hypertension with goal blood pressure of less than 130/80 mm Hg
  - β-Blockers and diuretics are alternatives if ACE inhibitors or ARBs not tolerated or contraindicated
  - Non-dihydropyridine calcium channel-blockers should be used as second-line agents
- Behavioral therapy
  - Sodium restriction: Approximately 2000 mg/day
  - Weight loss, moderately intense physical activity (30–45 minutes of brisk walking daily), smoking cessation, moderation of alcohol consumption

Diabetic Retinopathy

Basic Information

- Diabetic retinopathy is the leading cause of blindness in adults aged 20 to 74 years, and its presence is strongly related to the duration of diabetes
- Factors that increase the risk of retinopathy
  - Hyperglycemia
  - Presence of nephropathy
  - High blood pressure
  - Pregnancy in patients with type 1 diabetes

Clinical Presentation

- Classification of diabetic retinopathy (Table 38-7; Fig. 38-5)
- Usually asymptomatic unless vitreous hemorrhage occurs (causing visual loss)

Diagnosis and Evaluation

- Ophthalmologic evaluation should be performed starting 5 years after diagnosis of type 1 diabetes and on initial diagnosis of type 2 diabetes (Table 38-8)

38

TABLE 38-7	*Definition of Diabetic Retinopathy*
Nonproliferative	Microaneurysms, increased vascular permeability
Preproliferative	Soft exudates representing ischemic infarcts to the retina (cotton wool spots), beading of retinal veins, tortuosity of retinal capillaries
Proliferative	Neovascularization (fibrous contraction from previous hemorrhage may lead to retinal detachment)
Rubeosis	Neovascularization of the iris
Macular edema	Suspect if hard exudates in proximity of macula

TABLE 38-8	*Ophthalmologic Examination Schedule*	
Patient Group	**Recommended First Examination**	**Minimum Routine Follow-Up**
≤29 yr	Within 3–5 yr after diagnosis once patient ≥ 10 yr of age	Yearly
≥30 yr	At diagnosis	Yearly
Pregnancy in patient with pre-existing diabetes	Before conception and 1st trimester	Physician discretion after 1st trimester

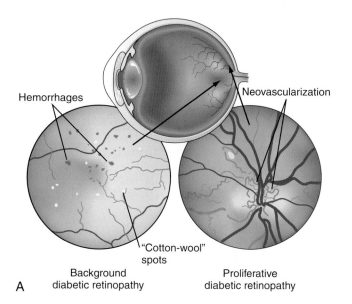

A

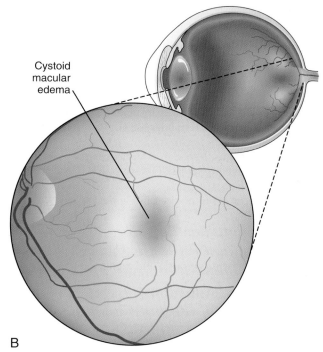

B

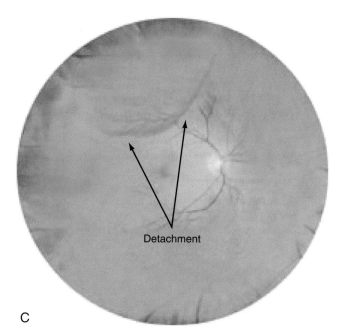

C

FIGURE 38-5 **A,** Background and proliferative diabetic retinopathy. **B,** Cystoid macular edema. **C,** Retinal detachment.

- Continue annual screening unless retinopathy warrants more intense follow-up
- Less frequent exams (every 2–3 years) can be considered in those with several normal eye exams

Treatment

- Laser photocoagulation therapy to prevent visual loss
  - Panretinal/scatter photocoagulation therapy is treatment to reduce risk of visual loss in patients with high-risk characteristics (neovascularization or vitreous hemorrhage with any retinal neovascularization) and in older-onset patients with severe nonproliferative diabetic retinopathy or less than high-risk proliferative diabetic retinopathy
  - Focal laser photocoagulation surgery for eyes with clinically significant macular edema

Diabetic Neuropathy and Diabetic Foot Disease

- Diabetic neuropathy can take many different forms
- Useful classification
  - Generalized symmetrical polyneuropathies: Acute sensory, chronic sensorimotor
  - Focal and multifocal neuropathies: Cranial, truncal, focal limb, proximal motor (amyotrophy), coexisting chronic inflammatory demyelinating polyneuropathy (CIDP)
  - Autonomic: Cardiac, gastrointestinal, genitourinary
- Chronic sensorimotor distal symmetrical polyneuropathy (DPN) and diabetic autonomic neuropathy (DAN) are the two most common neuropathies
- DPN
  - Up to 50% of DPN cases may be asymptomatic, increasing the patient's risk of insensate foot injuries, which can ultimately lead to ulcers and amputations
  - About 50% of patients have symptoms: Burning pain, electrical or stabbing sensations, paresthesias, hyperesthesia, deep aching pain occurring in the feet and lower limbs; symptoms worse at night
  - Diabetic ulcer (Fig. 38-6)
  - Patients at increased risk for ulcers and amputations
    - Duration of diabetes of 10 years or more
    - Male
    - Poor glucose control
    - Cardiovascular, retinal, or renal complications
    - Peripheral neuropathy with loss of protective sensation
    - Altered foot biomechanics, bony deformity
    - Presence of peripheral vascular disease
    - History of ulcers or amputation
    - Severe nail pathology
  - Diagnosis
    - Careful clinical exam with annual screening by examining pinprick, temperature, and vibration perception (using 128-Hz tuning fork), 10-g monofilament pressure sensation at distal halluces, and ankle reflexes
    - Examination in DPN shows loss of vibration, pressure, pain, and temperature sensation, and absent reflexes

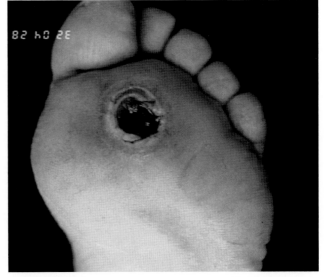

FIGURE 38-6 Stage 3 ulcer beneath second metatarsal head that extends into metatarsal head with presumptive contiguous osteomyelitis. (From Canale ST: *Campbell's operative orthopedics,* ed 10, St. Louis, Mosby, 2003, figure 82-2.)

- Signs of peripheral autonomic (sympathetic) dysfunction: Warm or cold feet, distended dorsal foot veins (in absence of peripheral arterial disease), dry skin, calluses in pressure-bearing areas
- Examine feet for ulcers, calluses, and deformities, and inspect footwear
- **Rule out other forms of neuropathy: CIDP, B_{12} deficiency, hypothyroidism, uremia (check B_{12}, thyroid function, blood urea nitrogen [BUN], and creatinine)**
- Treatment
  - Optimization of blood sugar control and avoiding extreme blood sugar fluctuations
  - Pharmacologic treatment
    - Tricyclic antidepressant drugs: Amitriptyline, imipramine; use limited by anticholinergic side effects, including fatigue and drowsiness
    - Selective serotonin re-uptake inhibitors: Paroxetine, citalopram
    - Anticonvulsants: Gabapentin, pregabalin, carbamazepine, topiramate; use limited by drowsiness
    - Opioid or opioid-like drugs: Tramadol, oxycodone CR
    - 5-hydroxytryptamine and norepinephrine uptake inhibitor: Duloxetine
    - Substance P inhibitor: Capsaicin cream
  - Podiatry referral to reduce the risk of foot ulcers
- Acute sensory neuropathy
  - Follows periods of poor metabolic control or sudden changes in glycemic control ("insulin neuritis")
  - Acute onset of severe sensory symptoms with marked nocturnal exacerbation
  - Few neurologic signs on exam
- Mononeuropathies
  - Focal nerves involved

38

- Percent of all diabetic neuropathies
  - Median (5.8%), ulnar (2.1%), radial (0.6%), common peroneal
  - Cranial (0.05%) III, IV, VI, and VII—usually resolve spontaneously
  - Entrapments: Median, ulnar, peroneal, medial plantar
  - Spinal stenosis
  - Diagnosis: Electrophysiologic studies useful in identifying conduction blocks at entrapment sites
- Diabetic amyotrophy
  - Occurs in older patients with type 2 diabetes
  - Severe neuropathic pain, unilateral or bilateral muscle weakness, atrophy in proximal thigh muscles
  - Diagnosis: Needs to be distinguished from CIPD and spinal stenosis; CIPD presents with progressive symmetrical or asymmetrical motor deficits, progressive sensory neuropathy despite optimal glucose control, and elevated cerebrospinal fluid protein
- DAN
  - Cardiovascular autonomic neuropathy (CAN)
    - Associated with morbidity and increased mortality
      - Limits exercise capacity and increases risk of adverse cardiovascular event during exercise
      - **May lead to sudden death or silent cardiac ischemia**
    - Presentation: Resting tachycardia (heart rate >100 beats/min), exercise intolerance, orthostatic hypotension (fall in systolic blood pressure > 20 mm Hg on standing)
    - Diagnosis: Three useful tests
      - R-R variation on electrocardiogram (ECG)
      - Valsalva maneuver
      - Postural blood pressure testing
    - Treatment of CAN
      - Graded supervised exercise, ACE inhibitors, and β-blockers for exercise intolerance
      - Mechanical measures, clonidine, midodrine, octreotide to treat postural hypotension
  - Gastrointestinal autonomic neuropathy
    - Presentation: Constipation (may alternate with diarrhea), gastroparesis, esophageal enteropathy, fecal incontinence; consider especially in individuals with erratic glucose control
    - Diagnosis: Evaluation with gastric emptying study, barium swallow, or referral for endoscopy
    - Treatment
      - Treat gastroparesis with frequent small meals and prokinetic agents (metoclopramide, domperidone, erythromycin)
      - Abdominal pain, early satiety, nausea, vomiting, and bloating treated with multiple approaches: Antibiotics, antiemetics, bulking agents, tricyclic antidepressants, pancreatic extracts, pyloric Botox, gastric pacing, enteral feeding
      - Constipation: High-fiber diet and bulking agents, osmotic laxatives, lubricating agents; prokinetics should be used with caution
      - Diarrhea: Soluble fiber, gluten and lactose restriction, anticholinergic agents, cholestyramine, antibiotics, clonidine, somatostatin, pancreatic enzyme supplements

- Genitourinary autonomic neuropathy
  - Presentation: Erectile dysfunction, retrograde ejaculation, bladder dysfunction (recurrent urinary tract infections, pyelonephritis, incontinence, palpable bladder)
  - Diagnosis: Medical and sexual history, psychological evaluation, measurement of hormone levels, measurement of nocturnal penile tumescence, assessment of penile, pelvic, and spinal nerve function; cardiovascular autonomic function tests; and measurement of penile and brachial blood pressure
  - Treatment
    - Erectile dysfunction: Sex therapy, psychological counseling, sildenafil, vardenafil, tadalafil, prostaglandin E_1 injection, device, or prosthesis
    - Bladder dysfunction/urinary retention and incontinence: Bethanechol, intermittent catheterization

Cardiovascular Disease

Basic Information

- Atherosclerosis accounts for approximately 80% of all diabetic mortality (75% from coronary atherosclerosis and 25% from cerebral or peripheral vascular disease) and more than 75% of all hospitalizations for diabetic complications
- More than 50% of patients with newly diagnosed type 2 diabetes already have coronary heart disease

Clinical Presentation

- Coronary artery disease may present with chest pain and/or silent ischemia
- Peripheral arterial disease may present with claudication or nonhealing extremity ulcers
- Cerebrovascular disease may present as transient ischemic attacks or stroke. Carotid bruits on physical exam may indicate underlying cerebrovascular disease.

Diagnosis and Evaluation

- Annual screening for dyslipidemia and hypertension
- **Recommended diabetic populations to undergo screening with an exercise stress test**
  - Symptomatic
    - Typical or atypical cardiac symptoms
    - Abnormal resting ECG
  - Asymptomatic
    - History of peripheral or carotid occlusive disease
    - Sedentary lifestyle, age older than 35 years, and plans to begin a vigorous exercise program

Treatment

- Aggressive management of hypertension and dyslipidemia, smoking cessation, and aspirin prophylaxis
- Blood pressure targets in patients with diabetes (see earlier section on diabetic nephropathy)

TABLE 38-9	*Cholesterol Targets in Patients with Diabetes*			
	MEDICAL NUTRITION TREATMENT		**DRUG TREATMENT**	
Status	**Initiation Level**	**LDL Goal**	**Initiation Level**	**LDL Goal**
With CHD, PVD, or CVD	>100 mg/dL	≤100 mg/dL	>100 mg/dL	≤100 mg/dL
Without CHD, PVD, or CVD	>100 mg/dL	≤100 mg/dL	≥130 mg/dL	≤100 mg/dL

CHD, coronary heart disease; CVD, cerebrovascular disease; LDL, low-density lipoprotein; PVD, peripheral vascular disease.

- Lipid targets in individuals with diabetes (Table 38-9)
- In individuals with a prior history of cardiovascular disease (coronary heart, cerebrovascular, or peripheral arterial disease), treat with statin to achieve LDL reduction of 30% to 40%, regardless of baseline LDL, a lower LDL goal of below 70 mg/dL using high-dose statin is also an option.
- In individuals without a history of cardiovascular disease who are older than 40 years, treat with statin to achieve 30% to 40% reduction in LDL regardless of baseline LDL
- Treatment options for dyslipidemia; see Chapter 3

REVIEW QUESTIONS

For review questions, please go to www.expertconsult.com.

SUGGESTED READINGS

American Diabetes Association: Diagnosis and classification of diabetes mellitus, *Diabetes Care* 32(Suppl 1):S62–S67, 2009.

American Diabetes Association: Standards of medical care in diabetes, *Diabetes Care* 32(Suppl 1):S13–S61, 2009.

Boulton AJM, Vinik AI, Arezzo JC, et al: Diabetic neuropathies, *Diabetes Care* 28:956–962, 2005.

Efendic S, Portwood N: Overview of incretin hormones, *Horm Metab Res* 36:742–46, 2004.

Kimmel B, Inzucchi SE: Oral agents for type 2 diabetes: an update, *Clin Diabetes* 23:64–76, 2005.

Nathan DM, Buse JB, Davidson MB, et al: Medical management of hyperglycemia in type 2 diabetes: a consensus algorithm for the initiation and adjustment of therapy, *Diabetes Care* 32:193–203, 2009.

Yki-Jarvinen H: Thiazolidinediones, *N Engl J Med* 351:1106–1118, 2004.

38

Thyroid Disease

DAVID S. COOPER, MD

Thyroid disorders can be classified into two categories: thyroid dysfunction (hyperthyroidism and hypothyroidism, which are generally autoimmune in etiology) and anatomic abnormalities such as goiter, nodules, and cancer. These problems often occur together in the same patient. In addition, they are extremely common, occurring in up to 10% of adults and 20% of women over age 65.

Thyroid Function Testing

- Many of the symptoms and signs of thyroid dysfunction are nonspecific; laboratory testing is an important part of the assessment (Table 39-1)

- Most common tests: thyroid-stimulating hormone (TSH), free thyroxine (T_4), and triiodothyronine (T_3); TSH is the most useful starting point (Fig. 39-1)
- Thyroid function tests in nonthyroidal illness (NTI)
  - Results in numerous changes in thyroid hormone metabolism and protein binding
  - The serum TSH may be low or normal in severely ill patients
    - Low values are caused by medications that are used in the intensive care unit that decrease pituitary TSH secretion, such as high doses of glucocorticoids and dopamine, as well as suppressive effects of endogenous cytokines, such as tumor necrosis factor

TABLE 39-1	**Thyroid Function Tests**	
Test	**Use**	**Comments**
Thyroid-stimulating hormone (TSH)	Produced by pituitary; stimulates thyroid to produce T_3 and T_4 (which feedback on pituitary) ↑ Suggests hypothyroidism ↓ Suggests hyperthyroidism	Very sensitive; normal TSH effectively excludes disease in asymptomatic patients Exceptions: Patients with severe nonthyroidal illness (NTI), patients on dopamine or high-dose glucocorticoids TSH will be low in central hypothyroidism
Total thyroxine (T_4) and triiodothyronine (T_3)	Helpful to quantitate the degree of hormone deficiency or excess T_3 is active form in tissues T_4 is converted to T_3 in thyroid and peripherally >99% bound to TBG Free fraction (<1%) determines biologic action	Routine assays measure the total levels; need to take into account TBG status

Thyroid-binding globulin (TBG)	Binds T_4 and T_3	Causes of ↑ TBG
		  Drugs (estrogen, oral contraceptives, tamoxifen, heroin, methadone, 5-fluorouracil)
		  Pregnancy
		  Acute hepatitis
		  Congenital
		  Acute intermittent porphyria
		Causes of ↓ TBG
		  Drugs (androgens, glucocorticoids, slow-release nicotinic acid)
		  Severe illness or malnutrition
		  Chronic liver disease
		  Protein-losing states (e.g., nephritic syndrome)
		  Congenital

T_3 resin uptake (T_3RU)	An indirect measure of the binding capacity of patient's serum proteins (measures unoccupied T_4-binding sites) Used in conjunction with serum T_4	↑ T_3RU: Hyperthyroidism, low TBG states ↓ T_3RU: Hypothyroidism, high TBG states
Free thyroxine index (FTI)	Product of serum T_4 and T_3 resin uptake Corrects for changes in binding protein concentration	Highly correlated with free T_4
Free T_4 (fT_4)	Direct measurement of free hormone; bypasses interfering effects of disease or drugs on TBG levels	Preferable over FTI

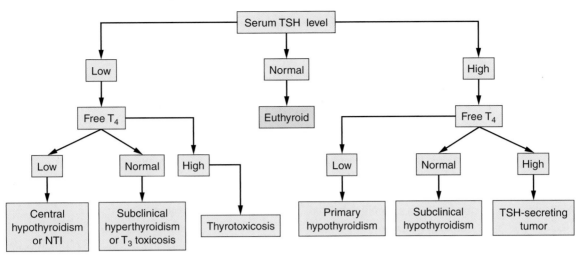

FIGURE 39-1 Sequential thyroid function testing using the serum thyroid-stimulating hormone (TSH) as a starting point. This strategy is useful in asymptomatic individuals. If symptoms are present, both the free thyroxine (T_4) and TSH should be assessed. NTI, nonthyroidal illness; T_3, triiodothyronine.

- High TSH values are typically seen in the recovery phase of illness, although the levels usually do not rise above 20 mU/L
  - **Therefore, the diagnosis of thyroid disease can be quite difficult in acutely ill individuals**
  - If the TSH is normal, the patient is probably euthyroid
  - If the TSH is increased and the patient is not recovering from an illness, hypothyroidism can be diagnosed
  - If the TSH is low, as occurs in up to 20% of hospitalized patients, the diagnosis of hyperthyroidism should not be made in the absence of supporting clinical and laboratory data

Thyrotoxicosis

Basic Information

- Definition: Thyrotoxicosis is a state of increased tissue exposure to elevated circulating thyroid hormone concentrations; it is a syndrome, not a diagnosis
- It is very common; lifetime prevalence is approximately 2% in women, 0.2% in men
- *Thyrotoxicosis* **is the term used to refer to all conditions associated with increased serum levels of thyroid hormone, regardless of the cause**
- *Hyperthyroidism* **usually refers to those diseases in which the thyroid gland is actually synthesizing and secreting excessive thyroid hormones**
- Etiology
  - **Graves' disease and toxic multinodular goiter probably account for more than 90% of all hyperthyroidism cases**
  - See Table 39-2 for other causes
- *Subclinical hyperthyroidism* refers to a state of mild thyroid overactivity in which the serum TSH levels are low (subnormal to undetectable) but the levels of free T_4 and T_3 are normal
- A low TSH and normal free T_4 are seen physiologically at the end of the first trimester of pregnancy as a result of increased placental secretion of human chorionic gonadotropin, which stimulates the thyroid

Clinical Presentation

- General symptoms and signs (Table 39-3; Figs. 39-2 and 39-3)
  - Reflect an increased metabolic rate and augmentation of adrenergic activity
  - Manifestations of thyrotoxicosis are quite variable and do not necessarily correlate with circulating thyroid hormone concentrations
    - Elderly patients may have few symptoms or may only present with weight loss or atrial fibrillation
    - **"Apathetic thyrotoxicosis": No signs of thyrotoxicosis except for weight loss and depression in elderly persons**
- Most patients with subclinical hyperthyroidism are asymptomatic

Diagnosis and Evaluation

- Often suspected from history and physical
- Drugs such as amiodarone and interferon-α can cause hyperthyroidism
- Thyroid examination (see Table 39-2)
- Laboratory studies
  - Low TSH (negative feedback with pituitary); usually undetectable (<0.1 mU/L)
    - Rare exception: Patients with TSH-secreting pituitary tumors, in whom the TSH levels are increased or are inappropriately normal in the face of elevations of serum free T_4
  - Increased free T_4 or free T_4 index
  - Subclinical hyperthyroidism: A low TSH with normal levels of free T_4 and T_3
  - Measurement of serum T_3 is also helpful because it can be increased in about 5% of patients with hyperthyroidism when the levels of T_4 are still normal (T_3 thyrotoxicosis)
  - In Graves' disease, serum T_3:T_4 ratio is increased because thyroid secretes relatively more T_3 than T_4

39

TABLE 39-2	Causes of Thyrotoxicosis		
Etiology	**Mechanism**	**Thyroid Examination**	**Radioiodine Uptake**
Graves' disease	Stimulatory anti-TSH receptor antibodies May be induced by interferon-α	Diffuse goiter	↑
Toxic multinodular goiter or solitary nodule	Activating gene mutations	Nodule(s)	↑
Thyroiditis	Follicular destruction causing release of stored hormone; viral (subacute), autoimmune ("silent" or postpartum), or drug-induced (amiodarone)	Tender goiter in subacute; nontender goiter in "silent"	↓
Iodine-induced	Iodine surplus (IV dye or amiodarone-induced thyrotoxicosis type 1)	Nodular or diffuse goiter	↓
Choriocarcinoma	Secretes hCG, a thyroid stimulator	Minimal goiter	↑
Pituitary tumor	TSH overproduction	Minimal goiter	↑
Struma ovarii	Ectopic thyroid tissue in ovarian tumor	Normal	↓ (over thyroid)
Exogenous thyrotoxicosis Iatrogenic Factitious	Oversupplementation of thyroxine Surreptitious ingestion of thyroxine	Normal in both	↓

hCG, human chorionic gonadotropin; TSH, thyroid-stimulating hormone.

TABLE 39-3	Clinical Manifestations of Thyrotoxicosis
Organ System	**Symptoms and Signs**
Constitutional	Weight loss, heat intolerance
Cardiovascular	Palpitations, atrial arrhythmias, congestive heart failure, systolic hypertension
Respiratory	Dyspnea
Gastrointestinal	Hyperdefecation, increased appetite, nausea
Musculoskeletal	Proximal muscle weakness, osteopenia, hypercalciuria, hypercalcemia, extraocular muscle weakness,* myasthenia gravis*
Neuropsychiatric	Nervousness, anxiety, tremor, insomnia, impaired mentation, delirium, psychosis
Endocrine	Hypomenorrhea, amenorrhea, gynecomastia, decreased libido
Hematologic	Splenomegaly,* enlarged thymus,* lymphadenopathy, neutropenia*
Ophthalmologic	Stare, lid lag,* proptosis,* diplopia,* visual loss*
Dermatologic	Warm, moist, velvety skin, palmar erythema, onycholysis, thinning hair, pruritus, hives, pretibial myxedema,* vitiligo,* thyroid acropachy*

* Denotes findings only seen in Graves' disease.

compared with the euthyroid state; in various forms of thyroiditis, $T_3:T_4$ ratio is normal
- In Graves' disease, circulating antibodies may be present but are not necessary for diagnosis
  - Thyroid-stimulating antibodies, or TSAbs, stimulate the TSH receptor
  - May be helpful to measure in pregnancy and in euthyroid patients with Graves' eye disease

- Other antibodies: antithyroperoxidase (antiTPO) antibodies and antithyroglobulin antibodies (together called *antithyroid antibodies*)
- 24-hour radioiodine uptake test
  - Should not be used as a thyroid function test (can also be increased in hypothyroid patients)
  - **Uptake will be high in Graves' disease**
  - **Uptake will be low in diseases associated with excessive release of thyroid hormone, but not increased synthesis, as in all forms of thyroiditis (see Table 39-2)**

Treatment

- Treatment of thyrotoxicosis due to Graves' disease
  - No ideal treatment for Graves' disease: Antithyroid drugs, radioiodine, and surgery are all effective and have specific advantages and disadvantages (Table 39-4)
  - **β-Adrenergic blocking agents**
    - **Used to control symptoms of palpitations, tremor, heat intolerance, and nervousness**
    - **Will not alleviate some symptoms (weight loss, myopathy) and are not considered to be a primary mode of therapy**
    - Best to use a long-acting agent that is cardioselective
  - **Antithyroid drugs**
    - **Methimazole (Tapazole) and propylthiouracil (PTU)**
    - **Act primarily to diminish thyroid hormone synthesis by interfering with the intrathyroidal use of iodine**
      - PTU also inhibits peripheral conversion of T_4 to T_3
      - Methimazole is the drug of choice
    - Typical starting doses: Methimazole 10 to 30 mg/day as a single daily dose; PTU 100 mg three times a day
    - Remission rate less than 50%
    - Best used as primary therapy in patients with relatively mild disease (highest likelihood of remission when the drug is discontinued)

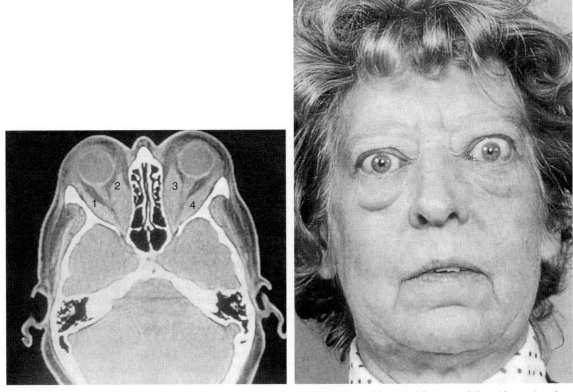

FIGURE 39-2   A, CT scan of orbits showing enlarged extraocular muscles. **B,** Patient with typical features of thyroid-associated ophthalmopathy showing lid retraction, exophthalmos, and periorbital edema. Patients may also have diplopia and strabismus due to edema and fibrosis of the extraocular muscles. (From Souhami R: *Textbook of medicine,* New York, Churchill Livingstone, 2002, figure 17.23B.)

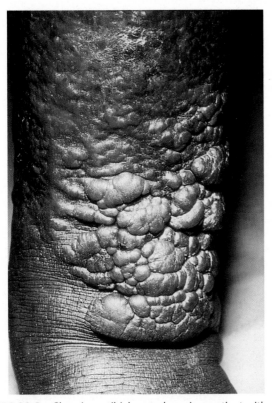

FIGURE 39-3   Chronic pretibial myxedema in a patient with Graves' disease and orbitopathy. The lesions are firm and nonpitting, with a clear edge to feel. (From Larsen PR, Kronenberg HM, Melmed S, Polonsky, KS: *Williams' textbook of endocrinology,* ed 10, Philadelphia, WB Saunders, 2003, figure 82-2.)

TABLE 39-4	Drugs Used in the Management of Thyroid Storm	
Drug	**Dose**	**Comments**
Propylthiouracil	200–400 mg every 4–6 hr	Must be given PO (or rectally)
Methimazole	30–80 mg/day	Must be given PO (or rectally)
Propranolol	PO: 20–100 mg every 4 hr	The very short-acting agent esmolol may be used
Hydrocortisone	100 mg every 6–8 hr or equivalent	"Stress doses"— unclear whether use affects outcome
Potassium iodide (SSKI)	3–5 drops 3 times daily	Blocks release of thyroid hormone

- Dose is adjusted to maintain serum free T$_4$ and T$_3$ levels within the normal range
- Usually takes 4 to 12 weeks to achieve euthyroid state
- Serum TSH may remain suppressed for 2 to 3 months after the patient has become euthyroid because of the chronic suppressive effects of the previous hyperthyroidism
- Usually treat for 1 to 2 years, then taper or discontinue to see whether a remission has been

39

achieved; if TSAbs are still positive at this point, remission is unlikely

- **If remission achieved, lifelong follow-up is required because remissions are not necessarily permanent and spontaneous hypothyroidism can also develop many years later**
- Relapse typically occurs in the first 6 months; another course of drug therapy can be undertaken, or the patient may opt for definitive therapy with radioiodine
- Common side effects: Rashes, fever, arthralgias, transient leukopenia
- **Major drug reaction is reversible agranulocytosis**
  - Develops in 0.2% to 0.3% of patients
  - Almost always within 90 days of starting the medication
- Liver damage and antineutrophil cytoplasmic antibody-positive vasculitis are very rare adverse effects, especially with PTU
- PTU is preferred in pregnancy, as it does not cause rare congenital anomalies
- **Radioiodine**
  - Radioactive iodine (^{131}I) is the treatment most often used in the United States
  - **Approximately 80% of patients will be cured after a single dose; overall cure rate is greater than 95%**
  - **Works slowly; euthyroid state may not be achieved for 3 to 6 months**
  - May be a transient worsening of thyroid function resulting from radiation-related thyroiditis or an increase in TsAb resulting from thyroid injury
    - May need to pretreat elderly patients or those with cardiac disease with antithyroid drugs, which will theoretically deplete the thyroid of hormonal stores
    - Should be stopped 3 to 7 days prior to therapy
  - **Hypothyroidism is almost inevitable after radioiodine**
  - No immediate side effects and no evidence of long-term sequelae, such as infertility, birth defects, cancer, or other neoplasms either in patients or their offspring
  - Only contraindication is pregnancy
  - Severe thyroid eye disease is a relative contraindication because radioiodine can exacerbate it; radioiodine can be given with concomitant glucocorticoid therapy to prevent worsening of the ophthalmopathy
- Surgery
  - Rarely used to treat Graves' disease in the United States
  - Cure rate greater than 95%
  - Reserved for patients who are allergic to antithyroid drugs, who refuse or cannot take radioiodine (e.g., in pregnancy), patients with a concomitant malignant or suspicious nodule, or patients with very large goiters, who generally have lower success rates with radioiodine
  - Complications may include: Recurrent laryngeal nerve damage, hypoparathyroidism
- Treatment of Graves' ophthalmopathy

- Local symptoms (irritation, tearing, photophobia) can be managed with artificial tears and lubricating eye ointments
- Ophthalmology consultation for severe degrees of inflammation, diplopia, severe proptosis leading to corneal exposure, or decreased visual acuity
  - May require high-dose glucocorticoids, retro-orbital radiotherapy, and/or surgical decompression of the orbits
- **Radioiodine may exacerbate ophthalmopathy if severe, especially in patients who smoke**
- Treatment of thyroid storm
  - Represents a rare, exaggerated, or accelerated form of hyperthyroidism
  - **Classic definition of thyroid storm includes fever, severe tachycardia or atrial fibrillation, and altered mental status (agitation, delirium, coma)**
  - Is usually precipitated by a stress (e.g., surgery, infection, childbirth) in a patient with poorly controlled hyperthyroidism
  - Drugs used in thyroid storm treatment (see Table 39-4)
    - **Antithyroid drugs are the mainstay and should be started at least several hours before iodine or iodine-containing drugs are given**
    - **PTU may be preferred because of its inhibitory effects on T_4 to T_3 conversion**
  - Supportive measures
    - Attention to fluid and electrolyte balance
    - Search for an underlying cause (e.g., occult infection)
    - Sedatives for agitation
    - Cooling blankets and acetaminophen for fever (aspirin should not be used because it binds to thyroid-binding globulin and can displace T_4, causing the free T_4 to rise)
- **Treatment of toxic multinodular goiter (Plummer's disease) and solitary toxic nodules**
  - These entities are less frequent than Graves' disease, but they make up a higher proportion of hyperthyroidism in older individuals
  - Little chance for spontaneous remission
  - Antithyroid agents have little role in the management except in preparation for definitive therapy with radioiodine or surgery
  - **Radioactive iodine is the treatment of choice**
  - **Surgery is a reasonable therapy, especially in patients with large goiters or nodules and compressive symptoms, such as dysphagia or hoarseness**
- Treatment of subclinical hyperthyroidism
  - In untreated patients, may be related to osteopenia and fractures in postmenopausal women and may be a predisposing factor for atrial fibrillation in individuals over age 60 years
  - Recent guidelines recommend treatment in older patients if TSH less than 0.1 mU/L. It is reasonable to treat women who have osteoporosis or patients who have known heart disease with antithyroid drugs or radioiodine.
  - In untreated patients, periodic follow-up is necessary to monitor for the development of overt hyperthyroidism

Hypothyroidism

Basic Information

- **Definition: A clinical state in which the circulating levels of thyroid hormone are insufficient for normal cellular function**
- Extremely common, especially in women
- Prevalence: Approximately 8% in women and 2% in men, most of which is very mild (subclinical)
- **Primary failure of the thyroid due to autoimmune disease (chronic lymphocytic thyroiditis or Hashimoto's thyroiditis) is the most common cause of hypothyroidism**
  - Patients will usually, but not always, have positive antithyroid antibodies
  - AntiTPO antibodies are more sensitive and specific than antithyroglobulin (AntiTg) antibodies
- Other causes (Box 39-1)
- **Subclinical hypothyroidism**
  - **Refers to a state of mild thyroid dysfunction, in which the serum TSH levels are slightly increased (usually <10 mU/L) and the serum levels of free T_4 and T_3 are normal**
  - Prevalence is up to 15% to 20% in individuals over age 60
  - Causes similar to those of overt hypothyroidism

Clinical Presentation

- Symptoms and signs may be nonspecific and overlap with many other conditions (Table 39-5; Fig. 39-4)
- Development of symptoms depends on the severity of disease, its duration, and individual factors, such as the age of the patient (elderly have fewer symptoms than younger individuals)

- Typical patient notes fatigue, mild constipation, cold intolerance, and mild weight gain
  - A weight gain of more than 5 to 10 pounds cannot be attributed to hypothyroidism
- Myxedema coma
  - Typically occurs in patients with long-standing untreated severe hypothyroidism
  - Often precipitated by stress, such as systemic disease, surgery, and sedative drugs or narcotics; occurs more frequently in the winter months
  - Clinical manifestations: Hypothyroidism with mental status changes, such as lethargy, stupor, or seizures, hypoventilation, and hypothermia
  - Mortality may be as high as 50%; should be treated as a medical emergency

TABLE 39-5	Clinical Manifestations of Hypothyroidism
Organ System	**Symptoms and Signs**
Constitutional	Weight gain, cold intolerance, fatigue, weakness, hypercholesterolemia
Cardiovascular	Bradycardia, decreased contractility, pericardial effusion
Respiratory	Hoarseness, dyspnea, hypoventilation, sleep apnea, pleural effusion
Gastrointestinal	Constipation, ileus, macroglossia
Musculoskeletal	Myalgias, arthralgias, nonpitting edema
Neuropsychiatric	Depression, psychosis, carpal tunnel syndrome, delayed reflex relaxation
Endocrine	Growth failure, menorrhagia, galactorrhea (hyperprolactinemia), precocious puberty
Hematologic	Anemia, platelet defect
Dermatologic	Dry skin, pallor, yellowing of skin (carotinemia)

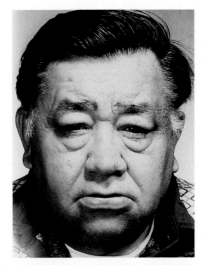

FIGURE 39-4 Advanced hypothyroidism. Note dulled expression, facial puffiness, and periorbital edema. (From Noble J, Green HL, Levinson W, et al: *Textbook of primary care medicine,* ed 3, St. Louis, Mosby, 2001, figure 97-2.)

BOX 39-1	*Causes of Hypothyroidism*

Associated with Goiter

Chronic lymphocytic (Hashimoto's) thyroiditis

Silent (postpartum) thyroiditis (transient)

Subacute thyroiditis (transient)

Iodine deficiency (not seen in North America)

Goitrogenic drugs (lithium, iodine-containing drugs [amiodarone], antithyroid agents, sunitinib [mechanism uncertain])

Congenital biosynthetic enzyme deficiencies

Not Associated with Goiter

Post thyroidectomy

Post ablation for hyperthyroidism

Congenital absence of the thyroid

Atrophic thyroiditis (variant of Hashimoto's thyroiditis)

Following radiation for head and neck tumors

Secondary Hypothyroidism

Pituitary or hypothalamic dysfunction

Peripheral Thyroid Hormone Resistance

Due to defective thyroid hormone receptor

39

Diagnosis and Evaluation

- Laboratory studies
  - **In all forms of hypothyroidism, circulating level of free T_4 will be low**
  - Serum level of T_3 is low as well in severe cases
  - Primary hypothyroidism: Serum level of TSH will be increased (due to the lack of negative feedback inhibition by thyroid hormone on pituitary TSH secretion)
  - Milder cases: TSH may be only slightly increased
  - Severe cases: TSH will be markedly increased (>50 mU/L)
  - Subclinical hypothyroidism: The degree of abnormality is so slight that the free T_4 is still within the broad range of normal, but the TSH level is high (usually 5–10 mU/L)
  - Autoantibodies are not necessary for diagnosis but may be helpful in subclinical hypothyroidism to help predict prognosis (see later discussion)
  - Hypothalamic or pituitary disease
    - The free T_4 is low and the TSH levels are either low or normal
    - Stimulation testing with the hypothalamic TSH secretagogue thyrotropin-releasing hormone (TRH) may show a preserved TSH secretory response in hypothalamic disease, whereas the TSH response to TRH is absent in pituitary disease (TRH is not currently available in the United States)

Treatment

- **Synthetic T_4 is the treatment of choice for all forms of hypothyroidism**
  - **Replacement dose is roughly 1.6 μg/kg/day, which is in the range of 100 to 200 μg/day for the average adult**
  - Treatment can be initiated with the full dose in younger patients
  - Replacement dose is 10% to 15% lower in patients over age 65 years
  - **Should start with lower doses (25–50 μg/day) in elderly patients who may have underlying coronary disease; titrate up the dose gradually**
- **Monitoring therapy with the TSH level**
  - **Goal TSH is between 0.5 and 3 mU/L**
  - **Because of its 7-day half-life, T_4 and TSH blood levels take at least 5 to 6 weeks to reach a steady state**
  - Dose adjustments should be made only every 6 weeks
  - May take weeks or even months for some of the hypothyroid symptoms to resolve
  - Over-replacement, as indicated by a low TSH level, should be avoided (may cause osteopenia in postmenopausal women and may predispose to atrial fibrillation in patients > 65 years of age)
  - In hypothyroidism secondary to pituitary or hypothalamic disease, the TSH level cannot be used as a guide to therapy; in this case, the free T_4 level should be maintained in the high-normal range
- Conditions necessitating thyroxine dose adjustment (Box 39-2)
- Treatment of myxedema coma
  - Standard treatment is T_4 given as a loading dose of 300 to 500 μg IV, followed by daily IV doses of 100 to 150 μg
  - If no improvement in patient's clinical status within 1 to 2 days, consider adding IV T_3 (10 μg every 8 hours)

BOX 39-2	*Clinical Situations in Which Thyroxine Doses May Need Adjustment*

Increased Dose

Pregnancy

Malabsorption

Certain drugs that

    Interfere with absorption (sucralfate, aluminum hydroxide, cholestyramine, colestipol, ferrous sulfate, calcium, raloxifene)

    Accelerate thyroxine metabolism (phenytoin, carbamazepine, phenobarbital, rifampin, sertraline, imatinib [Gleevec])

    Increase TBG (estrogen)

    Block T_4 to T_3 conversion in the pituitary gland (amiodarone)

Decreased Dose

Advanced age

Androgen therapy (decreases TBG)

- Acts more quickly than T_4
- However, may increase myocardial oxygen consumption and precipitate myocardial infarction or arrhythmias
- **Scrupulous attention to the patient's ancillary problems:** Ventilatory support for hypercarbia or hypoxemia, correction of electrolyte abnormalities (especially hyponatremia), and treatment of possible infection; occult infection should be suspected if the patient is normothermic because hypothyroid patients do not mount a normal febrile response
- Sedatives and narcotics are contraindicated because all drugs are metabolized slowly and may have prolonged and unpredictable effects
- Hypoadrenalism
  - Should be suspected in patients with hypothyroidism caused by autoimmune thyroiditis or in central hypothyroidism and in patients with myxedema coma who may have diminished adrenal reserve
  - If adrenal insufficiency is not treated first, administration of T_4 may precipitate an adrenal crisis; therefore, it is reasonable to administer hydrocortisone 100 mg every 8 hours IV for several days with rapid tapering as the clinical picture improves or until adrenal insufficiency can be ruled out with a cortisol determination or adrenocorticotropic hormone (ACTH) stimulation test
- Treatment of subclinical hypothyroidism
  - Treatment is controversial, since patients tend to be relatively asymptomatic
  - High rate of progression to overt hypothyroidism in those patients who have positive antithyroid antibodies (5–10% per year)
  - Some untreated patients with TSH levels less than 10 mU/L can revert to a euthyroid state, especially if they are antithyroid antibody negative
  - Treatment may result in an improvement of unfavorable lipid patterns, especially if the TSH level is greater than 10 mU/L
  - Relatively small doses of T_4 (50–100 μg/day) are needed

Thyroiditis

Basic Information

- **Definition: Thyroiditis is a group of diseases characterized by thyroid inflammation**
- Types
  - **Chronic lymphocytic (Hashimoto's) thyroiditis**
    - **Most common thyroid disease in the United States; most common cause of hypothyroidism** (see previous discussion)
  - Subacute (de Quervain's, granulomatous thyroiditis) thyroiditis
    - Fairly uncommon
    - Affects women aged 20 to 50 years, with a female-to-male ratio of 6:1
    - Associated with human leukocyte antigen (HLA) Bw35
    - Treatment: β-Blockers, NSAIDs; prednisone if NSAIDs are ineffective
  - Silent (painless, postpartum) thyroiditis
    - A variant of Hashimoto's thyroiditis
    - Women aged 20 to 60 years, with a female-to-male ratio of 2:1
    - When it occurs after pregnancy, silent thyroiditis is referred to as *postpartum thyroiditis*; approximately 5% of women develop postpartum thyroiditis
    - May cause permanent hypothyroidism in about 25% of patients
    - Treatment: β-Blockers
  - Acute bacterial (suppurative) thyroiditis: Rare; occurs in all age groups
  - Amiodarone-induced thyroiditis
    - Occurs more than 1 year after starting therapy
    - Treatment: Prednisone
- Etiology (Table 39-6)

Clinical Presentation, Diagnosis, and Treatment

See Table 39-6 for a summary of the presentation, diagnosis, and treatment of thyroiditis.

Goiter and Thyroid Nodules

Basic Information

- Goiter is a chronic enlargement of the thyroid gland
- Thyroid nodules are focal isolated lumps in the thyroid gland
- Thyroid nodules and goiter are extremely common
  - Prevalence on physical examination of one or more thyroid nodules ranges from 1% to 5%
  - **Frequency of small, nonpalpable nodules that are detected by ultrasound examination is as high as 50% to 70%** in older persons, especially women
  - The major clinical significance of thyroid nodules is the possibility of thyroid cancer, which is present in 5% to 10% of thyroid nodules
- Etiology
  - In most patients, the cause of goiter and thyroid nodules is not known
  - Iodine deficiency is the major cause of goiter in the world but probably does not exist in North America
  - Chronic lymphocytic thyroiditis accounts for 10% to 20% of goiters and thyroid nodules
  - Ionizing radiation and genetic factors are also important in the genesis of thyroid nodular disease

Clinical Presentation

- Most patients with thyroid nodules or goiter are asymptomatic and clinically euthyroid
- A large goiter may cause neck discomfort and pressure, dysphagia, hoarseness, and dyspnea (Fig. 39-5)
- Some multinodular goiters are substernal in location and may not be readily palpable, but they can cause significant airway obstruction or superior vena caval compression (with jugular venous distention and facial edema)
- Benign versus malignant nodules
  - The distinction of a benign from a malignant thyroid nodule is almost impossible on clinical grounds
  - A few features favor malignancy (Box 39-3)

Diagnosis and Evaluation

- Diffuse or multinodular goiter
  - Can be seen with a normal TSH (nontoxic goiter), increased TSH (probable chronic lymphocytic thyroiditis), or a decreased TSH (Graves' disease, toxic multinodular goiter, thyroiditis)
  - Thyroid radionuclide scanning will provide only general information about the size of the thyroid and whether certain areas within the gland concentrate the radioactive tracer (Fig. 39-6).
  - Thyroid ultrasound can accurately assess the size of the gland, the overall echotexture of the gland, and the echo characteristics, size, and number of nodules within the gland
- Solitary thyroid nodules
  - Measurement of serum TSH is useful
    - If the value is high, it suggests the presence of chronic lymphocytic thyroiditis
    - If the value is low, it suggests that the nodule is autonomous and one could consider radioiodine scan
    - If TSH is normal or high, an ultrasound should be strongly considered to confirm the presence of the nodule, its size, and its appearance
  - See Figure 39-7 for general approach
  - Thyroid ultrasonography cannot reliably differentiate benign from malignant nodules
    - However, certain sonographic features alone and especially in combination have reasonable sensitivity and specificity for predicting malignancy. These include hypoechogenicity, increased blood flow, microcalcifications, and irregular borders.
    - Can document the presence and size of a nodule and can define whether a nodule is solitary or whether it is one of many others
    - Good for follow-up of nodule size
  - **Fine-needle aspiration biopsy (FNAB) is the procedure of choice in the diagnosis of thyroid nodules (Fig. 39-8).**

TABLE 39-6	*Types of Thyroiditis*			
Type	**Etiology**	**Clinical Features**	**Diagnosis**	**Treatment**
Chronic lymphocytic thyroiditis (CLT)	Autoimmune Antithyroid antibodies: antithyroperoxidase (aka, antiTPO, antimicrosomal) and antithyroglobulin antibodies May be induced by interferon-α therapy	Most patients have symptoms of hypothyroidism Often with firm, nontender goiter Pyramidal lobe may be palpable May have other evidence of autoimmunity (prematurely gray hair, vitiligo)	Often see ↑ TSH Radioiodine uptake testing usually not necessary	Thyroxine for hypothyroid patients In euthyroid patients, may use higher doses of thyroxine to shrink goiter
Subacute thyroiditis (SAT)	Probably viral More likely to occur if HLA-Bw35 positive	Gradual or acute onset of thyroid pain; may be severe and disabling Pain may radiate to angle of jaw or ear May see systemic symptoms, such as fever, night sweats, fatigue, and weight loss On exam, thyroid is very tender, firm, and irregular Course: Pain and hyperthyroidism for 3–6 wk followed by transient hypothyroidism for several months	Acute inflammatory phase: ↑ T_4 ↓ TSH Radioiodine uptake is low High ESR (>30 mm/hr) Recovery phase: May see temporary mild ↓ T_4 and ↑ TSH for 1–3 mo	Salicylates or other nonsteroidals for neck discomfort Severe cases: Glucocorticoids are helpful Treat symptoms of hyperthyroidism with β-blocking drugs Full recovery is the rule
Silent thyroiditis (postpartum thyroiditis)	Autoimmune	Symptoms and signs of mild thyrotoxicosis Usually a firm, nontender goiter Triphasic course (as with SAT) May recur with successive pregnancies May present as postpartum depression	Similar to SAT ↑ T_4 and T_3 but T_3 not as high as seen in Graves' disease Radioiodine uptake is low	Treat symptoms of hyperthyroidism with β-blocking drugs Glucocorticoids rarely needed for severe hyperthyroidism 25% become permanently hypothyroid
Acute (suppurative) thyroiditis	Bacterial; most commonly *Staphylococcus aureus*, *Streptococcus pyogenes*, *Streptococcus pneumoniae*, and *Enterobacter* spp. Typically preceded by an upper respiratory or pharyngeal infection May also be due to opportunistic infections in immunocompromised hosts, especially *Aspergillus* and *Pneumocystis*	Anterior neck pain, fever, dysphagia May see erythema over thyroid or jugular venous phlebitis	Thyroid function usually remains normal Leukocytosis Fine-needle aspiration with stains to identify organism	Antibiotics Surgical drainage if abscess develops
Amiodarone-induced thyroiditis (type 2 amiodarone-induced thyrotoxicosis)	3% of patients on amiodarone More common in men	Thyrotoxicosis features develop rapidly May have recurrence of atrial fibrillation Thyroid is nontender; not enlarged Usually occurs after 1–3 yr of therapy	↑ T_4 and T_3 T_3 may also be normal ↓ TSH ↓ Radioiodine uptake Thyroid Doppler ultrasound will demonstrate "low" blood flow similar to euthyroid state	Prednisone 40 mg daily Slow taper over 2–3 mo

AntiTPO, antithyroperoxidase; ESR, erythrocyte sedimentation rate; HLA, human leukocyte antigen; T_3, triiodothyronine; T_4, thyroxine; TSH, thyroid-stimulating hormone.

Treatment

- Therapy of diffuse or multinodular goiters is based on two factors
  - Evidence of thyroid dysfunction
  - Symptoms and/or signs of tracheal, esophageal, or recurrent laryngeal nerve compression
- Pharmacologic therapy

- Diffuse or multinodular goiters
  - Hypothyroidism is treated with T_4
  - Hyperthyroidism is generally treated with radioiodine
  - The use of T_4 "suppression" therapy in euthyroid patients is controversial but may be effective in some patients with nontoxic goiter

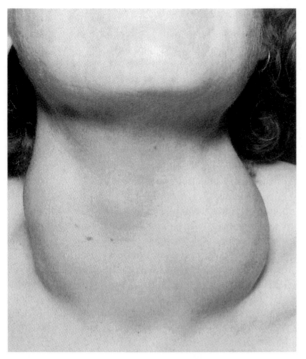

FIGURE 39-5 Dominant left-sided nodule in a multinodular goiter. (From Souhami R: *Textbook of medicine,* New York, Churchill Livingstone, 2002, figure 17.25.)

BOX 39-3	*Clinical Features Suggesting Malignancy in a Thyroid Nodule*

History
Rapid growth
Male sex
Older male or young child
Childhood neck irradiation
Family history of thyroid cancer

Physical Examination
Firm or rock-hard consistency
Ipsilateral cervical adenopathy
Fixation to surrounding structures

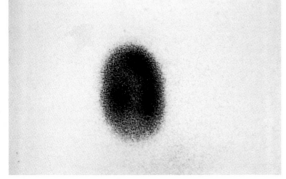

FIGURE 39-6 Toxic adenoma in the right thyroid (a hot nodule) demonstrated with radioiodine uptake scan. Remainder of gland does not take up the isotope. (From Forbes CD, Jackson WF: *Color atlas and text of clinical medicine,* ed 3, St. Louis, Mosby, 2003, figure 7.63.)

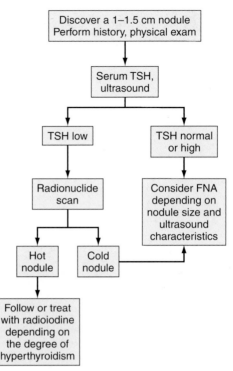

FIGURE 39-7 Evaluation of a thyroid nodule. FNA, fine-needle aspiration; TSH, thyroid-stimulating hormone.

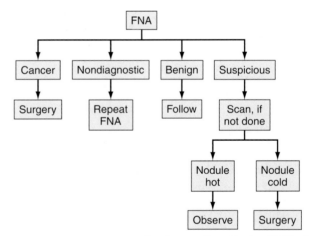

FIGURE 39-8 Management after fine-needle aspiration (FNA) of a thyroid nodule.

- Solitary thyroid nodules: Suppression therapy with T_4 is probably of little use
- Nonpharmacologic therapy
  - Diffuse or multinodular goiters: Surgery is usually required for large, obstructive goiters; radioiodine can be used in elderly patients who are not surgical candidates
  - Solitary thyroid nodules
    - Surgery is indicated for malignant and indeterminant nodules and for those nodules that are causing compressive symptoms
    - For "hot" nodules that produce hyperthyroidism, radioiodine therapy is the procedure of choice; surgery is also a reasonable option for large (>4 cm) nodules

39

TABLE 39-7	*Clinical Features and Therapy of Thyroid Cancer*					
Cancer Type	**% of All Cancers**	**Age at Diagnosis (yr)**	**Rate of Growth**	**Primary Therapy**	**Prognosis**	**Comment**
Papillary	70–80	30–60	Slow	Surgery	Excellent	Radioiodine used as adjunct
Follicular	10–15	50+	Slow	Surgery	Good to excellent	Radioiodine used as adjunct
Medullary	10	50+ (younger if MEN 2)	Moderate	Surgery	Good	RET germline mutation in 20% of cases; produces calcitonin
Lymphoma	<5	50+	Moderate	Radiotherapy, chemotherapy	Good	Seen in association with Hashimoto's thyroiditis
Anaplastic	<5	60+	Rapid	Surgery, radiotherapy, chemotherapy	Poor	Often prior history of goiter or papillary thyroid cancer

MEN, multiple endocrine neoplasia.

- In patients with biopsy-proven benign nodules, observation and follow-up ultrasound in 1 year are all that is required in most situations
- Rebiopsy if benign nodule enlarges on follow-up

Thyroid Cancer

Basic Information

- Definition: Primary malignancy arising from thyroid follicular cells or C cells
  - Histologic types (Table 39-7)
  - Papillary and follicular cancer are referred to collectively as *differentiated thyroid cancer* and account for 80% to 90% of all thyroid cancer
- Thyroid lymphomas may develop from lymphocytes within the thyroid gland in individuals with Hashimoto's thyroiditis
- Overall incidence of thyroid cancer in the United States is approximately 3 per 100,000 per year
- Etiology of most cancers is unknown; ionizing radiation is a risk factor for differentiated thyroid cancer
- Medullary thyroid cancer (MTC)
  - About 20% of patients belong to kindreds with multiple endocrine neoplasia 2 syndrome (see Chapter 42)
  - Autosomal dominant

Clinical Presentation

- Patients are usually asymptomatic, and a thyroid nodule is found on routine physical examination or incidentally on imaging done for other purposes (chest CT, neck MRI, carotid Doppler, etc.)

Diagnosis and Evaluation

- FNA required for diagnosis
- See Table 39-7 for histologic types

Treatment

- See Table 39-7

- Radioiodine ablation of thyroid remnants after thyroidectomy is usually performed in patients with differentiated thyroid cancer, especially in those patients at high risk for recurrence
- **Serum markers may be helpful for monitoring for disease recurrence**
  - **Serum thyroglobulin useful in patients with differentiated thyroid cancer**
  - **Serum calcitonin useful in patients with MTC**
- Factors influencing the prognosis in differentiated cancer include the patient's age (better in patients < 50 years of age), the tumor size, the degree of tumor invasiveness, and the presence of distant metastases

REVIEW QUESTIONS

For review questions, please go to www.expertconsult.com.

SUGGESTED READINGS

Basaria M, Graf H, Cooper DS: The use of recombinant thyrotropin in the follow-up of patients with differentiated thyroid cancer, *Am J Med* 112(9):721–725, 2002.

Basaria S, Cooper DS: Amiodarone and the thyroid, *Am J Med* 118:706–714, 2005.

Cooper DS: Antithyroid drugs, *N Engl J Med* 352:905–917, 2005.

Cooper DS: Clinical practice: subclinical hypothyroidism, *N Engl J Med* 345:260–265, 2001.

Cooper DS: Hyperthyroidism, *Lancet* 362:459–468, 2003.

Franklyn JA: The management of hyperthyroidism, *N Engl J Med* 330:1731–1738, 1994.

Hegedus L: Clinical practice: the thyroid nodule, *N Engl J Med* 351:1764–1771, 2004.

Mazzaferri EL: Management of a solitary thyroid nodule, *N Engl J Med* 328:553–559, 1993.

Mazzaferri EL, Kloos RT: Current approaches to primary therapy for papillary and follicular thyroid cancer, *J Clin Endocrinol Metab* 86:1447–1463, 2001.

Roberts CG, Ladenson PW: Hypothyroidism, *Lancet* 363:793–803, 2004.

Sherman SI: Thyroid carcinoma, *Lancet* 361:501–511, 2003.

Toft AD: Subclinical hyperthyroidism, *N Engl J Med* 345:512–516, 2001.

Weetman AP: Graves' disease, *N Engl J Med* 343:1236–1248, 2000.

CHAPTER 40

Calcium Disorders and Metabolic Bone Disease

REDONDA G. MILLER, MD, MBA

Calcium disorders are common, particularly in hospitalized patients. Malignancy accounts for the vast majority of hypercalcemia cases in hospitalized patients. In the outpatient setting, hyperparathyroidism is the leading cause, with an increase in the incidence of asymptomatic primary hyperparathyroidism, probably attributable to the frequent use of screening chemistry panels. Metabolic bone disease includes a heterogeneous group of disorders. Given the aging population, osteoporosis is the most prevalent and important of these. Every internist should be familiar with screening and treatment principles of this disease.

Hypercalcemia

Basic Information

- Calcium metabolism
  - Calcium is important for many physiologic processes, including bone matrix crystallization and muscle contraction
  - In the extracellular compartment it circulates in three forms:
    - "Ionized" or the free form: Maintained in very narrow limits (45%)
    - Bound to protein (albumin and globulin) (40%)
    - Bound to anions (bicarbonate, phosphate, citrate) (15%)
  - **Parathyroid hormone (PTH), produced by the four parathyroid glands, tightly regulates serum calcium levels**
    - PTH level is responsive to level of ionized calcium in the blood as well as to the levels of phosphate and magnesium
    - PTH actions (via G protein-coupled receptor; Fig. 40-1)
  - Vitamin D
    - A fat-soluble steroid obtained from diet or synthesized in skin in presence of ultraviolet light
    - Transported to the liver where it is 25-hydroxylated
    - Then transported to kidney where it is 1-hydroxylated (under the control of PTH); 1,25(OH)2D (calcitriol) is the active form
    - Actions of 1,25(OH)2D (see Fig. 40-1)
- Definition of hypercalcemia: An abnormal elevation in the ionized calcium (usually >1.32 mmol/L) or total calcium greater than 10.5 mg/dL

- Moderate hypercalcemia: Levels between 12 and 14 mg/dL; variable clinical manifestations
- Severe hypercalcemia: Levels of 14 mg/dL or greater; almost always associated with symptoms and requires immediate treatment
  - High levels should always be repeated to confirm and ionized calcium level also checked
  - **Calcium is bound to albumin (40%); a "normal" total calcium may actually be high if the albumin is low**
    - Rule of thumb: Adjust the total serum calcium level by 0.8 mg/dL for each 1 g by which the serum albumin level is above or below 4 g/dL
  - Acid-base status is also important because alkalosis increases calcium binding to albumin, whereas acidosis decreases it
- Causes of hypercalcemia (Box 40-1; Table 40-1)
  - **The two most common causes are hyperparathyroidism and malignancy, which make up more than 90% of cases**

Clinical Presentation

- The clinical presentation can be variable and often depends on factors other than total calcium level, such as:
  - Age of patient (older patients present more severely)
  - Comorbid conditions
  - Duration of hypercalcemia (the longer the duration, the better tolerated)
  - Rate of increase in calcium concentration (a more rapid increase leads to more severe symptoms)
- Malignancy tends to present most acutely and severely
  - 10% to 20% of cancer patients develop hypercalcemia at some point
  - Associated with a poor prognosis: 50% mortality at 1 month
- Main clinical manifestations of acute hypercalcemia
  - Gastrointestinal: Anorexia, nausea, vomiting, constipation (decreased GI motility)
  - Central nervous system: Confusion, weakness, lethargy, hyporeflexia, obtundation, coma
  - Cardiovascular: Hypertension (if not too dehydrated), shortened QT interval, occasional bradycardia, and first-degree atrioventricular block
  - Renal: Polyuria and polydipsia (via interference with antidiuretic hormone [ADH] action and inhibition

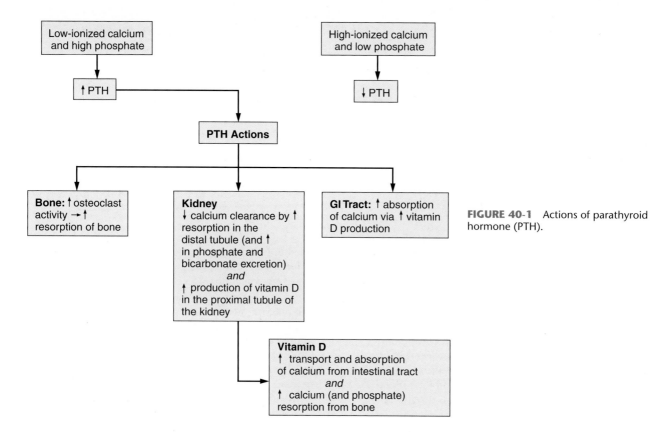

FIGURE 40-1 Actions of parathyroid hormone (PTH).

BOX 40-1   *Causes of Hypercalcemia*

Primary hyperparathyroidism

Malignancy

    Bone metastases

    Humoral hypercalcemia (related to PTH-rp)

    Conversion of 25(OH) vitamin D to 1,25(OH)

      vitamin D

Granulomatous disease

    Sarcoidosis

    Tuberculosis

Familial hypocalciuric hypercalcemia

Drugs

    Thiazide diuretics (stimulate renal resorption of calcium)

    Lithium (changes "set point" of PTH release)

Vitamin A or D intoxication

Immobilization

Other

    Thyrotoxicosis

    Pheochromocytoma

    Adrenal insufficiency

    Parenteral nutrition

    ■ Chondrocalcinosis
    ■ Pancreatitis (calcium deposition in the pancreas)
    ■ Hypertension

Diagnosis and Evaluation

- Often the cause of the hypercalcemia is readily apparent from a good history and physical examination
- **If not, the first step is to determine between PTH-mediated and non-PTH-mediated forms of hypercalcemia**
  - **Intact PTH (iPTH) is the test of choice**
  - **Diagnosis often suggested by iPTH level (Fig. 40-3)**

Treatment

- Treatment approach for acute, life-threatening hypercalcemia
  - Rapidity and aggressiveness of treatment depend on absolute calcium level and patient's symptoms
    - **All patients should receive aggressive IV fluids**
    - Calcitonin, pamidronate, and zoledronate are good first choices (calcitonin will take effect rapidly, but action is short-lived; pamidronate and zoledronate will have slower onset but will provide more durable response)
    - Definitive therapy, however, is to treat the underlying disorder (see Table 40-1)
- **Treatment options for acute, severe hypercalcemia**
  - If severe, acute, symptomatic hypercalcemia is present, institute treatment immediately
  - Saline infusion with diuresis
    - Volume expansion using isotonic saline initially (most patients are severely dehydrated) and delivered at a rapid rate
    - Improves renal blood flow and glomerular filtration rate (GFR) with increased filtration of calcium

of sodium resorption), azotemia (dehydration and afferent arteriolar constriction)
- Chronic manifestations of hypercalcemia ("stones, bones, abdominal groans, and psychic overtones"); most commonly associated with chronic hyperparathyroidism
  - Osteoporosis with bone pain
  - Nephrocalcinosis
  - Band keratopathy (deposition of calcium-phosphate in sun-exposed cornea; Fig. 40-2)

TABLE 40-1	*Selected Disorders Associated with Hypercalcemia*		
Disorder	**Pathophysiology**	**Clinical and Diagnostic Considerations**	**Treatment**
Primary hyperparathyroidism	Oversecretion of parathyroid hormone (PTH) by the parathyroid glands
Sporadic, solitary adenoma (85%)
Hyperplasia of all 4 glands (10–15%)
Carcinoma (<1%)	Most patients are asymptomatic; high calcium found on routine testing
Typical symptoms: fatigue, nausea, constipation
Associated with osteoporosis
Loss of trabecular bone > cortical bone
DXA should include forearm measurement for this reason (higher cortical bone percentage)
Advanced form: Osteitis fibrosa cystica (rare)
Preoperative sestamibi scan is helpful in localizing adenoma if present
If hyperplasia of all 4 glands present, consider MEN syndromes
Follow patients with serum calcium every 6 mo and yearly creatinine and DXA	All symptomatic patients should undergo surgery
Resection of adenoma, if nodule present
Removal of 3½ glands if hyperplasia present
Minimally invasive surgery if possible
Highly consider surgery in asymptomatic patients if:
Age < 50 yr
Calcium > 11.5 mg/dL
24-hr urine calcium > 400 mg
Low bone density
Nephrolithiasis
Medical therapy (if not a surgical candidate)
Estrogen and raloxifene will decrease serum calcium and decrease bone resorption
Cinacalcet: Calcimimetic that binds to calcium-sensing receptor in parathyroid gland
↓ sensitivity to serum calcium level
↓ PTH secretion
Not an FDA-approved indication
Malignancy	Three mechanisms
Bony metastases resulting in local resorption (e.g., breast, multiple myeloma, prostate, lymphoma, thyroid, lung)
Humoral hypercalcemia: Mediated by PTH-related peptide (PTH-rp); analogy with amino-terminus of PTH; usually squamous cell carcinomas (e.g., lung); also renal, bladder, ovarian
Conversion of 25(OH) vitamin D to active form (e.g., lymphoma)	More likely to present acutely and severely
Can measure PTH-rp via sensitive assay	Treat acute, symptomatic hypercalcemia as outlined in text
Treat underlying malignancy
Granulomatous diseases	Unregulated synthesis of $1,25(OH)_2$ vitamin D by granuloma-associated macrophages
Not sensitive to negative feedback suppression by ↑ calcium	Diseases such as sarcoidosis, tuberculosis, disseminated fungal infections, berylliosis
Serum Po_4 often elevated as well; may lead to soft tissue calcification and nephrocalcinosis	Steroids particularly useful
Treat underlying disease
Familial hypocalciuric hypercalcemia	Mutation in gene encoding calcium-sensing receptor
Kidneys cannot sense calcium level and resorb too much
Parathyroid glands also exhibit sensing defect and do not appropriately suppress PTH secretion
Autosomal dominant	Clinical manifestations are very benign; most patients asymptomatic
May have a family history of unsuccessful neck explorations
Urine calcium low (<100 mg/24 hr or urinary calcium/creatinine ratio <0.01)
PTH usually normal	No treatment necessary

DXA, dual-energy x-ray absorptiometry; FDA, Food and Drug Administration; MEN, multiple endocrine neoplasia.

40

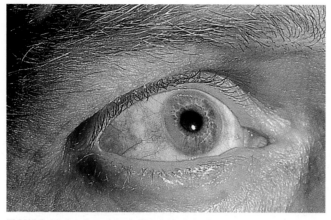

FIGURE 40-2 Ectopic calcification at the lateral and nasal margins of the right cornea (band keratopathy) in a patient with primary hyperparathyroidism. (From Forbes CD, Jackson WF: *Color atlas and text of clinical medicine,* ed 3, St. Louis, Mosby, 2003, figure 3.138.)

- Once volume is replete, loop diuretic can be added to enhance sodium excretion and protect against volume overload
  - Calcium follows sodium in the proximal tubule; the more sodium excreted, the more calcium excreted
  - Loop diuretics should be used because they also inhibit calcium resorption in the thick ascending limb of the loop of Henle
  - Thiazide diuretics do the opposite and should never be used in hypercalcemia
- Mobilization, if possible (immobility increases bone resorption because of lack of weight bearing)
- Pharmacologic options
  - Bisphosphonates
    - Are the gold standard
    - Bind to hydroxyapatite in bone and inhibit the dissolution of crystals; also inhibit osteoclast activity
    - **Pamidronate or zoledronate are drugs of choice; potent and effective**
    - **Poor oral absorption (<10%) means they must be given parenterally**
    - **Calcium level begins to decline within 2 days and hits nadir at 7 days**
    - Adverse effects include transient, mild increase in temperature and transient leukopenia
  - Calcitonin
    - Inhibits bone resorption and increases renal excretion
    - **Has some analgesic properties and can be effective at relieving bone pain**
    - **Quickest in onset; takes effect within a few hours**
    - Effect is often limited and transient (because of tachyphylaxis)
    - Very safe; patients may have mild nausea, abdominal cramps, and flushing; because of occasional allergic reactions, initial 1-unit skin test is recommended
  - Mithramycin and gallium nitrate: Rarely used because of their serious side effects
  - **Glucocorticoids**
    - **Most useful in treating vitamin D–mediated hypercalcemia (i.e., vitamin D intoxication, granulomatous diseases); work via inhibition of 1,25(OH)2D production**
    - Also useful in certain malignancies involving cytokine release (e.g., some myelomas)
    - Usual dose is prednisone 20 to 40 mg/day
- Treatment of other more chronic causes of hypercalcemia (see Table 40-1)

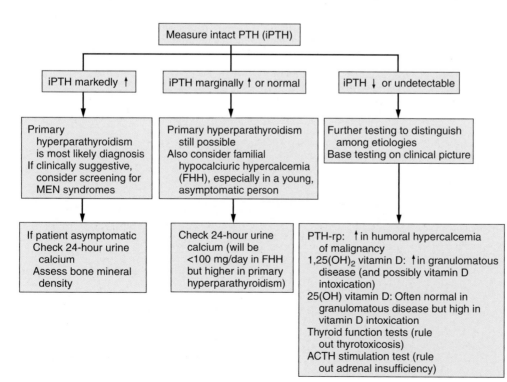

FIGURE 40-3 Approach to the patient with hypercalcemia. ACTH, adrenocorticotropic hormone; MEN, multiple endocrine neoplasia; PTH, parathyroid hormone.

Hypocalcemia

Basic Information

- Causes
  - Defect in action or metabolism of PTH
    - Hypoparathyroidism (after neck surgery, autoimmune, infiltrative diseases)
    - Resistance to action of PTH (pseudohypoparathyroidism)
  - Vitamin D deficiency (often low-normal calcium values) resulting from
    - Inadequate oral intake
    - GI malabsorptive disorders (celiac disease, pancreatic insufficiency, ileal bypass)
    - End-stage liver or renal disease
    - **May manifest as osteomalacia (Box 40-2)**
  - Large blood transfusions (citrate in transfused blood can bind calcium)
  - Magnesium depletion (decreased PTH release)
  - Acute respiratory alkalosis (increases binding of calcium to albumin)
  - Acute pancreatitis (calcium binds to free fatty acids released by lipase)
  - Excessive tissue breakdown resulting in calcium binding to excess phosphate (tumor lysis syndrome, rhabdomyolysis)

Clinical Presentation

- **Neurologic**
  - **Numbness, paresthesias (especially perioral), muscle irritability, tetany**
  - **Chvostek's sign (spasm of the facial nerve when tapped)**
  - **Trousseau's sign (carpopedal spasm elicited by inflating blood pressure cuff above systolic pressure; Fig. 40-4)**

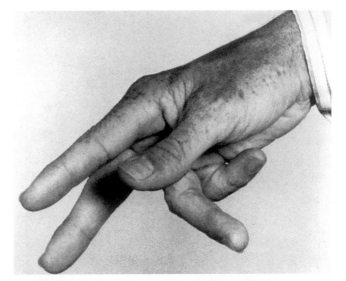

FIGURE 40-4 Trousseau's sign (carpopedal spasm). (From Larsen PR, Kronenberg HM, Melmed S, et al: *Williams textbook of endocrinology,* ed 10, Philadelphia, WB Saunders, 2002, figure 26-32.)

- Cardiovascular
  - Hypotension with decreased contractility
  - Prolonged QT interval on electrocardiogram
- Pulmonary
  - Bronchospasm

Diagnosis and Evaluation

- Measurement of serum calcium, phosphate, magnesium, iPTH, vitamin D levels
- Diagnosis often suggested by clinical presentation

Treatment

- Severe cases (symptomatic patients): IV repletion with calcium gluconate or calcium chloride slowly
  - Ensure magnesium is also replete
- Mild cases: Oral calcium carbonate or calcium citrate; usually vitamin D as well

---

BOX 40-2   *Osteomalacia*

Main defect: Undermineralized bone

Cause: Usually calcium +/− phosphorus deficiency due to
Dietary deficiency
Gastrointestinal malabsorption
Decreased vitamin D synthesis (liver disease, inadequate sun exposure, drugs such as phenytoin)

Clinical symptoms
Fatigue
Diffuse bone pain
Muscle weakness

Diagnosis
Labs often reveal low (or low-normal) calcium, significant hypophosphatemia, mildly elevated alkaline phosphatase, low vitamin D levels
Diagnosis confirmed by bone biopsy (with tetracycline labeling) showing undermineralization

Treatment: Repletion of calcium and vitamin D
Calcium: 1000–1500 mg by mouth per day in divided doses
Vitamin D: Often need 50,000 U of ergocalciferol by mouth once or twice weekly for up to 6–12 mo

---

Osteoporosis

Basic Information

- **Definition: A skeletal disorder characterized by compromised bone strength predisposing to an increased risk of fracture**
- Scope of the problem
  - Responsible for 1.5 million fractures per year
  - Lifetime risk for hip fracture of an average 50-year-old woman: 17.5% (with a 1-year mortality rate of 20%)
- Pathophysiology
  - Bone remodeling is a dynamic equilibrium between bone formation (by osteoblasts) and bone resorption (by osteoclasts)
  - Peak bone mass is achieved at age 30 years and is about 30% greater in men than women
  - Around the fourth or fifth decade, women and men start losing bone at a rate of 0.3% to 0.5% per year

40

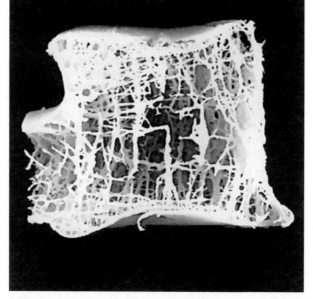

FIGURE 40-5 Cross-section of an osteoporotic vertebra showing extensive loss of trabecular bone architecture. (From Larsen PR, Kronenberg HM, Melmed S, et al: *Williams textbook of endocrinology,* ed 10, Philadelphia, WB Saunders, 2002, figure 27-15.)

- Loss is accelerated in women with loss of estrogen at menopause (can lose 3% to 5% per year for up to 5 years)
  - Leads to "postmenopausal" osteoporosis, the most common form
- Pathology reveals distortion in microarchitecture, loss of trabeculae, and microfractures (Fig. 40-5)
- **Risk factors**
  - **Major risk factors**
    - **Personal history of a fragility fracture**
    - **Family history of osteoporosis or fracture in a first-degree relative**
    - **Thin body habitus (<127 pounds)**
    - **Current smoking**
    - **Current use of glucocorticoid therapy for longer than 3 months**
  - Other risk fractures
    - Age
    - Premature menopause (age < 45 years) or hypogonadism
    - Predisposition to falls (vision loss, prior cerebrovascular accident, frailty)
    - Heavy alcohol intake
    - Sedentary lifestyle
    - Dietary deficiencies (calcium, vitamin D)
  - Secondary causes (Box 40-3)
    - **Glucocorticoid use is the most common secondary cause**
      - **Only small doses, equivalent to 7.5 mg or higher of prednisone per day, required for bone loss to occur**
      - **Occurs within 3 to 6 months of use**
    - In men with osteoporosis, consider checking testosterone level (hypogonadism is a fairly common cause)

BOX 40-3 *Selected Secondary Causes of Osteoporosis*

Endocrine Disorders
Hyperthyroidism
Hyperparathyroidism
Hypogonadism
Excess cortisol production (e.g., Cushing's disease)

Bone Marrow Disorders
Multiple myeloma
Leukemia/lymphoma

Gastrointestinal Diseases
Gastrectomy
Malabsorption syndromes

Connective Tissue Diseases
Rheumatoid arthritis
Osteogenesis imperfecta
Ehlers-Danlos syndrome
Marfan syndrome

Drugs
Glucocorticoids
Anticonvulsants
Cyclosporine
Prolonged heparin use

Clinical Presentation

- Most patients are asymptomatic
- Main causes of symptoms are vertebral and hip fractures
- Physical examination
  - Routine height measurement: Loss of height (>1 inch) may be only clue to vertebral fractures
  - Kyphosis: Decreases thoracic volume and can lead to dyspnea and restrictive lung disease (Fig. 40-6)
  - Look for clues to secondary causes of osteoporosis

Diagnosis and Evaluation

- Radiography: May see increased lucency of bone
  - Not helpful for detecting early disease; osteopenia not evident until 30% bone loss
  - Lateral films useful for visualization of spine compression fractures
- Dual-energy x-ray absorptiometry (DXA)
  - Calculates bone mineral density (BMD) on the basis of tissue absorption of photons from a radionuclide source or x-ray tube
  - **Measures BMD both at axial (spine) and at appendicular (hip) sites**
  - **Low BMD highly correlates with increased risk of fracture**
  - Is the gold standard for diagnosis
  - Results expressed as two scores
    - **T-score: BMD expressed as the number of standard deviations above or below the mean BMD of normal young adults (30-year-olds)**
    - Z-score: BMD expressed as the number of standard deviations above or below the mean BMD of adults of the same age and gender

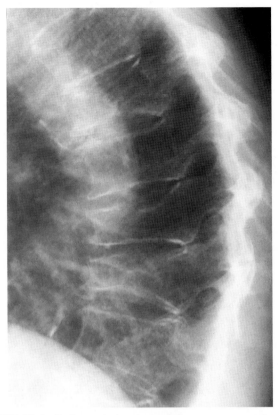

FIGURE 40-6 Radiograph showing radiolucency, compression fractures, and kyphosis in the spine of a patient with osteoporosis. (From Goldman L, Bennett JC, Ausiello D: *Cecil textbook of medicine,* ed 22, Philadelphia, WB Saunders, 2004, figure 258-4.)

TABLE 40-2	*World Health Organization Criteria for Diagnosis of Osteoporosis*
T-Score	**Assessment**
> –1	Normal bone mineral density
–1 to –2.5	Osteopenia
< –2.5	Osteoporosis
< –2.5 + fracture	Severe osteoporosis

- Other tests are not routinely sent unless history, physical, or initial laboratory test results suggest need: Serum protein electrophoresis (SPEP), urine protein electrophoresis (UPEP), 24-hour urinary calcium, PTH, testosterone (in men)

Treatment

- Traditional indications for instituting therapy (based predominantly on BMD):
  - History of a hip or vertebral fracture
  - History of other fragility fracture wtih T-score between –1 and –2.5
  - T-score less than –2 with no risk factors present
  - T-score less than –1.5 with at least one risk factor present
- **Newer treatment guidelines from the National Osteoporosis Foundation (NOF) recommend incorporating other risk factors in addition to BMD: Treat if**
  - **History of a hip or vertebral fracture**
  - **History of other fragility fracture wtih T-score between –1 and –2.5**
  - **10-year probability of hip fracture is 3% or greater**
  - **10-year probability of any major osteoporosis-related fracture is 20% or greater**
- 10-year probability of both hip and any major osteoporosis-related fracture is calculated using the FRAX algorithm
  - FRAX is an online tool developed by the World Health Organization
  - Incorporates nine clinical risk factors in addition to BMD
  - Tailored to nationality, gender, ethnicity
- All patients with osteoporosis should be prescribed the following:
  - Behavior modification
    - Exercise (particularly modest weight-bearing exercise)
    - Alcohol intake only in moderation
    - Smoking cessation
  - Calcium
    - Recommended dietary requirements (Table 40-3)
    - Average diet in the United States is deficient (~600 mg/day)
    - Major food sources: Milk and dairy products (~300 mg per serving)
    - Nonprescription supplements are helpful in those with deficient diets
      - Supplements better absorbed when taken with meals (presence of acid) and in small doses (500 mg or less at a time)

- **World Health Organization diagnostic criteria based on T-scores (Table 40-2)**
- **Indications for BMD measurement with DXA scan**
  - **All postmenopausal women 65 years of age or older**
  - **Women under age 65 years with one or more clinical risk factors**
  - **All men 70 years of age or older**
  - **Men under age 70 years with one or more clinical risk factors**
  - **Aid in decision regarding hormone replacement therapy**
  - **Radiologic evidence of osteopenia**
  - **Prior osteoporotic fracture**
  - **Monitoring therapy for osteoporosis**
  - Peripheral devices (e.g., heel ultrasonography, heel or wrist DXA) may not be as accurate but are less expensive and can predict fracture at one year; central DXA is preferable if possible
- Biochemical assessment once osteoporosis confirmed by DXA
  - Baseline CBC; chemistry panel including calcium, phosphorus, alkaline phosphatase; thyroid-stimulating hormone
    - Useful as a clue to secondary causes
  - Highly consider checking a 25-hydroxyvitamin D level
    - Many adults are deficient (minimal sun exposure, dietary insufficiencies)
    - If less than 30 ng/mL, may need to replete with high-dose ergocalciferol or cholecalciferol (see section on osteomalacia)

40

TABLE 40-3	Recommended Daily Calcium and Vitamin D Intake*	
Age (yr)	Calcium (mg/day)	Vitamin D (IU/day)
Adults < 50	1000	400–800
Adults ≥ 50	1200	800–1000

*Adapted from the National Osteoporosis Foundation guidelines.

- Calcium carbonate has highest calcium content and is cheapest
- Calcuim citrate may be better absorbed in patients with achlorhydria or in those who take H_2-receptor antagonists or proton-pump inhibitors
- **Vitamin D**
  - Recommended daily requirements (see Table 40-3)
  - Food sources similar to calcium (dairy products)
  - Many calcium supplements also contain vitamin D
- Estrogen
  - At menopause, falling estrogen levels contribute to rapid bone loss

- Prescribing estrogen will halt bone loss in menopausal women (and result in BMD gain of 3% to 5% in osteoporotic women)
- The earlier it is started, the bigger the effect on bone density
- Currently approved only for prevention because of lack of large, randomized controlled trials examining efficacy for treatment
- Pharmacologic options for the treatment of osteoporosis (Table 40-4)
  - Therapy must be tailored to individual wants and needs of the patient
  - All approved therapies, except teriparatide, work by inhibiting bone resorption
  - **First-line therapy is often a bisphosphonate because of potency, duration of effect, bone specificity (as opposed to hormonal therapies), and tolerability**
    - IV forms (pamidronate and zoledronic acid) are options for patients who cannot tolerate oral preparations

TABLE 40-4	Pharmacologic Options for Osteoporosis Treatment				
Medication	Mechanism	Advantages	Prevention of Vertebral Fractures	Prevention of Hip/Nonvertebral Fractures	Side Effects and Precautions
Raloxifene	Synthetic estrogen receptor agonist and antagonist Inhibits bone resorption	No effect on breast or endometrial tissue (unlike estrogen) Lowers LDL cholesterol	Yes	Not proven	Risk of thromboembolism comparable to estrogen No effect on menopausal vasomotor symptoms
Bisphosphonates (alendronate, risedronate, ibandronate, zoledronic acid)	Structural analogues of inorganic pyrophosphate Bind to hydroxyapatite and inhibit osteoclast activity	Very potent Long half-life: Allows for once weekly administration (once monthly for risedronate and ibandronate) Zoledronic acid may be administered IV once yearly	Yes	Yes (for alendronate, risedronate, zoledronic acid)	Poor oral absorption Upper GI irritation— have to take with 8 oz water on empty stomach then remain upright with no food for 30 min (60 min for ibandronate)
Calcitonin	Naturally occurring peptide Directly inhibits osteoclast activity	Intranasal administration Well tolerated with few side effects Analgesic effect; useful in compression fractures	Yes	Not proven	Limited effectiveness Tachyphylaxis may develop
Teriparatide	Is the amino terminus (1–34) of PTH Subcutaneous administration causes increase in bone formation with little effect on bone resorption	First drug to result in bone formation Large increases in bone mineral density	Yes	Yes	May see transient hypercalcemia Theoretical risk of osteosarcoma with prolonged use (use currently limited to 2 yr) Disadvantage: Daily subcutaneous administration

LDL, low-density lipoprotein; PTH, parathyroid hormone.

- IV forms given in high dose to cancer patients may be linked to osteonecrosis of the jaw
- Raloxifene and calcitonin; see Table 40-4
- Teriparatide: A recombinant N-terminus of parathyroid hormone
  - Delivered by daily subcutaneous injection
  - Intermittent delivery by injection, as opposed to continuous delivery in vivo by parathyroid glands, results in increased bone formation
  - Indicated for "severe" osteoporosis
- Monitoring therapy
  - Repeat densitometry is the standard method of follow-up
    - Need to wait sufficient time to avoid BMD changes that are simply margin of error of the test
    - **Usually reassessment by DXA at 2 years is reasonable**
      - Possible exceptions: Newly menopausal women, patients on corticosteroids, patients with other secondary causes of low BMD
  - **Treatment is probably successful if repeat DXA documents either modest increase in or stabilization of BMD**
    - Regardless of percent increase in BMD, most therapies (raloxifene, bisphosphonates) decrease fracture risk by roughly 50%

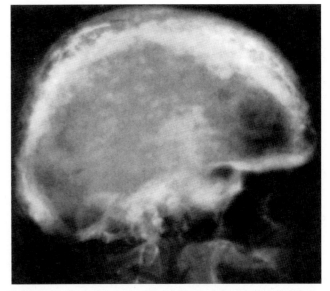

FIGURE 40-7 Radiograph of the skull of a patient with advanced Paget's disease showing thickening, disordered new bone formation (cotton-wool patches), and basilar impression. (From Larsen PR, Kronenberg HM, Melmed S, et al: *Williams textbook of endocrinology,* ed 10, Philadelphia, 2002, WB Saunders, figure 27-22.)

Paget's Disease

Basic Information

- Second most common bone disease
- Prevalent in the United Kingdom, Australia, South Africa, and the United States
- Pathophysiology: Chaotic osteoclast function with increased bone remodeling (both formation and resorption)
  - Many large osteoclasts with numerous nuclei
  - New bone formed is structurally weaker
  - Hypervascularity
- Etiology is unclear; possibly linked to a virus or genetic factors

Clinical Presentation

- **Pattern of bone involvement**
  - **May involve one bone or many bones asymmetrically**
  - **Most common sites: Pelvis, lumbar spine, skull, femur**
- Many patients have no symptoms (>90%)
- **Others experience bone pain, skeletal deformities**
  - **Enlarged skull, particularly frontal and occipital areas (Fig. 40-7)**
  - **Bowed lower extremities (Fig. 40-8)**
  - **Increased risk of fracture, particularly femur, tibia, radius**
  - **Impingement syndromes (e.g., inner ear with hearing loss and vertigo)**
  - Less common and occurs late in course

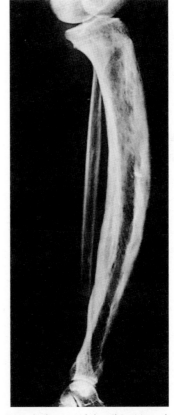

FIGURE 40-8 Paget's disease of the tibia. Note the bowing, marked irregularity of the anterior cortex, and flame-shaped lytic lesion of the posterior cortex. (From Larsen PR, Kronenberg HM, Melmed S, Polonsky, KS: *Williams textbook of endocrinology,* ed 10, Philadelphia, WB Saunders, 2003, figure 8-14.)

40

- High-output congestive heart failure from numerous vascular shunts
- Increased risk of osteosarcoma
- Hypercalcemia during immobilization

Diagnosis and Evaluation

- Lab studies show an isolated increase in alkaline phosphatase (can be quite high, >500 U/L)
- Plain films can reveal all three phases of disease; seeing all three is essentially diagnostic
  - First phase: Osteoporosis from osteolytic activity
  - Second phase (most commonly seen): Mixed phase with both sclerosis and osteolytic activity
  - Third phase: Mainly sclerosis with cortical thickening
- **Bone scan: Most sensitive test; can identify areas of increased uptake**

Treatment

- **Treatment is recommended for**
  - **All patients with symptoms**
  - **Asymptomatic patients with involvement of axial skeleton or weight-bearing long bones (high risk of progression to deformity)**
- Analgesics for pain
- **Bisphosphonates for severe disease (risedronate, alendronate, zoledronic acid)**
  - First-line therapy
  - Requires higher doses than those used for osteoporosis
  - Oral agents (risedronate, alendronate)
    - Can use until disease in remission (usual treatment course is 2 months), then discontinue drug with close monitoring of the alkaline phosphatase
  - IV agents (pamidronate, zoledronic acid)
    - Single infusion of zoledronic acid provides fast and sustained response

- Calcitonin is also useful but not first-line
  - Marked decrease in bone resorption, but disease recurs if drug is stopped
  - Significant bone pain relief, even when used intermittently
  - Some patients develop resistance to drug
- Prognosis is good; disease responds well to treatment with an increase in lamellar bone formation and a decrease in pain
- Disease activity can be monitored with biochemical markers (alkaline phosphatase and urine N-telopeptide)

REVIEW QUESTIONS

For review questions, please go to www.expertconsult.com.

SUGGESTED READINGS

Bilezikian JP: Management of acute hypercalcemia, *N Engl J Med* 36:1196–1203, 1992.

Bilezekian JP, Potts JP, Fuliehan Gel-H, et al: Summary statement from a workshop on asymptomatic primary hyperparathyroidism: a perspective for the 21st century, *J Bone Miner Res* 17(Suppl 2): N2–N11, 2002.

Calcium supplements, *Med Lett Drugs Ther* 42:29–31, 2000.

Delmas PD, Neunier PJ: The management of Paget's disease of bone, *N Engl J Med* 336:558–566, 1997.

Eastell R: Treatment of postmenopausal osteoporosis, *N Engl J Med* 338:737–746, 1998.

Ettinger B, Black DM, Mitlak BH, et al: Reduction of vertebral fracture risk in postmenopausal women with osteoporosis treated with raloxifene, *JAMA* 282:637–645, 1999.

Liberman UA, Weiss SR, Broll J, et al: Effect of oral alendronate on bone mineral density and the incidence of fractures in postmenopausal osteoporosis, *N Engl J Med* 333:1437–1496, 1995.

McClung MR, Geusens P, et al: Effect of risedronate on the risk of hip fracture in elderly women. Hip Intervention Program Study Group, *N Engl J Med* 344:333–340, 2001.

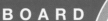
Reproductive Endocrinology

TODD T. BROWN, MD

This chapter focuses on the reproductive endocrine disorders the internist is most likely to encounter. Common problems for women include amenorrhea and hirsutism. Men may present with symptoms of gynecomastia, impotence, or other features of hypogonadism. Despite their prevalence, patients are often hesitant to discuss these symptoms. Therefore, internists may need to actively inquire about their presence.

Female Reproductive Disorders

FEMALE REPRODUCTIVE PHYSIOLOGY

- Normal menstrual cycle requires cyclic release of gonadotropin-releasing hormone (GnRH) from the hypothalamus, which leads to cyclic secretion of the pituitary gonadotropins: follicle-stimulating hormone (FSH) and luteinizing hormone (LH)
- The ovaries respond to FSH and LH by producing follicles containing ova
- Phases of the normal female menstrual cycle (Fig. 41-1)
  - Follicular phase of menstrual cycle: Ovarian follicle development
    - Estrogen predominantly produced by ovary
    - Causes thickening of uterine endometrium
  - Ovulation: LH surge induces release of egg from ovarian follicle
  - Luteal phase: Progesterone production by corpus luteum induces maturation of secretory endometrium
  - Menses: Decline in estrogen and progesterone results in endometrial shedding

AMENORRHEA

- Oligomenorrhea is defined as infrequent menses (>35 days between cycles or <6–8 periods per year)
- Amenorrhea is the absence of menses; may be physiologic or pathologic
  - Physiologic amenorrhea is normal and occurs with pregnancy, lactation, menopause
  - Pathologic amenorrhea can exist in either a primary or a secondary form
    - ***Primary amenorrhea* is defined as the persistent absence of menses by age 16 years**
    - ***Secondary amenorrhea* is the absence of menses for more than 6 months in a patient with a prior history of menses**

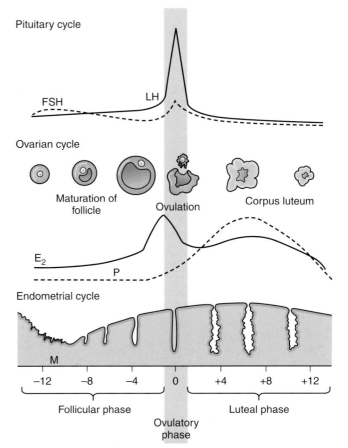

FIGURE 41-1 Hormone levels during the female menstrual cycle. The idealized cyclic changes observed in gonadotropins, estradiol (E_2), progesterone (P), and uterine endometrium during the normal menstrual cycle. The data are centered on the day of the luteinizing hormone (LH) surge (day 0). Days of menstrual bleeding are indicated by M. FSH, follicle-stimulating hormone. (From Goldman L, Bennett JC, Ausiello D: *Cecil textbook of medicine,* ed 22, Philadelphia, WB Saunders, 2004, figure 250-1.)

PRIMARY AMENORRHEA

Basic Information and Clinical Presentation

- Patients with primary amenorrhea may be grouped into those with and those without secondary sexual characteristics
- Primary amenorrhea with secondary sexual characteristics and normal sexual development
  - Usually indicates presence of ovaries

TABLE 41-1	**Causes of Primary Amenorrhea Without Secondary Sexual Characteristics**			
Disorder	**Features**	**Diagnosis**	**Fertility**	**Treatment**
Constitutional delay of puberty	Family history of delayed puberty	Family history Difficult to distinguish from GnRH deficiency	Will be present at maturity	Observation and reassurance
Pituitary and hypothalamic disorders	Hypogonadotropic hypogonadism Causes include destructive lesions (tumors) or isolated gonadotropin deficiency (Kallman's syndrome)	↓ FSH and LH No change in FSH and LH in response to GnRH stimulation	Variable, depending on underlying disorder	If malignancy, consider surgery or radiation Consider hormone replacement
Turner's syndrome (see Fig. 41-2)	45, XO karyotype Physical features include lack of sexual maturation, short stature, webbed neck, shield chest, and valgus deformity of the elbow	↑ FSH and LH XO karyotype	Usually absent unless mosaic of XO and XX cells	Hormone replacement
Gonadal dysgenesis	Absence of ovaries Congenital	↑ FSH and LH	Absent	Hormone replacement

FSH, follicle-stimulating hormone; GnRH, gonadotropin-releasing hormone; LH, luteinizing hormone.

- Etiologies include testicular feminization and müllerian defects
  - **Testicular feminization**
    - **Caused by androgen insensitivity**
    - **XY karyotype**
    - Normal male testosterone levels
    - Physical features: Breasts and feminine appearance, absence of axillary or pubic hair, and blind-ending vagina
  - Müllerian defects
    - Usually congenital
    - Physical features: Imperforate hymen, abnormal cervix, absence of vagina
- Primary amenorrhea without secondary sexual characteristics or other signs of puberty
  - Etiologies (Table 41-1)

Diagnosis and Evaluation

- Primary amenorrhea with signs of puberty
  - Many causes can be identified on physical examination and subsequent karyotype if needed
  - If physical examination findings are inconsistent with either testicular feminization or müllerian defects, then perform withdrawal bleed as described in the section on secondary amenorrhea
- Primary amenorrhea without signs of puberty
  - Check gonadotropin (FSH, LH) levels
    - If elevated, check karyotype to rule out Turner's syndrome (Fig. 41-2)
    - If low, perform GnRH stimulation testing to assess pituitary function and help differentiate delayed puberty from hypothalamic-pituitary disorder

Treatment

- Primary amenorrhea with signs of puberty
  - For patients with testicular feminization, inguinal testes must be removed at puberty because of risk of malignancy

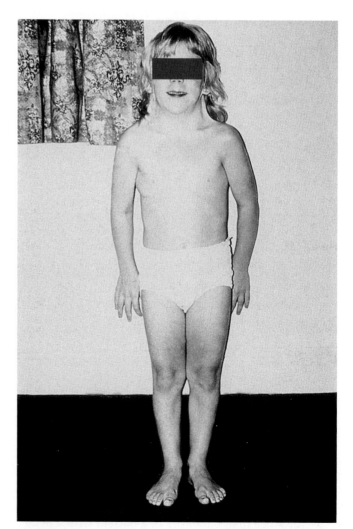

FIGURE 41-2 Girl with Turner's syndrome. Note the shield chest, widely spaced nipples, and webbed neck. (From Lowenstein EJ, Kim KH, Glick SA: Turner's syndrome in dermatology. *J Am Acad Dermatol* 50:767–776, 2004, figure 1.)

- For patients with müllerian defects, surgical repair is usually necessary
- Primary amenorrhea without signs of puberty
  - **Treat underlying disorder, if possible (see Table 41-1)**
  - Hormone replacement therapy
    - Start estrogen and progesterone in young patients to preserve bone density, improve well-being, prevent genitourinary atrophy, and promote breast development; long-term safety of hormone replacement in this setting has not been evaluated
    - Oral contraceptives often used for hormone replacement in young patients
- Patients who desire children should be referred to a reproductive endocrinologist

SECONDARY AMENORRHEA

Basic Information

- Most common causes are physiologic (e.g., pregnancy and menopause)
- **Differential diagnosis of pathologic secondary amenorrhea consists of four main disease states:**
  - **Hyperprolactinemia (e.g., prolactinoma, drugs)**
  - **Anovulatory states (e.g., most commonly, polycystic ovary syndrome; Box 41-1)**
  - **Androgen excess (e.g., androgen-secreting tumors)**
  - **Hypothalamic amenorrhea (e.g., physical or emotional stress, anorexia, excessive exercise)**
- Rarely caused by disorders of the outflow tract, such as:
  - Endometrial atrophy from prolonged use of progestins
  - Adhesions and obliteration of the uterine cavity (Asherman's syndrome)
  - Endometritis

Clinical Presentation

- **Symptoms and signs of hypoestrogenic state: Hot flashes, vaginal dryness, dyspareunia, osteopenia**
- Findings suggestive of underlying cause
  - Prolactin excess: Breast tenderness, galactorrhea
  - Androgen excess: Hirsutism, acne, increased muscle mass, clitoromegaly

Diagnosis and Evaluation

- **First step always: Rule out pregnancy**
- **Algorithm for evaluation (Fig. 41-3)**
- **Mechanics of inducing a withdrawal bleed with progesterone (see Fig. 41-3)**
  - If the endometrium is estrogenized, it should respond to progesterone challenge
  - Give 10 mg medroxyprogesterone daily for 5 to 7 days
  - Withdrawal bleeding should occur within 1 week of completion of progesterone challenge

Treatment

- Treat the underlying disorder (e.g., dopamine agonist for prolactinoma)
- **In young women (younger than 50 years), oral contraceptives are often used (see treatment of primary amenorrhea)**
- In older women (older than 50 years), postmenopausal hormone combinations may be used, but benefits versus risks need to be carefully considered

---

BOX 41-1	*Polycystic Ovary Syndrome*

Basic Information

Affects up to 10% of women

Thought to be caused by stimulatory effects of excess insulin on ovarian androgen production

Clinical Features

Amenorrhea, hirsutism, acne, obesity, and insulin resistance

Diagnosis

Is a clinical diagnosis; a diagnostic test with high sensitivity and specificity has not been identified

Ovarian ultrasound (for cysts) and LH:FSH ratio (often increased); do not always distinguish these patients from normal

Treatment

Metformin or thiazolidinediones (insulin sensitizers) may restore ovulation and fertility, thus confirming the role of insulin resistance

Oral contraceptives if fertility is not desired

Anti-androgens for hirsutism (spironolactone)

- In women with normal menopause, postmenopausal hormone therapy (HT) to prevent chronic medical conditions (such as coronary heart disease) is no longer recommended
  - **Indications for HT: Debilitating vasomotor symptoms**
  - Other benefits: Preservation of bone mineral density and possible reduced risk of colorectal cancer (but other specific treatments, such as bisphosphonates for osteoporosis, are considered first-line treatments)
  - Risks: Results from the Women's Health Initiative demonstrated that HT increases the risk of breast cancer, stroke, and venous thromboembolic disease and has no benefit in preventing heart disease
  - **If HT started, lowest dose for shortest duration (preferably <5 years) is generally recommended;** reassessment for continued need should be done at least yearly
  - Many forms available (oral, transdermal); none definitively shown to be superior
  - If uterus is present, must administer progestin with estrogen to avoid increased risk of endometrial cancer
    - Cycled if patient desires monthly withdrawal bleeding
    - Continuous if withdrawal bleeding is undesirable (more commonly used in postmenopausal women)
  - Vaginal spotting and bleeding may be a nuisance side effect
    - Usually resolves within 6 months
    - If heavy or first bleeding occurs 6 months after initiating therapy, endometrial biopsy should be performed to rule out hyperplasia or cancer

HIRSUTISM

Basic Information

- **Hirsutism is defined as the presence of terminal (coarse, pigmented) hairs on parts of a woman's body where terminal hairs are considered to be a**

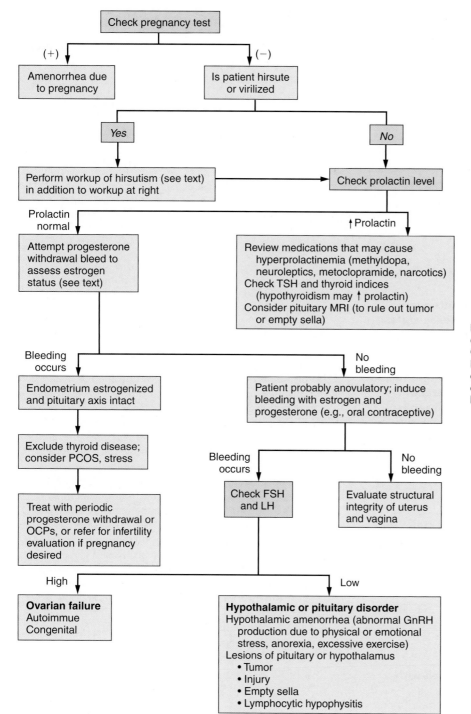

FIGURE 41-3 Algorithm for the diagnosis of secondary amenorrhea. GnRH, gonadotropin-releasing hormone; LH, luteinizing hormone; OCPs, oral contraceptive pills; PCOS, polycystic ovary syndrome; TSH, thyroid-stimulating hormone.

male secondary sexual characteristic (e.g., face, chest, back, lower abdomen, inner thighs; Fig. 41-4)
- **Virilization refers to signs of more severe androgen excess (e.g., deep voice, clitoromegaly, frontal balding, enhanced musculature, hirsutism)**
- Hirsutism may occur with or without virilization
- Androgens
  - Testosterone: Derived from the ovaries (25%), adrenals (25%), and peripheral conversion from androstenedione (50%)
    - Most potent androgen

- Circulates as free (1%) and bound (99%)
- Dihydroepiandrosterone-sulfate (DHEA-S) is predominantly derived from the adrenal cortex (95%)
- Causes of hirsutism include ovarian or adrenal causes, drugs, and physiologic (most common; Box 41-2)
  - **Idiopathic familial form (physiologic) is most common cause overall**
  - **Most common ovarian cause: Polycystic ovary syndrome (PCOS; see Box 41-1)**
  - **Most common adrenal cause: Congenital adrenal hyperplasia (Box 41-3)**

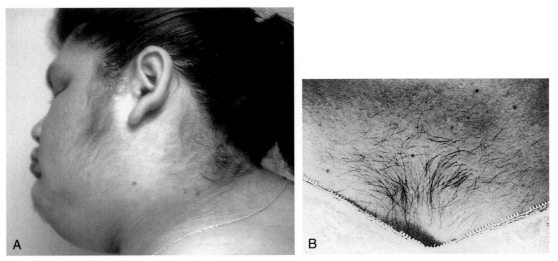

FIGURE 41-4   Examples of hirsutism. Male-pattern hair growth on the face (**A**), and on the chest (**B**). (From Larsen PR, Kronenberg HM, Melmed S, Polonsky, KS: *Williams textbook of endocrinology*, ed 10, Philadelphia, WB Saunders, 2003, figure 16-30.)

BOX 41-2	*Causes of Hirsutism*

Ovarian Causes
Polycystic ovary syndrome
Hyperthecosis (rests of ovarian stromal cells that produce testosterone)
Androgen-producing ovarian tumors

Adrenal Causes
Congenital adrenal hyperplasia
Androgen-producing adrenal tumors
Cushing syndrome

Elevated Prolactin
Unclear mechanism

Medications
Androgens (e.g., danazol)
Cyclosporine
Phenytoin

Physiologic Causes
Idiopathic familial
Postmenopausal

BOX 41-3	*Congenital Adrenal Hyperplasia*

Basic Information
Inherited defects in adrenal cortisol synthesis result in overproduction of other adrenal hormones, including androgens
Late-onset or nonclassical 21-hydroxylase deficiency is the most common form, occurring in 0.1–1% of women

Clinical Presentation
Hirsutism begins at menarche
Menstrual irregularities begin in adulthood

Diagnosis
17-hydroxyprogesterone will be elevated (stimulation with synthetic ACTH may be necessary to elicit the abnormality)

Treatment
Hydrocorticosone will decrease the excess androgen production

ACTH, adrenocorticotropic hormone.

- Look for signs of insulin resistance, including acanthosis nigricans (to suggest PCOS)
- Look for signs of Cushing's syndrome (e.g., dorsocervical fat pad, striae, proximal muscle weakness)

Clinical Presentation

- History
  - Assess onset, duration, and progression of hair growth
  - Look for symptoms of PCOS: Weight gain, acne, diabetes, menstrual irregularities
  - Inquire about family history of hirsutism (suggesting familial form)
  - Inquire about medications that might cause hirsutism (see Table 41-2)
- Physical examination
  - Assess extent of hirsutism
  - Look for signs of virilization (e.g., acne, clitoromegaly, deepened voice, muscle hypertrophy)

Diagnosis and Evaluation

- **Sudden onset, rapid course, and/or presence of virilization suggestive of a malignancy**
- Laboratory tests
  - Free and total testosterone
    - Often only free (not total) testosterone is elevated
    - Usually only mildly elevated with PCOS
    - **Total testosterone greater than 200 ng/dL raises concern for adrenal or ovarian tumor (DHEA-S helpful to distinguish source)**
  - DHEA-S
    - If level greater than 500 mg/dL, consider adrenal tumor or late-onset congenital adrenal hyperplasia

- Prolactin (hyperprolactinemia may cause hirsutism)
- 17-Hydroxyprogesterone
  - May be elevated in congenital adrenal hyperplasia
  - Adrenocorticotropic hormone (ACTH) stimulation test may be necessary to elicit elevation
- Imaging
  - Abdominal CT or sonogram if adrenal or ovarian tumors are suspected
  - MRI of the pituitary if prolactin is elevated and no medication is identified as the culprit

Treatment

- Treatment is directed toward correction of the underlying problem (if possible)
- Once a terminal hair has developed, it may not disappear, even if abnormal hormone levels resolve
- Spironolactone is useful for inhibiting effects of androgens on hair follicles but primarily prevents worsening of hirsutism
- **Insulin sensitizers, such as metformin or thiazolidinediones ("glitazones"), can induce ovulation, decrease hirsutism, and reduce insulin resistance in women with PCOS**
- Eflornithine cream may inhibit an enzyme needed for hair growth; often used for facial hair

Male Reproductive and Hormonal Disorders

GYNECOMASTIA

Basic Information

- *Gynecomastia* **refers to benign growth of glandular tissue of the male breast**
- **Considered normal in males at three life stages**
  - **Newborn (first 2–3 weeks of life)**
  - **Pubertal**
  - **Elderly**
- Causes of gynecomastia (Box 41-4)
  - Most causes induce gynecomastia by causing a change in the relative amounts of estrogens and androgens (e.g., the ratio favors estrogen excess)
  - Mechanisms include decrease in androgen or androgen effect or increase in estrogen (exogenous or endogenous)
  - Most common causes in adults are medications and alcoholic liver disease

Clinical Presentation

- Confirm gynecomastia: Concentric enlargement of the tissue deep to the nipple
  - May be unilateral or bilateral
  - May be asymmetrical
  - May be associated with pain and tenderness
  - Nipple discharge is rare; if presenst, consider malignancy
  - Distinguish from obesity by palpating for a ridge of tissue concentric with the nipple
- Assess for sexual dysfunction
- Perform a testicular examination to detect any masses

BOX 41-4	*Causes of Gynecomastia*

Medications
  ACE inhibitors
  Amiodarone
  Antipsychotics
  Calcium channel-blockers
  Diazepam
  Digoxin
  Efavirenz
  HIV nucleoside reverse transcriptase inhibitors
  Ketoconazole
  Omeprazole
  Opiates
  Phenytoin
  Ranitidine
  Spironolactone
  Tricyclic antidepressants
Endocrine disorders
  Hyperthyroidism
  Hypogonadism
  Hormone-secreting tumors
Chronic systemic illness
  Renal disease
  Hepatic disease
Marijuana
Idiopathic

Diagnosis and Evaluation

- Cause is often clear from history and physical examination
- **Highly consider malignancy if gynecomastia is unilateral, ulcerative, associated with bloody discharge or with axillary adenopathy; in this case, proceed directly to mammography and biopsy**
- Laboratory evaluation (if cause is not clear from the history and physical)
  - Check renal and hepatic function
  - Testosterone level (low level suggests hypogonadal cause)
  - FSH, LH
    - High levels associated with primary testicular failure
    - Low levels associated with exogenous steroids or hypogonadotropic hypogonadism
  - Prolactin (prolactinoma), thyroid-stimulating hormone (TSH; hyperthyroidism), hCG (human chorionic gonadotropin [hCG]-producing testicular tumor), estradiol (estrogen-producing testicular tumor)
- Mammogram: Perform if gynecomastia is unilateral or if the mass is not concentric with the nipple

Treatment

- Gynecomastia is primarily a cosmetic problem, although it can be a clue to underlying disease
- Men with gynecomastia may have a slight increase in risk of breast cancer
- **Treatment is aimed at eliminating the underlying disease**

- If treatment begins in the first few months after symptoms of gynecomastia appear, chance of regression of the gynecomastia is good
  - **Over time, the enlarged breast tissue becomes fibrotic and is not likely to shrink even if hormones return to normal**
- Options
  - Anti-estrogens (e.g., tamoxifen) may be useful
  - Surgery may be performed if gynecomastia does not resolve and is bothersome to the patient

MALE HYPOGONADISM

Basic Information

- *Hypogonadism* **in men is defined as an inappropriately low testosterone level for age**
  - Normal range for men ages 18 to 29 years is approximately 700 to 1300 ng/dL
  - Declines to approximately 150 to 500 ng/dL for men aged 70 to 79 years
- **Classification of male hypogonadism**
  - **Primary: Caused by dysfunction of the testes (hypergonadotropic hypogonadism)**
  - **Secondary: Caused by a disorder of the pituitary or hypothalamus** that impairs the ability of the pituitary to stimulate testosterone production (**hypogonadotropic hypogonadism**)
  - **Testosterone resistance: Inability of the target tissues to respond to testosterone**
- Causes of primary and secondary hypogonadism (Box 41-5)
- Most common cause of primary hypogonadism in men is Klinefelter's syndrome (Box 41-6; Fig. 41-5)

Clinical Presentation

- Symptoms
  - Decreased libido
  - Hot flashes if testosterone loss is sudden
- Signs
  - Sparse facial and body hair
  - Gynecomastia
  - Small penis, prostate, and testes
- Related conditions
  - Infertility
  - Osteoporosis
- **If hypogonadal during adolescence, may have complete failure of sexual maturation**
  - **Absence of growth spurt, high-pitched voice, and upper-to-lower body ratio of less than 1**

BOX 41-5   *Causes of Male Hypogonadism*

Primary Hypogonadism (Hypergonadotropic Hypogonadism)
Trauma to genital organs
Autoimmune destruction
Mumps orchitis
Medications
   Cyclosporine
   Chemotherapeutic agents
Congenital disorders
   Klinefelter's syndrome
   Bilateral anorchia

Secondary Hypogonadism (Hypogonadotropic Hypogonadism)
Chronic illness
Medications
   Opiates
   Glucocorticoids
   Leuprolide
Prolactinoma
Damage to hypothalamus or pituitary
   Radiation
   Tumor
   Trauma
Hereditary
   Hemochromatosis (pituitary iron deposition)
Congenital disorders
   Kallman's syndrome

BOX 41-6   *Klinefelter's Syndrome*

Basic Information
Incidence of 1 per 1000 live male births
XXY karyotype
↑ FSH and LH in response to low testosterone production; promotes estrogen production by the Leydig cells

Clinical Presentation
May be asymptomatic until puberty
Intellect may be subnormal throughout life
Physical examination
   Gynecomastia develops in response to the estrogen
     Variable secondary sexual characteristics ranging from no sexual development to normal development
   Infertility
   Testicular exam: During puberty, testes become small and firm
   Increased risk of breast cancer, autoimmune disorders, varicose veins, germ cell neoplasms

Diagnosis
History and physical
   Upper body segment to lower body segment ratio < 1
   High palate
   Above-average arm span
Labs
   Low testosterone
   Elevated FSH and LH
   XXY karyotype is needed to confirm the diagnosis

Treatment
Androgen replacement

FSH, follicle-stimulating hormone; LH, luteinizing hormone.

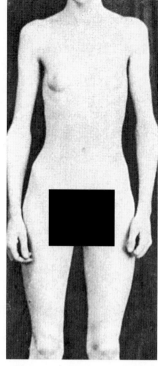

FIGURE 41-5 Klinefelter's syndrome. Note the narrow shoulders, long upper body segment, and gynecomastia. (From Ferri FF: *Ferri's clinical advisor: instant diagnosis and treatment,* ed 8, Philadelphia, Mosby, 2006, figure 1-133.)

- Consider possibility of
  - Klinefelter's syndrome (see Box 41-5 and Fig. 41-5)
  - Kallman's syndrome (congenital lack of development of the olfactory lobes and GnRH-producing cells leading to anosmia; hypogonadotropic hypogonadism; and, occasionally, cleft palate or color blindness)

Diagnosis and Evaluation

- **Low testosterone is diagnostic**
  - **Total testosterone less than 300 ng/dL is generally considered abnormal at any age when accompanied by clinical symptoms**
  - Check a free testosterone level to rule out an abnormality with sex hormone-binding globulin
- Semen analysis helpful (even if fertility not an issue): If normal, hypogonadism essentially ruled out
- FSH and LH: High in primary hypogonadism, low in secondary hypogonadism
- Other tests should be based on the clinical picture
  - Comprehensive metabolic panel and complete blood counts (to look for undiagnosed chronic disease, such as hepatic or renal failure)
  - Prolactin and brain MRI if pituitary tumor suspected
  - Estradiol, hCG, and testicular ultrasound if testicular tumor suspected
  - Iron studies if hemochromatosis suspected

Treatment

- Treatment of underlying problem if possible
- Androgen replacement with testosterone injection, patch, or gel

- Contraindication to replacement: History of androgen-dependent tumor (e.g., prostate cancer)
- **Hematocrit should be monitored regularly given the increased risk of erythrocytosis with testosterone replacement**
- **Prostate examination and prostate-specific antigen (PSA) testing should be done in men older than 40 years receiving androgen replacement**
- Therapy with FSH and hCG (by injection) may be used in those with hypogonadotropic hypogonadism who desire fertility

ERECTILE DYSFUNCTION

Basic Information

- **Definition: Inability to attain or maintain an erection to achieve penetration**
- Causes
  - Penile disorders
    - Peyronie's disease (penile induration): Stems from fibrotic plaques of unclear etiology that can result in penile curvature, painful erections, and impotence; treatment is surgical
    - Trauma
  - Nervous system disorders: Stroke, spinal cord injury, prostatectomy complicated by nerve injury
  - Vascular disorders
    - Atherosclerotic vascular disease
    - **Leriche's syndrome (impotence associated with distal aortic atherosclerosis resulting in claudication of the lower back, buttocks, and thighs)**
  - Endocrine disorders: Diabetes, hypogonadism
  - Psychogenic disorders (common in young men)
  - Medications (see Box 41-4 for male hypogonadism), as well as β-blockers, antidepressants, and antipsychotics
  - Substance abuse

Clinical Presentation

- Difficulty with obtaining or maintaining an erection
- May or may not have features of hypogonadism (see previous section)

Diagnosis and Evaluation

- History and physical examination
  - Look for clues to an underlying diagnosis (e.g., presence of peripheral vascular disease, complications of diabetes)
  - **Sudden onset of impotence favors psychogenic cause**
- Check testosterone levels, FSH, LH, estradiol
- Psychiatric evaluation if psychogenic cause suspected

Treatment

- Directed at underlying cause
- **Sildenafil, vardenafil, and tadalafil are phosphodiesterase-5 (PDE-5) inhibitors that prolong vasodilatation by nitric oxide and are considered first-line drugs after underlying causes have been investigated**
  - Sildenafil and vardenafil should be taken 1 hour before intercourse; duration of effect is approximately 4 hours

- Tadalafil has a faster onset of action and longer duration (36 hours)
- **Warn patients about potential side effects**
  - **Color vision changes**
  - **Headaches**
  - **Sudden blindness from nonischemic anterior optic neuropathy (case reports)**
- **Avoid in patients on nitrates (may induce hypotension) and those with recent or unstable coronary artery disease**
- All PDE-5 inhibitors are metabolized by cytochrome P450 CYP3A4; doses should be reduced when combined with inhibitors of CYP3A4 (erythromycin, ketoconazole, protease inhibitors, and grapefruit juice)
- Other treatment options
  - Vasodilators such as prostaglandin E, papaverine, intraurethral alprostadil
- Vacuum devices (avoid in patients at risk for bleeding)
- Penile prostheses (associated with risk of infection)

REVIEW QUESTIONS

For review questions, please go to www.expertconsult.com.

SUGGESTED READINGS

Fraser IS, Kovacs G: Current recommendations for the diagnostic evaluation and follow-up of patients presenting with symptomatic polycystic ovary syndrome, *Best Pract Res Clin Obstet Gynaecol* 5:813–823, 2004.

Rosenfield RL: Clinical practice: hirsutism, *N Engl J Med* 353:2578–2588, 2005.

Warren MP, Hagey AR: The genetics, diagnosis and treatment of amenorrhea, *Minerva Ginecol* 56:437–455, 2004.

Neuroendocrine and Adrenal Disease

ROBERTO SALVATORI, MD

Protein hormones, most of which are **produced or stored in the pituitary gland,** and **steroid hormones,** many of which are **produced in the adrenal glands,** have profound impact on growth, development, and metabolism. Overproduction or underproduction of a single hormone may result in signs or symptoms that range from minimal to life threatening.

Neuroendocrine Disorders

OVERVIEW OF THE PITUITARY GLAND AND PITUITARY MASSES

- The pituitary gland includes the anterior and posterior parts (Fig. 42-1)
  - **Anterior pituitary produces prolactin (PRL), thyroid-stimulating hormone (TSH, also known as thyrotropin), adrenocorticotropic hormone (ACTH), luteinizing hormone (LH), follicle-stimulating hormone (FSH), and growth hormone (GH)**
    - ACTH is synthesized as part of a larger protein, pro-opiomelanocortin. Any stimulation of ACTH production will result in increased production of pro-opiomelanocortin.
  - **The posterior pituitary stores antidiuretic hormone (ADH) and oxytocin, which are produced in the hypothalamus**
- Pituitary/sellar masses: **Neuroendocrine disorders commonly present in the setting of a sellar mass**
  - **Approximately 45% of sellar masses are hormone-secreting pituitary tumors**
  - **Approximately 45% of sellar masses are non–hormone-secreting pituitary tumors**

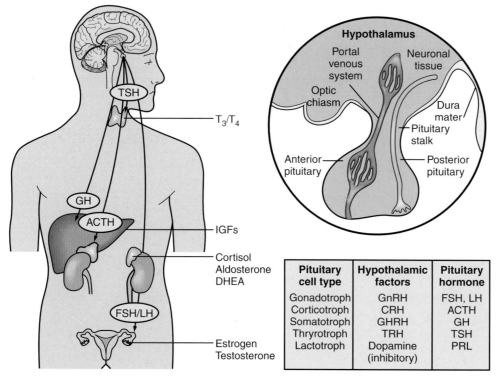

Pituitary cell type	Hypothalamic factors	Pituitary hormone
Gonadotroph	GnRH	FSH, LH
Corticotroph	CRH	ACTH
Somatotroph	GHRH	GH
Thryrotroph	TRH	TSH
Lactotroph	Dopamine (inhibitory)	PRL

FIGURE 42-1 The hypothalamic-pituitary axis. ACTH, adrenocorticotropin hormone; CRH, corticotropin-releasing hormone; DHEA, dehydroepiandrosterone; FSH, follicle-stimulating hormone; GH, growth hormone; GHRH, growth hormone–releasing hormone; GnRH, gonadotropin-releasing hormone; IGF, insulin-like growth factor; PRL, prolactin; T_3, tri-iodothyronine; T_4, thyroxine; TRH, thyroid-releasing hormone. TSH, thyroid-stimulating hormone. (From Page C: *Integrated pharmacology,* ed 3, Philadelphia, Mosby, 2006, figure 15.2.)

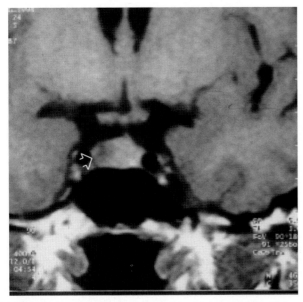

FIGURE 42-2 An MRI scan of pituitary demonstrating the typical appearance of a pituitary microademona. A hypodense lesion is seen in the right side of the gland with deviation of the pituitary stalk away from the lesion *(arrow)*. After a biochemical diagnosis of Cushing's disease, this patient was cured following trans-sphenoidal hypophysectomy. (From Larsen PR, Kronenberg HM, Melmed S, Polonsky, KS: *Williams textbook of endocrinology,* ed 10, Philadelphia, WB Saunders, 2003, figure 14-23.)

- The remainder of sellar masses are not tumors of anterior pituitary origin, and they represent craniopharyngiomas, Rathke's cleft cysts, meningiomas, metastatic tumors, lymphoma, granulomatous diseases, or the increasingly recognized autoimmune lymphocytic hypophysitis
- **Pituitary tumors smaller than 10mm are referred to as** *microadenomas* **(Fig. 42-2).** If the adenoma is equal to or larger than 10mm, it is referred to as a *macroadenoma.*
- Pituitary incidentaloma: A pituitary mass discovered in a patient without endocrine symptoms; prevalence of incidentalomas has increased because of increased use of brain imaging
  - **All patients with a pituitary adenoma should be evaluated for hormone hypersecretion syndromes that cannot be excluded by history or physical examination (see following discussion)**
  - **Incidental microadenomas grow in less than 10% of cases**
    - If nonsecreting, conservative management with periodic MRIs at progressively increasing intervals is performed
  - **Incidental macroadenomas should also be evaluated for hypopituitarism. Visual field testing should be performed as well.**
    - **Further growth occurs in about 50% of macroadenomas**
    - **Surgery is indicated if optic chiasm is compressed, if the patient is symptomatic (e.g., headaches), or if the tumor is growing**

Pituitary Hormone Excess States

- General principles
  - Disorders of the pituitary may present **with three classes of signs and symptoms**
    - Syndromes of **hormone excess** (e.g., acromegaly, Cushing's disease, hyperprolactinemia)
    - Symptoms of **hormone deficit** (partial or complete hypopituitarism, discussed in the next section)
    - **Compressive symptoms**
      - Frontal headaches
      - Visual changes (typically a bitemporal hemianopsia)
      - If cavernous sinus invaded by expanding tumor, cranial nerve palsies develop (cranial nerves III, IV, VI)
- The clinical presentation of a neuroendocrine disorder will also vary based on the actions of the hormone that is either undersecreted or oversecreted (Table 42-1; see following discussion)
- Pituitary tumors may exist as part of syndromes
- In conjunction with other endocrine tumors; this is known as the **multiple endocrine neoplasia** (MEN)-I syndrome (Box 42-1)
- As part of the **"Carney complex"** (autosomal dominant complex of cardiac myxomas, cutaneous myxomas, spotty pigmentation of the skin, and hyperendocrine states)
- As the syndrome of familial isolated pituitary adenomas (FIPA)
  - A thorough family history is indicated for all patients diagnosed with a pituitary adenoma
    - **All patients should be asked about personal or family history of hypercalcemia or kidney stones because hyperparathyroidism is the most common feature of MEN-1**
    - **All patients should be examined for perioral hyperpigmentation, tumors of the heart, and hyperendocrine states, which may suggest Carney complex**

Prolactinoma

Basic Information

- **PRL is produced by lactotroph cells in the anterior pituitary**
  - **Dopaminergic pathways inhibit PRL production**
- Elevations in serum PRL levels may be physiologic (e.g., pregnancy) or pathologic (Box 42-2)
- **Prolactinomas are the most common hormone-secreting pituitary adenomas (see Box 42-2)**

Clinical Presentation

- **Elevated PRL levels inhibit gonadotropin secretion** (by inhibiting release of luteinizing hormone-releasing hormone) and decrease gonadal responsiveness to gonadotropins (Fig. 42-3)
- **Galactorrhea can be seen in premenopausal women and in postmenopausal women if they are taking hormone replacement, but it is seen rarely in men**

TABLE 42-1	*Pituitary Hormones: Key Details*			
Hormone	**Major Actions**	**Secretagogue**	**Inhibitor**	**Deficiency Syndrome**
Prolactin (PRL) Growth hormone (GH)	Lactation Linear growth (via insulin-like growth factors)	Thyrotropin-releasing hormone (TRH) Growth hormone–releasing hormone	Dopamine Somatostatin Insulin-like growth factor-1 (IGF-1)	Inability to lactate Children: Dwarfism Adults: Loss of bone mass, hypoglycemia, hypercholesterolemia
Adrenocorticotropic hormone (ACTH)	Release of cortisol from adrenal gland	Corticotropin-releasing hormone (CRH)	Glucocorticoids	Secondary adrenal insufficiency (no hyperpigmentation or electrolyte disturbances seen)
Thyroid-stimulating hormone (TSH)	Production and release of thyroid hormones	TRH	Thyroid hormones (thyroxine or triiodothyronine)	Central hypothyroidism (see Chapter 39)
Follicle-stimulating hormone (FSH)	Women: Growth of granulose cells and estradiol production in ovarian follicle Men: Stimulates seminiferous tubules to produce sperm	Gonadotropin-releasing hormone (GnRH) GnRH is also known as luteinizing hormone–releasing hormone (LHRH)	Inhibin Estradiol Testosterone (PRL inhibits GnRH release)	Children: Delayed puberty Women: Amenorrhea Men: Impotence, testicular atrophy Kallmann's syndrome: Gonadotropin deficiency caused by congenital GnRH deficiency
Luteinizing hormone (LH)	Women: Stimulates ovarian theca cells to produce androgens; LH surge stimulates ovulation Men: Stimulates testosterone production in Leydig cells	Same as FSH	Estradiol Testosterone (PRL inhibits GnRH release)	Same as FSH
Antidiuretic hormone (ADH) (arginine vasopressin [AVP])	Makes collecting ducts in renal tubules permeable to water Stimulates thirst	Increases in osmolality Decreases in volume	Decreases in osmolality	Diabetes insipidus
Oxytocin	Contraction of uterine and breast muscles	Estrogen Suckling	None	None

- **Menstrual irregularities are common and result in women being diagnosed earlier than men. Women most commonly present with microadenomas.**
- **Men present with decreased libido and impotence or visual loss and are more likely to present with macroadenomas, sometimes very large**

Diagnosis

- Exclude other causes of elevated PRL levels (see Box 42-2)
  - **If PRL level is greater than 200 ng/mL, prolactinoma is very likely**
- MRI of sella obtained
  - High serum PRL level and pituitary mass by MRI typically used to diagnose prolactinoma
    - **However, a sellar mass in the presence of elevated serum PRL levels is not definitive proof of prolactinoma. A large, nonsecreting adenoma may cause elevated PRL levels by compressing pituitary stalk and inhibiting hypothalamic dopaminergic regulation of PRL.**
    - **Suspect this if macroadenoma seen with only moderate elevation of PRL level (i.e., <100 ng/mL)**

- If PRL is elevated but the patient has no clinical symptoms, the presence of "macroprolactinemia" must be suspected
- In macroprolactinemia, PRL molecules bind to circulating immunoglobulins, causing marked increase in serum half-life
- Serum PRL is high, but this is not biologically active
- Condition can be identified by repeating serum PRL measurement after precipitating immunoglubulins with polyethylene glycol
- Requires no treatment

Treatment

- Normalization of PRL is usually required to normalize menses and to restore eugonadism
- First-line treatment is with dopaminergic agonists
  - **Bromocriptine (Parlodel) and cabergoline (Dostinex) are agents most commonly used**
- If medical therapy fails, surgery is performed via transsphenoidal approach
- Radiation used if tumor recurs after surgery (rare)

BOX 42-1 Multiple Endocrine Neoplasia Syndromes

MEN-1 (Autosomal Dominant)

Parathyroid hyperplasia/adenoma (high penetrance)

Pancreatic islet cell hyperplasia/adenoma/carcinoma (usually Zollinger-Ellison syndrome*; insulinoma; or, rarely, glucagonoma)

Pituitary adenoma

(Rarely includes carcinoid, pheochromocytoma)

MEN-2A (Autosomal Dominant)

Medullary thyroid carcinoma

Pheochromocytoma

Parathyroid hyperplasia or adenoma

MEN-2B (Autosomal Dominant)

Medullary thyroid carcinoma

Pheochromocytoma

Mucosal/gastrointestinal neuromas

Marfanoid body habitus

Carney Complex (Autosomal Dominant)

Pituitary tumors (mostly GH secreting)

Cushing's syndrome due to bilateral micronodular adrenal hyperplasia

Thyroid tumors

Atrial myxomas

Perioral hyperpigmentation

*Overproduction of gastrin, resulting in recurrent multiple peptic ulcers.
GH, growth hormone; MEN, multiple endocrine neoplasia.

BOX 42-2 Causes of Elevated Serum Prolactin Level

Endocrine

Pituitary adenoma

Hypothalamic disease

    Sarcoidosis

    Craniopharyngioma

    Empty sella syndrome

Primary hypothyroidism

Pregnancy

Drugs

CNS active

    Risperidone (associated with very high prolactin levels)

    Phenothiazines

    Haloperidol

Metoclopramide

Antihypertensives

    Methyldopa

    Reserpine

    Verapamil

Estrogens

Opiates

Other

Stress

Nipple stimulation

Chest wall trauma

Renal failure

Macroprolactinemia: Artifactual elevation of measured serum prolactin while actual level is normal

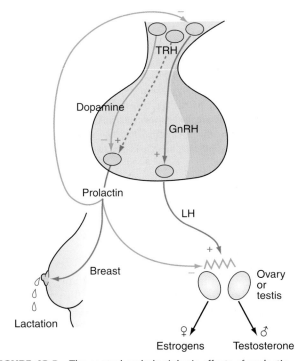

FIGURE 42-3 The control and physiologic effects of prolactin secretion, demonstrating inhibition of luteinizing hormone (LH) secretion and action. GnRH, gonadotropin-releasing hormone; TRH, thyroid-releasing hormone. (From Kumar P, Clark M: *Clinical medicine,* ed 5, Philadelphia, WB Saunders, 2005, figure 18-11.)

Growth Hormone–Secreting Tumors

Basic Information

- **Excess growth hormone (GH) results in gigantism in children, whose epiphyseal bone plates have not closed (Fig. 42-4), or acromegaly in adults (Fig. 42-5)**
- **GH acts on tissues both directly and indirectly by stimulating the production of other hormones that stimulate growth (somatomedin C or insulin-like growth factor-1 [IGF-1])**
- Onset of acromegaly is insidious and often missed

Clinical Presentation

- Most common features are **acral growth, excessive sweating, and weakness/fatigue**
  - Also seen are **sleep apnea, arthralgias, glucose intolerance, teeth malocclusion, and carpal tunnel syndrome**
  - Incidence of colonic polyps two to three times higher than age-matched controls and may correlate with presence of skin tags
- **Characteristic physical appearance includes coarse facial features with frontal bossing; prognathism; and deep, sonorous voice**
  - Hand, foot, and hat sizes are increased

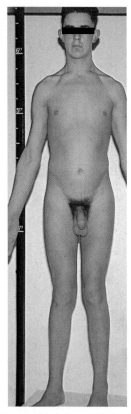

FIGURE 42-4 A 16-year-old patient suffering from gigantism. Growth hormone is raised, and bone age is not advanced, indicating that the boy's eventual stature will be abnormally tall. (From Besser GM, Thorner M: *Comprehensive clinical endocrinology,* ed 3, Mosby, 2002, figure 24B.31.)

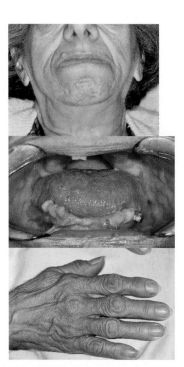

FIGURE 42-5 Acromegaly of the jaw and hand. (From Regezi JA, Sciubba JJ, Jordan RCK: *Oral pathology: clinical pathological correlations,* ed 4, Philadelphia, WB Saunders, 2003, figure 15-8.)

Diagnosis

- Because GH levels fluctuate according to a diurnal pattern (and significant overlap exists between normal and abnormal individuals), **GH levels alone are not used to diagnose acromegaly**
- **IGF-1 (also called somatomedin C) levels are more consistently elevated in acromegaly and are the initial test of choice in screening for acromegaly**
- **To confirm the diagnosis in dubious cases, a glucose suppression test is performed**
  - **In normal subjects, a 75-g oral glucose load suppresses GH levels to less than 1 ng/mL**
  - **In acromegaly, a 75-g oral glucose load does not suppress GH levels and may paradoxically increase GH levels**
- Brain imaging is typically done after serologic evaluation

Treatment

- Goal of treatment is **normalization of IGF-1 and GH levels** because non-cured acromegalic patients have a reduced life expectancy
- **Surgery is initial management** (transsphenoidal)
  - Curative in 50%; cure less likely with macroadenoma
  - **Somatostatin analogue (octreotide) used with postsurgical recurrence, with hormonal response in 60% of patients**
  - Some (20%) may respond to cabergoline (particularly if they co-secrete PRL)
  - GH receptor antagonist (pegvisomant) normalizes IGF-1 in 90% of patients
  - **Radiation also used with postsurgical recurrence; it requires several years to be effective**

Hypercortisolism

Basic Information

- **Cushing's disease: Hypercortisolism as a result of ACTH-producing pituitary adenoma**
- **Cushing's syndrome: Hypercortisolism caused by adrenal adenoma or carcinoma, by ectopic ACTH production, or by the administration of exogenous glucocorticoids**

Clinical Presentation

- See Figure 42-6 for an example of Cushing's syndrome
- Patients present with hypertension, central obesity, moon facies, dorsal fat pad, purple striae on skin, and muscle weakness
  - Psychiatric symptoms also common
- Secondary amenorrhea may develop in women, along with hirsutism or other evidence of masculinization
- Osteoporosis also develops in women and men
- Common laboratory abnormalities may include glucose intolerance (or diabetes) and metabolic alkalosis with hypokalemia

Diagnosis

- Diagnosis of hypercortisolism (Fig. 42-7): **Begin by measuring 24-hour urine free cortisol or 11 PM**

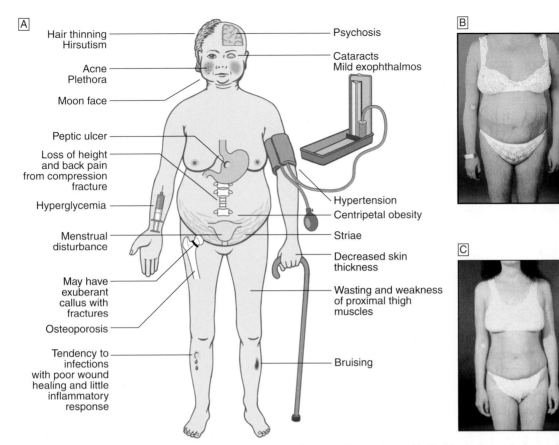

FIGURE 42-6 Cushing's syndrome. **A,** Clinical features common to all causes. **B,** A patient with Cushing's disease before treatment. **C,** The same patient 1 year after successful removal of an adrenocorticotropin hormone–secreting pituitary microadenoma by transsphenoidal surgery. (From Haslett C, Chilvers ER, Boon NA, et al: *Davidson's principles and practice of medicine,* ed 19, New York, Churchill Livingstone, 2002, figure 16.17.)

salivary cortisol or performing a 1-mg overnight dexamethasone suppression test
- Plasma ACTH levels differentiate between ACTH-dependent and independent Cushing's
- If ACTH-independent, adrenal imaging is necessary
- Localization of source of ACTH in ACTH-dependent conditions (i.e., pituitary versus ectopic ACTH) requires sequential testing
- Sequential testing based on the following principles:
  - In normal host, **glucocorticoids inhibit ACTH** secretion (Fig. 42-8)
  - **ACTH-secreting pituitary adenomas are partially autonomous but can be inhibited with high doses of glucocorticoids (e.g., dexamethasone)**
- In difficult cases of differentiation of pituitary versus ectopic ACTH, bilateral inferior petrosal sinus sampling is done after administration of corticotropin-releasing factor (CRF)

Treatment

- **For pituitary source, transsphenoidal resection, sometimes followed by irradiation, is used**
- **For adrenal source, adrenalectomy performed**
- **When surgical cure is not obtainable, medical adrenalectomy can be achieved with administration of medications that inhibit production of cortisol (e.g., ketoconazole, metyrapone, mytotane)**

Syndrome of Inappropriate Antidiuretic Hormone

See Chapter 33.

Uncommon Disorders of the Anterior Pituitary

- **Pituitary hyperthyroidism, caused by a TSH-producing adenoma, is rare**
- **Gonadotropin-secreting tumors (i.e., LH, FSH) typically present as macroadenomas and may be asymptomatic**
  - Many "nonfunctioning" macroadenomas may actually produce nonbiologically active gonadotropins (e.g., α-subunits of gonadotropins)

Pituitary Hormone Insufficiency States

Basic Information

- Hypopituitarism is **most commonly caused by pituitary adenoma,** with destruction or compression of normal pituitary cells
  - **With pituitary tumors/mass effect, GH typically is affected first, followed by gonadotropins, then TSH; ACTH is affected last**

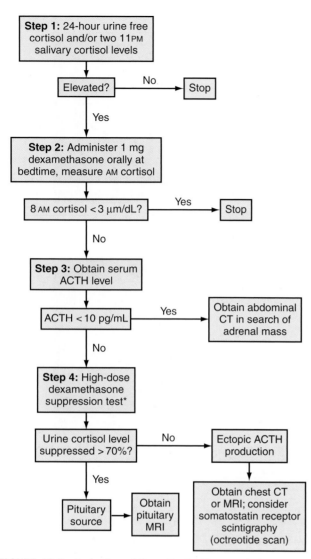

FIGURE 42-7 Evaluation of the patient with suspected hypercortisolism. *Dexamethasone 2 mg every 6 hours for 2 days; collect urine on day 0 and day 2. ACTH, adrenocorticotropin hormone.

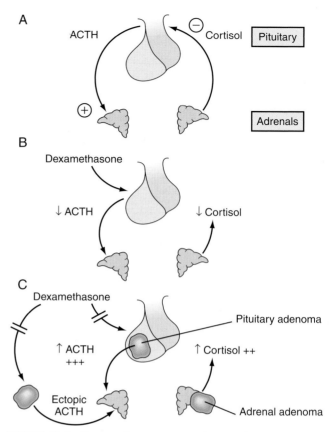

FIGURE 42-8 Dexamethasone suppression test. **A,** Normal feedback mechanism for cortisol production. **B,** Normally, dexamethasone suppresses adrenocorticotropin (ACTH) and hence cortisol production. **C,** In Cushing's syndrome resulting from pituitary or ectopic ACTH excess, or adrenal adenoma, dexamethasone has no effect, and cortisol is not suppressed. (From Souhami R: *Textbook of medicine,* New York, Churchill Livingstone, 2002, figure 17.30.)

- Order may change with other causes of hypopituitarism (e.g., radiation)
- Other causes of hypopituitarism include pituitary apoplexy; pituitary infarction; inflammation of the pituitary (lymphocytic hypophysitis, typically but not exclusively in postpartum women); CNS radiation; surgery; head trauma (single or multiple repeated traumas); or replacement of the pituitary or hypothalamus with infectious, granulomatous, or malignant disease
- Clinical manifestations depend on which hormone or combination of hormones is affected (Fig. 42-9) and to what extent they are affected (see Table 42-1)
- **Pituitary apoplexy: The acute development of pituitary insufficiency,** most commonly from sudden hemorrhage or infarction of the pituitary gland
  - Most commonly occurs in patients with **previously undiagnosed pituitary tumor**

- Symptoms include **sudden headache, visual deficit, ophthalmoplegia** (cranial nerves III, IV, or VI may be affected), and altered mental status
- **Most dangerous result is lack of ACTH** and therefore secondary adrenal insufficiency (see following section on adrenal insufficiency)
- **Sheehan's syndrome:** Pituitary infarction **caused by blood loss during childbirth;** presents within first days or week following childbirth; classic presentation is a **new mother who is unable to produce milk**

Prolactin Deficiency

Basic Information

- **Usually occurs in the setting of other pituitary hormone deficiencies**

Clinical Presentation

- **Asymptomatic in men**
- Women will note lack of lactation (i.e., with pregnancy)

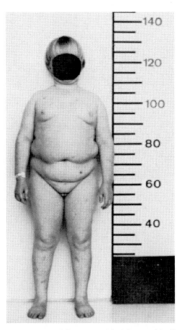

FIGURE 42-9 A 20-year-old man with idiopathic hypopituitary dwarfism and deficiencies of gonadotropins, thyrotropin, corticotropin, and growth hormone, who had a history of arrested hydrocephalus. Note the extreme atrophy of the genitalia, the absence of body hair, and apparent gynecomastia associated with obesity. (From Yen SCC, Jaffe RB: *Reproductive endocrinology*, ed 2, Philadelphia, WB Saunders, 1986, figure 24-52.)

Diagnosis

- Low serum PRL level in the appropriate host

Treatment

- There is **no treatment** for PRL deficiency

Growth Hormone Deficiency

Basic Information

- Patients with panhypopituitarism have a 99% likelihood of being GH deficient

Clinical Presentation

- Symptoms of GH deficiency depend on the age of onset
  - In children, stunted growth occurs
  - In adults, symptoms of GH deficiency are usually overshadowed by other manifestations of pituitary insufficiency but include a **decreased sense of well-being, decreased muscle mass, increased fat mass, osteopenia, and an abnormal lipid profile** (increased total and low-density lipoprotein [LDL] cholesterol)

Diagnosis

- **To diagnose, a low serum IGF-1 is typically seen,** but this is not sensitive or specific
- Large overlap exists in serum IGF-1 between GH-deficient and normal subjects, particularly in patients older than 40 years
- If IGF-1 is normal but suspicion is high, testing of GH-reserve by insulin-induced hypoglycemia or growth hormone–releasing hormone (GHRH) and arginine or glucagon is used

Treatment

- Although in the past GH deficiency in fully grown adults was not treated, adult patients with severe GH deficiency should be considered for GH-replacement therapy to improve muscle mass, bone density, quality of life, and lipid profile

ACTH Deficiency

ACTH deficiency is known as secondary adrenal insufficiency and is discussed in the section on adrenal insufficiency that follows.

Central Hypothyroidism

Basic Information

- A rare cause of hypothyroidism
- As with other disorders noted, most commonly occurs in association with other causes of pituitary insufficiency

Clinical Presentation

- Patient presents with the typical signs and symptoms of hypothyroidism, **often milder than primary hypothyroidism** (see Chapter 39)

Diagnosis

- Diagnosed by **low serum free thyroxine levels in setting of low (or inappropriately normal) TSH level**

Treatment

- TSH cannot be followed for medication dosing in individuals with central hypothyroidism
- Treatment is repletion with thyroxine, adjusted to **symptoms and serum free thyroxine (T$_4$) levels**
- **In patients with central hypothyroidism, never replace thyroid hormone before assessing adrenal function because pharmacologically induced euthyroidism may trigger adrenal crisis (T$_4$ accelerates cortisol catabolism)**

Central Hypogonadism

Basic Information

- Central hypogonadism, or secondary hypogonadism, is caused by **insufficient production of LH and/or FSH**
- **Secondary hypogonadism is less common than primary hypogonadism (primary hypogonadism is testicular or ovarian failure associated with elevated levels of LH and FSH)**
- Occurs with other causes of hypopituitarism as well as other clinical settings
  - **Kallmann's syndrome (Fig. 42-10): Lack of GnRH secretion, resulting in central hypogonadism**
    - Additional features may include neurosensory hearing loss, red-green color blindness, urogenital tract abnormalities, and lack of sense of smell

42

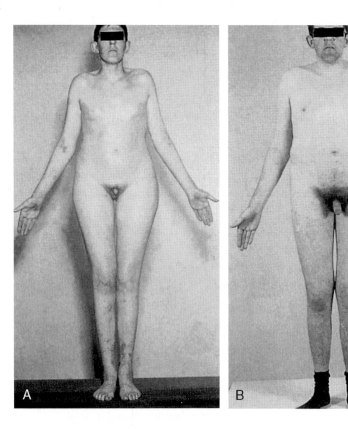

FIGURE 42-10 Grossly eunuchoidal 31-year-old man with Kallmann's syndrome. **A,** Before androgen replacement. **B,** After 2 years of androgen replacement. (From Souhami R: *Textbook of medicine,* New York, Churchill Livingstone, 2002, figure 17.36.)

Clinical Presentation

- **Determined in large part by the age of onset of secondary hypogonadism**
  - **Prepubertal boys and girls will fail to develop secondary sexual characteristics**
  - **In adults infertility and decreased sexual drive are common (in both men and women) as well as amenorrhea (females)**
    - Men may have eunuchoid body habitus (arm span greater than height; lower body segment longer than upper body segment) and gynecomastia

Diagnosis

- **Diagnosed by low sex hormone levels in setting of low (or inappropriately normal) LH and FSH levels**

Treatment

- **In men, treatment is with testosterone, titrated to normal serum levels**
  - If fertility in men is desired, LH and FSH can be administered as intramuscular injections
  - May take several months of therapy to reach normal sperm count
- **In women, treatment is with estrogen and progesterone**
  - If fertility is desired, LH and FSH can be administered under the care of a reproductive endocrinologist

Diabetes Insipidus

Basic Information

- **Neurogenic diabetes insipidus (DI):** Lack of production and release of ADH from **posterior pituitary**

- **Caused by either hypothalamic disease (e.g., sarcoidosis, tuberculosis) or following neurosurgery;** pituitary adenomas do not cause DI unless there has been a surgical treatment
  - Rare forms include familial DI, traumatic DI, or idiopathic DI
- **Nephrogenic DI:** Lack of **renal response** to ADH (no disorder of posterior pituitary implied)
  - May be congenital or acquired
    - Acquired form may result from hypercalcemia, hypokalemia, or medications (e.g., lithium; nephrogenic DI may persist after discontinuation of lithium)

Clinical Presentation

- Patients present with impaired renal conservation of water and production of dilute urine
  - **Polyuria, polydipsia, and sometimes hypernatremia result**

Diagnosis

- Suspect if increased serum osmolarity present, or in an individual who produces high volume (up to 16 L) of inappropriately dilute urine
- Water deprivation test is test of choice (Fig. 42-11)

Treatment

- Treatment of neurogenic diabetes insipidus is dDAVP (a synthetic vasopressin analogue, administered either intranasally or orally)
- Thiazide diuretics are used for treatment of nephrogenic DI to reduce intravascular volume and polyuria

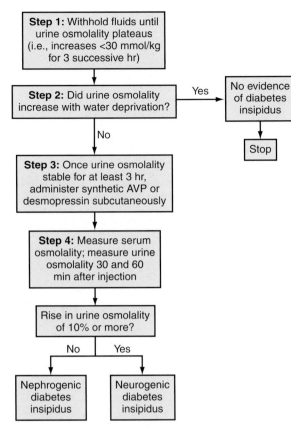

Step 1: Withhold fluids until urine osmolality plateaus (i.e., increases <30 mmol/kg for 3 successive hr)

Step 2: Did urine osmolality increase with water deprivation? — Yes → No evidence of diabetes insipidus → Stop

No ↓

Step 3: Once urine osmolality stable for at least 3 hr, administer synthetic AVP or desmopressin subcutaneously

Step 4: Measure serum osmolality; measure urine osmolality 30 and 60 min after injection

Rise in urine osmolality of 10% or more?

No → Nephrogenic diabetes insipidus

Yes → Neurogenic diabetes insipidus

FIGURE 42-11 Water deprivation test. AVP, arginine vasopressin.

Adrenal Disease

OVERVIEW OF THE ADRENAL GLAND

- The adrenal glands are the major site of synthesis and secretion of steroid hormones
- There are **three categories** of steroid hormones produced in the adrenal glands
  - **Glucocorticoids, such as cortisol (sometimes referred to as *hydrocortisone*)**
  - **Mineralocorticoids, such as aldosterone**
  - **Adrenal androgens, such as dehydroepiandrosterone (DHEA)**
- Major actions of adrenal hormones are shown in Table 42-2
- Adrenal incidentalomas: Increases in imaging of abdomen result in incidental detection of adrenal mass in 0.1% to 1.5% of scans
  - **Most adrenal incidentalomas (67–94%, depending on the case series) are nonhypersecretory adrenal adenomas**
  - Clinically significant incidentally discovered masses may be hormonally active, malignant, or both
    - **In absence of clinical signs or symptoms of Cushing's syndrome or hyperaldosteronism (see following discussion), no further investigation for these disorders is indicated**
    - **If any signs or symptoms of hormone excess are present, further evaluation is needed**
  - **Pheochromocytoma may be asymptomatic and may be present in the nonhypertensive patient;**

screening for pheochromocytoma with 24-hour urine total and fractionated metanephrines collection or plasma free metanephrines should always be performed, unless radiologic appearance (very low density) rules it out
- Mass size determines management; **size greater than 4 cm increases the suspicion for malignancy**
  - **Biopsy cannot differentiate between benign and malignant primary adrenal tumors; therefore all masses greater than 4 cm in diameter should be removed**
- If mass less than 4 cm in diameter, repeat imaging done in 3 to 6 months
  - If no change, imaging repeated annually for 3 years
  - If mass increases in size, surgery should be performed
- Management is different if patient has known primary cancer that risks spread to adrenals; fine-needle aspiration biopsy may be performed if metastatic disease suspected

Adrenal Hormone Excess States

CORTISOL EXCESS (CUSHING'S SYNDROME)

- See preceding section

ALDOSTERONE EXCESS

Basic Information

- **Most common cause is a functional adrenal adenoma (Conn's syndrome, Fig. 42-12);** aldosterone-producing adrenal carcinoma is rare
- Bilateral adrenal cortex hyperplasia will also result in aldosterone excess

Clinical Presentation

- **Patients present with hypertension (caused by sodium retention), metabolic alkalosis, and hypokalemia**
- Hypokalemia is not invariably present; may be unveiled by the use of diuretics
- Hypokalemia may result in muscle weakness

Diagnosis

- Because patients with hyperaldosteronism are typically hypertensive, the diagnosis is suggested by the presence of **hypokalemia in the hypertensive patient** (although normal potassium does not exclude the diagnosis)
  - Potassium should be normalized before evaluating for hyperaldosteronism because hypokalemia suppresses aldosterone secretion
- If the patient is taking a potassium-wasting diuretic, this must be discontinued, and potassium supplementation should be given
  - If hypokalemia resolves, hyperaldosteronism is less likely, **but it is not ruled out**
- If hyperaldosteronism still considered, screening may be performed with **serum aldosterone-plasma renin ratio**
  - **If ratio (aldosterone in ng/dL, and plasma renin activity in ng/mL/hour) less than 20, this is normal, and hyperaldosteronism is not suggested**

TABLE 42-2	*Adrenal Hormones: Key Details*		
Hormone	**Secretagogues**	**Inhibitor**	**Major Actions**

Cortisol	ACTH	Cortisol inhibits CRH release (and thus ACTH release) in negative feedback loop
		Exogenous steroids also inhibit CRH release
			Increases serum glucose levels
			  Opposes insulin
			  Stimulates hepatic gluconeogenesis
			Creates catabolic protein state
			  Stimulates protein breakdown
			  Stimulates mobilization of amino acid precursors from muscle, bone, skin, and connective tissue
			  Inhibits protein synthesis
			Opposes inflammatory response
			  Opposes increased vascular permeability and other actions of inflammatory mediators
			  Decreases eosinophils and T-cells
			Mobilizes polymorphonuclear lymphocytes

Aldosterone	Renin-angiotensin system activation Hyperkalemia ACTH	Sodium	Stimulates sodium retention, impacting extracellular fluid volume Stimulates potassium excretion
DHEA	ACTH	Inhibitors of ACTH release	Stimulates secondary sexual characteristics in men (or virilization in women)

ACTH, adrenocorticotropic hormone; CRH, corticotropin-releasing hormone; DHEA, dehydroepiandrosterone.

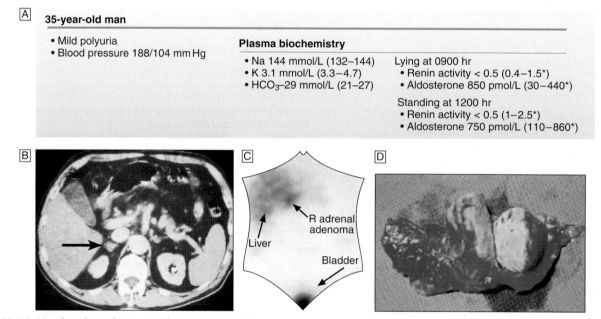

FIGURE 42-12 Conn's syndrome. **A,** Characteristic biochemical results, including hypernatremia, hypokalemia, and metabolic alkalosis. Plasma renin activity is suppressed, and aldosterone levels are elevated. **B,** Right adrenal adenoma *(arrow).* **C,** Uptake of radiolabeled cholesterol in right adrenal gland. **D,** Pathologic specimen of the right adrenal gland in part **C.** (From Haslett C, Chilvers ER, Boon NA, et al: *Davidson's principles and practice of medicine,* ed 19, New York, Churchill Livingstone, 2002, figure 16.19.)

- **If ratio greater than 20, next step is to demonstrate nonsuppressible levels of aldosterone** in presence of sodium load
  - 2 L of normal saline administered over 4 hours
  - If aldosterone levels do not suppress to less than 8 ng/dL, hyperaldosteronism is present
  - Alternatively, 24-hour urine aldosterone can be measured during oral salt loading

- Adrenal imaging then performed to differentiate adrenal adenoma from bilateral adrenal hyperplasia

Treatment

- **If hyperaldosteronism is caused by a functional adrenal adenoma (i.e., Conn's syndrome), treatment is surgical excision of adenoma**

- If hyperaldosteronism is caused by bilateral adrenal hyperplasia, treatment is with a potassium-sparing diuretic (e.g., spironolactone or eplerenone)

ADRENAL ANDROGEN EXCESS

Basic Information

- **DHEA and DHEA-sulfate are the most common adrenal androgens that may be produced in excess**
- **Adrenal androgens may be produced because of adrenal tumors, congenital adrenal hyperplasia (CAH), and Cushing's syndrome**
  - **In the most common form of CAH (21-hydroxylase deficiency, Fig. 42-13), cortisol synthesis is impaired, with overproduction of 17-hydroxyprogesterone**
  - **Mineralocorticoid production may also be impaired, resulting in hypoaldosteronism**
- **Androgen synthesis is intact,** resulting in overproduction of androstenedione

Clinical Presentation

- Clinical manifestations result from conversion of DHEA and DHEA-S to androstenedione and testosterone
- **Men are typically asymptomatic from overproduction of DHEA and DHEA-S**
- **Women are most likely to present with signs and symptoms of androgen excess (Fig. 42-14), including**
  - Hirsutism (i.e., hair growth in a male pattern, such as on the chest, face, or back)
  - Virilization (e.g., clitoromegaly)
  - Oligomenorrhea
  - Acne

Diagnosis

- Clinical manifestations typically prompt imaging of abdomen, along with evaluation of androgen levels (DHEA and testosterone)
- Adrenal tumor may be noted on imaging
- **If congenital adrenal hyperplasia suspected, 17-hydroxyprogesterone levels (the cortisol precursor that cannot be further metabolized) are assessed and will be elevated**
- Adrenal androgen excess often associated with Cushing's disease; less commonly it is associated with cortisol-producing adrenal adenomas

Treatment

- If caused by adrenal tumor, treatment is excision of tumor
- If caused by Cushing's syndrome, treatment is focused on treatment of Cushing's
- **Congenital adrenal hyperplasia is treated with glucocorticoid and mineralocorticoid replacement (the latter not always needed) as in adrenal insufficiency (see following discussion)**

PHEOCHROMOCYTOMA

Basic Information

- **Most pheochromocytomas occur in the adrenal medulla, where catecholamines are produced and stored**
- **Rarely, pheochromocytomas develop from the wall of the urinary bladder or in the retroperitoneal space**
- **Pheochromocytoma may occur as part of MEN-2A or 2B syndrome (see Box 42-1) and is also seen with**

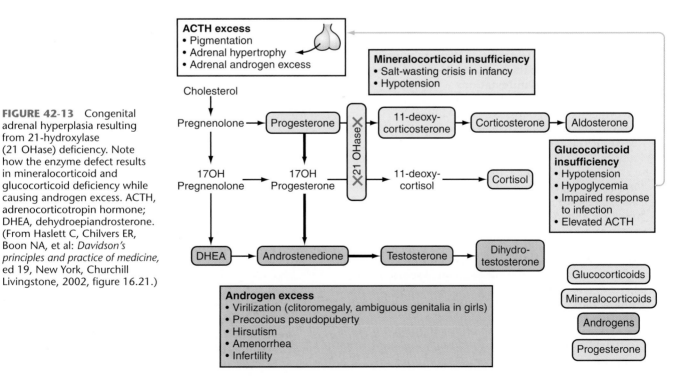

FIGURE 42-13 Congenital adrenal hyperplasia resulting from 21-hydroxylase (21 OHase) deficiency. Note how the enzyme defect results in mineralocorticoid and glucocorticoid deficiency while causing androgen excess. ACTH, adrenocorticotropin hormone; DHEA, dehydroepiandrosterone. (From Haslett C, Chilvers ER, Boon NA, et al: *Davidson's principles and practice of medicine,* ed 19, New York, Churchill Livingstone, 2002, figure 16.21.)

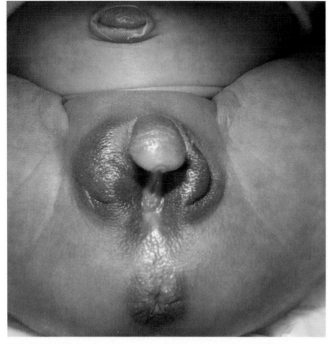

FIGURE 42-14 Ambiguous genitalia of a newborn female infant with virilizing congenital arenal hyperplasia. An enlarged clitoris (phallic-like structure), genital hyperpigmentation, empty labioscrotal folds, and a single perineal opening into a urogenital sinus were present. (From Shah BR, Laude TA: *Atlas of pediatric clinical diagnosis,* Philadelphia, WB Saunders, 2000, figure 8-14.)

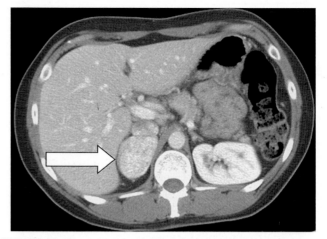

FIGURE 42-15   A CT scan of the abdomen with IV administration of a contrast agent demonstrating peripartum discovery of pheochromocytoma *(arrow).* (From Goldman L, Ausiello D: *Cecil textbook of medicine,* ed 23, Philadelphia, WB Saunders, 2008, figure 246-2.)

von Hippel-Lindau syndrome, neurofibromatosis, MEN-2, or succinyl dehydrogenase mutations
- **Most pheochromocytomas produce both norepinephrine and epinephrine.** Epinephrine-only secreting tumors are rare and are usually seen in the presence of an MEN syndrome.

Clinical Presentation
- Release of catecholamines results in clinical manifestations
  - **Most common manifestation is hypertension**
  - **Headache, diaphoresis, tachycardia, and anxiety are also common manifestations**
  - Less common are orthostatic hypotension, polycythemia, and congestive heart failure
- **Symptoms classically described as paroxysmal, caused by episodic release of catecholamines from tumor**
  - Pressure on abdomen or urination (if tumor in bladder wall) can precipitate symptoms
  - **Paroxysms more common early in disease; larger tumors lead to more sustained elevations in blood pressure and symptoms**

Diagnosis
- **Diagnosis made by collection of 24-hour urine sample for total and fractionated metanephrines**
- Yield may be increased in the intermittently symptomatic patient by **initiating the urine collection at the onset of a paroxysm**
- Other tests used include 24-hour urine collection for vanillylmandelic or measurement of plasma free metanephrines

- Once diagnosed, pheochromocytoma must be located
  - Imaging of abdomen with CT or MRI is first step, with attention to adrenal glands (Fig. 42-15)
    - **90% of pheochromocytomas are located in the adrenal glands;** those external to the adrenal glands are usually elsewhere in the abdomen (including the bladder)
  - If initial imaging of abdomen negative, further localization is done, usually with iodinated metaiodobenzylguanidine (MIBG) scan
  - **If a pheochromocytoma is suspected to be malignant, MIBG scan should be performed before surgery to detect metastatic disease**

Treatment
- Treatment consists of **surgical excision** of tumor
  - **Because surgery can precipitate hormonal release, preventive treatment with the β-blocker phenoxybenzamine often started before surgery**

Adrenal Hormone Deficiency States

ADRENAL INSUFFICIENCY

Basic Information
- **Adrenal insufficiency may occur because of failure of the adrenal glands (primary adrenal insufficiency) or pituitary disease (secondary adrenal insufficiency)**
  - Autoimmune primary adrenal insufficiency is often associated with other autoimmune disorders (e.g., hypothyroidism, vitiligo)
  - Other causes of primary adrenal insufficiency include infection (e.g., tuberculosis), surgical excision, and bilateral hemorrhage of the adrenal glands
    - **Hemorrhagic destruction of the adrenal glands is described in disseminated meningococcal infection (Waterhouse-Friderichsen syndrome), as well as with anticoagulation or lupus anticoagulant**

- **Secondary adrenal insufficiency is much more common than primary adrenal insufficiency and is most often caused by suppression of the hypothalamic-pituitary-adrenal axis by the administration of exogenous steroids**

Clinical Presentation

- **Clinical manifestations of adrenal insufficiency differ based on whether or not the cause is primary adrenal insufficiency or secondary adrenal insufficiency**
  - **With primary adrenal insufficiency, hypothalamus will respond by increasing CRH production, resulting in increased production of pro-opiomelanocortin (the ACTH precursor) and increased serum levels of ACTH**
  - **Because of increased production of pro-opiomelanocortin in primary adrenal insufficiency, skin and mucous membrane hyperpigmentation results.** Skin hyperpigmentation does not result from secondary adrenal insufficiency.
  - **With primary adrenal insufficiency, mineralocorticoid deficiency is also seen and hyponatremia and hyperkalemia result**
  - Hyponatremia is less common with secondary adrenal insufficiency and is seen more often if concomitant central hypothyroidism is present
- Clinical manifestations shared by all patients with adrenal insufficiency include weakness, hypotension, nausea, vomiting, diarrhea, and weight loss
  - **Acute adrenal insufficiency, which is a medical emergency, can be precipitated in patients with chronic adrenal insufficiency who are exposed to stress (e.g., surgery, infection) or by rapid destruction of the adrenal glands (such as with hemorrhage) or pituitary apoplexy**

Diagnosis

- **Recall that in primary adrenal insufficiency, plasma ACTH levels will be elevated, whereas in secondary adrenal insufficiency, plasma ACTH levels will be low (or inappropriately normal)**
  - ACTH levels are used in conjunction with other tests to determine presence of primary or secondary adrenal insufficiency
- A random morning cortisol measurement may be insufficient to diagnose partial adrenal insufficiency because **normal levels overlap with levels seen in mild adrenal insufficiency**
  - **However, if a patient is under significant stress (e.g., hypotensive or in the ICU) and a random cortisol (taken any time of day) is less than 18 µg/dL, the patient should be considered adrenally insufficient unless serum albumin is less than 2.5 g/dL**
    - All patients diagnosed with adrenal insufficiency based on a low serum cortisol while in the ICU should be retested after the acute problem is solved
  - A very low serum morning cortisol level (<3 µg/dL) in an ambulatory patient is presumptive evidence of adrenal insufficiency
- Gold standard test of adrenal function is insulin-induced hypoglycemia or insulin tolerance test (ITT)

- Test performed by administering insulin (0.1–0.15 U/kg) intravenously, with measurement of cortisol levels during symptomatic hypoglycemia
  - A normal response is considered to be a peak cortisol level greater than 18 mg/dL
- ITT contraindicated in presence of coronary artery disease, seizure disorder, or age greater than 60 years
- Most commonly used test is ACTH stimulation test
  - Low-dose ACTH stimulation test
    - Administer ACTH (cosyntropin) **1 µg IV**
    - Measure serum cortisol just before injection and **30 min** following injection
    - **If cortisol level 18 µg/dL or more at either measure, patient does not have adrenal insufficiency**
      - **If cortisol levels stay below 15 µg/dL, adrenal insufficiency is present**
      - A value between 15 and 18 should prompt repeating the test or using alternative testing
    - Results then combined with results of ACTH levels to determine whether adrenal insufficiency is primary (high ACTH levels) or secondary (low or inappropriately normal ACTH levels)
  - High-dose ACTH stimulation test
    - Administer ACTH (cosyntropin) **250 mg IV**
    - Measure serum cortisol just before injection and **60 minutes** following injection
    - If **cortisol level 20 µg/dL** or more at either measure, patient does not have adrenal insufficiency
      - If cortisol levels stay **below 20 µg/dL, adrenal insufficiency is present,** and results are combined with ACTH levels as described previously

Treatment

- Adrenal insufficiency: Treatment differs based on cause of adrenal insufficiency (e.g., primary versus secondary) as well as whether or not adrenal insufficiency is acute or chronic (Fig. 42-16)
  - Usual dose is hydrocortisone 10 to 12.5 mg/m²/day
  - The lowest dose that improves patient's symptoms should be used
  - Dose should be **increased during intercurrent illnesses**
  - **Mineralocorticoid (fludrocortisone 0.05–0.2 mg/day) is used primarily only in primary adrenal insufficiency**

HYPOALDOSTERONISM

Basic Information

- Most common presentation is hyporeninemic-hypoaldosteronism
  - **Common in patients with renal insufficiency and in those with long-standing diabetes**
  - Results in type **IV renal tubular acidosis** (see Chapter 32)
  - **Other causes of hyporeninemic-hypoaldosteronism include angiotensin-converting enzyme (ACE) inhibitors, NSAIDs, cyclosporine, and heparin**
  - AIDS may also be associated with hyporeninemic-hypoaldosteronism

42

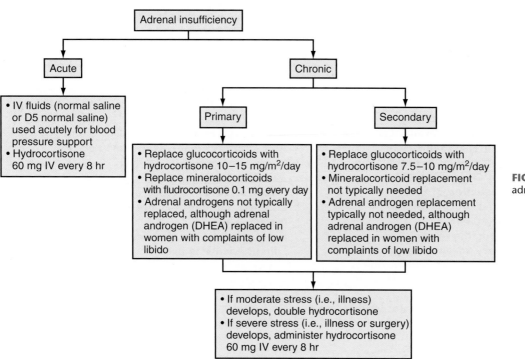

FIGURE 42-16 Treatment of adrenal insufficiency.

- Hypoaldosteronism also occurs in patients with primary adrenal insufficiency and congenital adrenal hyperplasia (see preceding discussion)
  - Rare causes include isolated enzyme defects in synthesis of aldosterone and are usually diagnosed in children

Clinical Presentation

- **Hyperkalemia** is the major clinical feature of patients with hypoaldosteronism

Diagnosis

- First step is to exclude obvious causes of hyporeninemic-hypoaldosteronism (noted previously)
- With these causes excluded, major differential is between hyporeninemic-hypoaldosteronism, adrenal insufficiency, congenital adrenal hyperplasia, or rare enzyme defect
  - **After patient is upright for 3 hours, check plasma renin activity, serum aldosterone, and serum cortisol levels**
    - With hyporeninemic-hypoaldosteronism, plasma renin activity and aldosterone levels will be low; cortisol will be normal
    - With adrenal insufficiency, plasma renin activity will be high, whereas serum aldosterone and cortisol will be low
- Further evaluation of the patient with suspected adrenal insufficiency or congenital adrenal hyperplasia is discussed previously

Treatment

- Treatment may or may not be given, based on the cause of hypoaldosteronism and presence or absence of symptoms

- Hypoaldosteronism in the presence of adrenal insufficiency is treated with fludrocortisone (see Fig. 42-16)
- Hypoaldosteronism from hyporeninemic-hypoaldosteronism may be treated with fludrocortisone
- If hypertension or fluid retention is present and prevents treatment with fludrocortisone, potassium-wasting diuretics and a low potassium diet may be used

REVIEW QUESTIONS

For review questions, please go to www.expertconsult.com.

SUGGESTED READINGS

Aron DC, Howlett TA: Pituitary incidentalomas, *Endocrinol Metab Clin North Am* 29:205–221, 2000.

Biochemical assessment and long-term monitoring in patients with acromegaly: statement from a Joint Consensus Conference of The Growth Hormone Research Society and The Pituitary Society, *J Clin Endocrinol Metab* 89:3099–3102, 2004.

Dekkers OM, Pereira AM, Romijn JA: Treatment and follow-up of clinically nonfunctioning pituitary macroadenomas, *J Clin Endocrinol Metab* 93:3717–3726, 2008.

Doga M, Bonadonna S, Gola M, et al: Current guidelines for adult GH replacement, *Rev Endocr Metab Disord* 6:63–70, 2005.

Freda PU, Post KD: Differential diagnosis of sellar masses, *Endocrinol Metab Clin North Am* 28:81–117, 1999.

Gordon RD, Laragh JH, Funder JW: Low renin hypertensive states: perspectives, unsolved problems, future research, *Trends Endocrinol Metab* 16:108–113, 2005.

Mantero F, Arnaldi G: Management approaches to adrenal incidentalomas, *Endocrinol Metab Clin North Am* 29:107–125, 2000.

Raff H, Finding JW: A physiologic approach to diagnosis of the Cushing syndrome, *Ann Intern Med* 138:980–991, 2003.

Salvatori R: Adrenal insufficiency, *JAMA* 294:2481–2488, 2005.

Verbalis JG: Diabetes insipidus, *Rev Endocr Metab Disord* 4:177–185, 2003.

Young WF Jr: Adrenal causes of hypertension: pheochromocytoma and primary aldosteronism, *Rev Endocr Metab Disord* 8: 309–320, 2007.

SECTION SEVEN

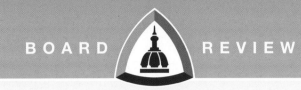

BOARD REVIEW

Rheumatology

CHAPTER 43

Arthritis

ALLAN C. GELBER, MD, PhD

Arthritis encompasses a number of conditions that are cumulatively the leading cause of disability in the United States. More than 60% of the population can expect to develop some form of arthritis in their lifetime.

Approach to the Patient with Joint Symptoms

Basic Information

- Strictly speaking, the term *arthritis* refers to joint inflammation, but it is commonly used more loosely to denote more than a hundred musculoskeletal conditions, both inflammatory and mechanical.
- It is important to distinguish true arthritis from conditions that mimic it (Box 43-1)

Clinical Presentation

- A careful history and detailed physical examination should be directed at answering the following five key diagnostic questions:
  - Is the process truly **articular?**
  - Is the process **inflammatory** or **mechanical?**
  - Who is the **host?**
  - What is the pattern of joint involvement?
  - Are there **extra-articular manifestations?**
- Features that suggest an articular process
  - Symptoms (pain) localized to the joints
  - Physical findings (swelling, erythema, heat, or tenderness) localized to the joints
  - Joint range of motion is painful
  - Joint range of motion is restricted
- Features that suggest an inflammatory process
  - Morning stiffness longer than 60 minutes (versus worsening in the evening in mechanical processes)
  - Gel phenomenon (stiffness after prolonged inactivity)
  - Symptoms improve with use (versus worsening with use in mechanical processes)

BOX 43-1	*Processes That Mimic Arthritis*
Bursitis	Myositis
Tendinitis	Vasculitis
Fasciitis	Neuropathy
Enthesitis	Thyroid disease
Periostitis	Parathyroid disease
Fibromyalgia	Osteoporosis

- Joint swelling, erythema, heat, or tenderness
- Constitutional manifestations (e.g., fever, malaise, or weight loss)
- Relevant host factors
  - Age
  - Gender
  - Race
  - Comorbidities
  - Occupational exposures
  - Family history
- Relevant patterns of joint involvement
  - **Acute onset** (e.g., microcrystalline) versus insidious onset (e.g., osteoarthritis [OA])
  - **Episodic** (e.g., microcrystalline) versus **migratory** (e.g., disseminated gonococcal infection and acute rheumatic fever) versus **additive** (e.g., rheumatoid arthritis [RA])
  - **Monoarticular** (e.g., microcrystalline and septic) versus **oligoarticular** (e.g., human leukocyte antigen [HLA]-B27-associated) versus **polyarticular** (e.g., RA)
  - **Symmetrical** (e.g., RA) versus **asymmetrical** (e.g., HLA-B27-associated)
  - **Axial** (e.g., HLA-B27-associated) versus **peripheral** (e.g., RA)
- Relevant extra-articular features
  - Constitutional
  - Mucocutaneous (e.g., photosensitive and other cutaneous eruptions, alopecia, mucosal aphthous ulcers, and Raynaud's phenomenon)
  - Ocular (e.g., conjunctivitis, episcleritis, scleritis, and uveitis)
  - Renal (e.g., glomerulonephritis, renal tubular acidosis, and nephrolithiasis)
  - Neurologic (e.g., focal central and peripheral disease, seizures, and cognitive and psychiatric disorders)
  - Pulmonary (e.g., nodules, infiltrates, interstitial fibrosis, pulmonary embolism and hypertension, alveolar hemorrhage, bronchiolitis, and pleuritis)
  - Gastrointestinal (e.g., inflammatory bowel disease and autoimmune liver disease)
  - Hematologic
    - Anemia (e.g., anemia of "chronic disease" and hemolytic anemia)
    - Leukopenia (e.g., neutropenia in Felty's syndrome and lymphopenia in systemic lupus erythematosus [SLE])
    - Thrombocytopenia (e.g., SLE with antiphospholipid antibodies)

Diagnosis and Evaluation

- The judicious use of laboratory, synovial fluid, and imaging studies serves to test and confirm the diagnostic hypothesis, to assess the severity and prognosis of the disease process, and to guide therapy
- Obtain relevant laboratory studies as indicated
  - Kidney and liver function
  - CBC and differential WBC
  - Urinalysis
  - Erythrocyte sedimentation rate and C-reactive protein
  - Thyroid function
  - Autoantibodies
- Obtain and evaluate synovial fluid as indicated
  - Check cell count, Gram stain and culture, and polarized microscopy for crystals
  - WBC less than 200/mm^3 (normal), greater than 2000/mm^3 (inflammatory), and greater than 75,000/mm^3 (microcrystalline or septic)
- Obtain relevant imaging studies
  - Conventional radiography is the starting point in imaging studies due to widespread availability, low cost, and high resolution, but may reveal only nonspecific soft tissue swelling in early inflammatory disease
  - CT is widely available and a good choice for assessment of the spine and pulmonary parenchyma
  - MRI has replaced CT in many situations (e.g., disc herniation, sacroiliac joints, osteonecrosis, and soft tissue processes)
  - Arthrography (e.g., evaluation for rotator cuff tears)
  - Angiography (e.g., evaluation for vasculitis)
  - Both mechanical and inflammatory joint disease cause increased tracer uptake so that nuclear medicine scans have a limited role in the evaluation of arthritis
  - Ultrasound is useful in differentiating thrombophlebitis from pseudothrombophlebitis (ruptured Baker's cyst), and is seeing an expanding role in the assessment of synovitis and erosive joint disease

Osteoarthritis

Basic Information

- **Prototypical and most prevalent mechanical (noninflammatory) joint disorder**
- One third of individuals 65 years and older have radiographic knee OA
- **Primarily a disease of the cartilage, with secondary bony changes**
- There are a variety of risk factors for OA (Box 43-2)
  - Even though advancing age is a risk factor for OA, it should not be considered a "normal" part of aging

Clinical Presentation

- Typically presents insidiously in middle-aged or elderly patients
- Most commonly seen in the **hands** (e.g., first carpometacarpal, proximal interphalangeal [PIP], and distal interphalangeal [DIP] joints) and **weight-bearing joints** (e.g., hips, knees, and spine)
- **Joints ache and are painful, worsening with use and at the end of the day**

BOX 43-2	*Risk Factors for Osteoarthritis*

Advanced age
Female gender
Developmental
Collagen polymorphisms
Types II, IX, and XI
Obesity
Trauma
　Acute and repetitive
Neuropathy
Inflammatory arthritis
Osteonecrosis
Paget's disease
Endocrine/metabolic
　Acromegaly
　Alkaptonuria
　Chondrocalcinosis
　Hemochromatosis

- Rest and nocturnal pain may be seen with severe disease
- Patients may experience minimal morning stiffness and gelling
- No constitutional or other extra-articular manifestations with primary OA
- May have a variety of clinical presentations that are not mutually exclusive
  - First carpometacarpal joint
  - Interphalangeal joints (often familial and affects primarily older women; Fig. 43-1)
    - **Bouchard's nodes** represent bony enlargement of the PIP joints
    - **Heberden's nodes** represent bony enlargement of the DIP joints
  - Erosive osteoarthritis
    - Affects the DIP and PIP joints
    - Characterized by recurrent flares of pain, swelling, and tenderness
    - Joint destruction occurs, leading to bony ankylosis and joint deformity
    - May be associated with microcrystalline disease and can be confused with RA
  - Hip
    - Symptoms often localize to the groin and anterior thigh
    - Distinguish from trochanteric bursitis (pain over the lateral aspect of the hip)
    - Symptoms provoked by use (e.g., weight bearing) and internal rotation
    - May be associated with congenital malformations (e.g., hip dysplasia, slipped capital femoral epiphysis, and Legg-Calvé-Perthes disease)
  - Knee
    - All three joint compartments may be affected (e.g., medial tibiofemoral, lateral tibiofemoral, and patellofemoral)
  - Spine
    - Characterized by pain, stiffness, and (sometimes) radicular symptoms

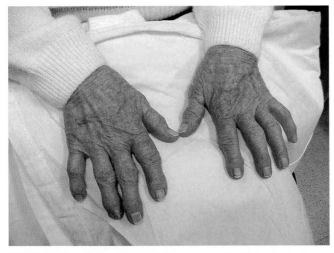

FIGURE 43-1 Osteoarthritis of the hands, with Heberden's nodes (distal interphalangeal joints) and Bouchard's nodes (proximal interphalangeal joints). (Courtesy of Don R. Martin, MD.)

- Most commonly affects the lower cervical and lumbar spine
- Diffuse idiopathic skeletal hyperostosis (DISH)
  - Variant of OA with axial and peripheral skeletal manifestations
  - Radiographic diagnosis (Fig. 43-2) characterized by
    - Flowing calcification or ossification along the anterolateral aspect of at least four contiguous vertebrae
    - Relative preservation of the intervertebral disk space at the involved levels (in contrast to classical OA)
    - Absence of apophyseal or sacroiliac joint involvement (in contrast to ankylosing spondylitis)

Diagnosis and Evaluation

- Clinical presentation highly suggestive in classic cases
- History characterized by
  - Insidious onset
  - Absence of inflammatory manifestations
- Physical examination reveals
  - Variable pattern of joint involvement as detailed previously
  - Bony hypertrophy
  - Bony deformity
  - Joint line tenderness
  - Crepitus
  - Limited joint mobility or laxity/pseudolaxity
  - Muscle (disuse) atrophy
- Laboratory findings
  - Renal and hepatic function normal unless due to drug toxicity
  - Normal erythrocyte sedimentation rate (aside from age-associated changes)
  - Seronegative (aside from age-associated changes)
  - **Synovial fluid is noninflammatory with less than 2000 WBC/mm³**
- Radiographic findings
  - Symptoms and radiographic findings may be discordant (e.g., significant symptoms or functional limitation with minimal radiographic findings, and vice versa)

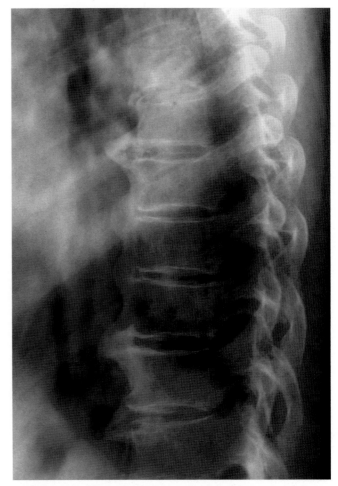

FIGURE 43-2 Radiographic findings in diffuse idiopathic skeletal hyperostosis (DISH), with flowing ossification along the anterolateral aspect of at least four contiguous vertebral bodies and relative preservation of the disk spaces. (From Harris ED, Budd RC, Genovese MC, et al, editors: *Kelley's textbook of rheumatology,* ed 7, Philadelphia, WB Saunders, 2005, figure 51-66.)

- May be normal in early disease
- Radiographic hallmarks include
  - Joint space narrowing (often asymmetrical; Fig. 43-3)
  - Subchondral bone sclerosis (or eburnation)
  - Subchondral cysts
  - Joint margin osteophytes

Treatment

- Principles
  - Provide symptomatic relief
  - Maintain and maximize function
  - Minimize medication-associated toxicity
- Nonpharmacologic treatment
  - Patient education, weight loss (if overweight), exercise (low-impact, conditioning, and range of motion), occupational therapy, physical therapy, and assistive devices (e.g., cane)
- Pharmacologic treatment
  - Topical therapy
    - Capsaicin (depletes substance P in sensory nerve endings)

43

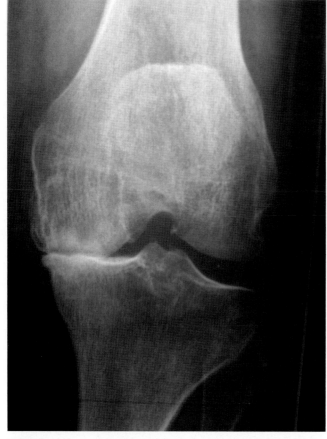

FIGURE 43-3 Radiographic findings in osteoarthritis of the knee, with asymmetrical narrowing of the medial joint space. (From Harris ED, Budd RC, Genovese MC, et al, editors: *Kelley's textbook of rheumatology,* ed 7, Philadelphia, WB Saunders, 2005, figure 92-1.)

- Methylsalicylate
- Oral therapy
  - Acetaminophen (considered first-line oral pharmacologic therapy)
  - NSAIDs
    - Therapeutically equivalent, although individual responses may vary
    - **Nonselective cyclooxygenase (COX)-1 and -2 inhibitors reduce pain and improve function, but carry significant potential for GI and other toxicities**
    - Selective COX-2 inhibitors may be safer with respect to GI toxicity and do not block platelet activity but have been associated with increased risk for cardiovascular and cerebrovascular morbidity and mortality and are not more effective. Only celecoxib remains available in the United States.
  - Other pure analgesics (e.g., propoxyphene, tramadol, and opioids)
  - Glucosamine and chondroitin sulfate may provide symptomatic relief in some patients, but the results of clinical trials vary. Marketing claims of joint protection and restoration remain unproven.

- Intra-articular therapy may provide temporary relief of symptoms when topical and oral regimens are ineffective or not tolerated
  - Joint aspiration may provide temporary relief when a large effusion is present
  - Corticosteroid injections may be particularly helpful in patients who have signs of joint inflammation
  - There is no role for systemic corticosteroid therapy
  - Hyaluronan injections have demonstrated efficacy, but individual responses are quite variable
- Surgical treatment
  - Arthroscopic débridement is indicated when internal derangements (e.g., meniscal tears) cause joint catching, locking, instability, or pain
  - **Total joint replacement is indicated in patients with symptoms and functional impairment that are unresponsive to medical intervention**
  - Tidal irrigation of joints has not been demonstrated to be effective

Prevention

- Diagnosis and treatment of risk factors for OA may result in prevention of articular damage
- **The relative risk of developing knee OA is higher in obese individuals, so weight loss may have a major role in prevention of disease**

Rheumatoid Arthritis

Basic Information

- **Prototypical and most prevalent inflammatory joint disorder in women**
- Affects 1% of the population
- Peak incidence in the 30s to 50s
- Female-to-male ratio 3:1
- Familial predisposition, with HLA-DR4 association and amino acid motif QKRAA susceptibility shared epitope

Clinical Presentation

- **Additive, symmetrical polyarthritis affecting both small and large joints**
  - **Wrists, metacarpophalangeal (MCP) and PIP joints prominently involved; DIP joints spared**
  - Shoulders, elbows, hips, knees, ankles, and feet commonly involved
  - Cervical spine (atlantoaxial joint) may be involved; lumbar spine is spared
- Presentation is consistent with its inflammatory character
  - **Fatigue, fever, and weight loss may be present reflecting systemic nature of the disease**
  - Joint pain, swelling, erythema, heat, and tenderness may develop acutely or insidiously
  - Morning stiffness lasts more than 1 hour, and "gel" phenomenon present after inactivity
- **Untreated, RA can cause joint destruction and disability, beginning in the first year of disease**
  - Ulnar deviation and subluxation of the fingers at the MCP joints, with radial deviation at the wrist
  - Swan-neck deformity (hyperextension of the PIP and flexion of the DIP joints; Fig. 43-4)

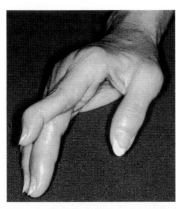

FIGURE 43-4 Swan-neck deformity in advanced rheumatoid arthritis. (From Harris ED, Budd RC, Genovese MC, et al, editors: *Kelley's textbook of rheumatology,* ed 7, Philadelphia, WB Saunders, 2005, figure 33-6.)

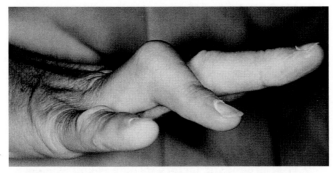

FIGURE 43-5 Boutonnière deformity in advanced rheumatoid arthritis. (From Townsend CM, Beauchamp RD, Evers BM, Mattox KL: *Sabiston textbook of surgery,* ed 17, Philadelphia, Saunders, 2004, figure 73-17.)

- Boutonnière deformity (flexion of the PIP and hyperextension of the DIP joints; Fig. 43-5)
- **Extra-articular manifestations**
  - Rheumatoid nodules
    - Typically appear on extensor surfaces and pressure points (e.g., olecranon process and Achilles tendon) but may also affect internal organs
    - Occur in approximately 25% of patients with RA
    - Associated with rheumatoid factor (RF) seropositivity and more severe disease
    - Nodules are not specific for RA and can occur in other rheumatic diseases
    - Histology marked by central necrosis, surrounded by palisading fibroblasts, and a collagenous capsule with a chronic inflammatory infiltrate
    - **Methotrexate can worsen nodulosis, even as inflammatory joint disease improves**
  - Ocular
    - Episcleritis, scleritis, and scleromalacia perforans
    - Keratoconjunctivitis sicca (secondary Sjögren's syndrome)
  - Pulmonary
    - Pleural disease (effusions exudative and pleural fluid glucose typically low)
    - Interstitial lung disease and fibrosis
    - Bronchiolitis obliterans
    - Pulmonary nodules

- Single or multiple
- Nodules may cavitate and pleural nodules cause bronchopleural fistulae
- **Caplan's disease (nodules with underlying RA and pneumoconiosis)**
- Cardiac
  - Pericarditis and effusions are common but rarely symptomatic
  - Constrictive pericarditis, myocarditis, and conduction defects develop rarely
- Hematologic
  - Anemia due to iron deficiency (NSAID-associated GI loss) and "chronic disease"
  - **Felty's syndrome (RA associated with splenomegaly, neutropenia, and leg ulcers)**
  - Thrombocytosis or thrombocytopenia
  - Increased risk for non-Hodgkin's lymphoma independent of tumor necrosis factor (TNF)-inhibitor use
- Neurologic
  - Atlantoaxial (C1-C2) instability and subluxation
  - Peripheral neuropathy
    - Compressive associated with synovitis (e.g., carpal tunnel syndrome)
    - Ischemia-associated with vasculitis (e.g., mononeuritis multiplex)
- Vasculitis
  - Leukocytoclastic vasculitis, cutaneous ulcers, visceral involvement, and mononeuritis multiplex
  - **Associated with high-titer RF and severe disease**

Diagnosis and Evaluation

- Clinical presentation highly suggestive in classic cases
- History characterized by
  - Acute or subacute onset
  - Inflammatory manifestations
- Physical examination reveals
  - Synovitis
  - Symmetrical polyarthritis as detailed previously
- Laboratory findings
  - Renal and hepatic function normal unless due to drug toxicity
  - Normochromic normocytic anemia
  - Elevated sedimentation rate and C-reactive protein
  - **RF**
    - Immunoglobulin (Ig)M autoantibody directed against the Fc fragment of IgG
    - IgM-RF is 60% to 80% sensitive and 80% to 90% specific for RA
    - RF is also seen in a wide variety of other rheumatic diseases (Sjögren's syndrome, juvenile arthritis, SLE, and cryoglobulinemia) and nonrheumatic diseases (interstitial lung disease, endocarditis, tuberculosis [TB], hepatitis, and malignancy)
    - Prevalence increases with age
  - **Anticyclic citrullinated peptide (anti-CCP) antibodies**
    - Anti-CCP antibody is 68% to 80% sensitive and 98% specific for RA
    - Anti-CCP is more likely to be present in early RA than RF
  - Synovial fluid inflammatory with greater than 2000 WBC/mm^3

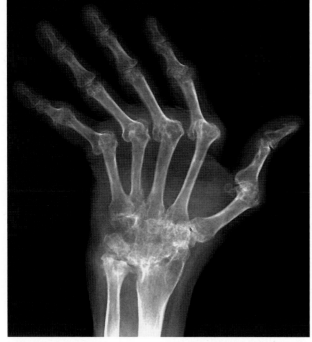

FIGURE 43-6 Radiographic findings in rheumatoid arthritis of the hand, with erosions and ulnar deviation. (From Harris ED, Budd RC, Genovese MC, et al, editors: *Kelley's textbook of rheumatology*, ed 7, Philadelphia, WB Saunders, 2005, figure 51-6.)

BOX 43-3	*Criteria for the Classification of Rheumatoid Arthritis*

Morning stiffness (≥1 hr)
Arthritis in three or more joint areas (simultaneously)
Arthritis of hand joints (wrist, MCP, or PIP joints)
Symmetrical arthritis
Rheumatoid nodules
Serum rheumatoid factor
Radiographic changes (consistent with RA)

MCP, metacarpophalangeal; PIP, proximal interphalangeal; RA, rheumatoid arthritis.
From Arnett FC, Edworthy SM, Bloch DA, et al: The American Rheumatism Association 1987 revised criteria for the classification of rheumatoid arthritis, *Arthritis Rheum* 31:315–324, 1988.

- Radiographic findings (Fig. 43-6)
  - May reveal only soft tissue swelling in early disease, but with advanced disease show
    - Periarticular osteopenia
    - **Uniform joint space narrowing**
    - Joint margin erosions
    - Ulnar styloid erosions
    - Atlantoaxial (C1-C2) instability and subluxation
- Criteria for the classification of RA (Box 43-3)
  - Developed to classify patients for study purposes
  - Need four of the seven criteria to classify patient with RA
  - May still consider the diagnosis of RA if two or more criteria are present

Treatment

- Principles
  - Provide symptomatic relief
  - Prevent joint destruction

- Maintain and maximize function
- Minimize medication-associated toxicity
- **Tailor approach to the individual patient given heterogeneity in clinical course and outcome**
- Nonpharmacologic treatment
  - Patient education, exercise (low-impact, conditioning, and range of motion), occupational therapy, physical therapy, and assistive devices (e.g., cane)
- **Pharmacologic treatment**
  - NSAIDs
    - Analgesic and anti-inflammatory effects reduce pain and improve function
    - **NSAIDs are not "disease-modifying"**
  - Corticosteroids
    - Anti-inflammatory effect helps to control symptoms and maintain function
    - **Most effective as "bridging therapy" while disease-modifying antirheumatic drugs (DMARDs) take effect**
    - Toxicity (e.g., weight gain, hypertension, glucose intolerance, hyperlipidemia, osteoporosis, etc.) makes prolonged use undesirable, but sometimes it is unavoidable
    - Regimens vary (IV or PO "pulse," daily low dose, and intra-articular)
  - **DMARDs** (Table 43-1)
    - DMARD use improves long-term outcomes
    - Early use advised for patients with the potential for progressive disease or poor prognostic factors
    - **Poor prognostic factors include young women, more than 20 involved joints, rheumatoid nodules, high sedimentation rate, high-titer RF-positive, and radiographic erosions**
    - Time for maximal effect varies from **4 weeks to 6 months** depending on the agent
    - Often used with NSAIDs or corticosteroids (or both)
    - **Combination therapy (>1 DMARD) used when disease unresponsive to single agents**
    - Gold, D-penicillamine, azathioprine, cyclophosphamide, and cyclosporine C rarely used anymore
- Surgical treatment
  - Synovectomy may be indicated when synovitis fails to respond to medical therapy
  - Joint replacement is indicated when joint destruction occurs despite medical therapy, and the resultant pain is no longer responsive to medical management

Prevention

- RA is not currently preventable

Gout

Basic Information

- **Intensely inflammatory arthritis caused by deposition of monosodium urate crystals**
- Peak incidence in the 50s to 60s
- Most common in postpubertal males (uric acid rises after puberty)

TABLE 43-1 *Disease-Modifying Anti-Rheumatic Drugs (DMARDs)*

Drug	Indication	Toxicity/Precautions	Monitoring
Hydroxychloroquine	Mild disease	Nausea, rash, and retinal damage (rare)	Eye exam every 6–12 mo
Sulfasalazine	Mild disease	Nausea, hepatitis, renal, G6PD-associated anemia, myelosuppression, and oligospermia	Initial G6PD; LFTs and CBC monthly ×3, then every 3 mo
Methotrexate (MTX)	First-line DMARD	Stomatitis, nausea, diarrhea, hepatitis, hepatic fibrosis, myelosuppression, interstitial pneumonitis, and teratogenic; may require folate supplement	Creatinine, LFTs, and CBC monthly until dose stable, then every 2–3 mo
Leflunomide	Alternative to MTX	Stomatitis, nausea, diarrhea, hepatitis, myelosuppression, and teratogenic	LFTs and CBC monthly until dose stable, then every 2–3 mo
Adalimumab	TNF inhibitor, used if MTX ineffective	Injection site reactions; avoid in patients with active or chronic infections or multiple sclerosis	Baseline PPD
Etanercept	TNF inhibitor, used if MTX ineffective	Injection site reactions; avoid in patients with active or chronic infections or multiple sclerosis	Baseline PPD
Infliximab	TNF inhibitor, used if MTX ineffective	Injection site reactions; avoid in patients with active or chronic infections or multiple sclerosis	Baseline PPD
Anakinra	IL-1 receptor antagonist used if TNF inhibitors ineffective	Injection site reactions and neutropenia; avoid in patients with active or chronic infections	Neutrophil count monthly ×3, then every 3 mo
Abatacept	Inhibitor of T-cell activation; used if TNF inhibitors ineffective	Avoid in patients with active or chronic infections; increased adverse respiratory effects in patients with COPD; do not combine with TNF inhibitors or anakinra	Baseline PPD; no live vaccines during treatment
Rituximab	Anti-CD20 monoclonal antibody; used if TNF inhibitors ineffective	Avoid in patients with active or chronic infections; infusion reactions (especially first) common; hepatitis B reactivation reported	Effective contraception required

CBC, complete blood count; COPD, chronic obstructive pulmonary disease; G6PD, glucose-6-phosphate dehydrogenase; IL-1, interleukin-1; LFTs, liver function tests; PPD, purified protein derivative; TNF, tumor necrosis factor.

- Incidence rises in postmenopausal females (uric acid rises after menopause)
- Hyperuricemia is due to increased production (10%) and diminished excretion (90%; Box 43-4)
  - Limit of solubility of uric acid is approximately 7 mg/dL
  - Primary hyperuricemia caused by polygenic factors
  - Secondary hyperuricemia caused by familial or acquired conditions

Clinical Presentation

- Asymptomatic hyperuricemia
  - Found at some point in about 5% of adult Americans
  - **More than 75% of individuals remain asymptomatic**
- Acute gout
  - Acute onset of joint pain, swelling, erythema, and heat
  - Fever (systemic manifestation of inflammation) may be present
  - 50% of patients present with first metatarsophalangeal joint involvement (podagra)
  - **75% to 90% of patients develop podagra at some point in their course**

- Gout may also affect the ankles, midfoot, knees, wrists, shoulders, and hands
- Attacks are usually monoarticular or oligoarticular (two to three joints); rarely polyarticular
- **Early attacks are self-limited and will resolve over 3 to 10 days, even without treatment**
- Intercritical gout
  - Asymptomatic period between acute attacks
  - May be years in duration
  - Uric acid levels are generally persistently elevated
- Chronic (tophaceous) gout (Fig. 43-7)
  - After years of recurrent attacks, joints develop persistent pain, swelling, and deformity
- Extra-articular disease
  - Tophi
    - Deposits of monosodium urate crystals in soft tissue
    - Typically found in the synovium and subchondral bone, on the pinna of the ear, and over extensor surfaces (e.g., forearm) and pressure points (e.g., Achilles tendon)
    - Typically appear after years of repeated episodes of acute gout

BOX 43-4	*Causes of Hyperuricemia*

Increased Production
Hypoxanthine-guanine phosphoribosyltransferase deficiency
Glycogen storage diseases
Increased purine intake
Increased nucleic acid turnover
   Myeloproliferative disorder
   Tumor lysis syndrome
   Hemolytic disorder
   Psoriasis
Accelerated adenosine triphosphate degradation
   Tissue hypoxia
   Sustained exercise
Ethanol

Reduced Excretion
Intrinsic renal disease
Drugs
   Diuretics
   Low-dose aspirin
   Cyclosporin A
   Ethambutol
   Pyrazinamide
Ketoacidosis and lactic acidosis
Dehydration
Hyperparathyroidism
Lead nephropathy
Ethanol

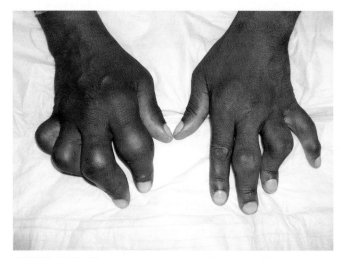

FIGURE 43-7 Chronic tophaceous gout involving the hands. (Courtesy of Don R. Martin, MD.)

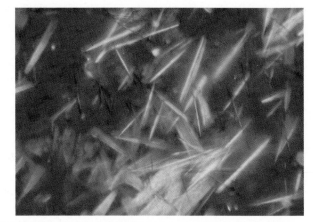

FIGURE 43-8 Polarized light microscopy demonstrating the strongly negative birefringence of needle-shaped uric acid crystals. (From Forbes CD, Jackson WF: *Color atlas and text of clinical medicine,* ed 3, St. Louis, Mosby, 2003, figure 3.13.)

- May be confused with rheumatoid nodules
- Renal disease
  - Parenchymal urate nephropathy associated with tumor lysis syndrome (acute) and comorbid conditions (chronic)
  - Nephrolithiasis risk 50% with serum uric acid greater than 13 mg/dL or urinary uric acid excretion greater than 1100 mg/day

Diagnosis and Evaluation

- Clinical presentation highly suggestive in classic cases
- History characterized by
  - Acute onset
  - Intermittent nature with asymptomatic intercritical phase
  - Inflammatory manifestations
- Physical examination reveals
  - Intensely inflammatory arthritis
  - Tophi may be present
- Laboratory findings
  - **Serum uric acid level elevated more than 80% of the time during acute gout, but can be normal**
  - Arthrocentesis (joint aspiration), for polarized microscopy and culture, at onset to rule out septic arthritis
  - Synovial fluid inflammatory with greater than 2000 WBC/mm³, and as high as 100,000/mm³
  - **Crystals are needle-shaped, are negatively birefringent, and may be intracellular (Fig. 43-8)**

- Crystals may be found in asymptomatic joints
- Radiographic findings
  - May reveal only soft tissue swelling in early disease, but with advanced disease shows
    - Early relative joint space preservation
    - Joint margin erosions with overhanging edges (**"parrot's beak"**; Fig. 43-9)
  - Uric acid is radiolucent

Treatment

- Acute
  - NSAIDs
    - Effective and rapid, especially if started early
    - Indomethacin has traditionally been used, but there is no evidence that one NSAID is superior to another
  - Corticosteroids
    - Effective when NSAIDs are contraindicated
    - Must rule out infection
    - Carry risk of "rebound" arthritis after taper
    - Administered as an oral taper, parenteral infusion, or intra-articular injection

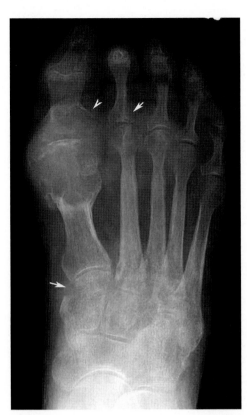

FIGURE 43-9 Radiographic findings in tophaceous gout, with extensive bony destruction of the first metatarsophalangeal joint. *Arrows* indicate erosions; *arrowhead* shows overhanging edge ("parrot's beak"). (From Harris ED, Budd RC, Genovese MC, et al, editors: *Kelley's textbook of rheumatology*, ed 7, Philadelphia, WB Saunders, 2005, figure 51-28.)

- Colchicine
  - Administered PO or IV, but potential for significant toxicity (GI, hepatic, renal, bone marrow, myopathy, and neuropathy), so use only if NSAIDs or corticosteroids not an option
- Prophylaxis
  - **Low-purine diet, discontinue aspirin and diuretics, and limit alcohol as feasible**
  - **Colchicine 0.6 mg once or twice daily reduces or eliminates attacks in approximately 95% of patients**
    - Caution advised in patients with impaired renal function due to risk for toxicity
  - Uric acid-lowering agents
    - Indicated for failure of colchicine prophylaxis or inability to correct hyperuricemia
    - Do not treat asymptomatic hyperuricemia
    - **Do not start uric acid-lowering agents during acute gout or without prophylaxis, as any change in the uric acid concentration (up or down) may precipitate an acute gout attack**
    - Uricosuric agents (e.g., probenecid and sulfinpyrazone) have limited usefulness due to these constraints
      - Use in patients with reduced uric acid excretion, but need GFR greater than 50 mL/min
      - If used in patients with high excretion may lead to stone formation
      - Must have no history of nephrolithiasis

- Must maintain daily fluid intake of more than 2 L to avoid stone formation
- Must avoid low-dose salicylates
- Xanthine oxidase inhibition (e.g., allopurinol, febuxostat)
  - Blocks xanthine oxidase enzyme in production of uric acid
  - **Indicated for "extreme" hyperuricemia, tophi, stones, and tumor lysis syndrome**
  - Adjust dose for renal function
  - **Lower dose of azathioprine and mercaptopurine by 75% when used in conjunction with allopurinol**
  - Titrate dose to uric acid level of 5 to 6 mg/dL
  - Adverse effects include fever, rash, hepatitis, and leukopenia

Prevention

- Correct causes of hyperuricemia (see Box 43-4)

Calcium Pyrophosphate Dihydrate Deposition Disease

Basic Information

- **Inflammatory arthritis caused by deposition of calcium pyrophosphate dihydrate (CPPD) crystals**
- Incidence increases with age; 50% of population has chondrocalcinosis by 80s
- Most cases are idiopathic, but some are associated with other diseases (Box 43-5)

Clinical Presentation

- Acute (pseudogout)
  - Inflammatory arthritis of large joints
  - **Knees involved in 50% of cases**
  - Wrists, metacarpophalangeal joints, hips, shoulders, elbows, and ankles also affected
  - Resembles an acute gout attack with monoarticular inflammation
  - Attacks may be recurrent
- Subacute (RA-like) presentation is uncommon
- Chronic (OA-like) presentation is generally more destructive than is typical of OA

Diagnosis and Evaluation

- History characterized by
  - Varied onset and course
  - Inflammation often less intense than in gout
- Physical examination reveals
  - Varied patterns and intensity of disease

BOX 43-5	*Diseases Associated with Pseudogout*

Osteoarthritis
Gout
Hemochromatosis
Hypothyroidism
Hyperparathyroidism
Wilson's disease

43

- Laboratory findings
  - Synovial fluid inflammatory with greater than 2000 WBC/mm^3 in acute arthritis
  - **Crystals are rhomboid-shaped and positively birefringent (Fig. 43-10)**
- Radiographic findings
  - Chondrocalcinosis (Fig. 43-11)
    - Linear calcifications in the cartilage
    - Most commonly found in the wrist, symphysis pubis, and knee

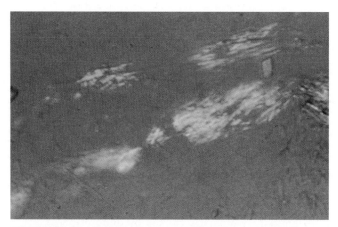

FIGURE 43-10   Polarized light microscopy demonstrating the weakly positive birefringence of rhomboidal crystals of calcium pyrophosphate dihydrate. (From Forbes CD, Jackson WF: *Color atlas and text of clinical medicine,* ed 3, St. Louis, Mosby, 2003, figure 3.14.)

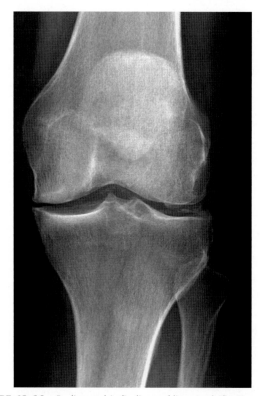

FIGURE 43-11   Radiographic findings of linear calcification of the hyaline cartilage and lateral meniscus in calcium pyrophosphate dihydrate deposition (CPPD) disease. (From Harris ED, Budd RC, Genovese MC, et al, editors: *Kelley's textbook of rheumatology,* ed 7, Philadelphia, WB Saunders, 2005, figure 51-30.)

Treatment

- Acute
  - NSAIDs
  - Corticosteroids
- Chronic
  - NSAIDs
- Prophylaxis
  - Chronic administration of low-dose colchicine or NSAIDs may be effective
  - No CPPD-lowering agents are currently available

Prevention

- Treat associated diseases (see Box 43-5)

Seronegative Spondyloarthropathies

Overview

- Four diseases grouped together by overlapping clinical features and molecular evidence of a common etiology
  - Ankylosing spondylitis
  - Enteropathic arthritis
  - Psoriatic arthritis
  - Reactive arthritis
- Common clinical features
  - Enthesopathy (inflammation at the site of ligamentous and tendinous insertion to bone)
  - Inflammatory back disease/sacroiliitis
  - Mucocutaneous manifestations
  - Inflammatory eye disease
  - Inflammatory bowel disease
  - HLA-B27 association
  - RF-seronegative

Ankylosing Spondylitis

Basic Information

- Inflammatory arthritis that predominantly affects the axial skeleton
- Affects 0.5% to 1% of whites; less common in blacks
- Peak incidence in the 20s to 30s
- Male to female ratio is 5:1

Clinical Presentation

- **Presents with insidious onset of low back or buttock pain and stiffness**
- Symptoms typically inflammatory (e.g., worse in the morning and with rest; improve with use)
- **Begins as sacroiliitis, progressing to the lumbar spine and cephalad, resulting in fusion**
- Thoracic spine disease may present as chest pain
- Extra-axial disease
  - Limb-girdle joints (e.g., shoulders and hips) commonly affected
  - Peripheral joints less commonly affected and usually asymmetrical
  - Enthesopathy (e.g., Achilles tendinitis and plantar fasciitis)
  - Anterior uveitis

- Aortitis and aortic insufficiency
- Pulmonary fibrosis (upper lung fields)
- Subclinical colitis

Diagnosis and Evaluation

- Clinical presentation highly suggestive in classic cases
- History characterized by
  - Localization of symptoms to sacroiliac joints and lumbar spine
  - Inflammatory manifestations
  - **Anterior uveitis may be initial manifestation**
- Physical examination reveals
  - Sacroiliac and lumbar spine tenderness
  - Loss of lumbar lordosis
  - Loss of lumbar spine range-of-motion
    - **Schober test measures lumbar spine distraction with flexion (<5 cm is significant)**
  - Chest expansion is limited in patients with thoracic involvement
- Laboratory findings
  - Inflammatory markers may be elevated
  - **90% of patients are HLA-B27-positive; nearly 100% of those with uveitis or aortitis**
  - **However, HLA-B27 is nondiagnostic, as 6% to 8% of white population is positive**
- Radiographic findings
  - Symmetrical sacroiliitis (e.g., iliac margin sclerosis and fusion; Fig. 43-12)
  - Early findings include squaring and sclerosis of the corners of the vertebrae
  - Later findings include ossification of the anterior longitudinal ligament and bridging syndesmophytes resulting in "bamboo spine" (Fig. 43-13)
  - Typical radiographic findings may take months or years to become apparent
  - CT and MRI are sensitive for early sacroiliitis

Treatment

- Nonpharmacologic
  - Thin or no pillow
  - Physical therapy to maintain posture and prevent progressive thoracic kyphosis and loss of mobility
  - Breathing exercises to maintain chest wall expansion
- Pharmacologic
  - NSAIDs
    - Analgesic and anti-inflammatory effects relieve pain and stiffness
    - NSAIDs are not "disease-modifying"
    - Indomethacin has traditionally been used, but there is no evidence that one NSAID is superior to another
  - Sulfasalazine
    - May slow disease progression
    - Potential for significant toxicity (e.g., GI, hepatic, renal, glucose-6-phosphate dehydrogenase [G6PD]-associated anemia, myelosuppression, and oligospermia)
  - **TNF-inhibitors appear to be the first truly "disease-modifying" agents for this disease**
    - Etanercept and infliximab Food and Drug Administration (FDA)-approved for this indication

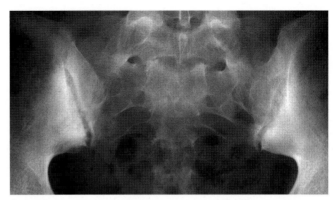

FIGURE 43-12 Radiographic findings of sacroiliitis in ankylosing spondylitis, with both erosions and sclerosis along the iliac sides of the sacroiliac joints. (From Harris ED, Budd RC, Genovese MC, et al, editors: *Kelley's textbook of rheumatology*, ed 7, Philadelphia, WB Saunders, 2005, figure 51-54.)

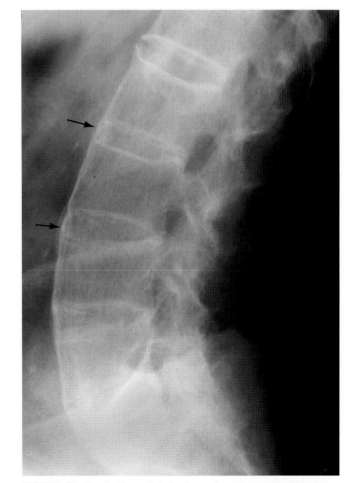

FIGURE 43-13 Radiographic findings of syndesmophytes in ankylosing spondylitis, with bony bridging (*arrows*) extending from the edge of one vertebral body to the next. (From Harris ED, Budd RC, Genovese MC, et al, editors: *Kelley's textbook of rheumatology*, ed 7, Philadelphia, WB Saunders, 2005, figure 51-56.)

Prevention

- Ankylosing spondylitis is not currently preventable

Enteropathic Arthritis

Basic Information

- Inflammatory arthritis associated with inflammatory bowel disease (IBD): Crohn's disease or ulcerative colitis
- Peripheral arthritis occurs in 10% to 20% of patients with IBD; spondylitis in 10%
- Male-to-female ratio is 3:1 in those with spondylitis

Clinical Presentation

- Axial skeletal disease clinically indistinguishable from ankylosing spondylitis
- Peripheral joint disease most commonly affects the knees, ankles, and feet
- **Peripheral joint disease activity correlates with GI disease activity; axial skeletal disease is independent**
- Extra-axial disease
  - Anterior uveitis
  - Oral aphthous ulcers
  - Erythema nodosum
  - Pyoderma gangrenosum

Diagnosis and Evaluation

- Clinical presentation highly suggestive in classic cases
- History characterized by
  - Coexistence of IBD and arthritis
- Physical examination reveals
  - Manifestations of IBD
  - Inflammatory axial or peripheral joint disease
  - Consider occult IBD in cases of "typical" articular pattern (e.g., isolated knee arthritis) without otherwise symptomatic GI involvement
- Laboratory findings
  - Inflammatory markers may be elevated
  - 50% of patients with spondylitis are HLA-B27-positive
- Radiographic findings are indistinguishable from ankylosing spondylitis

Treatment

- **Treat underlying IBD medically or surgically as indicated**
- NSAIDs must be used cautiously as they may provoke flare of bowel inflammation
- Corticosteroids may be used intravenously, orally, or intra-articularly
- TNF-inhibitors
  - Infliximab FDA-approved for this indication

Prevention

- Enteropathic arthritis is not currently preventable, beyond treatment of the underlying IBD

Psoriatic Arthritis

Basic Information

- Inflammatory arthritis associated with psoriatic skin disease
- At least 15% of patients with psoriatic skin disease are affected
- Male-to-female ratio is 1:1

Clinical Presentation

- Psoriasis may precede (70%), present with (15%), or follow (15%) onset of arthritis
- Patterns of joint involvement (not mutually exclusive)
  - Peripheral
    - Symmetrical polyarticular (30–50%; may be clinically indistinguishable from RA, but RF-negative)
    - Asymmetrical oligoarticular (30–50%; "classic" spondyloarthropathy pattern)
    - Distal interphalangeal joints (25%) (frequently associated with nail changes)
    - Arthritis mutilans (5%) (highly destructive)
  - Axial (5%)
    - Sacroiliitis (may be asymptomatic or asymmetrical)
    - Spondylitis (may be discontinuous)
  - Enthesitis
    - Dactylitis ("sausage digit"; Fig. 43-14)
- Extra-articular disease
  - Nail pitting, onycholysis, and "oil drop" sign (yellow-orange discoloration of the nail)
  - Anterior uveitis, aortitis, and pulmonary fibrosis are rare

Diagnosis and Evaluation

- Clinical presentation highly suggestive in classic cases
- History characterized by coexistence of psoriasis and arthritis
- Physical examination reveals
  - Manifestations of psoriatic skin disease
  - Inflammatory axial or peripheral joint disease

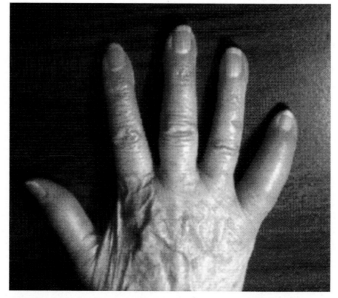

FIGURE 43-14 "Sausage digit" (dactylitis) of the fifth finger in psoriatic arthritis. (From Harris ED, Budd RC, Genovese MC, et al, editors: *Kelley's textbook of rheumatology,* ed 7, Philadelphia, WB Saunders, 2005, figure 71-S169.)

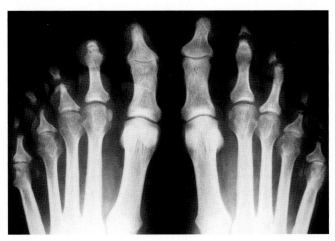

FIGURE 43-15 Bony resorption and osteophyte formation involving the phalanges in psoriatic arthritis creating "pencil-in-cup" changes. (From Harris ED, Budd RC, Genovese MC, et al, editors: *Kelley's textbook of rheumatology*, ed 7, Philadelphia, WB Saunders, 2005, figure 72-9.)

- Laboratory findings
  - Inflammatory markers may be elevated
  - 50% of patients with spondylitis are HLA-B27-positive
- Radiographic findings marked by both bony destruction and proliferation
  - Erosive arthritis
  - Osteolysis
  - Sacroiliitis
  - Ankylosis
  - Spondylitis
  - Enthesopathy
  - Periostitis
  - **"Pencil-in-cup"** (i.e., erosion of the distal end of one phalanx with bony proliferation of the proximal end of the adjacent phalanx; Fig. 43-15)

Treatment

- Treat underlying psoriasis as indicated
- NSAIDs
  - Analgesic and anti-inflammatory effects relieve pain and stiffness
- **Systemic corticosteroids may provoke flare of skin disease with taper**
- Methotrexate effective for both skin and joint disease
- Sulfasalazine
- TNF-inhibitors
  - Adalimumab, etanercept, and infliximab all FDA-approved for this indication

Prevention

- Psoriatic arthritis is not currently preventable, beyond treatment of the underlying skin disease

Reactive Arthritis

Basic Information

- Sterile inflammatory arthritis occurring following a genitourinary or enteric infection

- Reiter's disease (arthritis, conjunctivitis, and history of urethritis or enteritis) is a subset
- Etiologic agents: *Chlamydia, Campylobacter, Salmonella, Shigella,* and *Yersinia*
- Typically affects young males
- Male-to-female ratio is 9:1

Clinical Presentation

- **Manifestations typically appear 2 to 4 weeks after genitourinary or enteric infection**
- Patterns of joint involvement
  - Peripheral
    - Lower extremity oligoarthritis (particularly knees, ankles, and feet)
  - Axial
    - Sacroiliitis (may be asymmetrical)
  - Enthesitis
    - Achilles tendinitis
    - Plantar fasciitis
    - Dactylitis ("sausage digit")
- Extra-articular disease
  - Inflammatory eye disease (i.e., conjunctivitis or uveitis)
  - Mucocutaneous manifestations
    - Oral aphthous ulcers
    - Circinate balanitis
    - Keratoderma blenorrhagicum (clinically indistinguishable from psoriasis)
- Epidemiologic association with HIV/AIDS

Diagnosis and Evaluation

- Clinical presentation highly suggestive in classic cases
- History characterized by
  - **Classic triad of arthritis, conjunctivitis, and history of recent urethritis or enteritis**
  - Partial triad raises possibility of forme fruste
- Physical examination as detailed previously
- Laboratory findings
  - Inflammatory markers may be elevated
  - 50% to 80% of patients are HLA-B27-positive; 90% of those with uveitis or sacroiliitis
  - **Urethral swab may be positive for *Chlamydia trachomatis***
  - Stool cultures are usually negative for enteric infections
- Radiographic findings
  - Sacroiliitis
  - Erosions or spurring at insertion of Achilles tendon into plantar fascia (Fig. 43-16)

Treatment

- Disease is usually self-limited, lasting 3 to 12 months, but
  - Up to 50% of patients may experience relapse (possible reinfection)
  - 15% of patients may experience chronic, destructive, and disabling disease
- NSAIDs
  - Analgesic and anti-inflammatory effects relieve pain and stiffness

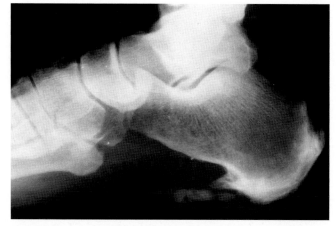

FIGURE 43-16 Calcaneal spur formation at the plantar fascial insertion in reactive arthritis. (From Harris ED, Budd RC, Genovese MC, et al, editors: *Kelley's textbook of rheumatology,* ed 7, Philadelphia, WB Saunders, 2005, figure 71-6.)

- Doxycycline (3-month course) may be beneficial in patients with persistent disease
- Sulfasalazine may be beneficial in patients with persistent disease
- Methotrexate has been used in patients whose disease is refractory to other measures

Prevention

- Avoidance and early treatment of genitourinary and enteric infections

Septic (Pyogenic/Nongonococcal) Arthritis

Basic Information

- Intensely inflammatory and rapidly destructive arthritis associated with bacterial joint infection
- Populations at risk
  - Chronically ill (e.g., diabetes mellitus, chronic renal failure, and malignancy)
  - Elderly
  - Immune-suppressed (e.g., AIDS and immunosuppressant medications)
  - Diseased or prosthetic joints
- Routes of infection
  - Direct inoculation
  - Local extension from an adjacent process
  - Hematogenous spread
- Etiology
  - Common agents
    - *Staphylococcus aureus* (~40%)
    - Group A *Streptococcus* (~30%)
    - Gram-negative (~30%)
  - Injection drug users may become infected with *Pseudomonas*
  - Sickle cell anemia patients may become infected with *Salmonella*

- **Prosthetic joints are susceptible to infection with *Staphylococcus epidermidis***
- Cat scratches or animal bites may cause *Pasteurella multocida* joint infections

Clinical Presentation

- **Most patients present with a monoarticular arthritis**
- Oligo- or polyarthritis may be seen with bacteremia
- **Injection drug users may present with sternoclavicular, sacroiliac, or disc space infections**
- Both systemic (fever/chills) and local (joint pain, swelling, erythema, and heat) manifestations
- Distinguish primary cellulitis from that due to an underlying septic joint

Diagnosis and Evaluation

- Clinical presentation highly suggestive in classic cases
- History as in preceding discussion
- Physical findings as in preceding discussion
- Laboratory findings
  - Synovial fluid analysis is critical
    - Arthrocentesis for cell count, Gram stain, and culture
    - **Highly inflammatory, often with greater than 75,000 cells/mm³ (predominantly neutrophils)**
    - **60% to 80% of patients have positive Gram stain**
    - **Approximately 90% of patients have positive synovial fluid culture**
    - Approximately 50% of patients have positive blood culture
- Radiographic findings
  - May reveal only soft tissue swelling in early disease
  - Joint space narrowing and bony erosions indicate severe and advanced disease
  - CT and MRI may detect fluid in deep joints (e.g., hip and sacroiliac joints)

Treatment

- **Drainage is essential in the management of infected joints**
  - Repeated needle aspiration is adequate for easily accessible joints without loculation
  - Arthroscopy or arthrotomy is required if repeated aspirations do not clear the infection
  - Arthrotomy is indicated as the initial mode of drainage for the hip
- Antibiotics
  - **Broad-spectrum antibiotics must be promptly administered (after arthrocentesis) and continued until the results of the Gram stain and culture are available**
  - Host risk factors (as detailed previously) are taken into consideration with empirical coverage

Prevention

- Avoid risk factors for infection, and treat infections promptly

Disseminated Gonococcal Infection

Basic Information

- Gonococcal (GC) infection is responsible for most cases of septic arthritis in young adults
- Female-to-male ratio is 3:1, as women are more likely to have asymptomatic GC infection
- Congenital complement deficiency is a risk factor

Clinical Presentation

- **May present as migratory arthritis or tenosynovitis, with or without rash**
- **May also present as purulent arthritis most commonly involving the wrist, knee, or ankle**
- Systemic manifestations (fevers and chills) may be present
- Macular, papular, or pustular rash may be present on the trunk or extremities

Diagnosis and Evaluation

- Clinical presentation highly suggestive in classic cases
- History characterized by
  - Sexually active young adult
  - Pharyngeal, urethral, cervical, and anal symptoms are frequently absent
- Physical findings as in the previous discussion
- Laboratory findings
  - Synovial fluid analysis
    - Arthrocentesis for cell count, Gram stain, and culture
    - Highly inflammatory with greater than 2000 WBC/mm³
    - **Gram stain usually negative**
    - Culture less than 50% positive
  - Blood and skin lesion cultures rarely positive
  - **Culture pharynx, urethra, cervix, and anus as potential sources of infection**
- Radiographic findings
  - May reveal soft tissue swelling

Treatment

- Repeated needle aspiration may be necessary, but arthroscopy and arthrotomy are rarely needed
- Sensitive to third-generation cephalosporins

Prevention

- Avoid risk factors for infection, and treat infections promptly

Viral Arthritis

Basic Information

- Common agents
  - Parvovirus B19
  - Rubella virus
  - Hepatitis B and C viruses
- Both children and adults affected

Clinical Presentation

- **May present as migratory arthralgias/arthritis or polyarthritis**
- Most commonly affects the wrists, hands, and knees
- Frequently symmetrical
- Rash may be present
- Hepatitis-associated arthritis may precede icterus

Diagnosis and Evaluation

- There may be a history of recent vaccination or exposure to sick contacts

Treatment

- **Most viral arthritides are self-limited, and are best managed supportively**
- Parvovirus may occasionally cause a chronic arthropathy

Prevention

- Avoid risk factors for infection

Lyme Disease

See also Chapter 16.

Basic Information

- Multisystem inflammatory disease caused by the tick-borne spirochete *Borrelia burgdorferi*
- 90% of cases reported from eight states (NY, NJ, CT, RI, MA, PA, WI, and MN)

Clinical Presentation

- Early localized disease (<30 days after infection)
  - Fever, malaise, headache, arthralgias, myalgias, and erythema migrans (50–90%)
- Early disseminated disease (weeks to months after infection)
  - Cardiac (e.g., heart block) and neurologic (e.g., Bell's palsy)
- Late disseminated disease (months to years after infection)
  - Cutaneous, neurologic, fibromyalgia-like, and articular (chronic knee arthritis in 10%)

Diagnosis and Evaluation

- **5% of the population has false-positive enzyme-linked imunnosorbent assay (ELISA)**
- Confirmation by Western blot

Treatment

- Arthritis treated with
  - Doxycycline (100 mg PO bid × 14–21 days)
  - Amoxicillin (500 mg PO tid daily × 21–30 days)
  - Ceftriaxone (2 g IV once daily × 14–28 days)

Prevention

- Avoid risk factors for infection, and treat infections promptly

43

Tuberculous Arthritis

Basic Information

- Develops in only a small percentage of cases of tuberculosis

Clinical Presentation

- Chronic granulomatous arthritis
  - Monoarticular
  - Usually involves the hips, knees, or ankles
  - Chronic joint pain and swelling
  - Usually not associated with active pulmonary TB
- Poncet's disease (tuberculous rheumatism; rare)
  - Symmetrical polyarthritis
  - Seen in conjunction with active disseminated infection

Diagnosis and Evaluation

- Chronic granulomatous arthritis
  - Acid-fast stain and culture of synovial fluid may be positive
  - Synovial biopsy may demonstrate granulomatous inflammation
  - Synovial tissue culture is usually positive
- Poncet's disease
  - Acid-fast stain and mycobacterial culture are negative

Treatment

- Six to nine months of combination antituberculous therapy

REVIEW QUESTIONS

For review questions, please go to www.expertconsult.com.

SUGGESTED READINGS

Harris ED, Budd RC, Genovese MC, et al, editors: *Kelley's textbook of rheumatology*, ed 7, Philadelphia, WB Saunders, 2005.

Klippel JH, Stone JH, Crofford LJ, White PH, editors: *Primer on the rheumatic diseases*, ed 13, Atlanta, Arthritis Foundation, 2008.

Levine SM, Gelber AC: Infectious monoarthritis. In Cheng A, Zaas A, editors: *The Osler medical handbook*, Philadelphia, Mosby, 2003.

Tehlirian C, Gelber AC: Connective tissue diseases. In Nilsson KR Jr, Piccini JP, editors: *The Osler medical handbook*, ed 2, Philadelphia, Saunders, 2006.

Acknowledgment

This chapter is adapted from a chapter previously written by Alan K. Matsumoto, MD, and later modified by Don R. Martin, MD, for earlier editions of the *Johns Hopkins Internal Medicine Board Review*.

CHAPTER 44

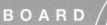
Office Orthopedics

JOHN A. FLYNN, MD, MBA, FACP, FACR, and KRISTI MIZELLE, MD, MPH

Office orthopedics covers a broad spectrum of disorders, many of which are not primarily articular and are variously characterized as "regional, soft tissue, or musculoskeletal pain syndromes." These disorders are common; occur in isolation or as part of a systemic process; involve any of the articular or periarticular soft tissues; cause pain; and may cause progressive functional disability. **In addition, few if any specific diagnostic laboratory tests apply to these disorders, with the diagnosis depending instead on a detailed history and physical examination.**

Shoulder

Figure 44-1 illustrates normal shoulder range of motion.

Basic Information

- Shoulder pain is one of the most common musculoskeletal complaints
- In younger patients (<40 years), symptoms are often caused by acute (e.g., sports-related) injuries
- In older patients, symptoms are more likely caused by chronic, degenerative changes of the rotator cuff
- Table 44-1 compares the most common disorders

Elbow

LATERAL EPICONDYLITIS ("TENNIS ELBOW")

Cause

- Repetitive wrist extension and forearm rotation

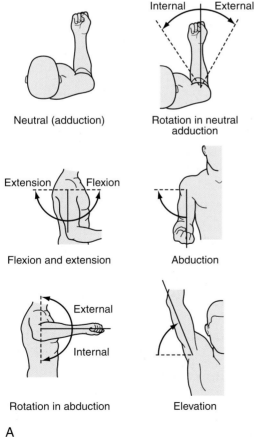

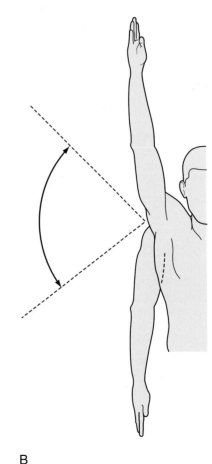

A   B

FIGURE 44-1   A and **B,** Normal shoulder range of motion. (From Swash M: *Hutchison's clinical methods,* ed 21, Philadelphia, WB Saunders, 2001, figure 10.30.)

TABLE 44-1	*Common Disorders of the Shoulder*			
	Rotator Cuff Tendinitis	**Rotator Cuff Tear**	**Adhesive Capsulitis**	**Bicipital Tendinitis**
Cause	Overuse	Trauma Recurrent rotator cuff tendinitis	Prolonged shoulder immobilization	Overuse
Clinical presentation	Anterolateral shoulder pain	Anterolateral shoulder pain	Shoulder pain Loss of motion	Anterior shoulder pain

Diagnosis and evaluation	Pain with
	  Abduction < resisted abduction
	  Internal and external rotation
	  Lateral palpation
	Positive "impingement test"*
		Same as rotator cuff tendinitis
		Positive "drop test"†
		  with full-thickness tear
			Painful and limited active and passive motion	Tenderness over bicipital groove
				Positive "Speed's test"‡
				Positive "Yergason's sign"§

Treatment	Rest NSAIDs Steroid injection Physical therapy	Orthopedic evaluation for repair	Physical therapy Steroid injection Possible orthopedics referral	Rest NSAIDs Steroid injection Physical therapy

*Relief of pain after injection of the subacromial bursa.
†Unable to maintain active shoulder abduction.
‡Pain with resisted shoulder flexion.
§Pain with resisted forearm supination.

Clinical Presentation

- Lateral elbow pain

Diagnosis and Evaluation

- Tenderness over lateral epicondyle
- Pain elicited by resisted wrist extension and forearm supination (Fig. 44-2)

Treatment

- Rest
- NSAIDs
- Steroid injection
- Bracing
- Physical therapy

MEDIAL EPICONDYLITIS ("GOLFER'S ELBOW")

Cause

- Repetitive wrist flexion and forearm rotation

Clinical Presentation

- Medial elbow pain

Diagnosis and Evaluation

- Tenderness over medial epicondyle
- Pain elicited by resisted wrist flexion and forearm pronation (see Fig. 44-2)

Treatment

- Same as for lateral epicondylitis

ULNAR NEUROPATHY

Cause

- Trauma to the ulnar nerve as it traverses the elbow joint

Clinical Presentation

- Posteromedial forearm and hand pain and paresthesias

Diagnosis and Evaluation

- Tenderness with percussion over the cubital tunnel
- Decreased sensation in the ulnar nerve distribution

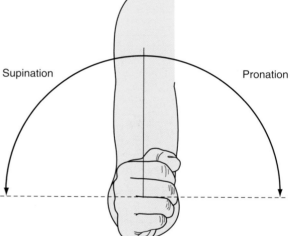
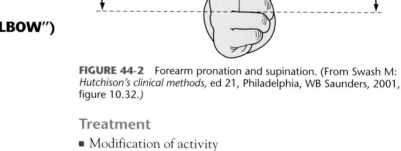

FIGURE 44-2 Forearm pronation and supination. (From Swash M: *Hutchison's clinical methods,* ed 21, Philadelphia, WB Saunders, 2001, figure 10.32.)

Treatment

- Modification of activity
- NSAIDs
- Surgery is sometimes required for decompression

OLECRANON BURSITIS

Cause

- Trauma
- Infection secondary to overlying cellulitis (most commonly gram-positive bacteria, especially *Staphylococcus aureus*)
- Gout and pseudogout
- Rheumatoid arthritis

Clinical Presentation

- Pain and swelling over olecranon process

Diagnosis and Evaluation

- Inflamed olecranon bursa
- Pain with flexion, but not extension

- Examination of bursa fluid critical to diagnose infection

Treatment
- Rest and treatment of the underlying cause
- NSAIDs for gout
- Drainage and antibiotics for infection

Hand and Wrist

Basic Information
- The hand and wrist are subject to a number of common conditions, many of which may be attributed to overuse or repetitive use (Fig. 44-3)
- Table 44-2 compares the most common disorders

Hip

Figure 44-4 illustrates normal range of motion in the hip.

TROCHANTERIC BURSITIS

Cause
- Overuse
- Trauma
- Associated with obesity

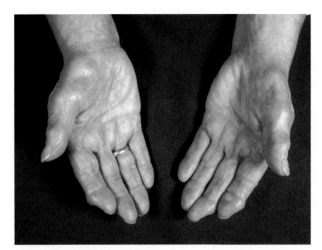

FIGURE 44-3 Thenar eminence wasting due to carpal tunnel syndrome. (From Swash M: *Hutchison's clinical methods*, ed 21, Philadelphia, WB Saunders, 2001, figure 10.13.)

Clinical Presentation
- Deep aching lateral hip pain extending to buttock or lateral knee
- Painful to lie in lateral decubitus position

Diagnosis and Evaluation
- Pain on palpation over greater trochanter
- Pain with resisted hip abduction

TABLE 44-2	Common Disorders of the Wrist and Hand				
	Carpal Tunnel Syndrome	**Ulnar Tunnel Syndrome**	**De Quervain's Tenosynovitis**	**Trigger Finger**	**Dupuytren's Contracture**
Cause	Median nerve compression at wrist	Ulnar nerve compression at wrist	Abductor policis longus and extensor policis brevis tendon inflammation	Inflammation and stenosis of digital flexor tendon	Contracture of palmar fascia
Precipitating factors	Overuse Synovitis Hypothyroidism Amyloidosis Acromegaly Pregnancy	Overuse Trauma Ganglion cyst	Overuse RA	Overuse RA	Heredity Alcoholism Diabetes Epilepsy
Clinical presentation	Numbness and paresthesias in median nerve distribution* Nocturnal exacerbation Wasting of thenar eminence (see Fig. 44-3)	Numbness and paresthesias in ulnar nerve distribution§	Wrist pain extending from thumb	Tendon catches with flexion of digit	Unable to fully extend digits
Diagnosis and evaluation	Median nerve Tinel's sign† Phalen's sign‡ Abnormal nerve conduction test and electromyography	Ulnar nerve "Tinel's sign"† Abnormal nerve conduction test and electromyography	Tender over radial styloid Finkelstein test#	Pain and palpable "catch" with digit flexion Nodule may be palpable	Flexion deformity of fourth > fifth > third > second digits Palpable thickening of palmar fascia
Treatment	Wrist splint NSAIDs Steroid injection Surgical release	Wrist splint NSAIDs Surgical release	Wrist/thumb splint NSAIDs Steroid injection Surgery	Occupational therapy Steroid injection Surgical release	Surgical excision in extreme cases

*First–third fingers and radial half of the fourth.
†Provoke pain and paresthesia with percussion over nerve at the wrist.
‡Provoke pain and paresthesia, and numbness with forced wrist flexion (reversed "prayer position").
§Fifth finger and ulnar half of the fourth.
#Provoke pain with forced ulnar deviation of the wrist, with thumb enclosed by fist.

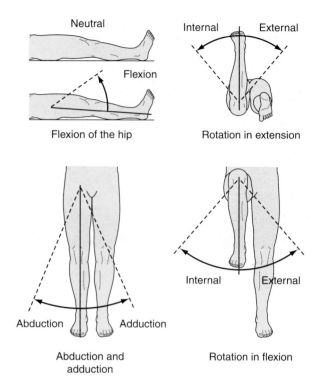

FIGURE 44-4 Normal hip range of motion. (From Swash M: *Hutchison's clinical methods,* ed 21, Philadelphia, WB Saunders, 2001, figure 10.39.)

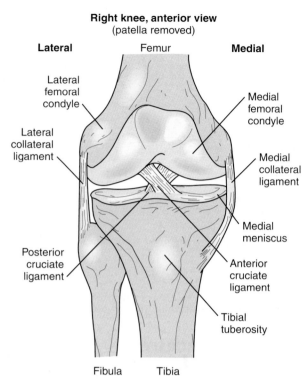

FIGURE 44-5 Anterior view of the knee demonstrating the anterior and posterior cruciate ligaments. (From Gosling J, Willan PLT, Whitmore I, Harris PF: *Human anatomy: color atlas and text,* ed 4, St. Louis, Mosby, 2002, figure 6.78.)

Treatment

- Rest
- NSAIDs
- Steroid injection
- Physical therapy

MERALGIA PARESTHETICA

Cause

- Entrapment of lateral femoral cutaneous nerve
- Associated with obesity, pregnancy, diabetes, and tight clothing

Clinical Presentation

- Numbness and paresthesias over anterolateral thigh

Diagnosis and Evaluation

- Anterolateral thigh sensory deficit
- Tender over inguinal ligament

Treatment

- NSAIDs
- Treat underlying condition

Hip and Knee

ILIOTIBIAL BAND SYNDROME

Cause

- Overuse of iliotibial band (e.g., running)

Clinical Presentation

- Pain over lateral thigh above the joint line of the knee

Diagnosis and Evaluation

- Tender over lateral femoral condyle
- Pain when standing on flexed knee

Treatment

- Rest
- NSAIDs
- Steroid injection
- Physical therapy

Knee

See Figure 44-5 for ligaments of the knee joint.

Basic Information

- The knee, by virtue of its weight-bearing status, is subject to a variety of disorders
- Table 44-3 compares the most common disorders
- McMurry test
  - Flex the knee as much as possible
    - Medial meniscus evaluated by externally rotating the foot and extending the knee
    - Lateral meniscus evaluated by internally rotating the foot and extending the knee
    - A positive test occurs when maneuver provokes pain at the appropriate meniscus; occasionally a click may also be palpated

TABLE 44-3   *Common Disorders of the Knee*

	Chondromalacia Patellae	Meniscal Injury	Collateral Ligament Injury	Anterior Cruciate Ligament Injury	Posterior Cruciate Ligament Injury	Prepatellar Bursitis	Anserine Bursitis	Ruptured Baker's Cyst (Pseudothrombophlebitis)
Cause	Patellofemoral cartilage degeneration	Trauma	Overuse Trauma	Twisting injury to knee with foot planted	Hyperextension injury to knee	Overuse Trauma Infection Gout	Overuse Osteoarthritis	One-way flow of knee effusion to gastrocnemius–semimembranosus bursa
Clinical presentation	Anterior knee pain when climbing stairs	Pain Swelling Catching Locking Buckling	Medial or lateral knee pain	Pain Swelling Instability	Pain Swelling Instability	Anterior knee pain Swelling	Anteromedial pain 4–5 cm below joint line	Popliteal fullness Calf pain, swelling, and ecchymosis on rupture
Diagnosis and evaluation	Tender with patellar compression	Tender joint margin Pain with motion Pain with McMurray test	Tenderness over affected ligament Provoke pain with medial or lateral stress in 20° of flexion	Swelling Anterior instability of the tibia at the knee (anterior drawer sign)	Swelling Posterior instability of the tibia at the knee (posterior drawer sign)	Swollen and tender prepatellar bursa Aspirate to diagnose cause	Tender with palpation Pain with knee flexion	Rule out deep venous thrombosis with ultrasound (Fig. 44-6)
Treatment	Quadriceps strengthening exercises NSAIDs Rarely surgery	Rest NSAIDs Physical therapy Possible surgical meniscectomy	Rest Physical therapy Surgery if unstable	Orthopedic evaluation	Orthopedic evaluation	Rest NSAIDs Antibiotic if needed	Rest NSAIDs Steroid injection Physical therapy	Rest Elevation Steroid injection

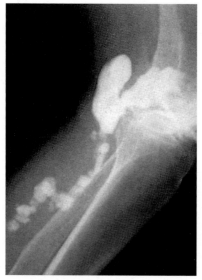

FIGURE 44-6 Arthrogram demonstrating a ruptured Baker's cyst. (From Forbes CD, Jackson WF: *Color atlas and text of clinical medicine*, ed 3, St. Louis, Mosby, 2003, figure 3.28.)

Ankle

ACHILLES TENDINITIS

Cause

- Overuse, poor training habits, and improper footwear in athletes
- Fluoroquinolone antibiotics
- Associated with spondyloarthritis

Clinical Presentation

- Pain along the Achilles tendon

Diagnosis and Evaluation

- Tenderness and thickening along the tendon
- Dorsiflexion of foot is painful

Treatment

- NSAIDs
- Heel lift
- Stretching program
- If underlying spondyloarthritis is detected (ankylosing spondylitis, psoriatic arthritis, reactive, or inflammatory bowel disease-related), treatment is directed at underlying condition

ACHILLES TENDON RUPTURE

Cause

- Forced dorsiflexion of the foot as the gastrocnemius muscle contracts
- Males affected more than females

Clinical Presentation

- Tearing and popping sensation in the calf

Diagnosis and Evaluation

- Swelling of the calf
- Weakness of foot flexion
- Palpation of gap caused by tendon rupture
- Abnormal Thompson test (failure of the foot to plantarflex when squeezing the gastrocnemius muscle)

Treatment

- Orthopedic evaluation and possible repair

TARSAL TUNNEL SYNDROME

Cause

- Posterior tibial nerve entrapment behind the medial malleolus
- Associated with pes planus (flat feet), ganglion cyst, and lipomata

Clinical Presentation

- Burning pain over the medial and plantar aspects of the foot
- Aggravated by activity

Diagnosis and Evaluation

- Posterior tibial nerve (Tinel's sign) posterior to the medial malleolus
- Decreased sensation over medial and plantar aspects of the foot
- Nerve conduction study if examination equivocal

Treatment

- Orthotics
- Surgery occasionally necessary

Foot

PLANTAR FASCIITIS

Cause

- Overuse, causing inflammation of plantar fascia
- Heel spur
- Associated with spondyloarthritis

Clinical Presentation

- Heel and posterior foot pain
- Sensation of "walking on pebbles"
- Classically, with the first steps of the morning and after prolonged sitting
- Improves with use

Diagnosis and Evaluation

- Tenderness on plantar aspect of heel

Treatment

- Stretching
- Orthotics
- NSAIDs
- Steroid injection
- Rarely surgery

MORTON'S NEUROMA

Cause

- Neuroma formation causing compression of digital nerve in foot

Clinical Presentation

- Pain and paresthesias
- Most commonly between third and fourth toes

Diagnosis and Evaluation

- Tenderness to deep palpation between toes
- Neuroma may be palpable

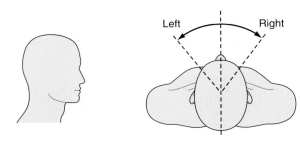

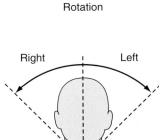

Neutral

Rotation

Extension | Flexion

Right | Left

Flexion and extension

Lateral bending

FIGURE 44-7 Normal cervical spine range of motion. (From Swash M: *Hutchison's clinical methods,* ed 21, Philadelphia, WB Saunders, 2001, figure 10.26.)

Treatment

- Metatarsal bar orthotic
- Steroid injection
- Surgical excision of neuroma

Cervical Spine

Figure 44-7 shows normal cervical spine range of motion.

CERVICAL SPINE STRAIN

Cause

- Overuse
- Poor posture
- Hyperextension injury

Clinical Presentation

- Neck pain and stiffness
- No symptoms or signs of radiculopathy

Diagnosis and Evaluation

- Localized tenderness over cervical musculature
- Absence of neurologic deficits (Table 44-4)

Treatment

- NSAIDs
- Soft cervical collar
- Physical therapy

CERVICAL DISK DISEASE

Cause

- Disk herniation

Clinical Presentation

- Neck pain and stiffness
- Radicular complaints (weakness, numbness, paresthesias along involved nerve root)
- Worse with straining

Diagnosis and Evaluation

- Symptoms exacerbated with neck compression
- Abnormal neurologic examination (Fig. 44-8; see also Table 44-4)

Treatment

- Initially conservative
- NSAIDs
- Soft collar
- Surgical evaluation for intractable pain or progressive neurologic deficits

Lumbar Spine

Figure 44-9 shows normal lumbar spine range of motion.

Basic Information

- Low back pain is one of the most common musculoskeletal complaints
- 80% of the population experience low back pain at some time in their life
- Low back pain is generally a self-limited condition
  - 50% are better in 1 week
  - 90% are better in 6 weeks
  - Sciatica can have a more protracted course, but 50% recover in 4 weeks

TABLE 44-4	**Cervical and Lumbar Spine Neurologic Examination**		
Nerve Root	**Motor Function**	**Sensory Function**	**Reflex**
C5	Deltoid and biceps (elbow flexion)	Shoulder and lateral aspect of arm	Biceps
C6*	Biceps and wrist extensors	Lateral forearm and thumb	Biceps
C7	Triceps (elbow extension)	Middle finger	Triceps
C8	Finger flexors	Medial forearm and little finger	None
T1	Intrinsic muscles of the hand	Medial aspect of arm	None
L4	Quadriceps (knee extension)	Medial aspect of calf and ankle	Quadriceps (knee)
L5	Tibialis anterior (ankle dorsiflexion)[†]	Dorsum of foot	None
S1	Gastrocnemius (ankle plantarflexion)[‡]	Lateral aspect of ankle and foot	Gastrocnemius (ankle)

*May be confused with carpal tunnel syndrome.
[†]Cannot stand on heels.
[‡]Cannot stand on toes.

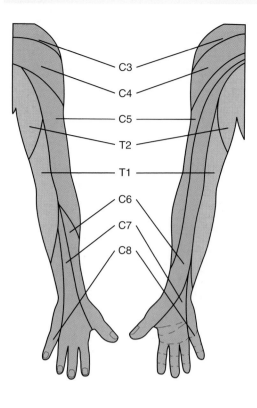

FIGURE 44-8 Cervical nerve root dermatomal distribution in the upper extremity. (From Gosling J, Willan PLT, Whitmore I, Harris PF: *Human anatomy: color atlas and text,* ed 4, St. Louis, Mosby, 2002, figure 3.6.)

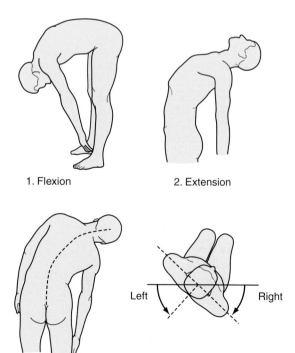

1. Flexion   2. Extension

3. Lateral bending   4. Rotation

FIGURE 44-9 Normal lumbar spine range of motion. (From Swash M: *Hutchison's clinical methods,* ed 21, Philadelphia, WB Saunders, 2001, figure 10.28.)

BOX 44-1	*Low Back Pain*

Local Causes
Muscle strain
Lumbar spine osteoarthritis
Degenerative disk disease
Hip osteoarthritis
Vertebral body infection
Vertebral body malignancy
Disk space infection

Distant Causes
Ulcer disease
Pancreatitis
Nephrolithiasis
Prostatitis
Aortic dissection
Subacute bacterial endocarditis
Pelvic pathology

Worrisome Findings
Nocturnal pain
   Cancer
   Infection
Writhing pain
   Aneurysm
   Perforated viscus
Evolving neurologic deficits
   Epidural abscess
   Hemorrhage
   Disk herniation
Fever
   Infection

Clinical Presentation

- Acute low back pain (Box 44-1)
- Spinal stenosis
  - Caused by impingement on lumbosacral spinal cord
  - Associated with degenerative arthritis
  - Pseudoclaudication (nonvascular claudication improving with flexion at the waist)

Diagnosis and Evaluation

- Lumbar spine examination (Fig. 44-10; see also Table 44-4)
- Straight-leg-raising test
  - Sensitive (>90%) but not specific
  - Pain should be radicular
  - Helpful in ruling out sciatica
  - Crossed straight-leg-raising test less sensitive (25%) but more specific (80%)
- Indications for radiographic evaluation
  - Preceding significant trauma
  - Evolving neurologic findings
  - Suggestion of malignancy or infection
  - Suspect lumbar spinal stenosis
  - Older age
  - Persistent pain

Treatment

- Rest
- Heat and cold
- NSAIDs
- Physical therapy
- Surgery may be indicated (e.g., infection, intractable pain, neurologic defects, and spinal stenosis)

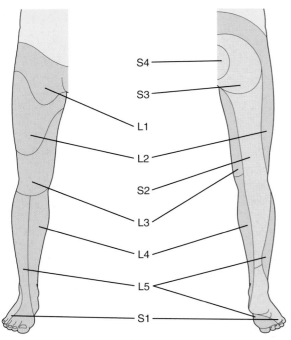

FIGURE 44-10 Lumbar nerve root dermatomal distribution in the lower extremity. (From Gosling J, Willan PLT, Whitmore I, Harris PF: *Human anatomy: color atlas and text,* ed 4, St. Louis, 2002, Mosby, figure 6.10.)

REVIEW QUESTIONS

For review questions, please go to www.expertconsult.com.

SUGGESTED READINGS

Biundo JJ: Musculoskeletal signs and symptoms: regional rheumatic pain syndromes. In Klippel JH, editor: *Primer on the rheumatic diseases,* ed 12, Atlanta, Arthritis Foundation, 2001.

Borenstein D: Musculoskeletal signs and symptoms: disorders of the low back and neck. In Klippel JH, editor: *Primer on the rheumatic diseases,* ed 12, Atlanta, Arthritis Foundation, 2001.

Ruddy S, Harris ED, Sledge CB: Musculoskeletal pain and evaluation. In Ruddy S, Harris ED, Sledge CB, editors: *Kelley's textbook of rheumatology,* ed 6, Philadelphia, WB Saunders, 2001.

44

Vasculitis

PHILIP SEO, MD, MHS

The primary systemic vasculitides (vasculitis) are autoimmune disorders characterized by inflammation of the blood vessels. The vasculitides can affect almost any organ system and often lead to significant morbidity. There are at least 15 currently recognized individual disorders, differentiated clinically by (1) the size of blood vessel typically involved; (2) their predilection for certain organ systems; and (3) characteristic pathologic features. The traditional way of classifying the vasculitides by the size of the predominant vessels involved remains a valuable method of approaching these diseases. One classification scheme based on blood vessel size is depicted in Box 45-1.

Hypersensitivity vasculitis—which may appear as a reaction to a drug, virus, or other antigen—is often seen in a primary care setting. **Giant-cell arteritis** (GCA) is the most common form of primary (idiopathic) systemic vasculitis. It may be most helpful to study these syndromes first and then review **cryoglobulinemic vasculitis, Henoch-Schönlein purpura** (HSP), and **Wegener's granulomatosis,** any of which may be encountered by an internist. Learning these relatively common forms of vasculitis well will provide an excellent foundation that can be used to approach the other diseases described in this chapter.

Behçet's Disease

Basic Information

- Widest range of blood vessel involvement of all the vasculitides: Small, medium, and large vessels, in both the venous and arterial circulations
- Found most commonly in the regions that once made up the old Silk Route: Turkey, Iran, China, and Japan
- Associated with human leukocyte antigen (HLA)-B51

Clinical Presentation

- **Classic triad of signs is oral ulcers (Fig. 45-1), genital ulcers, and ocular inflammation**
  - Oral ulcers: Painful and virtually pathognomonic of Behçet's disease
  - Genital ulcers: Commonly heal with scarring
  - Ocular inflammation
    - Anterior uveitis: May manifest as a hypopyon (pus in the anterior chamber); asymmetrical pupils may also be present because of synechiae formation between the lens and iris
    - Posterior uveitis: May manifest as retinal vasculitis
  - Folliculitis
  - Erythema nodosum

| BOX 45-1 | *Classification of the Vasculitides* |

Predominantly or Exclusively Small-Vessel Vasculitides
Immune complex-mediated
  Cutaneous leukocytoclastic angiitis (hypersensitivity vasculitis)
  Henoch-Schönlein purpura
  Urticarial vasculitis
  Cryoglobulinemia*
  Connective tissue disorders*
  Erythema elevatum diutinum
ANCA-associated disorders
  Wegener's granulomatosis*
  Microscopic polyangiitis*
  Churg-Strauss syndrome*
Miscellaneous small-vessel vasculitides
  Behçet's disease†
  Paraneoplastic
  Infection
  Inflammatory bowel disease

Predominantly or Exclusively Medium-Vessel Vasculitides
Classic polyarteritis nodosa
Cutaneous polyarteritis nodosa
Rheumatoid vasculitis*
Kawasaki disease
Buerger's disease (thromboangiitis obliterans)

Predominantly Large-Vessel Vasculitides
Giant-cell (temporal) arteritis
Takayasu's arteritis
Cogan's syndrome

*Common overlap of small- and medium-sized blood vessel involvement.
†May involve small-, medium-, and large-sized blood vessels.

- In contrast to erythema nodosum associated with other conditions, they may ulcerate and heal with scarring
- Biopsy often reveals medium-vessel vasculitis rather than septal panniculitis
- **Pathergy: Development of sterile pustules at sites of needle stick; only a minority of patients demonstrate the pathergy phenomenon, but when present this lesion is highly suggestive of Behçet's disease**

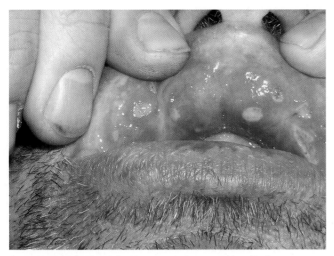

FIGURE 45-1 Aphthous oral ulcers in Behçet's disease.

- Superficial and deep venous thrombophlebitis
- Cerebral venous thrombosis
- Aseptic meningitis
- Brainstem involvement: May mimic multiple sclerosis because of its tendency to involve white matter
- Arthritis: Typically nondeforming

Diagnosis and Evaluation

- No specific laboratory or histologic findings are diagnostic
- Manifestations may occur simultaneously or be separated by several years
- **Diagnosis based on physician observation of the various clinical manifestations and recognition of the characteristic constellation of physical findings, guided by the International Study Group criteria, which require recurrent oral ulceration plus two of the following four manifestations:**
  - **Recurrent genital ulceration**
  - **Eye lesions**
  - **Skin lesions**
  - **Positive pathergy test**

Treatment

- A variety of regimens have been used, based on the extent and severity of involvement
  - For mucocutaneous disease:
    - Colchicine: First-line therapy for oral ulcers; effective only in milder cases; may be used up to three times per day if tolerated gastrointestinally
    - Topical glucocorticoids: Limited efficacy for oral and genital ulcers
  - For more refractory disease:
    - Low-dose systemic glucocorticoids
    - Thalidomide: For mucocutaneous lesions
    - Azathioprine
    - Tumor necrosis factor inhibitors
  - For the most serious disease manifestations, including CNS and uveitis (because of the risk for blindness):
    - High-dose systemic glucocorticoids
    - Cyclophosphamide

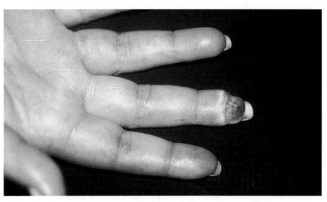

FIGURE 45-2 Digital ischemia in Buerger's disease.

Buerger's Disease (Thromboangiitis Obliterans)

Basic Information

- Manifestations primarily caused by involvement of medium-sized arteries, but veins affected as well
- Should not be confused with Berger's disease (IgA nephropathy)

Clinical Presentation

- **Typical patient is young male smoker with digital infarction, although it may also occur in female smokers**
- **Striking contrast between the severity of digital vasculitis and absence of internal organ disease**
- Does not involve smallest vessels (i.e., capillaries) and therefore more likely to be associated with digital infarction (Fig. 45-2) than with purpura

Diagnosis and Evaluation

- Superficial thrombophlebitis may be the first sign
- Should be considered high on the differential diagnosis when there is severe digital ischemia involving two or more extremities but no other organ dysfunction
- **Angiography reveals distinctive "corkscrew" collateral vessels in blood vessels at the level of the wrists and ankles**

Treatment

- **Smoking cessation is the only effective form of treatment**
- No form of immunosuppression (including glucocorticoids) provides control or cure
- Continued smoking may result in progression of ischemia and the need for amputation

Churg-Strauss Syndrome (Allergic Granulomatosis and Angiitis)

Basic Information

- Characterized by necrotizing inflammation within small arteries, veins, and capillaries
- Classically described as a clinical triad of asthma, hypereosinophilia, and vasculitis

Clinical Presentation

- **Typical patient presents with the recent onset of allergy or asthma, followed by eosinophilic tissue infiltration and the subsequent development of symptoms and signs of vasculitis**
- Asthma associated with Churg-Strauss syndrome may improve as the vasculitic phase begins
- Typical symptoms and signs include:
  - **Sinusitis: Nondestructive, in contrast to Wegener's granulomatosis**
  - Wheezing
  - **Mononeuritis multiplex: Neuropathy involving named motor and sensory nerves, often acute in onset, which manifests as the inability to dorsiflex or to hyperextend the wrist (i.e., "foot drop" or "wrist drop")**
  - Cutaneous nodules: Cutaneous extravascular necrotizing granuloma
    - May mimic rheumatoid nodules
    - Also known as Churg-Strauss granuloma or Winkelman's granuloma
    - Usually occurs over extensor surfaces (e.g., the olecranon)

Diagnosis and Evaluation

- In addition to the characteristic clinical features, distinctive diagnostic features include the following:
  - **Fleeting pulmonary infiltrates (30% of cases)**
  - **Eosinophilia (up to 60,000 eosinophils/mm³)**
  - **Positive antineutrophil cytoplasmic antibody (ANCA) (50% of cases):** When present, the antigen specificity for ANCA is usually myeloperoxidase (MPO) rather than proteinase-3 (PR-3) and is associated with peripheral ANCA (P-ANCA; peripheral) rather than C-ANCA (cytoplasmic) immunofluorescence
- Biopsy may help confirm the diagnosis

Treatment

- **Usually responds dramatically to glucocorticoids alone**
- Eosinophilia disappears with glucocorticoids (eosinophilia of the hypereosinophilic syndrome is more refractory to treatment)
- Cyclophosphamide may be required for refractory cases

Cogan's Syndrome

Basic Information

- Large-vessel vasculitis (e.g., aortitis) occurs in approximately 10% of patients
- The ocular inflammation and sensorineural hearing loss are presumed secondary to small-vessel vasculitis

Clinical Presentation

- **Typical patient presents with ocular disease (interstitial keratitis) and sensorineural hearing loss**
- Eye and ear disease do not always begin simultaneously, but usually occur within a few months of each other

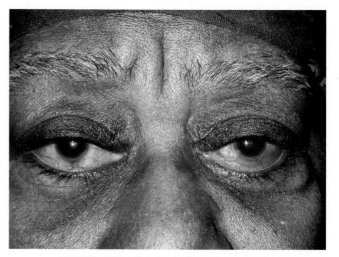

FIGURE 45-3 Scleritis in Cogan's syndrome.

- Symptoms and signs may include:
  - Ocular manifestations:
    - Interstitial keratitis (pain, photophobia, decreased visual acuity, and red eye) is most common
    - Episcleritis
    - Scleritis (Fig. 45-3)
    - Retinal disease
    - Uveitis
  - Sensorineural manifestations:
    - Tinnitus
    - Hearing loss
    - Vertigo
    - Oscillopsia
  - Constitutional symptoms present in 50% of patients
- 10% of patients present with a large-vessel vasculitis mimicking Takayasu's arteritis

Diagnosis and Evaluation

- Diagnosis based on distinctive combination of eye and ear inflammation
- **Important to exclude syphilis and acoustic neuromas**

Treatment

- Topical glucocorticoids used for interstitial keratitis
- Systemic glucocorticoids required for other manifestations
- Sensorineural hearing loss must be treated promptly and aggressively to avoid permanent hearing loss and may require cyclophosphamide

Cryoglobulinemia (Essential Mixed Cryoglobulinemia)

Basic Information

- **Cryoglobulins are immunoglobulins that precipitate out of serum in cold conditions**
- Cryoglobulinemia affects small- to medium-sized arteries, capillaries, and veins

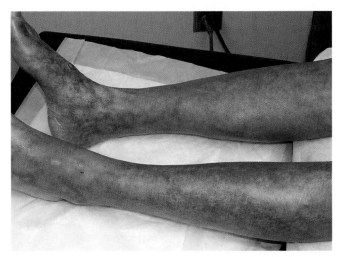

FIGURE 45-4 Hyperpigmentation and ulceration of the legs due to mixed cryoglobulinemia associated with hepatitis C.

TABLE 45-1	*Subtypes of Cryoglobulinemia*		
	Type I	**Type II**	**Type III**
Monoclonality of immunoglobulin component?	Yes (usually IgG)	Yes (IgM)	No
Rheumatoid factor activity?	No	Yes	Yes
Clinical syndrome	Hyperviscosity	Vasculitis	Vasculitis
Disease association	Hematopoietic malignancy	Hepatitis C Rheumatic diseases Malignancies Idiopathic	Hepatitis C Rheumatic diseases Idiopathic

Clinical Presentation

- **Typical patient has hepatitis C virus infection (causes 90% of cases)**
- Symptoms and signs:
  - Recurrent purpura
  - Hyperpigmentation that results from repeated bouts of purpura (Fig. 45-4)
  - Brawny induration that mimics venous stasis disease
  - Livedo reticularis
  - Raynaud's phenomenon
  - Digital infarction
  - Mononeuritis multiplex (e.g., foot drop)
  - Glomerulonephritis (seen only with type II cryoglobulinemia)
  - Occasional CNS vasculitis

Diagnosis and Evaluation

- Based on clinical presentation and isolation of cryoglobulins (from blood samples kept at body temperature until transport to the lab)
- Classification (and clinical manifestations) based on properties of cryoproteins present (Table 45-1)

- **Hypocomplementemia is a hallmark of cryoglobulinemic vasculitis because the disorder is mediated by immune complex deposition**
- **Pattern of hypocomplementemia is distinctive: C4 levels are decreased out of proportion to C3**
- Patients with cryoglobulinemia are often initially misdiagnosed as having either rheumatoid arthritis or lupus for the following reasons:
  - Vast majority are positive for rheumatoid factor (IgM component of mixed cryoglobulins has rheumatoid factor activity)
  - Majority are antinuclear antibody (ANA)-positive
  - Hypocomplementemia is also commonly seen in lupus

Treatment

- Interferon-α and ribavirin for hepatitis C-related cases
- Glucocorticoids and cyclophosphamide for refractory, organ-threatening cases
- **Plasmapheresis should also be considered in acutely ill patients with severe disease**

Giant-Cell Arteritis (Temporal Arteritis)

Basic Information

- Medium to large arteries of the head and neck affected
- **Never occurs in people younger than 50 years of age**

Clinical Presentation

- Typical patient is elderly person with new-onset headaches and inflamed temporal arteries
- Typical symptoms and signs
  - **New headaches of any type**
  - **Jaw claudication (most specific symptom) may manifest itself as pain in the face or throat, particularly with chewing**
  - Visual symptoms
    - Possible manifestations include amaurosis fugax, blurriness, or diplopia
    - **Once visual loss occurs in GCA, it is usually permanent**
  - Large-vessel symptoms (e.g., arm claudication and aortic dissection); symptomatic large-vessel disease occurs in at least 20% of patients with GCA
  - Polymyalgia rheumatica (50% of cases)
- **Atypical manifestations include fever of unknown origin; weight loss; nonproductive cough; and nonspecific pains in the neck, throat, or tongue**

Diagnosis and Evaluation

- Diagnosis based on typical clinical presentation and these additional findings
  - The temporal arteries may be abnormal (swollen, tender, nodular) on examination (Fig. 45-5), but arteries are normal in up to one third of biopsy-proven cases
  - **Elevated erythrocyte sedimentation rate in the great majority of cases (90% of cases >50 mm/hour)**

45

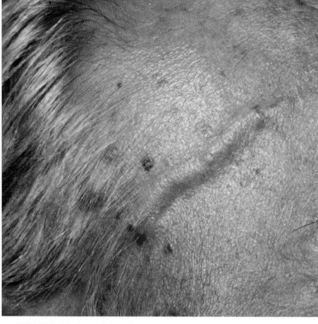

FIGURE 45-5 Inflamed temporal artery in giant-cell arteritis.

- Disruption of internal elastic lamina evident on temporal artery biopsy
  - Giant cells not always present; earliest finding is lymphoplasmacytic inflammation in the adventitia
  - Bilateral temporal artery biopsies that do not reveal GCA have a negative predictive value of 90%
  - **Temporal artery biopsy specimen may be positive for up to 2 weeks (or longer) after treatment with high-dose glucocorticoids is started**
- Despite the importance of the temporal artery biopsy, the diagnosis of GCA and the initiation of treatment ultimately remain clinical decisions

Treatment

- **Systemic glucocorticoids, initially 1 mg/kg/day**
  - **Glucocorticoid treatment should begin at the time the diagnosis is strongly suspected, without awaiting biopsy results**
  - **However, the initiation of therapy does not invalidate the importance of tissue confirmation of the diagnosis as soon as possible**
- Studies of methotrexate efficacy as a steroid-sparing agent give conflicting results
- Flares occur with tapering of medication in at least 25% to 50% of patients
- GCA tends to run a self-limited course, and glucocorticoids may be tapered off over 1 to 2 years; as many as one third of patients, however, may require chronic low-dose glucocorticoids

Henoch-Schönlein Purpura

Basic Information

- Small arterioles and venules affected
- 90% of cases occur in children
- Majority of cases resolve within a few weeks
- Chronic cases do occur, particularly in adults
- Characterized by immunoglobulin (Ig)A deposition in biopsies

Clinical Presentation

- Typical patient is child with recent upper respiratory tract infection, followed by the onset of the typical tetrad of symptoms and signs:
  - Palpable purpura, occasionally with pustular lesions
  - Arthritis
  - Crampy abdominal pain (with or without GI bleeding)
  - Hematuria or proteinuria (renal insufficiency in <5% of cases)

Diagnosis and Evaluation

- IgA deposition on tissue biopsy specimen
  - Two forms of IgA (IgA1 and IgA2)
  - HSP associated only with abnormalities of IgA1
- Serum and urine protein electrophoresis studies should be performed in chronic cases to exclude IgA paraproteinemia

Treatment

- **Usually self-limited illness that requires no therapy**
- Treatment with glucocorticoids needed only in cases of advancing glomerulonephritis or mesenteric ischemia

Hypersensitivity Vasculitis

Basic Information

- A hypersensitivity response to exogenous antigen
- Postcapillary venules affected

Clinical Presentation

- **Typical patient presents with palpable purpura on shins and buttocks (dependent regions)**
- An array of skin lesions may be seen but are not distinctive for hypersensitivity vasculitis
  - Nonpalpable purpura
  - Palpable purpura (Fig. 45-6)
  - Livedo reticularis
  - Urticaria

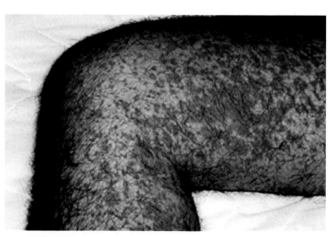

FIGURE 45-6 Palpable purpura in hypersensitivity vasculitis.

- Erythematous papules or plaques
- Vesiculobullous lesions
- Nodules
- Ulceration
- Necrotic lesions
- **Vasculitic lesions occur in "crops" (i.e., lesions of approximately same age, corresponding to time of exposure to inciting antigen)**
- Hypersensitivity vasculitis usually starts 7 to 14 days after exposure to the offending agent
- In the case of drug-induced hypersensitivity vasculitis, no new lesions appear after roughly 3 weeks after removal of the offending agent

Diagnosis and Evaluation

- High index of clinical suspicion necessary
- Impossible to distinguish skin lesions from those of HSP without immunofluorescence testing of biopsy specimens, confirming IgA deposition in HSP
- Important to exclude underlying systemic involvement (e.g., pulmonary, renal, peripheral nerve)

Treatment

- Colchicine or dapsone may be tried for milder cases
- Systemic glucocorticoids
- Leg elevation helpful

Microscopic Polyangiitis

Basic Information

- Small- and medium-sized arteries and veins affected (distinct from polyarteritis nodosa, which involves only medium-sized arteries)

Clinical Presentation

- **Typical patient presents with pulmonary renal syndrome**
  - **Alveolar hemorrhage caused by pulmonary capillary alveolitis, and**
  - **Rapidly progressive glomerulonephritis caused by necrotizing, crescentic renal lesion**
- More common than Goodpasture's syndrome as cause of pulmonary renal syndrome

- Typical symptoms and signs
  - Glomerulonephritis
  - Weight loss
  - Mononeuritis multiplex
  - Fever
  - Pulmonary hemorrhage

Diagnosis and Evaluation

- **May mimic Wegener's granulomatosis clinically, but no granulomatous inflammation evident on pathology**
- Associated with ANCA in most cases (70%), usually directed against myeloperoxidase (MPO) that on immunofluorescence staining demonstrates a P-ANCA (perinuclear) pattern (Table 45-2)

Treatment

- Glucocorticoids and cyclophosphamide
- It is appropriate to use cyclophosphamide from the outset of treatment in microscopic polyangiitis

Polyarteritis Nodosa

Basic Information

- Medium-sized muscular arteries affected (veins spared)
- **The classic medium-vessel vasculitis**
- May be found in patients chronically infected with hepatitis B

Clinical Presentation

- **Typical patient presents with subacute onset of multisystem inflammatory illness**
- Typical symptoms and signs
  - Constitutional symptoms
  - Livedo reticularis
  - Cutaneous nodules or ulcers, particularly over distal lower extremities
  - Intestinal angina (abdominal pain after eating)
  - Mononeuritis multiplex
  - Hypertension
  - Congestive heart failure
  - Elevated hepatic transaminases
  - Aneurysms of involved blood vessels (Fig. 45-7)
  - Classic polyarteritis nodosa (PAN) spares the lung

TABLE 45-2 *Correlation Between Immunofluorescence and Enzyme Immunoassay in Patients with ANCA-associated Vasculitis*

Immunofluorescence Pattern	Enzyme Immunoassay	Disease Association
C-ANCA	Anti-proteinase 3 (90%*)	Wegener's granulomatosis
P-ANCA	Anti-myeloperoxidase (90%†)	Wegener's granulomatosis Microscopic polyangiitis Churg-Strauss syndrome Renal-limited vasculitis

*90% of vasculitis patients who are C-ANCA-positive have antibodies to proteinase-3.
†90% of vasculitis patients who are P-ANCA-positive have antibodies to myeloperoxidase.
C-ANCA, cytoplasmic antineutrophil cytoplasmic antibody; P-ANCA, protoplasmic antineutrophil cytoplasmic antibody.

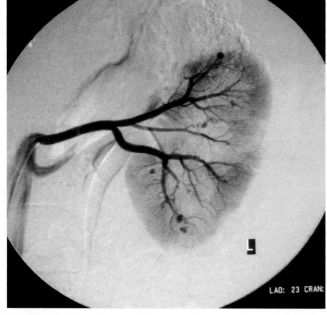

FIGURE 45-7 Angiogram demonstrating renal microaneurysms in polyarteritis nodosa.

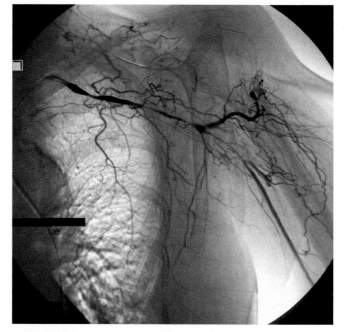

FIGURE 45-8 Angiogram demonstrating subclavian artery narrowing in Takayasu's arteritis.

Diagnosis and Evaluation

- **Biopsy of affected organ or tissue**
- Blind tissue biopsy rarely useful
- **Mesenteric angiogram may reveal aneurysms even without GI symptoms**
- Classic PAN is ANCA-negative (i.e., PR-3 and MPO-ANCA assays are negative in this disease)

Treatment

- Glucocorticoids
- Cyclophosphamide

Takayasu's Arteritis

Basic Information

- Involves large arteries, including the aorta and branches of the aortic arch (Fig. 45-8)

Clinical Presentation

- **Typical patient is a young (<40 years old) woman**
- Typical symptoms and signs:
  - Nonspecific complaints in the prepulseless (inflammatory) stage
  - Symptoms and signs of extremity or organ ischemia, although loss of digit or limb very rare
    - Postural dizziness
    - Visual disturbance
    - Claudication
    - Intrascapular back pain
    - Absence of distal pulses in one or more extremities (arms more often than legs)
    - Asymmetrical (or undetectable) blood pressures
      - **Because of subclavian artery involvement, at times the only way to measure blood pressure accurately is during aortic catheterization**

- **Hypertension (usually caused by renal artery stenosis)**
- Bruits
  - Subclavian arteries nearly always involved
  - **Auscultate for bruits above and below clavicle**
- Erythema nodosum-like lesions (20% of cases)

Diagnosis and Evaluation

- **Angiography reveals stenoses that are long, smooth, and concentrically tapered (in contrast to short, irregular, and eccentric vascular narrowing caused by atherosclerotic disease)**
  - Involves thoracic aorta more than abdominal aorta (10–15% of cases affect the latter)
  - Exuberant collateral circulation in extremities is characteristic, often making mechanical revascularization attempts (stents, balloon dilatation, bypass) unnecessary
- Magnetic resonance angiography is potentially useful in gauging disease activity through demonstration of thickening of aorta and its branches, and through perivascular edema; the full application of this technique to large-vessel vasculitis, however, remains incompletely understood

Treatment

- Glucocorticoids, if there is evidence of active inflammation

Wegener's Granulomatosis

Basic Information

- Small- to medium-sized arteries, veins, and capillaries affected

Clinical Presentation

- **Typical patient is middle-aged individual with long-standing upper respiratory tract or ear complaints (often lasting months or years), who develops symptoms and signs of a systemic inflammatory illness**
- Typical symptoms and signs
  - Skin: Palpable purpura and nodules (often over elbows); nodules are identical to the Churg-Strauss granulomas
  - Eye: Episcleritis, scleritis, peripheral ulcerative keratitis, uveitis, and orbital pseudotumor
  - Ear: Conductive hearing loss caused by serous otitis media or granulomatous inflammation in middle ear; less commonly, sensorineural hearing loss
  - **Nose: Septal perforation and saddle nose deformity (Fig. 45-9)**
  - Trachea: Subglottic stenosis
  - **Lungs: Nodular lesions (with a tendency to cavitate) and pulmonary hemorrhage (Fig. 45-10)**
  - Cardiac: Pericarditis (rare)
  - Kidney: Segmental, necrotizing crescentic glomerulonephritis; the glomerulonephritis that occurs in ANCA-associated vasculitis (Wegener's granulomatosis, microscopic polyangiitis, and the Churg-Strauss syndrome) is pauci-immune (i.e., characterized by the deposition of few immunoreactants—IgG, IgM, C3, and so on—within the kidney)
  - CNS: Chronic meningitis and cranial nerve lesions
  - Peripheral nerve: Mononeuritis multiplex
  - Extremities: Arthralgias or myalgias and frank arthritis (often rheumatoid factor-positive)

Diagnosis and Evaluation

- Diagnosis based on three histopathologic hallmarks
  - Granulomatous inflammation
  - "Geographic" (extensive) necrosis
  - Vasculitis
- **Majority of cases associated with C-ANCA pattern on immunofluorescence staining (see Table 45-2), usually caused by antibodies to PR-3**
  - The sera of 10% to 15% of patients with Wegener's granulomatosis, however, may demonstrate P-ANCA pattern, typically caused by antibodies to MPO
  - PR-3 and MPO-ANCA never both occur in the same patient
  - Despite rigorous testing, 10% of patients with severe Wegener's granulomatosis and 20% of those with limited disease may be ANCA-negative

Treatment

- Limited disease: Systemic glucocorticoids and methotrexate
- Severe (organ- or life-threatening) disease: Systemic glucocorticoids and (daily) cyclophosphamide
- **Disease appears to accelerate when serum creatinine begins to rise; detection of renal involvement signals medical emergency that must be treated swiftly**
- ANCA serologies useful in making the diagnosis, but serial testing of ANCA titers not useful in predicting disease flares
- Reflecting dramatic improvements in treatment, there is now 90% survival at 5 years

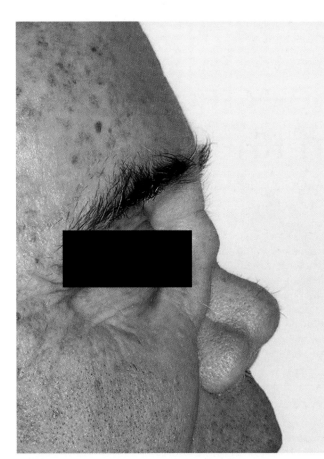

FIGURE 45-9 Saddle nose deformity in Wegener's granulomatosis.

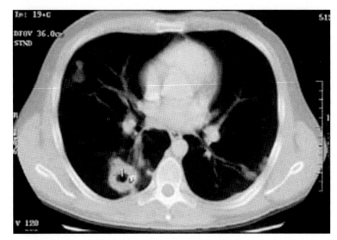

FIGURE 45-10 CT demonstrating nodular and cavitary pulmonary lesions in Wegener's granulomatosis.

SUGGESTED READINGS

Sakane T, Takeno M, Suzuki N, Inaba G: Behçet's disease, *N Engl J Med* 341:1284–1291, 1999.

Seo P, Stone JH: ANCA-associated vasculitis, *Am J Med* 117:39–50, 2004.

Seo P, Stone JH: Large-vessel vasculitis, *Arthritis Care Res* 51:128–139, 2004.

Seo P, Stone JH: Small-vessel and medium-vessel vasculitis, *Arthritis Care Res* 57:1552–1559, 2007.

Stone JH, Calabrese LH, Hoffman GS, et al: Vasculitis: pearls and myths, *Rheum Dis Clin North Am* 27:677–728, 2001.

Stone JH, Nousari HC: "Essential" cutaneous vasculitis: what every rheumatologist should know about vasculitis of the skin, *Curr Opin Rheumatol* 13:23–34, 2001.

45

Selected Topics in Rheumatology

CAROL M. ZIMINSKI, MD

Clinical presentation is the key element in the diagnosis of rheumatic diseases. The diagnosis of a specific disorder is suggested by a particular constellation of what may individually be nonspecific signs and symptoms. The diagnosis is then confirmed by obtaining a detailed history, physical examination, and appropriate laboratory and imaging studies.

Systemic Lupus Erythematosus

Basic Information

- **Systemic lupus erythematosus (SLE) is the prototypical autoimmune disease, in which the production of autoantibodies is associated with a multisystem inflammatory process**
- Epidemiology and risk factors
  - Incidence greatest from ages 18 to 45 years
  - Female-to-male ratio is 9:1
  - Four times more prevalent in African-American women than in white women
  - Regulation of the clearance of immune complexes is a common feature of many associated genes
    - Human leukocyte antigen (HLA) associations: DR2 and DR3
    - Congenital deficiency of complement components: C1, C2, and C4
- Pathogenesis
  - **Cardinal feature is the production of autoantibodies directed against nuclear, cytoplasmic, and cell-surface antigens**
  - Process is antigen-driven and T cell-dependent
  - Antigens to which patients with SLE respond are packaged in "blebs" on the cell surface during the process of apoptosis (programmed cell death)
  - Mechanisms of tissue injury involve both immune complex deposition and cell-specific antibodies
    - Most commonly identified immune complex is double-stranded DNA (dsDNA)–anti-dsDNA that can form in the circulation and deposit in the kidney, or form in situ
    - Cell-specific antibodies do not usually destroy cells directly but mark cells for premature destruction by the reticuloendothelial system (e.g., hemolytic anemia, leukopenia, and thrombocytopenia)
  - A recent study from the Department of Defense found that 115 of 130 patients with SLE had at least one

autoantibody present before diagnosis (mean, 3.3 years). In 78%, antinuclear antibodies (ANAs) were present in a titer of greater than or equal to 1 to 120. Anti-dsDNA was found in 58%.
  - Implication of these data is that **SLE is the culmination of compound and complex autoimmune abnormalities that may begin simply, then spread and multiply until manifesting as clinical disease**

Clinical Presentation

- Cutaneous lupus
  - Common presenting feature
  - **Rash occurs at some time in 90% of cases of SLE**
  - Most rashes are photosensitive
  - Types
    - Malar "butterfly" rash (nonscarring) over cheeks and bridge of nose (Fig. 46-1)
    - Discoid lesions (often scarring) are deeper, but rarely (around 5%) evolve to systemic lupus (Fig. 46-2)
    - Subacute cutaneous lupus (nonscarring) presents with annular, polycyclic lesions (Fig. 46-3); occasional arthritis and serositis; but no CNS or renal disease
    - Bullous lupus (blistering rash) is rare
- Lupus arthritis
  - Episodic and migratory
  - Distribution often symmetrical, similar to rheumatoid arthritis
  - **Rarely erosive or destructive**
  - Jaccoud's arthropathy characterized by reversible, nonerosive, "swan-neck" deformities
- Lupus nephritis
  - Occurs in one-half to two-thirds of SLE patients
  - More common in African Americans
  - Associated with antibodies to native dsDNA
  - Diffuse proliferative glomerulonephritis is the most serious form and can lead to rapidly progressive renal failure
- Drug-induced lupus (Box 46-1)
- Age effect
  - "Young" SLE manifests with more adenopathy; splenomegaly; and cutaneous, CNS, and renal disease
  - 10% of SLE patients have an onset at 50 years of age or older. Their disease is milder, with more serositis and pulmonary manifestations, but it rarely is associated with CNS and renal disease.

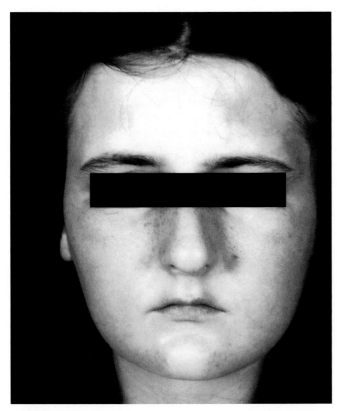

FIGURE 46-1 Malar "butterfly" rash demonstrating the typical distribution over the bridge of the nose and cheeks, sparing the nasolabial folds. (Courtesy of Carol M. Ziminski, MD.)

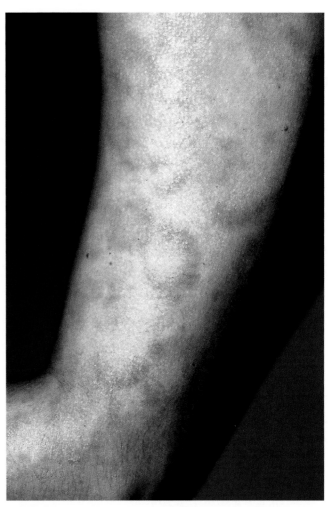

FIGURE 46-3 Subacute cutaneous lupus. The annular polycyclic lesions have an erythematous, slightly scaling border with central clearing. The distribution in light-exposed areas suggests photosensitivity. (Courtesy of Carol M. Ziminski, MD.)

46

BOX 46-1	*Drug-Induced Lupus*

Many drug associations (e.g., hydralazine, procainamide, sulfonamides, and INH)

Primarily older patients

No CNS or renal disease

ANA (antihistone) (+); antinative DNA (−)

Clinical features improve after discontinuing drug, though ANA may persist for years

ANA, antinuclear antibody; INH, isoniazid.

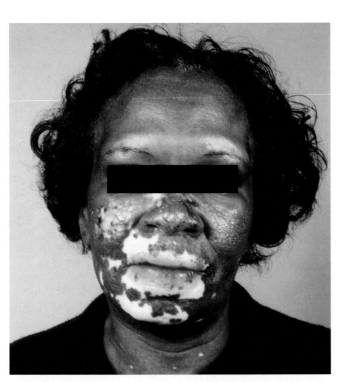

FIGURE 46-2 Discoid lupus lesions typically occur over exposed areas, such as the face or scalp. This patient demonstrates characteristic features including telangiectasias, erythema, follicular plugging, atrophy, and postinflammatory hypo- and hyperpigmentation. (Courtesy of Carol M. Ziminski, MD.)

Diagnosis and Evaluation

- SLE often suggested based on initial presentation with fever, rash, and polyarthritis
- **Diagnosis clinical but aided by the American College of Rheumatology SLE criteria (Table 46-1)**
- These criteria date from 1982 and are currently undergoing reevaluation and reassessment
- Serology (Table 46-2)

TABLE 46-1	*Criteria for the Classification of Systemic Lupus Erythematosus*
1. Malar rash	
2. Discoid rash	
3. Photosensitivity	
4. Oral ulcers	
5. Arthritis	
6. Serositis	Pleuritis *or* Pericarditis
7. Renal disorder	Persistent proteinuria > 0.5 g/day or >3+ if no quantitation *or* Cellular casts—RBC, hemoglobin, granular, tubular, or mixed
8. Neurologic disorder	Seizures *or* Psychosis—in absence of offending drugs or known metabolic derangements (e.g., uremia, ketoacidosis, or electrolyte imbalance)
9. Hematologic disorder	Hemolytic anemia—with reticulocytosis *or* Leukopenia: <4000/mm^3 on two or more occasions *or* Lymphopenia: <1500/mm^3 on two or more occasions *or* Thrombocytopenia: <100,000/mm^3, absent offending drugs
10. Immunologic disorder	Positive LE cell preparation *or* Anti-DNA: to native (double-stranded) DNA *or* Anti-Sm: Presence of antibody to Smith nuclear antigen *or* False-positive serologic test for syphilis known to be positive for at least 6 months and confirmed by *Treponema pallidum* immobilization or fluorescent treponemal antibody absorption test
11. Antinuclear antibody	Abnormal titer of antinuclear antibody by immunofluorescence or an equivalent assay at any point in time, and in the absence of drugs known to be associated with the "drug-induced lupus" syndrome

Presence of at least 4 of 11 criteria is sensitive and specific for diagnosis of SLE.
Patients may not achieve four criteria until several years into course of disease.
Criteria developed for enrollment of patients in research studies; therefore should not be adhered to rigorously for diagnosis in the individual patient.
From Tan EM, Cohen AS, Fries JF, et al: The 1982 revised criteria for the classification of systemic lupus erythematosus (SLE), *Arthritis Rheum* 25:1271, 1982.

Treatment

- Rationale for treatment
  - Survival 85% to 90% at 10 years and 68% at 20 years, with treatment
  - 50% have relapsing-remitting course
  - Poor prognostic signs: Poverty, advanced age, male gender, and increased creatinine at onset
  - Bimodal mortality curve
    - **Early deaths caused by active disease (renal and CNS) or infection**
    - **Late deaths caused by accelerated coronary artery disease;** imaging techniques to measure carotid intimal-medial thickness and coronary artery calcification have shown coronary artery calcification and carotid plaques in women with SLE, presumably the result of both disease and side effects of corticosteroid therapy
- Principles
  - **Treat the disease, not the serologic activity**
  - Use the lowest effective dose of steroids or immunosuppressives for the shortest time necessary
  - Minimize morbidity/mortality of SLE and its therapy by reducing risk factors or treating hypertension, hyperlipidemia, coronary artery disease, osteoporosis, and osteonecrosis
  - In all patients with SLE, traditional cardiovascular risk factors (high blood pressure, hyperlipidemia, elevated fasting blood glucose levels, cigarette smoking, obesity, lack of exercise) should be addressed
- Pharmacotherapy
  - Cutaneous manifestations: Sunscreen, topical steroids, and hydroxychloroquine
  - Arthritis: NSAIDs, hydroxychloroquine, and low-dose steroids
  - Fever and serositis: NSAIDs and low-dose steroids
  - Major organ system involvement (e.g., hematologic, myopathy, renal, and CNS): High-dose steroids and immunosuppressives (mycophenolate mofetil, cyclophosphamide)
- Infections
  - Prednisone (>20 mg/day) and other immunosuppressives increase risk for fatal infections
  - **50% of fatal infections involve opportunistic organisms (e.g., *Pneumocystis jiroveci* and *Candida*)**

Antiphospholipid Syndrome

Basic Information

- Antiphospholipid syndrome (APS) results from the long-term persistence of serum antiphospholipid antibodies, a **family of autoantibodies that may be seen in patients who have a hypercoagulable state marked by arterial or venous thromboses, recurrent pregnancy loss, or thrombocytopenia**
- Interference with coagulation in vitro contrasts with the thrombogenic effect in vivo
- **50% of cases of APS are seen in patients who have no associated diseases ("primary"). Most other cases are seen in patients with SLE ("secondary").**
- Antibodies may be produced transiently after infections (e.g., HIV) or following exposure to certain drugs (e.g., chlorpromazine and procainamide)

TABLE 46-2	*Serology in the Rheumatic Diseases*	
Autoantibody	**Disease Association**	**Comment**
ANA	SLE Polymyositis/dermatomyositis Scleroderma CREST syndrome Sjögren's syndrome Mixed connective tissue disease	Antibody to multiple nuclear antigens (see below) Immunofluorescence: Multiple patterns (see below) (+) in 95–99% of SLE (+) in 10–20% of healthy young women
Antihistone	SLE Drug-induced lupus	Antibody to DNA/protein complex Immunofluorescence: Homogeneous
Antinative DNA	SLE	Antibody to double-stranded DNA Immunofluorescence: Rim (+) in 70% of SLE More specific for SLE than ANA, but less sensitive Associated with renal disease
Anti-Smith (Sm)	SLE	Antibody to nuclear ribonucleoprotein Immunofluorescence: Speckled (+) in 20–30% of SLE More specific for SLE than ANA, but less sensitive
Anti-RNP	SLE Mixed connective tissue disease	Antibody to nuclear ribonucleoprotein Immunofluorescence: Speckled

Anti-Ro/La	SLE
	Subacute cutaneous lupus
	Neonatal lupus
	Sjögren's syndrome
		Antibody to nuclear ribonucleoprotein
		Immunofluorescence: Speckled
		Associated with
		  Photosensitivity
		  Congenital heart block

Anti-Scl 70	Diffuse scleroderma	Antibody to DNA topoisomerase I Immunofluorescence: Nucleolar (+) in 40% of patients with scleroderma
Anticentromere	CREST syndrome	Antibody to centromere/kinetochore Immunofluorescence: Centromere (+) in >50% of patients with CREST
Anti-PM-Scl	Polymyositis/scleroderma overlap	Antibody to nuclear protein Immunofluorescence: Nuclear or nucleolar
Anti-Jo-1	Polymyositis Dermatomyositis	Antibody to histidyl-tRNA synthetase Immunofluorescence: Diffuse Associated with interstitial lung disease
Anti-SRP	Polymyositis	Antibody to signal recognition particle (cytoplasmic ribonucleoprotein) Associated with resistance to therapy
Anti-Mi-2	Dermatomyositis	Antibody to nuclear protein Immunofluorescence: Homogeneous Associated with V (anterior neck/upper chest rash) and "shawl" (posterior neck/shoulder rash) signs

ANA, antinuclear antibody; CREST, calcinosis, Raynaud's syndrome, esophageal dysmotility, sclerodactyly, telangiectasia; SLE, systemic lupus erythematosus.

Clinical Presentation

- Cutaneous: Livedo reticularis (see Fig. 66-37), splinter hemorrhages, leg ulcers, and gangrene
- Hematologic: Thrombocytopenia and hemolytic anemia (especially with anticardiolipin immunoglobulin [Ig]M)
- Venous thrombosis: Superficial or deep venous thrombophlebitis, retinal vein thrombosis, cerebral venous thrombosis, Budd-Chiari syndrome, and pulmonary hypertension
- Neurologic: Transient ischemic attacks, ischemic cerebral infarction, chorea, and transverse myelitis
- Gynecologic: Recurrent pregnancy loss (antiphospholipid antibodies found in up to 10% of women with three or more consecutive pregnancy losses)

Diagnosis and Evaluation

- **Patients may have antiphospholipid antibodies but not develop the thrombotic manifestations required for the diagnosis of the APS**
- Diagnosis is based on the presence of at least one of the following autoantibody types:
  - Biologic false-positive serologic test for syphilis
  - Lupus anticoagulant
    - IgM or IgG that prolongs phospholipid-dependent coagulation in vitro by binding to the prothrombin activator complex, impairing conversion of prothrombin to thrombin
    - Assayed by phospholipid-dependent coagulation tests (e.g., activated partial thromboplastin time and Russell viper venom time)

- Anticardiolipin antibodies (ACA)
  - Directed against the complex of phospholipid and β_2-glycoproteins
  - High-titer ACA IgG is most strongly associated with thrombosis and pregnancy loss
  - Low titers are found in up to 5% of healthy young women
  - Autoantibodies cannot be assayed in patients taking heparin or warfarin

Treatment

- Directed by clinical features
- Serologic abnormalities alone
  - **No treatment, although some advocate low-dose aspirin prophylaxis**
- Patients who have had a thrombotic event
  - Heparin, then warfarin with target internationalized ratio of 3 to 4
  - Some suggest the addition of low-dose aspirin to warfarin for those who have had an arterial event
  - Steroids, rather than anticoagulation, with thrombocytopenia (e.g., platelets < 50,000/mm³)
  - Warfarin is not used during pregnancy because of potential teratogenicity
  - Prednisone and aspirin, or subcutaneous heparin and aspirin, have been used successfully in pregnancy with APS

Scleroderma and Systemic Sclerosis

Basic Information

- **A multisystem autoimmune disease characterized by vasculopathy, excessive collagen deposition, and tissue fibrosis**
- Epidemiology
  - Usual onset in 20s or 30s
  - Female-to-male ratio is between 3:1 and 4:1
  - More common in African Americans than whites

Clinical Presentation

- Raynaud's phenomenon (Fig. 46-4)
  - One of earliest clinical manifestations
  - Classic phases: White (ischemic), leads to blue (cyanotic), leads to red (hyperemic)
  - Primary Raynaud's phenomenon
    - Occurs in the absence of another rheumatic disease
    - Benign and common
    - Onset: 14 to 35 years
    - Affects 5% to 10% of young women
  - Secondary Raynaud's phenomenon
    - Occurs in the setting of another rheumatic disease (e.g., scleroderma or SLE)
    - Should be considered if
      - Onset in childhood or after age 35 years
      - Patient is male
      - Abnormal nail-fold capillary loops are present (Fig. 46-5)
      - Episodes cause digital tip ulceration or gangrene
      - Patient has symptoms and signs of another disease
- Organ system manifestations (Table 46-3)

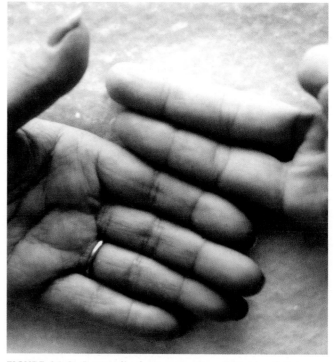

FIGURE 46-4 Raynaud's phenomenon manifested by digital cyanosis in a patient with scleroderma. (Courtesy of Carol M. Ziminski, MD.)

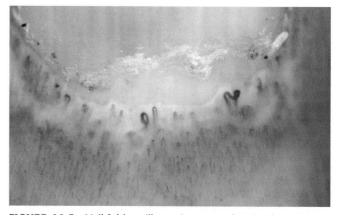

FIGURE 46-5 Nail-fold capillary microscopy showing busy capillaries. (From Habif TB: *Clinical dermatology: a color guide to diagnosis and therapy*, ed 4, St. Louis, Mosby, 2004, figure 17-24.)

Diagnosis and Evaluation

- **Skin changes suggest the diagnosis, but internal organ involvement determines survival**
- Clinical subsets
  - Limited scleroderma (CREST syndrome)
    - **C**alcinosis
    - **R**aynaud's phenomenon
    - **E**sophageal dysmotility
    - **S**clerodactyly (Fig. 46-6)
    - **T**elangiectasia

TABLE 46-3	*Organ System Manifestations in Scleroderma*			
Cutaneous	**Gastrointestinal**	**Pulmonary**	**Renal**	**Cardiac**

Early
  Edematous phase
    (scleredema) may
    last several months
Subsequent
  Induration
    and skin tightening
    may last several years
Late
  Atrophic changes
  Also telangiectasias,
    calcification, and
    pruritis
	Esophageal dysmotility,
	  with reflux
	Gastroparesis, with
	  early satiety
	Small-bowel involvement,
	  with pseudo-obstruction
	Colonic involvement, with
	  wide-mouthed diverticulae
		Interstitial
		  pneumonitis with
		  bibasilar interstitial
		  infiltrates
		Pulmonary
		  hypertension
		May manifest as
		  cough or dyspnea
			Renal crisis presents with
			  malignant hypertension
			  and rapidly progressive
			  renal failure
			Biopsy reveals transmural
			  microangiopathy (not
			  vasculitis) with intimal
			  proliferation, medial
			  hypertrophy, and
			  adventitial fibrosis
				Cardiomyopathy with
				  contraction band
				  necrosis or myocardial
				  fibrosis
				Pericarditis

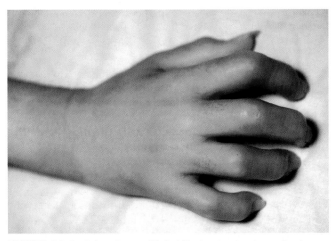

FIGURE 46-6 Scleroderma. Digital flexion contractures due to thickened, indurated skin (sclerodactyly). (Courtesy of Carol M. Ziminski, MD.)

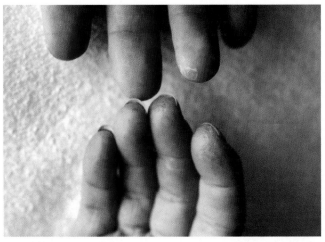

FIGURE 46-7 Scleroderma. Pitting scars on the pulps of the index and middle fingers due to microvascular disease. (Courtesy of Carol M. Ziminski, MD.)

46

- Diffuse scleroderma (progressive systemic sclerosis [PSS])
  - Scleroderma involving not only the fingers but also the dorsum of the hand proximal to the metacarpophalangeal joints or on forearms, legs, face, and trunk, or
  - Sclerodactyly associated with either digital pulp pitting (Fig. 46-7) or basilar pulmonary fibrosis
  - Localized scleroderma: Morphea and linear scleroderma
- The presence of a tendon friction rub is highly specific (although not sensitive) for the diagnosis of scleroderma
- **Autoantibodies are found in most affected patients: ANA (+) in up to 98% of patients (see Table 46-2)**
- Bronchoalveolar lavage may identify patients with active inflammatory pulmonary disease, who may benefit from immunosuppressive agents

Treatment

- **There is no cure for scleroderma, but many of its problems and complications can be treated (Table 46-4)**
- In the future, therapy may focus on inhibiting the release of cytokines that induce fibrosis
- Many of the major advances in management today are directed toward preventing damage to endothelial cells

TABLE 46-4	*Management of Scleroderma*
Manifestation	**Intervention**
Raynaud's phenomenon	Cold avoidance Calcium channel blockers
Digital ulcers	IV iloprost (prostaglandin analogue)
Interstitial pneumonitis	Steroids Cytotoxic agents (e.g., cyclophosphamide)
Gastroesophageal reflux	Proton-pump inhibitors
GI immotility	Prokinetic agents (e.g., metoclopramide)

GI bacterial
  overgrowth/
  malabsorption
	Broad-spectrum antibiotics

Renal crisis	ACE inhibitor

ACE, angiotensin-converting enzyme.

- **There is no role for systemic steroids except in pneumonitis or myositis**
- Poor prognostic factors
  - Older age
  - Male gender

- African-American race
- Diffuse scleroderma
- Early visceral involvement

Polymyositis and Dermatomyositis

Basic Information

- **Immune-mediated inflammatory myopathy affecting striated muscle and resulting in symmetrical proximal (i.e., shoulder and pelvic girdle) weakness**
- Incidence 1 in 100,000
- Bimodal distribution of incidence: Ages 10 to 15 years and 45 to 60 years
- Female-to-male ratio is 2:1

Clinical Presentation

- Muscle manifestations
  - **Weakness is pathognomonic**
    - **Proximal and symmetrical**
    - May also affect the neck, pharyngeal, respiratory, and trunk muscles, but spares the facial muscles
  - Dysphagia may occur (due to involvement of striated pharyngeal muscle)
  - Muscle pain (25% of cases)
- Cutaneous manifestations
  - **Heliotrope rash: Periorbital edema with violaceous discoloration of eyelids**
  - Erythematous, sometimes scaling rash may occur over face, upper chest (V sign), and upper back ("shawl" sign)
  - **Gottron's papules: Erythematous or violaceous scaling papules over knuckles** (Fig. 46-8)
  - Mechanic's hand: Scaling skin over palms, with "dirty" discoloration of creases
  - Calcinosis (especially in children)
  - Vasculitis
- Pulmonary involvement with interstitial lung disease occurs in 30% to 50% of patients
- Clinical patterns
  - Polymyositis (PM)
  - Dermatomyositis (DM)
  - Juvenile dermatomyositis
  - Myositis associated with another rheumatic disease
  - Myositis associated with malignancy

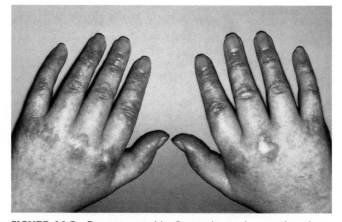

FIGURE 46-8 Dermatomyositis. Gottron's papules manifested by a rash accentuated over interphalangeal joints, with variable manifestations including erythematous or violaceous induration, papules, or nodules. (Courtesy of Carol M. Ziminski, MD.)

Diagnosis and Evaluation

- **Clinical suspicion based on presentation with symmetrical proximal muscle weakness**
- Elevated muscle enzymes
  - **Creatine phosphokinase (CPK) is the most specific and sensitive for muscle injury**
  - Aldolase, aspartate aminotransferase, alanine aminotransferase, and lactate dehydrogenase may also reflect muscle inflammation
- Autoantibodies may allow better definition of subsets but may not be widely available (see Table 46-2)
  - Tests are positive for ANAs in 20% to 30% of patients with PM, more frequently in patients who have myositis in the setting of other rheumatic diseases
  - Approximately 30% of patients have antibodies directed against cytoplasmic ribonucleoproteins; found only in myositis and are known as myositis-specific antibodies
  - Antigens define three subgroups of patients that differ in clinical features and prognosis (Table 46-5)
- Complement system
  - PM: No evidence of complement activation
  - DM: Vascular deposition of complement membrane attack complex

TABLE 46-5	Syndromes Associated with Myositis-Specific Autoantibodies	
Autoantibody	**Clinical Features**	**Prognosis**
Aminoacyl-tRNA synthetases (anti-Jo-1, PL-7, and others)	Acute onset Interstitial lung disease Arthritis Hyperkeratotic rash ("mechanic's hands") HLA-DR3, -DR52	Variable Significant mortality
Signal recognition peptide	Hyperacute onset Cardiac involvement Onset in autumn More prevalent in black women	Poor 5-year mortality rate 75%
Components of histone acetylase complexes (MI2)	Dermatomyositis Shawl sign of rash Cuticular overgrowth	Good

HLA, human leukocyte antigen.

- Electromyography (EMG) reveals inflammatory myopathy with short duration, low-amplitude and polyphasic potentials, and irritative features
- Muscle biopsy may confirm the diagnosis
  - Negative in up to 30% of cases, but abnormal EMG supports diagnosis of myositis in appropriate clinical setting
  - PM: Inflammatory cell infiltrate found between muscle fibers, with varying stages of muscle fiber necrosis and regeneration, but vessels spared
  - DM: Inflammatory cells surround the small endomysial vessels
- MRI adds important dimension and is noninvasive
  - T1-weighted images provide excellent anatomic detail, useful in assessing changes resulting from damage and chronicity
  - T2-weighted images with fat suppression or STIR (short tau inversion recovery) sequences identify edema, which is indicative of active inflammation
- Differential diagnosis
  - Drugs: Colchicine, penicillamine, "statins," corticosteroids, and zidovudine
  - Endocrine: Hypothyroidism
  - Malignancy-associated: Perform age-appropriate cancer screening
  - Neuromuscular: Muscular dystrophies and myasthenia gravis
  - Inclusion body myositis (Box 46-2)
  - Infections
    - Viral: Coxsackie virus, influenza, and HIV
    - Parasitic: *Trichinella*
    - Protozoan: *Toxoplasma*
  - Other: Electrolyte disorders and metabolic myopathies

Treatment

- **High-dose steroids (80% response)**
- **Methotrexate and azathioprine useful as steroid-sparing agents**
- Intravenous immunoglobulin (IV Ig) is sometimes used successfully in dermatomyositis refractory to steroids because IV Ig can inhibit complement activation
- Search for and treat associated malignancy

Polymyalgia Rheumatica

Basic Information

- **Clinical syndrome marked by proximal limb girdle muscle pain and stiffness**
- May be prodrome for rheumatoid arthritis
- **May be associated with giant-cell arteritis (see Chapter 45)**
- Epidemiology
  - Rarely diagnosed at ages younger than 50 years
  - Female to male ratio is 2:1
  - Predominantly whites (especially patients of northern European descent)

Clinical Presentation

- Proximal limb girdle pain and morning stiffness in the appropriate host

---

| BOX 46-2 | *Inclusion Body Myositis* |

Basic Information

Unique subset of the inflammatory myopathies

Typical patient is a man older than 50 years

Clinical Presentation

Weakness may be both proximal and distal, and less symmetrical

Typical course is chronic, with slow progression over years, or even decades

Diagnosis and Evaluation

Consider in setting of atypical distribution of weakness

Mild elevation in creatine phosphokinase (up to 5× normal)

Muscle biopsy specimen reveals characteristic rimmed vacuoles with inclusions and occasional ragged red fibers

Treatment

Poor response to steroids

- Constitutional manifestations include fever, malaise, and weight loss

Diagnosis and Evaluation

- **Examination reveals muscle tenderness but no true muscle weakness**
- Laboratory features
  - Elevated erythrocyte sedimentation rate
  - Elevated C-reactive protein
  - Normochromic normocytic anemia
  - Elevated platelets

Treatment

- Steroids
  - Treatment of choice
  - Low-dose (10–20 mg of prednisone daily)
  - Rapid and dramatic symptomatic improvement is characteristic
  - Taper guided by symptoms
- NSAIDs may give partial relief of symptoms in mild cases

Fibromyalgia Syndrome

Basic Information

- **Chronic syndrome marked by multifocal musculoskeletal pain and fatigue, in the setting of a noninflammatory physical examination and laboratory studies**
- Epidemiology
  - May affect 2% of population
  - Peak age 30 to 50 years
  - 80% to 90% of patients are female

Clinical Presentation

- May include the following
  - Chronic, diffuse pain
  - Morning stiffness
  - Subjective swelling

- Raynaud's-like symptoms
- Sleep disturbance
- Fatigue
- Headache
- Dry mouth
- Paresthesias
- Irritable bowel syndrome
- Urinary urgency
- Dysmenorrhea
- Anxiety
- Depression

Diagnosis and Evaluation

- American College of Rheumatology definition: **Chronic widespread pain (bilateral, above and below the waist, and axial) and at least 11 of 18 specified tender points**
- Consider possible contributing events
  - Physical trauma: Physical abuse or motor vehicle accident
  - Emotional trauma: Sexual abuse
  - Infections: Hepatitis C, Lyme disease, parvovirus, and HIV

Treatment

- Goals
  - Decrease pain
  - Decrease distress
  - Improve sleep
  - Increase energy level
  - Improve function
  - Treat associated symptoms including anxiety and depression
- Methods
  - Patient education and reassurance
  - Stress reduction
  - **Aerobic conditioning exercise**
  - Pharmacologic intervention
    - **Low-dose tricyclic antidepressant (e.g., amitriptyline or nortriptyline)**
    - Cyclobenzaprine

- Anticonvulsants (e.g., pregabalin)
- Serotonin reuptake inhibitors (e.g., fluoxetine)
- Dual-receptor inhibitors inhibit serotonin and norepinephrine (e.g., venlafaxine, milnacipran)
- **Pitfalls**
  - Psychosocial issues not addressed
  - Benefit of exercise undervalued
  - Exercise program too rigorous or advanced too quickly
  - Tricyclic therapy discontinued prematurely
  - Unrealistic expectations for improvement

REVIEW QUESTIONS

For review questions, please go to www.expertconsult.com.

SUGGESTED READINGS

Burkham J, Harris ED: Fibromyalgia: a chronic pain syndrome. In Harris ED, Budd RC, Genovese MC, et al, editors: *Kelley's textbook of rheumatology*, ed 7, Philadelphia, WB Saunders, 2005, pp 522–536.

Edworthy SM: Clinical manifestations of systemic lupus erythematosus. In Harris ED, Budd RC, Genovese MC, et al, editors: *Kelley's textbook of rheumatology*, ed 7, Philadelphia, WB Saunders, 2005, pp 1201–1224.

Hahn BH: Management of systemic lupus erythematosus. In Harris ED, Budd RC, Genovese MC, et al, editors: *Kelley's textbook of rheumatology*, ed 7, Philadelphia, WB Saunders, 2005, pp 1225–1247.

Hahn BH, Karpouzas GA, Tsao BP: Pathogenesis of systemic lupus erythematosus. In Harris ED, Budd RC, Genovese MC, et al, editors: *Kelley's textbook of rheumatology*, ed 7, Philadelphia, WB Saunders, 2005, pp 1174–1200.

Hellmann DB, Hunder GG: Giant cell arteritis and polymyalgia rheumatica. In Harris ED, Budd RC, Genovese MC, et al, editors: *Kelley's textbook of rheumatology*, ed 7, Philadelphia, WB Saunders, 2005, pp 1343–1356.

Lockshin MD: Antiphospholipid antibody syndrome. In Harris ED, Budd RC, Genovese MC, et al, editors: *Kelley's textbook of rheumatology*, ed 7, Philadelphia, WB Saunders, 2005, pp 1248–1257.

Seibold JR: Scleroderma. In Harris ED, Budd RC, Genovese MC, et al, editors: *Kelley's textbook of rheumatology*, ed 7, Philadelphia, WB Saunders, 2005, pp 1279–1308.

Wortmann RL: Inflammatory diseases of muscle and other myopathies. In Harris ED, Budd RC, Genovese MC, et al, editors: *Kelley's textbook of rheumatology*, ed 7, Philadelphia, WB Saunders, 2005, pp 1309–1335.

SECTION EIGHT

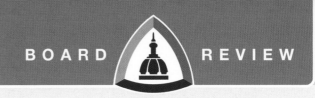

Hematology

Anemia

BIMAL H. ASHAR, MD, MBA

Anemia, a reduction in the proportion of red blood cells, is one of the most common conditions seen by internists. Although patients are often asymptomatic, the presence of anemia is indicative of an underlying disorder. From a laboratory perspective, anemia is somewhat arbitrarily defined as a hemoglobin (Hgb) concentration of less than 12 g/dL in women and less than 13 g/dL in men. This chapter provides a general framework for approaching patients with anemia in order to uncover their underlying disorders.

Overview

Basic Information

- Normal erythropoiesis (Fig. 47-1)
  - Regulated by the production of erythropoietin (EPO) in the kidney
    - EPO production increases as a result of hypoxia, as sensed by the kidney
    - EPO then stimulates RBC production by the bone marrow
- Mechanisms of anemia
  - Decreased production of RBCs (hypoproliferation)
  - Increased destruction of RBCs (hemolysis)
  - Acute blood loss (hemorrhage)

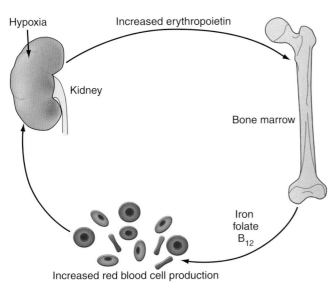

FIGURE 47-1 Regulation of red cell production. (Adapted from Hoffman R, Heidrick E, Benz E, et al: *Hematology: basic principles and practice,* ed 4, Philadelphia, Churchill Livingstone, 2005, figure 29-2.)

Clinical Presentation

- Often asymptomatic
- When symptomatic, weakness and fatigue are the most common
- Angina, congestive heart failure, dyspnea, tachycardia, and cerebral insufficiency can occur
- **Severity of symptoms is dependent on rapidity of development of anemia, degree of anemia, and the ability of the body to compensate**

Diagnosis

- Laboratory evaluation begins with a CBC
  - Hgb and hematocrit (Hct) values determine the presence of anemia
  - WBC and platelet counts should be examined to determine the presence or absence of pancytopenia
  - Mean corpuscular volume (MCV)—serves as an estimate of RBC size
  - RBC count—low in most cases of anemia but can be normal or high in some conditions (e.g., thalassemia trait)
  - Red cell distribution width (RDW)—estimates the degree of variation in red cell size
- Reticulocytes—immature RBCs
  - Correct the reticulocyte count for the degree of anemia as follows

Corrected reticulocyte count = Percent reticulocytes × (Patient's hematocrit/normal hematocrit)

  - **A corrected reticulocyte count greater than 2% suggests hemolysis or acute blood loss**
  - **A corrected reticulocyte count of less than 2% suggests a hypoproliferative process**
- Peripheral smear
  - Can help confirm the MCV and potentially identify mixed disorders (e.g., concomitant iron deficiency and folate deficiency presenting with a normal MCV)
  - Can be suggestive of specific diagnoses (see Chapter 52)
- Basic approach to anemia (Fig. 47-2)

Treatment

- Blood transfusions
  - **Not routinely indicated in asymptomatic patients**
  - Transfusion is currently recommended for patients with
    - Rapid acute blood loss
    - Cardiovascular disease and an Hgb less than 10 g/dL
    - Symptomatic patients with an Hgb between 7 and 9 g/dL
    - Stable patients with an Hgb less than 7 g/dL
  - Can cause a number of immunologic reactions (Table 47-1)

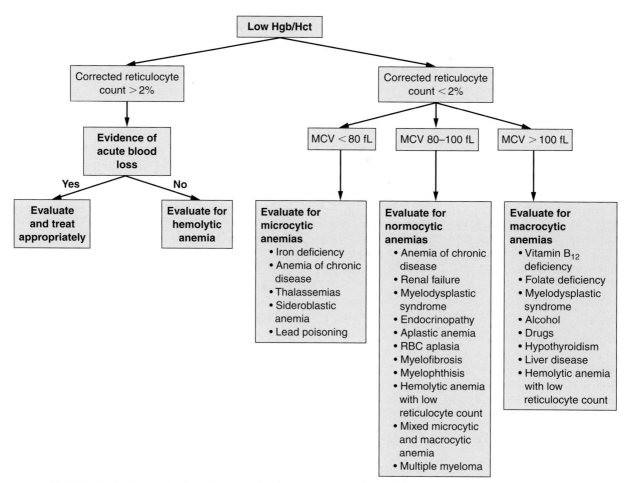

FIGURE 47-2 Basic evaluation of anemia. Hct, hematocrit; Hgb, hemoglobin; MCV, mean corpuscular volume.

- Erythropoiesis-stimulating agents (ESA)
  - Beneficial for patients with renal failure and Hgb levels less than 11 g/dL
  - Increases quality of life in some patients with anemia of chronic disease (e.g., caused by rheumatoid arthritis)
  - Controversy exists regarding risks and benefits in cancer patients
    - Recommended for symptomatic patients with anemia (Hgb $\leq$ 10 g/dL) resulting from chemotherapy for nonhematologic malignancies
    - Not routinely recommended for patients with anemia caused by a nonhematologic malignancy who are not receiving chemotherapy
  - Reduces the need for postoperative transfusion in some patients
  - May ultimately reduce transfusion requirements in critically ill patients
  - Side effects
    - Hypertension
    - Arthralgias
    - Thrombosis
    - Seizures (rare)
    - Polycythemia—if Hct not followed closely
    - Some data suggest that it can lead to greater disease progression of certain solid tumors
    - Anemia

- Iron deficiency can occur if iron levels are not monitored and repleted when necessary
- Pure RBC aplasia has been reported

Microcytic Anemia

Basic Approach

- Obtain and interpret iron studies (Table 47-2)
  - Serum iron: Not very helpful by itself because there is significant variation in values
  - Total iron-binding capacity (TIBC): Reflects the total amount of transferrin (iron transport protein) available in the blood; is a measure of aggregate iron-binding sites; elevated if iron is low
  - Transferrin saturation: Normally between 20% and 45%
  - Ferritin—correlates with total iron stores; can be normal in iron deficiency if there is concomitant inflammation; even with inflammation, level is usually less than 100 mg/L
  - Serum transferrin receptor level: Measure of tissue iron; levels typically go up in iron deficiency but do not change in anemia of chronic disease
- Look at the peripheral smear
- Consider Hgb electrophoresis if studies suggest thalassemia or other hemoglobinopathy
- Bone marrow biopsy with iron staining—gold standard if etiology unclear

TABLE 47-1	Immunologic Blood Transfusion Reactions
Reaction	**Description**
Febrile nonhemolytic	Fever ± chills 1–6 hr after start of transfusion Sometimes can be confused with acute hemolytic reactions so transfusion may need to be temporarily halted Treat with antipyretics and/or meperidine (if chills predominate)

Acute hemolytic	Caused by preformed antibodies in patient's serum that bind and lyse transfused cells
	Most cases are caused by ABO incompatibility
	Can present with fevers and chills with or without flank pain, hypotension, DIC shortly after starting the transfusion
	Management includes
	  Discontinuing the transfusion
	  Notifying the blood bank
	  Starting IV fluids
	  Obtaining blood for direct antiglobulin test, plasma free hemoglobin, coagulation times, renal function

Delayed hemolytic	Caused by an amnestic response in patients who have previously undergone transfusion and have developed low levels of alloantibodies that go undetected during crossmatch Seen 2–10 days after transfusion Direct and indirect antiglobulin tests are positive with identification of the antigen Treatment is supportive
Anaphylactic	Anaphylaxis and shock seconds to minutes after start of the transfusion Commonly caused by anti-IgA antibodies in patients who are IgA deficient Treat by stopping the transfusion, administering epinephrine, and supporting airway and blood pressure
Urticarial	Can continue transfusion after treating with diphenhydramine
Transfusion-related acute lung injury (TRALI)	Dyspnea, hypoxemia, and pulmonary infiltrates that develop within 6 hr after the end of transfusion of a blood product Can cause death in some cases but usually resolves within 96 hr with adequate supportive care (which may include intubation)
Post-transfusion purpura	Causes thrombocytopenia 5–10 days after transfusion of any blood product containing platelets Usually occurs in women Treat with IV immune globulin

DIC, disseminated intravascular coagulation; IgA, immunoglobulin A.

IRON DEFICIENCY ANEMIA

Basic Information

- Present in 2% of the population
- Etiologies
  - **Blood loss is the most common cause**
  - Decreased iron intake
  - Increased iron utilization (e.g., with EPO therapy, chronic hemolysis)
  - Atransferrinemia—rare autosomal recessive disorder

TABLE 47-2	Interpretation of Iron Studies			
	Serum Iron	**TIBC**	**Transferrin Saturation**	**Ferritin**
Iron deficiency	↓	↑	↓	↓ or N
Anemia of chronic disease	↓	N or ↓	N or ↓	N or ↑
Thalassemia trait	N	N	N	N or ↑
Sideroblastic anemia	N or ↑	N or ↑	N or ↑	N or ↑

N, normal; TIBC, total iron-binding capacity.

- Malabsorption
  - From partial gastrectomy—iron deficiency develops almost 50% of time
  - From malabsorption syndromes (e.g., celiac sprue) if the disease affects the proximal small intestine

Clinical Presentation

- Paresthesias
- Sore tongue, cheilosis
- Brittle nails or koilonychias ("spoon nails")
- Pica—desire to eat unusual substances (e.g., ice, clay, starch)

Diagnosis

- **Iron studies classically show reduced iron, increased TIBC, reduced transferrin saturation, and reduced ferritin**
- Peripheral smear should show hypochromic, microcytic cells (Fig. 47-3)
- Evaluation of iron-deficient patients
  - Search for evidence of blood loss (e.g., uterine bleeding, GI bleeding, genitourinary [GU] bleeding)
    - If there are no clinical signs or symptoms suggesting a potential cause, start with GI evaluation (esophagogastroduodenoscopy [EGD]/colonoscopy)
    - If EGD and colonoscopy are negative, small bowel capsule endoscopy may be helpful
  - Consider malabsorption if the evaluation for blood loss is negative

Treatment

- Transfusions—only if there is hemodynamic compromise or acute hemorrhage

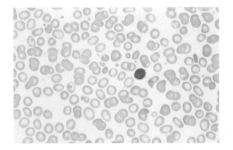

FIGURE 47-3 Iron-deficiency anemia. Hypochromic, microcytic blood cells (smaller than the lymphocyte in the center). (From Goldman L, Bennett JC, Ausiello D: *Cecil textbook of medicine,* ed 22, Philadelphia, WB Saunders, 2004, figure 167-1.)

47

- Oral iron
  - Normal dose is 50 mg elemental iron three times a day between meals
  - Vitamin C administration may improve absorption
  - Should see reticulocytosis within 7 days
  - Correction of anemia in about 6 weeks if dose is adequate
  - **If anemia does not improve, consider noncompliance or insufficient dosing, malabsorption, incorrect diagnosis, coexisting disease (e.g., anemia of chronic disease), or continued blood loss**
- Parenteral iron
  - May be indicated in refractory cases
  - Three formulations currently available for use:
    - Iron dextran (IV or IM): Easy to use because total dose can be given in one infusion, but anaphylaxis occurs in 1% of patients
    - Ferric gluconate (IV) and iron sucrose (IV): Need repeat infusions (over weeks) to deliver total dose, but side effects and risk of anaphylaxis lower

ANEMIA OF CHRONIC DISEASE

Basic Information

- **Most cases are actually normocytic, not microcytic**
- Etiologies
  - Malignancy
  - Chronic infections (e.g., osteomyelitis, tuberculosis, AIDS)
  - Chronic inflammatory disorders (e.g., rheumatoid arthritis [RA], systemic lupus erythematosus [SLE], ulcerative colitis)
  - Congestive heart failure
- Mechanisms
  - Decreased RBC survival
  - Impaired EPO production
  - Impaired marrow response to EPO
  - Impaired mobilization of iron (i.e., increased iron uptake and retention within the reticuloendothelial system)

Clinical Presentation and Diagnosis

- Iron studies (see Table 47-2)
- Peripheral smear usually shows normocytic, normochromic cells but can be microcytic in 30% to 40% of cases; **MCV is rarely less than 75 fL**
- Bone marrow biopsy may be helpful if the diagnosis is unclear; it should reveal normal or increased iron stores
- Soluble transferrin receptor (sTfR) level can help distinguish pure anemia of chronic disease from anemia of chronic disease with concomitant iron deficiency in patients with normal ferritin levels
  - If the sTfR/log ferritin index is greater than 2, iron deficiency probably coexists with anemia of chronic disease
  - If the sTfR/log ferritin index is less than 1, iron deficiency is likely not present with anemia of chronic disease

Treatment

- Treat the underlying disorder (if possible)
- Transfusion rarely indicated because anemia is usually not severe
- EPO/darbepoietin has been shown to increase quality of life and reduce the need for transfusion in some patients

with anemia of chronic disease (ACD) but is very costly and may be harmful in some cases (e.g., treatment of anemia due to certain solid tumors)

THALASSEMIA

Basic Information

- Defined as a decrease in production of one of the two globin chains
  - Normal Hgb A has 2 α and 2 β chains ($\alpha_2\beta_2$)
  - In β-thalassemia, there is partial or complete suppression of β-globin chain synthesis resulting in a relative excess of α-globin chains
  - In α-thalassemia, there is suppression or absence of α chains resulting in a relative excess of β chains
- Seen predominantly in people of African, Asian, or Mediterranean descent
- There are a number of genetic variations seen clinically
  - β-Thalassemia
    - β-Thalassemia major: Presents in the first year of life; patients are transfusion dependent
    - β-Thalassemia intermedia: Regular transfusions unnecessary until second, third, or fourth decade; can develop iron overload independently of transfusions
    - β-Thalassemia minor (β-thal trait): Causes mild anemia and significant microcytosis
  - α-Thalassemia
    - Hydrops fetalis and Hgb Barts: Usually fatal in utero
    - Hgb H: Significant anemia, hemolysis, splenomegaly are usually diagnosed in late childhood
    - α-Thalassemia trait (α-thalassemia minor): Causes mild anemia and significant microcytosis
    - Asymptomatic carrier (α-thalassemia minima): No significant anemia

Clinical Presentation and Diagnosis

- Most cases of clinically severe anemia present in childhood
- Patients with thalassemia trait are commonly asymptomatic
- Several clues may be present that can help distinguish thalassemia trait from iron-deficiency anemia (Table 47-3)
- Peripheral smear can show basophilic stippling, microcytosis, and target cells (Fig. 47-4)

TABLE 47-3	Clues to Differentiating Thalassemia Trait from Iron Deficiency Anemia	
	Thalassemia Trait	**Iron Deficiency Anemia**
RBC count	N or ↑	↓
MCV	Lower than would be expected with iron deficiency	↓
RDW	N	↑
Ferritin	N or ↑	↓
Bone marrow iron	N	↓

MCV, mean corpuscular volume; N, normal; RDW, red blood cell distribution width.

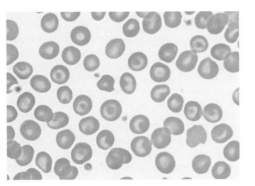

FIGURE 47-4 β-Thalassemia trait. Hypochromic, microcytic red blood cells with frequent targeting. Mild anemia. (From McPherson RA, Pincus MR: *Henry's clinical diagnosis and management by laboratory methods,* ed 21, Philadelphia, WB Saunders, 2006, figure 31-27.)

- Hgb electrophoresis can be helpful in some cases
  - Normal—Hgb A ($\alpha_2\beta_2$) 97%; Hgb A$_2$ ($\alpha_2\delta_2$) 2% to 3%; Hgb F ($\alpha_2\gamma_2$) 0% to 1%
  - **β-Thal trait: Increased Hgb A$_2$ and Hgb F**
  - α-Thal trait: Usually normal but may possibly show a decreased Hgb A$_2$ concentration

Treatment

- Thalassemia trait—none indicated
- β-Thalassemia intermedia, β-thalassemia major, and Hgb H
  - Chronic transfusion
  - Splenectomy
  - Treatment for iron overload
  - Management of complications including leg ulcers, pulmonary hypertension, gallstones, aplasia

SIDEROBLASTIC ANEMIAS

- Consist of inherited or acquired defects that result in impaired heme biosynthesis
- **Characterized by iron-positive granules surrounding the nucleus of RBCs (ringed sideroblasts) in the bone marrow**
- Hereditary sideroblastic anemia
  - Most cases are X-linked and present in childhood
  - Usually presents with a fairly stable anemia
  - **Iron overload develops in all patients because of increased absorption of iron**
  - Iron studies show an increased transferrin saturation and ferritin level
  - Genetic studies should help confirm the diagnosis
  - Anemia responds to pyridoxine in most cases
  - Need to treat iron overload with phlebotomy or chelation
- Acquired idiopathic sideroblastic anemia
  - Usually occurs in older individuals
  - Anemia is usually normocytic or macrocytic
  - Iron studies reveal overload
  - Risk of transformation to acute leukemia
  - **Considered one of the myelodysplastic syndromes** (MDS; see Chapter 51)
  - Typically does not respond to treatment with pyridoxine

- Reversible sideroblastic anemia
  - Can be caused by a number of different precipitants including alcohol, isoniazid, and chloramphenicol
  - Anemia improves with removal of the drug
- Lead poisoning
  - It is controversial whether it truly causes sideroblastic changes
  - Some causes include ingestion of lead-based paint, ingestion of contaminated dietary supplements, consumption of moonshine from lead-lined stills, and inhalation of fumes
  - **Clinical manifestations include microcytic anemia, autonomic and motor neuropathy, and abdominal pain**
  - Diagnosed by finding elevated blood lead levels
  - Treat with EDTA chelation

Normocytic (Nonhemolytic) Anemia

- Basic approach
  - Can result from a number of different processes (see Fig. 47-2)
  - Clues to the diagnosis may be present in the history, physical, and other laboratory tests
    - The presence of pancytopenia suggests a primary bone marrow disorder
    - An elevated creatinine level suggests the possibility of anemia caused by renal insufficiency or failure
    - The presence of cancer, infection, or other inflammatory disorder suggests the presence of anemia of chronic disease

ANEMIA OF CHRONIC DISEASE

See the previous discussion of ACD in the microcytic anemia section.

ANEMIA OF RENAL INSUFFICIENCY OR FAILURE

- Usually manifests when creatinine clearance falls to below 50 mL/min
- **The primary abnormality is EPO deficiency**
- Uremia can also contribute to anemia
  - Can cause blood loss usually through the GI tract
  - Decreases RBC survival
- Folate deficiency, aluminum overload, and hyperparathyroidism (causing bone marrow fibrosis) can all potentially contribute to anemia
- Treatment
  - Standard of care is now subcutaneous or IV ESA
  - ESAs can potentially delay the progression of renal disease in patients with renal insufficiency and anemia
  - **Goal is to maintain Hct between 33% and 36% (Hgb between 11 and 12 g/dL)**
  - Iron therapy indicated for ferritin levels below 100 mg/L

APLASTIC ANEMIA

- Characterized by pancytopenia and a reticulocyte index less than 2
- Fanconi's anemia (short stature, café-au-lait spots, GU abnormalities, microphthalmia, mental retardation, and

BOX 47-1   *Causes of Aplastic Anemia*

Drugs
    Chemotherapeutic agents
    Chloramphenicol
    Gold
    Sulfonamides
    Phenylbutazone
Chemicals (e.g., benzene, insecticides)
Radiation
Viruses
    Parvovirus B19
    Non-A, non-B, non-C hepatitis
    HIV, Epstein-Barr virus, cytomegalovirus
Connective tissue disease
Paroxysmal nocturnal hemoglobinuria

skeletal abnormalities seen in association with aplastic anemia) is the most common congenital form
- Most acquired cases are idiopathic, but a number of other causes have been described (Box 47-1)
- Usually occurs between the ages of 15 and 25 years with a second peak after age 60 years
- Thought to be an autoimmune disease
- Bone marrow is hypocellular with fat replacement of bone marrow elements (Fig. 47-5)
- Cytogenetic studies may help to distinguish from hypocellular MDS (i.e., abnormalities can be seen in MDS but not in aplastic anemia)
- Treatment
  - Withdraw the offending agent (if identified)
  - Support with transfusions as needed; mild forms of disease may not need definitive treatment
  - **Bone marrow transplantation (BMT) is the treatment of choice in all patients under the age of 45 years with severe aplastic anemia when there is a human leukocyte antigen (HLA)-matched donor**
  - Antithymocyte globulin (ATG) plus cyclosporine is used when BMT not possible
- Is associated with future development of myelodysplasia and paroxysmal nocturnal hemoglobinuria in 10% to 15% of patients

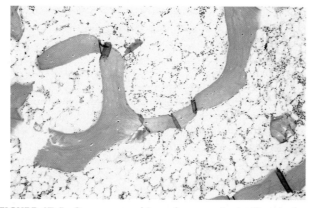

FIGURE 47-5 Bone marrow biopsy from a patient with aplastic anemia. (From Kumar V, Fausto N, Abbas A: *Robbins and Cotran's pathologic basis of disease*, ed 7, Philadelphia, WB Saunders, 2004, figure 13-27.)

PURE RED CELL APLASIA
- Characterized by selective absence of RBCs in the marrow
- Can be idiopathic or associated with a number of conditions
  - Thymoma
  - Lymphoproliferative disease (e.g., chronic lymphocytic leukemia [CLL], large granular lymphoma [LGL], chronic myelogenous leukemia [CML])
  - Collagen vascular disease
  - Drugs (similar to aplastic anemia)
  - EPO
    - Can induce antibodies to EPO, resulting in anemia
      - Most cases have been seen with subcutaneous administration from a formulation not sold in the United States, although cases in the United States have been reported
  - Parvovirus B19
    - Usually a transient process in normal hosts
    - Can cause severe transient aplastic crisis in patients with underlying hemolytic disorders
    - Can cause chronic aplasia in immunodeficient patients
- CBC reveals anemia with normal WBC and platelets
- Bone marrow reveals few or absent erythroid precursors
- **CT scan should be ordered to look for thymoma in all idiopathic cases**
- Treatment
  - Initial treatment is supportive with transfusions, if needed
  - Cases caused by parvovirus infection may respond to IV immune globulin
  - Cases caused by thymoma may respond to tumor removal
  - Immunosuppressive drugs are used in refractory cases (e.g., corticosteroids, cyclosporine, cyclophosphamide)

Macrocytic Anemia
- Basic approach
  - Confirm that the anemia is hypoproliferative (corrected reticulocyte count < 2%)
  - Consider the two basic types of macrocytic anemia: Megaloblastic and nonmegaloblastic
  - The history and physical examination can suggest certain etiologies
    - Use of certain medications (e.g., methotrexate, hydroxyurea, zidovudine, phenytoin, triamterene)
    - Alcohol use
    - History of GI surgery (i.e., gastrectomy, ileal resection)
    - Signs or symptoms of liver disease
    - Signs or symptoms of hypothyroidism
  - Clues on the peripheral smear
    - Macro-ovalocytes—suggestive of megaloblastic anemias (Fig. 47-6)
    - Hypersegmented neutrophils (more than six lobes)
      - Has a high sensitivity and specificity for megaloblastic anemias (see Fig. 47-6)
      - Can appear before macrocytosis or anemia
    - Target cells—can be suggestive of liver disease

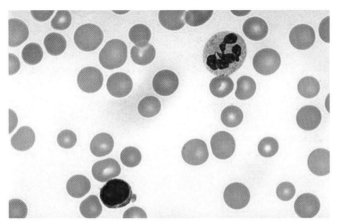

FIGURE 47-6 Megaloblastic anemia. Macrocytes, macro-ovalocytes, and a hypersegmented neutrophil.

- Pseudo Pelger-Huet anomaly—hyposegmented neutrophils suggestive of myelodysplasia
- Laboratory evaluation
  - **A very high MCV (>110 fL) is suggestive of vitamin B$_{12}$ or folate deficiency**
  - Vitamin B$_{12}$ and RBC folate levels
  - Liver function tests
  - Thyroid-stimulating hormone
- Bone marrow examination is necessary if etiology is unclear or if MDS is being considered

MEGALOBLASTIC ANEMIA

- Characterized by abnormal nuclear maturation of red cell precursors (megaloblasts) in the bone marrow
- Causes include vitamin B$_{12}$ deficiency, folate deficiency, myelodysplastic syndromes (occasionally), and chemotherapy

VITAMIN B$_{12}$ (COBALAMIN) DEFICIENCY

Basic Information

- Vitamin B$_{12}$ is absorbed in the terminal ileum
- Parietal cells in the stomach secrete intrinsic factor that facilitates absorption
- **Usually takes years to develop**
- Most cases result from food–cobalamin malabsorption whereby stomach acids are unable to cleave vitamin B$_{12}$ bound to food
- Numerous other causes exist (Table 47-4)

Clinical Presentation

- Symptoms of anemia are nonspecific
- **Neurologic symptoms may be present before anemia develops**
  - Symmetrical paresthesias
  - Ataxia, spasticity
  - Memory loss, irritability, dementia
- Asymptomatic patients may present with only laboratory abnormalities
  - Pancytopenia
  - Elevated low-density lipoprotein (LDL) and indirect bilirubin caused by destruction of cells within the bone marrow

TABLE 47-4	*Etiologies of Vitamin B$_{12}$ Deficiency*
Pernicious anemia	Autoimmune disease that results in achlorhydria and the absence of intrinsic factor Associated with other autoimmune processes (e.g., vitiligo, hypothyroidism, Addison's disease) Associated with increased risk of gastric cancer Anti-intrinsic factor antibodies are specific but not sensitive for the diagnosis Antiparietal cell antibodies are sensitive but not specific for the diagnosis
Gastrectomy	Can result in deficiency in intrinsic factor Can cause impaired ability to cleave cobalamin from food
Atrophic gastritis	Thought to be a major cause of subclinical deficiency in elderly patients Results in inability to cleave cobalamin from food
Intestinal disorders (e.g., ileal resection, Crohn's disease, celiac disease, tropical sprue, bacterial overgrowth syndromes)	Look for other signs of malabsorption Can coexist with iron deficiency
Pancreatic insufficiency	Look for signs of chronic pancreatitis
Diet	Strict vegans have decreased intake of vitamin B$_{12}$
Medications (e.g., metformin, proton-pump inhibitors)	Cause impaired intestinal absorption

Diagnosis

- Peripheral smear may show macro-ovalocytes and hypersegmented neutrophils
- Serum vitamin B$_{12}$ level is the standard diagnostic test, but it might not accurately represent true tissue levels in some patients
- Metabolic testing may be useful in patients who present with clinical evidence of deficiency and borderline serum levels (200–300 pg/mL)
  - Methylmalonic acid—elevated levels are sensitive and specific for vitamin B$_{12}$ deficiency in patients with normal renal function; this elevation is not seen in folate deficiency
  - Homocysteine: Elevated levels are very sensitive but not specific; elevations are also seen in folate deficiency
- Antibody testing for the diagnosis of pernicious anemia (see Table 47-4)
- The Schilling test can be done if a cause for the deficiency is not evident (Table 47-5)

Treatment

- Intramuscular vitamin B$_{12}$ injections are usually the initial treatment of choice for pernicious anemia
- Oral vitamin B$_{12}$ can also be equally effective in raising serum levels
  - Must be given in very large doses (1 mg/day) in patients with pernicious anemia

47

TABLE 47-5	*Schilling Test*

Stage I: Oral radioactive free B$_{12}$ is given, followed by intramuscular unlabeled B$_{12}$ to saturate tissue receptors and displace bound radiolabeled B$_{12}$. A 24-hr urine is then obtained to look for absorbed oral B$_{12}$. If <9% of the administered oral dose is found in urine, the test is considered abnormal.

Stage II: Oral radioactive B$_{12}$ plus oral intrinsic factor is given, followed by intramuscular unlabeled B$_{12}$. A 24-hr urine is again obtained. Excretion should correct to >9% if the problem is an intrinsic factor deficiency (e.g., pernicious anemia).

Stage III: Done if the first two stages are abnormal. A gluten-free diet (to diagnose celiac sprue), administration of antibiotics (to diagnose bacterial overgrowth), or administration of pancreatic enzymes (to diagnose pancreatic insufficiency) is done before repeating stage I.

TEST INTERPRETATION

Condition	Stage I	Stage II
Normal	Normal	
Dietary deficiency (veganism)	Normal	
Inadequate dissociation of cobalamin from food* (e.g., atrophic gastritis)	Normal	
Pernicious anemia	Low	Normal
Gastrectomy	Low	Normal
Ileal resection/malabsorption	Low	Low
Bacterial overgrowth of the ileum	Low	Low
Pancreatic insufficiency	Low	Low

*A modified version of stage I of the test can be done to diagnose food–cobalamin malabsorption. This test utilizes radiolabeled B$_{12}$ bound to food rather than free B$_{12}$. Patients with food–cobalamin malabsorption should have abnormally low urine B$_{12}$ excretions.

- Lower oral doses (250 mcg/day) may be sufficient to treat food–cobalamin malabsorption
- Consider the risk of noncompliance if choosing the oral route
- Hematologic abnormalities should normalize within 2 months
- Neurologic abnormalities normalize within 6 months

FOLATE DEFICIENCY

- **Can develop rapidly (within months)**
- Causes
  - Nutritional deficiency
  - Alcoholism
  - Malabsorption (e.g., celiac sprue, tropical sprue)
  - Excess demands (e.g., pregnancy, chronic hemolytic states)
  - Drugs that interfere with folate metabolism (e.g., methotrexate, phenytoin, trimethoprim)
- Pancytopenia, elevated lactate dehydrogenase (LDH), and elevated bilirubin can occur
- The peripheral smear will be identical to that seen in vitamin B$_{12}$ deficiency
- Red cell folate levels may more accurately measure true tissue status because normal serum folate levels are a reflection of short-term intake
- Treat with oral folic acid (1 mg/day is usually sufficient)

BOX 47-2	*Effect of Alcohol on Red Blood Cells*

Macrocytosis without anemia can occur with regular intake of as little as a half bottle of wine per day

Anemia may result from a number of different mechanisms
  Direct toxic effect on the bone marrow
  Iron deficiency caused by GI bleeding
  Folic acid deficiency
  Liver disease causing splenic sequestration hemolysis
  Liver disease resulting in acanthocyte (spur cell) formation and hemolysis

MYELODYSPLASTIC SYNDROMES

- Peripheral smear can have ovalocytes, but hypersegmented neutrophils are not typically seen
- Bone marrow may or may not show megaloblastic changes
- Vitamin B$_{12}$ and folate levels should be normal
- See Chapter 51 for diagnostic and treatment information

CHEMOTHERAPEUTIC AGENTS

- Hydroxyurea and azathioprine are examples
- Peripheral smear should not show hypersegmented neutrophils
- Bone marrow may or may not show megaloblastic changes

NONMEGALOBLASTIC MACROCYTIC ANEMIA

- Alcohol is the most common cause and may affect red cells through several different mechanisms (Box 47-2)
- Hypothyroidism, multiple myeloma, liver disease, aplastic anemia, drugs, and MDS may also present with macrocytic anemia

Hemolytic Anemia

Basic Approach

- Defined as the premature destruction of RBCs
- Occurs by two different mechanisms:
  - Extravascular hemolyis: RBCs are prematurely removed from the circulation by the liver and spleen (most cases)
  - Intravascular hemolysis: RBCs lyse in the circulation
- Laboratory studies
  - **Reticulocyte count (corrected) is greater than 2%**
  - Indirect bilirubin is elevated
  - LDH is elevated
  - Haptoglobin is low or absent; haptoglobin binds free Hgb and is then taken up by the reticuloendothelial system; during hemolysis the rate of haptoglobin catabolism exceeds the liver's ability to produce it, resulting in a low or absent level
  - Urine hemosiderin: Present in intravascular hemolysis only
  - Urine Hgb: Present in severe intravascular hemolysis; urine dip is positive for blood but no RBCs seen on microscopic examination
  - Direct antiglobulin test (direct Coombs'; Fig. 47-7)
    - Useful in diagnosing immune hemolytic anemia (>95% sensitivity), where there is antibody coating a patient's RBCs

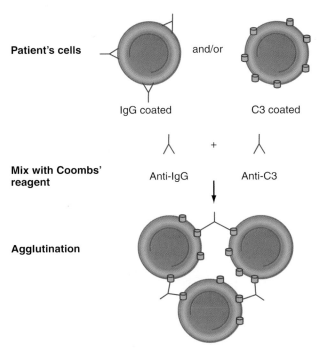

FIGURE 47-7 Direct antiglobulin (Coombs') test. IgG, immunoglobulin G.

- Done by mixing the patient's erythrocytes with antihuman globulin (which contains antibody to immunoglobulin G [IgG] and C3)
- If agglutination occurs, the test is positive and the diagnosis of immune hemolysis is made
- **Once a positive test is found, further testing is done to determine whether IgG and/or C3 are coating the patient's erythrocytes**
- Indirect antiglobulin test (indirect Coombs')
  - Useful to detect antibodies present in a patient's serum
  - Helpful in detecting alloantibodies that were induced by prior transfusion or by fetal transfer of RBCs to the mother
- The peripheral smear can assist in developing a systematic approach to patients (Fig. 47-8)

IMMUNE HEMOLYTIC ANEMIA

- Autoimmune hemolytic anemia (a positive direct antiglobulin [Coombs'] test)
  - Warm-antibody autoimmune hemolytic anemia
    - Autoantibodies optimally reactive at 37°C
    - **Almost always has IgG identified on red cell surface (Table 47-6)**
    - May also have C3 identified
    - Most cases are idiopathic
    - Can be a complication of an underlying disease
      - Lymphoproliferative disorder—CLL, lymphoma
      - Collagen vascular disease—SLE, RA
      - Ulcerative colitis
      - Congenital immunodeficiency
    - Findings include anemia, reticulocytosis, splenomegaly, and spherocytosis
    - Rarely patients may have separate antibodies directed at platelets causing concomitant thrombocytopenia (Evan's syndrome)
    - Treatment
      - Initial: Prednisone 1 mg/kg/day with or without IV immunoglobulin (IgG)
      - Splenectomy: If refractory to prednisone
      - Immunosuppressives: If refractory to splenectomy and prednisone
  - Cold agglutinin syndrome
    - **Caused by an IgM complement-fixing antibody that binds to C3 on the red cell surface at low temperatures (4°C)**
    - Patients may have worsening of hemolysis and acrocyanosis when exposed to the cold
    - Direct antiglobulin test (Coombs') is positive for C3
    - Associated with a number of infections
      - *Mycoplasma* pneumonia self-limited hemolysis can occur 5 to 10 days after recovery from infection
      - Infectious mononucleosis (Epstein-Barr virus, or EBV)
    - Also associated with lymphoproliferative disorders and monoclonal gammopathy
      - Disease may be mild and chronic
      - Reticulocytosis may be minimal

47

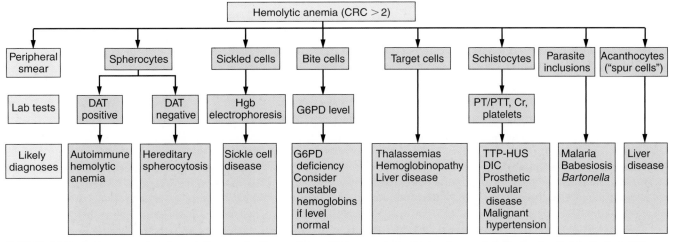

FIGURE 47-8 Basic approach to hemolytic anemia. Cr, creatinine; CRC, corrected reticulocyte count; DAT, direct antiglobulin test; DIC, disseminated intravascular coagulation; G6PD, glucose-6–phosphate dehydrogenase; Hgb, hemoglobin; PT/PTT, prothrombin time/partial thromboplastin time; TTP-HUS, thrombotic thrombocytopenic purpura–hemolytic uremic syndrome.

TABLE 47-6	Interpretation of Antiglobulin Tests in Immune Hemolytic Anemia		
Condition	**DAT-IgG**	**DAT-C3**	**IAT**
Warm Ab	+	±	± No specific Ab
Cold agglutinin	−	+	± No specific Ab
Drug— methyldopa	+	−	± No specific Ab
Drug—PCN, ceph	+*	−	± No specific Ab
Drug—quinine, sulfa	−	+	± No specific Ab
Delayed transfusion reaction	+	±	+ With alloantibody found

*Positive only during exposure to drug.
Ab, antibody; DAT, direct antiglobulin test (Coombs'); IAT, indirect antiglobulin test; PCN, penicillin.

- Diagnosed by IgM cold agglutinin antibody titers
  - Low titers (<1:32) can be found in normal serum
  - **Most patients with disease have titers in excess of 1:1000 at 4°C**
  - Treatment is usually supportive, but chlorambucil and cyclophosphamide have been used, especially in patients with monoclonal gammopathy
- Paroxysmal cold hemoglobinuria
  - Very rare disorder historically associated with tertiary syphilis
  - Most cases in adults are autoimmune
  - Caused by IgG (Donath-Landsteiner) antibody that can induce hemolysis (and often hemoglobinuria) with cold exposure
  - Direct antiglobulin test can be positive with anti-C3 during episodes of hemolysis but negative between episodes
  - Initial treatment is with prednisone
- Drug-induced hemolytic anemia
  - Drug-independent autoantibody induction
    - Presents identically to warm-antibody hemolytic anemia
    - Seen with methyldopa, procainamide, ibuprofen
    - Red cells coated with IgG but not C3
    - Hemolysis decreases weeks after cessation of drug
  - Drug-dependent drug adsorption
    - Antibody is directed against the drug and the membrane protein to which it is attached
    - Direct antiglobulin test is positive for IgG during the period of drug administration
    - Seen most commonly with cephalosporins and high-dose penicillin
  - Drug-dependent immune complex
    - Drugs loosely bind to RBC membrane with formation of antibodies reacting to both drug and membrane components
    - Results in stimulation of complement cascade
    - Direct antiglobulin test is positive for C3 but not IgG
    - Seen most commonly with cephalosporins, quinine, quinidine, sulfa drugs

- Nonimmunologic protein adsorption
  - Hypothesized that drug induces change in RBC membrane properties
  - Associated with prolonged exposure to high-dose cepahalothin, although other drugs have been implicated as well
- Transfusion-related hemolysis (see Table 47-1)

NONIMMUNE HEMOLYTIC ANEMIA (DIRECT COOMBS' NEGATIVE)

- Inherited nonimmune hemolytic anemia
  - RBC membrane disorders
    - Hereditary spherocytosis
      - More common in patients of northern European ancestry but occurs in all racial groups
      - Clinical manifestations include anemia, splenomegaly, and jaundice
      - Disease severity can range from mild (no anemia) to death in utero
      - Gallstone formation is common
      - Aplastic crises can develop during viral infections (e.g., parvovirus)
      - Diagnosis is made by finding spherocytes on peripheral smear (Fig. 47-9) and a negative direct antiglobulin test
      - The mean cell Hgb concentration is commonly elevated
      - Splenectomy is the treatment of choice in symptomatic patients
    - Hereditary elliptocytosis
      - Similar in presentation to spherocytosis
      - More than 75% of cells are elliptical
  - RBC enzyme defects
    - Glucose-6-phosphate dehydrogenase (G6PD) deficiency

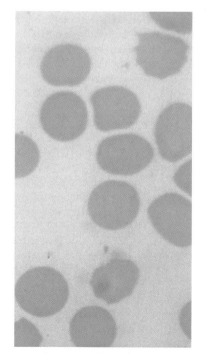

FIGURE 47-9 Hereditary spherocytosis. (From Stevens A, Lowe J: *Pathology*, ed 2, St. Louis, Mosby, 2000, figure 15.23.)

- G6PD helps protect Hgb from oxidation on exposure to a drug or toxin that results in the generation of free radicals
- Drugs that have been implicated include primaquine, sulfa, dapsone, and nitrofurantoin
- Favism is the acute hemolysis seen in some patients with G6PD deficiency after ingestion of fava beans
- Patients present with an acute hemolytic reaction of varying severity 2 to 4 days after exposure to a drug
- Infections and diabetic ketoacidosis can also trigger hemolysis
- Can see "bite" cells on peripheral smear
- Can also see Heinz bodies (precipitated Hgb) with a reticulocyte stain
- **Diagnosis is made by measuring the level of the G6PD enzyme, but this may be normal when there is active hemolysis**
- Treatment is supportive
- Sickle cell disorders (SS, Sβ-thal, SC)
  - Characterized by a chronic hemolytic state in which vaso-occlusion is caused by a deformity of RBCs
  - Sickle trait rarely has clinical implications
  - Hgb SC disease is usually milder than Hgb SS disease
  - Functional asplenia results from SS disease
  - Most common presentation is acute pain crisis but can affect virtually every organ system (Table 47-7)
  - The most life-threatening complications include acute chest syndrome, stroke, and infections
  - **Pulmonary hypertension occurs in about 30% of adults with sickle cell disease and is a strong predictor for near-term mortality**
  - Hgb electrophoresis establishes the diagnosis
  - Treatment
    - Pain crises: Hydration and analgesics; transfusion usually not needed
    - Acute chest syndrome: Antibiotics, oxygen, exchange transfusion
    - Stroke: Exchange transfusion
  - Prevention of complications
    - Vaccination: Pneumococcal, *Haemophilus influenzae* B, *Meningococcus*, influenza
    - Folate and iron may be necessary to keep up with cell turnover
    - Regular retinal examinations
    - **Hydroxyurea: Has been shown to decrease the incidence of acute chest syndrome, decrease the number of pain crises, decrease transfusions, and possibly decrease mortality**
    - Preoperative transfusion: To an Hgb level of 9 to 11 mg/dL can improve outcome in surgical patients
- Acquired nonimmune hemolytic anemia
  - Splenomegaly (sequestrational hemolysis)
    - Can lead to destruction of normal RBCs
    - Causes include lymphoproliferative disorders, myeloproliferative disorders, inflammatory diseases, infection, portal hypertension, and hemolytic anemia
  - March hemoglobinuria
    - Intravascular hemolysis with hemoglobinuria
    - Seen after prolonged physical activity
    - Anemia is usually not present
  - Microangiopathic hemolytic anemia
    - Cardiac hemolysis

TABLE 47-7	*Clinical Manifestations of Sickle Cell Disease*
Organ System	**Type of Complication**
CNS	Stroke Subarachnoid hemorrhage
Eye	Retinopathy Hyphema

Lung	Acute chest syndrome
	  Most common cause of death in adults
	  Patients present with fever, chest pain, and an infiltrate on chest radiography
	  Treat with antibiotics and oxygen
	  Exchange transfusion indicated if there is progressive hypoxemia
	Fat emboli
	Restrictive lung disease
	Pulmonary hypertension/cor pulmonale

Heart	MI CHF (rare)
Renal	Nephrotic syndrome Hypertension Chronic renal failure Hyposthenuria Hematuria Hyperuricemia
Urologic	Priapism
Bone	Joint effusions Avascular necrosis
Skin	Hyperpigmentation Leg ulcers
Liver/GB	Acute/chronic liver disease Gallstones
Infectious disease	Pneumonia (*Streptococcus pneumoniae, Haemophilus influenzae*) Osteomyelitis (*Salmonella* spp., *Staphylococcus aureus*) Urinary tract infection Sepsis
Heme	Chronic hemolytic anemia Splenic sequestration crisis Acute aplastic crisis

CHF, congestive heart failure; GB, gallbladder; MI, myocardial infarction.

- Occurs in about 10% of patients with mechanical aortic valve replacements
- Severity of the anemia is variable but can cause significant hemoglobinuria
- Hemosiderin can be detected in the urine
- Schistocytes seen on peripheral smear
- Need to watch for iron deficiency because of Hgb loss in urine
- New-onset (or worsening) hemolysis in a patient with a prosthetic valve warrants an evaluation with an echocardiogram to assess for perivalvular leak and valve failure
- Thrombotic thrombocytopenic purpura: Hemolytic uremic syndrome (see Chapter 48)
- Disseminated intravascular coagulation (see Chapter 49)

47

- Direct toxic effects on RBCs
  - Infections
    - Parasites—malaria, *Babesia*, *Bartonella*
    - *Clostridium welchii*—produces a phospholipase that can lead to membrane rupture
  - Snake and spider bites
  - Copper—seen in Wilson's disease
- Paroxysmal nocturnal hemoglobinuria
  - Caused by an acquired mutation of the X-chromosome gene *PIGA*
  - Ultimately found in 10% to 20% of patients with aplastic anemia
  - Mutation results in impaired synthesis of glycosyl phosphatidylinositol-anchored proteins (GPI-APs)
  - Clinical presentation includes hemolytic anemia (intravascular), venous thrombosis (particularly at unusual sites), and/or deficient hematopoiesis
  - Some patients may also develop esophageal spasm and erectile dysfunction from a deficiency in nitric oxide during hemolytic episodes
  - Laboratory features
    - Normocytic anemia usually; can be microcytic if iron deficiency develops from loss of Hgb in the urine
    - Hemoglobinuria: Present only intermittently
    - Hemosiderinuria: Present in virtually all patients
    - Leukopenia and thrombocytopenia: Usually mild but can develop into aplastic anemia
  - Diagnosis
    - Flow cytometry is the test of choice with demonstration of deficiency of GPI-APs CD55 and CD59
  - Treatment
    - Supportive care with iron, folate, and blood transfusions
    - Humanized monoclonal antibody against complement protein C5 (e.g., eculizumab) reduces the need for transfusion, ameliorates (but does not eliminate) the anemia, and improves quality of life
      - Does not affect the underlying stem cell disorder
      - Treatment is lifelong
      - **Increases the risk of *Neisseria meningitides* infection, so need to vaccinate before therapy begins**
    - Prednisone may decrease hemolysis
    - Androgenic hormones may be beneficial
    - Anticoagulation if thrombosis is present
    - Bone marrow transplantation should be considered if a donor is available and severe disease is present

REVIEW QUESTIONS

For review questions, please go to www.expertconsult.com.

SUGGESTED READINGS

Brodsky RA, Jones RJ: Aplastic anaemia, *Lancet* 365:1647–1656, 2005.
De Montalembert M: Management of sickle cell disease, *BMJ* 337:a1397, 2008.
Gladwin MT, Vichinsky E: Pulmonary complications of sickle cell disease, *N Engl J Med* 359:2254–2265, 2008.
Johnson CS: The acute chest syndrome, *Hematol Oncol Clin North Am* 19:857–879, 2005.
Parker CJ: Bone marrow failure syndromes: paroxysmal nocturnal hemoglobinuria, *Hematol Oncol Clin North Am* 23:333–346, 2009.
Rund D, Rachmilewitz E: Beta-thalassemia, *N Engl J Med* 353:1135–1146, 2005.
Sawada K, Hirokawa M, Fujishima N: Diagnosis and management of acquired pure red cell aplasia, *Hematol Oncol Clin North Am* 23: 249–259, 2009.
Weiss G, Goodnough LT: Anemia of chronic disease, *N Engl J Med* 352:1011–1023, 2005.

Platelet Disorders

ELIZABETH A. GRIFFITHS, MD, and SOPHIE M. LANZKRON, MD

Platelet disorders may result in life-threatening consequences. They may be due to an isolated defect in the platelet's role in clot formation or evidence of systemic disease. A stepwise approach in the evaluation of a patient with a suspected platelet disorder is essential to make the diagnosis and initiate treatment.

Basic Information

- Normal platelet function requires four steps to result in clot formation: Activation, adhesion, aggregation, and secretion (Fig. 48-1)
- Platelet dysfunction can be categorized as caused by quantitative defects (i.e., the number of platelets), by qualitative defects (i.e., how well they function), or by both
  - Quantitative assessment of platelets is performed by machine counters and by visualization of the peripheral smear
    - **Automated tests identifying thrombocytopenia should be confirmed with visual inspection of a peripheral smear**
  - Bleeding complications may be associated with thrombocytosis if the platelets produced

are dysfunctional or if there is an acquired von Willebrand's factor (vWF) deficiency
  - Qualitative assessment for defects in platelet function is evaluated by obtaining a bleeding history, bleeding time, platelet function analyzer (PFA-100), and aggregometry (see following discussion)

Clinical Evaluation

- The medical history
  - Clues in the history suggestive of platelet dysfunction include the following
    - **Bleeding that is limited to superficial sites such as skin or mucosa (hemarthroses are uncommon with platelet disorders and usually represent defects in the clotting cascade)**
    - **Bleeding that starts immediately after trauma or surgery**
    - Excessive menstrual bleeding
    - Other family members with bleeding histories suggest an inherited platelet disorder
    - Because many medications may result in thrombocytopenia or dysfunctional platelets, medication (and toxin) exposure should be reviewed in any patient with a suspected platelet disorder

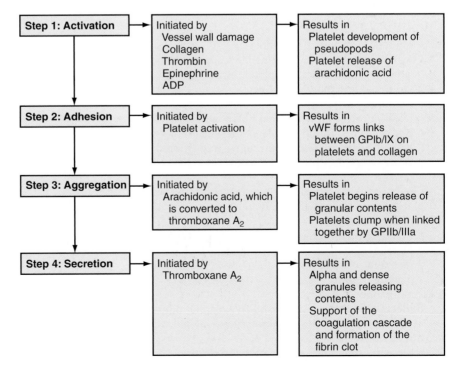

FIGURE 48-1 Steps in normal platelet function. ADP, adenosine diphosphate.

Step 1: Activation	Initiated by Vessel wall damage Collagen Thrombin Epinephrine ADP	Results in Platelet development of pseudopods Platelet release of arachidonic acid
Step 2: Adhesion	Initiated by Platelet activation	Results in vWF forms links between GPIb/IX on platelets and collagen
Step 3: Aggregation	Initiated by Arachidonic acid, which is converted to thromboxane A_2	Results in Platelet begins release of granular contents Platelets clump when linked together by GPIIb/IIIa
Step 4: Secretion	Initiated by Thromboxane A_2	Results in Alpha and dense granules releasing contents Support of the coagulation cascade and formation of the fibrin clot

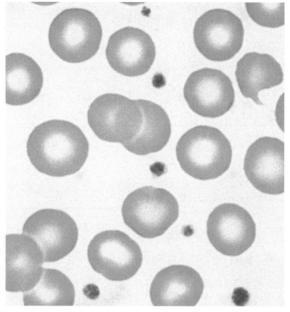

FIGURE 48-2 Normal platelets in a normal peripheral blood smear. (From Young B, Stevens A, Heath JW, Lowe JS: *Wheater's functional histology,* ed 5, Philadelphia, Churchill Livingstone, 2006, figure 3.10.)

- Disorders of platelet excess (e.g., thrombocytosis) are most commonly reactions to other illnesses (e.g., acute hemorrhage, iron deficiency, infection), which should be sought in the history (see following discussion)
- The physical examination
  - **Clues in the physical examination suggestive of platelet dysfunction include the following**
    - **Petechiae**
    - **Mucosal bleeding**
  - Splenomegaly
    - May suggest an underlying bone marrow process or liver disease that may be causing platelet abnormalities

Laboratory Evaluation

- Peripheral blood smear (Fig. 48-2)
  - Great importance in evaluating both qualitative and quantitative deficiencies in platelets
  - Used to confirm platelet number
    - Spuriously low platelet counts may occur as a result of interaction between EDTA and platelet glycoproteins, leading to platelet aggregation. Repeating the platelet count drawn in a citrated (rather than an EDTA) tube will verify that the platelet count is normal.
  - Used to evaluate platelet morphology; both the size of platelets and the presence of platelet granularity may aid in the diagnosis
    - Many disorders can produce large platelets, but platelets that approximate the size of RBCs are seen almost exclusively in the context of inherited platelet disorders
- Bleeding time
  - Reflects quantitative and qualitative platelet disorders as well as some vascular defects that are related to interactions with platelets
    - **Bleeding time does not involve the clotting cascade**

- Most common technique is Ivy technique, in which a blood pressure cuff is inflated to 40 mm Hg and a small, standardized incision is made in the forearm with a lancet; filter paper or cotton is used to absorb blood at regular intervals, and the time until cessation of bleeding is recorded
  - **Bleeding time is not useful in predicting bleeding risk, does not predict excessive surgical bleeding, and cannot predict bleeding risk in patients who have ingested aspirin**
- Patients with uremia often have a bleeding diathesis and platelet dysfunction. No controlled study has demonstrated that patients with uremia and prolonged bleeding time have more surgical bleeding than those with normal bleeding time.
- The PFA-100 is an in vitro test that has been used by some rather than the standard bleeding time to evaluate platelet function
  - This test is now being done in lieu of a bleeding time as it is more convenient and less invasive
  - **As with the bleeding time, the PFA-100 has not been shown to predict bleeding risk**
- Classic platelet aggregation assays
  - Platelet-rich plasma or whole blood is exposed to adenosine diphosphate (ADP), epinephrine, collagen, and ristocetin. The patterns of aggregation suggest specific platelet defects.
- Ristocetin activity
  - Ristocetin is an antibiotic that induces platelet agglutination in the presence of vWF
  - This test is abnormal in patients deficient in vWF (i.e., von Willebrand's disease) or in the receptor for vWF (glycoprotein IbIX; i.e., Bernard-Soulier syndrome)
- **Laboratory testing for liver disease, hepatitis C, HIV, and pregnancy should be sent as all of these can manifest as thrombocytopenia**

Inherited Disorders of Platelets

Basic Information

- **Inherited platelet disorders are rare**
- There are four major inherited platelet disorders (Table 48-1)
- Glanzmann's thrombasthenia and Bernard-Soulier syndrome are autosomal recessive
- Gray platelet syndrome (Fig. 48-3) and storage pool disease are of poorly defined inheritance patterns, in part because of their heterogeneous nature

Clinical Presentation

- Bleeding abnormalities may be present at birth or may become evident later in life
- Aspirin may exacerbate bleeding abnormalities
- **Common early manifestations include easy bruising, gingival bleeding, and epistaxis**
- **Menorrhagia with menarche is also common**
- Bleeding with trauma may be severe and life threatening
  - Patients with gray platelet syndrome or storage pool disease often have only mild bleeding manifestations

TABLE 48-1	*Inherited Platelet Disorders*						
Platelet Disorder	**Defect**	**Bleeding Time**	**Aggregation with Ristocetin?**	**Confirmatory Test**	**Treatment**	**Notes**	
Glanzmann's thrombasthenia	Platelets lack functional IIb-IIIa receptor (needed to bind fibrinogen and cross-link platelets)	Prolonged	Yes	Flow cytometry, demonstrating absence of receptor	Local measures to stop bleeding; ε-aminocaproic acid. If severe bleeding, transfuse platelets (at risk of developing IIb-IIIa antibodies)	Platelets are normal in quantity and appearance	
Bernard-Soulier syndrome	Platelets lack GP IbIX complexes (needed to bind subendothelial vWF)	Markedly prolonged	No	Flow cytometry, demonstrating absence of receptor	Local measures; ε-aminocaproic acid; platelet transfusion	Thrombocytopenia common	
Gray platelet syndrome	Deficiency of α granules	Prolonged	Yes	Electron microscopy demonstrates absence of α granules	DDAVP; ε-aminocaproic acid; platelet transfusions rarely needed	Large, pale platelets Thrombocytopenia	
Storage pool disease	Deficiency of dense granules	Normal or prolonged	Yes	Electron microscopy confirms absence of dense granules	DDAVP; ε-aminocaproic acid; cryoprecipitate; platelet transfusions rarely needed	First wave of platelet aggregation occurs, but second wave does not	

DDAVP, desmopressin; Gp, glycoprotein; vWF, von Willebrand's factor.

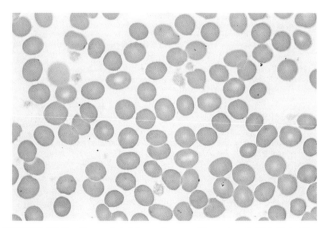

FIGURE 48-3 Gray platelet syndrome. (From Lewis SM, Bain BJ, Bates I: *Dacie and Lewis practical haematology,* ed 10, Philadelphia, Churchill Livingstone, 2006, figure 5-97.)

Diagnosis

- **Bleeding time is prolonged in all these disorders, except some mild forms of storage pool disease**
- Ristocetin aggregation
  - Absent in Bernard-Soulier syndrome and von Willebrand's disease
  - Present in Glanzmann's thrombasthenia
- For other results of diagnostic testing, see Table 48-1

Treatment

- Treatment is determined by severity of bleeding; **mild bleeding episodes treated with local measures (e.g., compression)**

- **Platelet transfusion should be reserved for major episodes of bleeding** because transfusion increases risk of alloimmization and development of platelet receptor antibodies
- Aminocaproic acid
  - Antifibrinolytic agent
  - Useful for treatment of all inherited platelet disorders
- Desmopressin (DDAVP)
  - Analogue of arginine vasopressin but with no activity on blood pressure or vasoconstriction
  - Through unclear mechanism, increases plasma levels of factor VIII and vWF
  - Effective for treatment of gray platelet syndrome and storage pool disease

Acquired Disorders of Platelets

Basic Information

- **Acquired platelet disorders more common than inherited platelet disorders**
- Acquired platelet disorders may result from medications, medical disorders, or hematologic disorders (including immune disorders; Table 48-2). These should all be considered in the history, physical, and laboratory evaluation of the patient with a suspected acquired platelet disorder.

Clinical Presentation

- Clinical presentation varies but **typically results in bleeding**

48

TABLE 48-2	*Common Acquired Platelet Disorders*
Category of Disorder	**Examples**
Medication-related	Aspirin NSAIDs Heparin Penicillin Quinine/quinidine GP IIb/IIIa inhibitors Clopidogrel/ticlopidine
Medical disease–related	Uremia Liver disease Cardiopulmonary bypass
Hematologic or immunologic disease–related	Paraproteinemia ITP TTP HELLP Myeloproliferative disorders Myelodysplasia Disseminated intravascular coagulation
Infection-related	HIV CMV, EBV, Hantavirus, *Mycoplasma* Viral hepatitis

CMV, cytomegalovirus; EBV, Epstein-Barr virus; HELLP, hemolysis, elevated enzymes, low platelets; GP, glycoprotein; ITP, idiopathic thrombocytopenic purpura; TTP, thrombotic thrombocytopenic purpura.

- **Exceptions include the following**
  - Heparin-induced thrombocytopenia (HIT) type 2 is associated with thrombosis (Table 48-3)
  - Myeloproliferative disorders, in which patients may have bleeding or thrombosis
- Medication-related platelet disorders (Box 48-1; see also Table 48-3) may result in immediate increase in risk of bleeding by deactivating platelets or delayed impact on bleeding risk if pathogenesis includes development of autoantibodies
- Medical disease–related platelet disorders (specifically liver disease; Table 48-4) may result in apparent thrombocytopenia caused by sequestration but no clinical bleeding disorder. Other causes are included in Table 48-4.
- **Hematologic/immunologic disease–related platelet disorders might be associated with normal numbers of abnormally functioning platelets, decreased platelet counts, or both**
  - Paraproteinemias may cause destruction or dysfunction of platelets
  - Myeloproliferative disorders may be associated with thrombocytopenia or thrombocytosis; one third of these patients have bleeding complications, and one third have thrombosis
  - Myelodysplasia may result in decreased platelet production or in production of abnormal platelets

TABLE 48-3	*Medication-Related Platelet Disorders*	
Medication	**Mechanism**	**Notes**
Aspirin	Irreversibly acetylates COX-1 and COX-2	COX-1 needed for production of thromboxane A_2, which is needed for platelet aggregation Impact present for lifetime of platelet (7–10 days)
NSAIDs	Reversibly acetylates COX-1 and COX-2	Impact present only for half-life of drug
Heparin	HIT type 1: Nonimmune-mediated; begins a few days after initiation of heparin and will spontaneously resolve if heparin is continued HIT type 2: Immune-mediated development of antibodies against heparin: platelet factor 4 complex; **begins 5–10** days after initiation of heparin	Type 2 associated with thrombosis (type 1 is not) Suspect a type 2 process if the platelet count falls by >50% within 5–10 days of heparin initiation **Heparin must be discontinued immediately in HIT type 2** Anticoagulation with a direct thrombin inhibitor should be started immediately if HIT type 2 is suspected An earlier onset of thrombocytopenia is possible if there has been exposure to heparin in the prior 3 mo Thromboses can present 40 days after heparin exposure Type 2 HIT confers significant risk in hospital mortality
Penicillin	Drug binds covalently to platelet membrane and acts as hapten	Typically occurs on reexposure to drug, with rapid drop in platelets Treated by discontinuing drugs
Clopidogrel/ ticlopidine	Drug induces platelet clumping in the microvasculature and results in TTP Inhibits ADP-induced platelet aggregation	Treated by discontinuing the drug and plasmapheresis Peripheral blood smear is essential for diagnosis Impact present for lifetime of platelet (7–10 days)
GP IIB/IIIa inhibitors	Drug binds directly to the GP IIb/IIIa receptor exposing neoantigens which are bound by preformed antibody. Thrombocytopenia occurs rapidly following initiation of the drug	Treated by discontinuing the drug. Platelets should recover at a rate of about 20,000 per day (rate of bone marrow production). Peripheral blood smear should be performed to demonstrate isolated thrombocytopenia without schistocytes May be safely treated with platelet transfusions
Quinine/ quinidine, procainamide, gold salts	Drug induces production of autoantibodies to platelet membrane	Treated by discontinuing drug May require treatment with IVIG or steroids

ADP, adenosine diphosphate; COX, cyclooxygenase; GP, glycoprotein; HIT, heparin-induced thrombocytopenia; IVIG, intravenous immune globulin; TTP, thrombotic thrombocytopenic purpura.

BOX 48-1	*Medications Associated with Platelet Dysfunction*

Aspirin
NSAIDs
Quinine/quinidine
Calcium channel blockers
Ticlopidine
Clopidogrel
Nitroglycerin
Nitroprusside
Thrombolytic agents
β-Lactam antibiotics
Abciximab
Heparin
Dextran
Lepirudin
Alcohol
Dipyridamole
Antipsychotics
Prostacyclin

For a complete list of drugs associated with thrombocytopenia, see Pedersen-Bjergaard U, Andersen M, Hansen PB: Drug-specific characteristics of thrombocytopenia caused by non-cytotoxic drugs. *Eur J Clin Pharmacol* 54:701–706, 1998; and Pedersen-Bjergaard U, Andersen M, Hansen PB: Drug-induced thrombocytopenia: clinical data on 309 cases and the effect of corticosteroid therapy. *Eur J Clin Pharmacol* 52:183–189, 1997.

- Post-transfusion purpura develops when alloantibodies are produced against platelet surface antigens, resulting in a decline in platelet count 7 to 10 days after RBC transfusion; treatment is with intravenous immunoglobulin (IVIG)
- Immune thrombocytopenic purpura (ITP), thrombotic thrombocytopenic purpura (TTP), hemolysis/elevated liver enzymes/low platelets (HELLP), and disseminated intravascular coagulation (DIC) are described in Table 48-5
- **HIV and hepatitis C can cause thrombocytopenia directly**
  - HIV can infect the stromal cells of the bone marrow, leading to decreased platelet production
    - HIV can also be associated with ITP
  - Hepatitis C appears also to have a direct effect on platelets that is not well understood. Recent literature suggests that clearance of hepatitis C virus infection can result in resolution of thrombocytopenia.

Diagnosis

- This group of disorders is **distinguished by onset of a new platelet-related bleeding disorder in a patient without a preexisting platelet-related bleeding disorder**
- Diagnosis requires a thorough review of all medications that affect either platelet function or production because medications are a common cause of acquired platelet disorders

TABLE 48-4	*Medical Disease–Related Platelet Disorders*	
Medical Disease	**Mechanism**	**Notes**
Uremia	Multifactorial, with uremic toxins causing defect in platelet aggregation	Treatment options include dialysis, DDAVP, cryoprecipitate, or estrogen DDAVP increases release of factor VIII: von Willebrand factor from endothelial cells Cryoprecipitate includes factor VIII: von Willebrand factor Mechanism of estrogen not understood; given IV it can be efficacious in 24 hr Erythropoietin or transfusions should be given to maintain a hematocrit of 30% Dialysis improves platelet adhesion to the vessel wall and can decrease bleeding
Liver disease	Dysfibrinogenemia, not thrombocytopenia, leads to bleeding risk	Sequestered platelets will be available should need arise Platelet transfusion, DDAVP, and cryoprecipitate may be used
Cardiopulmonary bypass	Destruction of platelets in bypass circuit as well as platelet dysfunction from activation of platelets	50% drop in platelets common postoperatively Platelet dysfunction a minor cause of postoperative bleeding Prophylactic administration of platelets preoperatively not indicated
Sepsis	Increased platelet phagocytosis mediated by increased concentration of macrophage colony-stimulating factor	Sepsis can also precipitate DIC
HIV	ITP is a major cause, also direct infection of marrow stromal cells contributing to hematopoiesis	1.7% of patients with HIV and 8.7% of patients with AIDS will be asymptomatically thrombocytopenic Increased risk associated with IVDA, anemia, lower CD4 Treatment is the same as for conventional ITP but with the addition of HAART AZT seems to improve platelet count and so should be considered in selecting a regimen Response to prednisone is 80–90%
Hepatitis C	Unknown mechanism	Recent research has demonstrated a correlation between clearance of viremia and platelet count recovery

AZT, zidovudine; DDAVP, desmopressin; DIC, disseminated intravascular coagulation; HAART, highly active antiretroviral therapy; ITP, idiopathic thrombocytopenic purpura; IVDA, intravenous drug abuse.

48

TABLE 48-5	*Selected Hematologic or Immunologic Disease–Related Platelet Disorders*		
Disease	**Basic Information**	**Diagnosis**	**Treatment**
ITP	Most commonly affects women in second and third decade of life Mechanism is autoantibodies against platelet membrane glycoproteins	Diagnosis of exclusion Antiplatelet antibodies demonstrated in 80% of cases Bone marrow shows normal or increased megakaryocytes May be secondary to HIV, SLE, thyroid disease, CLL, lymphoma, and solid tumors	Corticosteroids 1–2 mg/kg/day IVIG in refractory cases Splenectomy rarely needed Transfuse platelets only if severe thrombocytopenia (platelet count < 20,000/mm³) and bleeding
TTP	More common in women, typically in their fourth decade of life 10–40% report viral URI in 2 wk before onset Due to autoantibodies against ADAMSTS 13: Metalloproteinase that cleaves ultralarge vWF multimers	Pentad of symptoms: Microangiopathic hemolytic anemia, thrombocytopenia, neurologic symptoms, fever, renal dysfunction Most have hemolytic anemia, thrombocytopenia, and neurologic symptoms; only 40% have complete pentad Neurologic symptoms may range from headache to coma Renal symptoms may include hematuria or proteinuria, with or without renal insufficiency	Plasmapheresis is treatment of choice; done daily until neurologic symptoms, platelet count, and LDH have been normal for 3 consecutive days 30% will relapse Corticosteroids have a questionable role in treatment Splenectomy reserved for refractory cases
HELLP	One of several causes of thrombocytopenia in pregnant women Normal pregnancy associated with mild thrombocytopenia (100,000–150,000/mm³) ITP, TTP, and DIC also may be associated with pregnancy	Patient typically presents with right upper quadrant pain Often associated with eclampsia/preeclampsia Hematologic findings include hemolysis and low platelets	Delivery of fetus is definitive treatment, although abnormalities may persist Some evidence that corticosteroids are effective if delay of delivery desired
DIC	Process may be initiated by infection (especially gram-negative bacteria), obstetric complications, tissue injury, burns, or certain malignancies Generation of thrombin is central to pathogenesis; this allows consumption of fibrinogen, factor V, and factor VIII	Coagulopathy usually overshadowed by symptoms of illness that initiated DIC, but bleeding is major clinical manifestation, with thrombosis less common Common laboratory markers include elevated D-dimer, elevated fibrin degradation products, prolongation of PT and PTT, low fibrinogen, and low platelets	Treat underlying disorder while initiating aggressive supportive measures Platelet transfusions, cryoprecipitate, and FFP may be used if bleeding predominates, especially if associated with very low fibrinogen or platelet counts Heparin indicated if thrombotic complications predominate

CLL, chronic lymphocytic leukemia; DIC, disseminated intravascular coagulation; FFP, fresh-frozen plasma; ITP, idiopathic thrombocytopenic purpura; IVDA, intravenous drug abuse; IVIG, intravenous immune globulin; LDH, lactate dehydrogenase; PT, prothrombin time; PTT, partial thromboplastin time; SLE, systemic lupus erythematosus; TTP, thrombotic thrombocytopenic purpura; URI, upper respiratory infection; vWF, von willebrand factor.

- Because the life of a platelet is 7 to 10 days, exposure to a medication that affects platelet function would have to occur within this time
- Medications (and toxins) that affect platelet production may have a longer interval between exposure and clinical presentation
- **Evaluation of the peripheral blood smear remains essential in this group of disorders to exclude TTP in any patient with an acquired platelet disorder (Fig. 48-4)**
- Antibodies
  - Antiplatelet antibodies are seen in 80% of individuals with ITP
  - Antiheparin/platelet factor 4 complex antibodies are seen in heparin-associated thrombocytopenia (type 2) and mediate platelet activation, which results in increased thrombosis

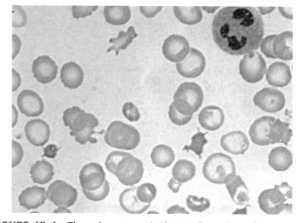

FIGURE 48-4 Thrombocytopenia due to disseminated intravascular coagulation. Note that platelets are nearly absent. (From Forbes CD, Jackson WF: *Color atlas and text of clinical medicine,* ed 3, St. Louis, Mosby, 2003, figure 10.115.)

- Evaluation of the bone marrow may be needed in ITP in elderly patients to exclude myeloproliferative, lymphoproliferative, or myelodysplastic disorders

Treatment

- Treatment is based in part on the presence or absence of immediate complications, including either bleeding or thrombosis. If life-threatening bleeding is present, platelet transfusion should be considered.
  - An exception is patients with thrombocytopenia resulting from TTP. **Patients with TTP should not receive platelet transfusions; treatment is plasmapheresis.**
    - **If plasmapheresis is not immediately available, patients should receive fresh-frozen plasma**
- At times, correction of the underlying disorder (e.g., dialysis in a patient with uremia and dysfunctional platelets) may be all that is needed to correct the bleeding disorder
- Medications that are used to treat platelet disorders include the following
  - DDAVP: A synthetic form of arginine vasopressin that increases plasma levels of vWF factor and factor VIII
  - Corticosteroids are used in disorders in which an immune component predominates; they are the initial treatment of choice for ITP
  - Rho(D) immune globulin (rhogam) can also be used effectively in Rh-positive patients with ITP and bleeding, inducing splenic sequestration of Rh-positive antibody–coated RBCs, thereby sparing platelets
  - Thrombopoietin (TPO) mimetics: Two new drugs that mimic the effect of TPO available to treat thrombocytopenia; both increase the platelet count in more than 80% of patients with ITP
- Plasmapheresis separates plasma from RBCs via centrifugation, allowing preservation of RBCs while plasma can be discarded
  - Plasmapheresis is essential treatment for TTP but is also used for some paraproteinemias
- Cryoprecipitate is a fraction of plasma that is frozen and then thawed (hence the name); the freeze–thaw process results in high concentrations of factor VIII, vWF, and fibrinogen
  - Cryoprecipitate can be used in patients who have depleted fibrinogen as a result of DIC and can be useful in patients with bleeding from uremia

Thrombocytosis

Basic Information

- Thrombocytosis is most commonly diagnosed when the **platelet count is greater than 600,000/mm³**
- Thrombocytosis may occur either in response to medical illness (i.e., reactive thrombocytosis) or as a clonal disorder
  - **Reactive thrombocytosis is much more common than clonal disorders**

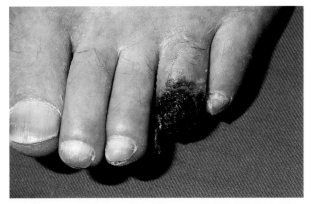

FIGURE 48-5 Thrombocytosis causing vessel occlusion and gangrene. (From Haslett C, Chilvers ER, Boon NA, et al: *Davidson's principles and practice of medicine,* ed 19, New York, Churchill Livingstone, 2002, figure 19.15.)

Clinical Presentation

- Reactive thrombocytosis may occur in response to infections (e.g., pneumonia, osteomyelitis, tuberculosis) or chronic inflammatory conditions (e.g., vasculitis, rheumatoid arthritis)
  - Other causes of reactive thrombocytosis include iron deficiency, acute hemorrhage, hemolysis, and splenectomy; some nonhematologic malignancies may also be accompanied by thrombocytosis
  - Clinical manifestations of reactive thrombocytosis are rarely seen, and symptoms of the underlying illness predominate
- Clonal thrombocytosis may be caused by an isolated clonal overproduction of platelets (i.e., essential thrombocytosis, Fig. 48-5), but is also commonly seen in polycythemia vera. Other clonal disorders include idiopathic myelofibrosis, myelodysplastic syndromes, and chronic granulocytic leukemia.
  - Hemorrhagic complications, although mild, are seen in up to 20% of individuals with essential thrombocytosis or polycythemia vera but rarely unless the platelet count exceeds 1,000,000/mm³
  - **Thrombotic complications may be venous or arterial and are not predicted by the platelet count (see Fig. 48-5)**
    - Advanced age and previous thrombosis are the greatest predictors of increased risk of thrombosis

Diagnosis

- As reactive thrombocytosis is by far more common, **efforts should be made to exclude infection, chronic inflammation, and iron deficiency (among others) in any patient with thrombocytosis**
- Clonal thrombocytosis is confirmed by associated clinical features and by bone marrow aspirate and biopsy, often with cytogenetic markers. Clonal thrombocytosis may be associated with the phenomenon of erythromelalgia (painful erythema, typically of the feet and hands), mediated by platelet thrombi in the peripheral vasculature.
  - Aspirin is the treatment of choice for this symptom

48

Treatment

- Reactive thrombocytosis is treated by treating the underlying illness
- Clonal thrombosis treatment is dictated by the type of clonal disorder
  - Aspirin therapy reduces risk of thrombosis and may be used prophylactically in patients with essential thrombocytosis or polycythemia vera, provided they do not have acquired von Willebrand's disease
- Cytotoxic agents including hydroxyurea and cytoxan may be used short term to reduce platelet counts, even when cure is not possible
  - Prolonged use of cytoxan is associated with an increased incidence of secondary leukemia
  - Anagrelide is an agent that prevents the maturation of megakaryocytes into platelets. This is used to decrease the platelet count in those with essential thrombocytopenia. Caution is recommended with use in elderly patients because side effects can include heart failure, myocardial infarction, and pulmonary hypertension.

REVIEW QUESTIONS

For review questions, please go to www.expertconsult.com.

SUGGESTED READINGS

George JN: Platelets, *Lancet* 355:1531–1539, 2000.

George JN, Woolf SH, Rashkob GE, et al: Idiopathic thrombocytopenic purpura: a practice guideline developed by explicit methods for the American Society of Hematology, *Blood* 88:3–40, 1996.

Pedersen-Bjergaard U, Andersen M, Hansen PB: Drug-induced thrombocytopenia: clinical data on 309 cases and the effect of corticosteroid therapy, *Eur J Clin Pharmacol* 52:183–189, 1997.

Pedersen-Bjergaard U, Andersen M, Hansen PB: Drug-specific characteristics of thrombocytopenia caused by non-cytotoxic drugs, *Eur J Clin Pharmacol* 54:701–706, 1998.

Peterson P, Hayes TE, Arkin CF, et al: The preoperative bleeding time test lacks clinical benefit: College of American Pathologists and American Society of Clinical Pathologists position article, *Arch Surg* 133:134–139, 1998.

Warkentin TE, Kelton JG: A 14-year study of heparin-induced thrombocytopenia, *Am J Med* 101:502–507, 1996.

Williams WJ: *Hematology*, New York, McGraw-Hill, 1995.

Coagulation Disorders

MICHAEL B. STREIFF, MD

Normal hemostasis is achieved by the cooperative function of coagulation proteins, platelets, and the vessel wall. Qualitative or quantitative abnormalities of any one of these components can precipitate excessive bleeding or thrombosis. Coagulation disorders are fairly common; therefore internists should be familiar with the components of the hemostatic system, the tests used to evaluate their function, and the diseases that affect hemostasis. This chapter focuses on the coagulation system. Platelet disorders are covered in Chapter 48.

Bleeding Disorders

Basic Information

- Bleeding disorders vary in frequency and severity
- To understand and diagnose these conditions, one needs an understanding of the coagulation cascade (Fig. 49-1)
  - Intrinsic pathway: Factors XII, XI, IX, and VIII, pre-kallikrein, and high-molecular-weight kininogen
  - Extrinsic pathway: Factor VII, tissue factor
- Can be categorized as congenital or acquired disorders
- **Congenital disorders include coagulation factor deficiencies such as hemophilia A (factor VIII deficiency), hemophilia B (factor IX deficiency), and hemophilia C (factor XI deficiency), as well as von Willebrand disease (vWD; Table 49-1)**
  - **vWD, the most common inherited bleeding disorder, may affect as many as 0.1% of the population**

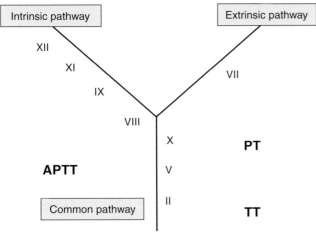

FIGURE 49-1 A simplified view of the coagulation cascade. APTT, activated partial thromboplastin time; PT, prothrombin time; TT, thrombin time.

- von Willebrand factor (vWF) serves two functions in hemostasis:
  - It mediates the adhesion of platelets to damaged vessel walls
  - It binds to and protects factor VIII from degradation by activated protein C, thus prolonging factor VIII half-life in the plasma
- Several types of vWD exist:
  - Type I vWD (75% of all vWD) is caused by a mutation that results in a quantitative deficiency of functional vWF
  - Type II vWD subtypes (20–25%) are due to mutations that result in the production of a dysfunctional vWF protein
  - Type III vWD (<5%) is rare and results in a severe quantitative deficiency of vWF
  - **Bleeding symptoms in vWD patients tend to be in mucosal sites (epistaxis, gum bleeding, menorrhagia, etc.) and mild to moderate in severity;** the exception is patients with type III disease, who can develop severe bleeding similar to hemophilia (hemarthroses, etc.)
- **Acquired coagulation disorders include the following:**
  - **Liver disease**
    - **Results in decreased synthesis of all coagulation factors except for factor VIII**
    - Laboratory tests typically show prolongation of the prothrombin time (PT), the activated partial thromboplastin time (aPTT), and the thrombin time (TT) (the last one caused by decreased or dysfunctional fibrinogen)
    - Treatment
      - Fresh-frozen plasma (FFP) for bleeding
      - Recombinant human factor VIIa [rhFVIIa or Novo Seven, Novo Nordisk, Princeton, NJ] has been used off-label for life-threatening bleeding refractory to FFP, but it may be associated with an increased risk of thrombotic complications
      - Liver transplantation for long-term management
  - **Disseminated intravascular coagulation (DIC; Box 49-1)**
  - **Vitamin K deficiency**
    - Vitamin K is required for the synthesis of active forms of factors II, VII, IX, and X, as well as the natural anticoagulant proteins C and S
    - Vitamin K deficiency is common with the following
      - Poor nutrition (especially diets deficient in green, leafy vegetables)

TABLE 49-1	*Selected Congenital Bleeding Disorders*

Disorder	Deficiency	Inheritance	aPTT	Laboratory Findings	Clinical Issues	Treatment
Hemophilia A	Factor VIII	X-linked recessive (1:10,000 male births)	↑	Reduced factor VII level	Mild: Factor VIII > 5%; bleed after significant trauma Moderate: Factor VIII = 1–5%; bleed after minor trauma Severe: Factor VIII < 1%; spontaneous bleeding	Factor VIII concentrate
Hemophilia B (Christmas disease)	Factor IX	X-linked recessive (1:50,000 male births)	↑	Reduced factor IX level	Clinically similar to hemophilia A Same severity scale as hemophilia A	Factor IX concentrate
Hemophilia C (Rosenthal's disease)	Factor XI	Autosomal-recessive; rare except among Askhenazi Jews	↑	Reduced factor XI level	Variable severity, but usually mild; bleeding usually in response to trauma	FFP
von Willebrand's disease (vWD)	Quantitative or qualitative defect in von Willebrand factor (vWF)	Autosomal dominant or recessive (1:1000 live births)	Normal or ↑	vWF antigen detects the quantity of vWF protein Ristocetin cofactor activity measures vWF function Factor VIII activity may be low or normal Tests of platelet function (e.g., bleeding time) may also be abnormal	Function of vWF: Aids in platelet adhesion and protection of factor VIII from inactivation Types of vWD: Type I: Partial deficiency of vWF; 75% of vWD Type II: Qualitative defect in vWF Type III: Complete deficiency of vWF	DDAVP causes the release of preformed vWF multimers from endothelium Factor VIII concentrates that contain vWF (e.g., Humate P)
Factor XIII deficiency	Factor XIII	Autosomal recessive (rare: <1:1,000,000 live births)	Normal	Factor XIII screen Tests for clot solubility in 5 M urea (clot will dissolve because of lack of fibrin cross-links)	Factor XIII is important for cross-linking fibrin strands to make a clot more resistant to fibrinolysis Clinical symptoms include delayed bleeding after trauma or surgery, poor wound healing	FFP

aPTT, activated partial thromboplastin time; DDVAP, 1-desamino-8-D-arginine vasopressin; FFP, fresh-frozen plasma.

- Broad-spectrum antibiotics (which kill intestinal bacteria, a significant source of vitamin K)
- Antibiotics with an *N*-methylthio-tetrazole (MTT) side chain (e.g., moxalactam, cefamandole, cefaperazone), which can interfere with vitamin K metabolism and potentiate the deficiency state
- Malabsorption (e.g., biliary disease, which interferes with delivery of bile necessary for absorption of fat-soluble vitamins)
- Vitamin K deficiency is characterized by a prolonged PT initially (factor VII has the shortest half-life of the coagulation factors, factors X and II also influence the PT), then prolonged aPTT (reflects factors IX, X, and II deficiency)

- Coagulation factor inhibitors: Antibodies directed against specific coagulation factors
- Factor VIII inhibitors are the most common inhibitors that result in bleeding
- Develop in 10% to 15% of hemophilia A patients because of chronic exposure to exogenous factor VIII
- Rarely occur in nonhemophiliacs (1:1,000,000); most common associations are with tumors, pregnancy, drugs, and rheumatologic conditions
- Inhibitor titer (concentration of the antibody) measured by the Bethesda assay
- Low-titer inhibitors (<5 Bethesda units) can be transiently overcome with large doses of factor VIII
- High-titer inhibitors (>5 Bethesda units) require alternative plasma products, such as factor VIII inhibitor bypassing activity (FEIBA VH, Baxter, Westlake Village, CA) or

| BOX 49-1 | *Disseminated Intravascular Coagulation* |

Unbridled activation of the coagulation and fibrinolytic cascades because of excessive tissue factor expression

Exuberant thrombin production results in excess fibrin clot formation, platelet activation, and secondary fibrinolysis

Results in bleeding because of consumption of coagulation factors (including fibrinogen) as well as thrombocytopenia

If fibrinolysis is inadequate or inhibited, thrombosis may predominate

Causes: Infections, neoplasms, snake venoms, endothelial disruption and abnormalities, tissue factor release (from trauma, obstetric complications)

Clinical presentation

　May see bleeding from wounds and venipuncture sites, petechiae, ecchymoses, hematuria, hematemesis, and other diffuse bleeding

　Thromboembolic phenomena may include pulmonary emboli, necrotic skin lesions, and stroke

Lab diagnosis (suggestive but not diagnostic)

　Prolonged aPTT, PT

　Low fibrinogen concentration

　Elevated D-dimer or fibrin degradation products are most sensitive tests

　Thrombocytopenia and schistocytes on the peripheral blood smear are supportive but nonspecific

Treatment: Treat underlying disorder; supportive care (FFP, platelets); heparin may be worthwhile if thrombosis predominates (contraindicated if CNS lesions present)

Mortality rate: 50–80% in severe cases

aPTT, activated partial thromboplastin time; FFP, fresh-frozen plasma; PT, prothrombin time.

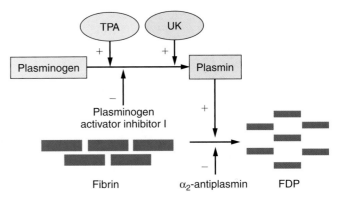

FIGURE 49-2 Regulation of the fibrinolytic system. FDP, fibrin degradation products; TPA, tissue plasminogen activator; UK, urokinase.

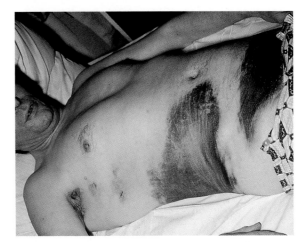

FIGURE 49-3 Massive hematomas in the absence of major trauma suggest hemophilia, Christmas disease, von Willebrand's disease, or supratherapeutic anticoagulant therapy. (From Forbes CD, Jackson WF: *Color atlas and text of clinical medicine,* ed 3, St. Louis, Mosby, 2003, figure 10.104.)

Rh factor VIIa, which can activate the coagulation cascade in the presence of a factor VIII inhibitor

- Hemophilia B patients have a lower incidence of inhibitor formation (2–4%)
- **Vessel wall disorders**
  - Immune complex-mediated destruction (cryoglobulinemia)
  - Inflammation (infection, vasculitis)
  - Destructive infiltration with proteins (amyloidosis)
  - Defective connective tissue structure (Ehlers-Danlos syndrome, vitamin C deficiency)
- **Fibrinolytic disorders can also result in bleeding**
  - Fibrinolytic system is responsible for clot digestion and remodeling (Fig. 49-2)
  - Excessive amounts of plasmin (the primary fibrinolytic enzyme) or its activators (tissue plasminogen activator, urokinase) or deficiency of inhibitors (PAI-I, α_2-antiplasmin) can result in bleeding
  - These are rare disorders characterized by delayed bleeding

Clinical Presentation

- **Bleeding history**
  - Easy bruisability is very common and not always pathologic
  - More specific indicators of a bleeding disorder are excessive bleeding with surgical procedures, an excessive transfusion requirement, a history of

reoperation for bleeding, a positive family history of bleeding, and chronic iron deficiency anemia

　- Hemarthroses and soft tissue bleeds suggest a coagulation factor deficiency (Fig. 49-3)
　- Skin (petechiae) and mucosal bleeding (epistaxis, gingival bleeding, menorrhagia) are more suggestive of vWD or platelet disorders (Fig. 49-4)
　- Delayed bleeding is typical of factor XIII deficiency or fibrinolytic defects; factor XIII deficiency is also associated with poor wound healing
- Physical examination findings for bleeding
　- Ecchymoses at inaccessible sites suggest a coagulation disorder (Fig. 49-5)
　- **Palpable purpura indicates vessel wall inflammation (e.g., vasculitis)**
　- Nonpalpable purpura suggests vessel wall disorders, such as scurvy (vitamin C deficiency) or connective tissue disorders (e.g., Ehlers-Danlos syndrome)

Diagnosis and Evaluation

- Basic laboratory evaluation
　- PT: Measures factors in the extrinsic and common pathways (see Fig. 49-1)

49

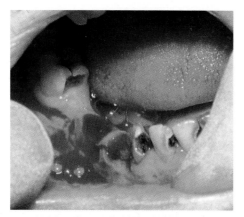

FIGURE 49-4 Hemorrhage after dental extraction may be the first clue to more minor degrees of coagulation disorder and is a common presentation in von Willebrand's disease. (From Forbes CD, Jackson WF: *Color atlas and text of clinical medicine,* ed 3, St. Louis, Mosby, 2003, figure 10.105.)

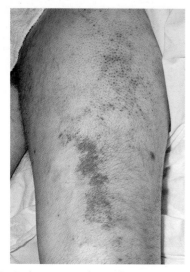

FIGURE 49-5 Ecchymoses and petechiae on lateral thigh of a patient with septicemic plague complicated by disseminated intravascular coagulation. (From Mandell GL, Bennett JE, Dolin R: *Principles and practice of infectious diseases,* ed 6, Philadelphia, Churchill Livingstone, 2005, figure 226-7.)

- **International normalized ratio (INR): A method for reporting PT results in patients on vitamin K antagonists (e.g., warfarin) that helps to normalize interlaboratory differences in reagent sensitivity**
- aPTT: Measures factors in the intrinsic and common pathways
- TT: Measures fibrinogen function
- Basic coagulation test scenarios
  - Isolated prolonged PT: Extrinsic pathway defect (e.g., factor VII deficiency; see Fig. 49-1)
  - Isolated prolonged aPTT: Intrinsic pathway defect, in order of frequency, are VIII greater than IX greater than XI greater than XII, prekallikrein, or high-molecular-weight kininogen (the latter two accelerate factor XII activation)
  - Isolated prolonged aPTT (usually markedly prolonged) in the absence of clinical bleeding suggests factor XII, prekallikrein, or high-molecular-weight kininogen deficiency

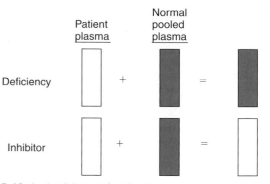

FIGURE 49-6 A mixing study. *Blue* denotes normal clotting activity; *white* denotes abnormal clotting activity.

  - Both PT and aPTT prolonged: Common pathway defect (e.g., factor X, factor V, or prothrombin deficiency)
  - Isolated prolonged TT: Fibrinogen deficiency or dysfunction, heparin or presence of a heparin-like factor (e.g., monoclonal proteins, fibrin degradation products), thrombin inhibitor
  - Prolonged PT, aPTT, TT: Generally the same considerations as isolated prolonged TT except heparins do not consistently prolong the PT
  - Normal PT and aPTT: Think of platelet disorders, vWD, factor XIII deficiency, fibrinolytic disorders, and vessel wall disorders
- **Distinguishing between a factor deficiency or inhibitor**
  - **Factor deficiency: The clotting time will correct when 1 part patient plasma is mixed with 1 part normal pooled plasma (NPP; 1:1 mix; Fig. 49-6)**
  - **Factor inhibitor: The clotting time fails to correct when 1 part patient plasma is mixed with 1 part normal pooled plasma (see Fig. 49-6)**
    - Weak inhibitors may only be identified in a mix of 3 parts patient plasma with 1 part NPP

Treatment

- Goal is to stop active bleeding
- Treatment of individual factor deficiencies (see Table 49-1)
- Recombinant products (e.g., recombinant factor VIII concentrate) are preferred because they are less likely to transmit blood-borne infectious agents (e.g., HIV, hepatitis B and C)
- **DDAVP (1-desamino-8-D-arginine vasopressin)**
  - An analogue of arginine vasopressin that may be administered intravenously or nasally
  - **Induces factor VIII and vWF release from liver and endothelial cells**
  - **Useful in type I vWD, mild hemophilia A (minor bleeds), and acquired and congenital platelet disorders**
  - Side effects may include flushing, headache, hyponatremia, hypertension, and mild hypotension
  - Doses may be repeated every 12 to 24 hours up to three or four doses, after which tachyphylaxis develops
- Acquired coagulation disorders: Usually treat the underlying cause
  - **Vitamin K deficiency: FFP for rapid correction; administer oral or IV vitamin K (correction begins in 8–12 hours) for more gradual but definitive correction**

- Liver disease: FFP for bleeding; RhFVIIa has been used for life-threatening bleeding unresponsive to FFP, eventual liver transplantation

Thrombotic Disorders

Basic Information

- The procoagulant function of the coagulation proteins is opposed by natural anticoagulants and the fibrinolytic system
- Defects or deficiencies in anticoagulant proteins or excessive function of coagulation proteins predisposes patients to thrombosis (thrombophilia; Table 49-2)
- **Extravascular risk factors for venous thromboembolism: Surgery, trauma, cancer, limb paresis or immobility, pregnancy/postpartum, obesity, smoking, estrogen use** (including oral contraceptives; see Chapter 22)

Clinical Presentation

- Patients generally have symptoms suggestive of venous thromboembolism
  - Pain, erythema, swelling of an extremity
  - Dyspnea, pleuritic chest pain
- Headache and mental-status changes (suggesting cerebral vein sinus thrombosis) and abdominal pain, heptomegaly, and ascites (suggesting Budd-Chiari syndrome or mesenteric vein thrombosis) are less common presentations

Diagnosis and Evaluation

- **Whom do you test for thrombophilia?**
  - Not all patients with thrombosis require a workup
  - Consider workup in patients with
    - Age younger than 50 years
    - Recurrent thrombosis
    - Positive family history
    - Thrombosis in unusual sites
    - Thrombosis with minimal provocation
    - Unexplained, recurrent pregnancy loss
- PT and aPTT will most often be normal
- Initial workup should include factor V Leiden, prothrombin gene (20210) mutation, antiphospholipid antibody testing, homocysteine, antithrombin (III) activity, protein C activity, protein S activity
- Thrombophilia evaluation: Factor V Leiden, prothrombin gene mutation, antiphospholipid antibody testing, protein C, and protein S may be tested in the acute setting
  - Antithrombin (III) activity may be affected by acute thrombosis and heparin therapy
- Protein C and S activity and antigen levels and the dilute Russell viper venom time are affected by warfarin therapy
  - Homocysteine levels should be measured after fasting

Treatment

- General principles
  - Modify risk factors
  - Treat symptomatic patients (with thrombosis) with anticoagulation
- Treat underlying disorder, if one is found (see Table 49-2), often with anticoagulation

- **If patient is asymptomatic, may defer treatment (because some will never develop thrombosis)**
- **If patient develops thrombosis, indefinite anticoagulation may be necessary (for combined thrombophilic defects; antiphospholipid antibody syndrome; homozygous factor V Leiden; antithrombin III, protein C, and protein S deficiencies)**
- For asymptomatic patients with thrombophilia, it is reasonable to provide aggressive deep venous thrombosis (DVT) prophylaxis during periods of increased risk
- For hyperhomocysteinemia, vitamin supplementation (with folate, vitamins B_{12} and B_6) can lower homocysteine levels, but supplementation does not reduce the risk of clinical events
- Anticoagulation options
  - **Unfractionated heparin**
    - Binds to antithrombin III and potentiates its inhibition of thrombin (factor IIa), factor Xa, factor IXa, and factor XIa
    - Quick onset of action (within minutes to hours)
    - Delivered intravenously to treat thromboembolism; may be used subcutaneously (5000 units subcutaneously two or three times daily) for prophylaxis
    - **Monitor aPTT (goal is 1.5–2.5 times control): Therapeutic range should be correlated with heparin levels**
    - Safe during pregnancy
    - Side effects include bleeding, osteoporosis with prolonged use, thrombocytopenia (see Chapter 48)
    - Reversal with IV protamine infusion (1 mg/100 units of heparin)
  - **Low-molecular-weight heparin**
    - Enzymatically/chemically fractionated form of heparin that can be administered subcutaneously in fixed weight-based doses
    - Useful for prophylaxis or treatment
    - Examples: Enoxaparin, dalteparin, tinzaparin
    - **Blood monitoring of therapy is usually not necessary; aPTT is not useful for monitoring**
    - Lower risk of heparin-induced thrombocytopenia
    - Partially reversible with protamine (1 mg/100 units or 1 mg)
    - **Use with caution in patients with severe renal insufficiency (creatinine clearance < 30 mL/min)**
    - Use actual body weight for dosing as dose capping may increase the risk of recurrent thrombosis (e.g., enoxaparin 150 mg subcutaneously every 12 hours for 150-kg patient)
  - **Warfarin**
    - A vitamin K antagonist that interferes with synthesis of vitamin K–dependent coagulation factors (II, VII, IX, and X), protein C, and protein S
    - Oral bioavailability
    - **Requires at least 96 to 120 hours for onset of antithrombotic effects (reduction in thrombin and factor X levels)**
    - Overlap initiation of warfarin with heparin to prevent initial depletion of protein C (before factors II, IX, and X) and theoretical risk of temporary hypercoagulability

49

| **TABLE 49-2** | *Selected Disorders Leading to Hypercoagulability* |

Disorder	Pathogenesis	Importance	Increase in Relative Risk of Thrombosis	Laboratory Findings
Factor V Leiden (activated protein C resistance)	Mutation in the first protein C cleavage site in factor V Prevents down-regulation of factor V activity	Common: 5% of white U.S. population Less common in African Americans and Asians Is synergistic with other thrombophilic states (e.g., prothrombin 20210 mutations)	Heterozygotes: 8× Homozygotes: 50×	Screening test: Activated protein C resistance assay DNA-based test for confirmation
Prothrombin 20210 gene mutation	Mutation beyond the coding region of the prothrombin gene Results in a 25% increase in prothrombin levels	Common: 1–2% of white U.S. population Less common in African Americans and Asians	2–3×	DNA-based test for mutation
Hyperhomocysteinemia	Homocysteine is a sulfur-containing amino acid produced during methionine metabolism Elevated in folate or vitamin B_{12} deficiency, homocysteinuria (autosomal recessive inherited enzyme deficiency state associated with dislocated lenses, mental retardation, vascular thrombosis), renal failure Pathophysiology of thrombosis is unclear	Mild hyperhomocysteinemia (15–30 µmol/L) is present in 5–10% of the general population	2×	Serum fasting homocysteine level >15 µmol/L is considered abnormal
Antiphospholipid antibody syndrome	Antibodies directed at phospholipid-binding proteins Associated with rheumatic disease (SLE, rheumatoid arthritis), neoplasms, drugs (procainamide, phenothiazines), viral infections (HIV), or idiopathic Pathophysiology of thrombosis is unclear	Predisposes to venous *and* arterial thrombosis Recurrence rate off therapy as high as 50% May also see thrombocytopenia and recurrent fetal loss	10×	Prolonged aPTT; no correction with 1:1 mix with normal plasma Prolonged dilute Russell's viper venom time (dRVVT) Detectable anticardiolipin or β_2-glycoprotein 1 antibodies
Antithrombin (AT) III deficiency	In the presence of endogenous or exogenous heparins, AT III binds and inactivates thrombin, factors Xa, IXa, and XIa	Heterozygous deficiency present in 1:2000 to 1:5000	15–20×	Can measure AT III activity in the absence of heparin and acute thrombosis Family studies can be diagnostically useful
Protein C deficiency	In complex with protein S, it inactivates the activated forms of factors V and VIII	Heterozygous deficiency present in 1:250 to 1:500	5–10×	Protein C activity can be measured in the absence of warfarin, vitamin K deficiency, and acute thrombosis Family studies may be helpful
Protein S deficiency	Cofactor of protein C in the inactivation of activated forms of factors V and VIII	Heterozygous deficiency in 1:1000	5–10×	Protein S activity can be measured in the absence of warfarin, acute thrombosis, vitamin K deficiency, inflammation, pregnancy, and estrogen therapy

aPTT, activated partial thromboplastin time; SLE, systemic lupus erythematosus.

- **Monitor with INR**
  - **Standard therapeutic range for venous thromboembolism (VTE), aortic bi-leaflet mechanical heart valves, atrial fibrillation (INR 2–3)**
  - **Mitral bileaflet mechanical valves, recurrent VTE (INR 2.5–3.5); antiphospholipid syndrome with recurrent thromboembolism (INR 3–4)**
- Contraindicated in pregnancy
- Many drug interactions (Box 49-2)
- Avoid use with nonsteroidal anti-inflammatory drugs, aspirin, or platelet inhibitors (increase bleeding risk)
- **Warfarin reversal**
  - INR less than 5, no bleeding: Hold dose, monitor INR closely; restart at lower dose when approaching therapeutic range
  - INR 5 to 9, no bleeding: Hold dose, monitor INR closely; may give 1 to 2.5 mg oral vitamin K if at high risk for bleeding, restart at lower dose when approaching therapeutic range
  - INR greater than 9, no bleeding: Hold dose, monitor INR closely; may give 2.5 to 5 mg oral vitamin K if at high risk for bleeding; restart at lower dose when approaching therapeutic range

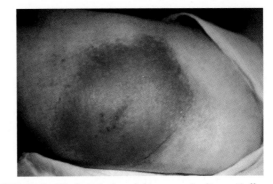

FIGURE 49-7   Warfarin-induced skin necrosis. (From Hoffman R, Benz EJ Jr, Shattil SJ, et al: *Hematology: basic principles and practice,* ed 4, Philadelphia, Churchill Livingstone, 2005, figure 112-19.)

- Any INR, life-threatening bleeding: Reverse warfarin with 10 mg vitamin K IV; use prothrombin complex concentrate (e.g., Bebulin or Profilnine) or rhFVIIa or FFP for rapid INR reversal; monitor INR closely
- Warfarin skin necrosis (Fig. 49-7)
  - A rare hypercoagulable state most commonly seen in association with the use of large loading doses of warfarin (10 mg or more daily) in the absence of concomitant heparin anticoagulation
  - Results from rapid decrease in protein C levels (plasma half-life, 6–8 hours) preceding the decline of procoagulant factors II (prothrombin half-life, 72 hours) and X (half-life, 42 hours), which tips the hemostatic balance toward thrombosis
  - Timing: Usually within 1 to 10 days of warfarin initiation
  - Histopathology: Dermal microvascular thrombosis typically involving the breast, buttocks, or thighs
  - Hypercoagulable states such as factor V Leiden, prothrombin gene mutation, antiphospholipid antibody syndrome, antithrombin (III), protein C, and protein S deficiencies: Increase the risk of warfarin skin necrosis
  - Treatment: Heparin anticoagulation, protein C concentrate (Ceprotin), or FFP; skin grafting in severe cases

---

BOX 49-2	*Selected Drug Interactions with Warfarin**

Drugs That Potentiate Warfarin Effects

Acetaminophen
Allopurinol
Amiodarone
Azole antifungals
Broad-spectrum antibiotics
Cimetidine
Ciprofloxacin
Clarithromycin
Disulfiram
Erythromycin
Isoniazid
Metronidazole
Norfloxacin
Omeprazole
Phenylbutazone
Propafenone
Quinidine
Sulfa-containing medications
   (e.g., trimethoprim-sulfamethoxazole)

Drugs That Decrease Absorption of Warfarin

Cholestyramine and other bile acid resins

Drugs That Increase the Hepatic Metabolism of Warfarin

Azathioprine
Barbiturates
Carbamazepine
Phenytoin
Rifampin

*This list is not all-inclusive. The international normalized ratio should be monitored whenever a patient's medical regimen is modified.

SUGGESTED READINGS

Ansell J, Hirsh J, Poller L, et al: The pharmacology and managment of vitamin K antagonists: the Seventh ACCP Conference on Antithrombotic and Thrombolytic Therapy, *Chest* 126(Suppl 3): 204S–233S, 2004.

Buller H, Agnelli G, Hull RS, et al: Antithrombotic therapy for venous thromboembolic disease: the Seventh ACCP Conference on Antithrombotic and Thrombolytic Therapy, *Chest* 126(Suppl 3): 401S–428S, 2004.

Hirsh J, Raschke R: Heparin and low molecular weight heparin: the Seventh ACCP Conference on Antithrombotic and Thrombolytic Therapy, *Chest* 126(Suppl 3):188S–203S, 2004.

Hoffman R, Benz EJ Jr, Shattil SJ, et al, editors: *Hematology: basic principles and practice,* ed 4, Philadelphia, Churchill Livingstone, 2005.

Kitchens CS, Alving BA, Kessler CM, editors: *Consultative hemostasis and thrombosis,* Philadelphia, WB Saunders, 2002.

Levine MN, Raskob G, Beyth RJ, et al: Hemorrhagic complications of anticoagulant treatment: the Seventh ACCP Conference on Antithrombotic and Thrombolytic Therapy, *Chest* 126(Suppl 3): 287S–310S, 2004.

Seligsohn U, Lubetsky A: Genetic susceptibility to venous thrombosis, *N Engl J Med* 344:1222–1231, 2001.

49

Acute and Chronic Leukemias

B. DOUGLAS SMITH, MD, and ERICA WARLICK, MD

Leukemias arise from malignant transformation of hematopoietic cells and proliferate primarily in the bone marrow. In general, leukemias are classified as "acute" based on the rapidity of presentation and the progression versus "chronic" in those disorders that are more insidious. In addition, acute leukemias are often morphologically poorly differentiated, whereas chronic leukemias show a more normal differentiation pattern of the malignant cells. Finally, leukemias are further classified by the cell of origin being either myeloid or lymphoid. A comparison of the clinical aspects of the various leukemias is seen in Table 50-1. This chapter focuses on three of these types: acute myelogenous leukemia (AML), acute lymphocytic leukemia (ALL), and chronic myelocytic leukemia (CML). Chronic lymphocytic leukemia is discussed in Chapter 56.

Acute Myelogenous Leukemia

Basic Information

- **AML is a clonal disorder of a primitive stem cell that results in excess proliferation of immature cells and suppression of normal hematopoiesis**
- Leukemic cells infiltrate the marrow and other organs (e.g., gums, skin, CNS) and suppress normal cell lines, resulting in cytopenias

- Classification of AML (Table 50-2) has traditionally relied on morphology to break this group of disorders into eight types according to the French-American-British (FAB) classification system. Recently, this schema has undergone changes—the so-called World Health Organization (WHO) classification system—based on new molecular characteristics of the individual disorders within AML.
- Epidemiology
  - Median age: 62 to 65 years
  - Five cases per 100,000 at age 60 years
  - 1% of cancer deaths
- Risk factors
  - Exposure to ionizing radiation
  - Exposure to chemicals: Benzene
  - Exposure to drugs
    - Alkylating agents (cyclophosphamide, chlorambucil, melphalan)
    - Topoisomerase II inhibitors (etoposide)
  - Genetic factors
    - Identical twins of leukemic patients have higher rates of leukemia
    - Increased rates of leukemia in Down's syndrome, Bloom's syndrome, Fanconi's anemia, ataxia-telangiectasia, Klinefelter's syndrome
  - Myelodysplastic syndromes

TABLE 50-1	Comparison of the Different Types of Leukemia			
	AML	**ALL**	**CML**	**CLL**
Median age (yr)	60	4	50	60
Initial remission rate	50–70%?	Adult: 70% Child: 90%	90%	90%
Median survival with treatment (yr)	1	Adult: 2 Child: 5	>5	5
Splenomegaly	Usually not	Often	Yes	Yes
Adenopathy	Usually not	Often	No	Yes
Infection risk	Yes	Yes	No	Yes
Hct	Low	Low	Normal	Low
WBC/μL	Variable	Variable	100,000–300,000 granulocytes	>20,000 lymphocytes
Platelet count	Low	Low	Normal or high	Normal or low

ALL, acute lymphocytic leukemia; AML, acute myeloid leukemia; CLL, chronic lymphocytic leukemia; CML, chronic myelogenous leukemia; Hct, hematocrit.

TABLE 50-2	*Classification Systems for Acute Myeloid Leukemias (AMLs)*
AML FAB Classification	**AML Proposed WHO Classification**

M0 = Minimal differentiation
M1 = Without differentiation
M2 = With maturation
M3 = APL
M3m = APL microgranular variant
M4 = Myelomonocytic
M4eos = Myelomonocytic
M4eos = Myelomonocytic with eosinophil
M5a,b = Monocytic
M6a,b = Erythroblastic leukemia
M7 = Megakaryocytic
	AML with specific cytogenetic defects
	  AML with features of t(8;21)
	  AML with features of inv(16)
	  Promyelocytic leukemia with t(15;17)
	  Promyelocytic leukemia with t(v;17)
	  AML with t(6;9)
	AML with trilineage dysplasia (>50% of all cell lineages)
	Classify using FAB subgroups (M0–M7)
	AML without defining cytogenetic defects of dysplasia
	AML M1–M6
	Myeloid sarcoma
	Acute panmyelosis with myelofibrosis
	AML arising in a previously MDS
	Therapy-related AML (alkylating agent or topoisomerase II inhibitor related)

APL, acute promyelocytic leukemia; FAB, French-American-British; MDS, myelodysplastic syndrome.

- Prognostic factors: In general, prognosis is worse with age over 60 years, poor functional status, AML secondary to prior chemotherapy or arising from another marrow disorder (i.e., myelodysplastic syndrome or myeloproliferative disorder), WBC greater than 50,000/μL or the presence of an FLT3-ITD molecular mutation
  - **Cytogenetics (Table 50-3) and FLT3-ITD mutations are the most critical prognostic factors**

Clinical Presentation

- The main presenting symptoms are caused by decreased production of normal cells:
  - Anemia: pallor, fatigue, and dyspnea
  - Thrombocytopenia: petechiae, hematoma, and bleeding (oral, GI)
    - Neutropenia: recurrent infections (sepsis, cellulitis, pneumonia)
- **Splenomegaly is uncommon**
- Individual subtypes of AML may have unique features (see Table 50-2)
- Leptomeningeal involvement is most common with elevated WBC at diagnosis or M4/M5 morphology
  - **Headache and altered mental status are the most common symptoms**
  - Cranial nerve palsies are the most common signs
- Hyperleukocytosis is seen when increased WBC (can be noted at 35,000–50,000/μL, common if WBC > 100,000/μL) results in obstruction of capillaries and small blood vessels causing widespread ischemic changes and can result in the following
  - Stroke and/or mental status changes
  - Congestive heart failure and/or myocardial ischemia
  - Pulmonary congestion and/or hypoxia
  - Renal failure

- Tumor lysis syndrome (see Chapter 58)
- **DIC (disseminated intravascular coagulopathy) is seen most commonly with M3 AML, or acute promyelocytic leukemia (APL) and is an oncologic emergency**

Diagnosis

- Diagnosis depends on identification of myeloblasts in peripheral blood smear or bone marrow preparations
  - Peripheral smear may vary from pancytopenia without circulating blasts to marked leukocytosis and leukostasis (Fig. 50-1)
  - **Auer rods, which can be present and are considered pathognomonic for AML are cytoplasmic inclusions of aggregated lysosomes (Fig. 50-2)**
- Morphology and immunologic or cytologic markers define the AML subtypes
- Other laboratory features
  - Hematologic
    - WBC can be low or high (low WBC raises suspicion of M3-APL)
    - Blast count may be low or high
    - Hematocrit usually low
    - Platelet count is usually low

TABLE 50-3	*Acute Myeloid Leukemia Cytogenetic Risk Groups*	
Good	t(8;21), inv 16, t(15;17)	
Intermediate	"Normal," +8	
Poor	−5/5q−, −7/7q−, t(6;9), 3q, 11q23, multiple/complex	

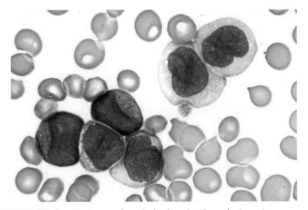

FIGURE 50-1 Acute myelocytic leukemia (French-American-British AML-M4) bone marrow. This category is typified by nearly equal numbers of myeloblasts and monoblasts plus promonocytes. (From Henderson ES, Lister A, Greaves MF: *Leukemia,* ed 7, Philadelphia, WB Saunders, 2002, figure 11-14.)

50

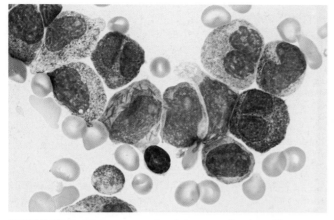

FIGURE 50-2 Bone marrow showing promyelocytes with azurphilic granules. The cell in the center of the field reveals numerous needle-like Auer rods. (From Kumar V, Fausto N, Abbas A: *Robbins and Cotran pathologic basis of disease,* ed 7, Philadelphia, WB Saunders, 2004, figure 14-29.)

- Increased cell turnover can increase serum potassium, phosphate, and uric acid
- Spurious abnormalities are related to utilization (oxygen, glucose) by the high WBC count or excessive cell death (potassium) in the phlebotomy tube

Treatment

- **Chemotherapy treatment consists of two parts: Induction and consolidation**
- Induction chemotherapy: Based on a combination of cytarabine (typically believed to be the most important and active agent for AML) and an anthracycline (daunomycin or idarubicin); has the goal of stabilizing the sick patient and restoring bone marrow function to state of morphologic remission
  - In patients with M3/APL, all-*trans* retinoic acid (ATRA) is added to the induction phase
    - A syndrome called *retinoic acid syndrome* or *differentiation syndrome* can occur and is associated with increasing leukocyte counts and a clinical picture of capillary leak syndrome/cytokine release and often consists of increased weight gain, respiratory distress, serous effusions (pulmonary, pericardial), potentially resulting in respiratory, cardiac, and renal failure
    - It can occur in up to 15% of patients receiving ATRA and can be fatal (M3/APL presenting with high WBC is of particular risk)

- **Hyperleukocytosis is treated with leukophoresis (temporizing measure) and emergent lowering of counts with chemotherapy (more longitudinal measure) before full induction**
- Consolidation therapy: Consists of either several additional cycles of intensive cytarabine-based chemotherapy or stem cell transplant with a goal of curing the patient of AML by eradicating remaining microscopic disease
- **Allogeneic stem cell transplantation (SCT) is potentially curative but is often reserved for younger patients (<60–65 years) considered incurable by routine chemotherapy (i.e., those patients with poor risk cytogenetics or leukemias related to previous therapy or arising from previous bone marrow disorders)**
- Expected results from treatment
  - 35% to 40% of the patients will be alive and free of disease at 5 years
  - The relapse rate declines sharply after 3 to 4 years

Acute Lymphocytic Leukemia

Basic Information

- Occurs mainly in children
- **Worse prognosis with increasing age, Philadelphia chromosome, WBC greater than 30,000/μL, and prolonged time to remission**
- Recently classification schema has been updated by WHO (Table 50-4)

Clinical Presentation

- Usually acute onset of symptoms (<2 weeks)
- Presents with fatigue, pallor, bleeding or bruising, or infection
- 50% present with fever because of either pyrogenic cytokine release or concurrent infection
- 50% have lymphadenopathy and splenomegaly on examination
- Anterior mediastinal mass is common with T-cell infiltration of the thymus
- CNS involvement is common in all types of ALL

Diagnosis

- Lymphoblasts are seen on peripheral smear and bone marrow preparations (Fig. 50-3)

TABLE 50-4	Classification of Acute Lymphocytic Leukemia	
ALL FAB Classification	**ALL WHO Classification**
ALL L1 = Fine to slightly condensed chromatin ALL L2 = Variable nuclear size, moderate amount cytoplasm ALL L3 = Homogeneous, round nucleus, deeply basophilic, highly vacuolated	Precursor B-cell ALL, ± noted cytogenetics: t(9;22)(q34;q11) = *BCR/ABL* t(v;11q23) = MLL rearrangement t(1;19)(q23;p13) = E2A/PBX1 t(12;21)(p12;q22) = ETV/CBF–α Precursor T-cell ALL Burkitt's cell leukemia

ALL, acute lymphoblastic leukemia; CBF, cerebral blood flow; ETV, endoscopic third ventriculostomy; FAB, French-American-British; MLL, malignant lymphoblastic lymphoma; WHO, World Health Organization.

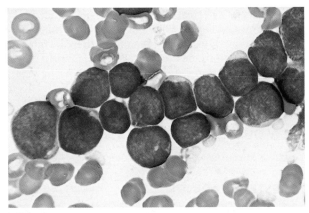

FIGURE 50-3 Acute lymphoblastic leukemia/lymphoma. Lymphoblasts with condensed nuclear chromatin, small nucleoli, and scant agranular cytoplasm. (From Kumar V, Fausto N, Abbas A: *Robbins and Cotran: pathologic basis of disease,* ed 7, Philadelphia, WB Saunders, 2005, figure 14-5.)

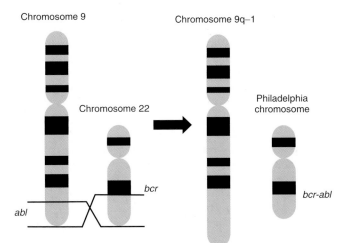

FIGURE 50-4 The Philadelphia chromosome. A reciprocal translocation involving the long arms of chromosomes 9 and 22 results in the production of the Philadelphia chromosome. The t(9;22) translocation results in the fusion of the c-abl oncogene on chromosome 9 with the *bcr* gene on chromosome 22. (From Rakel RE: *Conn's current therapy,* ed 57, Philadelphia, WB Saunders, 2005, figure 1.)

- May be difficult to differentiate from myeloblasts on morphology alone
- Flow cytometry is helpful in distinguishing ALL and AML
- **Evaluation always includes analysis of cerebrospinal fluid for CNS involvement**

Treatment

- Standard treatment is multiple cycles of multiagent chemotherapy; maintenance therapy required for at least 2 years
- **CNS chemoprophylaxis with intrathecal chemotherapy with or without CNS radiation is critical to reduce the chance of CNS relapse**
- Allogeneic SCT is often performed if poor prognostic factors are found

Chronic Myelogenous Leukemia

Basic Information

- CML is a malignant clonal disorder classified as one of the myeloproliferative syndromes
  - **Defined by the presence of the 9;22 translocation (the Philadelphia chromosome), which produces a *bcr:abl* gene fusion resulting in constitutively active tyrosine kinase, causing uncontrolled cell proliferation and blocked apoptosis (Fig. 50-4)**
- In general, prognosis is better with age younger than 40 years, in early stage, with a low percentage of blasts, in the absence of thrombocytopenia, and with only mild splenomegaly
- Natural progression of untreated disease moves from a relatively benign chronic phase to fatal blast crisis in 3 to 5 years
  - Blasts typically myeloid (70%) but can be lymphoblastic (20%) or undifferentiated
  - Prognosis after blast crisis is very poor, with median survival of a few months

Clinical Presentation

- Asymptomatic elevation in peripheral blood counts occurs nearly 50% of the time
- Symptoms, when present, include early satiety, left upper quadrant fullness, fatigue
- Splenomegaly on examination present in more than 50% of patients
- CBC typically shows WBC count greater than 100,000/μL with left-shifted differential, anemia, and thrombocytosis (in CML, the mature WBCs are functional and there does not appear to be an increased risk of infection in patients with chronic-phase presentations)
- Blast crisis may present with constitutional symptoms such as fever, night sweats, bone pain, and easy bruising

Diagnosis

- Peripheral smear typically shows the presence of virtually all cells of the neutrophilic series, from mature neutrophils to myeloblasts (Fig. 50-5)

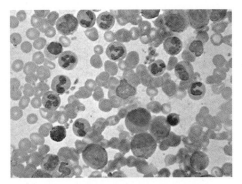

FIGURE 50-5 Chronic myelogenous leukemia. Note the abundance of granulocytes at all stages of maturation. (From Forbes CD, Jackson WF: *Color atlas and text of clinical medicine,* ed 3, St. Louis, Mosby, 2003, figure 10.77.)

50

- Diagnosis is established by demonstration of the Philadelphia chromosome and can be made by traditional marrow karyotyping or detection by peripheral blood fluorescent in situ hybridization (FISH) testing; molecular testing for the *bcr/abl* fusion by polymerase chain reaction is the most sensitive test

Treatment

- **Allogeneic SCT remains only known curative therapy**
  - Cure rates as high as 70% are reported with human leukocyte antigen (HLA)-matched donors
  - Graft versus leukemia effects are critical for success in CML and are weighed against the potential risks of graft-versus-host disease, which remains the most critical component of morbidity and mortality
  - In general, transplantation has better outcome when done on patients early in the course of their disease or during chronic phase
- Medical management: Considered the standard first line in most patients (exception being patients who present with advanced-phase CML)
  - **Imatinib mesylate (Gleevec) is a tyrosine kinase inhibitor that blocks the effects of *bcr/abl* on the cell and results in marked clinical improvements**
  - Complete hematologic remissions in more than 90% of patients treated up front
  - Complete cytogenetic remissions in more than 80% of patients treated up front
- Also effective in treating patients with advanced CML (accelerated, blast crisis) and all with the Philadelphia chromosome; however, remissions in these advanced diseases are often measured in weeks to months
- Second-generation tyrosine kinase inhibitors are now available (dasatinib and nilotinib) and are often effective treatments for many cases of imatinib-resistant CML

REVIEW QUESTIONS

For review questions, please go to www.expertconsult.com.

SUGGESTED READINGS

Burns CP, Armitage JO, Frey AL, et al: Analysis of the presenting features of adult acute leukemia: the French-American-British classification, *Cancer* 47:2460–2469, 1981.

Cassileth PA, Harrington D, Appelbaum F, et al: Chemotherapy compared with autologous or allogeneic bone marrow transplantation in the management of acute myeloid leukemia in first remission, *N Engl J Med* 339:1649–1656, 1998.

Druker DJ, Talpaz M, Resta D, et al: Efficacy and safety of a specific inhibitor of the BCR-ABL tyrosine kinase in chronic myeloid leukemia, *N Engl J Med* 344:1031–1042, 2001.

Hoelzer D, Thiel E, Loffler H, et al: Prognostic factors in a multicenter study for treatment of acute lymphoblastic leukemia in adults, *Blood* 71:123–131, 1988.

Jones R: Biology and treatment of chronic myeloid leukemia, *Curr Opin Oncol* 9:3–7, 1997.

National Comprehensive Cancer Network (NCCN): NCCN guidelines for acute myeloid leukemia. Available at: www.NCCN.org.

Pui CH, Robison LL, Look AT: Acute lymphoblastic leukemia, *Lancet* 37:1030–1043, 2008.

Myelodysplastic Syndrome

ERICA WARLICK, MD, and B. DOUGLAS SMITH, MD

Myelodysplastic syndromes (MDSs) are a complex and heterogeneous group of disorders characterized by ineffective hematopoiesis in the absence of nutritional deficiencies, dysplasia, cytopenias, and increased risk of infection. In the general population, the incidence is approximately 2 to 10 cases per 100,000 people; however, as age increases, the incidence rises to approximately 50 cases per 100,000 people older than 70 years.

Basic Information

- Etiology
  - Idiopathic: No known or explained cause of MDS development
  - **Secondary: Accounts for 20% to 30% of cases;** risk factors:
    - Benzene
    - Ionizing radiation
    - Tobacco/ethanol (ETOH)
    - Immunosuppressive therapy
    - Viral infections
    - Treatment-related or chemotherapy-related MDS
      - Topoisomerase II inhibitors (e.g., etoposide, topotecan): Associated with 11q23 cytogenetic abnormality; typical onset between 1 to 3 years after chemotherapy
      - Alkylating agents (e.g., cyclophosphamide): Associated with unbalanced cytogenetic changes including abnormalities of chromosome 5 or 7; typical onset is 5 to 7 years after chemotherapy
- Pathophysiology
  - Complete understanding of the MDS pathophysiology has not yet been achieved
  - Inciting genetic event occurs within an early hematopoietic progenitor in a milieu of inflammation with increased levels of the cytokines tumor necrosis factor-α and interferon-γ
    - **Detectable cytogenetic abnormalities are evident in approximately 40% to 70% of patients with primary MDS and in more than 90% with treatment-related MDS.** The cytogenetic abnormality predicts the outcome.
  - Early MDS → increased levels of apoptosis + increased proliferation → hypercellular bone marrow with peripheral cytopenias
  - Later MDS → apoptosis decreases and proliferation increases → more aggressive disease and possible transformation to acute myelogenous leukemia (AML)
- Classifications
  - Subtle differences exist between a number of classification systems that have been developed

- Staging systems follow the natural progression of the disease by describing the number of cell lines affected, cellularity of the bone marrow, and percentage of blasts within the bone marrow and blood
  - The French-American-British (FAB) classification system (Table 51-1) focuses mainly on morphologic descriptions and is less accurate for predicting prognosis for an individual patient
  - The World Health Organization (WHO) classification system (see Table 51-1) focuses more specifically on the biology of MDS and takes into account blast percentage, estimation of degree of dysplasia, and establishment of genetic subclassifications

Clinical Presentation

- Patient symptoms usually depend on the bone marrow cell line or lines most affected
  - Anemia can present with fatigue, pallor, dyspnea, or weakness
  - Thrombocytopenia can present with bruising or bleeding
  - Neutropenia can present with infection
- **RBCs are typically the first cell line affected followed by WBCs and then platelets**
- Splenomegaly can be seen in some cases, usually in chronic myelomonocytic leukemia (CMML)

Diagnosis

- Anemia or pancytopenia is typically seen
- **The mean corpuscular volume is usually increased, indicating macrocytosis**
- Differential diagnosis
  - Vitamin B_{12} or folate deficiency
  - Viral infections (e.g., HIV)
  - Alcohol abuse
  - Benzene exposure
  - Chemotherapy
  - Aplastic anemia or paroxysmal nocturnal hemoglobinuria (PNH) (in settings of a hypoplastic marrow)
- Peripheral blood smear
  - Hypersegmented (five or six lobes) neutrophils (Fig. 51-1)
  - Macrocytosis of RBCs
  - **Presence of Pseudo-Pelger Huet cells: Hyposegmented "dumbbell"-shaped nuclei of neutrophils (Fig. 51-2)**
- Bone marrow biopsy
  - Required for diagnosis

TABLE 51-1	*Classification Systems for Myelodysplastic Syndromes (MDSs)*

FAB Morphologic Classification	**WHO Biologic Classification**	**IPSS Prognostic Classification**

Refractory anemia (RA)
  Cytopenia of one PB lineage
  Normocellular or hypocellular BM
  <1% PB blasts
  <5% BM blasts
Refractory anemia with ringed
  sideroblasts (RARS)
  Cytopenia, dysplasia, and same blast
    percentage as RA but >15% ringed
    sideroblasts
Refractory anemia with excess blasts (RAEB)
  Cytopenia of two or more lineages
  Dysplasia in all three lineages
  <5% PB blasts or 5–20% BM blasts
  Refractory anemia with excess blasts in
    transformation (RAEB-t)
  Same hematologic parameters as RAEB
  >5% PB blasts or 21–30% BM blasts
Chronic myelomonocytic
  leukemia (CMML)
  Monocytosis in PB
  <5% PB blasts
  ≤20% BM blasts
	1. Refractory anemia (RA)
	2. Refractory cytopenias with
	   multilineage dysplasia (RCMD)
	3. RARS
	4. RCMD RS
	5. RAEB-1: 5–10% blasts
	6. RAEB-2: 11–20% blasts
	7. 5q– syndrome
	8. MDS unclassified
	Acute myelogenous leukemia
	   (AML): >20% BM blasts
	  1. AML with recurrent
	     genetic abnormalities
	  2. AML with multilineage
	     dysplasia
	  3. AML and MDS
	  4. AML NOS
		Blasts in bone marrow (%)
		  <5%—score 0
		  5–10%—score 0.5
		  11–20%—score 1
		  21–30%—score 2
		Cytogenetics
		  Good: normal, –Y, 20q–, 5q– syndrome—score 0
		  Intermediate: trisomy 8—score 0.5
		  Poor: abnormal 7, complex—score 1
		Cytopenias: number of lineages
		  0–1—score 0
		  2–3—score 0.5
		Overall score
		  Low risk
		    Score (0)—survival 5.7 yr
		  Intermediate 1
		    Score (0.5–1)—survival 3.5 yr
		  Intermediate 2
		    Score (1.5–2)—survival 1.2 yr
		  High risk
		    Score (≥2.5)—survival 0.4 yr

BM, bone marrow; FAB, French-American-British; IPSS, International Prognostic Staging System; NOS, not otherwise specified; PB, peripheral blood; WHO, World Health Organization.
Adapted from Catenacci DV, Schiller GJ: Myelodysplastic syndromes: a comprehensive review, *Blood Rev* 19:301–319, 2005.

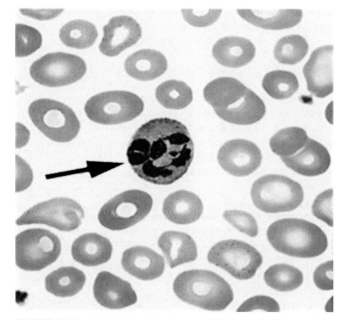

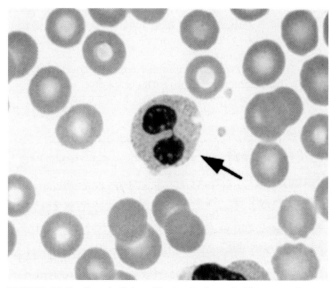

FIGURE 51-2   Pseudo Pelger-Huet cells *(arrow)*. (Courtesy of Thomas Kickler, MD.)

FIGURE 51-1   Hypersegmented neutrophils *(arrow)*. (Courtesy of Thomas Kickler, MD.)

- Cellularity: Typically normocellular to hypercellular
  - Hypocellular MDS (<20% of cases) can occur and can be difficult to distinguish from aplastic anemia or paroxysmal nocturnal hemoglobinuria (PNH). However, **because cytogenetic abnormalities are typically seen in MDS and not in aplastic anemia or PNH, chromosome analysis can assist in defining the disorders.**
- Dysplasia: 1+ cell lines

- White blood cells: Hypogranular, poor maturation, abnormal segmentation of nuclei
- Red blood cells: Binucleate or multinucleate forms, megaloblastic changes, nuclear-cytoplasmic asynchrony
- Platelets: Small, monolobated
- Cytogenetic abnormalities: Helpful in determining prognosis:
  - Good prognosis: 20q–, 5q– syndrome, normal, –Y
  - Intermediate prognosis: Trisomy 8, other
  - Poor prognosis: Abnormality of chromosome 7, complex cytogenetics

- Prognosis
  - The International Prognostic Staging System (IPSS) (Table 51-1)
    - Scoring system that assigns a point scale for three categories
      - Number of cell lines affected
      - Percentage of blasts within the bone marrow (blasts are usually distinguished by an increase in CD34-positive cells)
      - Cytogenetic abnormalities
    - Calculations based on these categories risk stratify patients into low risk, intermediate-1, intermediate-2, and high-risk categories

Treatment

- Regardless of stage of disease of MDS patients, there are four major generalizable goals of medical treatment
  - Control the symptoms caused by cytopenias and minimize transfusion needs
  - Improve overall quality of life
  - Decrease risk of progression to AML
  - Improve overall survival
- Supportive care
  - Careful count monitoring with transfusion support
    - Iron overload can occur with repeated transfusions
    - Iron chelation recommended for patients who have had more than 20 to 30 transfusions: Monitor ferritin levels with goal ferritin level below 1000 ng/mL
  - Growth factor support
    - Erythropoietin (EPO) effective only when levels are low; response seen in less than 20% of patients
    - Granulocyte colony-stimulating factor (G-CSF) indicated only in setting of repeated infections or in combination with EPO to boost RBC response (the combination is especially important for refractory anemia with ringed sideroblasts)
- Allogeneic stem cell transplantation
  - **Only curative approach to treatment**
  - Best outcome generally seen in younger patients with a matched donor (either sibling or unrelated) and with good performance status
    - Numerous studies now confirm that nonmyeloablative, or "mini," transplants are feasible in elderly MDS patients with decreased treatment-related mortality (15–20%) but at the expense of slightly increased relapse rates
  - Approximately 30% to 50% disease-free survival at 3 years
  - Treatment-related mortality can be as high as 30% or more with standard myeloablative transplants
- Medical management
  - Numerous new agents have been approved by the Food and Drug Administration for the treatment of MDS over the last 5 years

- Hypomethylating agents (azacitidine or decitabine): Traditionally studied in higher-risk patients (intermediate-1, intermediate-2, and high IPSS)
  - Overall response rate is about 40% to 60% (includes complete response, partial response, and hematologic improvement)
  - Trilineage responses are common and expected with transfusion independence rates ranging from 40% to 60%
  - **Azacitidine shown to delay time to AML and prolong overall survival in phase III studies**
- Lenalidomide is a new thalidomide analogue with immunomodulatory effects recently found with significant activity in MDS patients with 5q– syndrome
  - **5q– syndrome:** This syndrome typically occurs in older women. It is characterized by anemia, bone marrow findings of small hyposegmented megakaryocytes, and less than 5% blasts. Treatment is typically supportive care only, as transformation to acute leukemia rarely occurs. This is a separate entity from deletions of 5q.
  - **Best responses seen in patients with anemia only, 5q– abnormality, and low or intermediate-1 IPSS risk score**
    - **Response aim is to decrease or eliminate transfusion requirements**
- Conventional chemotherapy (cytarabine-based)
  - High-dose chemotherapy targets the abnormal clonal cells
  - Results are often short-lived and toxicity is high
  - Overall survival is not improved by intense chemotherapy, but this treatment is sometimes needed for patients with high blast percentage

REVIEW QUESTIONS

For review questions, please go to www.expertconsult.com.

SUGGESTED READINGS

Aul C, Giagounidis U, Germing U: Epidemiological features of myelodysplastic syndrome: real or factitious? *Int J Hematol* 73: 405–410, 2001.

Bennett JM, Catovsky D, Daniel MT, et al: Proposals for the classification of the myelodysplastic syndromes, *Br J Haematol* 51:189–199, 1982.

Catenacci DV, Schiller GJ: Myelodysplastic syndromes: a comprehensive review, *Blood Rev* 19:301–319, 2005.

Fenaux P, Mufti GJ, Hellstrom-Lindberg E, et al: Efficacy of azacitidine compared with that of conventional care regimens in the treatment of higher-risk myelodysplastic syndromes: a randomized, open-label, phase III study, *Lancet Oncol* 10(3):223–232, 2009.

Mufti GJ: Pathobiology, classification, and diagnosis of myelodysplastic syndromes, *Best Pract Res Clin Haematol* 17:543–57, 2004.

National Comprehensive Cancer Network (NCCN): NCCN guidelines for myelodysplastic syndromes. Available at: www.NCCN.org.

Blood Smear and Bone Marrow Review

JONATHAN M. GERBER, MD, and LAWRENCE B. GARDNER, MD

An internist should be familiar with the key components of a peripheral blood smear (PBS). Findings on a PBS, coupled with information obtained from the CBC, will aid the internist in narrowing the differential diagnosis. Uncertainties not answered by the PBS and CBC may necessitate an examination of the bone marrow.

Peripheral Blood Smear

- Role of PBS in the evaluation of a patient
  - Part of the initial evaluation for any abnormality in the CBC
  - Useful in narrowing the differential diagnosis
    - Sometimes what is not seen on the PBS can be of great value in ruling in or out a specific diagnosis
- Two components of evaluation of a PBS are the descriptive report and the prepared slide
  - In describing the PBS, terms often used to describe RBCs include the following:
    - **Anisocytosis: Differently sized RBC (Fig. 52-1B and C)**
    - **Poikilocytosis: Differently shaped RBC (Figs. 52-1A and 52-2B, D, and F)**
    - **Polychromasia: Indicating an increase in young RBCs (see Fig. 52-2E)**
    - **Microcytosis: Small RBCs (see Figs. 52-1C and 52-2A)**
    - **Macrocytosis: Large RBCs (see Fig. 52-1B)**
    - **Schistocytes: Fragmented RBC forms (see Fig. 52-1A)**
- The prepared slide may provide the diagnosis or narrow the differential diagnosis (Figs. 52-3 and 52-4; Tables 52-1 and 52-2; see also Figs. 52-1 and 52-2)
  - Poor slide preparation may result in artifacts such as rouleaux (stacked RBCs), which may be caused by an overly thick smear but also may be a sign of inflammation (e.g., infection, hepatitis, or HIV) or myeloma
- The normal PBS
  - RBCs should be round, **the size of a lymphocyte nucleus, with one-third central pallor**
  - **Lymphocytes should have small, compact nuclei**
  - **Polymorphonuclear neutrophils (PMNs) should have three to four lobes**
  - **Platelets should number 15 to 20 per high-powered field (1 platelet on PBS equals ~10,000 in CBC)**
- In addition to a microscopic examination, peripheral blood may also be sent for the following

- **Flow cytometry:** Quantitates cell surface markers and can also establish clonality
- **Fluorescent in situ hybridization (FISH):** A sensitive method of determining specific cytogenetic abnormalities; does not require proliferating cells and can thus be done on peripheral blood but limited to specific probes for known abnormalities
- **Polymerase chain reaction (PCR):** A highly sensitive method for looking at mutations; can be qualitative or quantitative, but limited to known mutations for which there are primers

Bone Marrow Analysis

- A bone marrow examination consists of two components: (1) a bone marrow aspirate and (2) a bone marrow biopsy
  - **The aspirate is a smear of the marrow elements;** it is stained and examined for cell morphology, such as when considering myelodysplastic syndrome, vitamin deficiency, and other conditions
  - Tests performed on a bone marrow aspirate include the following:
    - **Iron staining:** The gold standard for diagnosis of iron deficiency
    - **Culture:** Note that the sensitivities of bone marrow culture and blood culture are similar
    - **Flow cytometry, FISH, and PCR** (as stated previously with peripheral blood)
    - **Cytogenetics:** Often used in the evaluation of leukemias; used to detect chromosomal aberrations, including translocations (such as 9;22 in chronic myeloid leukemia or 15;17 in acute promyelocytic leukemia [the M3 variant of acute myelogenous leukemia]). *Note:* Cytogenetic analysis requires dividing cells, which are usually found only in the marrow (as opposed to peripheral blood); it is less sensitive than FISH or PCR but not limited by specific probes
  - The bone marrow biopsy is a core biopsy that is then decalcified
    - **The bone marrow biopsy is most helpful in determining cellularity** (e.g., hypocellular, as in aplastic anemia, or hypercellular, as in myelodysplastic syndrome), in assessing fibrosis or marrow replacement by tumor (mestastatic or hematologic), and in determining the relative

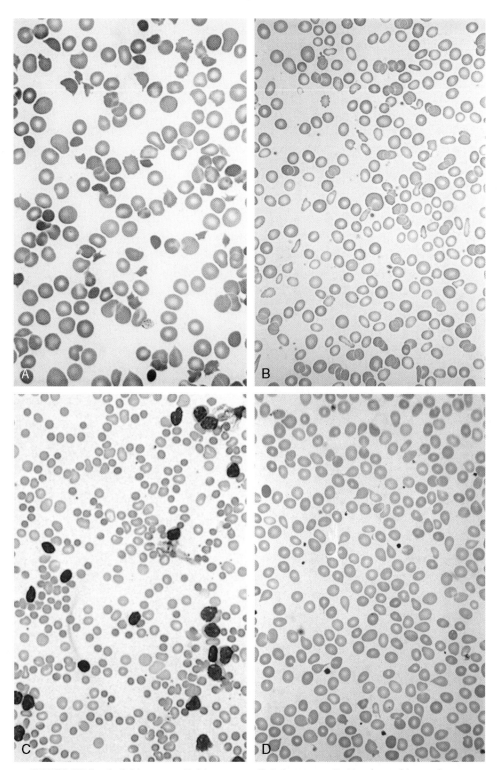

FIGURE 52-1 **A,** Schistocytes. **B,** Macrocytes. **C,** Spherocytes. **D,** Teardrops, bizarre shapes.

quantities of cell populations in a marrow (e.g., increased number of plasma cells in myeloma and normal to increased megakaryocytes in idiopathic thrombocytopenic purpura [ITP])

- Tests performed on the biopsy include the following:
  - Immunohistochemical stains for specific cell populations (such as κ or λ)
  - Special stains for fibrosis (reticulin) or amyloid (Congo red)
  - Stains for infections (fungal, acid-fast bacilli, some viral antigens)
- Indications for bone marrow analysis
  - **Bone marrow aspirate** is used for evaluation of:
    - Pancytopenia
    - Unexplained anemias (especially with teardrops or bizarre forms on PBS)
    - Isolated thrombocytopenia (if the patient > 50 years, if there are any other abnormalities in the CBC

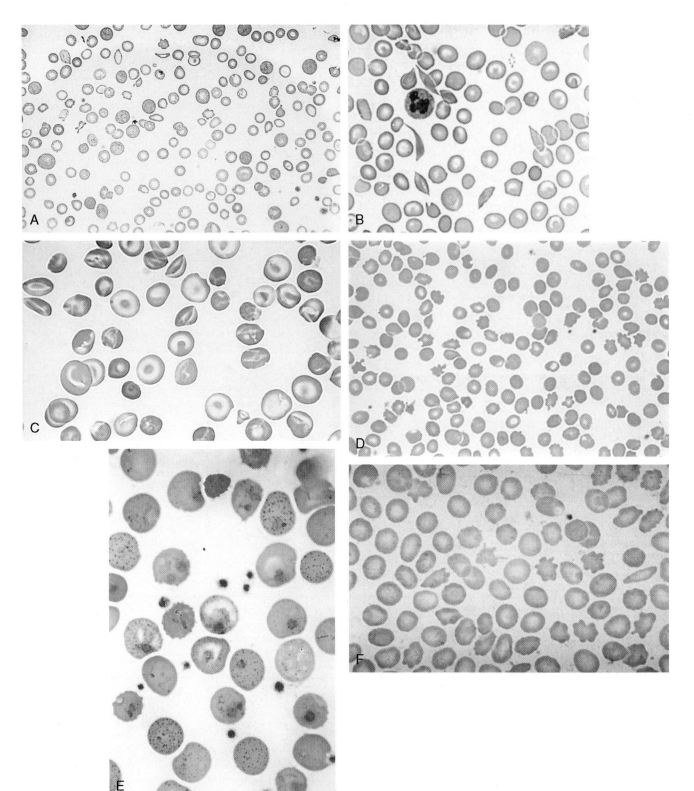

FIGURE 52-2 **A,** Hypochromic, microcytic. **B,** Sickle cells. **C,** Target cells. **D,** Burr cells. **E,** Basophilic stippling. **F,** Acanthocytes.

or in the PBS, or if there are other concerns for myelodysplasia)
- Suspected hematologic malignancy
- *Note:* Bone marrow aspirate has a relatively low yield for evaluation of fever of unknown origin or aggressive lymphoma (excisional biopsy of an affected lymph node is preferred)

- **Bone marrow biopsy** is used for evaluation of:
  - **Overall cellularity** of bone marrow (normal overall cellularity can be approximated by 100 minus the patient's age; so for a 70-year-old patient, the bone marrow should be 30% cellular)
  - **Diagnosis (and staging) of a suspected clonal process:** The biopsy can be stained for cell markers

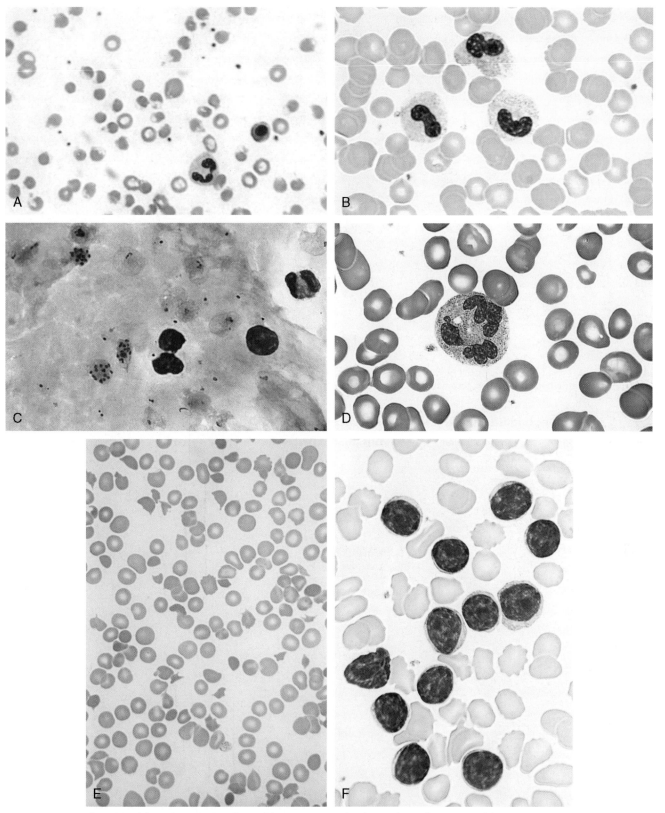

FIGURE 52-3 Leukopenia with nucleated RBCs (**A**) and hyposegmented polymorphonuclear neutrophils (PMNs) (**B**). **C,** Parasite inclusions. **D,** Leukopenia with hypersegmented PMNs. **E,** Microangiopathic hemolytic anemia with schistocytes and thrombocytopenia. **F,** Lymphocytosis with normal-appearing lymphocytes.

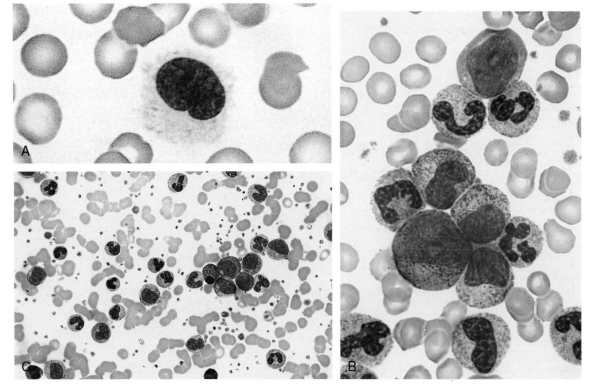

FIGURE 52-4 **A,** Lymphocytosis with cell membrane projections. **B** and **C,** Leukocytosis with wide range of immature forms, including blasts. (Note the large nuclei with open chromatin and prominent nuclei, seen well in part B.)

TABLE 52-1	*Abnormalities on Peripheral Blood Smear (PBS): Red Blood Cells*		
Findings on PBS	**Appearance**	**Differential Diagnosis**	**Further Testing***
Hypochromic, microcytic		Iron deficiency Thalassemia Anemia of chronic disease	Iron studies; Hb electrophoresis
Target cells		Hemoglobin C Liver disease Thalassemia	Hb electrophoresis; studies of liver function
Basophilic stippling		Hemolysis Lead poisoning Thalassemia	Coomb's testing; lead levels; Hb electrophoresis; reticulocyte count
Sickle cells		Sickle cell syndromes	Hb electrophoresis
Burr cells		Renal disease	Studies of renal function

TABLE 52-1	*Abnormalities on Peripheral Blood Smear (PBS): Red Blood Cells (Continued)*		
Findings on PBS	**Appearance**	**Differential Diagnosis**	**Further Testing***
Acanthocytes		Liver disease Abetalipoproteinemia	Studies of liver function; lipid profile
Schistocytes		Microangiopathic hemolytic anemia (e.g., TTP, DIC) Malignant hypertension Prosthetic heart valve	See Chapter 47
Spherocytes		Immune hemolytic anemia Spherocytosis	See Chapter 47

Macrocytes		Vitamin B_{12} deficiency
		Folate deficiency
		Myelodysplastic syndrome
		Liver disease
		Hypothyroidism
			Serum vitamin B_{12} levels, RBC folate;
			  TSH; liver function tests; bone
			  marrow examination

Teardrops, nucleated RBC,
  bizarre forms
		Myelofibrosis
		Marrow infiltration (e.g., tumor,
		  tuberculosis)
			Bone marrow examination;
			  splenomegaly suggests
			  extramedullary hematopoiesis

Bite cells		G6PD deficiency Unstable hemoglobinopathy	Enzyme assays; drug history; Heinz body preparation; heat stability test

Parasite inclusions		Malaria (shown)
		Babesiosis
			Thick and thin blood smear remains
			  gold standard for diagnosis of
			  malaria; polymerase chain reaction
			  and antibody testing now available
			  for babesiosis

*See also Chapter 47.
DIC, disseminated intravascular coagulopathy; G6PD, glucose-6-phosphate dehydrogenase; Hb, hemoglobin; TSH, thyroid-stimulating hormone; TTP, thrombotic thrombocytopenic purpura.

(e.g., if most plasma cells stain κ positive, not λ, a monoclonal process such as myeloma is suggested). Bone marrow biopsy is part of the staging workup for lymphoma.

- Bone marrow biopsy can also be examined for fungus, acid-fast bacilli, or granuloma, which may greatly facilitate the diagnosis of some infectious disorders

SUGGESTED READINGS

Hoffbrand AV, Pettit JE: *Clinical haematology*, London, Gower Medical Publishing, 1988.
Hoffbrand AV, Pettit JE: *Color atlas of clinical hematology*, ed 3, London, Mosby, 2000.
Tkachuk DC, Hirschmann JV, McArthur JR: *Atlas of clinical hematology*, Philadelphia, WB Saunders, 2002.
Zucker-Franklin D: *Atlas of blood cells: function and pathology*, ed 2, Philadelphia, Lea & Febiger, 1988.

TABLE 52-2	Abnormalities on Peripheral Blood Smear (PBS): Platelet and Leukocyte Disorders		
Findings on PBS	**Appearance**	**Differential Diagnosis**	**Further Testing**
Thrombocytopenia		Idiopathic thrombocytopenic purpura (if RBC fragments present, suspect microangiopathic hemolytic anemia)	Bone marrow examination if patient > 50 yr old, other cytopenias present, or any other abnormality seen on the PBS; immature platelet fraction (typically high if destructive cause)
Leukopenia with hyposegmented PMNs		Myelodysplastic syndrome Stress, infection Pelger-Huët anomaly	Bone marrow examination with cytogenetics/FISH if myelodysplastic syndrome suspected
Leukopenia with hypersegmented PMNs		Vitamin B_{12} deficiency Folate deficiency	Serum B_{12} and RBC folate levels
Lymphocytosis with normal-appearing lymphocytes		Chronic lymphocytic leukemia	Flow cytometry
Lymphocytosis with cell membrane projections		Hairy cell leukemia	Flow cytometry
Lymphocytosis with open nuclei/nucleoli		Activated lymphocytes (e.g., seen in viral infection)	Clinical correlation and viral serologies as appropriate; flow cytometry to rule out leukemia/lymphoma
Leukocytosis with wide range of immature forms		Reactive bone marrow (i.e., leukemoid reaction) Chronic myelogenous leukemia Myeloproliferative neoplasm	Clinical correlation and bone marrow examination (with additional studies) as appropriate
Immature cells (blasts)		Leukemia	Bone marrow examination with flow cytometry; cytogenetics/FISH/PCR (see also Chapter 57)
Blasts with Auer rods		Acute myeloid leukemia	Bone marrow examination with flow cytometry; cytogenetics/FISH/PCR (see also Chapter 57)

FISH, fluorescent in situ hybridization; PCR, polymerase chain reaction; PMNs, polymorphonuclear neutrophils.

SECTION NINE

 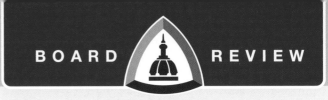

Oncology

Colorectal Cancer

MARK LEVIS, MD, PhD

Colorectal cancer (CRC) is the third most common malignancy seen in both men and women. Over 100,000 cases of colon cancer are diagnosed each year, making it a disease that ultimately affects 6% of the population in the United States.

Basic Information

- Epidemiology
  - Starting at age 40 years, CRC incidence increases with age, with a mean presentation between ages 60 and 65 years
  - Incidence higher in developed countries
  - Third leading cause of cancer deaths
    - 57,000 deaths each year in the United States
  - African Americans have a higher incidence and mortality from CRC than any other ethnic group
- Etiology
  - CRC development proceeds in stepwise fashion from adenoma to invasive carcinoma, with accumulation of oncogenic mutations (Fig. 53-1)
- Classification by location
  - Rectal cancers are those arising below the peritoneal reflection or less than 12 to 15 cm from the anal verge
  - Cancers arising proximal to this area are designated as colon cancers
  - Incidence of CRC by anatomic location (Table 53-1)

- Risk factors
  - Polyposis syndromes are associated with a higher risk of CRC (Table 53-2)
  - **Familial adenomatous polyposis (FAP) increases risk to almost 100% unless prophylactic total colectomy is performed (Fig. 53-2)**
  - Hereditary nonpolyposis colon cancer (HNPCC)— also known as the Lynch syndromes (Table 53-3)—can increase risk as much as seven times that of the general population
    - Lynch syndromes are associated with *mutHLS* gene complex leading to genetic instability; 4% of CRC cases
      - Usually right-sided lesions
      - Median age 44 years
      - Prognosis not worse than in sporadic tumors
      - Caused by germ-line mutations of DNA mismatch repair genes (*MLH1, MSH2, PMS1, PMS2*)
      - Total colectomy recommended by some authorities after diagnosis of this syndrome; most recommend total colectomy after a recurrence
  - Risk increases in patients with personal or family history of sporadic CRC or adenoma
  - **Sporadic CRC occurs in 80% of the cases, with mutations of adenomatous polyposis coli (APC) gene found in 70% of sporadic tumors**
  - There is also a higher incidence of CRC in patients with inflammatory bowel disease (IBD), either ulcerative colitis or Crohn's disease

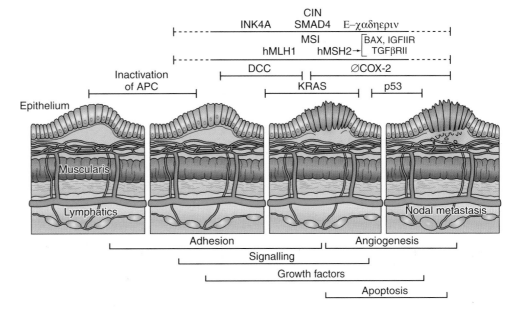

FIGURE 53-1 Adenoma-to-carcinoma sequence and the associated molecular alterations involved in colon cancer development. (From Abeloff MD, Armitage JO, Niederhuber JE, et al: *Clinical oncology,* ed 3, Philadelphia, Churchill Livingstone, 2004, figure 80-3.)

TABLE 53-1	*Location of Colorectal Cancers*
Location	**Incidence (%)**
Cecum	12.5
Ascending colon	9
Transverse colon	11
Descending colon	6.1
Sigmoid colon	23.6
Rectosigmoid junction	8.6
Rectum	22.1

- Risk is associated with duration of IBD, extent of disease, and development of mucosal dysplasia
- Weaker risk factors include environmental, nutritional, and lifestyle factors
  - Increased risk of CRC is associated with higher total calories, animal fat, and protein in diet
  - Lower risk is associated with increased calcium; vitamins A, C, D; folate; and selenium
  - Dietary fiber is currently an area of controversy
- ***Streptococcus bovis* bacteremia: Patients who develop this condition have a high incidence of occult CRC**

Clinical Presentation

- Clinical presentations may differ depending on the tumor location
- Right-sided lesions commonly produce the following
  - Vague abdominal aching
  - Abdominal mass
  - Anemia from chronic blood loss (Fig. 53-3)
  - Fatigue
- Left-sided tumors more commonly produce the following
  - Obstructive symptoms
  - Colicky abdominal pain
  - Changes in bowel habits, with or without rectal bleeding
- Rectal tumors commonly present with the following
  - Change in caliber of stools

- Sensation of rectal fullness
- Urgency
- Hematochezia, tenesmus
- **Pelvic pain usually indicates local extension into pelvic nerves (later stage of disease)**

Diagnosis and Evaluation

- Screening
  - Because the only definitive cure is via surgical resection, detection at an early stage is imperative
  - The American Cancer Society (ACS) recommends the following tests and precautions:
    - Fecal occult blood test (FOBT) annually beginning at age 50 years
    - Plus flexible sigmoidoscopy every 3 to 5 years, colonoscopy every 10 years, or a double-contrast barium enema every 5 to 10 years
    - Although there are no proven screening recommendations for high-risk patients, it is reasonable to begin screening at an earlier age and conduct it with increased frequency in these populations
  - The United States Preventive Services Task Force (USPSTF) recommends:
    - Annual high-sensitivity FOBT or sigmoidoscopy every 5 years combined with high-sensitivity FOBT every 3 years or screening colonoscopy at intervals of 10 years
    - **Against routine screening in patients older than age 75 years**
    - Definitive evidence to support screening with CT colonography or fecal DNA tests is currently lacking
- Initial diagnostic evaluation for suggested CRC
  - Complete history and physical examination is warranted
  - Preoperative staging includes the following
    - Complete blood count
    - Liver function tests
    - Renal function studies
    - Urinalysis
    - Serum carcinoembryonic antigen (CEA)
    - Chest radiograph
    - CT scans of the abdomen and pelvis
    - TNM staging (Table 53-4)

TABLE 53-2	*Polyposis Syndromes*	
Syndrome	**Inheritance Pattern**	**Clinical Features**
Familial adenomatous polyposis 1% of colorectal cancer (CRC) cases	Autosomal dominant	Pancolonic adenomatous polyposis by late adolescence; almost all patients will develop CRC unless prophylactic colectomy is performed
Gardner's syndrome	Autosomal dominant	Small- and large-bowel adenomas, extracolonic tumors of soft tissue (desmoid tumors, fibromas, lipomas), bone (osteomas), and ampulla; epidermoid and sebaceous cysts also associated; almost all patients will develop CRC
Turcot's syndrome	Autosomal recessive	Bowel polyposis associated with malignant CNS tumors; CRC commonly develops
Peutz-Jeghers syndrome	Autosomal dominant	Hamartomas of the small intestine and colon; also associated with mucocutaneous pigmented lesions of the hands, feet, and mouth; tumors of ovary, breast, pancreas, and endometrium can be seen; rarely transforms to malignancy
Juvenile polyposis	Autosomal dominant	Hamartomas may be limited to the stomach or colon or may be distributed throughout the GI tract; low malignant potential

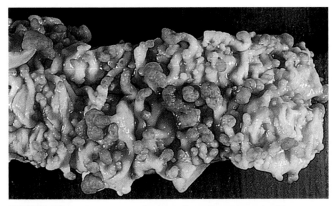

FIGURE 53-2 A segment of a large intestine covered with adenomatous polyps in a patient with familial adenomatous polyposis. The entire colon is covered with hundreds of polyps. (From Skarin AT, Shaffer K, Wieczorek T, editors: *Atlas of diagnostic oncology,* ed 3, St. Louis, Mosby, 2003, p 153. In Abeloff MD, Armitage JO, Niederhuber JE, et al: *Clinical oncology,* ed 3, Philadelphia, Churchill Livingstone, 2004, figure 80-7.)

TABLE 53-3	*Lynch Syndromes (HNPCC)*
Lynch I	Autosomal dominant trait, early-onset trait; early development of primarily proximal colon cancers; colon specific
Lynch II	Associated with colonic and extracolonic adenocarcinomas of the ovary, breast, stomach, small bowel, endometrium, pancreas, bile duct, kidney, and urinary tract

Treatment

- Surgical treatment
  - The primary goal of surgery is resection for cure
  - In the setting of known metastatic disease, the need for surgery depends on the presence or risk of obstruction or bleeding
  - Types of surgical resections performed also depend on location and extent of tumor. Right, transverse, or left hemicolectomy; wide sigmoid resection; or a low anterior resection with end-to-end anastomosis for proximal rectal cancers may be performed.
  - For distal rectal tumors, when unable to spare the sphincter, abdominoperineal resection with permanent colostomy is often necessary
  - An alternative procedure for tumors 2 to 5 cm from the anal verge is a coloanal anastomosis
  - In selected rectal cancer cases with tumors smaller than 3 to 4 cm, T1, well to moderately differentiated, and without lymphovascular involvement, local excision alone may be performed with a full-thickness negative margin
  - Preoperative endorectal ultrasound is an extremely useful tool in defining lesions that are amenable to local excision alone
- Postoperative adjuvant therapy
  - Offered to those at high risk for recurrence because approximately 50% of CRC patients die secondary to metastatic disease
  - For colon cancer
    - The current standard adjuvant chemotherapy regimen in the United States is 5-fluorouracil (5-FU) and leucovorin, with or without oxaliplatin

53

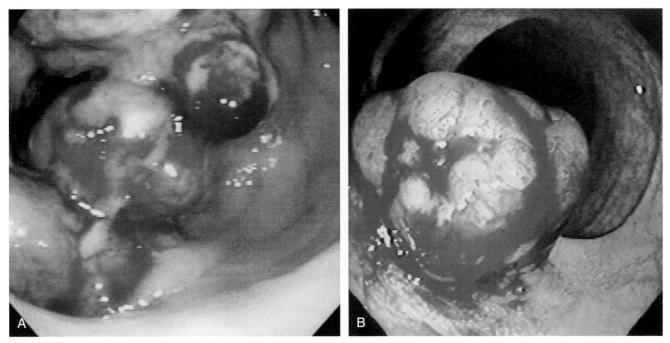

FIGURE 53-3 Colonoscopic view of bleeding carcinomas of the sigmoid colon (**A**) and cecum (**B**). Carcinomas of the colon often bleed intermittently. Patients may present with evidence of microcytic anemia or with red blood per rectum (hematochezia), depending on tumor site and amount of blood loss. (From Feldman M: *Sleisenger and Fordtran's gastrointestinal and liver disease,* ed 7, Philadelphia, WB Saunders, 2002, figure 115-22.)

TABLE 53-4 *TNM Staging for Colorectal Cancer*

TNM Stage	Distant Metastasis	Primary Tumor	Lymph Node Classification	Duke's Metastasis
0	Tis (carcinoma in situ)	N0 (no regional lymph node metastasis)	M0 (no distant metastasis)	—
I	T1 (tumor invades the submucosa) T2 (tumor invades the muscularis propria)	N0	M0	A B1
II	T3 (tumor invades through the muscularis propria)	N0	M0	
IIA	Any T	N1 (metastasis in 1–3 pericolic or perirectal lymph nodes)	M0	C
IIIB	Any T	N2 (metastasis in ≥4 pericolic or perirectal lymph nodes along the course of a named vascular trunk)	M0	C
IV	Any T	Any N	M1 (distant metastasis)	D

TABLE 53-5 *Surveillance of Patients after Treatment for Colon Cancer*

Surveillance Method	Frequency/Comment
Colonoscopy	At 1 yr after surgery, then every 3 yr if no polyps on previous endoscopy
Physical examination including rectal examination	Every 3 mo for 2 yr, then every 6 mo until 5 yr post-therapy (for stage II and III disease)
Fecal occult blood testing	Every 3 mo for 2 yr, then every 6 mo until 5 yr post-therapy (for stage II and III disease)
CBC and chemistries	Every 3 mo for 2 yr, then every 6 mo until 5 yr post-therapy (for stage II and III disease)
Carcinoembryonic antigen	Every 6 mo for 2 yr, then annually for 5 yr if it was elevated at diagnosis or after surgery
Chest radiograph	Every 12 mo for 5 yr in patients who received adjuvant therapy
Chest and abdominal CT	Every 6 mo for 2 yr, then annually for 3 yr in patients who have undergone resection or liver or lung metastases

- **Adjuvant chemotherapy has been demonstrated to significantly improve survival in stage III disease**
- Benefit of chemotherapy in stage II patients is currently unclear
- Radiation therapy is not routinely used adjuvantly; however, it may be useful in achieving better local control in T4 tumors
- For rectal cancer
  - The combination of radiation therapy and 5-FU does increase locoregional control, disease-free survival, and overall survival for stages II and III
  - With the preoperative use of combined-modality treatment, locally advanced (T3 or T4) or unresectable cancer may be rendered resectable and sphincter preservation can be achieved
- Recurrence patterns
  - Sites of colon cancer recurrence
    - Peritoneum
    - Liver
    - Other distant sites
  - Rectal cancer commonly associated with locoregional recurrences; in these cases, radiation therapy is important for local control
  - Recurrence evaluation

- If a patient is found to have only an elevated CEA, colonoscopy and CT scans of chest, abdomen, and pelvis should be performed
- If imaging is negative, repeat CT scans should be ordered every 3 months
- If imaging is positive, patients should undergo salvage therapy
- Treatment of local recurrence and metastatic disease
  - Local recurrences
    - Whenever possible, resection is recommended
    - Recurrence to regional or retroperitoneal lymph nodes is associated with poor prognosis
    - Pelvic recurrences may be cured by pelvic exenteration in some patients
  - Recurrences in the liver
    - If the liver is the only site of recurrence, resection of liver metastasis is a viable treatment option in selected patients
  - In the setting of metastatic disease
    - 5-FU-based chemotherapy (preceded by leucovorin) is still the standard systemic palliative treatment, with other agents such as anti-epidermal growth factor receptor monoclonal antibodies, irinotecan, and oxaliplatin available

- Palliative radiation therapy in situ regionally recurrent rectal cancer
    - Can decrease pain and bleeding in 70% to 80% of patients
- Prognosis
    - At diagnosis, 25% of colon cancers have extended through the bowel wall. Of all rectal cancers, up to 60% have extended through the bowel wall or to regional lymph nodes.
    - **The most common site of distant metastasis is the liver**
    - The most commonly affected extra-abdominal organ is the lung
    - Stage of disease is the single most significant prognostic factor
    - Other unfavorable clinical prognostic factors include the following
        - Long duration of symptoms
        - Bowel obstruction or perforation
        - Elevated preoperative CEA level
    - Surveillance after therapy (Table 53-5)

REVIEW QUESTIONS

For review questions, please go to www.expertconsult.com.

SUGGESTED READINGS

Engstrom PF, Arnoletti JP, Benson AB, et al: Colon cancer clinical practice guidelines in oncology, *J Natl Compr Canc Netw* 5:884–925, 2007.

Kemeny N: Management of liver metastases from colorectal cancer, *Oncology* 20:1161–1176, 1179, 2006.

Krook JE, Moertel CG, Gunderson LL, et al: Effective surgical adjuvant therapy for high-risk rectal carcinoma, *N Engl J Med* 324:709–715, 1991.

Mamounas EP, Wieand S, Wolmark N, et al: Comparative efficacy of adjuvant chemotherapy in patients with Duke's B versus Duke's C colon cancer: results from four National Surgical Adjuvant Breast and Bowel Project adjuvant studies (C-01, C-02, C-03, and C-04), *J Clin Oncol* 17:1349–1355, 1999.

Vasen HF, Moslein G, Alonso A, et al: Guidelines for the clinical management of familial adenomatous polyposis (FAP), *Gut* 57: 704–713, 2008.

53

Breast and Ovarian Cancer

DEBORAH K. ARMSTRONG, MD

Breast cancer is the most commonly diagnosed malignancy in women, affecting 1 out of every 8 women in the United States. It is the second most common cause of cancer deaths in women. Ovarian cancer is less prevalent, affecting 1 out of every 50 to 70 women, but it is associated with high mortality rates because of difficulties in diagnosing early-stage disease. This chapter provides an overview of these two very important malignancies.

Breast Cancer

Basic Information

- Affects 12% of the female population in the United States
  - Less than 1% of breast cancer cases occur in men
- There are significant variations in breast cancer incidence and mortality between countries. This is thought to be due to variations in genetic, reproductive, environmental, dietary, and social factors.
  - Japan and other Asian countries have the lowest death rates
  - England and Wales have the highest death rates
- A number of breast cancer risk factors have been identified (Box 54-1)
- Genetics of breast cancer
  - **More than 90% of breast cancer cases appear to be sporadic without an apparent familial or genetic predisposition**
  - Approximately 10% of breast cancers appear to be familial
  - Factors suggestive of a familial or genetic inheritance of breast cancer

- Multiple affected family members
- Multiple generations involved
- Early age of onset (before age 50)
- Bilateral disease
- Presence of ovarian cancer within the family
- Male breast cancer (associated with *BRCA2*)
  - *BRCA* mutations
    - The two *BRCA* genes account for the vast majority of identified genetic mutations associated with breast cancer
    - Lifetime breast cancer risk in women with a deleterious *BRCA* mutation is 40% to 85%
    - Lifetime risk of male breast cancer is 6% for *BRCA2* carriers
    - The inheritance pattern is autosomal dominant
    - The *BRCA* genes are not sex-linked, but they are silent in most males
    - There is a high penetrance of disease in female carriers
    - Certain *BRCA* mutations are seen more often in specific populations (i.e., three founder mutations in people of Ashkenazi Jewish descent)
    - **Hormonal prevention with tamoxifen or raloxifen, oophorectomy, and mastectomy are all possible prophylactic measures in *BRCA*-positive patients**
- Breast cancer screening (Table 54-1)
- Pathology
  - Generally classified by the anatomic area of the breast that is affected (ducts versus lobules), by the level of tumor invasion (carcinoma in situ versus invasive carcinoma) and grade of the tumor cells
    - Ductal carcinoma in situ (DCIS) is a marker for development of subsequent invasive disease at the same site

BOX 54-1	Risk Factors Associated with Breast Cancer

Known carrier of a deleterious *BRCA-1* or *BRCA-2* mutation
Personal history of prior breast, endometrial, or ovarian cancer
Family history of breast or ovarian cancer
Increasing age
Nulliparity or late age at first pregnancy (age 30 yr or older)
Absence of breast feeding
Early menarche
Late menopause
Hormone replacement therapy
Prior breast biopsy, especially with documented hyperplasia
Prior radiation to breast area (e.g., mantle radiation for lymphoma)

TABLE 54-1	American Cancer Society Breast Cancer Screening Recommendations*

Age (yr)	Examination	Frequency
20–39	Breast self-examination Clinical breast examination	Monthly Every 3 yr
≥40	Breast self-examination Clinical breast examination Mammography	Monthly Yearly Yearly

*Women at increased risk due to family history, genetic risk, or prior breast cancer should have individualized recommendations that may include starting mammography earlier, additional screening tests such as breast ultrasound or MRI, or having more frequent exams.

- **Lobular carcinoma in situ (LCIS) is a marker for development of invasive cancer in either breast, so close surveillance of both breasts is required**
- Infiltrating (invasive) ductal carcinoma is the most common histologic type of breast cancer

Clinical Presentation and Diagnosis

- **Most cases manifest as a palpable breast mass or abnormality on mammogram**
  - Palpable breast mass
    - **A mammogram should be obtained after discovering a mass; however, the absence of a mammographic abnormality does not eliminate the need for tissue diagnosis of a new palpable mass**
  - Tissue diagnosis
    - Fine-needle aspiration does not preserve tissue architecture and is most appropriate for possible benign cystic lesions
    - **Incisional (core) biopsy maintains tissue architecture of the sample and is the best approach for diagnosis, but the lesion is not completely removed**
    - Excisional biopsy involves complete removal of the lesion
  - Mammographic abnormality
    - Risk of the abnormality is stratified based on patient history, exam findings, and imaging characteristics
    - A core biopsy of a mammographic abnormality is frequently done by the radiologist with the assistance of imaging

Treatment

- DCIS
  - Requires complete excision (goal of attaining negative margins)
  - May be treated with lumpectomy and radiation therapy (RT) or mastectomy
  - Lymph node evaluation not required for pure DCIS without invasion
  - **Tamoxifen decreases local recurrence after lumpectomy, and RT and decreases risk of a contralateral cancer**
- LCIS
  - The optimal treatment strategy is unknown at this time and may involve careful surveillance of both breasts, with or without tamoxifen therapy, or bilateral prophylactic mastectomies
  - Excision of the lesion is recommended to rule out invasion, but negative margins are not required
  - Lymph node evaluation not required for pure LCIS without invasion
- Invasive breast cancer
  - Local control of disease in the breast
    - Removal of the tumor
      - Modified radical mastectomy (MRM) involves removal of the breast and draining axillary lymph nodes, sparing the musculature of the chest wall
      - Lumpectomy involves removal of tumor with the goal of attaining pathologically negative margins and requires RT for optimal control; contraindicated in patients who are pregnant,

have a history of prior radiation to the breast, have evidence of diffuse breast calcifications, have certain connective tissue disorders, or have more than one distinct tumor
    - Pathologic evaluation of the regional lymph nodes can be done by sentinel lymph node biopsy. Complete axillary lymph node dissection is required if the sentinel node is positive for cancer or when nodes are known to be involved with cancer.
    - RT is used after lumpectomy and for selected node-positive patients after mastectomy
    - Choosing between lumpectomy plus RT and MRM
      - **Survival is equivalent**
      - Most patients (>80%) are good candidates for lumpectomy plus RT; patient preference is a critical element
      - In patients with large tumors, large breast size, or tumors under the nipple, mastectomy may be preferable because of poor cosmetic outcome
      - Approximately 9% risk of local recurrence in the conserved breast with lumpectomy plus RT (0.5–1% per year)
      - Local recurrences after lumpectomy can be salvaged with MRM
  - Staging (Box 54-2)
  - Poor prognostic factors
    - Larger tumor size
    - Axillary lymph node metastases
    - Absent estrogen/progesterone receptor (ER/PR)
    - Poor nuclear grade
    - Elevated measures of proliferation (S-phase fraction, Ki67)
    - Molecular markers such as *Her-2/neu* are increasingly used to aid in prognosis and to direct treatment
      - **Tumors that have negative ER, PR, and *Her-2/neu* carry an especially poor prognosis and are referred to as "triple-negative" breast cancer**
  - Adjuvant systemic therapy
    - Even though 90% of women present with apparently localized disease (i.e., breast and regional lymph nodes), only about 70% will be free of disease 5 years later, despite adequate local therapy

---

BOX 54-2 — *Simplified Staging Schema for Invasive Breast Cancer*

Stage I: Small primary tumor (≤2 cm), negative nodes, no distant metastases

Stage II: Involved axillary lymph nodes *or* large primary tumor (>2 cm), no distant metastases

Stage III: Locally advanced disease

Large tumor and involved nodes

Matted or fixed axillary nodes

Tumor with direct extension to the skin or chest wall

Inflammatory breast cancer: Redness, warmth, peau d'orange skin changes

Stage IV: Distant metastases; common sites (in order of frequency) are bone, lung, liver, adrenals, and brain/cerebrospinal fluid

TABLE 54-2 *Adjuvant Therapy for Breast Cancer*

	Node-Negative	Node-Positive	Node-Positive and *Her-2* Positive
Premenopausal			
Estrogen receptor-positive	Hormone Rx ± chemotherapy	Chemotherapy + hormone Rx	Chemotherapy + trastuzumab + hormone Rx
Estrogen receptor-negative	Chemotherapy	Chemotherapy	Chemotherapy + trastuzumab
Postmenopausal			
Estrogen receptor-positive	Hormone Rx	Hormone Rx ± chemotherapy	Chemotherapy + trastuzumab + hormone Rx
Estrogen receptor-negative	Chemotherapy	Chemotherapy	Chemotherapy + trastuzumab

- **Adjuvant therapy is given when no disease is apparent, with the goal of eradicating potential micrometastatic disease and thereby reducing the risk of relapse**
- Important factors to keep in mind with regard to adjuvant therapy:
    - The higher the risk of relapse, the greater the absolute reduction in the risk of relapse with adjuvant therapy
    - The choice of the type of adjuvant therapy is based on patient factors (age, comorbidities and menopausal status) and on disease factors (nodal status, hormone receptor status [ER/PR], and *Her-2/neu* status) (Table 54-2)
    - In certain clinical situations a genetic profile of the tumor (e.g., oncotype DX) can aid in predicting relapse risk and has the benefit of adding chemotherapy
- See following sections for types of adjuvant therapy (e.g., hormone therapy, chemotherapy, antibody therapy)
    - Hormonal therapy
        - Used when the tumor expresses ER, PR, or both
        - The highest response rates seen when both receptors expressed
        - Response rate negligible when neither receptor expressed
        - Generally recommended for 5 years; sequential use of different agents may extend duration of therapy
        - Postmenopausal patients
            - Tamoxifen: Mixed ER antagonist/agonist (Box 54-3)
            - Aromatase inhibitors (e.g., anastrozole, letrozole, exemestane)—prevent conversion of androgens to estrogen thereby suppressing plasma estrogen levels
        - Premenopausal patients
            - Surgical removal of the ovaries
            - Radiation of the ovaries (rarely used in the United States)
            - Inhibition of the pituitary-hypothalamic-gonadal axis with gonadotropin-releasing hormone analogues (goserelin, leuprolide acetate)
            - Tamoxifen: Mixed ER antagonist/agonist (see Box 54-3)
            - The toxic effect of chemotherapy drugs on ovarian follicular cells frequently results in cessation of menses. The closer a woman is to natural menopause, the more likely that amenorrhea will be permanent.

- Chemotherapy
    - Considered for tumors that are more than 1 cm in size and occasionally for smaller aggressive tumors
    - **Shown to increase survival for women younger than 70 years regardless of node or receptor status**
    - The effects of chemotherapy are additive with hormonal therapy when used sequentially. However, they may have antagonistic effects when used together.
    - Breast cancer is responsive to a variety of cytotoxic chemotherapeutic agents, including anthracyclines (doxorubicin, epirubicin), taxanes (paclitaxel, docetaxel), alkylating agents (cyclophosphamide), antimetabolites (5-fluorouracil, capecitabine, gemcitabine), and plant alkyloids (vinorelbine)
    - Combination multiagent chemotherapy for 3 to 6 months standard
- Trastuzumab (Herceptin)
    - *HER-2/neu* proto-oncogene is overexpressed in 20% to 30% of human breast cancers
    - Cell surface localization of *HER-2/neu* allows for immunotherapeutic targeting
    - Trastuzumab: Recombinant humanized anti-*HER-2* monoclonal antibody
        - Synergistic cardiac toxicity when used with doxorubicin

---

BOX 54-3 *Tamoxifen Therapy for Breast Disease*

It is a nonsteroidal antiestrogen when acting on breast tissue

It binds to the estrogen receptor protein and competitively inhibits estrogen action in breast and breast tumors

In some tissues it acts as a partial estrogen agonist

   Uterus: Estrogenic activity of tamoxifen increases endometrial cancer risk (increase of 1–2:1000)

   Bone: Increases bone density and delays bone loss

   Cardiovascular: Lowers low-density lipoprotein and total cholesterol

Side effects

   Hot flashes and other vasomotor symptoms

   Weight gain

   Thromboembolic disease (rare)

   Increased risk of endometrial cancer (rare)

   Keratopathy and optic neuritis (very rare)

- Single-agent activity in *HER-2/neu* overexpressing breast cancer
- At least additive effects in combination with chemotherapeutic agents
- **Significantly improves survival when used with adjuvant chemotherapy in patients with *Her-2* overexpressing tumors**
- Follow-up after diagnosis and treatment of localized breast cancer
  - Regular history and physical examination
  - Standard blood work: CBC, calcium, and liver function testing
  - Yearly mammography; every 6 months for 3 years in involved breast after lumpectomy plus RT
  - CT, nuclear scanning, and tumor markers should not be routinely employed unless specific symptoms or indications dictate their use
- Advanced or recurrent disease
  - Treatment goals for the patient with disseminated breast cancer are to prolong life, improve the quality of life, and palliate symptoms
  - Treatment of advanced disease depends on several factors including prior therapy, time from diagnosis, sites of metastases, hormone receptor status, and *Her-2/neu* status
  - Two-thirds of metastatic breast cancer patients respond to chemotherapy
  - Quality of life is improved for some advanced breast cancer patients receiving chemotherapy
  - Response rates are higher for patients who have received no prior chemotherapy or who have had a long treatment-free interval since prior chemotherapy
  - Patients with lytic bone metastases have decreased skeletal morbidity (pain and fractures) with the use of IV bisphosphonate therapy

Epithelial Ovarian Cancer

Basic Information

- Cancers that arise from the epithelium of the ovary (not germ cell or stromal tumors)
- Fourth leading cause of cancer deaths in American women
- **High mortality because of difficulty in diagnosing localized (early-stage) disease**
- Risk factors
  - Clear-cut cause has not been established for most cases of ovarian cancer
  - Family history
    - Risk of ovarian cancer significantly increased in patients with a familial predisposition (Table 54-3)
    - Patients with *BRCA1* mutations appear to have ovarian cancer onset about 10 years earlier (median age 54 years) than patients with *BRCA2* mutations or sporadic ovarian cancer (64 years)
    - Three inherited genetic mutations currently are associated with an increased risk of ovarian cancer
      - *BRCA1* is associated with a lifetime risk of 14% to 45%

TABLE 54-3	*Familial Risk of Ovarian Cancer**
Relationship	**Risk**
One second-degree relative	1:25 (4%)
One first-degree relative (any age)	1:20 (5%)
Age < 55 yr	1:10 (10%)
Age < 45 yr	1:5 (20%)
Two first-degree relatives	1:2 (50%)

*Familial ovarian cancer accounts for only 5–10% of all cases.

- *BRCA2* is associated with a lifetime risk of 10% to 20%
- Hereditary nonpolyposis colorectal cancer (HNPCC, or Lynch syndrome II, or familial cancer syndrome) associated with increased risk of GI, ovarian, and endometrial cancers (see Chapter 53)
- Direct relationship between number of lifetime ovulations and the risk of ovarian cancer
  - Ovulation causes injury to the epithelial surface of the ovary
  - Repeated injury or the process of repairing injury may contribute to malignant transformation
  - **Conditions that cause a relative increase in the number of ovulations (e.g., early menarche, late menopause, and infertility) associated with an increased risk of ovarian cancer**
  - Conditions that cause a relative decrease in the number of ovulations (e.g., oral contraceptive use, multiple pregnancies, early pregnancy, and breast-feeding for more than a year) associated with a decreased risk of ovarian cancer
- Risk reduction for high-risk patients
  - Oral contraceptives can reduce the risk by more than 50% when used for over 5 years
  - Bilateral oophorectomy
    - The degree of risk reduction is estimated to be 90% to 95%
    - Risk of peritoneal cancer remains and is not reduced by removal of the ovaries
    - Oophorectomy results in premature menopause for menstruating women, thus reducing the risk of breast cancer in these women, but may result in vasomotor symptoms and an increased risk of heart disease and osteoporosis
    - Premenopausal *BRCA* mutation carriers who have undergone prophylactic oophorectomy may take low-dose, short-term hormone replacement therapy to manage hormone withdrawal symptoms without apparent excess risk of breast cancer
  - Close surveillance and screening
- Screening
  - **No ovarian cancer screening techniques have sufficient sensitivity, specificity, or cost-effectiveness to routinely recommend their use for the general population**
  - Screening (with transvaginal ultrasound or cancer antigen 125 [CA-125]) is commonly used in women at high risk for ovarian cancer based on personal or family history

54

Clinical Presentation

- Specific symptoms are uncommon when disease localized to the ovary
- Symptoms of advanced disease vague and nonspecific for ovarian cancer but usually present
  - Abdominal fullness or bloating
  - Pelvic heaviness or pressure
  - Pain with intercourse
  - Vaginal bleeding or discharge
  - GI symptoms such as lack of appetite, nausea, vomiting, constipation
- Tumor spread can occur by a number of different mechanisms
  - Local shedding of tumor cells into the peritoneal cavity followed by implantation on the peritoneal surfaces
  - Local invasion of bowel or bladder
  - Lymphatic spread to local or distant lymph nodes
  - Hematogenous spread to distant sites (parenchyma of liver, lungs, pleura)

Diagnosis

- Not commonly diagnosed by pelvic examination
- Can be found incidentally on ultrasound or CT scan
- Surgical laparotomy necessary for diagnosis, staging, and tumor debulking
- CA-125 tumor marker
  - CA-125 common to most ovarian tumors
  - **82% of advanced ovarian cancer patients have an elevated CA-125, but less than 50% with stage I disease show an elevation**
  - Rising or falling titers correlate with disease in 93% of patients, making it a useful tool for monitoring disease
  - Persistent elevation of CA-125 after treatment strongly associated with residual disease
  - Doubling or an absolute value greater than 100 usually indicates recurrence
  - Even though an elevation of CA-125 may antedate appearance of disease or recurrence, it is not a useful screening tool in unaffected women because of its lack of sensitivity and specificity

Treatment

- Surgery
  - **Aggressive tumor debulking usually indicated even in advanced disease**
  - Volume of tumor after surgery and before chemotherapy major prognostic factor for survival
    - After surgical debulking patients categorized as
      - Optimally debulked (≤1 cm postoperative residual disease)
      - Suboptimally debulked (>1 cm postoperative residual disease)
- Staging (Box 54-4)
- Chemotherapy
  - Chemotherapy is not used in borderline, low malignant potential (LMP), or atypical proliferating tumors

---

BOX 54-4	*Simplified Staging Schema for Ovarian Cancer**

Stage I: Disease limited to the ovaries: 5-year survival, 80–90%

Stage II: Disease confined to the pelvis: 5-year survival, 60–70%

Stage III: Disease spread to upper abdomen or regional lymph nodes: 5-year survival, 15–30%

Stage IV: Distant metastases (liver parenchyma, lung, pleura): 5-year survival, 5–10%

*Stages I and II are considered early ovarian cancer; stages III and IV, advanced ovarian cancer.

- Use of chemotherapy in early stage (stage I or II) invasive ovarian cancer based on risk
  - Patients with well-differentiated stage I tumors have a 5-year disease-free survival rate of over 90% and do not benefit from chemotherapy
  - Chemotherapy justified for patients with high-grade stage I tumors, tumors involving the surface of the ovary, or when there is ascites, positive peritoneal washings, or stage II disease
    - Postoperative, platinum-based chemotherapy, usually in combination with a taxane
    - Three to six courses standard
- Advanced-stage disease (stage III or IV)
  - All patients receive systemic, platinum-based chemotherapy
  - Usually receive six courses of treatment
  - Combination of a taxane (paclitaxel or docetaxel) plus platinum (carboplatin or cisplatin) standard
  - Intraperitoneal administration of chemotherapy improves survival in selected low-volume patients
  - Small percentage of patients (10–15%) will be cured
- Recurrent ovarian cancer
  - High rate of response to therapy but is generally not curable
  - Noncurative treatment can prolong life
  - Number of chemotherapeutic options available

REVIEW QUESTIONS

For review questions, please go to www.expertconsult.com.

SUGGESTED READINGS

Armstrong DK, Bundy B, Wenzel L, et al: Intraperitoneal cisplatin and paclitaxel in ovarian cancer, *N Engl J Med* 354(1):34–43, 2006.

Cannistra SA: Cancer of the ovary, *N Engl J Med* 351(24):2519–2529, 2004.

Gradishar WJ: Safety considerations of adjuvant therapy in early breast cancer in postmenopausal women, *Oncology* 69(1):1–9, 2005.

Kuhl CK, Schrading S, Leutner CC, et al: Mammography, breast ultrasound, and magnetic resonance imaging for surveillance of women at high familial risk for breast cancer, *J Clin Oncol* 23(33):8469–8476, 2005.

Romond EH, Perez EA, Bryant J, et al: Trastuzumab plus adjuvant chemotherapy for operable HER2-positive breast cancer, *N Engl J Med* 353(16):1673–1684, 2005.

Genitourinary Cancer

MICHAEL A. CARDUCCI, MD, FACP, and HANS HAMMERS MD, PhD

Cancers of the genitourinary system are commonly seen in the United States and result in significant morbidity and mortality. Neoplasms of the prostate and testicle are the leading causes of cancer in elderly and young men, respectively. This chapter describes the clinical features of these two cancers, as well as cancers of the bladder and kidney.

Prostate Cancer

Incidence

- Most common cancer for men in the United States
- **One in six lifetime risk for a man to develop invasive prostate cancer**
- For 2008, it is estimated that 186,320 new cases were diagnosed, and 28,660 deaths were attributed to this disease. Second most common cause of cancer death in men after lung cancer

Epidemiology

- The Japanese and mainland Chinese have the lowest rates of invasive prostate cancer
- Incidence of prostate cancer is highest in Scandinavian countries
- Socioeconomic status appears unrelated to risk
- Risk may be inversely related to UV light exposure (vitamin D) because the incidence increases the farther one lives from the equator

Etiology and Risk Factors

- **Age: Nearly 60% of men will have prostate cancer by age 80**
- Family history: Men with a first-degree relative with prostate cancer have a twofold increased risk; an individual with two first-degree relatives with prostate cancer has a ninefold increased risk; hereditary prostate cancer may account for 5% to 10% of all prostate cancers and tends to develop at a very early age (<55 years)
- Race: African Americans have a 9.8% lifetime risk
- Intake of dietary fat may increase the risk of prostate cancer
- Vasectomy, sexual activity, and sexually transmitted disease are not associated with an increased risk in prostate cancer. Some studies have shown a lower risk of prostate cancer with a higher frequency of ejaculation.

Signs and Symptoms

- Early-stage disease
  - **Most are asymptomatic**
  - Some present with bladder outlet obstruction

- Locally advanced disease
  - Bladder outlet obstruction causing urinary frequency, urgency, irritative voiding symptoms, hematuria, or urinary tract infections most commonly seen
  - Extension to seminal vesicles may manifest with hematospermia
  - Extension to the periphery of the gland and involvement of the neurovascular bundles may manifest as impotence or erectile dysfunction
- Advanced disease
  - Bulky lymph node metastasis can manifest with bilateral lower extremity edema
  - **Men with bony metastasis may have bone pain or lower extremity weakness or paralysis from spinal cord compression**

Screening and Diagnosis

- If prostate cancer is detected early, treatment can be effective and result in minimal morbidity
- No universally agreed-on strategic plan for its diagnosis and management
- Digital rectal examination (DRE)
  - 7% to 15% of men older than 50 years will have suggestive results on DRE
  - Positive predictive value of DRE for prostate cancer is 15% to 30%, and varies little with age
  - DRE has 1% to 2% detection rate when used alone
  - **A normal DRE does not reduce the odds of clinically significant prostate cancer**
- Prostate-specific antigen (PSA)
  - Serine protease specific to prostate tissue, not just cancer
  - **Can be elevated from benign prostate hypertrophy, acute prostatitis, transrectal needle biopsy, acute urinary retention, prostate surgery, and ejaculation**
  - In general, DRE does not increase serum PSA
  - It doubles the detection rate of DRE
  - It detects nearly 70% of prostate cancer cases
  - PSA and DRE are complementary as screening tests for prostate cancer
  - PSA levels greater than 4 ng/mL are seen in 15% of men older than 50 years; the probability that this PSA level indicates cancer is 20% to 30%
  - In recent Prostate Cancer Prevention Study, 16% of men diagnosed with prostate cancer had a PSA below 1 ng/mL
  - **Most men with PSA greater than 10 ng/mL and prostate cancer have extracapsular disease that is much less likely to be curable**

- PSA rises of more than 2 ng/mL in year prior to diagnosis is associated with high-risk disease
- American Cancer Society screening recommendations
  - Annual examination with DRE and PSA beginning at age 50 years in patients with an anticipated survival of 10 years
  - Begin earlier (age 40 years) in high-risk groups (e.g., African-American men, those men with a positive family history)
- American College of Physicians recommends that the decision to screen be individualized after discussion with the patient
- The U.S. Preventive Services Task Force (USPSTF) recently concluded that current evidence is insufficient to assess the balance of benefits and harms of prostate cancer screening in men younger than age 75 years. The USPSTF recommends against screening for prostate cancer in men age 75 years or older.
- Transrectal biopsy
  - Should be done only in those patients who would require therapy, either definitive or palliative
  - Men with PSA values greater than 4 ng/mL or an abnormal DRE suggestive of prostate cancer should consider prostate biopsy. Age-specific thresholds and rate of rise within the normal range may be reason to consider biopsy in younger or high-risk men.
  - Side effects of the transrectal biopsy include hematuria, hematochezia, and hematospermia
  - **If the biopsy specimen is negative, the patient should be followed conservatively with serial PSAs and DREs.** Consideration for an earlier repeat biopsy depends on the number of cores taken initially and the pretest likelihood of finding cancer.

Pathology

- Adenocarcinomas make up the vast majority of tumors, although ductal adenocarcinoma, transitional cell carcinoma, and small-cell neuroendocrine tumors can occur
- Most (70%) occur in the peripheral zone of the gland; only 10% occur in the area surrounding the prostatic urethra
- Histologic grade is summarized using the Gleason system
  - Based on architectural patterns of the tumor
  - A score for each cancer based on the sum of the grade assigned to the most predominant (1–5) and secondary (1–5) architectural patterns (Fig. 55-1)
  - Gleason grades 2 to 6 are associated with a better prognosis
  - **The risk of developing metastatic disease with a Gleason grade of 8 to 10 is 75%**
- Adenocarcinoma may spread locally to periprostatic fat, seminal vesicles, and regional lymph nodes; hematogenous spread is predominantly to bone, particularly the lumbosacral spine and the axial skeleton

Staging and Prognosis

- Prognosis depends on tumor stage, Gleason score, and pretreatment PSA value
- Table 55-1 summarizes the basic staging for prostate cancer
- **In general, cure is anticipated for men with organ-confined disease and local treatments.** Men with

recurrence despite local treatment can have a long survival. Median survival for men with PSA recurrence after local therapy is 13 to 15 years. Median survival for men presenting with metastatic disease approaches 7 years.

Treatment

- Needs to be individualized; decisions are based on the disease stage and grade, on pretreatment PSA, and on the patient's age and life expectancy
- Physiologic age is of greater importance than chronologic age
- **Patients with short life expectancy (<10 years) should probably be observed because there is little evidence to support a prolonged life expectancy with interventions**
- Localized disease (stages A and B): Radical prostatectomy and radiation therapy are clearly effective forms of treatment in the attempt to cure tumors limited to the prostate for appropriately selected patients; comparisons across studies suggest comparable 10-year survival rates with either form of management
- Locally advanced disease (stage C): Improved survival may be seen with androgen deprivation (see following discussion) plus radiation
- Advanced disease: First-line therapies include surgical or medical castration (androgen deprivation)
  - Advanced symptomatic or metastatic disease requires medical or surgical castration. Men with PSA recurrence after local therapy have a high likelihood of micrometastatic disease. Use of androgen ablation in the absence of clinically evident or radiographically evident metastasis is commonplace, although this approach has not been clearly shown to improve survival.
  - Androgen ablation is effective in 80% to 90% of patients, with an average duration of response of 18 to 24 months
  - Surgical castration (bilateral orchiectomy) removes testicular androgens. It is a safe and inexpensive procedure that ensures patient compliance; however, the psychological impact can be severe.
  - Medical castration is primarily in the form of luteinizing hormone-releasing hormone (LHRH) agonists. These regulate the release of luteinizing hormone (LH), thereby producing chemical castration by ultimately decreasing testosterone levels.
  - **Androgen ablation is associated with significant hot flashes, sexual dysfunction (e.g., loss of libido, erectile dysfunction, and microgenitalia), decreases in bone and muscle mass, gynecomastia, fatigue, anemia, metabolic syndrome, as well as neurocognitive effects. Use of early androgen ablation for men with PSA recurrence and no radiographic metastasis potentially exposes men to these negative aspects of hormonal therapy without known survival benefit.**
  - Second-line hormonal therapies include the addition and subtraction of antiandrogens, ketoconazole, or estrogens such as diethylstilbestrol. Antiandrogens (e.g., flutamide, nilutamide, bicalutamide) block the effects of androgens at the prostate tissue level by interfering with receptor binding of active androgens. Some experts suggest the addition of antiandrogens to either medical or surgical castration.

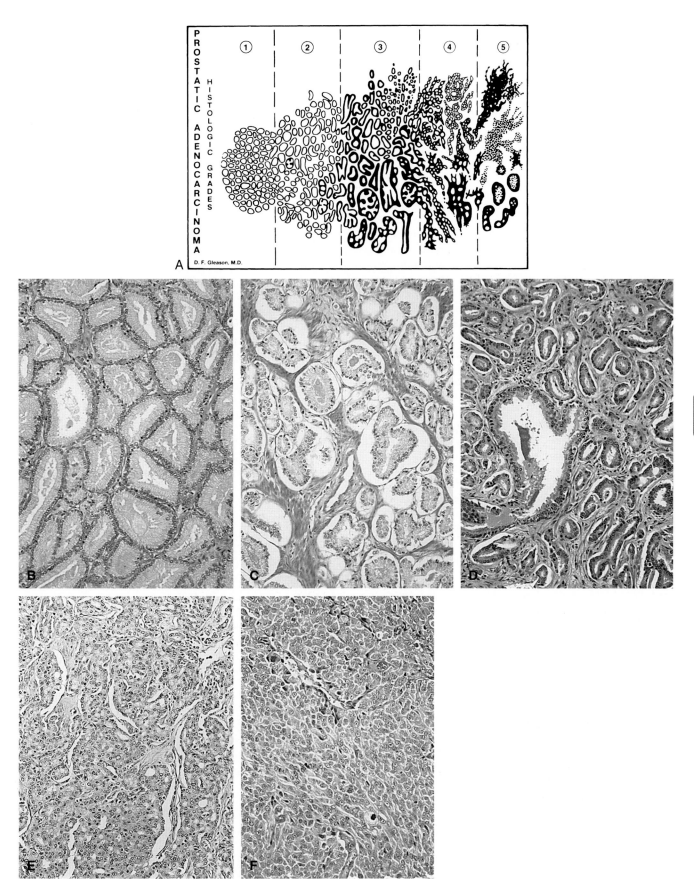

FIGURE 55-1   Gleason scoring system for grading of adenocarcinoma of the prostate. **A,** Schematic of the system. **B** to **F,** Histologic sections showing Gleason patterns 1 through 5, respectively. (From Walsh PC: *Campbell's urology,* ed 8, Philadelphia, WB Saunders, 2002, figure 86.2.)

TABLE 55-1	Simplified Staging System for Prostate Cancer
Stage	**Description**
A	Incidental finding of localized tumor
B	Tumor confined within the prostate capsule
C	Extracapsular disease
D	Disseminated disease to lymph nodes or distant sites

- Antiandrogens are reported to act as agonists in up to 25% of treated men. In these cases, the removal of the antiandrogen may be associated with a clinical response and is receommended for men with a rising PSA or progressive disease while on an antiandrogen.
- Disease progression (rising PSA, new lesions, or new symptoms) while on androgen ablation (castrate levels of testosterone) defines hormone-refractory disease
- Docetaxel and predisone in combination is FDA-approved for men with metastatic hormone-refractory prostate cancer based on randomized, phase III clinical trials demonstrating an improvement in overall survival. Median survival for men receiving docetaxel approximates 19 months.
- Radiopharmaceuticals (strontium-89 and samarium) may be beneficial for men with symptomatic metastatic hormone-refractory cancer. External beam radiation remains an important method to improve pain and reduce fracture at isolated painful bone metastasis.
- The bisphosphonate zolendronic acid is FDA-approved to reduce skeletal-related events (fractures, cord compression) in men with metastatic hormone-refractory prostate cancer. Increases in creatinine and osteonecrosis of the jaw are concerns associated with long-term use of this bisphosphonate.

Urothelial (Bladder, Ureteral, and Renal Pelvis) Cancer

Incidence

- In 2008, an estimated 68,810 cases were diagnosed and 14,100 deaths were attributed to cancer of the bladder
- Bladder cancer is much more common than ureteral cancer or cancer of the renal pelvis
- When cancer of the upper urinary tract is diagnosed there is a 30% to 50% chance of cancer of the bladder developing
- When bladder cancer is diagnosed there is a 2% to 3% chance of developing cancer of upper urinary tract

Epidemiology

- More common in men (3:1); incidence in women increasing secondary to tobacco use
- Peak incidence in the seventh decade of life
- More common in whites than in African Americans

Etiology and Risk Factors

- **Cigarette smoking**
- Analgesic abuse, phenacetin use
- Chronic urinary tract inflammation (stones in upper tract, recurrent infections)
- Occupational exposures (exposure to aryl amines in organic chemicals, rubber, paint, and dyes)
- Balkan nephropathy: A familial nephropathy of unknown cause that results in progressive inflammation of the renal parenchyma, leading to renal failure and multifocal, superficial, low-grade cancers of the renal pelvis and ureters
- *Schistosoma haematobium* infection usually associated with squamous cell carcinoma of the bladder

Signs and Symptoms

- Hematuria: Often painless
- Urinary voiding symptoms (e.g., frequency, urgency, or dysuria)
- Vesical irritation without hematuria: Common in carcinoma in situ of bladder
- Symptoms of advanced disease: Pain from metastatic sites, edema of lower extremities, cough or dyspnea from lung metastases

Diagnosis

- **Excretory urography/IV pyelogram (Fig. 55-2) followed by cystoscopy**
- Retrograde pyelography is best for detecting upper tract lesions
- Urine cytology may be helpful; brush biopsies may increase the diagnostic yield

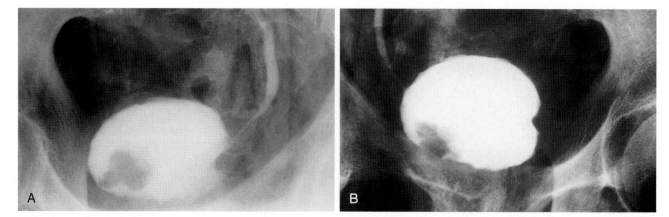

FIGURE 55-2 **A** and **B**, Excretory urography in a patient with a bladder tumor. Note the filling defect in the right inferior portion of the bladder. (From Bragg DG, Rubin P, Hricak H: *Oncologic imaging*, ed 2, Philadelphia, WB Saunders, 2002, figure 30-1.)

- Biopsies of any lesion must be of adequate size to include bladder wall muscle
- CT scan of abdomen: Evaluate for local extension and nodal involvement
- Obtain bone scan if bony symptoms are present
- Chest radiograph completes staging evaluation

Pathology

- Transitional cell carcinoma: 90% to 95% of all urothelial cancers
  - Superficial lesions most commonly low-grade papillary lesions that rarely become invasive
  - Carcinoma in situ (CIS)
    - Often accompanies higher stages of disease
    - Has high likelihood of progressing to muscle-invasive disease
- Squamous cell carcinoma: 3% to 7% of urothelial cancers, mostly renal pelvis and ureters
- Adenocarcinomas: Less than 3% of urothelial cancers; those arising from the dome of the bladder are urachal in origin

Staging and Prognosis

- Most important prognostic factors are T stage (Table 55-2) and differentiation pattern
- Superficial bladder cancer: Papillary tumors that involve only the mucosa (Ta) or submucosa (T1) and flat carcinoma in situ (Tis) (Note: This is different from CIS)
  - Natural history is unpredictable; recurrences are very common
  - Most superficial tumors recur within 6 to 12 months and are the same stage and grade
  - 10% to 15% of superficial cancers develop into invasive or metastatic disease
  - Well-differentiated lesions have a 95% survival rate, whereas high-grade (less differentiated) T1 lesions have a 10-year survival of 50%
- Muscle invasive carcinoma (T3) carries a 5-year survival of 20% to 50%; with regional node involvement and metastatic disease (T4), the 5-year survival is 0% to 20%

Treatment

- Localized disease
  - Superficial bladder cancer
    - Surgical approaches
      - Transurethral resection: Removes existing tumor; patients require close follow-up
      - Laser: Not adopted for general use because of limitations of obtaining stage and grade

TABLE 55-2	Simplified Staging System for Bladder Cancer
Stage	**Description**
Tis, Ta	Noninvasive (superficial) carcinoma
T1	Tumor invades lamina propria
T2	Tumor invades muscle
T3	Tumor invades through muscle into perivesicular fat
T4	Invasion of other structures/organs

- Partial cystectomy: If tumor not accessible or amenable to transurethral resection
- **Radical cystectomy: Generally not used for superficial bladder cancer; indications are unusually large tumors, some high-grade tumors, multiple tumors or frequent recurrences, symptomatic diffuse CIS, prostatic stromal involvement**
- Intravesical therapy
  - Indications are: Stage T1 tumors, multifocal papillary Ta lesions, rapidly recurring superficial disease
  - Agents used: Bacille Calmette-Guérin (BCG), thiotepa, or mitomycin; BCG has the greatest efficacy
- Invasive bladder cancer
  - Surgical approaches
    - Radical cystectomy is the gold standard; indicated in patients with muscle-invasive tumors (regardless of grade), diffuse CIS, or recurrent superficial cancers not responding to intravesical therapy
    - Patients can undergo urinary reconstruction with intestinal conduits, continent cutaneous diversions, or orthotopic reconstruction
  - Surgical approaches to ureteral and renal pelvic tumors: Nephroureterectomy with resection of cuff of bladder
  - Role of radiation therapy
    - Therapy of choice for patients with clinical condition precluding surgery
    - Addition of chemotherapy as radiosensitizing agent of benefit if patient can tolerate chemotherapy
    - Palliative radiation therapy is quite effective in controlling pain from local or metastatic disease
- Treatment of advanced disease is palliative; cisplatin-based regimens are commonly used; gemcitabine and paclitaxel appear most active as single agents and in combination with cisplatin/carboplatin. Median survival is 14 to 20 months depending on prognostic factors, such as performance status, sites of metastasis, and laboratory measures.

Renal Cell Carcinoma

Incidence

- Estimated new cases in 2008 were 54,390 (increasing in incidence)
- Estimated deaths in 2008 were 13,010

Epidemiology

- Twice as common in men as in women
- **Most cases diagnosed in fourth to sixth decades of life**
- More common in persons of northern European ancestry

Etiology and Risk Factors

- Sporadic form
  - Etiology unclear
  - Associated with smoking, obesity, and renal dialysis
  - Sporadic renal cell carcinomas of the nonpapillary type are associated with deletions or hypermethylation on chromosome 3
- Familial form
  - Von Hippel-Lindau disease: **Autosomal dominant disease, deletions of short arm on chromosome 3; associated with retinal angiomas, central nervous**

system hemangioblastomas, and renal cell carcinomas (sometimes bilateral); carries the same prognosis as sporadic disease
- Signs and symptoms
  - Classic triad of hematuria, flank mass, and flank pain occurs in only 10% of patients and is associated with a poor prognosis
  - Hematuria: More than 50% of patients describe hematuria
  - Normocytic/normochromic anemia, fever, and weight loss are other common manifestations
  - Less common manifestations: Paraneoplastic syndromes (polycythemia from excess erythropoietin production, thrombocytosis from increased interleukin [IL]-6, hypercalcemia from release of parathyroid hormone-related peptide), hepatic dysfunction not associated with metastases (Stauffer's syndrome)
  - **Varicocele: If acute in onset, right-sided, or does not decrease in size in the supine position, consider renal cell carcinoma with obstruction of the venous system**
  - With wide use of CT and ultrasound, renal cell cancer is being diagnosed more commonly as an incidental finding

Diagnosis

- **Standard evaluation includes CT scan of abdomen and pelvis, chest radiograph, urinalysis, urine cytology**
- Contrast-enhanced CT scan differentiates solid from cystic masses; supplies information on nodal or renal vein or inferior vena cava (IVC) involvement
- Venography or MRI: Best test to look at IVC involvement
- Evaluation of extra-abdominal disease: Bone scan if symptoms suggestive; CT of chest if plain film suggestive of metastasis

Pathology

- Tumor cells arise from proximal renal tubular epithelium
- Histologic cell types include clear cell, papillary, and sarcomatoid
- **Clear cell carcinomas are the most common**
- Sarcomatoid variants are more aggressive and associated with a worse prognosis

Staging and Prognosis

- Staging based on tumor size and extension from the kidney (Table 55-3)

TABLE 55-3	Simplified Staging System for Renal Cell Carcinoma	
Stage	**Description**	
I	Tumor ≤ 7 cm and limited to kidney	
II	Tumor >7 cm and limited to kidney	
III	Tumor extension outside of kidney but within Gerota's fascia or one regional lymph node involved	
IV	Tumor extends beyond Gerota's fascia or more than one regional lymph node involved or distant metastasis	

- Approximately 30% of patients have metastatic disease at diagnosis
- Five-year survival rates for tumors confined to the kidney are greater than 80%; renal vein involvement does not affect survival
- Prior to the introduction of approved targeted therapies, patients with metastatic disease had a median 1-year survival rate of 0% to 20%. Survival is improving for patients with metastatic disease.

Treatment

- Surgery
  - Radical nephrectomy is the established therapy for localized disease
  - **In the presence of metastatic disease, nephrectomy should be considered to debulk the primary tumor and is associated with a 4-month improvement in survival.** Not all patients are surgical candidates, or the burden of metastatic disease may be too great and the nephrectomy may delay other systemic therapies.
- Radiation therapy to metastatic sites may provide benefit
  - Most commonly used for palliation of bony metastasis
- Systemic therapy of advanced disease
  - Metastatic renal cell carcinoma is relatively resistant to chemotherapeutic agents, although chemotherapy agents like gemcitabine and capecitabine are rarely used in select patients
  - Immunotherapy remains the most tested approach to therapy
  - Patients with best response to immunotherapy are those with excellent performance status, lung-only disease, history of nephrectomy, nephrectomy longer than 1 year from treatment, and a long interval history from diagnosis to recurrence and need for treatment
  - IL-2 is FDA-approved treatment for metastatic renal cell carcinoma
    - Response rates range from 15% to 30%
    - Major toxicity is sepsis-like syndrome
  - Interferon-α had been used commonly in the past, but has been surpassed by newer targeted agents
    - Response rate as a single agent ranges from 15% to 20%
    - Responses are often short-lived, but there is some suggestion of improved survival in interferon-treated patients
    - The combination of interferon and bevacizumab improves progression-free survival over interferon alone by approximately 6 months
  - More recently, targeting vascular endothelial growth factor (VEGF) and other tyrosine kinases has demonstrated clinical benefit. Both sorafenib and sunitinib are FDA-approved for advanced renal cancer.
    - Sorafenib, a multitargeted tyrosine kinase, has been approved for advanced metastatic disease based on randomized data demonstrating a 12-week improvement in time to disease progression for sorafenib over interferon. The overall response rate for sorafenib is reported at 2%.

- Sunitinib, another multitargeted kinase, has also been approved for advanced metastatic disease based on randomized data demonstrating a 6-month improvement in progression-free survival and a higher response rate for sunitinib over interferon. Response rates range from 30% to 45% depending on the study. Recent data suggest that survival of patients receiving sunitinib for first-line metastatic disease approaches 28 months.
  - Common side effects of these agents include hypertension, hand-foot syndrome, and fatigue
- Temsirolimus and everolimus are mammalian target of rapamycin (mTOR) inhibitors, and both are FDA-approved. Temsirolimus demonstrated a 3-month improvement in survival over interferon alone in patients with metastatic renal cell cancer and poor risk features. Everolimus demonstrated a 3-month improvement in progression-free survival over best supportive care in patients who had disease progression after sunitinib, sorafenib, or both.
- At this time, the most effective sequence or combinations of agents have not been defined. Clinical trials remain an appropriate first step for patients with metastatic disease.

Testicular Cancer

Incidence

- Estimated new cases in 2008 were 8090 (increasing in incidence)
- Estimated deaths in 2008 were 380

Epidemiology

- **Most common cancer in men in the 20- to 34-year age group**
- There is a secondary peak after age 60 years (mostly seminoma)
- Incidence is rare in African Americans

Etiology and Risk Factors

- Prior testicular cancer (500-fold increase in risk)
- Cryptorchidism (20- to 40-fold increase in risk)
- High prevalence (90%) have isochromosome 12p
- Association of extragonadal germ cell tumors with Klinefelter's and possibly Marfan's syndromes
- Association of extragonadal germ cell tumors with hematologic malignancy
- Prior trauma, elevated scrotal temperature, wearing briefs instead of boxer shorts, sleeping with electric blankets, and activities like horseback and motorcycle riding are not related to development of testicular cancer

Pathology

- **Vast majority are germ cell tumors: Seminomas and nonseminomas**
- Seminoma: 30% of all germ cell tumors
- Nonseminoma cell types: Embryonal, endodermal sinus, teratoma, choriocarcinoma
- Other non–germ cell tumors are rare: Leydig cell tumors, Sertoli cell tumors

Presentation

- Most germ cell tumors manifest in the testis (90%)
- Extragonadal (10%) tumors typically manifest in the retroperitoneum, mediastinum, or pineal gland; primary tumor in the testis may be occult
- Classically manifests as an enlargement or mass within testicle
  - Pain and swelling commonly occur
  - An associated hydrocele may be present in 20% of patients
- Gynecomastia (usually bilateral) caused by excess β-human chorionic gonadotropin (β-hCG) production can be seen
- **Inguinal lymphadenopathy is usually not a presenting feature because the regional lymph nodes for the testis are in the retroperitoneum**
- Metastatic spread may present with low back pain (retroperitoneal adenopathy), chest pain, cough, dyspnea, or hemoptysis (mediastinal adenopathy or lung metastases)

Diagnosis

- Testicular ultrasound can easily distinguish extratesticular from testicular abnormalities, and solid from cystic lesions
- **All solid intratesticular lesions should be removed by an inguinal orchiectomy. Biopsy or scrotal orchiectomy is contraindicated because it is associated with local spread of tumor cells.**

Staging

- Tumor marker studies should be obtained pre- and postorchiectomy
  - Elevation of β-hCG or α-fetoprotein (AFP) is seen in 80% to 90% of nonseminomatous germ cell tumors
  - Pure seminoma may have elevated β-hCG, but not AFP
  - **Elevated AFP indicates presence of nonseminomatous elements**
  - False-positive β-hCG elevations can be seen with hypogonadism and use of marijuana. AFP may be elevated in patients with liver disease.
  - Lactate dehydrogenase (LDH) levels may also be elevated in patients with bulky disease and can serve as a useful tumor marker
- CT scan of chest, abdomen, and pelvis should be obtained to search for metastatic sites
- CT of head and bone scan unnecessary unless symptoms or signs are suggestive of spread to those areas
- Overall staging is based on extent of spread (Table 55-4)

TABLE 55-4	Simplified Staging System for Testicular Cancer
Stage	**Description**
I	Tumor limited to testis, epididymis, or spermatic cord
II	Tumor extends to but not beyond the regional (retroperitoneal) lymph nodes
III	Disseminated disease

55

Treatment

- Seminomas
  - Very sensitive to radiation therapy (XRT), so very low doses (25 Gy) should be used; acute side effects include nausea, vomiting, diarrhea; late side effects include peptic ulcers, infertility, and second malignancies
  - Stage I and II disease: Treat with XRT after inguinal orchiectomy
  - Stage III disease: Chemotherapy with bleomycin/ etoposide/cisplatin (BEP)
- Nonseminomas
  - Stage I: Inguinal orchiectomy with or without retroperitoneal lymph node dissection (RPLND)
  - Stage II: Inguinal orchiectomy followed by RPLND with or without adjuvant chemotherapy (BEP)
  - Stage III: Chemotherapy with BEP
- Recurrent disease: Treat with salvage chemotherapy

Prognosis

- **Five-year survival of all patients is approximately 95%**
- Cure rates high for disease with minimal-to-moderate spread
- Infertility is common in all stages of testicular cancer, but risk of permanent infertility increases with therapy and stage; sperm banking must be considered in all patients undergoing therapy for testis cancer.

REVIEW QUESTIONS

For review questions, please go to www.expertconsult.com.

SUGGESTED READINGS

Aparicio AM, Elkhouiery AB, Quinn DI: The current and future application of adjuvant systemic chemotherapy in patients with bladder cancer following cystectomy, *Urol Clin North Am* 32:217–230, 2005.

Chee KG, Cambio A, Lara PN Jr: Recent developments in advanced urothelial cancer, *Curr Opin Urol* 15:342–349, 2005.

Hellerstedt BA, Pienta KJ: The current state of hormonal therapy for prostate cancer, *CA Cancer J Clin* 52:154–157, 2002.

Hudson MA, Herr HW: Carcinoma in situ of the bladder, *J Urol* 153: 564–572, 1995.

International Germ Cell Cancer Collaborative Group: International germ cell consensus classification: a prognostic factor-based staging system for metastatic germ cell cancers, *J Clin Oncol* 15:594–603, 1997.

Jemal A, Siegal R, Ward E, et al: Cancer statistics 2008, *CA Cancer J Clin* 58:71–96, 2006.

Kanda S, Miyata Y, Kanetake H: Current status and perspective of antiangiogenesis therapy for cancer: urinary cancer, *Int J Clin Oncol* 11:90–107, 2006.

Montie JE: Observations on the epidemiology and natural history of prostate cancer, *Urol Sympos* 44:2, 1994.

Motzer RJ, Bander NE, Nanus DM: Renal cell carcinoma, *N Engl J Med* 335:865–875, 1996.

Nelson WG, DeMarzo AM, Isaacs WB: Prostate cancer, *N Engl J Med* 349:366–381, 2003.

Pienta KJ, Smith DC: Advances in prostate cancer chemotherapy: a new era begins, *CA Cancer J Clin* 55:300–318, 2005.

Rini BI, Campbell SC, Escudier B: Renal cell carcinoma, *Lancet* 373(9669):1119–1132, 2009.

Sarvis JA, Thompson IM: Prostate cancer chemoprevention: update of the prostate cancer prevention trial findings and implications for clinical practice, *Curr Oncol Rep* 10:529–532, 2008.

CHAPTER 56

Lymphoma and Chronic Lymphocytic Leukemia

YVETTE L. KASAMON, MD

Leukemia and lymphoma are both hematologic malignancies. Whereas leukemias proliferate primarily in the blood and bone marrow, lymphomas are characterized by uncontrolled proliferation of cells residing in the lymphoid tissues. Some diseases, like chronic lymphocytic leukemia, can have features of both.

Classic Hodgkin's Lymphoma

Basic Information

- Usually arises from B cells
- Bimodal age distribution (third and seventh decades)
- Subset associated with Epstein-Barr virus infection

Clinical Presentation

- **Patients often present with "B symptoms" (fever, weight loss, night sweats) and pruritus**
- Most patients present with an asymptomatic enlarged lymph node or mass found on chest radiograph (Fig. 56-1A and B)
  - Nodes are usually painless and rubbery
  - Most common sites are the neck and mediastinum
  - Hodgkin's lymphoma starts at a single site within the lymphatic system and then progresses to adjacent lymph nodes
  - Alcohol-induced pain is a rare symptom of Hodgkin's lymphoma
- **A mediastinal mass in a young person is most often Hodgkin's lymphoma,** followed in frequency by non-Hodgkin's lymphoma
  - Mediastinal masses may be incidental findings on chest film or produce chest pain, cough, dyspnea, or superior vena cava syndrome
- Common laboratory findings include
  - Elevated WBC count
  - Lymphopenia
  - Thrombocytosis
  - Elevated erythrocyte sedimentation rate

Diagnosis

- Diagnosed via lymph node biopsy
  - Reed-Sternberg cells (giant "owl eye" cells) are characteristic and are surrounded by a dense inflammatory infiltrate (see Fig. 56-1C)

- **Fine-needle aspiration is usually insufficient because of limited architecture**
- Mediastinoscopy may be performed to sample a mediastinal tumor
- Staging (Table 56-1) requires CT of chest, abdomen, and pelvis
  - Exploratory laparotomy is now rarely performed for staging
  - Bone marrow biopsy is not always necessary; consider especially if B symptoms or cytopenias
  - Positron emission tomography (PET) scan is a useful adjunct to CT

Prognosis

- Majority are curable
- Adverse prognostic factors include
  - Age older than 45 years
  - Male gender
  - Stage IV disease
  - Abnormal CBC (WBC ≥ 15,000/µL, lymphopenia, anemia)
  - Albumin less than 4 g/dL

Treatment

- Treatment is based on staging
  - Stages I and II are usually treated with combination chemotherapy followed by radiation. Some cases may be treated with radiation alone or chemotherapy alone.
  - Stages III and IV are treated with full-course chemotherapy. Localized radiation may be added afterward to areas of bulky tumor.
  - Doxorubicin, bleomycin, vinblastine, dacarbazine (ABVD) is the standard regimen; full-course is six to eight cycles
  - Mechlorethamine, vincristine, prednisone, and procarbazine (MOPP) is an older regimen with higher risk of sterility and treatment-related leukemias, and is rarely used
- CT scans are repeated during treatment, and chemotherapy is often continued for two cycles beyond remission
- Autologous bone marrow transplant (BMT) is considered for most patients who relapse after first-line treatment
- Sequelae from treatment are common. Toxicities of treatment are leading considerations because most Hodgkin's lymphoma patients are cured.
  - Pulmonary toxicity from bleomycin can occur, usually during treatment. Patient may be

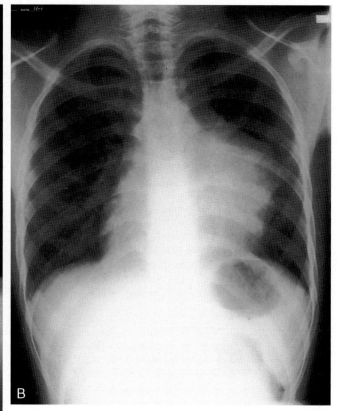

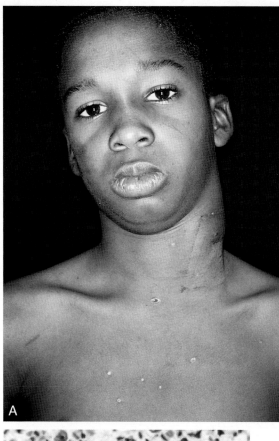

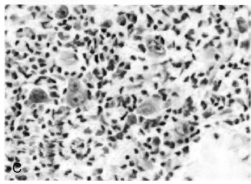

FIGURE 56-1 Hodgkin's lymphoma. Most patients present with an asymptomatic enlarged lymph node (**A**) or mediastinal mass (**B**). Binucleate Reed-Sternberg cells or "owl's eye" cells are characteristic pathologic findings (**C**). (A and B, From Shah B, Laude T: *Atlas of pediatric clinical diagnosis,* Philadelphia, Saunders, 2000, figure 7-32. C, From Hoffman R, Benz EJ Jr., Shattil SJ, et al: *Hematology: basic principles and practice,* ed 4, Philadelphia, Churchill Livingstone, 2005, figure 74-36.)

TABLE 56-1	*Staging of Lymphoma**
Stage I	Disease in one nodal area
Stage II	Two or more nodal areas on the same side of diaphragm
Stage III	Nodes on both sides of diaphragm
Stage IV	Disseminated disease involving one or more extranodal sites; or an extranodal site and nonadjacent lymph node

*Stages are designated as: A, absence of constitutional symptoms (unexplained fever > 38°C, drenching sweats, or unexplained >10% weight loss in preceding 6 months), or B, presence of constitutional symptoms.

asymptomatic, or bleomycin may cause cough, fever, dyspnea, and infiltrates
- Anthracyclines can cause late cardiomyopathy
- Radiation significantly increases risk of solid tumors (including lung, breast, thyroid)

- Mediastinal radiation also causes cardiac
  **complications, including premature coronary
  artery disease, constrictive pericarditis, restrictive
  cardiomyopathy, and valve disease**
- Thyroid function tests should be monitored for hypothyroidism after radiation
- Chemotherapy increases the risk of myelodysplastic syndrome and acute leukemia

Non-Hodgkin's Lymphoma

Basic Information

- Incidence
  - **Diffuse large B-cell lymphoma is the most common
    non-Hodgkin's lymphoma (NHL), followed by
    follicular (low-grade) lymphoma**
  - Incidence of lymphoma rises with age

- Histology
  - Most lymphomas arise from B cells
  - Cutaneous lymphomas are usually T cell
  - Broadly divided into "low-grade" (indolent) or "high-grade" (aggressive) lymphomas (Box 56-1)
- Risk factors
  - Altered immunity (HIV infection, organ transplantation, autoimmune diseases, congenital immunodeficiency)
    - Aggressive B-cell lymphoma is an AIDS-defining illness
  - Infections
    - Epstein-Barr virus (especially in African Burkitt's lymphoma and AIDS-related lymphomas)
    - HTLV-1 in adult T-cell leukemia/lymphoma
    - Hepatitis C virus in some low-grade lymphomas
    - *Helicobacter pylori* in gastric mucosa-associated lymphoid tissue (MALT) lymphoma **(H. pylori treatment can eradicate the lymphoma)**
    - Consider antibiotics as first line for low-grade, localized gastric lymphoma that is positive for *H. pylori*, with radiation as second line
  - Chemical exposure (pesticides)

Clinical Presentation

- Low-grade lymphomas (e.g., follicular lymphomas) manifest subtly
  - The lymph nodes can wax and wane, possibly for years
  - Often in multiple locations, small, soft, and moveable
- More aggressive lymphomas (like diffuse large B-cell lymphoma) usually manifest with firm, enlarging lymph node(s) or widespread lymphadenopathy, with or without B symptoms
- **Very high-grade lymphomas (like Burkitt's lymphoma) can grow extremely rapidly, usually manifesting with a single large mass in the chest or abdomen and an elevated lactate dehydrogenase (LDH)**

Diagnosis

- Excisional lymph node biopsy is generally preferable to needle biopsy
- Staging (see Table 56-1) includes chest/abdomen/pelvis CT and a bone marrow biopsy

BOX 56-1	*Examples of Non-Hodgkin's Lymphomas*

Indolent

Follicular lymphoma, grade 1 (follicular small-cleaved)

Follicular lymphoma, grade 2 (follicular mixed)

Marginal zone lymphoma, including mucosa-associated lymphoid tissue lymphoma

Chronic lymphocytic leukemia/small lymphocytic leukemia

Most skin lymphomas

Aggressive

Follicular lymphoma, grade 3 (follicular large cell)

Diffuse large B-cell lymphoma

Mediastinal large B-cell lymphoma

Mantle cell lymphoma

Peripheral T-cell lymphoma

Burkitt's lymphoma*

Lymphoblastic lymphoma/leukemia*

*These lymphomas are highly aggressive.

- PET scan often helpful
- Consider HIV antibody in most patients with aggressive NHL
- Consider lumbar puncture for cytopathology in high-grade lymphomas

Prognosis

- Stage is relatively poor indicator of outcome, because spread is hematogenous
- Adverse prognostic features in aggressive lymphomas include
  - Age older than 60 years
  - Elevated LDH
  - Stage III or IV disease
  - More than one extranodal site
  - Poor performance status
- In AIDS-related lymphomas
  - CD4 count is most important prognostic feature
  - Addition of highly active antiretroviral therapy (HAART) improves survival

Treatment

- Low-grade lymphomas are treatable but are virtually impossible to cure
  - Many treatment options (e.g., watchful waiting, chemotherapy, monoclonal antibodies such as rituximab, radiation)
  - **No benefit to early or aggressive treatment if patient is asymptomatic; consider observation**
  - Transformation to high-grade lymphoma may occur
  - In follicular lymphoma
    - Median survival is 8 to 10 years
    - Radiation may cure limited-stage disease
    - Most have disseminated disease at diagnosis
    - Transformation occurs in 40% and is treated like high-grade lymphoma
- Aggressive lymphomas are treated promptly with combination chemotherapy, with or without radiation, and are potentially curable (~50% cure rate)
  - Cyclophosphamide, doxorubicin, vincristine, prednisone (CHOP) is a widely used regimen
  - Addition of rituximab (monoclonal anti-CD20 antibody) to chemotherapy (e.g., rituximab-CHOP) improves outcomes in B-cell lymphomas
  - **Monitor for tumor lysis syndrome due to rapid cell breakdown**
    - Hyperuricemia
    - Hyperkalemia
    - Hyperphosphatemia
    - Hypocalcemia
    - Acute renal failure
  - **Dissemination into the CNS may occur**
    - Usually leptomeningeal disease, rather than brain mass
    - Risk factors include
      - HIV infection
      - Extranodal sites, such as bone marrow
      - Sinus, tonsillar (Waldeyer's ring), or testicular involvement
      - High LDH
      - Burkitt's lymphoma or lymphoblastic histology
    - CNS lymphoma requires directed therapy
      - Intrathecal chemotherapy, with or without radiation, is the mainstay

56

- Most systemic chemotherapies are ineffective
- Autologous BMT is considered for most patients with relapsed aggressive lymphoma

Chronic Lymphocytic Leukemia

Basic Information

- Chronic lymphocytic leukemia (CLL) is the most common leukemia in the United States
- Median age of diagnosis is 65 years, with male predominance
- Arises from B cells
- Most common cause of death is infection

Clinical Presentation

- Patients are often asymptomatic on diagnosis
  - About 25% present with **lymphocytosis** found on routine labs
    - **WBC greater than 50,000/μL can be asymptomatic and not require therapy**
- May also present with lymphadenopathy (usually painless), splenomegaly, anemia, thrombocytopenia, or B symptoms
- **Hypogammaglobulinemia increases infection risk**
- **Autoimmune complications may occur,** including hemolytic anemia and immune-mediated thrombocytopenia

Diagnosis

- Lymphocytosis in blood
  - At least 5000/μL circulating B cells
  - Peripheral smear shows small, mature lymphocytes, some appearing as "**smudge cells**" (an artifact) (Fig. 56-2A)
  - Cells have a characteristic phenotype

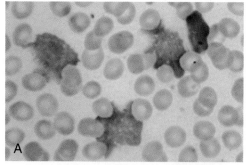

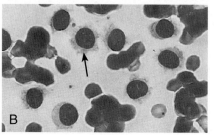

FIGURE 56-2 A, Peripheral blood smear showing "smudge cells" in chronic lymphocytic leukemia. **B,** Lymphocytes with fine surface projections or "hairs" (*arrow*) in hairy cell leukemia. (A, From Hoffman R, Benz EJ Jr, Shattil SJ, et al: *Hematology: basic principles and practice,* ed 4, Philadelphia, Churchill Livingstone, 2005, figure 79-5. B, From Rodak BF: *Diagnostic hematology,* Philadelphia, Saunders, 1995.)

- Lymphocytosis in bone marrow is common (often >30% lymphocytes)
- Staging (Table 56-2) based on CBC and presence of enlarged lymph nodes, spleen, or liver
- Small lymphocytic lymphoma (SLL) is the same disease as CLL, but with more lymphadenopathy than leukemia

Prognosis

- Virtually incurable
- Variable natural history
  - Median survival ranges from less than 4 years to more than 20 years, depending on risk factors
- Adverse features include
  - Rapid lymphocyte doubling time (12 months)
  - Advanced stage at diagnosis
  - Cytogenetics (17p deletion, 11q deletion are unfavorable; isolated 13q deletion is most favorable)
  - Immunoglobulin gene mutation status (unmutated immunoglobulin heavy-chain variable region [*IgVH*] gene is unfavorable)
- **Richter's syndrome (transformation to aggressive histology, usually large-cell lymphoma) occurs in 5% and is difficult to treat**
  - Suspect if rapid growth in one lymph node area

Treatment

- **Observation is appropriate for early-stage or asymptomatic CLL**
  - No proven advantage to early chemotherapy if patient is asymptomatic
- Indications for treatment
  - Bulky lymphadenopathy or organomegaly
  - Constitutional symptoms (weakness, night sweats, fever, weight loss)
  - Bone marrow failure (anemia or thrombocytopenia) from progressive CLL
  - Autoimmune hemolysis or autoimmune thrombocytopenia failing usual therapy
  - Rapidly progressive disease or Richter's transformation
- Active drugs include
  - Purine analogues: Fludarabine
  - Antibodies: Rituximab, alemtuzumab (Campath-anti-CD52 antibody)

TABLE 56-2		Rai Staging of Chronic Lymphocytic Leukemia	
Risk Group	**Stage**	**Features**	**Median Survival (yr)**
Low	0	Lymphocytosis only (blood or marrow)	>12
Intermediate	I II	Lymphadenopathy Hepatomegaly or splenomegaly	7
High	III	Any of the above + anemia (hemoglobin < 11 g/dL)	2.5
	IV	Any of the above + thrombocytopenia (platelets < 100,000/μL)	

- Alkylating agents: Chlorambucil (commonly used as single agent), cyclophosphamide
  - Other: Bendamustine
- **IVIG may be given for hypogammaglobulinemia and frequent infection**

Hairy Cell Leukemia

Basic Information

- Rare B-cell leukemia
- Median age of onset 55 years, with strong male predominance
- Indolent course, but progressive

Clinical Presentation

- **Manifests with pancytopenia and massive splenomegaly**
- A **"dry" bone marrow tap** despite marrow hypercellularity is characteristic

Diagnosis

- Peripheral smear may show small- to medium-sized lymphocytes with hairlike projections (Fig. 56-2B)
- Cells have characteristic staining and phenotype

Treatment

- Cladribine (2-CDA, a purine analogue) induces complete remission in most patients

REVIEW QUESTIONS

For review questions, please go to www.expertconsult.com.

SUGGESTED READINGS

Ansell SM, Armitage JO: Management of Hodgkin lymphoma, *Mayo Clin Proc* 81:419–426, 2006.

Armitage JO: How I treat patients with diffuse large B-cell lymphoma, *Blood* 110:29–36, 2007.

Chiorazzi N, Rai KR, Ferrarini M: Chronic lymphocytic leukemia, *N Engl J Med* 252:804–815, 2005.

Hasenclever D, Diehl VA: A prognostic score for advanced Hodgkin's disease. International Prognostic Factors Project on Advanced Hodgkin's Disease, *N Engl J Med* 339:1506–1514, 1998.

The International Non-Hodgkin's Lymphoma Prognostic Factors Project: a predictive model for aggressive non-Hodgkin's lymphoma, *N Engl J Med* 329:987–994, 1993.

56

Plasma Cell Dyscrasias

AMY DeZERN, MD, and CAROL ANN HUFF, MD

Plasma cell dyscrasias are **clonal B-cell disorders characterized by the overproduction of monoclonal immunoglobulins**. Patients with plasma cell dyscrasias may present with any of a number of symptoms, but many patients are asymptomatic at the time of diagnosis.

Basic Information

- Definition
  - There are seven categories of plasma cell dyscrasias (Table 57-1)
  - Each has an immunohistochemically identical production of antibody

TABLE 57-1	*Plasma Cell Dyscrasias*
Disorders	**Disease Definition**
Monoclonal gammopathy of undetermined significance (MGUS)	Overproduction of monoclonal immunoglobulin (<3g/dL) with <10% clonal plasma cells on bone marrow aspiration and biopsy and absence of end-organ damage (hypercalcemia, renal insufficiency, anemia, bone lesions)
Multiple myeloma	Clonal plasma cells ≥ 10% in the bone marrow and/or presence of serum and/or urinary monoclonal protein; when associated evidence of lytic bone lesions, anemia, hypercalcemia, or renal insufficiency, it is active myeloma. In the absence of associated symptoms, termed smoldering or asymptomatic
Plasmacytoma	Biopsy-proven solitary lesion with clonal plasma cells and insufficient criteria to diagnose multiple myeloma (see above)
POEMS	Presence of monoclonal plasma cells; **p**olyneuropathy, **o**rganomegaly, **e**ndocrinopathy, **m** protein, and **s**kin changes
AL amyloidosis	Presence of monoclonal plasma cells creating a syndrome where insoluble proteins deposit in tissues and cause end-organ damage
Waldenström's macroglobulinemia	IgM monoclonal gammopathy with >10% bone marrow lymphoplasmacytic infiltration
Cryoglobulinemia	Group of disorders associated with overproduction of monoclonal or polyclonal protein production: defining characteristic is that proteins precipitate when cooled and dissolve when heated

- Autoimmune disorders and chronic inflammatory conditions may lead to the production of monoclonal immunoglobulins; this is not malignant and is separate from plasma cell dyscrasias; examples include
  - Systemic lupus erythematosus, Sjögren's syndrome, and cold agglutinin disease
  - Infections such as tuberculosis, endocarditis, hepatitis; carcinoid tumors, polycythemia rubra vera, and pyoderma gangrenosum
  - **Monoclonal immunoglobulins seen in 1% of adults;** prevalence increases with increasing age
    - Prevalence: IgG > IgM > IgA
- Evaluation of the patient with possible monoclonal immunoglobulin production (Figs. 57-1 and 57-2)
  - Diagnostic clues to initiate evaluation
    - Asymptomatic individual: Elevated total protein; elevated globulin fraction of protein; normochromic, normocytic anemia
    - Symptomatic individual: Normochromic, normocytic anemia; recurrent bacterial infections; renal insufficiency; bone pain; pathologic fracture or osteolytic lesion on radiograph; osteoporosis; sensorimotor neuropathy; pyoderma gangrenosum

Multiple Myeloma

Basic Information

- **Second most common hematologic malignancy** (after non-Hodgkin's lymphoma [NHL]) resulting in 1% of cancer deaths each year
- Male predominance
- Twice as common in African Americans as whites
- Median age at diagnosis: 68 years
- Median survival after diagnosis is 3 to 5 years, but improving
- Poor prognostic indicators include renal insufficiency, hypercalcemia, anemia, elevated β_2-microglobulin, hypoalbuminemia, cytogenetic abnormalities including hypodiploidy, 13q deletion, or complex karyotype, or t[4;14], t[14;16], or p53 deletions detected with fluorescent in situ hybridization (FISH) or cytogenetics

Clinical Presentation

- Most common presenting features are calcium elevation, renal insufficiency, anemia, and bone pain (group of findings referred to as CRAB)
- Figure 57-3 illustrates the clinical manifestations of multiple myeloma

Step 1	Define and quantitate abnormal immunoglobulin production	Serum protein electrophoresis and immunofixation
		Urine protein electrophoresis and immunofixation* If both negative and high index of suspicion, check serum light chain assay
Step 2	Define and quantitate organ system dysfunction	CBC and differential—rule out anemia, pancytopenia
		Rule out renal dysfunction with BUN/creatinine; obtain serum calcium
Step 3	Rule out multiple myeloma	Bone marrow aspirate and biopsy
		Skeletal X-ray series to rule out lytic or sclerotic bone lesions†
Step 4	Define other characteristics of disorder	Serum viscosity if IgM gammopathy, or suggestive symptoms
		Rule out connective tissue disease or chronic inflammatory disorder if no plasma cell dyscrasias found

*Spot urine for qualitative assesment: 24-hr collection for quantitative assessment.
†Bone scan evaluates for blastic lesions and will be normal in multiple myeloma.

FIGURE 57-1 Evaluation of a monoclonal immunoglobulin. *Spot urine for qualitative assessment: 24-hour collection for quantitative assessment. BUN, blood urea nitrogen; IgM, immunoglobulin M.

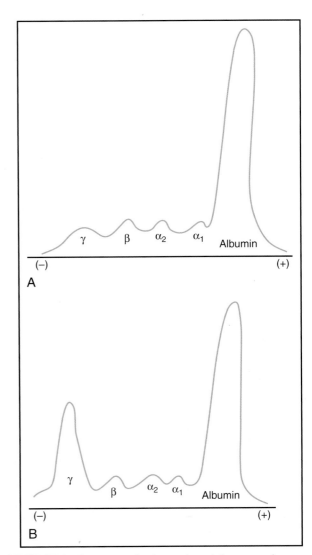

FIGURE 57-2 Serum protein electrophoresis in a normal individual (**A**) and in an individual with a monoclonal gammopathy (**B**). (From Waldman SD: *Interventional pain management,* ed 2, Philadelphia, WB Saunders, 2001, figure 9-1A, C.)

Diagnosis and Evaluation

- Diagnostic criteria for multiple myeloma
  - Smoldering/asymptomatic (Box 57-1)
    - Clonal bone marrow plasma cells greater than or equal to 10% or
    - Presence of serum and/or urinary monoclonal protein greater than or equal to 3 g/dL
  - Active
    - Above criteria with the addition of end-organ damage that can be attributed to the underlying plasma cell proliferative disorder, specifically the CRAB criteria
      - **C**alcium greater than 11.5 g/dL
      - **R**enal insufficiency (creatinine > 2 mg/dL)
      - **A**nemia (hemoglobin [Hbg] < 10 or 2 g < normal)
      - **B**one disease (osteopenia or lytic lesions)

- Common complications include the following:
  - **Hypercalcemia:** Present in 25% of patients; results from lytic bone disease; treated with saline hydration, loop diuretics, and bisphosphonates
  - **Anemia:** Normochromic, normocytic with an Hbg value of greater than 2 g/100 mL below the lower limit of normal or an Hbg value less than 10 g/100 mL
  - **Renal insufficiency:** Occurs in 50% of patients; usually progresses insidiously, but acute renal failure may be present
    - **Bence Jones proteinuria** (may be missed on routine urine dipstick, which detects albumin; sulfosalicylic acid effectively precipitates light chains), tubular casts, glomerular lesions
  - Hyperviscosity syndrome: Results from elevated serum proteins; symptoms usually not seen until serum viscosity greater than 4 cP (centiPoises; Box 57-2)
  - Neurologic: Sensory or sensorimotor neuropathy
  - Immunodeficiency: Increased risk of recurrent bacterial infections due to suppression of normal immunoglobulins

57

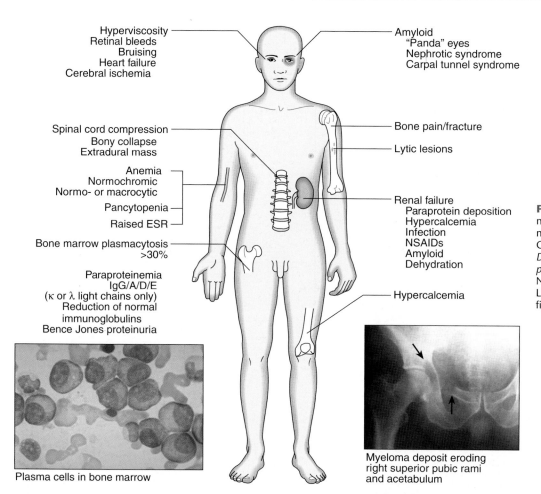

Hyperviscosity
Retinal bleeds
Bruising
Heart failure
Cerebral ischemia

Amyloid
"Panda" eyes
Nephrotic syndrome
Carpal tunnel syndrome

Spinal cord compression
Bony collapse
Extradural mass

Bone pain/fracture

Lytic lesions

Anemia
Normochromic
Normo- or macrocytic

Pancytopenia

Raised ESR

Bone marrow plasmacytosis
>30%

Paraproteinemia
IgG/A/D/E
(κ or λ light chains only)
Reduction of normal
immunoglobulins
Bence Jones proteinuria

Renal failure
Paraprotein deposition
Hypercalcemia
Infection
NSAIDs
Amyloid
Dehydration

Hypercalcemia

FIGURE 57-3 Clinical manifestations of multiple myeloma. (From Haslett C, Chilvers ER, Boon NA, et al: *Davidson's principles and practice of medicine*, ed 19, New York, Churchill Livingstone, 2002, figure 19.33.)

Plasma cells in bone marrow

Myeloma deposit eroding right superior pubic rami and acetabulum

---

| **BOX 57-1** | *Diagnostic Criteria for Multiple Myeloma* |

Smoldering

M protein ≥ 3 g/dL and/or clonal plasma cells on bone marrow ≥ 10%

No evidence of end-organ impairment and asymptomatic

Active

Requires one or more of the following in addition to the criteria for smoldering disease:

Calcium > 11.5 g/dL

Renal insufficiency (creatinine > 2 mg/dL)

Anemia (hemoglobin < 10 or 2 g < normal)

Bone disease (osteopenia or lytic lesions)

- Bone lesions: Lytic lesions, severe osteopenia or pathologic fractures (most commonly vertebral compression fractures)
  - To diagnose: Obtain skeletal survey to identify high-risk areas and consider prophylactic radiotherapy or surgical pinning of areas at high risk
  - Positron emission tomography (PET) scans and spine MRI are not routinely recommended at this point but are useful in certain situations
  - Bone scan is normal in myeloma patients because it only shows blastic lesions

---

| **BOX 57-2** | *Hyperviscosity Syndrome* |

Symptoms

Neurologic: Headache, dizziness, ataxia, paresthesias, somnolence, coma

Visual: Diplopia, blurred vision, loss of vision

Cardiac: Congestive heart failure, myocardial ischemia

Hematologic: Spontaneous bleeding, particularly from nose and gums; GI bleeding described

Physical Findings

Flame-shaped retinal hemorrhages

Papilledema

"Boxcar" formation of RBCs in retinal vessels

Treatment

Plasmapheresis until symptoms resolve (may be needed daily if symptoms persist)

Therapy directed at underlying cause

Caution if RBC transfusion needed, because this will expand volume and worsen symptoms

- Spinal cord compression serious complication that could present with pain, lower extremity paresthesias or weakness, and urinary retention or fecal incontinence; treatment with IV dexamethasone and radiation therapy and, sometimes, with urgent surgical decompression

Treatment

- **Chemotherapy: Not curative; should be instituted when patients are symptomatic or demonstrate end-organ dysfunction as described earlier**
  - Melphalan and prednisone; inferior results when compared to melphalan/prednisone combinations listed below
  - Melphalan, prednisone, thalidomide
  - Melphalan, prednisone, bortezomib
  - Thalidomide and dexamethasone
  - Lenaldiomide and dexamethasone
  - Bortezomib and dexamethasone
  - Bortezomib, liposomal adriamycin, and dexamethasone
  - Vincristine, adriamycin, and dexamethasone older regimen, with greater toxicities, rarely used now
- Bone marrow transplantation
  - **Autologous:** Increases survival by 12 to 18 months on average; all patients eventually relapse
  - **Allogeneic: Potentially curative (25–30%)** but with greatest toxicities
- Symptomatic management
  - Bone lesions: **Bisphosphonates** decrease risk of fracture and improve quality of life; surgical intervention for pathologic fractures; vertebroplasty or kyphoplasty for symptomatic vertebral lesions
  - Anemia: **Erythropoietin** in symptomatic patients who are not hyperviscous
  - Infectious: **Vaccinate** against *Pneumococcus*, *Haemophilus influenzae*, and influenza; consider prophylactic antibiotics if on long-term corticosteroids, varicella-zoster prophylaxis if on bortezomib

Plasmacytomas

Basic Information

- **Plasmacytomas are proliferations of monoclonal plasma** cells forming a mass at extramedullary or osseous sites
- No evidence of multiple myeloma or end-organ dysfunction (hypercalcemia, renal insufficiency, anemia, or other bone lesions, and no evidence of plasmacytosis on bone marrow biopsy)
- 50% of osseous plasmacytomas develop into overt myeloma; only 15% of extraosseous lesions develop overt myeloma

Clinical Presentation

- **Solitary plasmacytoma:** Single tumor of plasma cells resulting in localized complaints (bone pain, pathologic fracture); no evidence of diffuse plasma cell overgrowth throughout remainder of bone marrow (Fig. 57-4); most common sites are vertebrae, ribs, skull, and pelvis
- **Extramedullary plasmacytoma:** Tumor of plasma cells arising outside of the bone marrow; most **commonly found in the upper respiratory tract** (nasal passages, sinuses, nasopharynx, larynx); occasionally described in the lower extremity, GI tract, lung, lymph nodes; can be associated with HIV infection

Diagnosis and Evaluation

- **Diagnosis made by biopsy,** typically when mass or structural abnormality noted on imaging study
- Serum protein electrophoresis (SPEP), urine protein electrophoresis (UPEP), bone marrow aspiration, and

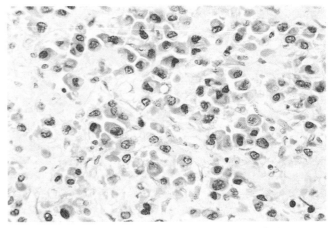

FIGURE 57-4 Bone marrow replaced with plasma cells. (From Stevens A, Lowe J: *Pathology,* ed 2, St. Louis, Mosby, 2000, figure 15.16.)

biopsy, as well as skeletal survey should be done at diagnosis to rule out extramedullary spread of multiple myeloma; if negative, consider spine MRI and PET scan to exclude occult lesions elsewhere; if truly isolated, follow serially in case of progression to myeloma

Treatment

- **Radiation therapy to the involved area;** 15% to 25% are disease-free at 10 years

Monoclonal Gammopathy of Undetermined Significance

Basic Information

- Most common plasma cell dyscrasia (3% of population older than age 50 years)
- Asymptomatic premalignant disorder
- Rate of progression of monoclonal gammopathy of unknown significance (MGUS) to myeloma or related malignancy is 1% per year
- Characterized by **overproduction of a monoclonal immunoglobulin without other abnormalities**; diagnosis of exclusion, usually made retrospectively, when one demonstrates stability over time in the quantity of M protein and the absence of other findings

Clinical Presentation

- **No symptoms associated with MGUS; diagnosed entirely on laboratory criteria**
- Evaluation: SPEP and immunofixation electrophoresis (IFE); 24-hour UPEP and IFE; CBC and differential, creatinine, calcium, albumin, serum light-chain assay, skeletal survey, bone marrow aspiration, and biopsy recommended for all patients with M protein greater than 1 g/dL and in those with non-IgG paraprotein, regardless of quantification of M protein

Diagnostic Criteria

- **M protein less than 3g/dL** (as determined by SPEP)
- **Less than 10% plasma cells on bone marrow** (biopsy recommended for all patients with M protein > 1 g/dL

and in those with non-IgG paraprotein, regardless of quantification of M protein)
- Normal Hgb, creatinine, calcium
- Absence of lytic bone disease
- Asymptomatic

Treatment/Follow-up

- **Observation alone, without therapy**
- **No formal guideline for follow-up:** Serial laboratories including SPEP, UPEP, CBC, and metabolic panel for creatinine and calcium at least yearly
- **Increased risk of progression to myeloma:** High monoclonal protein concentration; high percentage of plasma cells in the bone marrow, a non-IgG paraprotein, an abnormal serum-free κ/λ light-chain ratio

POEMS Syndrome

Basic Information

- **Syndrome resulting from overproduction of light chains, usually λ,** without significant overgrowth of plasma cells in the bone marrow; many organ systems involved, with characteristic abnormalities
- Also called osteosclerotic myeloma

Clinical Presentation

Table 57-2 summarizes the clinical presentation of POEMS syndrome.
- **Polyneuropathy is an inflammatory demyelinating process with predominantly sensory symptoms**
- **Organomegaly most common in spleen and liver**

TABLE 57-2	Criteria for the Diagnosis of POEMS Syndrome
Major criteria	Polyneuropathy* Monoclonal plasma cell–proliferative disorder (95% are lambda)* Sclerotic bone lesions Castleman's disease Vascular endothelial growth factor elevation
Minor criteria	Organomegaly (splenomegaly, hepatomegaly, or lymphadenopathy) Extravascular volume overload (edema, pleural effusion, or ascites) Endocrinopathy (adrenal, thyroid,† pituitary, gonadal, parathyroid, pancreatic†) Skin changes (hyperpigmentation, hypertrichosis, white nails) Papilledema Thrombocytosis, polycythemia
Other signs and symptoms	Clubbing, weight loss, hyperhidrosis, pulmonary hypertension, restrictive lung disease, low vitamin B₁₂, diarrhea, thrombotic diatheses
Possible associations	Arthralgias, cardiomyopathy, fever

*Polyneuropathy and monoclonal plasma cell disorder must be present in all patients; to make diagnosis, at least one other major criterion and one minor criterion is required.
†Endocrinopathy other than isolated thyroid disease or diabetes mellitus is required to meet this criterion (due to the relative frequency of these in the general population).

- **Endocrinopathies seen include hypogonadism and hyperprolactinemia**
- **M protein is usually λ light chains**
- **Skin changes include hypertrichosis and thickening of the dermis**
- **Sclerotic bone lesions**
- **Elevated vascular endothelial growth factor**
- **Papilledema**
- **Thrombocytosis or polycythemia**

Diagnosis

- Based on clinical suspicion and constellation of findings (see Table 57-2); neuropathy is typically the most prominent symptom; SPEP/immunofixation/serum-free light-chain assay demonstrating **λ light chains**

Treatment

- **Includes radiation therapy to bone lesion if isolated; if diffuse changes, then systemic therapy with corticosteroids, low-dose alkylator therapy, and high-dose chemotherapy followed by consideration of stem cell transplantation**

Waldenström's Macroglobulinemia

Basic Information

- Also known as lymphoplasmacytic lymphoma
- **A rare lymphoma characterized by bone marrow infiltration by clonal B cells with production of M-protein (IgM)**

Clinical Presentation

- **Signs and symptoms commonly related to both tumor infiltration of the marrow and elevated monoclonal IgM**
- **Most dangerous: Hyperviscosity** (Fig. 57-5; see Box 57-2) because of high production of IgM

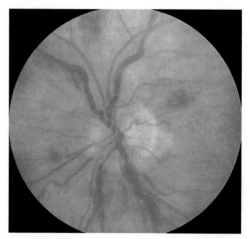

FIGURE 57-5 Waldenström's macroglobulinemia (hyperviscosity syndrome). The retina of a patient who presented with blurred vision, headache, and dizziness exhibits gross distention of vessels, particularly the veins, which show bulging and constriction (the "linked sausage" effect), as well as areas of hemorrhage. (From Skarin AT, editor: *Atlas of diagnostic oncology,* ed 3, Philadelphia, WB Saunders, 2003, figure 15.56.)

- Polyneuropathy, and cryoglobulinemia (with digital infarcts) also may be seen because of high production of IgM
- Tumor infiltration causing organomegaly, lymphadenopathy, B symptoms (fevers, night sweats, weight loss)
- Only 25% of patients with IgM monoclonal gammopathy have Waldenström's macroglobulinemia; others have MGUS, MM, chronic lymphocytic leukemia, NHL, or cold agglutinin disease

Diagnosis

- **Based on presence of IgM and evidence of B-cell lymphoma by pathology**

Treatment

- Plasmapheresis is performed to treat hyperviscosity and its related symptoms
- Chemotherapy: Use monoclonal antibody therapy, such as rituximab (anti-CD20) or nucleoside analogues (e.g., fludarabine) or oral alkylating agents (e.g., melphalan or cyclophosphamide)
- Some patients develop aggressive lymphoma (Richter's transformation)

Cryoglobulinemia

Basic Information

- **Group of disorders characterized by the production of soluble proteins that precipitate on cooling, typically associated with symptoms; often evidence of an underlying clonal disorder; divided into three subtypes (Table 57-3)**

Clinical Presentation

- Varies by subtype (see Table 57-3)

Diagnosis

- **Key to detection is proper transport of sample**—must be taken to lab at body temperature—(ideally in a warm-water bath); **diagnosis requires the demonstration of protein precipitation on cooling of blood**

Treatment

- Focused on **correcting underlying disease**
- Plasmapheresis for those symptomatic patients in which underlying disease is not treatable

Amyloidosis

Basic Information

- Relatively rare
- Characterized by **deposition of insoluble protein in organs and tissues**, resulting in organ dysfunction
- Disease classified by which protein precursor forms the fibril deposits
  - **AL amyloidosis: Amyloid protein is primarily the variable region of Ig light chains (λ > k)**
    - AL amyloidosis is a plasma cell dyscrasia related to myeloma
  - **AA amyloidosis: Secondary amyloidosis in which the amyloid protein is serum amyloid protein A (an acute-phase reactant produced in response to inflammation)**
    - Protein A is not related to a known immunoglobulin
    - **AA amyloidosis is associated with chronic infections (e.g., tuberculosis, osteomyelitis, bronchiectasis), chronic inflammatory disorders (e.g., rheumatoid arthritis, inflammatory bowel disease, and familial Mediterranean fever)**
  - **Familial amyloidosis:** Autosomal dominant disorder in which mutant protein (most commonly transthyretin) forms amyloid fibrils

Clinical Presentation

- Variable; **determined by the organs predominantly affected by protein deposition** and differs according to amyloid subtype (Table 57-4)

Diagnosis

- Requires demonstration of deposition of amyloid fibers, typically with a fat pad aspirate; staining with Congo red demonstrates **apple green birefringence under polarized light** (Fig. 57-6)

57

TABLE 57-3	*The Cryoglobulinemias*		
Subtype	**Immunoglobulin**	**Disease Association**	**Features**
I	Presence of isolated monoclonal immunoglobulin (usually IgG or IgM, less commonly IgA or free light chains)	Waldenström's macroglobulinemia, multiple myeloma	Many patients are asymptomatic; classic symptoms related to hyperviscosity: digital ischemia, Raynaud's phenomenon, purpura, livedo reticularis
II	"Essential mixed CG" is a mixture of polyclonal immunoglobulin with a monoclonal immunoglobulin (usually IgM or IgA); can also have RF activity	Persistent viral infectious—most often hepatitis C or HIV	Membranoproliferative glomerulonephritis, mononeuritis muliplex, vasculitis; classic Meltzer's triad of purpura, arthralgias, and weakness
III	Polyclonal immunoglobulins	Most often secondary to connective tissue disorders or chronic inflammatory conditions	Treatment directed at primary disorder

CG, cryoglobulinemia; Ig, immunoglobulin; RF, rheumatoid factor.

TABLE 57-4	*Clinical Presentation of Amyloidosis*		
Amyloid Subtype	Dominant Protein	Organ Deposit	Symptoms
AL	Immunoglobulin Light chains	Heart	Low-voltage ECG Right-sided heart failure with volume overload Echocardiogram shows classic myocardium speckled pattern; orthostatic hypotension
		Kidney	Nephrotic range proteinuria
		Tongue	Macroglossia
		GI tract	Infiltration of gut with malabsorptive process
		CNS	Peripheral neuropathy, carpal tunnel syndrome
AA	Serum amyloid protein A	Kidney	Most commonly involved with nephrotic range proteinuria
		Liver Spleen	Organomegaly
Familial	Transthyretin	CNS	Neuropathy with sensory or autonomic insufficiency
		Heart	Conduction abnormalities (see also symptoms of cardiac deposit of AL above)

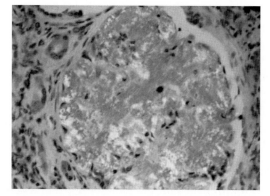

FIGURE 57-6 Amyloidosis. Congo red stain of a glomerulus that is largely replaced by amyloid demonstrates the characteristic birefringence under polarized light. (From Brenner BM: *Brenner and Rector's the kidney,* ed 7, Philadelphia, WB Saunders, 2004, figure 29-25.)

- **AL: Systemic chemotherapy shown to prolong survival—melphalan and prednisone**
  - Small studies suggest that autologous bone marrow transplantation may further improve survival in selected patients
  - Prognosis: Median survival is 1 to 2 years, depending on degree of organ involvement; median survival is 6 months if symptomatic cardiac involvement, 21 months with renal involvement
- **AA amyloidosis: Treat underlying infection or inflammatory disease**
- **Familial amyloidosis: Liver transplantation is curative;** often does not reverse the damage

REVIEW QUESTIONS

For review questions, please go to www.expertconsult.com.

SUGGESTED READINGS

Blade J: Clinical practice: monoclonal gammopathy of undetermined significance, *N Engl J Med* 355:2765–2770, 2006.

Comenzo RL: Amyloidosis, *Curr Treat Options Oncol* 7(3):225–231, 2006.

DeVita V, Hellman S, Rosenberg S, editors: *Cancer: principles and practice of oncology,* ed 8, Philadelphia, Lippincott-Raven, 2008.

Dispenzieri A: POEMS syndrome, *Blood Rev* 21:285–299, 2007.

Gertz M, Lacy MQ, Dispenzieri A, Hayman SR: Amyloidosis, *Best Pract Res Clin Haematol* 18:709–727, 2005.

Hoffman R, Benz EJ, Shattil SJ, et al, editors: *Hematology: basic principles and practice,* ed 4, New York, Churchill Livingstone, 2005.

Kyle R, Rajkumar S: Monoclonal gammopathy of undetermined significance and smouldering multiple myeloma: emphasis on risk factors for progression, *Br J Haematol* 139(5):730–743, 2007.

Kyle R, Rajkumar V: Multiple myeloma, *Blood* 15(111):2962–2972, 2008.

Rajkumar S, Dispenzieri A, Kyle R: Monclonal gammopathy of undetermined significance, Waldenstrom macroglobulinemia, AL amyloidosis and related plasma cell disorders: diagnosis and treatment, *Mayo Clin Proc* 81(5):693–703, 2006.

- Underlying plasma cell dyscrasias should be ruled out with SPEP/UPEP/serum IFE/urine IFE, bone marrow aspirate/biopsy, CBC and differential diagnosis, chemistry panel, and serum light chain assay
- Variant transthyretin (familial amyloidosis) should also be ruled out by DNA testing
- If no plasma cell dyscrasias, transthyretin normal, consider AA amyloidosis

Treatment

- **Directed at the underlying disease**, with goal to prevent further deposition of amyloid (**resorption of amyloid fibers usually does not occur**); management must also focus on control of symptoms from organ dysfunction

Selected Topics in Oncology

MARK LEVIS, MD, PhD

Previous chapters in this section have focused on the diagnosis and treatment of specific types of cancers. This chapter emphasizes other important aspects in the identification and care of oncologic patients. Specifically, the evaluation of patients with cancer of unknown primary, as well as the identification of oncologic emergencies and paraneoplastic syndromes, is emphasized. Although specific chemotherapeutic regimens are generally left to oncologists, basic toxicities and complications of chemotherapeutic agents should be recognized by all internists.

Cancer of Unknown Primary

Basic Information

- 3% to 5% of all patients with newly diagnosed cancers present with primary tumors of unknown origin
- Equal incidence in men and women
- Median age 60 years
- Most common primary site: Lymph nodes
- Only 20% of patients have a primary site identified after workup
- Cytopathology
  - Helpful in determining the primary tumor site
  - Histology
    - **Adenocarcinoma is the most commonly identified tumor type (60% of cases)**
      - Prostate-specific antigen stain may be helpful in identifying prostate cancer
    - Poorly or undifferentiated carcinoma is seen in about 30% of cases
    - Squamous cell carcinoma is seen in 5% to 10% of cases
    - Specific immunoperoxidase stains may be helpful in suggesting specific causes (Table 58-1)
  - Genetic studies may be helpful in identifying non-Hodgkin's lymphomas and sarcomas

TABLE 58-1	*Immunoperoxidase Stains*
Tumor Type	**Immunoperoxidase Stain**
Carcinoma	Cytokeratin, chromogranin
Melanoma	S100, HMB45
Sarcoma	Vimentin, desmin
Lymphoma	Leukocyte common antigen
Neuroendocrine	Cytokeratin, synaptophysin, chromogranin

Clinical Presentation

- Depends on site of organ involvement
- Weight loss and fatigue common
- Lymphadenopathy (cervical, supraclavicular, mediastinal, axillary, retroperitoneal) may be the only clinical abnormality

Diagnosis

- **Avoid the impulse to randomly order tumor markers and imaging studies**
  - Start with a thorough history and physical (including gynecologic examination or prostate examination) to guide your evaluation
  - Make sure appropriate cancer screening is up to date
- CBC, chemistry profile, liver function tests
- Chest radiograph and CT scan of abdomen and pelvis should be ordered routinely. A positron emission tomography/CT scan should be considered.
- Colonoscopy should be considered if clinical symptoms dictate or if screening measures are not up to date
- Mammography for women should be considered if indicated by symptoms or if screening measures are not up to date
- Order biopsy of mass and special studies (as described previously)
- Specific evaluation measures dictated by location of discovered tumor (Table 58-2)

Treatment

- Directed at the primary site of origin, if discovered
- In cases where the primary tumor is not identified, treatment is based on tumor histology and location (see Table 58-2)
- **In cases where the histology and location do not suggest a specific primary site (most cases), empirical chemotherapy can extend median survival by a few months**

Oncologic Emergencies

SPINAL CORD COMPRESSION

Basic Information

- More than 5% of patients who die from cancer have evidence of spinal cord compression
- The most common primary malignancies include lung cancer, breast cancer, prostate cancer, renal cell cancer, and multiple myeloma

TABLE 58-2	*Evaluation and Treatment of Specific Carcinomas*	
Clinical Finding	**Histology/Treatment***	**Evaluation**
Isolated axillary adenopathy in women	Breast examination	Adenocarcinoma Stage II breast cancer Mammogram Estrogen/progesterone receptor studies
Cervical adenopathy and neck cancer	Squamous cell carcinoma	Head and neck examination Panendoscopy of the aerodigestive tract CT scan of head and neck area
Inguinal adenopathy	Squamous cell carcinoma	Full gynecologic examination in women Evaluation of prostate, penis, and testes in males Rectal examinations Tumor markers (PSA, CA-125)
Bone metastases	Adenocarcinoma or poorly differentiated carcinoma	Physical examination Stage IV prostate cancer or breast cancer X-rays of spine/weight-bearing joints to rule out fracture PSA in men
Mediastinal/retroperitoneal adenopathy in young males	Extragonadal germ cell tumor	Poorly differentiated carcinoma Tumor markers (hCG, AFP, LDH)
Peritoneal carcinomatosis	Adenocarcinoma	Full gynecologic examination in women Colonoscopy

*Empirical treatment if the evaluation failed to confirm the primary site.
AFP, α-fetoprotein; CA-125, cancer antigen 125; hCG, human chorionic gonadotropin; LDH, lactate dehydrogenase; PSA, prostate-specific antigen.

- Compression most commonly caused by extradural metastases involving the spinal cord
- **Any delay in diagnosis and treatment may result in paralysis and incontinence of bowel and bladder that may be irreversible**
- Spinal cord compression (SCC) may be the initial manifestation of a malignancy
- Most cases (60%) involve the thoracic spine, but compression can occur at the lumbosacral (20%) and cervical (10%) regions as well

Clinical Presentation

- Back pain that continues to increase in intensity is the most common initial finding
  - Pain can be worsened by movement, coughing, sneezing
  - Radicular symptoms can develop (more common with lumbosacral lesions)
- Progressive motor weakness leading to instability of gait and paralysis is also common
- Sensory loss is seen in over half of patients
- Change in deep tendon reflexes (hyper- or hyporeflexia) and extensor plantar responses may be seen
- Incontinence of stool or urine is usually a late finding

Diagnosis

- History and physical examination should focus on neurologic abnormalities
- **Radiologic imaging should be immediately done in all cancer patients who present with persistent back pain with or without radicular symptoms**
  - Plain spinal radiographs may detect vertebral compression fractures or collapse or erosive spinal lesions, but there is a high false-negative rate

- MRI is now the test of choice given its widespread availability
- CT myelogram is an alternative for patients who cannot lie still for an MRI or who have a contraindication to MRI

Treatment

- Goal is to control pain and preserve neurologic function
- Options are surgical resection or decompression, radiation therapy, and, in some cases, systemic chemotherapy. Urgent surgical, radiation, and medical oncology consults should be obtained.
  - **Surgery, when feasible, has been shown to result in better clinical outcomes and possibly a survival benefit compared with radiation**
- Steroids should be given promptly
  - Initially, high-dose steroid therapy (dexamethasone 96 mg/day) may be given for palliation of pain and improvement of neurologic status, but this regimen may be associated with a higher treatment complication rate than a lower-dose regimen (16 mg/day)
- Surgery
  - Consider in patients who
    - Have tumors that are not sensitive to radiation
    - Have received prior radiation therapy to the affected area
    - Need a tissue diagnosis
    - Need spinal stabilization
- Chemotherapy should be considered in patients with chemosensitive tumors
- Overall, prognosis is poor; median survival after diagnosis is 6 months

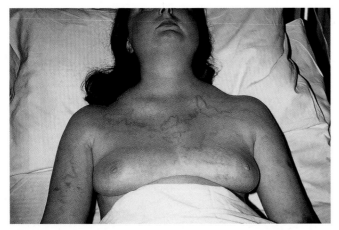

FIGURE 58-1 Superior vena caval obstruction in bronchial carcinoma. Note the swelling of the face and neck and the development of a collateral circulation in the veins of the chest wall. (From Goldman L, Bennett JC, Ausiello D: *Cecil textbook of medicine,* ed 22, Philadelphia, WB Saunders, 2004, figure 95-6.)

SUPERIOR VENA CAVA SYNDROME

- **Defined as obstruction of blood return to the heart by invasion, compression, or thrombosis of the superior vena cava (SVC)**
- Most cases are associated with lung cancer (small cell), lymphoma, thymoma, testicular, or breast cancer
- Can also result from venous thrombosis caused by indwelling venous access devices or fibrosing mediastinitis from infections (e.g., histoplasmosis, tuberculosis)
- Signs and symptoms include shortness of breath, facial swelling, fullness of face, cough, arm swelling, and prominent neck and chest veins (Fig. 58-1)
- CT scanning of the chest with contrast or MRI with gadolinium enhancement are the diagnostic modalities of choice
- If the cause is unknown, an evaluation that may include CT-guided biopsy, bronchoscopy, mediastinoscopy, or thoracotomy should be considered
- Treatment with radiation or chemotherapy may be indicated once the tumor type has been identified
- Intraluminal metal stents may provide palliation when cancer is refractory to chemotherapy or radiation
- Thrombolytics and anticoagulation may be necessary for patients with thrombosis

PERICARDIAL TAMPONADE

See also Chapter 8.
- Rarely occurs as the initial manifestation of a cancer
- Seen most commonly in patients with lung or breast cancer, lymphoma, or leukemia
- Cannot assume that all pericardial effusions in cancer patients are caused by metastasis
- Treatment options in symptomatic patients include prolonged catheter drainage, substernal pericardiotomy, pericardiectomy, or injection of a sclerosing agent
- **No need to treat asymptomatic pericardial effusions**

VENOUS THROMBOSIS

- Thromboembolism is the second leading cause of death in patients with malignancy
- Venous thrombosis is seen most commonly with visceral cancers from pancreas, lung, stomach, colon, breast, and ovary
- **Trousseau's syndrome refers to migratory superficial thrombophlebitis in the setting of visceral cancers**
- The risk of thrombosis is increased because of release of procoagulants by tumor cells, immobility of patients because of weakness, or obstruction of blood vessels by tumors
- Patients should be treated initially with heparin, then warfarin
- Sometimes the thromboembolism is resistant to warfarin and requires low-molecular-weight heparin therapy or inferior vena cava filter placement
- See Chapter 22 for detailed information regarding deep venous thrombosis and thromboembolism

METABOLIC EMERGENCIES

- Hypercalcemia of malignancy (see Chapter 40)
- Hyponatremia (see Chapter 33)

Paraneoplastic Syndromes

Basic Information

- Defined as conditions that arise as a result of factors produced by cancer cells
- **In some cases, the symptoms of these syndromes may precede the actual diagnosis of malignancy**
- Presence does not necessarily imply a poor prognosis
- Long-term treatment is geared toward the underlying malignancy

NEUROLOGIC SYNDROMES

- A number of specific syndromes have been described that may affect all parts of the nervous system (Table 58-3)
- Antineuronal antibodies may be helpful in diagnosis and in searching for particular neoplasms; however, they may not always be present

RHEUMATOLOGIC SYNDROMES

- Hypertrophic osteoarthropathy (Fig. 58-2)
  - Abnormal proliferation of bone and skin in the extremities
  - Most commonly associated with adenocarcinoma of the lung but sometimes seen with other lung cancers, lung infections, or conditions that result in right-to-left shunting of blood
  - Symptoms include joint pain with or without effusions
  - Examination may reveal new digital clubbing
  - Radiographs show periosteal new bone formation
  - **If the diagnosis is made, the thorax should be imaged to search for lung cancer**
- Dermatomyositis/polymyositis (see Chapter 46)
  - Presents with proximal muscle weakness with or without pain (polymyositis)

58

TABLE 58-3	*Selected Neurologic Paraneoplastic Syndromes*		
Syndrome	**Description**	**Most Commonly Associated Tumors**	**Antibody**
Encephalomyelitis	Precedes discovery of the tumor in most patients Symptoms vary because it can involve a number of different areas of the nervous system Subacute sensory neuronopathy causing asymmetrical paresthesias is the most common early symptom	SCLC	Anti-Hu (also called antineuronal nuclear antibodies or ANNA-1)
Cerebellar degeneration	Abrupt onset of dysarthria and ataxia Nystagmus and oculomotor dysfunction can occur	SCLC Ovarian cancer Breast cancer Uterine cancer Hodgkin's lymphoma	Anti-Yo Anti-Tr (in Hodgkin's lymphoma only)
Limbic encephalitis	Presents with memory loss, mood changes, emotional lability Hallucinations and seizures may occur	SCLC Testicular germ cell tumors Thymoma Hodgkin's lymphoma	Anti-Hu Anti-Ta (testicular or breast)
Stiff-person syndrome	Muscle stiffness or rigidity Usually begins asymmetrically Can cause significant pain EMG shows abnormal continuous firing of motor units	SCLC Breast cancer Thymoma Hodgkin's lymphoma	Anti-amphiphysin Anti-GAD (breast)
Lambert-Eaton myasthenic syndrome (LEMS)	Presents with proximal weakness that improves with exercise Bulbar weakness not seen (as opposed to myasthenia gravis) EMG shows motor unit potentials whose amplitude increases with exercise Treatment is geared to malignancy but plasmapheresis or immunosuppressives may be helpful	SCLC	LEMS antibody

EMG, electromyography; GAD, glutamic acid decarboxylase; SCLC, small-cell lung cancer.

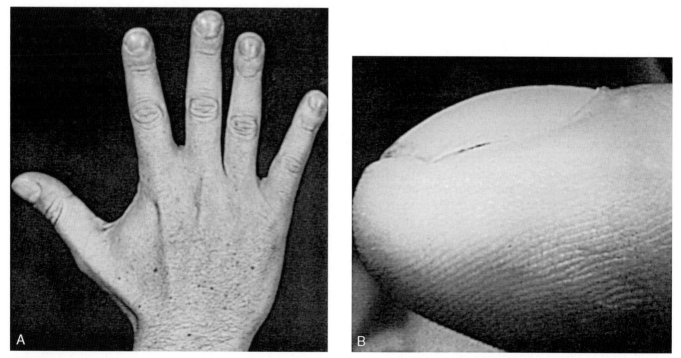

FIGURE 58-2 **A,** Dorsal view of the hand shows clubbing, with widening of the fingertips replacing the normally tapered appearance of the digits. **B,** A lateral view of the index finger demonstrates clubbing with loss of the normal 15-degree angle between the nail and the cuticle due to accentuated convexity of the nail. There is also enlargement of the distal finger pad and shininess of the nail and adjacent skin. (From Harris ED, Budd RC, Genovese MC, et al, editors: *Kelley's textbook of rheumatology,* ed 7, Philadelphia, WB Saunders, 2005, figures 110-2 and 110-3.)

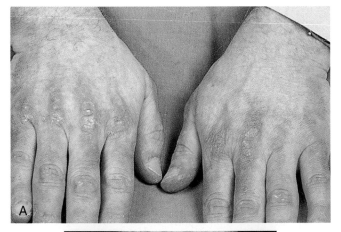

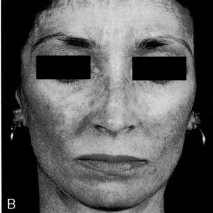

FIGURE 58-3 Dermatomyositis. **A,** Grotton's papules of the hands. **B,** Facial rash with periorbital and malar distribution. (From Albert RK, Spiro SG, Jett JR, editors: *Clinical respiratory medicine,* ed 2, St. Louis, Mosby, 2004, figure 48.6.)

- Dermatomyositis is diagnosed if skin involvement is also present (Fig. 58-3)
- Associated primarily with ovarian, breast, and lung cancers
- Tumors usually present within five years of the diagnosis
- Laboratory data reveal increased sedimentation rate, creatine phosphokinase level, and abnormal electromyogram
- Muscle biopsy confirms the diagnosis

ENDOCRINOLOGIC SYNDROMES

- Carcinoid syndrome
  - Associated with carcinoid tumors of the small intestine, cervix, stomach, rectum, and lung
  - **Usually presents when there is metastasis to the liver**
  - Clinical symptoms include flushing, diarrhea, abdominal pain, and wheezing
  - Fibrosis of the endocardium (predominantly tricuspid valve) is a late complication
  - Diagnose with 24-hour urine for 5-hydroxyindoleacetic acid (5-HIAA), or elevated serum or platelet serotonin levels
  - Treat with surgical resection whenever possible
  - Somatostatin analogues may help control symptoms

- Cushing's syndrome
  - Seen predominantly with small-cell lung cancer, pancreatic islet cell tumors, thymic cancer, and bronchial carcinoid
  - Usually caused by ectopic secretion of adrenocorticotropic hormones (ACTH) from cancer cells but can rarely occur secondary to ectopic secretion of corticotropin-releasing hormone (CRH)
  - Signs and symptoms include truncal obesity, fatigue, weakness, hypertension, abdominal striae, hyperpigmentation, hirsutism, polyuria, polydipsia
  - Laboratory evaluation (see Chapter 42)
  - Treatment is geared toward the underlying malignancy
  - Ketoconazole, metyrapone, or aminoglutethamide may be used to inhibit steroid production and provide symptomatic relief
- Acromegaly
  - Usually caused by ectopic release of growth hormone-releasing hormone (GHRH)
  - Associated with bronchial carcinoids, pancreatic islet cell tumors, lung cancer, breast cancer, and colon cancer
  - Signs and symptoms include increasing glove and shoe size, impotence, hypertension, amenorrhea, diabetes
  - Elevated insulin-like growth factor (IGF-1), GHRH, and glucose-suppressed growth hormone levels establish the diagnosis (see Chapter 42)
  - Treat the underlying malignancy
  - Bromocriptine and octreotide may be used to suppress growth hormone secretion from the pituitary
- Hypercalcemia (see Chapter 40)
  - Can be caused by parathyroid hormone-related protein (PTHrp), osteolytic metastases, and tumor production of calcitriol (seen mainly with lymphomas)
  - Most commonly occurs with lung cancer, breast cancer, and multiple myeloma
- Syndrome of inappropriate antidiuretic hormone (SIADH; see Chapter 33)
  - Caused by ectopic secretion of antidiuretic hormone (ADH)
  - Most commonly seen with small-cell lung cancer

NONBACTERIAL THROMBOTIC ENDOCARDITIS

- Caused by clotting and platelet activation by procoagulants released by tumors
- Associated primarily with adenocarcinomas (e.g., lung, GI tract)
- Sterile, verrucous lesions are seen, usually on left-sided heart valves
- Clinically may present as embolic stroke, seizure, confusion
- Can be associated with disseminated intravascular coagulation (DIC)
- Diagnose with echocardiogram and/or cerebral angiogram with negative blood cultures
- Treatment is geared to the underlying malignancy

CUTANEOUS SYNDROMES

See Chapter 66.

58

Cancer Chemotherapy

Basic Information

- Most drugs are designed to impair cell division
- Selectivity stems from the effect on cells that are more rapidly dividing (i.e., tumor cells)
- Normal cells that rapidly divide are also affected, causing common toxicities (e.g., bone marrow suppression, hair loss, mucosal sloughing)
- Chemotherapy toxicity may be acute or chronic, dose-dependent, or idiosyncratic

CHEMOTHERAPY TOXICITY

- Acute toxicities are common and include nausea, vomiting, diarrhea, headache, and fatigue
- Delayed toxicities
  - Bone marrow suppression is a common side effect of many agents
  - Some selective toxicities are listed in Table 58-4

TUMOR LYSIS SYNDROME

- Caused by rapid destruction of a large number of cancer cells
- **Results in hyperuricemia, hyperkalemia, hyperphosphatemia, lactic acidosis, hypocalcemia, and acute renal failure**
- Seen most commonly after treatment of leukemias and lymphomas
- Prevention of renal failure with fluid administration, allopurinol, and sodium bicarbonate should be attempted in high-risk patients (i.e., patients with high tumor burdens, baseline renal dysfunction, baseline hyperuricemia)
- Treatment with IV fluids, loop diuretics, alkalinization of the urine, and allopurinol can by tried initially in patients developing acute renal failure
- Treatment with rasburicase can lower the serum uric acid level rapidly, helping to prevent renal failure
- Hemodialysis may be necessary if the response is inadequate

TABLE 58-4	Delayed Toxicity of Selected Chemotherapeutic Agents
Drug	**Toxicity**
Bleomycin	Pneumonitis and pulmonary fibrosis
Cisplatin	Hearing loss, nephrotoxicity
Cyclophosphamide	Hemorrhagic cystitis
Daunorubicin	Cardiomyopathy
Doxorubicin	Cardiomyopathy
Fluorouracil	Severe diarrhea, oral or GI ulcers, palmar or plantar rash
Methotrexate	Oral/GI ulcers, pulmonary infiltrates and fibrosis, cirrhosis
Paclitaxel	Peripheral neuropathy
Vincristine	Peripheral neuropathy

FEBRILE NEUTROPENIA

Basic Information and Clinical Presentation

- Neutropenia is defined as absolute neutrophil count (ANC) less than 500/mL
- Fever usually defined as one temperature greater than 38.5°C or three temperatures above 38°C within 24 hours
- Usually occurs as a result of chemotherapy
- Patients may or may not have any localizing symptoms to suggest a source for infection
- Infectious agents to consider include *Staphylococcus aureus*, *Staphylococcus epidermidis*, *Escherichia coli*, *Klebsiella pneumoniae*, *Pseudomonas aeruginosa*, and fungi

Diagnosis

- History and physical examination
- Inspect rectal area but avoid digital rectal examination because it may introduce infection
- Obtain CBC and calculate ANC
- Obtain chest radiograph
- Panculture (i.e., blood, urine, sputum, throat, stool [including *Clostridium difficile*])

Treatment

- Empirical antibiotics should be administered immediately
- Evaluation usually identifies a primary source of infection in only 20% of patients
- Antibiotic choice depends on hospital practice, but in general should be broad-spectrum unless causal organism is clear
- Possible antibiotic regimens
  - Single-agent therapy: Cefipime, cefotetan, imipenem-cilastin, meropenem, ceftazidime
  - Combination therapy: β-Lactam (e.g., piperacillin, ticarcillin) plus an aminoglycoside (e.g., gentamicin, tobramycin) or ciprofloxacin
- In patients with persistent fever the addition of vancomycin or antifungal drugs (e.g., amphotericin or fluconazole) should be considered

TYPHLITIS

- Necrotizing infection of the cecum and colon
- Symptoms include fever, diarrhea, and right lower quadrant abdominal pain (mimics appendicitis)
- Seen predominantly after treatment for acute leukemia
- Treat with broad-spectrum antibiotics
- Surgery may be necessary

SUGGESTED READINGS

Abramowicz M: Treatment guidelines: drugs of choice for cancer, *Med Lett Drugs Ther* 1:41–52, 2003.

Dropcho EJ: Update on paraneoplastic syndromes, *Curr Opin Neurol* 18:331–336, 2005.

Ettinger DS, Aqulnik M, Cristea M, et al: Occult primary, *J Natl Compr Canc Netw* 6:1026–1060, 2008.

Hainsworth JD, Greco FA: Treatment of patients with cancer of an unknown primary site, *N Engl J Med* 329:257–263, 1993.

Picazo JJ: Management of the febrile neutropenic patient: a consensus conference, *Clin Infect Dis* 39(Suppl 1):S1–S6, 2004.

Rice TW, Rodriguez RM, Light RW: The superior vena cava syndrome: clinical characteristics and evolving etiology, *Medicine (Baltimore)* 85:37–42, 2006.

Schmidt MH, Klimo P Jr, Vrionis FD: Metastatic spinal cord compression, *J Natl Compr Canc Netw* 3:711–719, 2005.

Walji N, Chan AK, Peake DR: Common acute oncologic emergencies: diagnosis, investigation, and management, *Postgrad Med J* 84:418–427, 2008.

Lung Cancer and Head and Neck Cancer

MARK LEVIS, MD, PHD

Lung cancer is now the most common cause of death due to cancer in both men and women in the United States, claiming 160,000 lives per year. Given the well-established relationship between smoking and most types of lung cancer, it also remains the most preventable neoplastic disorder. Although head and neck cancer is less common than lung cancer, its relationship to tobacco use is similar, making it a highly preventable disease. This chapter will serve to highlight the features of these two smoking-related diseases.

Lung Cancer

Basic Information

- **Most common cause of death due to cancer in both genders**
- Incidence over the past decade has been declining in men but slowly increasing in women
- African-American males have highest incidence rates for lung cancer
- Risk factors
  - Tobacco
    - **80% to 90% of lung cancer cases result from cigarette smoking**
    - Risk is dependent upon total lifetime consumption of cigarettes
    - Risk of lung cancer begins to decrease 5 years after smoking has ceased, although the risk always remains higher than that for a nonsmoker
    - Passive or secondhand smoke associated with increased risk (3–5% of all lung cancer cases)
    - Smoking of cigars may also increase risk, although the association is highly variable
  - Asbestos
    - Increases risk of bronchogenic carcinoma and mesothelioma
    - A potential hazard for a number of occupations, including plumbers, pipefitters, carpenters, electricians, welders, and insulation workers
  - Radon
  - Uranium
  - Ionizing radiation
  - Nickel, chromium

- Screening
  - Prospective studies of lung cancer screening do not support use of chest radiograph or sputum cytology
  - Spiral CT scan of chest is more sensitive than chest film and is being evaluated in multiple clinical studies
- Pathology
  - Non-small-cell lung cancer (60–80% of cases)
    - Adenocarcinoma
      - **Most common type in nonsmokers**
      - Peripheral location
      - Bronchoalveolar carcinoma is a subtype that presents diffusely within the lungs
    - Squamous cell
      - Can be associated with hypercalcemia as a paraneoplastic syndrome (see Chapters 40 and 58)
      - Central location
      - 10% undergo cavitation
    - Large-cell lung cancer—usually peripheral location
  - Small-cell lung cancer (20% of cases)
    - Small primary tumors, but adenopathy may be bulky
    - Associated with a number of paraneoplastic syndromes, most commonly syndrome of inappropriate antidiuretic hormone (SIADH)
  - Mesothelioma (Box 59-1)

Clinical Presentation

- Cough, dyspnea, and chest pain are the most common presenting symptoms
- Hemoptysis is seen more commonly with central lesions

BOX 59-1	*Malignant Mesothelioma*

Most common risk factor is asbestos exposure

Male predominance

Disease manifests 20–30 yr after initial exposure; usually around age 60 yr

Presenting symptoms include dyspnea and chest pain

Chest imaging typically reveals pleural abnormality with a large pleural effusion

Diagnosis is made by thoracentesis and pleural biopsy

Treatment options are limited

   Extrapleural pneumonectomy with or without chemotherapy and radiation is one treatment strategy

Prognosis (even with treatment) is currently poor

- Recurrent or unresolving pneumonia caused by obstruction
- Hoarseness: Caused by recurrent laryngeal nerve compression
- **Horner's syndrome: Ptosis, miosis, ipsilateral anhydrosis from sympathetic chain involvement of tumor**
- Paraneoplastic syndromes (see Chapter 58)
- **Shoulder pain: Pancoast tumors—apical tumors locally invading the lower brachial plexus (C8–T2) and chest wall, resulting in shoulder pain and plexopathy—may be missed on chest radiograph**
- Poor prognostic factors
  - Weight loss of more than 5% body weight
  - Advanced stage (see following discussion)
  - Poor performance status
  - *K-ras* oncogene mutation (non-small cell)

Diagnosis

- All patients should have a history and physical examination, CBC, chemistry profile, liver function tests, and CT scan of chest and abdomen
- Bronchoscopy
  - 80% to 85% effective in establishing a diagnosis for centrally located tumors
  - Not as effective for peripheral lesions
- CT-guided biopsy is about 90% effective for establishing a diagnosis for peripherally located tumors
- Mediastinoscopy may be used for diagnosis or staging (especially for anterior mediastinal lymph nodes)
- Positron emission tomography (PET) scan
  - Hypermetabolic tumors enhance on scanning
  - Considered more sensitive than CT for mediastinal disease (Fig. 59-1)
  - Currently recommended to confirm the presence of resectable non-small-cell cancer

- Bone scan and head CT
  - For non-small-cell cancers: Obtain if symptoms are suggestive of bony metastasis or neurologic disease
  - For small-cell cancers: Obtain routinely as part of the staging workup
- Staging
  - Non-small-cell lung cancer: TNM staging criteria (Table 59-1)
  - Small-cell lung cancer
    - Limited stage: Disease confined to one hemithorax and can be encompassed within a single radiation therapy port
    - Extensive stage: Disease spread outside of the preceding area

Treatment

- Non-small-cell lung cancer
  - Stages I to IIIa
    - **Surgery is the treatment of choice if performance status is good and postresection pulmonary reserve is deemed to be adequate (forced expiratory volume in 1 second [FEV$_1$] > 0.8 L)**
    - Adjuvant chemotherapy or radiation may be beneficial for stage IIIa disease, but not for earlier stages
  - Stage IIIb: Radiation therapy with or without chemotherapy
  - Stage IV
    - Goal is palliation
    - Chemotherapy prolongs survival
    - Multitargeted receptor kinase inhibitors, which target the vascular endothelial growth factor receptor and platelet-derived growth factor receptor, may have a role in the future
- Small-cell lung cancer
  - Limited stage
    - Combined chemotherapy (platinum-/etoposide-based regimen) plus concurrent radiation
    - Consider prophylactic cranial irradiation (PCI)
      - Decreases risk of brain metastases

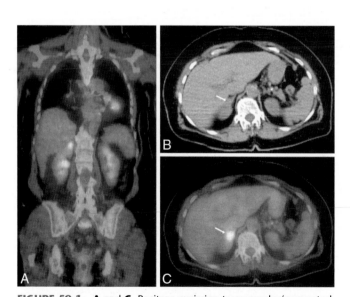

FIGURE 59-1 **A** and **C,** Positron emission tomography/computed tomography (PET/CT) scans demonstrate right adrenal mass (*arrow*). **B,** Less well-delineated on CT scan (*arrow*). (From Abeloff, MD, Armitage JO, Niederhuber JE, et al: *Clinical oncology,* ed 3, Philadelphia, Churchill Livingstone, 2004, figure 75-9.)

TABLE 59-1	Staging for Non–Small-Cell Lung Cancer	
Stage	**Description**	**5-Year Survival Rate (%)**
I	Any size tumor with or without extension into visceral pleura, at least 2 cm from carina, no nodal involvement	60–80
II	Any size, extension into intrabronchial lymph nodes	40–50
IIIa	Any size, extension into parietal pleura, chest wall, or mediastinal pleura, or into hilar or ipsilateral mediastinal lymph nodes	20–30
IIIb	Any size, extension into mediastinal structures, contralateral hilar, mediastinal, or supraclavicular lymph nodes	10–20
IV	Evidence of distant metastasis	<5

- No effect on survival
- Surgical resection may be an option in a small subset of patients after chemoradiation
- Median survival is 18 months
- Extensive stage
  - Chemotherapy with platinum/etoposide or irinotecan/etoposide
  - Median survival is 9 months

Head and Neck Cancer

Basic Information

- Responsible for as many as 11,000 cancer deaths per year, out of 48,000 cases diagnosed in the United States
- More common in men
- Median age is 60 years
- Can affect the oral cavity, larynx, pharynx, or nasopharynx
- Risk factors
  - Tobacco
    - Dose-response relationship between the occurrence of cancer and duration and amount of cigarette use
    - Secondhand smoke and cigars may also be risk factors
  - Alcohol
    - Increased risk with heavy use (>50 g/day)
    - No increased risk with moderate use (<19 g/day)
    - Risk is greatly increased in people who drink and smoke cigarettes heavily
  - Prior radiation therapy: Increased risk of salivary gland tumors
  - Plummer-Vinson syndrome
    - Characterized by dysphagia, iron deficiency anemia, and esophageal webs in women
    - Increased incidence of cancer of the hypopharynx and esophagus
  - **Epstein-Barr virus (EBV)**
  - **Strong association with nasopharyngeal carcinoma, which has a high incidence in southern China**
    - Pathology is usually undifferentiated rather than squamous cell type
  - Human papilloma virus (HPV)
    - Type 16 most strongly associated with invasive tumors of the oral cavity and oropharynx
    - Presence of HPV may confer a better prognosis
- Pathology
  - Most cancers in the United States are squamous cell carcinomas
  - Precancerous lesions
    - Leukoplakia (Fig. 59-2): Hyperkeratosis associated with a low malignant potential (<5% of cases)
    - Erythroplakia
      - Red, superficial patches adjacent to normal mucosa
      - Associated with dysplasia
      - Significant malignant potential (40% of cases)
    - Dysplasia
      - Presence of mitoses and prominent nucleoli
      - Can involve entire mucosa (carcinoma in situ)
      - Commonly progresses to invasive cancer

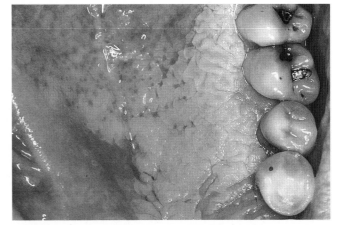

FIGURE 59-2 Leukoplakia of the hard palate. (From Cummings CW, Flint PW, Harker LA, et al: *Otolaryngology: head and neck surgery,* ed 4, Philadelphia, Mosby, 2005, figure 64-5B.)

- Lymphoepithelial: Undifferentiated tumors predominantly seen in nasopharyngeal carcinoma because of EBV (see preceding discussion)

Clinical Presentation

- Symptoms vary by the site of the tumor
  - Nasal cavity: Epistaxis, ulceration, nasal obstruction
  - Paranasal sinuses: Recurrent or persistent sinusitis
  - Nasopharyngeal: Mass, Eustachian tube dysfunction, serous otitis media
  - Oral cavity, tongue, lips: Mass with or without ulceration
  - Laryngeal/glottic: Hoarseness, dysphagia, odynophagia, hemoptysis
- Cervical lymphadenopathy may sometimes be the only finding on presentation

Diagnosis

- History and physical examination with emphasis on risk factors and direct visualization of tumor
- **Fiberoptic endoscopy is necessary to assess the extent of the tumor as well as vocal cord mobility**
- Diagnosis is usually made by direct biopsy of tumor or fine-needle aspiration of a metastatic lymph node
- CT scan of the head and neck aids in the staging process
- Chest CT and panendoscopy (e.g., laryngoscopy, esophagoscopy, bronchoscopy) are helpful for detecting distant metastases and second primary lesions
- PET scan is useful for detecting recurrent tumors in patients who have had surgery and may be useful in detecting occult head and neck cancers

Treatment

- Staging system and treatments vary depending on the primary tumor site
- Primary therapy of squamous cell carcinoma usually includes surgery (possibly neck dissection; Fig. 59-3) and radiation therapy, although the role of chemotherapy continues to expand
  - Early (stages I and II)
    - Goal is for cure with either radiation or surgery

59

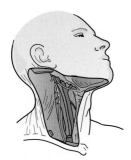

Radical neck dissection

A

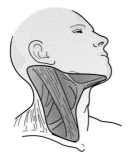

Modified radical neck dissection: one or more of the nonlymphatic structures are preserved

B

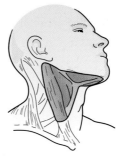

Supraomohyoid neck dissection

C

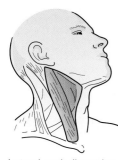

Lateral neck dissection

D

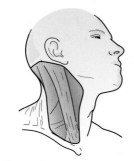

Posterolateral neck dissection

E

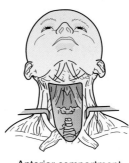

Anterior compartment neck dissection

F

FIGURE 59-3 Types of neck dissection. **A**, Radical. **B**, Modified radical: One or more of the nonlymphatic structures are preserved. **C**, Supraomohyoid. **D**, Lateral. **E**, Posterolateral. **F**, Anterior compartment. (From Abeloff MD, Armitage JO, Niederhuber JE, et al, editors: *Clinical oncology*, ed 3, Philadelphia, Churchill Livingstone, 2004, figure 71-6.)

- Advanced resectable (stages III and IV, without distant metastases)
  - Surgery and postoperative radiation plus chemotherapy
- Advanced unresectable
  - Treat with chemoradiotherapy
  - Prognosis is poor
- Metastatic disease
  - Radiation with or without chemotherapy
- Nasopharyngeal cancer is primarily treated with radiation therapy and chemotherapy
- Significant morbidity can be associated with treatment
  - Physical disfiguration
  - Loss of voice or hoarseness
  - Dysphagia or odynophagia leading to malnutrition
  - Xerostomia
    - Artificial saliva can provide temporary relief of symptoms
    - Oral pilocarpine is effective as a treatment and for prophylaxis
  - Osteoradionecrosis of the mandible
  - Fibrosis of neck, pharynx, temporomandibular joint, esophagus
  - Hypothyroidism
- Most tumor recurrences occur within 2 years of the initial treatment

- After 2 years, second primary aerodigestive tumors occur at 3% to 7% per year (field cancerization)
- **Recurrence risk higher in patients who continue to smoke**

REVIEW QUESTIONS

For review questions, please go to www.expertconsult.com.

SUGGESTED READINGS

Cognetti DM, Weber RS, Lai SY: Head and neck cancer: an evolving treatment paradigm, *Cancer* 113:S1911–S1932, 2008.

Department of Veterans Affairs Laryngeal Cancer Study Group: Induction chemotherapy plus radiation compared with surgery plus radiation in patients with advanced laryngeal cancer, *N Engl J Med* 324:1685–1690, 1999.

Hann CL, Rudin CM: Management of small-cell lung cancer: incremental changes but hope for the future, *Oncology* 22:1486–1492, 2008.

Jemal A, Siegel R, Ward E, et al: Cancer statistics, 2008, *CA Cancer J Clin* 58:71–96, 2008.

Molina JR, Yang P, Cassivi SD, et al: Non-small cell lung cancer: epidemiology, risk factors, treatment, and survivorship, *Mayo Clin Proc* 83:584–594, 2008.

Schiller JH, Adak S, Cella D, et al: Topotecan versus observation after cisplatin plus etoposide in extensive-stage small-cell lung cancer: E7593-a phase III trial of the Eastern Cooperative Oncology Group, *J Clin Oncol* 15:2114–2122, 2001.

Suzuki K, Nagai K, Yoshida J, et al: Prognostic factors in clinical stage I non-small cell lung cancer, *Ann Thorac Surg* 67:927–932, 1999.

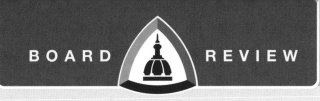

BOARD REVIEW

Neurology

Headaches

KIMBERLY S. PEAIRS, MD

It has been estimated that as many as 90% of individuals experience at least one headache per year. The presentation is much more common for younger women and is usually of benign origin, but may also be the hallmark of a more ominous illness. Certain characteristics of the headache pattern will help guide the clinician in assessing the cause.

Primary Headache Syndromes

Basic Information

- No obvious structural or metabolic cause
- More common in clinical practice than secondary headaches
- **Common primary headache disorders**
  - **Migraine** (see following section)
  - **Tension-type**
    - Episodic, occur less than 15 days a month
    - Chronic, occur more than 15 days a month
  - **Trigeminal autonomic cephalalgias (TACs)**
    - Short-lived attacks; unilateral pain in V1 distribution of trigeminal nerve (around eye) with autonomic features
    - **Cluster headache is most common subtype**
- Complete headache history is helpful in delineating headache type
- Complete physical exam should be done for a headache evaluation with the focus on
  - Blood pressure
  - Optic exam: Papilledema may suggest increased intracranial pressure
  - Visual fields: Field cut warrants imaging
  - Facial tenderness (sinuses, temporal artery): Structural etiology versus giant-cell arteritis
  - Complete neurologic exam: Focal changes are more worrisome for a secondary headache etiology and warrant neuroimaging

Clinical Presentation

- Important features of a history that are helpful to categorize the headache type are listed in Table 60-1
- Also consider comorbid medical diseases in a patient with a headache
  - Hypertension, pregnancy, depression, infection, etc.

Diagnosis and Evaluation

- Diagnosis is based on history and physical
- If history is consistent with a primary headache syndrome and the physical exam is unrevealing, then CNS imaging is usually unnecessary

Treatment

- Migraine (see following section)
- Tension-type headache
  - NSAIDs, acetaminophen, or aspirin
  - Antianxiety medications or antidepressants if concominant disorder exists
  - Biofeedback techniques to manage stress and tension (especially in chronic tension-type)
  - Avoid medication overuse as this may trigger a headache cycle
- Cluster headache
  - Abortive therapy
    - 100% oxygen inhalation (7 L/min) at onset of attack
    - Subcutaneous sumaptriptan
    - Dihydroergotamine (DHE-45) IV or IM
    - Intranasal lidocaine for anesthetic during attack
  - Preventive therapy (during cluster phase)
    - Calcium channel-blockers (verapamil)
    - Lithium
    - Prednisone taper
    - Valproate

Migraine Headache

Basic Information

- Pathophysiology involves neural excitation of the trigeminovascular system causing blood vessel dilatation and "neurogenic inflammation" from release of neurotransmitters, leading to pain and further neural activation
- In migraine with aura subtype, familial hemiplegic migraine, there is an association with mutations in at least three genes that encode for neuron transmembrane channels (i.e., P/Q-type calcium channel, Na/K pump)

Clinical Presentation

See Table 60-1 for clinical characteristics
- International Headache Society (IHS) classification scheme for migraine headache
  - **Migraine without aura (Box 60-1): This is nearly 80% of migraines**
  - Migraine with aura
    - Requires three of four criteria with at least two attacks
    - One or more aura symptoms are fully reversible
    - Aura symptoms develop over more than 4 minutes, or two or more in succession
    - No aura lasts more than 60 minutes

TABLE 60-1	*Clinical Presentations of Primary Headache Syndromes*		
Characteristic	**Migraine Headache**	**Tension-Type Headache**	**Cluster Headache**
Onset (age/sex)	Peak incidence in adolescence More common in females Family history	Variable age of onset More common in females	Age 20–50 yr Male to female ratio 5:1
Frequency	1–2 attacks per mo, may be more frequent Often near menses	Episodic type: <15 days/mo Chronic type: >15 days/mo	*Nightly* or daily for 6–12 wk Circadian association Periods of headache freedom may last months to years
Potential triggers	Stress Too much or too little sleep Hormonal changes Caffeine Red wine Foods: chocolate, cheese, MSG, nitrates	Fatigue Stress	Alcohol (in some or during a period of attacks)
Location	Unilateral > bilateral Bifrontal in 40%	Bilateral, neck, occipital	100% unilateral Temporal or orbital
Pain characteristics	Crescendo pattern Pulsating Moderate to severe pain Patient retreats to dark, quiet room	Pressure or squeezing Waxing/waning severity Patient may remain active	Quick onset of excruciating pain "Suicide headache" Deep and continuous (nonpulsating) Patient may pace or rock from severity of pain
Duration	4–72 hr	Minutes to days	30 min to 3 hr Average is 45–90 min
Associated symptoms	Nausea, vomiting, photophobia, phonophobia ± aura (visual, speech, or motor deficits)	None	*Ipsilateral* parasympathetic overactivity Ptosis, miosis, lacrimation, conjunctival injection Rhinorrhea, nasal congestion Cheek flushing, facial swelling

| BOX 60-1 | *Diagnostic Criteria for Migraine Without Aura* |

At least five attacks fulfilling the following criteria:
Untreated headache lasting 4–72 hr
Group A (2 of 4):
1. Unilateral headache
2. Throbbing or pulsating pain
3. Moderate to severe pain that inhibits ability to function
4. Pain aggravated by routine physical activity
Group B (1 of 2):
1. Presence of nausea or vomiting
2. Presence of photophobia and phonophobia
Underlying disorders that may cause secondary headaches must be ruled out

- Onset of headache within 60 minutes of aura termination
- Underlying cranial disorder must be ruled out
- Retinal migraine
- Monocular blindness with disc edema
- Peripapillary hemorrhage and slow resolution of the vision loss
- Complication of migraine
  - Chronic migraine
    - Migraines on more than 15 days a month
  - Infarction

Diagnosis and Evaluation
- Based on history, physical examination, and classification scheme
- CNS imaging may be warranted for atypical presentations

Treatment
- Therapy for acute migraine attack
  - Treat attacks rapidly and consistently
  - Restore patient's ability to function
  - **Choose drug based on severity of headaches (stratified care approach)**
  - May need to use different approaches for different headaches in same patient
  - Analgesics
    - NSAIDs (e.g., aspirin, ibuprofen, naproxen sodium, combination agent of acetaminophen + aspirin + caffeine)
      - Best for mild to moderate headaches but may be effective for severe attacks
      - Decreased gastric motility may limit effectiveness
    - Metoclopramide (Reglan)
      - Increases gastrointestinal motility and may help as antiemetic
      - Dopamine antagonist and may be used as monotherapy for treatment by IV route
    - Serotonin 5-HT$_{1B/1D}$ receptor agonists ("triptans")
      - **Drugs of choice for moderate or severe migraines or if no response to analgesics**

- Contraindications: Ischemic cardiac or cerebrovascular disease, uncontrolled hypertension, basilar or hemiplegic migraines, ergotamine use
- Use in pregnancy is class C drug: Inadequate data exist
- Sumatriptan: Subcutaneous form rapid onset of action
- Inhaled and oral forms also available: Vary in half-life, onset time, tolerability, efficacy, return of headache
- Ergotamine with or without caffeine
  - Nonspecific serotonin agonist and vasoconstrictor
  - Frequent adverse effects including medication-overuse headache
  - Contraindications: Vascular disease, liver disease, pregnancy (potent vasoconstrictor)
- Dihydroergotamine (DHE)
  - Available in intranasal form with evidence for efficacy and safety
  - Less vasoactive than ergotamine
- Combination agents (acetaminophen/dichloralphenazone/isometheptene)
- Preventive therapy for migraine
  - Behavioral modification
    - Avoid "triggers" (e.g., foods, alcohol, chocolate, caffeine, nicotine, nitrates)
    - Regular sleeping patterns
    - Minimize stress
  - Migraine diary to record patterns of headache and identify possible triggers
  - Consider prophylactic medication if
    - **Two or more attacks a month with three or more days of disability**
    - Failure or contraindication of acute therapy
    - Abortive medications required more than twice a week
  - Recommendations for use of prophylactic migraine medication
    - Start with low dose and titrate slowly
    - Titrate to maximum dose tolerated
    - Allow 6 to 8 weeks to ensure adequate trial
    - Avoid any interfering medications
    - After a period of headache stability, consider tapering or discontinuing medication
  - Migraine headache prevention medications
    - Antihypertensives
      - β-Blockers (propranolol, timolol, nadolol) demonstrate best evidence
      - Verapamil
      - Candesartan
      - Lisinopril (small trial showing efficacy)
    - Antidepressants
      - **Tricyclics (amitriptyline); effect is unrelated to antidepressant activity**
      - Venlafaxine, selective serotonin reuptake inhibitors may also be effective
    - Neuromodulators
      - Divalproex sodium (teratogenic)
      - Topiramate
    - NSAIDs (especially useful for menstrually related migraine)
    - Botulinum toxin injection is being evaluated for those with muscular stress as migraine trigger

- Acupuncture
  - No more effective than "sham acupuncture" for migraine prevention, but both groups had fewer headaches than the untreated group so may have a role in acute treatment and prophylaxis
- Riboflavin (vitamin B_2)

Secondary Headaches

Basic Information

- There is an underlying pathologic or metabolic cause of the headaches
- **Consider secondary headache when a patient with history of headache has new headache pattern**
- Often abnormal neurologic exam

Clinical Presentation

- "Red flags" of secondary headache syndromes (Box 60-2)
- Secondary headache types
  - Subarachnoid hemorrhage (SAH)
    - **Classic "worst headache of life" caused by ruptured intracranial aneurysm**
    - Warning or "thunderclap" headache in 20% to 50% of patients with SAH (severe headache lasting minutes in the days to weeks prior to major bleed)
    - Headache is severe and develops in seconds
    - Diagnosis
      - Noncontrast CT imaging is first choice (Fig. 60-1)
      - If CT done within 24 hours, blood seen in subarachnoid space in 92% of cases
      - Sensitivity begins to decline after 24 hours after bleed
      - Lumbar puncture if head CT negative
        Xanthochromia is criterion for SAH (RBCs break down, releasing hemoglobin, which is metabolized to reveal xanthochromia)
        May be negative if bleed less than 12 hours or more than 2 weeks old
  - Meningeal irritation or meningitis
    - Systemic symptoms, stiff neck, fever
    - Diagnosis made by lumbar puncture
  - Brain tumor
    - Usually other neurologic findings present (seizures, vomiting, papilledema)
    - Worse in morning or if supine
    - Diagnosis made by CNS imaging

BOX 60-2	*"Red Flags" of Secondary Headache Syndromes*

New-onset headache in absence of headache history
Onset age older than 40 yr
Unusually severe headache ("worst of life")
Headaches with progressive course
Significant change in headache pattern over prior 3 mo
Precipitation with exercise, Valsalva maneuver, head turning, supine position
Association with seizure or focal neurologic signs
Systemic symptoms (fever, weight loss, jaw pain)

60

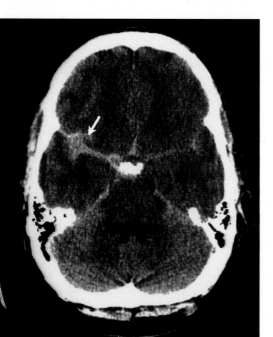

FIGURE 60-1 CT scan of the brain showing a subarachnoid bleed due to a middle cerebral artery aneurysm *(arrow)*. (From Townsend CM, Beauchamp RD, Evers BM, Mattox K: *Sabiston textbook of surgery,* ed 17, Philadelphia, WB Saunders, 2004, figure 71-1A.)

- Temporal arteritis (giant-cell arteritis)
  - Vasculitis of large and medium blood vessels
  - **Two thirds of patients with giant-cell arteritis have headache with localized temporal pain or jaw claudication**
  - Patients are typically older than 50 years
  - Other systemic features present (fever, fatigue, weight loss)
  - Diagnosis made by temporal artery biopsy
  - Other autoimmune illnesses (lupus, vasculitis) may present with headache
- Low-pressure headaches
  - Occurs from contraction of subarachnoid space from a CSF leak or lumbar puncture
  - Pain is worse with standing and relieved when supine
  - Bedrest, hydration, and analgesics are mainstay of therapy
  - Caffeine (PO or IV) may help relieve the pain
- Subdural hematoma
  - Gradual onset of headache often associated with fall
  - Often seen with elderly patients presenting with headache
  - Diagnosis made with CNS imaging
- Pseudotumor cerebri (idiopathic intracranial hypertension)
  - Increased intracranial pressure without mass
  - **More commonly presents in overweight young women**
  - Etiology unclear
  - Headache pattern similar to tension-type headache
  - **Neurologic exam normal except for papilledema, sixth nerve palsy, and possible vision loss**

- Diagnosis
  - Patient has normal head CT but elevated opening pressure on lumbar puncture without other cause for increased pressure
- Cerebral venous thrombosis
  - Rare cause of headache with increased intracranial pressure
  - CT scan may be normal in 30% of cases
  - MR venogram is gold standard

Chronic Daily Headache

Basic Information

- Category of headaches that represent primary and secondary types
- Headaches occur for more than 15 days of the month for longer than 3 months
- Chronic migraine and medication-overuse headaches are two of the more common types of chronic daily headache

Clinical Presentation

- Chronic migraine and medication-overuse headache patients are more frequently women and have history of episodic migraines
- Medications implicated in causing medication-overuse headache
  - Regular overuse of a headache medication for more than 3 months
  - Simple analgesic use more often than 15 days a month
  - Combination analgesics, narcotics, ergotamine, triptans more than 10 days a month

Treatment (Medication-Overuse Headache)

- Lifestyle modification (discontinue caffeine; exercise, regular sleep patterns, etc.)
- Stop all medications (taper opioids)
- If severe headache, try NSAIDs or dihydroergotamine (nonoral route)
- Consider preventive migraine therapy

SUGGESTED READINGS

Buse D, Rupnow M, Lipton R: Assessing and managing all aspects of migraine: migraine attacks, migraine-related functional impairment, common comorbidities, and quality of life, *Mayo Clin Proc* 84(5): 422–435, 2009.

Detsky M, McDonald D, Baerlocher M, et al: Does this patient with headache have a migraine or need neuroimaging? *JAMA* 296: 1274–1283, 2006.

Dodick DW: Chronic daily headache, *N Engl J Med* 354:158–165, 2006.

Edlow JA, Caplan LR: Avoiding pitfalls in the diagnosis of subarachnoid hemorrhage, *N Engl J Med* 342:29–36, 2000.

Goadsby PJ: Migraine—current understanding and treatment, *N Engl J Med* 346:257–270, 2002.

Kaniecki R: Headache assessment and management, *JAMA* 289: 1430–1433, 2003.

Lipton RB, Loder EW: Migraine: primary care challenges in diagnosis and treatment, *Am J Med* 118(Suppl 1):28S–35S, 2005.

Marks DR, Rapoport AM: Practical evaluation and diagnosis of headache, *Semin Neurol* 17:307–312, 1997.

Olesen J, Bousser MG, Diener H, et al: The international classification of headache disorders, ed 2, *Cephalalgia* 23(Suppl 1):1–160, 2004.

Snow V, Weiss K, Wall E, et al: Pharmacologic management of acute attacks of migraine and prevention of migraine headache, *Ann Intern Med* 137:840–849, 2002.

Cerebrovascular Disease and Seizure Disorders

RAFAEL H. LLINÁS, MD, and ROBERT J. WITYK, MD

Cerebrovascular disease is a common disorder in the United States, occurring at a rate of 1 per 1000 population. It is the third leading cause of medical deaths in developed countries. Stroke can be classified into ischemic disease (80%) and hemorrhagic disease (20%). Mortality from ischemic stroke has been declining in the United States because of an increased awareness and attention to modification of risk factors.

Seizures are electrical events of the brain, with varied clinical manifestations, that can be a cause of significant morbidity. Epilepsy is the chronic recurrence of seizures with a usual onset before age 20 years. Often, the underlying cause of epilepsy is unknown.

Cerebrovascular Disease

Basic Information

- Definitions
  - **Ischemic stroke: Focal neurologic deficit lasting more than 24 hours because of loss of blood flow to a portion of the brain that results in irreversible cell death (Fig. 61-1)**
    - Mechanisms
      - Large-vessel atherosclerosis
      - Embolic disease
  - **Transient ischemic attack (TIA): Transient focal neurologic deficit caused by loss of regional blood flow; lasts less than 24 hours, but typically only 10 to 60 minutes**
  - **Intracerebral hemorrhage: Bleeding into the brain parenchyma (Fig. 61-2)**
  - **Subarachnoid hemorrhage: Bleeding into the subarachnoid space around the brain**
- Classification of ischemic cerebrovascular disease (Table 61-1)

Clinical Presentation

- **Ischemic atherosclerotic stroke risk factors are similar to those of coronary artery disease (CAD)**
  - Increasing age
  - Male sex
  - African-American
  - Hypertension, diabetes, high cholesterol
  - Smoking
  - Drug abuse (cocaine, amphetamines)

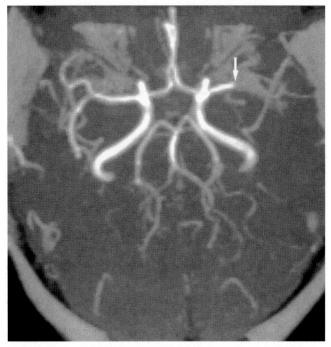

FIGURE 61-1 Magnetic resonance angiogram demonstrating occlusion of the left middle cerebral artery (*arrow*), consistent with a thromboembolic event. (From Forbes CD, Jackson WF: *Color atlas and text of clinical medicine,* ed 3, St. Louis, Mosby, 2003, figure 11.34.)

- Sedentary lifestyle, obesity
- Family history
- **Embolic stroke risk factors**
  - Cardiac arrhythmias: Atrial fibrillation, sick sinus syndrome
  - Dilated cardiomyopathy, including left ventricular aneurysm
  - Valvular disorders, including prosthetic valves, rheumatic heart disease
  - Infective and nonbacterial endocarditis
  - Left ventricular or left atrial thrombus
  - Cardiac myxoma
  - Atrial and ventricular septal defects, patent foramen ovale
- TIAs
  - Usually last 10 to 15 minutes; most resolve within 1 hour

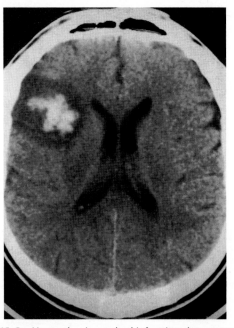

FIGURE 61-2　Hemorrhagic cerebral infarction demonstrated by a noncontrast CT scan. (From Forbes CD, Jackson WF: *Color atlas and text of clinical medicine,* ed 3, St. Louis, Mosby, 2003, figure 11.66.)

- High correlation with future stroke (lifetime risk is 33%)
- Amaurosis fugax is a common presentation
  - Temporary monocular blindness ("shade falling over vision")
  - Secondary to carotid artery atherosclerosis with embolization
- Classic (common) ischemic stroke presentations (see Table 61-1)
- Hemorrhagic stroke (Table 61-2)
  - **Subarachnoid hemorrhage (SAH)**
    - **Bleeding in the space between the brain and the pia arachnoid**
    - **Mortality 50%; prognosis particularly poor for patients who present in coma**
    - Often seen in younger patients (age, 35–65 years)
    - Causes, presentation, treatment (see Table 61-2)
    - Berry aneurysm is common cause (Fig. 61-3)
    - May occur with exertion, during rest, or even in sleep
  - **Complications of SAH**
    - **Rebleeding: Most common in first 2 weeks; 50% mortality**
    - **Hydrocephalus**
    - **Vasospasm: Cause of late ischemic infarctions**

TABLE 61-1	*Classification of Ischemic Cerebrovascular Disease*		
	Examples	**Clinical Presentation**	**Treatment**
Large artery atherosclerosis	Carotid stenosis (extra- or intracranial) Vertebrobasilar disease	Carotid stenosis Ipsilateral face and hand numbness/weakness Aphasia or dysarthria Amaurosis fugax Vertebrobasilar disease Dizziness Vertigo Ataxia "Drop attack"	For intracranial carotid disease: antiplatelet agent or anticoagulation For extracranial carotid disease: <30%: Antiplatelet agent 50–70%: Modest benefit of carotid endarterectomy (CAE) >70% and symptomatic: CEA For vertebrobasilar disease: Antiplatelet agent or anticoagulation
Lacune (small-vessel disease)	Atherosclerosis of small, penetrating vessels Associated with hypertension and diabetes	Pure motor ipsilateral hemiparesis (caused by internal capsule or pons lesion) Pure ipsilateral hemisensory stroke (caused by thalamic lesion)	Antiplatelet agents
Cardiac embolism	Atrial fibrillation Dilated cardiomyopathy Endocarditis	Presentation depends on site of embolization Often occurs at gray-white junction	Anticoagulation for primary or secondary prevention (except for endocarditis—bleeding risk too high Acute anticoagulation not advised because of bleeding risk
Nonatherosclerotic vasculopathy	Fibromuscular dysplasia (FMD) Arterial dissection Vasculitis	Depends on location FMD more common in women May have systemic symptoms with vasculitis May have neck pain with arterial dissection	Treat underlying cause (i.e., vasculitis) Antiplatelet agent for FMD Antiplatelet agent for anticoagulation for arterial dissection
Hematologic disorders/ coagulopathy	Antiphospholipid antibody Sickle cell disease	Depends on location	Treat underlying cause Consider anticoagulation for antiphospholipid antibodies
Watershed infarction	Caused by hypotension from various causes (e.g., shock)	Bilateral proximal weakness of arms and legs	Volume repletion Treat underlying cause
Other Drug abuse Migraine Venous infarction	Cocaine Saggital sinus thrombosis	Depends on location	Individualize treatment Consider anticoagulation for cerebral vein thrombosis

TABLE 61-2	*Hemorrhagic Cerebrovascular Disease*			
	Etiology	**Clinical Presentation**	**Diagnosis**	**Treatment**
Subarachnoid hemorrhage	Berry aneurysm (at bifurcation of vessels in circle of Willis) Trauma (dissecting aneurysm) Atherosclerosis (fusiform aneurysm) Infection (mycotic aneurysm) Arteriovenous malformation (AVM)	Sudden, severe headache —"worst of life" Meningismus Often decreased consciousness Focal neurologic deficits possible Oculomotor palsy (CN III) is clue to posterior communicating artery aneurysm (common location)	CT is most sensitive to blood; >90% accuracy If CT is negative but suspicion high, must perform LP with RBC counts in tubes 1 and 4, as well as spin for xanthochromia MRI relatively insensitive Cerebral angiography to detect underlying aneurysm	Supportive care Nimodipine for associated vasospasm Early surgical clipping of aneurysms in patients with minor deficits Endovascular therapy (coiling of aneurysms)
Intracranial hemorrhage (ICH)	Chronic hypertension (50–80% of ICH) Cerebral amyloid angiopathy (older patients with Alzheimer's disease) AVM (young patients) Tumor (renal cell, melanoma, glioma, choriocarcinoma) Drugs (cocaine, amphetamines, phenylpropanolamine) Other: vasculitis, coagulopathy, endocarditis, thrombocytopenia	Headache Vomiting Coma Seizures May be sudden onset or gradual progression of symptoms Lobar most common, followed by basal ganglia, thalamus, cerebellum, pons	CT most sensitive to blood MRI with gadolinium to detect underlying AVM, tumor Cerebral angiography if AVM suggested Avoid LP if mass effect from bleed	Control extreme hypertension Ventilation; airway protection Intracranial pressure management: Elevate head of bed, avoid hypotonic fluids, possibly mannitol and hyperventilation Surgical evacuation if possible
Subdural hemorrhage	Trauma (often minor in elderly)	Headache Confusion Seizures	CT: Concave-shaped bleed, may have mass effect	Supportive care Consider surgical evacuation
Epidural hemorrhage	Trauma	Headache Decreased level of consciousness	CT: Lens-shaped bleed between dura and skull, pushing on parenchyma	Often requires urgent surgical evacuation

CN, cranial nerve; LP, lumbar puncture.

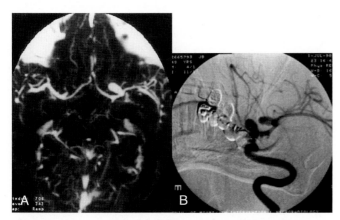

FIGURE 61-3 Proximal left middle cerebral artery aneurysm. Comparison of computed tomographic angiography (CTA) with conventional catheter angiography. **A,** Maximum intensity projection image from CTA of the circle of Willis shows a berry aneurysm of the M1 segment. **B,** Catheter angiography submentovertex view following left internal carotid artery injection, shows excellent correlation. (From Bradley WG, Daroff RB, Fenichel GM, Jankovic J: *Neurology in clinical practice,* ed 4, Philadelphia, Butterworth-Heinemann, 2004, figure 37B.16.)

- **Hyponatremia (caused by atrial natriuretic factor)**
- **Autonomic dysfunction**
- Intracerebral hemorrhage (ICH)
  - Numerous causes
  - Presentation and treatment (see Table 61-2)
- **Subdural hematoma**
  - **Classic "crescent" shape on CT underlying inner table of the skull (Fig. 61-4)**
  - Often seen in elderly after trauma, particularly if on anticoagulants
- Epidural hematoma
  - Often seen with trauma associated with skull fracture
  - Classic "lens" shape pushing on parenchyma by CT

Diagnosis and Evaluation

- **General diagnostic evaluation: Tailor to individual presentation**
  - Brain imaging
    - CT (high sensitivity for blood)
    - MRI (better for brainstem visualization or lacunar strokes)
  - Vascular imaging
    - Carotid duplex ultrasound
    - CT angiography

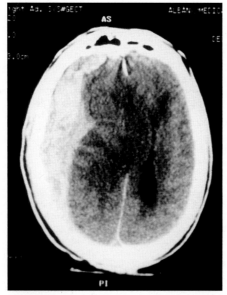

FIGURE 61-4　Head CT scan demonstrating an acute subdural hematoma. (From Ferrera PC, Couciello SA, Marx J, Verdile V: *Trauma management: an emergency medicine approach,* St. Louis, Mosby, 2001, figure 11-2.)

- Transcranial Doppler (ultrasound of intracranial vessels)
- Magnetic resonance angiography
- **Cerebral angiography (gold standard)**
  - **Better anatomic localization of disease**
  - **Involves dye load**
  - **1% risk of stroke with procedure**
- Cardiac evaluation
  - Electrocardiogram (examine rhythm, evidence of old CAD)
  - **Echocardiogram: Transesophageal preferred over transthoracic for better visualization of atria and aorta**
  - Holter monitor: Often low yield for arrhythmia
- Other
  - **Hypercoagulable evaluation (young stroke patients: Antithrombin III, protein C, and protein S deficiencies; antiphospholipid antibodies; lupus anticoagulant; homocysteine)**
  - Toxicology
  - Blood cultures
- Differential diagnosis of stroke or TIA
  - Focal seizure with Todd's paralysis (see following discussion)
  - Complicated migraine
  - Brain mass
  - Peripheral vestibular disorder
  - Cardiac arrhythmia

Treatment

- General treatment of ischemic stroke
  - Supportive medical care: Prevent aspiration, deep-vein thromboembolism, pressure sores
  - **Recommend against aggressive blood pressure control in the acute setting because this may lower cerebral perfusion**
  - **Aggressively control fever and hyperglycemia (may worsen stroke outcome)**

- Observe for cerebral edema (peaks typically at 48 hours)
- **Antiplatelet therapy: Reduction of future events by roughly 25%**
  - Aspirin: 81 to 325 mg/day
  - Clopidogrel: 75 mg/day
    - Rare cases of thrombotic thrombocytopenic purpura reported
  - Dipyridamole 200 mg plus aspirin 25 mg sustained-release PO bid
- Anticoagulants
  - **Heparin IV: No proven benefit and acutely increases bleeding risk**
  - Low-molecular-weight heparinoids: No proven benefit but alternative to IV heparin
  - **Warfarin for secondary prevention of cardioembolic stroke in atrial fibrillation**
- **Thrombolytic therapy**
  - FDA approval for tissue plasminogen activator (tPA) in 1996
  - For use in acute ischemic stroke
  - **Criteria for use**
    - **Suggested acute ischemic stroke**
    - **Administration of tPA within 3 hours from onset of symptoms**
    - **No contraindications for thrombolytic therapy (i.e., active GI bleeding and others as with thrombolysis for myocardial infarction)**
  - **Exclusions for use of tPA**
    - Time of onset uncertain or more than 3 hours
    - Minor stroke or resolving symptoms
    - Suggested or witnessed seizure
    - Blood pressure greater than 185/110 mm Hg or requiring aggressive treatment
    - Early hypodensity or other lesion on CT that would increase risk of bleeding (e.g., tumor)
  - Protocol
    - tPA dose 0.9 mg/kg, maximum dose of 90 mg (10% bolus followed by 60-minute infusion)
    - No invasive procedures for 24 hours
    - Strict blood pressure control to keep less than 185/110 mm Hg
- Carotid endarterectomy (CEA)
  - Useful for extracranial carotid stenosis
  - Helpful for long-term management and prevention of future events
  - **Indications (based on large trials)**
    - **50% to 70% symptomatic stenosis: Modest benefit from CEA; individualize treatment**
    - **Greater than 70% symptomatic stenosis: CEA superior to medical therapy in patients who are good surgical candidates**
    - **Greater than 60% asymptomatic stenosis: Modest benefit from CEA over medical therapy; individualize treatment**
- Carotid stenting
  - Useful for those patients who are not surgical candidates
  - Head-to-head trials versus CEA still pending
  - Surgery still preferred treatment for patients who are good surgical candidates

Seizure Disorders

Basic Information

- **Seizures do not necessarily imply epilepsy; may be caused by a temporary underlying disorder**
- In adults, the most common type of seizure is complex partial (40%), followed by generalized and simple partial seizures
- **The most common cause of epilepsy is "idiopathic" or "cryptogenic"**
- Up to 70% of patients can achieve remission; about half of these (35%) can remain seizure-free without medication

Clinical Presentation

- Classification of seizures (Table 61-3)
  - **Partial seizures: Onset is limited to one cerebral hemisphere**
    - May be motor, sensory, or psychoillusory ("déjà vu")
    - May generalize secondarily
    - "Jacksonian march": Focal seizure that begins in motor cortex and spreads to rest of motor area; clinically, clonic movements that spread proximally (usually up a limb)
  - **Primary generalized seizures (grand mal): Involve the cerebral cortex diffusely from the beginning**
- Each class of seizures can have varied clinical presentations (see Table 61-3)
- Todd's paralysis: A transient (not longer than 48 hours) neurologic deficit (e.g., motor weakness) after a seizure that reflects postictal depression of the involved area
- Tongue biting and incontinence can be hallmarks

TABLE 61-3	Classification of Seizures	
Class	**Definition**	**Examples**
Simple partial seizure	Normal consciousness	Simple motor (limb jerking) Simple sensory (paresthesias)
Complex partial seizure	Alteration of consciousness	"Temporal lobe epilepsy" Aura (strange odor, déjà vu, automatisms, lip-smacking, agitation, nondirected violence) May be associated with frontal or temporal lobe tumors, herpes encephalitis, hippocampal sclerosis
Generalized seizure	Complete impairment of consciousness	Primary generalized tonic–clonic (grand mal) Secondary generalized tonic–clonic (focal seizure that spreads) Absence (petit mal) Myoclonic (juvenile myoclonic epilepsy) Atonic (Lennox-Gastaut syndrome; "drop attack")

Diagnosis and Evaluation

- **Diagnosis depends on the clinical presentation and setting; electroencephalogram (EEG) findings are helpful but not definitive**
- Goals of diagnosis
  - Classify the type of seizure
  - Determine if epilepsy is truly present
  - Identify the underlying cause if possible
- Seizures may have underlying structural causes: Hippocampal sclerosis, glial tumors, cavernous malformations, encephalitis, trauma, hemorrhage
- **Consider metabolic and other causes of seizure (secondary seizure) in the right clinical setting**
  - Hyperglycemia (often focal seizures)
  - Hypoglycemia
  - Hyponatremia
  - Hypoxia
  - Uremia
  - Meningitis, encephalitis
  - Head trauma
- Drugs that can precipitate seizures
  - Antibiotics such as metronidazole, ciprofloxacin, acyclovir, high-dose penicillin and its derivatives
  - Bupropion
  - Methylphenidate
  - Rapid withdrawal of barbiturates, alcohol, benzodiazepines
- Differential diagnosis of seizures
  - Convulsive syncope
  - **Pseudoseizures**
    - **Also known as psychogenic seizures**
    - **Change in behavior not associated with abnormal brain electrical activity**
    - Often helpful to check prolactin 15 to 45 minutes after the event (will be normal in pseudoseizures, elevated in true seizure disorder)
  - Anoxic myoclonus
- Evaluation of new-onset seizures
  - History: Focality of onset, aura, family history (may need to talk with witnesses)
  - Brain imaging: MRI with gadolinium enhancement is best to rule out structural abnormalities
  - EEG (Fig. 61-5)
    - **"Spikes" or "sharp waves" help localize seizure focus and classify seizure type**
    - **Most useful if obtained during a clinical attack to avoid false negatives**
    - EEG in the setting of sleep deprivation enhances seizure detection
    - Video EEG for unusual symptoms or suggested pseudoseizures
  - **Serum prolactin may be elevated at 45 minutes with partial complex or generalized seizures**
  - Increased recurrent seizure risk: Focal neurologic deficit, brain lesion, abnormal EEG
  - **First isolated seizure: Recurrence rate is 50% within 2 years if untreated (25% if treated); risk drops to about 20% if physical examination, MRI, and EEG are all normal**

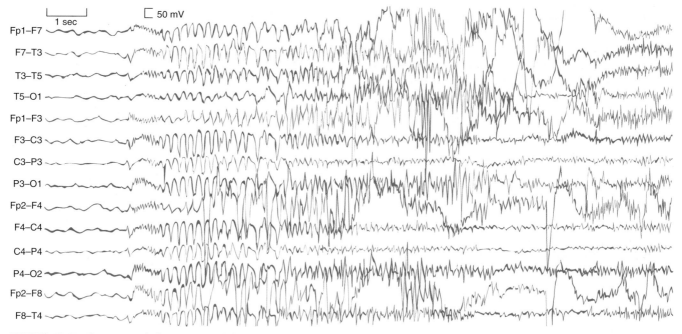

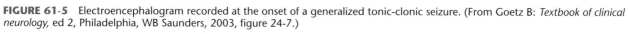

FIGURE 61-5 Electroencephalogram recorded at the onset of a generalized tonic-clonic seizure. (From Goetz B: *Textbook of clinical neurology,* ed 2, Philadelphia, WB Saunders, 2003, figure 24-7.)

TABLE 61-4	*Common Antiepileptic Drugs*		
Drug	**Indication**	**Typical Dose**	**Side Effect**
Lorazepam	Rapid treatment of acute seizures Not useful for long-term prophylaxis	0.5–1 mg PO every 6–8 hr	Sedation Respiratory compromise
Phenytoin	Partial seizures Generalized seizures	300 mg PO daily	IV dose may cause cardiac arrhythmias Nausea, ataxia, sedation Rash Hypersensitivity (mononucleosis-like) syndrome with rash, fever, lymphadenopathy Gingival hyperplasia Peripheral neuropathy Cerebellar degeneration Osteoporosis Fosphenytoin may be safer but is more costly
Carbamazepine	Partial seizures Generalized seizures Temporal lobe epilepsy	200 mg PO bid–tid	Nausea, ataxia, sedation Rash Leukopenia Aplastic anemia Hyponatremia Osteoporosis
Phenobarbital	Generalized seizures	30–120 mg PO daily	Sedation Respiratory depression with IV dosing
Valproic acid (valproate)	Partial seizures Generalized seizures Myoclonic seizures Lennox-Gastaut seizures	500–1000 mg PO bid–tid	Nausea Weight gain Birth defects Tremor Thrombocytopenia and platelet dysfunction Hair loss Pancreatitis
Gabapentin	Add-on to other therapy	300–900 mg tid	Sedation Ataxia

Treatment

- General principles
  - New seizure onset
    - **Workup as in preceding section; hospitalization is usually not necessary**
    - **Initiation of drug treatment for first seizure is controversial; must tailor to individual; assessing risk of further seizures is helpful**
      - Low risk: Normal physical examination, MRI, EEG, no history of brain trauma, and no family history of epilepsy
      - Higher risk (consider drug therapy): Two or more of preceding risk factors
  - Seizures that do not need long-term treatment: Drug- or alcohol-related, seizures immediately associated with head injury, convulsive syncope
  - Seizures from metabolic causes: Treat the underlying metabolic abnormality
- Common antiepileptic drugs (Table 61-4)
- Antiepileptic drugs of choice by diagnosis (Table 61-5)
- **Adverse effects common to most antiepileptic drugs**
  - **Dose-related side effects: Ataxia, nausea, sedation, diplopia**
  - "Allergic" effects (all except phenobarbital): Neutropenia, thrombocytopenia, aplastic anemia
  - **Drug interactions: Can be complex, but most antiepileptics induce cytochrome P450 and increase metabolism of other drugs (e.g., warfarin, other anticonvulsant drugs, folate, oral contraceptives)**
  - Birth defects
    - All antiepileptics increase birth defects twofold (3% increased to 6%)
    - Valproate felt to be worst offender
    - Patient should be on folic acid supplements at time of conception

- Surgical treatment
  - Consider when drug therapy fails (usually defined as two trials of high-dose monotherapy and one trial of combination therapy)
  - Most common procedure: Focal cortical resection
    - Must be able to identify focal epileptogenic region
    - Surgery must not leave patient with significant neurologic deficits
    - Most commonly used for refractory temporal lobe epilepsy
- **Treatment of status epilepticus**
  - Medical emergency
  - Untreated, a variety of complications may occur including aspiration, hypertension, cardiac dysrhythmias, lactic acidosis, rhabdomyolysis, hyperpyrexia, and, ultimately, death
  - Assess: Give oxygen; obtain IV access; send stat chemistry (glucose, calcium, magnesium)
  - Give IV normal saline, thiamine 100 mg, and 1 ampule of D50 empirically
  - Seizure-specific therapy (in usual order of preference)
    - Lorazepam 2 to 4 mg IV at 2 mg/min (0.05–0.2 mg/kg), maximum 8 mg for adults
    - Phenytoin 20 mg/kg IV in 50 mL normal saline at maximum rate of 50 mg/min (e.g., 1000 mg over 20 minutes for an adult), or fosphenytoin 20 "phenytoin equivalents" (PE)/kg IV at maximum rate of 150 PE/min (1 g IV over 10 minutes)
      - Monitor for hypotension, arrhythmia
    - Phenobarbital 20 mg/kg IV at 100 mg/min (5–10 mg/kg)
      - Monitor for respiratory depression
    - Pentobarbital coma
      - Last resort
      - Potential complications: Hypotension, hypothermia, decreased cardiac output

REVIEW QUESTIONS

For review questions, please go to www.expertconsult.com.

SUGGESTED READINGS

Brodie MJ, Dichter MA: Antiepileptic drugs, *N Engl J Med* 334:168–175, 1996.

International Stroke Trial Collaborative Group: The International Stroke Trial (IST): a randomized trial of aspirin, subcutaneous heparin, both, or neither among 19,435 patients with acute ischemic stroke, *Lancet* 349:1569–1581, 1997.

Moore WS, Barnett HJ, Beebe HG, et al: Guidelines for carotid endarterectomy: a multidisciplinary consensus statement from the Ad Hoc Committee, American Heart Association, *Circulation* 91:566–579, 1995.

The National Institute of Neurological Disorders and Stroke rt-PA Stroke Study Group: Tissue plasminogen activator for acute ischemic stroke, *N Engl J Med* 333:1581–1587, 1995.

Wityk RJ, Caplan LR: Hypertensive intracerebral hemorrhage: epidemiology and clinical pathology, *Neurosurg Clin North Am* 3: 521–532, 1992.

TABLE 61-5	*Antiepileptic Drugs of Choice*
Type of Seizure	**Drug of Choice**
Generalized seizure	Phenytoin Carbamazepine Valproate Phenobarbital
Partial complex seizure	Carbamazepine
Absence seizure	Ethosuxomide
Myoclonic seizure	Valproate
Add-on therapy	Gabapentin Lamotrigine Topiramate

Movement Disorders

RAINER VON COELLN, MD, PhD, H.A. JINNAH, MD, PhD, and JOSEPH SAVITT, MD, PhD

Movements of the body may be disrupted in a variety of ways and at a variety of levels in the nervous system. Primary practitioners should be aware of movement disorders because they are relatively common, and their diagnosis depends predominantly on **recognition of the clinical manifestations** rather than diagnostic testing. Movement disorders often signify an underlying medical illness, and many are treatable.

Tremor

Basic Information

- **Tremor: Rhythmic oscillations of any body part**
  - Potential causes: Physiologic tremor, medications, metabolic abnormalities (e.g., hyperthyroidism), other disorders of the nervous system (dystonic tremor, cerebellar tremor, psychogenic tremor)
- The cause of *essential tremor*, the most common of the tremor disorders, is unknown
  - Because half of patients with essential tremor have an affected first-degree relative, inherited factors likely play an important role

Clinical Presentation

- Tremors typically begin insidiously, in particular in essential tremor
- Tremors are typically exaggerated by physical or psychological stress
- Tremors typically attenuate with rest, relaxation, and modest amounts of alcohol
- Medications may also cause or exaggerate tremor
- *Essential tremor*: Most commonly manifests after the fourth decade of life, but may occur at any age, typically with a very slowly progressive course
  - Two types of essential tremor
    - **Postural tremor: Most prominent when the limbs are held in an active position**
    - **Kinetic tremor: Most prominent when the limbs are moving**
  - Other symptoms: Shaking of the head and neck, oscillations of the voice, or tremor of the lower limbs
    - Different manifestations are often combined in the same individual

Diagnosis and Evaluation

- Diagnosis based on history and physical examination
  - Evaluation focuses on discovering a potential cause (e.g., medications, hyperthyroidism)
- Most pressing issue: Distinguishing essential tremor from Parkinson's disease (Table 62-1)

TABLE 62-1	*Essential Tremor versus Parkinson's Disease–Associated Tremor*	
Clinical Feature	**Essential Tremor**	**Parkinson's Disease**
Family history	Positive in 50%	Usually negative
Response to alcohol	Tremor attenuates	No obvious effect
When does it occur?	With use	At rest
Speed	Fast (6–10 Hz)	Slow (4–6 Hz)
Appearance	Flexion–extension of wrists	Pill-rolling movement of fingers with pronation–supination of wrist
Location	Hands/arms (bilateral), head/neck, voice	Hands/arms (unilateral), jaw
Associated features	None	Masked face, cogwheel rigidity, bradykinesia, gait impairment

Hz, Hertz (cycles per second).

BOX 62-1	*Pharmacotherapy for Essential Tremor*

Propranolol (both short- and long-acting formulations)
Primidone (with or without propranolol)
Also effective
   Other β-blockers (e.g., metoprolol, atenolol)
   Anticonvulsants (e.g., gabapentin, topiramate)
   Benzodiazepines (e.g., lorazepam, clonazepam)

Treatment

- Depending on the underlying cause; treatment options for *essential tremor*:
  - Pharmacotherapy (Box 62-1)
  - Surgical treatment
    - **Patients with medically refractory and functionally disabling tremors are candidates for surgical treatments**
      - Thalamotomy: Placing a small lesion in the thalamus
      - Deep brain stimulation: Chronic electrical stimulation of the thalamus via implanted electrodes

Parkinsonism

Basic Information

- Parkinson's disease: Caused by **progressive degeneration of dopaminergic neurons within the substantia nigra**, along with the formation of characteristic pathologic cytoplasmic inclusions (Lewy bodies; Fig. 62-1), and neurodegeneration in other parts of the CNS
  - Parkinson's disease is a disorder of aging
    - Average age at diagnosis is 62 years
    - 4% to 10% of patients present before 40 years
    - By far most cases are idiopathic, but several rare monogenetic forms have been identified
  - **Onset is usually insidious,** and progression evolves over many months or years
- Parkinsonism: Neurologic syndromes resembling Parkinson's disease but caused by other processes
  - **Parkinsonism can result from drugs or medications, other neurodegenerative diseases (the Parkinson imitators), hydrocephalus, subcortical vascular disease, traumatic brain injury, and encephalitis**

Clinical Presentation

- Cardinal features
  - **Resting tremor**
  - Slowing of movements (bradykinesia)
  - Increased muscle tone with a cogwheeling quality (cogwheel rigidity)
- Early Parkinson's disease can be difficult to diagnose, because patients may present with only one of the cardinal features
  - Many present with resting tremor of one hand or arm, stiff or unnatural movements of one hand or arm, proximal pain or discomfort of one arm or leg, or a slowed or labored gait

- Asymmetry is a key feature in early stages, distinguishing Parkinson's disease from most of the Parkinson imitators (see later discussion)
- Majority of patients also experience one of many nonmotor features, including psychiatric difficulties (depression, anxiety, hallucinations), dementia, or autonomic dysfunction (orthostatic hypotension, sexual dysfunction, mild urgency with urination)
  - Dementia and autonomic dysfunction usually begin late in the disease, several years after onset
  - Psychiatric manifestations may occur at any time and sometimes precede motor signs and symptoms of Parkinson's disease
- Medications that can cause parkinsonism should be considered (Table 62-2)

Diagnosis and Evaluation

- Diagnosis based on history and physical examination
  - Secondary causes should be excluded (e.g., medications, see Table 62-2)
- Brain CT and MRI are usually unrevealing in Parkinson's disease, but they are useful to identify other causes of parkinsonism (i.e., hydrocephalus, vascular disease)
  - Other causes of parkinsonism typically have a worse prognosis and poor response to pharmacotherapy for Parkinson's disease
- The response to pharmacotherapy may be diagnostically useful. A positive response to medical therapy supports the diagnosis of Parkinson's disease, while a poor or transient response may provide the first clue to a Parkinson imitator.
- Red flags that suggest a Parkinson imitator (Table 62-3)
  - Early and prominent dementia (suggests dementia with Lewy bodies)
  - Early and prominent gait instability with falling (suggests any of the imitators)

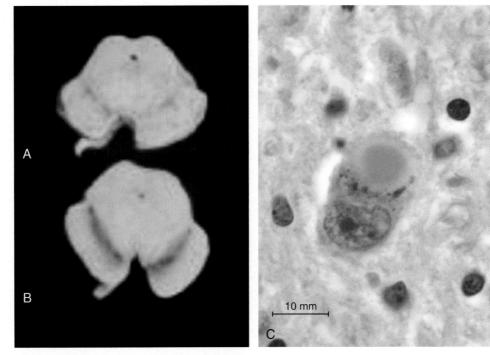

FIGURE 62-1 A, Substantia nigra in a patient with Parkinson's disease, showing area of depigmentation due to neuronal loss. **B,** Normal substantia nigra showing typical pigmentation for comparison. **C,** A large neuron showing a typical irregularly shaped nucleus and rounded cytoplasmic Lewy body with surrounding halo. Surrounding the Lewy body are the typical pigmentary granules of substantia nigra neurons.

10 mm

TABLE 62-2	Medications Associated with Secondary Parkinsonism
Class of Medication	**Drug(s)**
Cardiovascular drugs	Alpha methyldopa Reserpine
Dopamine antagonists for nausea	Prochlorperazine Metoclopramide
Dopamine antagonists for psychosis	Ziprasidone Haloperidol Thioridazine Pimozide Fluphenazine Risperidone Chlorpromazine Perphenazine Olanzapine (Quetiapine)*
Neurologic or psychiatric drugs	Valproic acid Lithium

*Much less so than the other atypical neuroleptics.

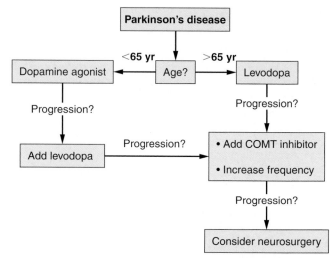

FIGURE 62-2 Algorithm for treatment of Parkinson's disease. COMT, catechol-O-methyl transferase.

- Early and prominent autonomic signs (suggests multiple system atrophy)
- Impairment of vertical eye movements (suggests progressive supranuclear palsy)
- Severe posturing of one limb (suggests corticobasal degeneration)

Treatment

See Figure 62-2 for a treatment algorithm for Parkinson's disease.

- Symptomatic medical therapies
  - **Levodopa/carbidopa**
    - Carbidopa inhibits peripheral metabolism and extends the half-life of the drug
    - Levodopa/carbidopa can also be combined with entacapone to further extend the half-life of the drug
      - Levodopa/carbidopa is still the most effective treatment ("gold standard of therapy")

- In later stages of the disease, levodopa therapy is typically complicated by fluctuation of effectiveness (wearing off) and dyskinesias (i.e., drug-induced choreoathetosis, see later section)
- **Other commonly used dopamine agonists include pramipexole, ropinirole, and pergolide**
  - Pergolide, once the most commonly used agonist, is now considered a third-line agent because it is an ergot derivative with a known risk for causing retroperitoneal and cardiac valve fibrosis
- Protective medical therapies
  - Designed to slow or stop progression of the disease
  - Concept of protective therapy is controversial, as evidence for protection is suggestive but not conclusive
  - Examples include coenzyme Q10, antioxidant vitamins, creatine, and monoamine oxidase inhibitors, such as selegiline or rasagiline, and others

TABLE 62-3	Red Flags for the Parkinson Imitators*		
Parkinson Imitator	**Characteristic Clinical Features**		**Brain MRI**
Progressive supranuclear palsy	Parkinsonism with difficulty with voluntarily directing eyes vertically downward, early gait impairment, dysarthria, or truncal dystonia		Normal or slight midbrain atrophy
Diffuse Lewy body disease	Parkinsonism with early dementia, fluctuating cognition, early visual hallucination		Diffuse atrophy
Corticobasal ganglionic degeneration	Parkinsonism with marked asymmetrical stiffness or dysfunction of one limb, impaired speech, limb apraxia, or alien limb phenomena		Normal or slightly asymmetrical cortical atrophy
Multiple system atrophy	Parkinsonism with early autonomic dysfunction, sometimes cerebellar ataxia		Normal or atrophy of brainstem and/or cerebellum
Normal pressure hydrocephalus	Parkinsonism with prominent gait disability, dementia, urinary incontinence		Enlarged lateral ventricles with normal cortical sulci
Vascular parkinsonism	Parkinsonism with prominent gait disability, dementia		Extensive patchy or diffuse white matter disease

*The Parkinson imitators are sometimes called Parkinson-plus syndromes or akinetic-rigid syndromes. The characteristic clinical features are combined with other features of parkinsonism.

- Surgical therapies
  - Treatment is **usually reserved for medically refractory cases** of idiopathic Parkinson's disease, since it does not appear to be helpful in the Parkinson imitator conditions
  - Deep brain stimulation: The most frequently used approach
    - Involves **stimulation of the globus pallidus or subthalamic nucleus**

Ataxia

Basic Information

- Many practitioners apply the term *ataxia* to any clumsy movement due to poor coordination, mild weakness, or other interfering movements such as dystonia (see following discussion)
- Among movement disorder specialists, ataxia is reserved for abnormalities of coordination that are not due to other motor defects (Fig. 62-3)
  - **Dysmetria ("poorly measured"): Irregular timing or trajectory of targeted movements**
  - **Dysdiadochokinesis: Breakdown of the normal timing and sequencing of rapid alternating movements (e.g., rapid succession of pronation and supination)**
- Ataxia often results from dysfunction of the cerebellum or its connections
  - However, ataxia is not synonymous with cerebellar dysfunction, as it can also arise from defects in sensory pathways and thalamus
- Causes of ataxia include ischemia or stroke, autoimmune disease, inherited diseases, toxic or metabolic insults, medications, and infections

Clinical Presentation

- Ataxia: Presentation best described as similar to that of an individual intoxicated with alcohol
  - Movements are poorly coordinated, but without frank weakness or other interfering movements
  - Repeated alternate touching of the tip of the nose and the tip of the examiner's finger is conducted with irregular timing with frequent overshoots or undershoots of the target (i.e., **dysmetria**)
  - Rapid alternating movements are performed irregularly or slowly (i.e., **dysdiadochokinesis**)
  - More complex movements (e.g., reaching for a drink) may lead to knocking over the glass or spilling the contents on the face due to poor timing and trajectory of hand and arm movements
  - **Gait is typically unbalanced** due to poor coordination of the legs and trunk during stepping
  - **Dysarthria** due to poor coordination of the muscles of mouth, pharynx, and larynx
  - Ataxia may also affect isolated body parts, such as one arm after stroke
    - Prominent gait ataxia without involvement of the arms is seen in chronic alcoholism and some neurodegenerative diseases because of selective involvement of the relevant parts of the cerebellum

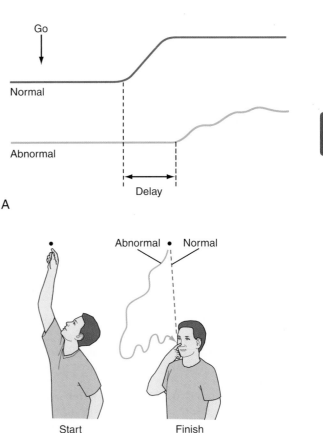

A

B

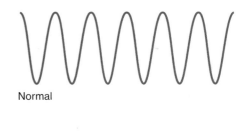

C

FIGURE 62-3 Typical defects in upper limb ataxia. **A,** Initiation of movement is delayed. **B,** Dysmetria (inaccuracy in range and direction) and kinetic tremor. **C,** Dysdiadochokinesis, an irregular pattern of alternating movements, can be seen in the abnormal position trace. (From Kandel ER, Schwartz JH, Jessell TM, editors: *Principles of neural science,* ed 3, Norwalk, CT, Appleton & Lange, 1991, figure 41-16, p 643. Adapted from Thach WT, Montgomery EB: Motor system. In Pearlman AL, Collins RC, editors: *Neurobiology of disease,* ed 3, New York, Oxford University Press, 1990, pp 168–196.)

Diagnosis and Evaluation

- Diagnosis based on history and physical examination, supplemented by neuroimaging and occasionally by laboratory testing
- **Brain MRI is useful for identifying focal lesions or atrophy of the cerebellum**

- Blood tests are needed to exclude autoimmune or metabolic diseases, and genetic tests are available for cases with suggested inherited cause
  - Autoimmune: Celiac disease, anti-glutamic acid decarboxylase syndrome, or paraneoplastic associated with anti-Hu or anti-Yo antibodies
  - Metabolic: Vitamin E deficiency, hypothyroidism, chronic alcoholism
  - Inherited: Spinocerebellar atrophy, Friedreich's ataxia

Treatment

- If found, treat the underlying cause
- No medical therapies have proven efficacy for ataxia
- Physical therapy and speech therapy play an important role along with assistive devices such as a cane, walker, or wheelchair

Dystonia

Basic Information

- Characterized by **involuntary and excessive muscle contractions that tend to be sustained and patterned, causing abnormal postures or twisting movements or both**
- **Most often associated with dysfunction of the neural circuits of the basal ganglia,** although it may arise from lesions in virtually any part of the nervous system
- Causes are varied and include, for example
  - Inherited diseases: Wilson's disease (dysfunction of copper metabolism), *DYT1*-associated Oppenheim's dystonia (gene identified, but mechanism unclear)
  - Ischemia or stroke: Putamen
  - Toxic or metabolic insults: Carbon monoxide poisoning
  - Medications: Neuroleptics
  - Infections: Viral encephalitis
- Cause cannot be determined for a large proportion of cases, which are labeled idiopathic

Clinical Presentation

- Varied nature of causes results in a broad range of clinical presentations
  - Dystonias may develop at any age
  - **Childhood cases are more likely to be genetic** with progression from regional to generalized involvement
  - **Adult cases are more likely to be idiopathic** with progression in a regional pattern over weeks or months followed by stabilization
  - Dystonias are often categorized according to the body part affected, with several well-recognized syndromes such as torticollis, blepharospasm, spasmodic dysphonia, and writer's cramp (Table 62-4)
- Clinical presentation depends on the severity and distribution of muscles involved
  - In some cases, dystonia presents merely as transient exaggeration or disruption of normal movements (e.g., golfer's yips, a task-specific dystonia)
  - In other cases, the result is slow, stiff, cramped, jerky, or twisting movements, or an abnormal posture that varies over time
  - In severe cases, distorted postures can be sustained and may lead to fixed deformities

TABLE 62-4	Subtypes of Dystonia Based on Involved Area
Dystonia Subtype	**Affected Region**
Focal	Limited body region
Torticollis	Neck muscles
Blepharospasm	Periocular muscles
Spasmodic dysphonia	Vocal cords
Writer's cramp	Hand muscles
Segmental	Two contiguous regions
Meige's syndrome	Periocular and perioral muscles
Oromandibular	Mouth, jaw, tongue
Hemidystonia	Half of the body
Generalized	Majority of the body

Diagnosis and Evaluation

- Diagnosis based on history and physical examination
- Further evaluation focuses on identifying a potential cause
  - Clues to the cause may be obtained from age of onset, manner of progression, family history, region affected, and any associated clinical features
- **Brain imaging (i.e., MRI) is indicated in virtually all cases**
- **In early-onset cases it is particularly important to test for reversible disorders**
  - Wilson's disease: Check for increased copper excretion in 24-hour urine, low serum ceruloplasmin, and the presence of Kayser-Fleischer rings by ophthalmologic examination
  - Dopa-responsive dystonia: Give diagnostic or therapeutic trial of levodopa/carbidopa
- Genetic testing for *DYT1* gene used to exclude the most common heritable form of generalized dystonia (reduced penetrance, so family history may be negative)

Treatment

- **Treat the underlying cause,** if present
- Symptomatic treatment determined by the region involved
  - Treatment of choice for most focal dystonias: Local injection of botulinum toxin
    - Botulinum toxin must be repeated every 3 to 6 months
    - Botulinum toxin not practical for patients with broader involvement, such as hemidystonia and generalized dystonia
  - Hemidystonia and generalized dystonia treated with trial of levodopa/carbidopa
    - If this is ineffective, palliative therapy may be offered with anticholinergics, benzodiazepines, or baclofen
- **Surgical procedures used for medically refractory cases**
  - Options include selective denervation, intrathecal baclofen, or deep brain stimulation of the globus pallidus

Chorea, Athetosis, and Ballismus

Basic Information

- **Chorea: Involuntary, irregular, unpatterned, and unsustained movements with variable timing and distribution**
- **Athetosis: Involuntary slow and irregular writhing movements most often affecting the distal limbs**
- **Ballismus: Fast, flinging movements, typically involving proximal muscles that move an entire limb**
  - The term *choreoathetosis* acknowledges the frequent co-occurrence of these types of movement
  - The preceding three movements often blend imperceptibly, with distinctions being the speed and location of movements
  - These movements are most often associated with dysfunction of neural circuits of the basal ganglia
  - Causes are varied and include inherited diseases, ischemia or stroke, toxic or metabolic insults, medications, infections, and autoimmune disorders
    - Medications: Stimulants such as amphetamines or methylphenidate, phenytoin (Table 62-5)
    - Autoimmune: SLE or anticardiolipin syndrome
    - Toxic or metabolic: Cocaine intoxication, hyperthyroidism

Clinical Presentation

- The mildest forms of chorea are **easily overlooked as occasional fidgeting movements**
  - Affected individuals often mask their problem by blending their abnormal movements into more purposeful-appearing movements
  - In its severest form, movements can be incessant and incapacitating
- Chorea may occur at any age
  - **Insidious onset of chorea and athetosis can signify an inherited disorder,** such as a metabolic disorder in a child or Huntington's chorea in an adult
  - **Abrupt onset of chorea and ballismus typically signify a stroke** (e.g., stroke of the subthalamic nucleus)
  - **Abrupt onset also can signify an autoimmune process** (e.g., systemic lupus erythematosus or the antiphospholipid syndrome)
    - Sydenham's chorea: Autoimmune process sometimes following rheumatic fever
    - Chorea gravidarum: Occurs in association with pregnancy

Diagnosis and Evaluation

- Diagnosis based on history and physical examination
- Evaluation focuses on discovering an underlying cause
- **Huntington's disease (autosomal dominant inheritance) is diagnosed with a genetic test that identifies abnormal expansion of a triplet nucleotide repeat in the Huntingtin gene**

Treatment

- Though chorea can present a dramatic picture of incessant movement, it does not need to be treated unless it is bothersome to the affected individual
- **Neuroleptic medications may be used with close monitoring** for development of tardive dyskinesia (which can be difficult to identify in a patient with a preexisting movement disorder)
- When resulting from stroke, chorea is often self-limited, resolving spontaneously after several weeks or months
  - Other forms of chorea respond to treatment of the underlying cause, such as those associated with medications, hyperthyroidism, or autoimmune disease

TABLE 62-5	**Drug-Induced Movement Disorders***				
Tremor	**Parkinsonism**	**Choreoathetosis**	**Acute Dystonia**	**Tardive Dyskinesia**
Stimulants	Dopamine antagonists	Stimulants	Dopamine antagonists	Dopamine antagonists
Amphetamine	Classical	Amphetamine	Classical	Classical
Pemoline	Atypical	Pemoline	Atypical[†]	Atypical[†]
Cocaine	Antiemetics	Cocaine	Antiemetics	Antiemetics
Caffeine	Metoclopramide	Theophylline	Metoclopramide	Metoclopramide
Adrenergics	Prochlorperazine	Adrenergics	Prochlorperazine	Prochlorperazine
Ephedrine	Cardiovascular	Ephedrine	Antihistamines	Antidepressants
β-Agonists	Reserpine	β-Agonists	Cimetidine	SSRI
Anticonvulsants	Alpha methyldopa	Anticonvulsants	Ranitidine	
Valproic acid	Calcium blockers	Carbamazepine	Antitussives	
Lamotrigine	Amiodarone	Phenytoin		
Phenytoin	Antidepressants	Others		
Others	SSRI	Lithium		
Cyclosporine	Lithium	Oral contraceptives		
Amiodarone		Levodopa		
Thyroxine				
Lithium				

*This is a partial list of the most common offenders.
[†]Exceptions: It is less likely for quetiapine, and extremely rare for clozapine, to cause these movement disorders, compared with the other atypical neuroleptics.
SSRI, selective serotonin reuptake inhibitor.

Myoclonus

Basic Information

- Definition: **Involuntary, abrupt, brief and jerky movement, either caused by a synchronous activation (positive myoclonus, more common) or by synchronous inhibition (negative myoclonus, i.e., asterixis/"flapping tremor") of a group of motor neurons**
  - A myoclonic muscle twitch can be distinguished from a brief voluntary muscle jerk by electromyography
  - The origin (i.e., the generator) of the myoclonus can be cortical, subcortical (basal ganglia, thalamus, or brainstem), or spinal
- Classification
  - Physiologic myoclonus (e.g., when falling asleep; startle reaction; singultus)
  - Essential myoclonus (rare benign genetic disorders)
  - Myoclonus epilepsy (rare fatal genetic disorders)
  - Symptomatic myoclonus (by far the most common form) from a variety of underlying conditions:
    - Metabolic encephalopathies (most commonly hepatic or renal encephalopathy), typically with asterixis
    - Toxic encephalopathies (cocaine, tetrahydrocannabinol, tricyclic antidepressants, levodopa, penicillin)
    - Neurodegenerative diseases (e.g., Wilson's disease, Creutzfeldt-Jakob disease)
    - Viral encephalitis
    - Posthypoxic myoclonus (Lance-Adams syndrome)

Clinical Presentation

- Myoclonic activity can be focal, segmental, multifocal, or generalized
- Muscle contractions can be arrhythmic, rhythmic (with a regular pattern), or oscillatory (resembling a tremor)
- Myoclonic jerks can occur spontaneously or may be triggered by either voluntary movements (action myoclonus, typical for posthypoxic brain damage) or by external stimuli
- Tremor-like myoclonus can be difficult to differentiate from actual tremor. An important clue can be sustained twitching during sleep, which is typically seen with myoclonus but not with tremor.

Diagnosis and Evaluation

- Diagnosis is based on history and physical examination
  - In a first step, the myoclonic activity needs to be characterized regarding distribution, triggering mechanisms (if any), and accompanying symptoms
- Electrophysiology might be helpful but may require referral to a specialized institution
- Evaluation focuses on discovering an underlying cause, including MRI of the brain or spine or both, lab workup including cerebrospinal fluid testing, routine electrophysiology (electroencephalogram, somatosensory evoked potentials)

Treatment

- The choice of drug depends on the type of myoclonus and the underlying condition
- Valproic acid, levetiracetam, and benzodiazepines (e.g., clonazepam) are most commonly used
- Treatment is difficult, and therapeutic response is usually partial at best

Tics and Tourette's Syndrome

Basic Information

- **Tic: Brief and often stereotyped movements that are preceded by an urge and followed by a sense of relief**
  - Tics are not entirely involuntary, but are instead called unvoluntary
    - Most patients who recognize the urge can suppress their tics for a few seconds or minutes
  - Suppression is accompanied by a buildup of tension, which is released when the tic is expressed
  - Tics can closely resemble other movement disorders such as chorea, dystonia, or myoclonus
    - **The features that distinguish them from these other disorders include the preceding urge, partial willful control, and buildup of tension during suppression**
- Tourette's syndrome: Multiple changing motor and audible tics beginning before age 18 and lasting for at least 6 months
- Tics and Tourette's syndrome are frequently associated with obsessive-compulsive disorder or attention-deficit hyperactivity disorder
  - The cause of these disorders is unknown

Clinical Presentation

- Clinical presentation is broad
  - May occur at any age, but more common in children
  - Symptoms may be chronic or have a waxing/waning course, which may remit for years
  - Common presentation is development of sudden and brief twitches (e.g., eye squinting, shoulder shrugging)
  - Tics also may manifest as more complicated mannerisms, such as neck rolling, brief ritualized sequences, or utterances of sounds or phrases
    - **Echolalia: Compulsive repeating of the words of others**
    - **Coprolalia: Compulsive blurting out of obscenities**

Diagnosis and Evaluation

- Diagnosis based on history and physical examination
- Additional diagnoses must be considered if tics first emerge during adulthood, as they can occasionally be early signs of degenerative disorders of the basal ganglia

Treatment

- **Neuroleptics** (haloperidol, pimozide, risperdal) are the most reliably effective medications, but must be used with caution because of the risk of tardive dyskinesia
- Other medications (e.g., clonidine, gabapentin, baclofen) are sometimes effective

Restless Legs Syndrome

Basic Information

- Restless legs syndrome (RLS) is defined by **discomforting sensations in the legs that are most prominent in the evening or at night when retiring to sleep** and relieved by specific activities
- **Common** in adults: Affects at least 1% of the population older than 50 years
  - Most commonly begins in early adulthood and progresses insidiously
- The disorder is not well recognized among patients or physicians, so the diagnosis is often delayed until later adulthood
- About **one third of affected patients** suffer from **secondary RLS**
- Well-documented underlying causes: Iron deficiency anemia, end-stage renal disease, and pregnancy
- Possible underlying causes: Peripheral neuropathy, rheumatoid arthritis, and diabetes
- The remaining **two thirds of cases** are considered to be **idiopathic RLS**
- About half of these patients report an affected first-degree relative, suggesting an **inherited predisposition**
  - The underlying pathophysiology is unclear for both idiopathic and secondary RLS, although dysfunction of CNS iron metabolism has been implicated
  - Certain medications, like tricyclic antidepressants, can worsen the symptoms

Clinical Presentation

- Patients complain of ill-defined discomfort in the legs that is most prominent at night
- Discomfort is variably described as restlessness, irritation, creeping or tingling sensations, or pain
- Symptoms temporarily **relieved by stretching, massaging, cycling the legs in bed, or getting up and walking it off**
  - These **problems disrupt sleep**, resulting in excessive daytime sleepiness
- In more seriously affected cases, the discomforting sensations may appear during any period of rest, such as sitting to read a book
  - Some patients find they are unable to take long car rides or airplane trips. The disorder can also spread to involve the trunk or arms.

Diagnosis and Evaluation

- Diagnosis based on history
  - Neurologic examination is usually normal in RLS
  - Overnight sleep study can be used to document coexisting periodic leg movements in sleep (PLMS), which are usually asymptomatic
- **Key differential is alternative diagnosis of akathisia** (a sense of inner restlessness often caused by neuroleptic medications)
  - Akathisia is not most prominent in the legs nor is it related to periods of rest or recumbency
- Peripheral neuropathy should also be excluded
- Laboratory evaluation focuses on identifying potential causes of secondary RLS (i.e., iron deficiency, renal dysfunction, diabetes)

Treatment

- Treatment of choice is a **dopamine agonist or levodopa/carbidopa,** usually used once in the evening, at doses far below those used to treat Parkinson's disease
- Some patients experience **rebound,** with symptoms worsening after the medication wears off in the morning
- Other patients experience **augmentation,** a phenomenon in which symptoms begin to intrude earlier in the evening, and eventually during much of the daytime
- **Gabapentin also is effective** in some cases
- Second-line agents include opiates (often effective at doses much lower than those required to treat pain) and certain antiepileptic drugs (carbamazepine, valproic acid)
- Benzodiazepines are useful to promote sleep if needed, but do not directly suppress symptoms of restlessness

Drug-Induced Movement Disorders

Basic Information

- Specific drugs or medications can have side effects that closely mimic movement disorders including tremor, parkinsonism, ataxia, chorea, dystonia, and tics (see Table 62-5)
- Drug-induced movement disorders are important to recognize, because many are effectively treated by eliminating the offending agent
- Some movement disorders arise only in the setting of specific medications, particularly neuroleptics and antiemetics (e.g., tardive dyskinesia, acute dystonic reactions, and neuroleptic malignant syndrome)

Clinical Presentation

- Drug-induced tremor: Typical manifestation as postural or kinetic tremor
- Clinical features of drug-induced ataxia, parkinsonism, chorea otherwise match the description in the respective paragraphs
- **Acute dystonic reaction: Sudden and forceful abnormal posturing; typically within an hour of receiving an offending medication** (including all neuroleptics such as haloperidol, fluphenazine, risperidone, and olanzapine; may also be seen with metoclopramide and prochlorperazine)
  - They often involve the neck and face, but can involve other regions; sometimes mistaken for seizures, except for preservation of consciousness
- **Tardive dyskinesia: Repetitive orolingual movements; typically follows chronic use of a dopamine antagonist (neuroleptic, antiemetic), even after the offending drug has been discontinued**
  - In early stages, movements are subtle and can appear as normal lip-wetting behaviors or chewing movements, except for their repetitive nature
  - In more advanced stages, repetitive tongue thrusting can interfere with speech and nutrition
  - Although the orolingual region is most commonly affected, some patients have involvement of the face, neck, or other regions
- **Neuroleptic malignant syndrome: A marked increase in muscle tone, hyperthermia, autonomic instability, depression of consciousness, and elevated serum creatine phosphokinase**

62

- Mortality can be as high as 50%
- May follow chronic or acute exposure to an offending medication, often after an increase in dose

Diagnosis and Evaluation

- Diagnosis based on history and physical examination
- Elimination of a suggested offending medication can help to establish a diagnosis
- Diagnosis of neuroleptic malignant syndrome is more challenging, because partial syndromes may occur, but early recognition is important for successful treatment

Treatment

- **Eliminate the offending agent,** if possible
  - Resolution of the movement disorder often follows within hours or days
  - Resolution may be delayed for weeks or months for some movement disorders such as drug-induced parkinsonism
  - Tardive dyskinesia, once fully established, may be permanent
- **Acute dystonic reactions**: IV diphenhydramine (Benadryl) is useful to speed resolution
- Neuroleptic malignant syndrome: Hospitalization with supportive care is often required because the syndrome can be life-threatening
  - Treatment includes **IV fluids, dantrolene and benzodiazepines to reduce muscle tone, bromocriptine, and antipyretics**

Psychogenic Movement Disorders

Basic Information

- Psychogenic movement disorders (PMDs, synonyms: functional or nonorganic disorders) are defined as physical symptoms that are brought on by psychological mechanisms
  - PMDs resemble organic movement disorders and are described based on phenomenology; however, they can typically be identified based on clinical criteria
  - About 2% to 3% of patients in a movement disorder clinic present with PMDs; women are more commonly affected (two thirds of cases)
  - PMDs encompasses a spectrum from conversion disorder to malingering
- Conversion disorder refers to a subconscious, nonwillful manifestation of a psychiatric disturbance, although the underlying pathophysiology is unclear
- Malingering refers to the deliberate production of symptoms for material gain
  - Established risk factors include sexual abuse, major emotionally stressful life events, and previous physical trauma (including surgery)

Clinical Presentation

- Most common manifestations are tremor, dystonia, gait disorder, and myoclonus
- Parkinsonism, chorea, ataxia, and tics are less commonly observed

- Criteria of PMDs versus organic movement disorders:
  - Acute onset and fast progression to maximal severity
  - Waxing and waning course; temporary complete remissions
  - Symptoms are incongruent with any established organic disease
  - Symptoms are inconsistent over time and regarding involved body parts
  - Symptoms are distractible and increase with attention to the affected body part
  - Association with "false neurologic symptoms" (e.g., weakness only with certain tasks)

Diagnosis and Evaluation

- PMD should be identified positively, and not primarily as diagnosis of exclusion, based on history, careful and thorough observation, and neurologic examination
- Ancillary workup, including imaging, electrophysiology, and lab tests, might be necessary depending on the presentation and the diagnostic certainty
- Psychiatric evaluation for comorbidity and possible underlying psychiatric or psychological factors
- **Delivery of the diagnosis is critical for the acceptance of and compliance with treatment**
  - Acknowledgement of the symptoms as "real and serious problem"
  - Unambiguous message that this is an established cause of movement disorders and that additional diagnostic tests are unnecessary
  - Emphasis of the "functional" character of the symptoms as an access path for therapeutic intervention
- **Avoid unnecessary workup, including aggressive and costly procedures, or administration of potentially harmful drugs, solely based on reluctance of the physician and the patient alike to accept the diagnosis of PMD**

Treatment

- Treatment of psychiatric comorbidity and underlying psychiatric mechanisms, if identified
  - Psychotherapy and concomitant medical treatment, if necessary (e.g., antidepressants)
  - Stress management and relaxation techniques (e.g., biofeedback, yoga, meditation)
- Physical therapy and occupational therapy to help reestablish healthy patterns of motor function

SUGGESTED READINGS

Janavs JL, Aminoff MJ: Involuntary movements in general medical disorders. In Aminoff MJ, editor: *Neurology and general medicine,* ed 3, New York, Churchill Livingstone, 2001, pp 983–1002. (This chapter describes many of the medical illnesses associated with movement disorders.)

Tolosa E, Koller WC, Gershanik OS: *Differential diagnosis and treatment of movement disorders,* Boston, Butterworth-Heinemann, 1998. (This is a short monograph covering the most common movement disorders, accompanied by videotape demonstrations.)

SUGGESTED WEB SITE

The following Web site provides useful basic information on many movement disorders for both practitioners and patients: www.wemove.com.

CHAPTER 63

Selected Topics in Neurology

RAFAEL H. LLINÁS, MD

This chapter reviews a selection of central and peripheral neurologic disorders involving the spinal cord, peripheral nerves, and neuromuscular junction and toxic myopathies. Inflammatory myopathies are reviewed in Chapter 46. Localization of neurologic lesions, based on clinical evaluation or imaging studies, is the diagnostic theme.

Spinal Cord

Basic Information

- The spinal column is made up of vertebrae separated by intervertebral disks (Fig. 63-1)
- The spinal cord is found within the spinal canal, beginning at the end of the brainstem and extending to L1
- Below L1 is the "cauda equina," which consists of nerve roots
- Spinal cord circulation
  - The anterior spinal cord is dependent on a single anterior spinal artery
  - The posterior spinal cord is fed by numerous posterior spinal arteries
  - **Spinal stroke preferentially affects the anterior spinal cord**
- Table 63-1 lists the most common entities affecting the spinal cord

Clinical Presentation

- Spinal cord lesions may be categorized by presentation
  - Upper motor neuron signs (long tract signs): **Weakness, spasticity, hyper-reflexia, and positive Babinski's sign** (Fig. 63-2)
  - **Sensory signs** (anterior or posterior columns or both): **Sensory level or loss of single modality** (pinprick/ temperature or light touch/proprioception)
  - **Bowel, bladder, and sexual dysfunction signs: Urinary overflow incontinence or bladder spasticity, and weak rectal tone with fecal incontinence**
  - **Local root dysfunction: Multimodal sensory and motor loss in a dermatomal distribution (Fig. 63-3)**
  - Caveats
    - No cranial nerve abnormalities should be present
    - In acute spinal cord trauma, weakness may be the only long tract sign present
    - The sensory level reveals only the lowest level possible for a lesion (e.g., a T10 sensory level may be caused by a cervical lesion)

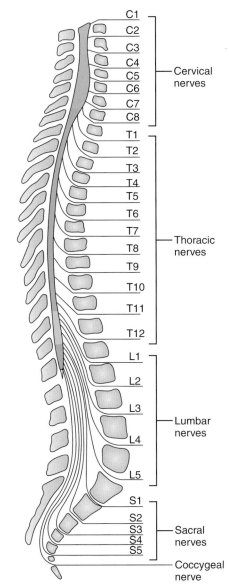

FIGURE 63-1 The spinal column, showing the relationships among the spinal cord, spinal nerves, and vertebral column. (From Crossman AR, Neary D: *Neuroanatomy*, ed 3, Philadelphia, Churchill Livingstone, 2006, figure 8.3.)

- Spinal cord lesions may be categorized by location
  - **Anterior** spinal cord lesions
    - Loss of **pain and temperature** sense (lateral spinothalamic tract)
    - Fine touch, proprioception, and vibration sense are spared

TABLE 63-1	Diseases Affecting the Spinal Cord				
	Multiple Sclerosis	**Vitamin B$_{12}$ Deficiency**	**Syringomyelia**	**Tabes Dorsalis**	**Epidural Abscess**
Basic information	Prototypical demyelinating disease "Transverse myelitis" when affects the spinal cord Most common presentation "optic neuritis"	Neurologic symptoms develop after prolonged B$_{12}$ deficiency (months to years) Neurologic symptoms occur in the majority of patients with pernicious anemia Anemia need not be present	Central cord cavitation, CSF accumulation and compression Often cervical cord Congenital (e.g., with Arnold-Chiari malformation) or post-traumatic	Onset many years after primary syphilitic infection	Often caused by *Staphylococcus aureus* May occur at any level
Clinical presentation	Two basic forms Chronic-progressive: Lesions develop, persist, and progress Relapsing-remitting: Lesions develop, resolve, and recur elsewhere	Loss of vibration and proprioception sense Loss of reflexes Mild weakness Mental status change Night blindness	Central cord syndrome (see Table 63-2) Atrophy, fasciculation, and lost reflexes	"Lightning shocks" in abdomen and legs Loss of vibration and proprioception sense Bladder dysfunction	Fever and chills Pain Cord or nerve root compression
Diagnosis and evaluation	Lesions "separated in time and space" Lhermitte's sign* MRI with contrast	Vitamin B$_{12}$ (low) Methylmalonic acid (high)	MRI	Argyll Robertson pupil† CSF VDRL (+)	Focal tenderness to percussion over spine Elevated WBC count
Treatment	Acute: Steroids Chronic: Immune modulators (e.g., interferon-β1a or -β1b, and glatiramer acetate)	Vitamin B$_{12}$ injections	Neurosurgical evaluation	IV penicillin	Antibiotics Urgent surgery for cord compression

*Sensation of an electric shock radiating to the arms or legs and provoked by neck movement or cough.
†Pupils react to convergence but not to light.
CSF, cerebrospinal fluid; VDRL, Venereal Disease Research Laboratory.

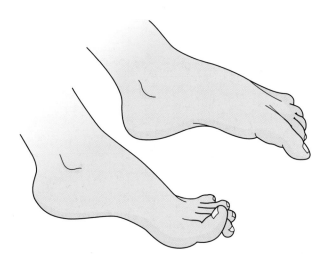

FIGURE 63-2 Babinski's sign. The normal adult response to stimulation of the lateral plantar surface of the foot (*top*). The abnormal adult response (*bottom*). (From Goetz B: *Textbook of clinical neurology,* ed 2, Philadelphia, WB Saunders, 2003, figure 15-13.)

- May occur with or without motor loss
- **Posterior** spinal cord lesions
  - Loss of **fine touch, proprioception, and vibration** sense (posterior columns)
  - Pain and temperature sense are spared
  - May occur with or without motor loss

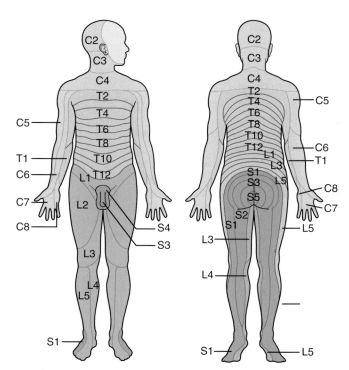

FIGURE 63-3 Dermatome map. (From FitzGerald MJT, Folan-Curran J: *Clinical neuroanatomy and related neuroscience,* ed 4, Philadelphia, WB Saunders, 2002, figure 11.10.)

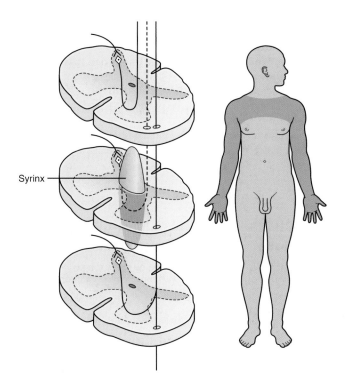

FIGURE 63-4 Central spinal cord lesion (in this case, syringomyelia), showing capelike distribution of analgesia. (From FitzGerald MJT, Folan-Curran J: *Clinical neuroanatomy and related neuroscience*, ed 4, Philadelphia, WB Saunders, 2002, figure 12.1.1.)

- ▪ **Central** spinal cord lesions (Fig. 63-4)
  - ▪ Lateral spinothalamic tract and local motor neurons disrupted
  - ▪ **Pain and temperature sense lost in "cape-like" distribution**
  - ▪ Fine touch, proprioception, and vibration sense spared
  - ▪ **Lower motor neuron weakness may be evident in the extremities**

Diagnosis and Evaluation

Table 63-2 provides a comparison of spinal cord syndromes.
- ▪ Anterior spinal cord syndromes are caused by the following:
  - ▪ Trauma
  - ▪ Rupture of disk, causing compression of the spinal cord (Fig. 63-5)
  - ▪ Occlusion of anterior spinal artery causing spinal stroke
  - ▪ Primary spinal cord tumors
  - ▪ Metastatic cancer
- ▪ Posterior spinal cord syndromes are caused by the following:
  - ▪ Cervical spondylosis (arthritis and ligamentous hypertrophy)
  - ▪ Epidural abscess
  - ▪ Vitamin B$_{12}$ deficiency
  - ▪ Syphilis
  - ▪ Multiple sclerosis
  - ▪ Primary spinal cord tumors
  - ▪ Metastatic cancer
- ▪ Central spinal cord syndromes are caused by the following:
  - ▪ Syringomyelia (congenital or post-traumatic)
  - ▪ Primary spinal cord tumors

TABLE 63-2	*Comparison of Spinal Cord Syndromes*
	Clinical Manifestations	**Possible Causes**

	Clinical Manifestations	**Possible Causes**
Anterior	Loss of pain and temperature sensation Motor weakness may or may not be present	Trauma Ruptured intervertebral disk Anterior spinal artery occlusion ("spinal stroke") Primary spinal cord tumors Metastatic cancer
Central	Loss of pain and temperature sensation Lower motor neuron weakness (in lower extremities)	Syringomyelia Primary spinal cord tumors Hyperextension injuries
Posterior	Loss of fine touch, vibratory sensation Loss of proprioception Motor weakness may or may not be present	Cervical spondylosis Epidural abscess Vitamin B$_{12}$ deficiency Syphilis Multiple sclerosis Primary spinal cord tumors Metastatic cancer

63

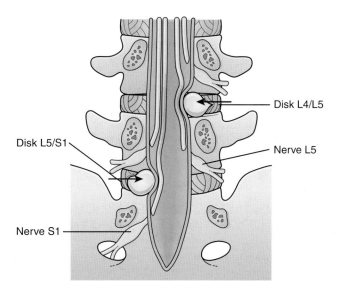

FIGURE 63-5 Nerve compression by rupture of intervertebral disks (*arrows*). (From FitzGerald MJT, Folan-Curran J: *Clinical neuroanatomy and related neuroscience*, ed 4, Philadelphia, WB Saunders, 2002, figure 11.2.2.)

- ▪ Hyperextension injuries that disrupt the central spinal cord gray matter
- ▪ Brown-Séquard's syndrome
  - ▪ Caused by hemisection of the spinal cord
  - ▪ Findings depend on where each tract decussates
    - ▪ Motor tract lesions give ipsilateral weakness (**motor fibers cross in the brainstem**)
    - ▪ Sensory tract lesions give ipsilateral fine touch, proprioception, and vibration loss (**posterior columns cross in brainstem**); and contralateral pain and temperature sense loss (**spinothalamic tracts cross in the spinal cord** through the gray matter)

Treatment

See Table 63-1.

Peripheral Nerves

Basic Information

- The peripheral nerves include the spinal roots, cauda equina, nerve plexus (brachial and lumbar), and named nerves (Tables 63-3 to 63-5)

Clinical Presentations

- **Lower motor neuron signs (Box 63-1)**
  - Acute: **Weakness, multimodal sensory loss, lancinating pain, and loss of reflexes**
  - Chronic: **Atrophy and fasciculation**
  - Not all features need to be present
- Spinal roots (Table 63-6)
- Cauda equina syndrome: Bowel and bladder dysfunction, flaccid paralysis of bilateral lower extremities, and saddle anesthesia

TABLE 63-3	**Compressive Neuropathies**		
	Carpal Tunnel Syndrome	**Ulnar Neuropathy**	**Peroneal Neuropathy**
Basic information	Caused by median nerve compression at wrist	Caused by ulnar nerve compression at elbow "funny bone"	Caused by peroneal compression at fibular head
Clinical presentation	Pain, numbness, and paresthesias in first through third fingers and radial half of fourth Weakness of thumb flexion, opposition, and abduction Nocturnal exacerbation	Pain, numbness, and paresthesias in fifth finger and ulnar half of fourth Weakness of finger abductors May resemble C8 radiculopathy	Foot drop Foot inversion spared
Diagnosis and evaluation	Positive median nerve "Tinel's sign"* and "Phalen's sign"† Abnormal EMG/NCS Rule out overuse, synovitis, hypothyroidism, amyloidosis, acromegaly, and pregnancy	Positive ulnar nerve "Tinel's sign" at the elbow‡ Rule out trauma caused by leaning on elbows or repetitive curls	May resemble L5 nerve root, but no sensory abnormalities Usually traumatic May be seen in diabetes
Treatment	Wrist splint, NSAIDs, steroid injection, and surgical release	Splinting, NSAIDs, and surgical transposition of the nerve	Splinting and physical therapy

*Provoke pain and paresthesias with percussion over nerve at the wrist.
†Provoke pain, paresthesias, or numbness with forced wrist flexion (reversed "prayer position").
‡Percussion between medial elbow epicondyle and olecranon process.
EMG/NCS; electromyography/nerve conduction study.

TABLE 63-4	**Inflammatory Neuropathies**	
	Acute Inflammatory Demyelinating Polyneuropathy (Guillain-Barré Syndrome)	**Chronic Inflammatory Demyelinating Polyneuropathy**
Basic information	Immune-mediated Onset 1–3 weeks after respiratory or GI illness, in two thirds of cases Herpesvirus (CMV and EBV) *Campylobacter jejuni* Nonseasonal, nonepidemic	Immune-mediated
Clinical presentation	Longest nerves affected first (presents with leg paresthesias and disordered gait) Motor > sensory Ascending pattern of progression Respiratory failure Bowel/bladder function preserved Dysautonomia Areflexia	Slowly progressive Atrophy and fasciculation Motor > sensory
Diagnosis and evaluation	Elevated CSF protein EMG/NCS normal early in course, except for loss of "F-waves"	EMG/NCS consistent with demyelination ↓ Conduction velocity Partial conduction block
Treatment	IVIG Plasmapheresis	Steroids IVIG Plasmapheresis

CMV, cytomegalovirus; EBV, Epstein-Barr virus; EMG, electromyography; NCS, nerve conduction study; IVIG, intravenous immunoglobulins.

TABLE 63-5 *Toxic Neuropathies*

	Diabetic Neuropathy	Lead Neuropathy	Alcoholic Neuropathy	Critical Illness Neuropathy
Basic information	Caused by hyperglycemia	Caused by lead toxicity	Caused by long-standing alcohol abuse	Associated with Prolonged stay in ICU Sepsis Exposure to steroids and paralytic agents
Clinical presentation	Distal symmetrical sensory or sensorimotor neuropathy Multimodal sensory loss	Unilateral or bilateral wrist drop (classic) Distal symmetrical sensorimotor neuropathy Abdominal pain	Pain Ataxia	Often difficult to wean from ventilator
Diagnosis and evaluation*	Host presentation	Host presentation Confirmed by serum and 24-hr urine lead measurement	Host presentation	Host presentation Nerve biopsy may be useful
Treatment	Glycemic control Symptomatic	Chelation therapy Symptomatic	Eliminate exposure Symptomatic	Remove offending agents Supportive care

*Axonal changes seen on electromyography/nerve conduction study.

BOX 63-1 *Upper and Lower Motor Neuron Signs*

Upper Motor Neuron Signs
Weakness
Spasticity
Hyper-reflexia
Positive Babinski's sign

Lower Motor Neuron Signs
Weakness
Multimodal sensory loss
Lancinating pain
Areflexia

- Plexus: Unilateral extremity affected without spinal cord signs; all sensory modalities are affected and upper motor neuron signs are absent
- Named nerves
  - **Compression neuropathies commonly present with pain** and are caused by repetitive or chronic external compression (see Table 63-3)
  - **Inflammatory neuropathies present with motor more than sensory involvement** and are caused by demyelination (see Table 63-4)
  - **Toxic neuropathies commonly present with lancinating pain** and are caused by axonal damage (see Table 63-5)

Diagnosis and Evaluation

- Electromyography (EMG) and nerve conduction studies (NCS) are helpful in localizing peripheral nerve lesions
  - **EMG evaluates for myopathy and denervation**
  - **NCS can differentiate axonal from demyelinating neuropathy**
- MRI most useful imaging study
- Peripheral nerve lesions have the lengthiest differential diagnosis in neurology, being subject to acute trauma,

TABLE 63-6 *Cervical and Lumbar Root Lesion Presentation*

Root Level	Weakness	Sensory Loss Distribution	Reflex Dropped?
C5	Deltoid	Top of shoulder	None
C6	Biceps	Lateral upper and lower arm including first finger and thumb	Biceps jerk
C7	Triceps	Medial arm and middle finger	Triceps jerk
C8	Grip strength	Lateral arm and little finger	Triceps jerk
L4	Knee extension	Posterolateral thigh	Knee jerk
L5	Foot dorsiflexion	Top of the foot	Hamstring jerk
S1	Foot plantarflexion	Sole of the foot and lateral foot	Ankle jerk

chronic compression, inflammation, demyelination, and toxic and infectious injury
  - Spinal nerve roots: Most commonly caused by compression by intervertebral disk; consider mass lesion
  - Cauda equina syndrome: Most common causes are disk herniation, tumor, and epidural hemorrhage
  - Plexus: Pancoast tumors present with brachial plexus lesion and Horner's syndrome

Treatment

- Eliminate or correct cause
- Symptomatic treatment with tricyclic antidepressants, gabapentin, and anticonvulsants
- See Tables 63-3 to 63-5

63

Neuromuscular Junction

Basic Information

- Myasthenia gravis is the prototypical disorder
- **Antiacetylcholine receptor autoantibodies block the postsynaptic receptor and block effect of acetylcholine** released from the presynaptic nerve ending to stimulate associated muscle cells

Clinical Presentation

- **Muscles fatigue and become weak with activity**
- **Present with fatigue with chewing, swallowing disorder, and diplopia**
- **Often associated with other autoimmune disorders or thymoma**
- Can be precipitated or worsened by aminoglycosides, clindamycin, erythromycin, tetracycline, procainamide, quinine, quinidine, β-blockers, and calcium channel-blockers (Box 63-2)

Diagnosis and Evaluation

- Neurologic examination is otherwise normal
- **Measure antiacetylcholine receptor antibodies in serum**
- Deficits improve transiently with edrophonium (Tensilon) test
- **EMG/NCS repetitive stimulation shows fatigue, but is otherwise normal**
- Differential diagnosis includes: Lambert-Eaton syndrome (see Chapter 58, Table 58-3), botulism, and drug toxicity

BOX 63-2	*Medications That Exacerbate Myasthenia Gravis*

Aminoglycosides
Clindamycin
Erythromycin
Tetracycline
Procainamide
Quinine
Quinidine
β-Blockers
Calcium channel-blockers

Treatment

- Prednisone, mestinon, IV immunoglobulin, and thymectomy

Toxic Myopathies

INFLAMMATORY MYOPATHIES

Basic Information

- Caused by a variety of agents including **alcohol, cimetidine, colchicine, D-penicillamine, heroin, prednisone, and statins**

Clinical Presentation

- **Prolonged, high-dose steroid use is associated with chronic progressive proximal muscle weakness**
- Other agents present with a classic myopathic examination

Diagnosis and Evaluation

- **Prednisone myopathy is unique in that it has normal creatine phosphokinase (CPK) levels** and is diagnosed by myopathic changes on EMG
- The other agents cause elevated CPK levels, and the EMG shows myopathic changes

Treatment

- Tapering the steroid dose or changing to a steroid-sparing immunosuppressive is the only effective treatment for steroid myopathy
- Likewise, the other inciting agents must also be stopped

REVIEW QUESTIONS

For review questions, please go to www.expertconsult.com.

SUGGESTED READINGS

Bradley WG, Daroff RB, editors: *Neurology in clinical practice*, ed 2, Philadelphia, WB Saunders, 1945.
Canale ST, editor: *Campbell's operative orthopedics*, ed 9, St. Louis, Mosby, 1998.
Collins RD: *Illustrated manual of neurological diseases*, Philadelphia, JP Lippincott, 1962.

Selected Topics in General and Internal Medicine

Selected Topics in Geriatric Medicine

COLLEEN CHRISTMAS, MD

The medical issues facing the elderly include those commonly seen in all adults, but also include issues that become increasingly prevalent with advancing age. With aging, people become increasingly less resilient, resulting in a lessened ability to withstand stress. These issues call on special skills when approaching elderly patients. With the aging of the U.S. population, internists will need to be familiar with the diagnosis and management of health issues common among the elderly. In this chapter, we review four syndromes commonly seen in older adults: Urinary incontinence, pressure ulcers, falls, and dementia.

Urinary Incontinence

Basic Information

- Definition: Involuntary loss of urine that causes a social, health, or hygiene problem
- Physiology of micturition involves the following:
  - Sympathetic innervation: Relaxes bladder and contracts bladder neck and urethra
  - Parasympathetic innervation: Contracts bladder (detrusor muscle) for emptying
  - Somatic innervation: Leads to voluntary contraction of external urethral sphincter
    - Helpful mnemonic: Sympathetics store, parasympathetics pee

Clinical Presentation

Table 64-1 summarizes the types of urinary incontinence.
- **Urge incontinence: The most common cause of incontinence** (accounts for 40–70% of cases)

- Results from detrusor overactivity, detrusor instability, or detrusor hyper-reflexia
- Characterized by a sudden urge and desire to void, a fear of leakage, and ultimately urine loss
- May lose small or large amounts of urine depending on sphincter function
- May result from defects of CNS inhibition (e.g., stroke, cervical stenosis, CNS masses, multiple sclerosis, Parkinson's disease, spinal cord injury, dementia) or local genitourinary irritants (e.g., infection, tumor, stone)
- **Stress incontinence: The second most common cause of incontinence in the elderly**
  - Characterized by small-volume losses of urine during times of increased intra-abdominal pressure (e.g., coughing, sneezing, laughing, exercising)
  - Usually seen in women who have lost pelvic support of the urethra, with resultant failure of the urinary sphincter mechanism during periods of increased intra-abdominal pressure
  - If seen in men, typically seen in those who have undergone urologic procedures
- **Overflow incontinence: Accounts for 10% of urinary incontinence among elderly patients**
  - Typically associated with some form of urinary outflow obstruction (e.g., prostatic enlargement, urethral stricture, or cystocele)
    - Also seen in diabetes mellitus, in part because of neurogenic bladder and in part because of nerve damage to control of detrusor contractility
  - Patients complain of reduced urinary stream, incomplete voiding, frequent or continuous dribbling, or leakage without warning

TABLE 64-1	Types of Urinary Incontinence		
Type	**Pathophysiology**	**Characteristic of Urine Lost**	**Common Causes**
Urge	Detrusor overactivity	Small to large without "warning"	UTI, fecal impaction, CVA, cord injury
Stress	Weak bladder outlet	Small, often with coughing or standing	Weakened pelvis from childbirth
Overflow	Bladder outlet obstruction	Small, frequently dribbling without "warning"	BPH, diabetes, cystocele
Functional	Can't or won't get to toilet	Can be small but usually large	Dementia, mobility problems, toilet inaccessible

BPH, benign prostate hypertrophy; CVA, cardiovascular accident; UTI, urinary tract infection.

- **Functional incontinence: Occurs when an individual is unable or unwilling to reach the toilet in time**
  - Associated factors include dementia, depression, physical impairments that impede mobility (e.g., degenerative arthritis, stroke, Parkinson's disease), or physical restraints or inaccessible toilets

Diagnosis

- Important historical features in the incontinent patient
  - Frequency, timing, and situations associated with incontinent episodes
  - Volume of urine loss
  - Comorbid medical and psychiatric conditions
  - Medications (Box 64-1)
  - Bladder (or voiding) record: Patient or caretaker records continent and incontinent voids over 48 hours; used to diagnose cause, assess effect on daily life, and track response to therapy
- The physical examination in the incontinent patient
  - Abdominal examination for bladder distention
  - Rectal examination for rectal tone, fecal impaction, and, in males, prostatic enlargement
  - In women, pelvic examination for cystocele, uterine prolapse, rectocele, atrophic vaginitis
  - Full neurologic examination including mental status and mobility assessment
- Laboratory examination in the incontinent patient should include measure of renal function as well as glucose and calcium (which cause osmotic diuresis)

- Urinalysis as well as urine culture to exclude infection as cause of incontinence
- Postvoid residual: Patient voluntarily empties bladder completely, followed by bladder catheterization to measure residual volume in bladder
  - Normal is less than 50 to 100 mL
  - **Postvoid residual of more than 100 mL suggests overflow incontinence** either from impaired detrusor contractility (e.g., neurogenic bladder) or outlet obstruction
- Urodynamic testing: Used to assess lower urinary tract function; tests commonly include cystometry, urinary flow measurement, and measurement of urethral pressure (some would add IV pyelography and cystourethrography to this list)
  - In majority of cases of incontinence, diagnosis can be made without testing
  - No clear guidelines exist on when to refer for testing
  - May help in the following situations
    - Failure of the initial treatment plan
    - Confusing or inconsistent history
    - To clarify need for surgery

Treatment

See Table 64-2.

Pressure Ulcers

Basic Information

- A pressure ulcer results when unrelieved pressure on skin and subcutaneous tissue results in infarction and necrosis
  - Moisture, friction, and body habitus may contribute to susceptibility and formation of ulcer
- Four stages of pressure ulcers (Table 64-3; Figs. 64-1 to 64-3)
  - **Stage I:** Damage to intact skin; apparent clinically as nonblanchable erythema of intact skin
  - **Stage II:** Partial-thickness skin loss involving epidermis or both epidermis and dermis; clinically apparent as a blister or superficial ulcer

---

BOX 64-1	*Medications That Exacerbate Incontinence*

Sedatives/hypnotics
Diuretics
α-Adrenergic agonists
α-Adrenergic antagonists
Anticholinergics
Narcotics
Alcohol
Calcium channel blockers

TABLE 64-2	*Treatment of Incontinence*	
Type	**Nonpharmacologic**	**Pharmacologic**

Urge incontinence	Pelvic muscle exercises (Kegel exercises)
	Bladder retraining
	Scheduled or prompted voiding
		Anticholinergics
		  Oxybutinin
		  Tolterodine
		  Imipramine

Stress incontinence	Pelvic muscle exercises
	Biofeedback
	Surgery
	  Colposuspension
	  Sling procedure
		α-Adrenergic agonists: Pseudoephedrine
		Anticholinergics: Imipramine
		Estrogen alone of no proven benefit;
		  may be of use in combination with
		  α-adrenergics

Overflow incontinence	Intermittent or chronic catheterization Surgical correction of obstruction	Discontinue medications that exacerbate overflow obstruction
Functional incontinence	Prompted or scheduled voiding Absorbent undergarments Remove barriers to bathroom Bedside commode when appropriate Optimize physical function	None

- **Stage III:** Full-thickness skin loss exposing subcutaneous tissue, with damage to subcutaneous tissue as well; underlying fascia is not affected;

<table>
<tr><td>TABLE 64-3</td><td colspan="2">Staging of Pressure Ulcers</td></tr>
<tr><td>Stage I</td><td>Nonblanchable erythema of intact skin</td></tr>
<tr><td>Stage II</td><td>Superficial ulcer extending through the epidermis or dermis or both</td></tr>
<tr><td>Stage III</td><td>Full-thickness skin loss exposing fat or subcutaneous tissue</td></tr>
<tr><td>Stage IV</td><td>Full-thickness skin loss exposing bone, muscle, tendon, or joint capsule</td></tr>
</table>

clinically apparent as a deep ulcer but **without exposure of bone, muscle, or joint capsule**
- **Stage IV:** Full-thickness skin loss extending to and including underlying fascia, **including muscle and bone**; clinically apparent as a crater with visibly involved underlying structures

Clinical Presentation

- Risk factors have been quantified into clinical prediction rules for likelihood of developing a pressure ulcer
  - Risk factors predictive of pressure ulcers include poor physical condition, decreased mental status, low level of activity, immobility, and incontinence

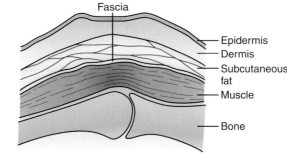
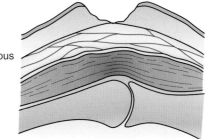
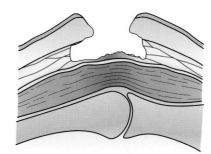
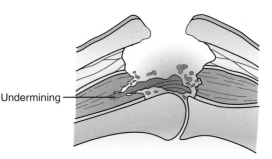

FIGURE 64-1 National Pressure Ulcer Advisory Panel classification of pressure ulcers. (From Bolognia JL, Jorizzo JL, Rapini RP: *Dermatology,* St. Louis, Mosby, 2003, figure 106.20.)

Stage I
Nonblanchable erythema with induration and warmth

Stage II
Irregular shallow ulceration; loss of epidermis, dermis, or both, with erythema, induration, and warmth

Stage III
Deep ulceration with necrotic base

Stage IV
Deep ulceration reaching underlying bone

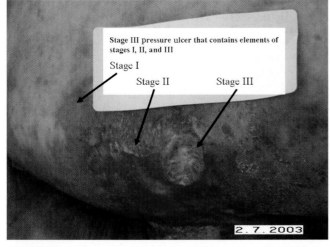

FIGURE 64-2 Pressure ulcer demonstrating stages I, II, and III of ulceration.

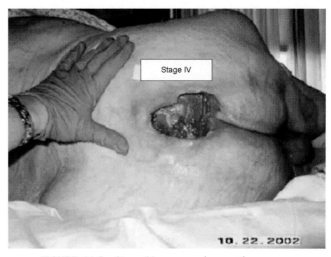

FIGURE 64-3 Stage IV pressure ulcer on the sacrum.

- Other clinical prediction rules add "poor nutritional status" (which is variably defined) and chronic skin moisture as risk factors for pressure ulcers
- Complications of pressure ulcers may accompany clinical presentation and include wound infection (manifesting as purulent drainage, often with foul odor, and surrounding erythema, warmth, and tenderness); osteomyelitis; and sinus tract formation
  - **Pressure ulcers are colonized with bacteria; a positive swab culture does not imply infection**
  - **Osteomyelitis is presumed if bone is grossly visible or can be reached with a probe**

Diagnosis

- Diagnosis based on preceding staging system
- If eschar overlies ulcer, staging cannot be performed

Treatment

Table 64-4 summarizes wound care products and information.

- Best treatment is identification of individuals at risk and prevention of ulcer development
  - Pressure reduction: Turn and reposition immobile patients **every 2 hours**
    - Specialized mattresses and beds may decrease risk of ulcer development, although it is unclear if they are superior to vigilant bedside care
  - Nutrition: It is unclear whether nutritional interventions improve pressure sore outcomes. Oral supplementation could play a role.
    - Despite this weak evidence, many authorities advise a diet providing 30 to 35 Cal/kg/day and 1.25 to 1.5 g protein/kg/day in undernourished individuals with pressure ulcers. If tube feeding is used and causes increased immobility and diarrhea, pressure sore outcomes may be worsened. The role of zinc supplementation is unclear.
    - Vitamin deficiencies should be corrected
- Débridement: To remove necrotic material and promote healing
  - Mechanical débridement is achieved with wet-to-dry dressings
    - Scalpel or scissor débridement may also be needed
  - Enzymatic débridement is achieved with collagenases

TABLE 64-4	Principles of Pressure Ulcer Management
Ulcer Appearance	**Management**
Infected or necrotic	Sharp or chemical débridement, Iodine product (e.g., Iodosorb) Bleach product (e.g., Chlorpactin)
Clean granulating	Supportive environment (e.g., Calginate, hydrogel)
Undermined	Fill tissue space with wick or vacuum device
Epithelializing	Petroleum gauze, collagen
Hypergranulating	Control granulation with salt foam (e.g., Mesalt) or silver nitrate

TABLE 64-5	Wound Care Products and Indications
Product	**Indication(s)**
Film covering (e.g., Opsite)	Stage I ulcer
Foam covering (e.g., Allevyn)	Noninfected stage II or III ulcer
Hydrocolloid covering (e.g., Duoderm)	Noninfected stage II ulcer; stage III ulcer with light exudate
Hydrogel (e.g., Carrington)	Stage II–IV ulcer with moderate drainage
Alginate (e.g., Sorbsan)	Stage II–IV ulcer with copious drainage

- Autolytic débridement achieved by covering ulcer with synthetic dressing, which allows enzymes in the wound to digest the necrotic but noninfected tissue
  - **Should not be used in infected wounds**
- Infection: As noted previously, colonization is common and does not represent infection; swab cultures of the wound base have no clinical utility
  - Use of topical antibiotics controversial; they may be toxic to fibroblasts
    - If used, topical antibiotics should be discontinued after 48 hours
  - **Systemic antibiotics are reserved for patients with signs of cellulitis, osteomyelitis, or systemic illness**
  - If a pocket of abscess is identified, culture of purulent contents may be useful in selecting antibiotics (Table 64-5)

Falls

Basic Information

- A fall represents an individual's unintentional coming to rest on the ground or other lower level without overwhelming intrinsic or extrinsic cause
- **Falls are distinct from syncope; with syncope, loss of consciousness occurs** (see Chapter 5)
- Incidence of falls increases with increasing age of patient
- Situational factors that predispose to falling include the type of activity and the environment
  - **70% of falls occur at home**
  - 10% of falls occur on the stairs
  - 50% of falls are associated with environmental hazards (e.g., ice, throw rugs)
- In addition to risks associated with trauma, falls are associated with a decline in the ability to perform activities of daily living (ADLs) and an increasing likelihood of nursing home placement

Clinical Presentation

- Among the tasks of the clinician is to differentiate a fall from a syncopal event
  - Evidence of trauma should also raise concern for abuse or neglect
- Otherwise, the clinical presentation is straightforward

Diagnosis

- The events surrounding the fall and other fall history should be reviewed
  - The frequency of falling and the location of falling (e.g., in the home, on the stairs) should be reviewed
    - Look for patterns to falls, such as timing in relation to medications or meals or directions of falling (e.g., falling backward would suggest parkinsonism)
- Risk factors for falling should be reviewed (Box 64-2)
  - More than one risk factor typically present in the patient who falls
  - **Medications such as sedatives, antidepressants, and neuroleptics are the greatest risk factors for falling**
    - Dementia increases the chances of falling fivefold
- Physical examination includes assessment of volume status (e.g., orthostatics), cognition, and the cardiovascular, musculoskeletal, and neurologic systems
  - Visual and auditory acuity should also be checked regularly
  - Many physicians informally evaluate fall risk with the "get up and go" test, in which they observe the patient rise from a chair and walk while paying attention to the speed and steadiness of the patient's gait

Treatment

- Prevention of falls for at-risk individuals
  - Exercise and balance training: Both have demonstrated effect at reducing falls
  - Home modification: Improve home lighting, maintain clutter-free passageways, install raised toilet seats, add grab bars in the bathroom, secure loose carpets, add stair rails (Box 64-3)
  - Adjust or avoid medications that increase risk of falling, **particularly psychotropic medications**
  - Cane or walker in those with imbalance or physical disability

---

BOX 64-2	*Risk Factors for Falling*

Medications
　　Benzodiazepines
　　Neuroleptics
　　Tricyclic antidepressants
　　Antihypertensives
　　Diuretics
Sensory impairment
　　Visual loss
　　Vestibular dysfunction
　　Decreased proprioception
Central nervous system disease
　　Stroke
　　Parkinson's disease
　　Cognitive disorders
Musculoskeletal disorders
　　Arthritis
Depression
Substance abuse
Past history of falling

- Prevention of injury in those at risk of falling
  - Osteoporosis screening
  - Hip protectors
  - Lifeline or other contact strategy if fallen

Dementia

Basic Information

- Dementia: A syndrome that results in a decline in memory and other cognitive abilities **to the point that it interferes with ADLs**
  - Impairment of daily living is an important distinction; age-related modest decline in intellectual function that does not impair function is normal and does not represent dementia
- At age 60 years, 1% of the population is demented
  - The age-related prevalence of dementia then doubles every 5 years
- Once diagnosed, estimates of average survival range from 5 to 9 years, but may be as short as 3 years
- Common causes of dementia
  - **Alzheimer's disease is the most common cause of dementia (70% of cases)**

BOX 64-3	*Home Environmental Modifications to Prevent Falls*

Stairs
Light switch at both ends
Clutter free
Tightly woven carpet or treads
Handrails

Kitchen
Avoid high shelves
Step stool with handrails
Keep floor dry

Living Area
Open pathway
No footstools, low tables, pets
Cords out of pathway
　　No throw rugs
　　Cordless phone

Bathroom
Night light
Nonskid rugs
Handrails in tub and toilet
Tub mat, chair

Bedroom
Clutter-free path
Night light
Sit on edge of bed before getting up

Footwear
Low-heel, nonskid soles
Appropriate fit
Keep laces tied/Velcro

64

- Vascular dementia is the second most common cause (10–20% of cases)
- Dementia with Lewy bodies may be more common than previously thought
- Alcohol-related causes are commonly associated with dementia; one out of five patients with dementia has a significant alcohol history
- Uncommon causes of dementia include infectious causes (e.g., HIV, neurosyphilis); endocrine or metabolic causes (e.g., hypothyroidism, hypercalcemia, vitamin B$_{12}$ deficiency); and neurologic disorders including Parkinson's disease, frontotemporal dementia (formerly known as Pick's disease), Creutzfeldt-Jacob disease, subdural hematoma, and normal pressure hydrocephalus
- **Only 2% of cases of dementia are caused by reversible causes**; even when found and treated (e.g., hypothyroidism, syphilis), dementia may not resolve

Clinical Presentation

- With dementia, family members or caregivers are usually the ones who initially raise concern for dementia
  - **A patient who complains of memory problems is more likely to be depressed or under stress than demented**
    - A psychiatric history should be taken in all patients with suggested dementia
  - **Consciousness is clear in the demented patient**; clouded consciousness (especially waxing and waning symptoms) suggests delirium
- Clinical features vary based on cause of dementia
  - Alzheimer's disease results in a gradual decline in cognitive function
    - **Language skills commonly affected**; motor skills typically spared
  - Vascular dementia is associated with **a stepwise, sudden progression** of decline in cognitive function
    - In this population, the medical history typically uncovers **other risk factors for vascular disease**
    - Abnormal motor signs are common including facial masking, rigidity, an extensor plantar reflex, and gait disturbances
  - Dementia with Lewy bodies is commonly associated with **fluctuations in alertness or cognition, visual hallucinations, and features of parkinsonism**

Diagnosis

- Diagnostic criteria for dementia are listed in Box 64-4
- Assessment of neurocognitive functioning
  - The mini-mental status examination (MMSE) or another similar test such as the mini-cog is used to provide a quantitative assessment of cognitive impairment and to provide a baseline for comparison over time
    - Age and education level affect score on MMSE
    - For English-speaking individuals with at least an eighth-grade education, **a score less than 24 in the appropriate clinical setting suggests the presence of dementia**
  - Functional status can also be assessed with standardized tests such as the functional activities questionnaire, which assess high-level activities (e.g., writing checks

---

| BOX 64-4 | *Diagnostic Criteria for Dementia* |

Part 1: The development of multiple cognitive defects, manifested by both

Memory impairment *plus*

One or more of the following cognitive (or cortical) disturbances

Aphasia (language disturbance)

Apraxia (impaired ability to carry out motor activities despite intact motor function)

Agnosia (failure to recognize or identify objects despite intact sensory function)

Disturbance in executive functioning (planning, organization, abstraction)

Part 2: The cognitive deficits must cause significant impairment in social or occupational functioning and represent a decline from a previous level of functioning

---

and balancing a checkbook, organizing tax records, shopping for groceries)
  - Formal neurocognitive testing is recommended when there is sufficient concern for the diagnosis of dementia
- Laboratory examination in the patient with suspected dementia (Box 64-5)
  - Increasing evidence has linked the apolipoprotein E ε4 allele with an increased risk of developing Alzheimer's disease
  - Until more medical evidence is available, routine testing of the apolipoprotein E genotype in the evaluation of the demented patient is not recommended
  - Testing for syphilis recommended if there is a history of prior infection, risk factors for syphilis, or the individual lives in an area with high prevalence of syphilis
- Neuroimaging is now recommended by the Academy of Neurology in the evaluation of all patients with dementia, though not all authorities agree with this approach and its cost-effectiveness has not been demonstrated

---

| BOX 64-5 | *Laboratory Evaluation of the Patient with Dementia** |

Complete blood count

Electrolytes

Blood urea nitrogen

Creatinine

Liver enzymes

Calcium

Thyroid-stimulating hormone

Rapid plasma reagin

HIV

Vitamin B$_{12}$

*Some clinicians would add homocysteine and methylmalonic acid to this list.

- Should be done in all patients, including those with a nonfocal neurologic examination
- Often performed to exclude identifiable causes such as tumors, mass lesions, subdural hematoma, or normal pressure hydrocephalus
- Neuroimaging normal or only shows atrophy in the patient with Alzheimer's disease

Management

- Overall goals of therapy are to **identify and treat reversible causes of dementia and to improve quality of life and maximize functional performance**
  - Caregiver and family education and counseling improves quality of life and delays the need for nursing home placement by as much as 1 year
- Symptomatic therapy focuses on treating cognitive impairment, mood disturbances, and behavioral disturbances
  - Pharmacotherapy for cognitive impairment limited; **all share mechanism of cholinergic augmentation by inhibiting cholinesterase**
    - Examples include tacrine, donepezil, rivastigmine, and galantamine
    - Best experience is in use in patients with mild to moderate Alzheimer's disease; no role in patients with severe Alzheimer's
    - Modest improvement in cognitive functioning may be demonstrable on neurocognitive testing, but improvement is often not evident to caregiver or clinician and **does not prevent the progression of disease**
    - The role of estrogen, NSAIDs, and 3-hydroxy-methylglutaryl coenzyme A (HMG-CoA) reductase inhibitors in the prevention and development of Alzheimer's disease has not been defined

- **Mood impairment, most commonly depression, should be anticipated and treated** in the patient with dementia
  - **Selective serotonin reuptake inhibitors** are preferred. The anticholinergic side effects of tricyclic antidepressants should be avoided.
- Behavioral therapy should be added if the patient becomes agitated or psychotic (seen in 50% of demented patients)
  - Haloperidol has been the drug of choice for behavioral management
    - Some use newer-generation antipsychotics that may have fewer extrapyramidal side effects (e.g., risperidone, olanzapine, and quetiapine), but at greater cost and without demonstration of enhanced efficacy
  - Benzodiazepines can worsen confusion and should be avoided

REVIEW QUESTIONS

For review questions, please go to www.expertconsult.com.

SUGGESTED READINGS

Boustani M, Peterson B, Hanson L, et al: Screening for dementia in primary care: a summary of the evidence for the U.S. Preventive Services Task Force, *Ann Intern Med* 138:927–937, 2003.

Cobbs EL, Duthie EH, Murphy JB, editors: *Geriatrics review syllabus: a core curriculum in geriatric medicine*, ed 5, Malden, MA, Blackwell, 2002.

Courtney C, Farrell D, Gray R, et al: Long-term donepezil treatment in 565 patients with Alzheimer's disease (AD2000 Collaborative Group): randomised double-blind trial, *Lancet* 363:2105–2115, 2004.

Executive summary of the American Geriatrics Society, British Geriatrics Society, and American Academy of Orthopaedic Surgeons: Clinical practice guideline: the prevention of falls in older persons, *J Am Geriatr Soc* 49:664–672, 2001.

64

CHAPTER 65

Selected Topics in Women's Health

PAULA KUE, MD, and REDONDA G. MILLER, MD, MBA

Internists provide care for women of all ages and often are faced with a variety of disorders specific to women. Familiarity with gynecologic disorders is crucial. In addition, pregnant women may have medical complications that require close evaluation and monitoring by the internist. This chapter covers many of these important issues, including cervical cancer screening, contraception, and medical complications of pregnancy.

Cervical Cancer Screening and Treatment

Basic Information

- Cervical cancer is highly prevalent, with 16,000 new cases reported each year in the United States. Early detection through the Papanicolaou (Pap) smear has greatly reduced mortality.
- **Risk factors for cervical cancer**
  - **Human papilloma virus (HPV)**
  - **Smoking**
  - **Multiple sexual partners**
  - **Early age of first intercourse**
  - **History of other STDs**
  - **HIV infection (see Chapter 12)**
  - **Other immunocompromised state**
- **Cervical cancer and its precursors are intimately linked to certain serotypes of HPV**
  - HPV exposure is already common and becoming more prevalent in humans
  - HPV serotypes 16, 18, 33, 35, and 39 confer highest risk and are often associated with high-grade neoplasia and invasive cancer
  - HPV serotypes 6, 11, and 42 are more often associated with low-risk lesions and condylomata
  - Cervical cancer in the absence of heterosexual activity is extremely rare, probably because sperm assist HPV infection of cervical epithelium
- HPV vaccine now available
  - Has excellent efficacy in prevention of infection with high-risk serotypes
  - Series of three injections at 0, 2, and 6 months
  - Recommended for women younger than 26 years of age
  - Avoid in pregnancy

Clinical Presentation

- The cervical epithelium most often affected by malignant transformation is where the columnar cells of the endocervical canal are undergoing transformation into the squamous cells of the exocervix (Fig. 65-1)
- Most women with precursors to cervical cancer are asymptomatic
- Invasive cervical cancer becomes symptomatic at a late stage
  - Abnormal bleeding (menorrhagia, postcoitally, or intermenstrual) may occur early in the disease
  - Late-stage symptoms are usually caused by local spread and may include pelvic, leg, or back pain; pedal edema; rectal bleeding; or hematuria
- Physical examination may show evidence of the following:
  - HPV infection: Condylomata acuminata (verrucous-like lesions; Fig. 65-2)
  - Invasive cancer: Induration, friable tissue, ulceration, exophytic (cauliflower-like) lesions

Diagnosis and Evaluation

- **Cervical cytology (the Pap smear) is the screening test of choice; screens for both dysplasia and cancer**
  - Involves exfoliative cytology of the uterine cervix

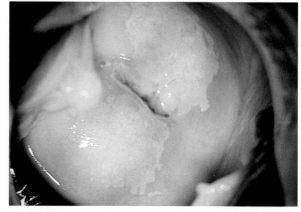

FIGURE 65-1 Cervix demonstrating abnormal epithelium on the anterior and posterior margins, demonstrating the white discoloration after the application of acetic acid. (From Oats J, Abraham S: *Llewellyn-Jones fundamentals of obstetrics and gynaecology*, ed 8, Philadelphia, Mosby, 2004, figure 37.6.)

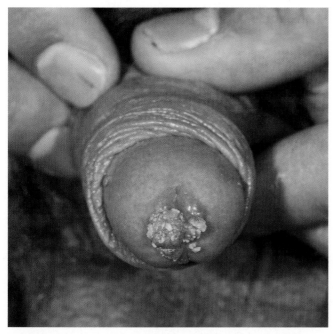

FIGURE 65-2 Genital warts at the urethral meatus associated with human papilloma virus. (From Habif TP: *Clinical dermatology: a color guide to diagnosis and therapy*, ed 4, Philadelphia, Mosby, 2004, figure 11-4.)

- Proven to reduce the incidence of squamous cervical cancer and resultant mortality
- Sensitivity is approximately 70% to 80%; specificity is 90% to 95%
  - **Proper interpretation of Pap smear is crucial to avoiding unnecessary testing (see following discussion)**
  - **Many lesions regress over time and do not portend a diagnosis of cancer**
  - **Management of abnormal Pap smears differs significantly in women with HIV infection; see Chapter 12 for details**
- Technique
  - Perform before bimanual examination
  - Visualize the entire cervix if possible
  - Remove any discharge carefully before obtaining specimen
  - Small amount of blood is acceptable; large amounts (i.e., menses) preclude adequate testing
  - Must include cells from the transformation zone to be deemed adequate
  - Conventional brush-and-scrape technique
    - Sample obtained with an endocervical spatula and brush (sequentially)
    - Scrape exterior cervix before endocervical canal
    - Must undergo rapid fixation on slide to avoid air-drying and subsequent artifact
  - Liquid-based sampling (preferred)
    - Specially designed round brush is inserted into the cervix and rotated clockwise five full rotations
    - Entire brush placed into liquid medium
    - Better sensitivity over conventional technique
    - HPV testing may be performed on the same sample (concurrently or retrospectively)

- Pap smear frequency
  - **Pap smear screening should be initiated in all women once sexually active or at age 21 years (whichever is first)**
    - **Should be repeated annually until at least three normal results are obtained**
    - **Thereafter, it may be repeated annually or as infrequently as every 3 years as long as normal results are obtained (and the patient remains at low risk)**
  - Women at high risk (see preceding risk factors) require annual Pap smear screening indefinitely, even if they never have an abnormal result
  - In women who have undergone hysterectomy without a cervical remnant, Pap smears are no longer required unless the hysterectomy was performed for cervical cancer
  - It is unclear whether screening beyond age 65 years is worthwhile
- The Bethesda System (1994) is used for classification of Pap smear adequacy and results (Table 65-1)
  - Descriptions may include the following
    - Benign cellular changes (e.g., infection)
    - Reactive cellular changes (e.g., inflammation)
    - Epithelial cell changes
  - **Infections found on Pap smear should be treated (i.e., *Candida*, *Trichomonas*)**
  - Squamous metaplasia is a normal finding
- **Consensus guidelines (2001) for management of abnormal Pap smears** (see Table 65-1)
  - Atypical squamous cells of unknown significance (ASCUS) and atypical glandular cells of unknown significance (AGUS) diagnoses are not normal, but do not meet the criteria for a more serious diagnosis
  - **ASCUS is the most common finding on abnormal Pap smears**
    - **Majority of these women have benign findings on colposcopy**
    - **HPV testing is a helpful option in triaging cases of ASCUS for colposcopy (see Table 65-1)**
      - Test for high-risk subtypes
      - Testing for low-risk subtypes is not helpful in triaging risk of more aggressive disease
    - ASCUS in an immunosuppressed woman should always prompt colposcopy
- Diagnosis is considered secured when Pap result, colposcopy, and biopsy histology are in agreement
- If the results of the Pap, colposcopic appearance, and biopsy histology are in significant disagreement, treatment can still be initiated if the histology is the most severe diagnosis
  - If the histology specimen indicates less severe results than Pap diagnosis, consider that the biopsy did not sample the region of the genital tract shedding the cells resulting in the Pap abnormality (sampling error)
    - Should obtain a larger biopsy specimen
    - Options to remove a larger portion of the cervix to include the entire exocervical portion of the transformation zone (identifiable by an applied stain) and part of the endocervical canal include
      - Cold knife conization (CKC) using a scalpel

65

TABLE 65-1	The Bethesda Classification of Pap Smear Results and Management Options	

Pap Smear Result	Risk of High-Grade Lesion (by Histology)	Management Options*
Normal	Essentially none	Continue routine screening
Atypical squamous cells of undetermined significance (ASCUS)	Low	Three options 　Repeat Pap smear in 4–6 mo 　　If two consecutive repeats are normal, continue yearly screening 　　If ASCUS obtained before two normal repeats, refer for colposcopy 　or 　Colposcopy 　　If normal, resume annual Pap screening 　　If abnormal, perform biopsies 　or 　DNA testing for human papilloma virus 　　If positive, refer for colposcopy 　　If negative, repeat Pap smear in 1 year
Atypical glandular cells of undetermined significance (AGUS)	More related to endometrial rather than cervical cancer	More aggressive follow-up because AGUS is more commonly related to serious disease than is ASCUS Colposcopy with directed biopsy is recommended Endometrial biopsy usually indicated as well If all normal, repeat Pap in 3–6 mo
Low-grade squamous intraepithelial lesion (LGSIL)	15–30%	Colposcopy and directed biopsies
High-grade squamous intraepithelial lesion (HGSIL)	70–75%	Colposcopy and directed biopsies
Invasive cancer	>99%	Colposcopy and directed biopsies

*See Chapter 12 for a discussion of women with HIV.

- Loop electrosurgical excision procedure (LEEP) using a heated wire loop
- Laser conization
- The biopsy sample is then considered adequate if the histologic diagnosis is at least as serious as the Pap diagnosis, and the margins of the biopsy are free of premalignant or malignant transformation

Treatment

- Low-grade squamous intraepithelial lesions (LGSIL) and high-grade intraepithelial lesions (HGSIL) are considered precursors of invasive squamous cell cancer of the cervix
- LGSIL treatment
  - **If LGSIL is confirmed by colposcopy and histology, treatment can be expectant with quarterly Pap smears because the majority revert to normal without treatment**
  - Once four quarterly Pap smears in a row have been normal, follow-up can be semiannual Pap smears for another year followed by annual testing (assuming all are normal)
  - Alternatively, if the patient prefers, or in older women or in women in whom follow-up may be problematic, treatment with LEEP or cryosurgery can be undertaken
- HGSIL treatment
  - May be treated in a variety of ways, all of which result in its removal from the cervix
  - If a conization procedure is performed in the evaluation, the cytology and histology do not include

invasive cancer, and the margins of the cone are free of disease, treatment is considered complete
- Otherwise, the affected region of the cervix can be removed by LEEP, CKC, laser conization, or cryosurgery (killing the affected cells using liquid nitrogen)
- Hysterectomy may be appropriate treatment for women with other problems (e.g., severe dysmenorrhea or menorrhagia)
- Follow-up is then quarterly Pap smears for a year, semiannual Pap smears for another year, and then annual Pap smears (assuming all are normal)
- Frequent follow-up is also indicated in women after a hysterectomy, in case part of the cervix remains or disease develops in the vaginal epithelium
- Treatment of invasive cervical cancer
  - Staging is first step: Requires pelvic examination, routine labs, chest radiograph, IV pyelogram; other studies as deemed necessary
    - Stage I: Confined to the cervix
    - Stage II: Extends beyond cervix but not to pelvic sidewall or lower third of vagina
    - Stage III: Involves pelvic sidewall or lower third of vagina
    - Stage IV: Metastatic disease (beyond pelvis) or involvement of bladder or rectum
  - Treatment based on stage
    - Stage I can usually be treated with hysterectomy with or without radiation
    - Stages II and III are predominantly treated with radiation

- Stage IV requires radical surgery, usually with radiation, or palliative chemotherapy or radiation
- Prognosis based on tumor size, stage, and nodal involvement
  - Stage I: 78% overall survival
  - Stage IV: 8% overall survival

Contraception

- Half of all pregnancies are unplanned; contraception is an important primary care issue
- Many different forms of contraception are available to women; choice is often based on personal preference
- **Contraceptive efficacy can be measured by the Pearl index**
  - **This is the number of women out of 100 using a particular method likely to be pregnant at the end of a year of usual use (Table 65-2)**
  - Actual failure rates of the techniques listed are higher than the values shown; usually caused by improper use of the method
- Specific types of contraception
  - Abstinence
  - Rhythm method (Fig. 65-3)

- Barrier methods
  - Condoms
    - Latex sheath that fits snugly over the penis during intercourse

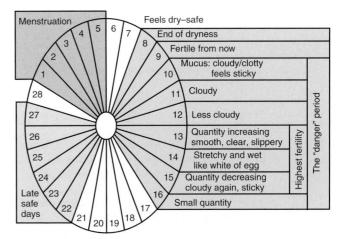

FIGURE 65-3 Periodic abstinence ("rhythm method"), using the mucus (ovulation) method. (From Oats J, Abraham S: *Llewellyn-Jones fundamentals of obstetrics and gynaecology,* ed 8, Philadelphia, Mosby, 2004.)

65

TABLE 65-2	*Contraceptive Options and Efficacy*	
Technique	**Pearl Index***	**Possible Side Effects**
Attempting conception	80	N/A
Withdrawal	40	None
Rhythm	40	None
Spermicidal suppositories or foam	20	Local irritation Allergic reactions
Condom	20	Skin irritation Latex allergy
Diaphragm	15	Pelvic irritation and discomfort Small increase in urinary tract infections
Intrauterine device	<1	Menorrhagia Dysmenorrhea Increased risk of salpingitis (leading to possible infertility) Uterine perforation
Combination oral contraceptive pills	1–2	Breakthrough bleeding (if occurs longer than 3 mo, deserves evaluation) Amenorrhea (not harmful) Headache, worsening migraines Breast tenderness Increase in blood pressure Increased risk of thromboembolism Increased risk of gallbladder disease
Progesterone-only contraceptive pills	5	Breakthrough or irregular bleeding Loss of bone density with prolonged use
Injected progesterone	<1	Breakthrough bleeding Weight gain Acne Loss of bone density with prolonged use
Female sterilization	<1	Risk of anesthesia

*Pearl index is the number of couples out of 100 using a particular method that are likely to be pregnant at the end of a year of usual use.

- **Advantages: Protection from STDs, easily obtained over the counter**
  - Efficacy greatly enhanced by addition of spermicides, which decrease sperm motility (e.g., nonoxynol-9)
- Diaphragm
  - Rubber dome-shaped cup that fits over the cervix
  - Inserted manually before intercourse
  - Major disadvantage is inconvenience
- Hormonal
  - Combination oral contraceptives
    - Most commonly used reversible method of contraception
    - Contain both estrogen and progestin in 21 tablets; remaining 7 tablets contain inert ingredients (to bring on withdrawal bleed)
      - **Estrogen: Serves mainly to inhibit ovulation by suppressing pituitary gonadotropin secretion; usually dosed between 20 µg ("low-dose") and 35 µg per tablet**
      - **Progestin: Causes changes in cervical mucus and endometrium that hinder fertility**
    - Many different formulations and combinations exist on the market
      - Choice of prescribed formulation often based on patient or doctor familiarity, cost, availability
      - Monophasic pill: Constant dose of estrogen and progestin in each tablet
      - Phasic pill: Changing dose of progestin (and sometimes estrogen) in the 21 active tablets; usually an escalating dose
    - **Combination oral contraceptives are highly effective; most common reason for failure is noncompliance**
      - **If a woman misses one or two tablets, she should take one tablet immediately on remembering followed by one tablet twice daily until missed tablets have been taken**
      - **If more than two tablets missed, another form of contraception should be used during that cycle**
    - Potential benefits: Improvement in dysmenorrhea, premenstrual symptoms, and benign breast disease; decreased risk of pelvic inflammatory disease and ectopic pregnancy; decreased risk of ovarian and endometrial cancer
    - Some women experience cessation of menses (not dangerous)
    - **Relative contraindications**
      - **History of thromboembolic disease or stroke**
      - **Active liver disease**
      - **History of breast or endometrial cancer**
      - **Smokers older than 35 years of age**
  - Newer progesterone options (in combination tablets)
    - Third-generation oral contraceptives contain newer progestins (i.e., norgestimate)
      - Fewer side effects and may improve acne
      - May also have a slightly higher thrombosis risk
    - Drosperidone
      - Has both antiandrogenic and antimineralocorticoid properties
      - Useful in polycystic ovary syndrome; reduces hirsutism and other clinical symptoms
      - Watch for hyperkalemia
    - Other dosing and administration options
      - May dose oral contraceptive to bring on withdrawal bleed every 3 months rather than monthly
        - Convenience for patient
        - Decrease in premenstrual migraines, premenstrual dysphoric disorder
      - Contraceptive patch
        - Apply patch once weekly for 3 weeks, then remove for 1 week
        - Some patients find it more convenient
        - Minor side effect of local irritation in a few
        - Contraindicated in women with weight greater than 200 pounds due to unpredictable absorption
      - Contraceptive ring
        - Inserted by patient for 3 weeks, then removed for 1 week
        - No need to remove during intercourse, but may remove for up to 3 hours if desired
        - Caution patients to watch for spontaneous expulsion
  - "Mini-pill"
    - Contains small doses of progestin only
    - Has 28 tablets of active hormone; no inert tablets
    - Less efficacious and more breakthrough bleeding than with combination pills
    - **Useful for women who cannot tolerate estrogen, lactating women, and older women with cardiovascular risk factors**
  - Injected progesterone (e.g., depot Provera)
    - Usually administered once every 3 months
    - Higher efficacy than combination oral contraceptive pills, possibly because of better compliance
    - Long-term use has been associated with reversible losses in bone mineral density
- Intrauterine device (IUD; Fig. 65-4)
  - Contraceptive device inserted into the lining of the uterus by a gynecologist
  - Interferes with fertilization and implantation
  - Underused option in the United States that confers excellent efficacy and convenience; consider particularly in perimenopausal women who desire convenient, nonsystemic contraception
  - Options
    - Copper-clad T-shaped IUD: Has an effective duration of 10 years
    - Levonorgestrel-releasing IUD: Inserted every 5 years; high rates of amenorrhea; no loss of bone mineral density
  - Whereas one third of failures with female sterilization result in an ectopic pregnancy, there is no increased risk of ectopia with the IUD
  - Disadvantages: Increased risk of infection leading to salpingitis (and possible infertility), uterine perforation
  - **Contraindications**
    - **Multiple partners**
    - **History of STDs**
    - **Need for anticoagulation**

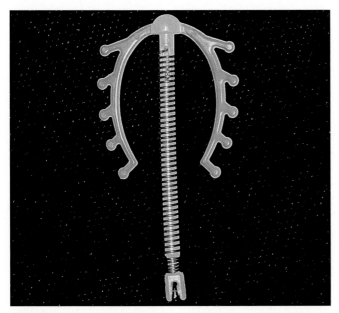

FIGURE 65-4 Copper 375 multiload intrauterine device. (From Oats J, Abraham S: *Llewellyn-Jones fundamentals of obstetrics and gynaecology,* ed 8, Philadelphia, Mosby, 2004, figure 38.9.)

- Sterilization
  - Tubal ligation or vasectomy are standard procedures
  - Most effective method of contraception
- **Emergency contraception (the "morning after" pill)**
  - Use of a contraceptive after unprotected intercourse to prevent pregnancy
  - Probably works by inhibiting ovulation and is 75% to 80% effective

- Is not considered to be an abortifacient
- Most common form is 0.75 mg of levonorgestrel given within 72 hours of intercourse and repeated once 12 hours later
  - Alternatively, a single dose of 1.5 mg of levonorgestrel is probably equally effective with fewer side effects
- Patient should expect usual menses within 21 days of treatment
- Main side effect is nausea and vomiting; consider simultaneous prescription of an antiemetic to take 1 hour before
- Contraindications: Pregnancy or undiagnosed pathologic genital bleeding

Medical Issues Related to Pregnancy

HYPERTENSIVE SYNDROMES IN PREGNANCY
- Can assume several different forms (Table 65-3)
- **Chronic hypertension**
  - **Definition: Blood pressure greater than 140/90 mm Hg observed before pregnancy or within the first 20 weeks**
  - Associated with an increased risk of intrauterine growth retardation, cesarean delivery, abruptio placentae, prematurity, and even fetal death
  - Unfortunately, therapy with antihypertensive drugs has not been proven to improve outcomes
  - In general, therapy should be started or altered when the maternal blood pressure is high enough that there

TABLE 65-3	*Hypertensive Complications of Pregnancy*	
Disorder	**Clinical Manifestations**	**Treatment**
Chronic hypertension	Usually asymptomatic If severe, may have headache, blurred vision, hematuria, pulmonary edema	Methyldopa is drug of choice Second-line choices: clonidine, calcium channel blockers
Preeclampsia	Classic triad Hypertension Proteinuria Edema "Severe" preeclampsia also may have Headache Visual disturbances Pulmonary edema Oliguria May also see elevated liver enzymes later in course	Delivery of fetus, if possible, is definitive therapy Antepartum Bed rest and observation Frequent fetal ultrasonography and surveillance Antihypertensives of unproven benefit Intrapartum Hydration with careful fluid monitoring Seizure prevention: Intravenous magnesium sulfate Hypertension: Intravenous hydralazine, labetalol, or nitroglycerin; sublingual nifedipine Postpartum Need to continue magnesium for 24–48 hr
Eclampsia	New-onset seizures or coma in preeclamptic patient	Similar to preeclampsia
HELLP syndrome	Hemolysis Elevated liver enzymes (AST and ALT up to 4000 U/L) Low platelets (as low as 6000/mm³) Other symptoms Epigastric pain Nausea, vomiting Headache Edema	Delivery is definitive Lab values (AST, ALT, platelets) normalize within 5 days postpartum

ALT, alanine aminotransferase; AST, aspartate aminotransferase; HELLP, hemolysis, elevated liver enzymes, low platelets.

65

is perceived risk in not treating it for the remaining duration of the pregnancy
- Some use a blood pressure of 160/100 mm Hg as a threshold for this purpose
- **Methyldopa is the most frequently used during pregnancy and is the drug of choice**
- Other options (in order of preference) are the following
  - Clonidine
  - Calcium channel blockers
  - Combined α-, β-blockers
  - Hydralazine
  - β-Blockers (associated with fetal growth restriction and inadequate neonatal response to hypoglycemia)
  - Diuretics (associated with fetal growth restriction and fetal distress if started or increased during pregnancy because the lack of uterine or placental autoregulation puts perfusion of the fetus at the mercy of maternal blood volume)
- **Angiotensin-converting enzyme (ACE) inhibitors and angiotensin receptor blockers are absolutely contraindicated in pregnancy**
- Once therapy is started, care should be taken to avoid large drops in maternal blood pressure because uterine, placental, and fetal perfusion will fall in proportion
- **A reasonable goal is to keep maternal blood pressures in the 140–160/90–100 mm Hg range**
- Preeclampsia and eclampsia
  - **Preeclampsia is defined as triad of hypertension occurring for the first time after 20 weeks' gestation with proteinuria (>300 mg/24 hour) and edema**
    - "Severe" preeclampsia: Blood pressure greater than 160/110 mm Hg, more than 5 g protein/24 hours, oliguria, retinal hemorrhages or papilledema, headache or visual disturbances, or pulmonary edema
  - Preeclampsia occurs in up to 7% of all pregnancies
    - More common in women during first pregnancy, with advanced maternal age, with twin gestation, with a prior history of preeclampsia, or with chronic hypertension or diabetes
  - **Eclampsia is diagnosed when a patient with preeclampsia develops seizures (not attributable to another cause)**
  - Preeclampsia and eclampsia may be related to maternal and fetal morbidity
    - Maternal: Intracranial hemorrhage, abruptio placentae with hemorrhage, renal cortical necrosis
    - Fetal: Intrauterine growth retardation, increased mortality
  - Management: Only "cure" is delivery of the fetus
- **Hemolysis, elevated liver enzymes, and low platelets (HELLP) syndrome**
  - **Variant of preeclampsia (10–15%), in which patients may also develop microangiopathic anemia, thrombocytopenia, or hepatocellular necrosis**
  - Can also develop in pregnant women without preeclampsia
  - May occur antepartum (two thirds of patients) and postpartum (one third of patients)
  - May be difficult to differentiate from hemolytic uremic syndrome and thrombotic thrombocytopenic purpura
  - Unlikely to recur in subsequent pregnancies
  - Clinical manifestations and management (see Table 65-3)

DIABETES MELLITUS IN PREGNANCY
- Most common medical complication of pregnancy, affecting approximately 5% of pregnancies
  - Half of these patients are pregestational diabetics
  - **Half develop diabetes during pregnancy because of the diabetogenic effects of the hormonal changes of pregnancy (gestational diabetes)**
    - **These women are at significant risk (about 50%) of developing overt diabetes later in life**
    - **Should have annual screening for diabetes indefinitely**
- Diabetes in pregnancy is associated with increased risks of the following:
  - Fetal death
  - Extremes of fetal growth (both macrosomia and growth restriction)
  - Neonatal problems including respiratory distress syndrome, hypercalcemia, hyperbilirubinemia, and polycythemia
  - Fetal anomalies: Primarily cardiac and skeletal
- If blood glucose values are kept normal, all of the risks associated with diabetes in pregnancy are no greater than those in the general population
- Screening for diabetes during pregnancy is with the 50-g glucose challenge test (GCT)
  - A positive screen is a serum glucose of 140 mg/dL or greater 1 hour after the oral ingestion of 50 g of hyperosmolar glucose irrespective of prior oral intake
  - If the screen is greater than 200 mg/dL, patient should be considered diabetic
  - If the screen is 140 to 200 mg/dL, a 3-hour glucose tolerance test (GTT) should be performed (more sensitive and specific)
- Management of diabetes in pregnancy involves maintaining glucose values approaching euglycemia
  - Insulin is usually started for fasting glucose values consistently above 100 mg/dL or values 2 hours postprandial consistently over 120 mg/dL
  - **Goals of glycemic control are a fasting value 60 to 80 mg/dL and a 2-hour postprandial value less than 120 mg/dL (1-hour value < 140 mg/dL)**

ASTHMA IN PREGNANCY
- Course in pregnancy is unpredictable: Some patients worsen, others improve
- Asthma exacerbations in pregnancy can result in maternal, and thus fetal, hypoxemia, leading to fetal death, prematurity, or low birth weight
- Benefit of continuing pharmacologic therapy for asthma far outweighs the risk
  - **All drugs in current general use for asthma are without major problems for the fetus**
  - This includes prednisone, which does not cross the placenta

THYROID DISEASE IN PREGNANCY

- Increased incidence of thyroid disease during pregnancy (see Chapter 39)
- Thyroid medications are generally safe in pregnancy
- Hypothyroid patients
  - Natural and synthetic thyroid hormones (thyroxine, triiodothyronine) do not cross the placenta and can be used during pregnancy
  - **Thyroid replacement requirements increase early in the first trimester—monitor aggressively to improve fetal outcomes**
  - **Goal is to maintain thyroid-stimulating hormone level between 1 and 2**
- Hyperthyroid patients
  - Antithyroid medications (propylthiouracil and methimazole) do cross the placenta; propylthiouracil is generally preferred
  - If too much antithyroid medication is given, the fetus may have developmental delay (including cretinism)
  - **Therefore, antithyroid therapy is directed at keeping the maternal serum free thyroxine at the upper limits of normal**

MEDICATIONS IN PREGNANCY

- No medication is proven to be absolutely safe; therefore, pregnant women should limit medication usage to true needs and minimize usage as much as possible
- **Classification of drugs regarding safety in pregnancy is as follows**
  - Category A: Controlled studies in women fail to demonstrate risk to fetus in first trimester; unlikely to cause fetal harm
  - Category B: Studies of animal reproduction have not demonstrated risk to fetus, but no controlled studies in pregnant women; or animal studies have shown effect, but no controlled studies in pregnant women
  - Category C: Animal studies have revealed adverse effects in fetus; no controlled studies in women; should be given only if potential benefit justifies risk
  - Category D: Evidence for fetal risk, but benefits may be acceptable in pregnant women despite risk
  - Category X: Studies in humans and animals demonstrate significant fetal risk; contraindicated in pregnancy
- Reasonable treatment for common symptoms in pregnancy (Table 65-4)
- Drugs contraindicated in pregnancy (Box 65-1)
- Vaccines
  - **"Dead" vaccines (using killed virus or bacterial or viral fragments) are considered safe**
    - Examples: Hepatitis A vaccine, hepatitis B vaccine, influenza (injected), polio (injected), pneumococcal, and meningococcal vaccines are considered safe
    - In appropriate cases, these are even indicated during pregnancy (e.g., influenza vaccine if patient will be in second or third trimester during influenza season)
  - **Only one attenuated live virus vaccine, the oral polio vaccine, is considered safe in pregnancy**
  - Although no reported problems are associated with measles, mumps, and rubella vaccines (MMR) during pregnancy, it is preferred to withhold until postpartum when they are considered safe

TABLE 65-4	Safe Drug Therapy for Common Pregnancy Symptoms
Symptom	**Drug**
Acne	Topical clindamycin, erythromycin, or benzoyl peroxide
Allergic rhinitis	Topical glucocorticoids and cromolyn Antihistamines, including loratadine, chlorpheniramine, and diphenhydramine Decongestants (pseudoephedrine)
Cough	Guaifenesin and dextromethorphan
Constipation	Docusate sodium, lactulose, and mineral oil
Gastrointestinal reflux	Calcium carbonate and ranitidine
Bronchitis	Amoxicillin and azithromycin
Urinary tract infection	Nitrofurantoin
Headache, generalized aches and pains	Acetaminophen
Thrombophlebitis	Heparin

BOX 65-1	Medications Contraindicated in Pregnancy

Antihypertensives

ACE inhibitors (birth defects in first trimester, decreased fetal renal perfusion and death if used in second or third trimester)

Angiotensin receptor blockers (same as ACE inhibitors)

Loop diuretics (fetal growth restriction and distress)

Diabetic Agents

Sulfonylureas

Thiazolidinediones

Antimicrobials

Tetracyclines (brittle bones and cartilage and yellow teeth)

Fluoroquinolones (arthropathies)

Anticonvulsants

Phenytoin

Carbamazepine

Other

Warfarin (fetal anomalies and fetal death)

ACE, angiotensin-converting enzyme.

65

- The varicella-zoster and smallpox vaccines are contraindicated during pregnancy

Menopause

- Each year, more than 31 million women experience menopause
- **Definition of menopause: The "last" menses; alternatively, the permanent cessation of menses following loss of ovarian activity**
  - Is a clinical diagnosis: **12 months of amenorrhea**

- Perimenopause is the entire time period from menstrual irregularity to the year after the menopause itself; usually lasts 2 to 8 years
- Average age of menopause is 51 years, with a range of 45 to 55 years; occurs earlier in smokers and nulliparous women
- An elevated follicle-stimulating hormone (FSH) level can provide supporting evidence, but is not useful for routine diagnosis (FSH fluctuates greatly during the perimenopause)
- **FSH may be useful in certain situations: Women with premature menopause, uncharacteristic clinical presentations, or hysterectomized women without classic symptoms**
- Loss of estrogen at the menopause greatly affects women and affects quality of life
  - Vasomotor symptoms (hot flashes) highly prevalent (≤75% of women in the United States); more frequent at night
  - Insomnia, fatigue
  - Genitourinary: Vaginal dryness, incontinence, recurrent urinary tract infections
  - Loss of bone mineral density (3–5% per year during the first 5 years after menopause)
  - Cardiac: Decrease in high-density lipoprotein, increase in low-density lipoprotein
  - Neurologic and psychological: Depressed mood, irritability, decreased libido
- Treatment of hot flashes
  - Layered, cotton clothing
  - Avoidance of known triggers (caffeine, alcohol, warm humid environments, spicy food)
  - Estrogen is by far the most effective therapy (reduces frequency and severity by >90%)
  - Available selective estrogen receptor modulators (SERMs) are not effective for hot flashes
  - Topical estrogen (delivered intravaginally) relieves vaginal mucosal atrophy and subsequent dryness; only one formulation (the estradiol ring) reaches high enough systemic levels to relieve hot flashes and preserve bone density
- **Indications for estrogen therapy (ET) or hormone therapy (HT): Moderate to severe vasomotor symptoms**
  - Other benefits: Preservation of bone mineral density, improvements in lipid profile (increased HDL, decreased LDL), possible reduced risk of colorectal cancer (but other disease-specific treatments, such as bisphosphonates for osteoporosis, are considered to be first line)
  - Risks: Results from the Women's Health Initiative demonstrated that hormone therapy increased the risk of breast cancer, stroke, and venous thromboembolic disease, and had no benefit in preventing heart disease
    - Caveat: WHI did not study a perimenopausal population
    - Methodologic limitations and high discontinuation rate limit generalizability of findings
  - **If HT started, lowest dose for shortest duration (preferably <5 years) generally recommended; reassessment for continued need should be done at least yearly**

TABLE 65-5	Alternatives to Estrogen for Vasomotor Symptoms	
Class	**Typical Agents**	**Side Effects**
SSRIs	Paroxetine Venlafaxine Fluoxetine	GI symptoms Decreased libido
α-Adrenergic agents	Clonidine Methyldopa	Fatigue, dizziness Dry mouth Constipation
Gabapentin		Drowsiness, lethargy
Progestins	Medroxyprogesterone acetate (oral, depot, or transdermal)	Breast tenderness Irritability, depression Headaches ? Long-term safety

SSRIs, selective serotonin reuptake inhibitors.

- Many forms available (oral, transdermal); none definitively shown to be superior
- **If uterus present, must administer progestin with estrogen to avoid increased risk of endometrial cancer**
  - Cycled use if patient desires monthly withdrawal bleeding
  - Continuous use if withdrawal bleeding undesirable (more commonly used in postmenopausal women)
- Vaginal spotting and bleeding may be a nuisance side effect
  - Usually resolves within 6 months
  - **If heavy or if first bleeding occurs 6 months after initiating therapy, endometrial biopsy should be performed to rule out hyperplasia or cancer**
- Other therapies for vasomotor symptoms
  - Certain selective serotonin reuptake inhibitors, gabapentin, clonidine, and methyldopa have shown efficacy (Table 65-5)
  - In general, these medications reduce frequency and severity of hot flashes by 50% (not as efficacious as estrogen)
  - Herbal therapies (soy products, black cohosh) are of questionable efficacy

SUGGESTED READINGS

Abalos E, Duley L, Steyn DW, et al: Antihypertensive drug therapy for mild to moderate hypertension during pregnancy (Cochrane Review). In *The Cochrane Library*, vol 2, Oxford, 2001, Update Software.

American College of Obstetricians and Gynecologists: gestational diabetes. ACOG *Practice Bulletin* 30, Washington, DC, ACOG, 2001.

Dekker G, Sibai B: Primary, secondary, and tertiary prevention of pre-eclampsia, *Lancet* 357:209–215, 2001.

Grimes DA, Raymond EG: Emergency contraception, *Ann Intern Med* 137:180–189, 2002.

Herndon EJ, Zieman M: New contraceptive options, *Am Fam Physician* 69:853–860, 2004.

Lonky NM, Navarre GL, Saunders S, et al: Low-grade Papanicolaou smears and the Bethesda system: a prospective cytohistopathologic analysis, *Obstet Gynecol* 85(Pt 1):716–720, 1995.

Treatment of menopause-associated vasomotor symptoms: position statement of the North American Menopause Society, *Menopause* 11:11–33, 2004.

Wright TC, Cox JT, Massad LS, et al: 2001 Consensus guidelines for the management of women with cervical cytological abnormalities, *JAMA* 287:2120–2129, 2002.

Dermatology for the Internist

MARY SHEU, MD, REBECCA A. KAZIN, MD, and THOMAS B. HABIF, MD

Internal medicine physicians often encounter patients complaining of skin eruptions. Even though some cutaneous diseases may require specialty referral, it is imperative for internists to be able to recognize common dermatologic conditions, serious conditions that may require urgent referral, and cutaneous manifestations that may signify other disease processes.

Common Dermatologic Conditions

ACNE VULGARIS

See Figure 66-1 for an example of acne vulgaris.

Basic Information

- Defined as a chronic inflammation of pilosebaceous units of the face and trunk
- Affects nearly all adolescents with varying severity
- The primary lesion in acne is the microcomedo, which is an accumulation of keratin and sebum within the follicle
- With androgenic stimulation during puberty, sebum production increases, providing the opportunity for *Propionibacterium acnes* to colonize and proliferate within the follicle, resulting in an inflammatory reaction
- Most patients with acne vulgaris do not overproduce androgens; however, they probably have a genetic hyper-responsiveness to androgens
- Acne formation can also be influenced by external factors
  - Oil-based cosmetics
  - Medications (e.g., steroids, phenytoin, lithium)

- Endocrine disorders (e.g., Cushing's disease, polycystic ovary syndrome)
- Chloracne: Severe acne occurring after exposure to halogenated hydrocarbons (e.g., herbicides, Agent Orange)

Clinical Presentation and Diagnosis

- Closed comedone ("whitehead"): Further accumulation of sebum within a microcomedo
- Open comedone ("blackhead"): Opening of the follicular orifice; follicle is packed with melanin and keratin, exposure to air results in oxidative darkening of sebum
- Inflammatory lesions: Rupture of follicular contents resulting in formation of cysts, papules
- Cutaneous nodules and scarring
- Emotional scarring (often permanent) is quite common; treatment has been shown to improve self-esteem

Treatment

- Comedonal acne
  - Topical retinoids (e.g., tretinoin, adapalene, tazerotene)
  - Salicylic acid
- Mild to moderate inflammatory acne
  - Topical retinoids (e.g., tretinoin, adapaline, tazarotene)
  - Topical benzoyl peroxide, clindamycin, or erythromycin
  - Oral antibiotics (doxycycline, minocycline usually; may also try erythromycin and trimethoprim/sulfamethoxazole)
  - In-office therapies (acne surgery—extraction of comedones; chemical peels with salicylic acid; photodynamic therapy—topical levulan followed by exposure to light source)
- Severe or resistant inflammatory acne
  - Oral antibiotics plus topical retinoids (anti-inflammatory property of antibiotics thought to play major role in action against acne)
  - Hormonal therapy (females only)
  - Isotretinoin
    - Synthetic vitamin A derivative
    - Common side effects include dry skin and hyperlipidemia
    - Rare side effects include pseudotumor cerebri, myalgias, alopecia
    - **Teratogenicity is a concern; therefore women of child-bearing age must be on two reliable means of birth control that should be continued for at least one menstrual period after the drug has been stopped; patients must be registered in the iPledge Program registry (www.ipledgeprogram.com).**

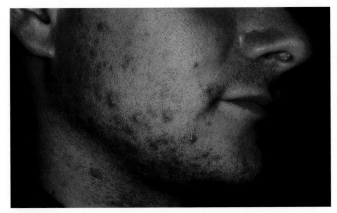

FIGURE 66-1 Acne vulgaris. (From Bolognia JL, Jorizzo JL, Rapini RP: *Dermatology*, St. Louis, Mosby, 2003, p 533.)

- In women with treatment-resistant acne, consider an endocrinopathy (e.g., polycystic ovary disease, Cushing's disease)

ACNE ROSACEA

See Figure 66-2 for an example of acne rosacea.

Basic Information

- Chronic inflammatory disorder of the face
- Lesions typically last days to weeks and recur
- Seen predominantly in middle-aged and older adults

Clinical Presentation

- Four subtypes; patients may have one or more than one manifestation: (1) erythrotelangiectatic, (2) papulopustular, (3) rhinophyma, (4) occular
- Earliest lesions include facial erythema and telangiectasias
- Vascular reactivity (flushing) can be triggered by food (caffeine, alcohol, spicy food, hot beverages), environmental exposure (heat and sun), or emotion (stress)
- Papules, pustules, cysts, and nodules can develop similarly to acne vulgaris but comedones are not present
- **Eye involvement can cause blepharitis, conjunctivitis, iritis, and keratitis**
- Hyperplasia of the soft tissues and sebaceous glands of the nose (rhinophyma) can be seen in severe cases (usually in men)

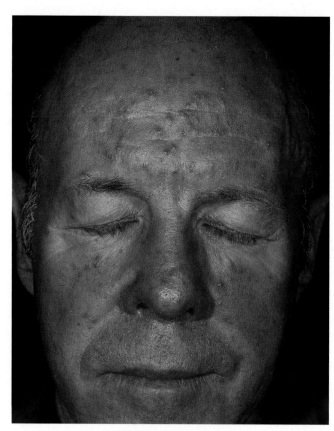

FIGURE 66-2   Rosacea.

TABLE 66-1	*Differential Diagnosis of Acne Rosacea*
Disease	**Clinical Differences**
Acne vulgaris	Comedones present Flushing not present Younger age group
Carcinoid syndrome	Rare Flushing is fleeting (lasts only seconds)
Systemic lupus erythematosus	Malar rash that spares the nasolabial folds No papules or pustules Systemic symptoms present
Seborrheic dermatitis	No papules or pustules Background erythema and telangiectasias are usually absent Can occur concurrently with rosacea

- Can easily be confused with a number of other conditions (Table 66-1)

Treatment

- Topical antibiotics (metronidazole), sulfacetamide/sulphur, azelaic acid, or benzoyl peroxide can be tried initially
- Oral antibiotics (e.g., tetracycline, doxycycline, erythromycin, or minocycline; mechanism of action also thought to be anti-inflammatory as in acne vulgaris treatment) or topical tretinoin (or both) can be used in cases that do not respond to the preceding treatments (Note: Topical retinoids have been reported to worsen telangiectasia in some patients)

ECZEMA

- Defined simply as an inflammation of the epidermis of the skin
- Can be caused by a number of different conditions (Table 66-2; Figs. 66-3 to 66-6)
- Broadly classified into three categories that define the approach to therapy
  - Acute eczema
    - Presentation: Edema, papules, vesicles, bullae, crusting, serous discharge, and scaling can be present
    - Initial treatment: Saline compresses or warm water bath, followed by medium-strength topical glucocorticoids (e.g., triamcinolone 0.1%) and emollients; use only low-potency steroids (e.g., desonide) for facial lesions; topical tacrolimus or pimecrolimus for maintenance
  - Subacute eczema
    - Presentation: Erythematous, scaling, and pruritic lesions, but no vesicles, bullae, or serous discharge
    - Initial treatment: High-potency corticosteroids (e.g., fluocinonide) and emollients; topical tacrolimus or pimecrolimus for maintenance
  - Chronic eczema
    - Presentation: Scaly thickening of the skin (lichenification); hypo- or hyperpigmentation can occur

TABLE 66-2	*Features of Eczematous Eruptions*	
Disease	**Description**	**Treatment**
Atopic dermatitis (see Fig. 66-3)	Patients usually have a history of allergic rhinitis, asthma, or family history of atopy Lesions often involve flexures of neck, wrist, legs, and arms; hands and face can be involved Secondary staphylococcal infections are common	Topical corticosteroids (medium to high potency) plus emollients Oral antibiotics if there is superinfection Topical nonsteroidal anti-inflammatory agents (e.g., pimecrolimus, tacrolimus)
Allergic contact dermatitis (see Fig. 66-4)	Caused by a delayed hypersensitivity reaction Most commonly caused by plant exposure (e.g., poison ivy, oak, sumac) Can also be caused by jewelry, cosmetics, and occupational exposures Diagnose by history or patch testing (or both)	Removal or avoidance of irritant Topical corticosteroids plus emollients Oral corticosteroids may sometimes be necessary
Irritant contact dermatitis	Caused by harsh cleansers and acids	Same as above
Dyshidrotic eczema (see Fig. 66-5)	Affects fingers, toes, palms, and soles Small, 1-mm vesicles, scaling, fissures Can be quite pruritic	Can be difficult to treat High-potency corticosteroids plus emollients
Seborrheic dermatitis	Epidermal inflammation in areas populated with sebaceous glands (e.g., scalp, face, ears, and chest) Scaling macules and plaques; can develop crusts or fissures *Pityrosporum* yeast may stimulate inflammation Increased incidence in patients with HIV and Parkinson's disease	Scalp: Ketoconazole, selenium sulfide, or tar shampoos plus corticosteroid topical solution Face: Low-potency corticosteroids and ketoconazole cream
Stasis dermatitis	Erythematous scaling plaques seen in the lower legs in persons with chronic venous insufficiency Can form ulcers Brown hemosiderin hyperpigmentation may also be present	Dermatitis: Wet dressings, topical corticosteroids, antibiotics (if needed) Ulcer: Wet dressings, leg elevation, compression bandages
Nummular eczema (see Fig. 66-6)	Sharply circumscribed, 1- to 5-cm diameter plaques on the extremities Can resemble tinea corporis but potassium hydroxide prep is negative Secondary staphylococcal infections are common	Topical corticosteroids and emollients Oral antibiotics if there is superinfection Skin should be kept lubricated after treatment to avoid recurrence
Asteotic eczema	Seen in winter in older adults Dry ambient air may predispose to disease Dry, cracked, fissured skin with or without pruritus most commonly seen on the lower legs	Humidify ambient air Tepid baths using oils or oil-based soaps Medium-potency corticosteroid ointment (not cream) plus emollients

66

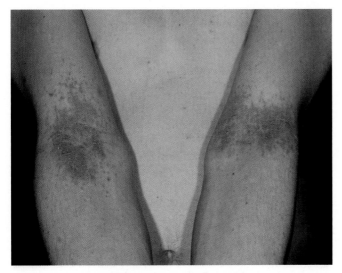

FIGURE 66-3 Atopic dermatitis.

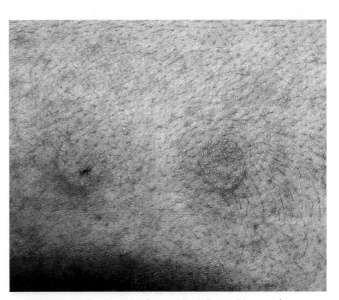

FIGURE 66-4 Contact dermatitis: A 2+ positive patch test.

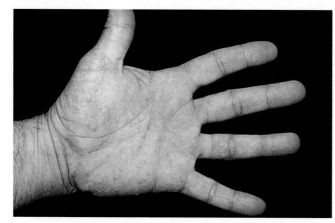

FIGURE 66-5 Dyshidrotic eczema.

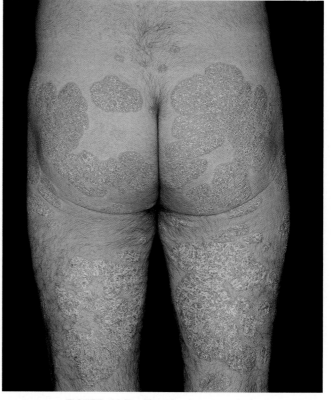

FIGURE 66-7 Chronic plaque psoriasis.

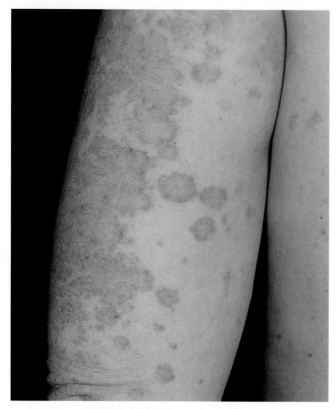

FIGURE 66-6 Nummular eczema.

- Treatment: High-potency topical steroids and emollients; topical tacrolimus or pimecrolimus for maintenance
- Subclassification of eczemas can be useful for guiding specific therapy in many instances (see Table 66-2)

PSORIASIS

Basic Information

- A T cell–mediated immune disorder in which CD4$^+$ and CD8$^+$ memory T cells stimulate the hyperproliferation of keratinocytes, causing chronic scaling papules or plaques
- **Average age of onset is in the third decade of life**
- Disease is characterized by periods of exacerbations and remissions

- Disease can be exacerbated by infections, drugs (e.g., lithium, antimalarials, β-blockers, corticosteroid withdrawal), alcohol, or stress

Clinical Presentation

- Skin disease
  - Chronic plaque psoriasis (Fig. 66-7): Sharply marginated, erythematous plaques with silvery-white scale, commonly seen on scalp and extensor surfaces of the knees and elbows
  - Guttate psoriasis (Fig. 66-8)
    - Presents as an acute exanthem over the trunk and proximal extremities
    - Lesions are small (<1 cm) and scaly
    - **Often follows streptococcal pharyngitis or viral infection**
    - May be self-limited, but in some cases may also herald the beginning of chronic psoriasis
  - Erythrodermic and pustular psoriasis are rare; more severe types that can be triggered by tapering of systemic corticosteroids
- Nail findings are seen in 30% of patients with psoriasis
  - Nail pitting, onycholysis (separation of nail from nail bed), and subungual hyperkeratosis can occur
- Arthritis can be seen in up to one third of patients and is more common in patients with psoriatic nail disease (see Chapter 43)

Treatment

- Limited chronic plaque psoriasis: Bland emollients with keratolytics, topical corticosteroids, calcipotriene

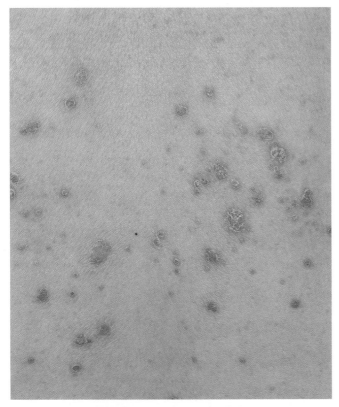

FIGURE 66-8 Guttate psoriasis.

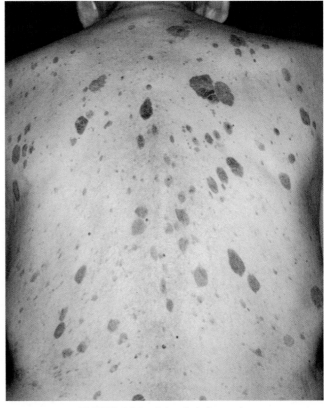

FIGURE 66-9 Seborrheic keratosis.

(topical vitamin D derivative), or tazarotene (topical vitamin A derivative)
- Generalized plaque psoriasis: Methotrexate, cyclosporine, acitretin, phototherapy (ultraviolet B radiation), photochemotherapy (psoralen plus ultraviolet A radiation, PUVA), biologics (e.g., alefacept, etanercept, infliximab, efalizumab)
- Guttate psoriasis: Phototherapy plus emollients and midpotency topical corticosteroids
- Erythrodermic and pustular psoriasis: Methotrexate, cyclosporine, or acitretin (synthetic retinoid); hospitalization may be necessary
- **Systemic corticosteroids should be avoided** because tapering predisposes to erythrodermic or pustular psoriasis

SEBORRHEIC KERATOSIS

Figure 66-9 illustrates seborrheic keratosis.
- Very common benign epidermal growth
- Usually occurs after the age of 30 years
- Starts as small papules or plaques with or without pigment
- Grows into fairly large (up to 6 cm) plaques with warty, "stuck on" appearance; variation in pigmentation (e.g., brown, black, gray) can be seen within individual lesions, may contain horn pseudocysts
- Commonly on the face, trunk, and upper extremities (light-exposed areas)
- Lesions may become irritated and resemble melanoma
- Therapy is not necessary
- Lesions can be destroyed with liquid nitrogen or electrocautery

PITYRIASIS ROSEA

See Figure 66-10 for an example of pityriasis rosea.
- **Self-limited, exanthematous eruption thought to be related to a viral illness**
- Predominantly seen in children and young adults
- Begins with a 2- to 5-cm oval, reddish pink lesion with a fine scale often found on the back or chest (herald patch)
- Similar smaller lesions then develop along the lines of cleavage of the skin (Christmas tree pattern on the back)
- Usually asymptomatic, but occasionally may be pruritic
- Differential diagnosis includes secondary syphilis, drug eruptions, guttate psoriasis, tinea corporis, HIV seroconversion illness

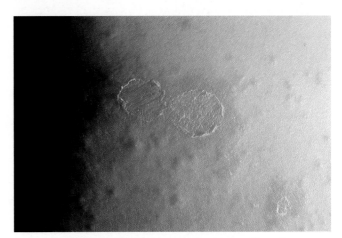

FIGURE 66-10 Pityriasis rosea with herald patch.

66

- Usually resolves without treatment in 2 to 3 months; if course is prolonged or pruritus is significant, treatment may include topical steroids or ultraviolet B phototherapy

ERYTHEMA NODOSUM

See Figure 66-11 for an example of erythema nodosum (EN).

Basic Information

- Proposed to be a delayed hypersensitivity reaction to antigens resulting from drugs, infections, or other inflammatory conditions
- More common in women
- Most commonly associated with streptococcal pharyngitis, but a number of other causes have been discovered
  - Sarcoidosis
    - **Lofgren's syndrome: Hilar lymphadenopathy, EN, and acute polyarthritis**
  - Tuberculosis, histoplasmosis, coccidioidomycosis
  - Hodgkin's lymphoma
  - *Chlamydia* infection
  - Inflammatory bowel disease
  - Behçet's disease
  - Medications (e.g., omeprazole, sulfonamides, oral contraceptives, hepatitis B vaccine)

Clinical Presentation

- Erythematous nodules that can develop into bruiselike lesions that can be tender and painful

- **Commonly seen on the lower extremities**
- Palpation of the subcutaneous tissue is often more sensitive than inspection of the rash
- Fever and arthralgias can accompany the eruption even in idiopathic cases

Diagnosis

- Usually made by clinical examination
- When the diagnosis is unclear, deep incisional biopsy (rather than punch biopsy) will show septal panniculitis with no evidence of vasculitis
- CBC, antistreptolysin O (ASO) titer, urinalysis, throat culture, intradermal tuberculin test, and chest radiograph should be obtained as part of the initial evaluation of a patient with EN

Treatment

- Rash is usually self-limited and improves with treatment of the underlying disease (if known)
- NSAIDs, potassium iodide, or systemic corticosteroids may alleviate discomfort

Bacterial Infections of the Skin

See Chapter 15.

Viral Infections of the Skin

HERPES SIMPLEX VIRUS TYPE 1

Figure 66-12 illustrates herpes simplex virus type 1 (HSV-1).
- Transmitted from person to person through oral secretions
- More than 90% of the world's population age 20 to 40 years is seropositive for HSV-1
- **Characterized by the sudden appearance of multiple grouped vesicles with an erythematous base**
- Infection can occur anywhere in the body but is often asymptomatic
  - Oral cavity
    - Primary infection: Exudative pharyngitis is commonly the primary infection and can be

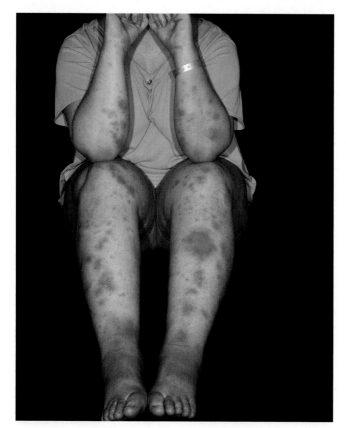

FIGURE 66-11 Erythema nodosum.

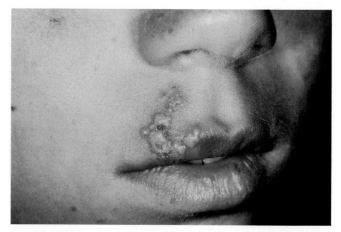

FIGURE 66-12 Herpes simplex virus type 1. (From Bolognia JL, Jorizzo JL, Rapini RP: *Dermatology*, St. Louis, Mosby, 2003, p 1237.)

associated with fevers, lymphadenopathy, and myalgias
  - Recurrent infections present as vesicles on the lips or in the oral cavity; associated systemic symptoms are usually absent
  - Skin: Any site on the skin, including the fingers (herpetic whitlow), and hips or buttocks
  - Other sites include the eye (see Chapter 67), lungs, liver, and CNS (see Chapter 15)
- **Diagnosis can be made by Tzanck preparation of vesicular fluid, which typically shows multinucleated giant cells; viral culture, immunofluorescence staining, and detection of HSV DNA by polymerase chain reaction may also be useful**
- Treatment of primary infections with oral (or IV) acyclovir may shorten the duration of illness and decrease viral shedding time
- Generalized treatment of all patients with recurrent herpes labialis with acyclovir has not been proven to be beneficial. However, for patients with a distinct prodrome, early administration of oral acyclovir, famciclovir, valacyclovir, or topical penciclovir may be useful.

HERPES SIMPLEX VIRUS TYPE 2

See Chapter 11 for a discussion of herpes simplex virus type 2.

HERPES ZOSTER

Figure 66-13 shows an example of herpes zoster.

Basic Information

- Primary varicella-zoster virus (VZV) infection occurs after inhalation of respiratory droplets and results in a generalized vesicular rash (chickenpox)
- **Primary infection is usually seen in children but can occur in adults and immunocompromised hosts**
- Following primary infection with VZV, latent infection is established in the dorsal root ganglia

- Reactivation of the infection results in a painful, unilateral vesicular rash limited to a restricted dermatomal distribution (herpes zoster, or "shingles")
- At times, neighboring dermatomes can be involved
- Risk factors include advancing age, immune suppression, and Hodgkin's disease

Clinical Presentation and Diagnosis

- Localized pain and systemic symptoms including fever, malaise, and headache may precede the vesicular rash by several days
- Crusting of the vesicular lesions usually occurs within 10 days, at which time the patient is no longer infectious
- A number of complications can result from infection
  - Postherpetic neuralgia: Persistence of pain more than 30 days after the rash began
  - Herpes zoster ophthalmicus: Can lead to blindness
  - **Ramsay Hunt syndrome (type 2): Ipsilateral facial paralysis caused by involvement of cranial nerve VII, ear pain, vesicles in the auditory canal; can lead to significant hearing loss**
  - Encephalitis/meningitis
  - Motor neuropathy
  - Transverse myelitis: More common in patients with HIV

Treatment

- Acyclovir, valacyclovir, or famciclovir can be used
- Starting therapy within 72 hours of appearance of the rash reduces pain and the incidence of postherpetic neuralgia
- The addition of prednisone may accelerate healing time
- **Postherpetic neuralgia pain can be severe and require treatment with opioids, tricyclic antidepressants, carbamazepine, gabapentin, pregabalin, or topical lidocaine**
- Shingles vaccine now recommended for disease prevention in patients older than 60 years

MOLLUSCUM CONTAGIOSUM

See Figure 66-14 for an example of molluscum contagiosum.

66

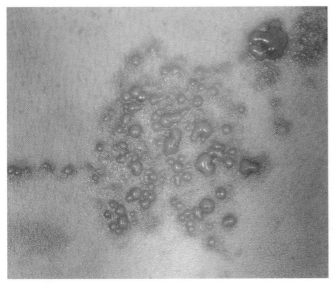

FIGURE 66-13 Herpes zoster.

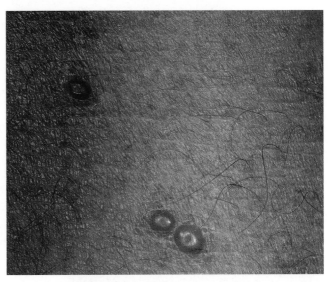

FIGURE 66-14 Molluscum contagiosum.

- A disease caused by a poxvirus spread by direct skin-to-skin contact
- Common in young children and in patients with HIV
- Lesions are usually small (2–5 mm), flesh-colored or white, umbilicated papules that can occur anywhere on the body except the palms and soles
- Diagnosis is made by clinical presentation or by histologic examination of a biopsied lesion
- Lesions are self-limited in immunocompetent hosts; curettage, cryotherapy, or laser therapy can be used, if needed; topical immune modulators (e.g., imiquimod) may also be effective
- In HIV patients, lesions can be long-lasting and extensive; there may be some improvement from treatment with antiretroviral therapy

Fungal Infections of the Skin

DERMATOPHYTOSIS

See Figure 66-15 for an example of dermaphytosis.
- **Caused by a group of fungi that penetrate the stratum corneum of the skin, hair, and nails**
- Symptoms usually consist of pruritus and burning
- Transmission is usually through direct contact
- Microscopic examination of the lesion with the addition of 1 or 2 drops of potassium hydroxide (KOH prep) usually reveals rod-shaped hyphae with branching
- Classification is based on location of the lesions (Table 66-3)

YEAST INFECTIONS

- Tinea versicolor (Fig. 66-16)
  - Recurrent superficial infection caused by *Pityrosporum orbiculare* (*Malassezia furfur*)
  - Most often seen in young adults
  - More commonly presents during warm, humid weather
  - Lesions are round and scaly; they can be hypopigmented, hyperpigmented, or erythematous
  - Occur predominantly on the trunk
  - **Diagnosis is made by KOH prep showing pseudohyphae and spores ("spaghetti and meatballs")**
  - Treatment is with topical antifungals, ketoconazole shampoo, selenium sulfide solution, or oral antifungals (e.g., fluconazole, itraconazole); griseofulvin is not effective
  - Patients experiencing frequent recurrences may benefit from prophylactic treatment with selenium sulfide solution, applied every 3 weeks; or oral ketoconazole, once per month
- Mucocutaneous candidiasis
  - Infection generally involving moist skin sites or mucosal surfaces
  - Most cases caused by *Candida albicans*
  - Predisposing factors include increased moisture at the site of the infection, diabetes, antibiotic therapy, and immunosuppression (e.g., HIV)
  - Infection seen at a number of different sites
    - Oral cavity: Whitish plaques on erythematous base (thrush)
    - Vulvovaginitis: Thick, creamy vaginal discharge with erythema of the vaginal skin and mucous membrane
    - Balanitis: Erosions, scaling, erythema along the penis
    - Diaper candidiasis: Erythema and edema caused by incontinence of urine or stool in the elderly
    - Interdigital candidiasis: Erythema and fissuring between the fingers
    - Intertriginous candidiasis: Erythema, edema, pustule formation beneath the breasts, in the groin, or around the scrotum
    - Paronychial candidiasis: Edema and erythema of the nail folds; creamy discharge may be present

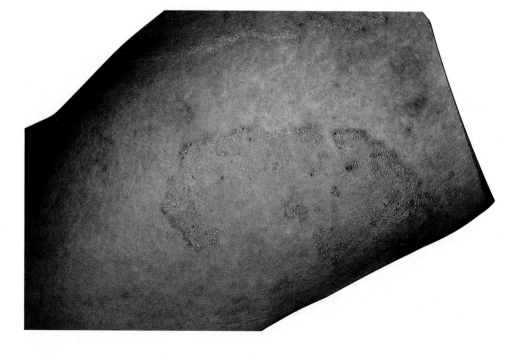

FIGURE 66-15 Dermatophytosis. (From Bolognia JL, Jorizzo JL, Rapini RP: *Dermatology*, St. Louis, Mosby, 2003, figure 2-8.)

TABLE 66-3	Dermatophyte Infections	
Disease	**Description**	**Treatment**
Tinea capitis	Usually occurs in children but can be seen in adults Commonly caused by *Trichophyton tonsurans* Starts as an erythematous, scaly patch on the scalp with broken-off hairs Can cause kerion formation (inflammatory pustular plaques with scarring) and permanent patches of hair loss	Topical antifungals usually not effective Griseofulvin is the treatment of choice Oral itraconazole and terbinafine can also be used Kerion treatment may require the addition of selenium sulfide shampoos and oral antistaphylococcal antibiotics
Tinea corporis ("ringworm")	Annular, scaling, papular lesions with an area of central clearing on the trunk, limbs, or face The presence of multiple lesions may be a sign of underlying immunosuppression	Topical antifungals (e.g., terbinafine) are usually effective Oral griseofulvin can be used in severe cases
Tinea cruris	Predominantly seen in men Associated with physical activity and sweating ("jock itch") Can occur with tinea pedis Semicircular erythematous, scaly lesion that begins on the thigh and can extend to the perineal area and buttocks Typically does not involve the scrotum	Topical antifungals (e.g., terbinafine) are usually effective Oral griseofulvin can be used in severe cases Groin area should be kept clean and dry to avoid recurrences Treat tinea pedis (if present)
Tinea pedis ("athlete's foot")	Lesions can range from having mild erythema and scale to maceration and bullae between the toes and on the soles of the feet Can be a point of entry of bacteria causing cellulitis	Topical antifungals (e.g., terbinafine) are usually effective Oral terbinafine or itraconazole can be used in resistant cases
Tinea unguium (onychomycosis)	Signs include white discoloration, crumbly debris from beneath the nail, and thickening of the nail	Topical therapy is generally ineffective Oral terbinafine or itraconazole for 6–12 wk is the most effective treatment Ciclopirox nail lacquer is effective in <10% of patients

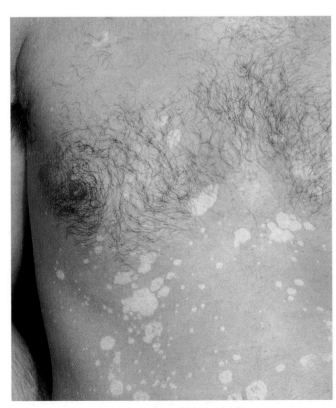

FIGURE 66-16 Tinea versicolor.

- Angular cheilitis: Fissures and erythema of the angles of the mouth
- Chronic mucocutaneous candidiasis
  - **Characterized by recurrent, severe mucocutaneous candidal infections caused by an underlying T-cell defect**
  - Usually presents in childhood
  - Suspect HIV in adult patients presenting with this syndrome
  - Treatment is with topical antifungal agents; long-term therapy may be necessary in patients with chronic disease

Infestations of the Skin

SCABIES

- Caused by infestation with the mite *Sarcoptes scabei*
- Transmission is from person to person by direct contact, although cases of transmission from clothing and bed linens have occurred
- In young adults, transmission commonly occurs during sexual contact
- **Intractable pruritus that is worse at night is the most prominent symptom**
- The primary lesion is usually a small, erythematous papule or vesicle that may be difficult to find
- Threadlike linear ridges that range from 2 to 15 mm in length (burrows) are pathognomonic for the disease

66

- **Vesicles, papules, and burrows are most commonly found on the hands, wrists, penis, nipples, axillae, and gluteal cleft; usually spares the scalp**
- The term *Norwegian scabies* describes an extensive scabies infestation involving the hands and feet, and elsewhere, with asymptomatic thick crusting. There is thick, subungual, keratotic material and nail dystrophy. It occurs in people with neurologic or mental disorders (especially Down syndrome), senile dementia, nutritional disorders, infectious diseases, leukemia, and immunosuppression (e.g., patients with AIDS).
- Diagnosis can be presumed on clinical grounds or be confirmed by microscopic examination of the lesion by scraping and applying 2 drops of mineral oil prior to covering with a coverslip. Identification of the mite, eggs, or feces confirms the diagnosis.
- **Treatment with permethrin cream over the entire body (washed off after 12 hours and repeated 1 week later) is usually effective**
- Family members and close contacts must also be treated
- Clothing and linens should be laundered
- Oral ivermectin may be considered to treat difficult cases and the elderly

PEDICULOSIS (LICE)

See Figure 66-17.
- Infestation with the human louse (*Pediculus humanus*)
- Characterized by the location of the infestation

- Pediculosis capitis (head lice)
  - Can be transmitted by hats and brushes
  - Epidemics can occur in schools
- Pediculosis pubis (pubic lice, crabs)
  - Most commonly occurs in young adults
  - Usually transmitted during sexual contact
- Pediculosis corporis: Seen in patients with poor hygiene with exposure to others with poor hygiene
- Predominant symptom is itching
- Diagnosed by visualization of nits attached to hair shafts or identification of the louse (usually by microscopy)
- **Treatment is with pyrethrin, permethrin, malthion, or lindane shampoos or lotions. Treatment should be followed by combing to remove all visible nits.**
- Ivermectin is also effective and may be used in cases resistant to topical medication

Benign, Premalignant, and Malignant Neoplasms of the Skin

MOLES

- Common moles (melanocytic nevi) are seen in everyone
  - They are small (<6 mm), tan or brown macules or papules
  - Develop in childhood, peak in early adulthood, and decline thereafter

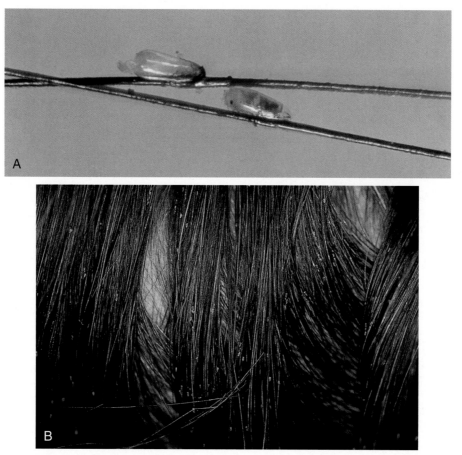

FIGURE 66-17 Pediculosis capitis. (From Bolognia JL, Jorizzo JL, Rapini RP: *Dermatology*, St. Louis, Mosby, 2003, p 1325.)

- Atypical moles (dysplastic nevi; Figure 66-18)
  - Are often larger (>6 mm) than common moles
  - Have irregular borders and variegated color
  - Surface may be complex and variable, with both macular and papular components; a characteristic presentation is a pigmented papule surrounded by a macular collar of pigmentation ("fried-egg lesion")
  - Can continue to appear after age 35 years, in contrast with common moles
  - Associated with an increased risk of melanoma
  - Biopsy often necessary to rule out melanoma
  - Familial atypical mole and melanoma (FAMM) syndrome (dysplastic nevus syndrome)
    - Patients have a large number of melanocytic nevi, often more than 50, some of which are atypical and often variable in size; and a positive family history of melanoma in one or more first- or second-degree relatives
    - Atypical lesions begin during puberty; melanoma often presents before the age of 40 years
    - **Lifetime risk of melanoma approaches 100% for those people with atypical moles from families with two or more first-degree relatives who have cutaneous melanoma**
    - Patients need to perform monthly self-examinations
    - Referral to a dermatologist is often necessary so that appropriate photographs and biopsies can be done at regular intervals (every 3–12 months)
- Evaluation of a mole
  - All pigmented skin lesions should be examined for the following features (ABCDEs):
    - **A**symmetry
    - **B**order irregularity
    - **C**olor variegation—variable degrees of black, brown, tan, or blue
    - **D**iameter greater than 6 mm
    - **E**volution—change in appearance or symptoms
  - Excisional biopsy should be considered for any lesion considered to be melanoma

MELANOMA

See Figure 66-19 for examples of melanoma.

Basic Information

- Sixth most common cancer in the United States, causing over 7000 deaths per year
- Affects whites more than African Americans
- Diagnosis most commonly made in the sixth decade of life
- Incidence in the United States is rising
- Risk factors (Box 66-1)
- Melanoma subtypes
  - Superficial spreading melanoma
    - Most common type
    - Deeply pigmented macules or papules usually greater than 6 mm in diameter; usually displays one of the ABCDE criteria (see under section on Moles)
  - Nodular melanoma
    - Dark black, tan, or brown (rarely amelanotic) dome-shaped papule or nodule
    - Typically do not present with the ABCDEs, making diagnosis difficult
  - Acral lentiginous melanoma
    - **Most common type found in African Americans and Asians**
    - Presents in palms, soles, or nail beds
    - Hutchinson's sign: Pigmented streak in nail with extension onto the nail fold skin

66

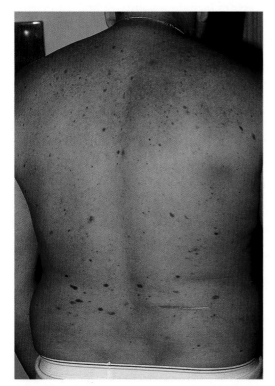

FIGURE 66-18 Atypical nevi. (From Bolognia JL, Jorizzo JL, Rapini RP: *Dermatology*, St. Louis, Mosby, 2003, p 1779.)

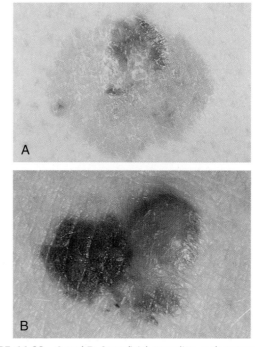

FIGURE 66-19 **A** and **B**, Superficial spreading melanomas.

BOX 66-1	*Risk Factors for the Development of Melanoma*

Sun exposure

Blond or red hair

Freckling on the upper back

Blistering sunburns in childhood

White race

Family history of melanoma

Therapy with psoralen and ultraviolet A radiation (PUVA) for psoriasis

Changing pigmented mole

Many (>50) common moles

Atypical mole

History of basal cell carcinoma or squamous cell carcinoma of the skin

Immunosuppression (e.g., after organ transplantation)

History of treated melanoma

- Lentigo maligna melanoma
  - Involves sun-exposed skin (usually the face)
  - Irregular pigmented macule that can develop papules within
  - One of the ABCDEs is typically present

Clinical Presentation

- Most melanomas exhibit one of the ABCDEs or have recently changed in size, shape, or color
- Bleeding, inflammation, or a sensory change at the site of the lesion should also suggest the possibility of malignancy
- In patients with numerous moles, an individual lesion that appears different from the others should be thoroughly evaluated
- Metastasis can occur (typically to the brain, liver, or lung)

Diagnosis

- Suggested by the clinical appearance
- Excisional biopsy of the lesion providing full-thickness skin sample that extends to the subcutaneous fat is the preferred diagnostic method
- **Staging is primarily based on tumor thickness**
- The presence of ulceration is the next most important histologic determinant of prognosis
- Sentinel lymph node biopsy is used for staging information in melanomas greater than 1.0 mm in depth
- Chest radiograph, liver function tests, and lactate dehydrogenase levels should also be obtained
- Scanning is indicated if metastatic disease is suggested

Treatment

- Excision with adequate margins is the treatment of choice for tumors without evidence of metastasis
- Elective lymph node dissection for patients with clinically enlarged lymph nodes and no evidence of distant disease
- Adjuvant chemotherapy may be employed for more advanced disease

BASAL CELL CARCINOMA

Figure 66-20 provides an example of basal cell carcinoma (BCC).

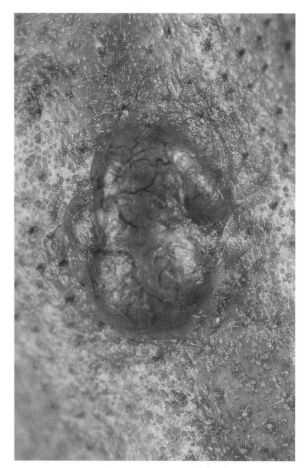

FIGURE 66-20 Basal cell carcinoma.

- **Risk factors include inability to tan, intermittent sun exposure, cumulative sun exposure, fair skin, and older age**
- Usually develop on the head and neck
- A patient typically complains of a red, peeling, eroded or bleeding lesion that may improve and then recur
- Subtypes of BCC
  - Nodular ulcerative
    - Most common type
    - Presents as a well-circumscribed pearly papule with telangiectasias; may ulcerate
  - Superficial
    - Well-circumscribed, erythematous, scaly patch
    - Resembles tinea, psoriasis, or dermatitis
    - Often occurs on non-sun-exposed skin
  - Sclerotic
    - Whitish plaque with sclerosis or fibrosis on palpation
  - Pigmented
    - Similar to nodular but are pigmented
    - Most common form seen in darker-skinned individuals
- Metastatic disease is very rare
- Diagnosis is made by clinical appearance or biopsy specimen
- Standard treatment options include electrodesiccation and curettage, surgical excision, radiation
- Superficial BCC may respond to topical treatment with the immune modulator imiquimod

- Mohs' micrographic surgery is used for sclerosing BCC and other BCC with poorly defined clinical margins, for tumors in areas of potentially high recurrence, such as the nose or eyelid, and for very large primary tumors and recurrent BCC

ACTINIC KERATOSIS

Figure 66-21 illustrates actinic keratosis.
- Premalignant lesions that develop on sun-exposed skin, usually in people older than 40 years
- **Low but significant risk of transformation to squamous cell carcinoma (SCC)**
- Fair-skinned individuals are more susceptible to developing actinic keratosis
- Present as erythematous, 2- to 8-mm macules with a whitish scale; or as hyperkeratotic plaques on the face, scalp, back of the hands, arms, chest, upper back, and lower legs
- Diagnosis is usually made by clinical appearance; lesions suggestive of SCC should be biopsied
- There is no way to determine which lesions will progress to SCC
- Patients who are immunosuppressed (especially transplant patients) are at high risk for the development of SCC from actinic keratosis
- Current treatment modalities include the following
  - Cryotherapy with liquid nitrogen or surgical curettage is effective for individual lesions
  - Topical 5-fluorouracil, imiquimod, and photodynamic therapy (topical aminolevulinic acid followed by exposure to a blue light source) may be useful in patients with multiple lesions
  - Excision or electrodesiccation and curettage should be performed for thicker or resistant lesions

SQUAMOUS CELL CARCINOMA

See Figure 66-22 for an example of SCC.
- More than half of cases arise from transformation of actinic keratoses
- Chronic exposure to ultraviolet sunlight and increasing age are the more important risk factors
- **Very common in patients after organ transplantation**
- In patients with chronic lymphocytic leukemia, the development of multiple SCCs may indicate deterioration of the leukemia
- Presents as an erythematous papule, nodule, or plaque with a hyperkeratotic scale; ulceration may also occur
- Clinical variants
  - Bowen's disease (SCC in situ): Reddish brown plaque that may have pigment or hyperkeratosis; has been associated with chemical exposures and human papilloma virus infection (SCC of the anogenital skin)
  - Keratoacanthoma: Hyperkeratotic nodule with a keratin plug; grows rapidly (over 3–6 weeks); most spontaneously regress
  - Cutaneous horns: Columns of hyperkeratosis on an erythematous base; can grow within an SCC
- 5% to 10% metastasize
- Surgical excision is the treatment of choice

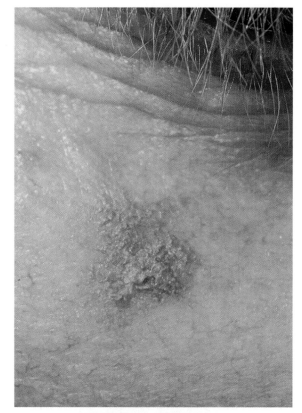

FIGURE 66-21 Actinic keratosis.

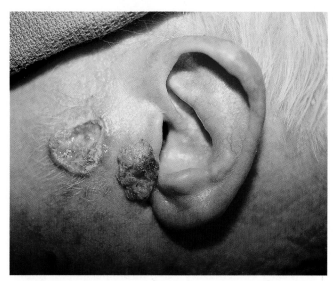

FIGURE 66-22 Squamous cell carcinoma. (From Bolognia JL, Jorizzo JL, Rapini RP: *Dermatology*, St. Louis, Mosby, 2003, p 1682.)

CUTANEOUS T-CELL LYMPHOMA

- Presents as erythematous, scaly plaques resembling psoriasis or eczema on sun-protected sites (i.e., buttock and covered areas of trunk and limbs); most common subtype is mycosis fungoides
- Fulminant lesions may be preceded by months to years by nonspecific scaly lesions that have been diagnosed as other dermatoses

66

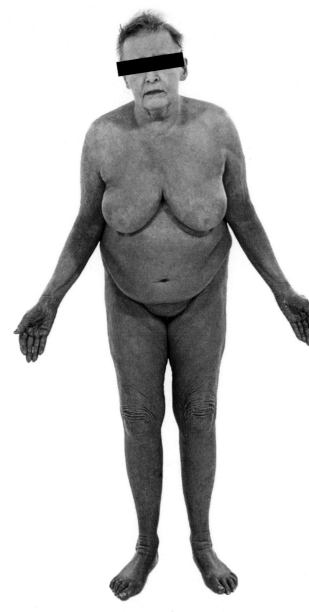

FIGURE 66-23   Sézary's syndrome.

- Significant pruritus, fever, and lymphadenopathy can be present
- **Sézary's syndrome (Fig. 66-23) is a leukemic variant characterized by generalized erythroderma, lymphadenopathy, pruritus, and leukocytosis with atypical T cells (Sézary cells) in the peripheral blood**
- Patients can be treated with topical nitrogen mustard, phototherapy, topical or oral retinoids, or radiation therapy

Cutaneous Drug Reactions

Basic Information

- Occur in up to 3% of hospitalized patients
- Antibiotics are responsible for most reactions
- Drug-induced skin eruptions can take many forms (the most common and significant ones are discussed in the following section)

EXANTHEMS

- **The most common acute drug-induced eruption, accounting for 75% of cases**
- Rash is generalized, pruritic, macular, and papular
- In some cases, exfoliative erythroderma can occur and can be an early sign for the development of toxic epidermal necrolysis (see following discussion)
- Onset of the rash is usually within 2 weeks of beginning drug therapy
- In patients who have been sensitized to the drug (by prior use), the rash typically develops within the first 3 days of therapy
- The most commonly implicated drugs include penicillins, cephalosporins, sulfonamides, quinidine, allopurinol, isoniazid, carbamazepine, and phenytoin
- Cessation of the drug usually leads to resolution of the rash; symptomatic treatment with topical corticosteroids, topical antipruritics, or oral antihistamines can be used

URTICARIA AND ANGIODEMA

See Chapter 69.

HYPERSENSITIVITY VASCULITIS

- Most commonly implicated drugs include penicillins, cephalosporins, sulfonamides, allopurinol, and phenytoin
- **Clinical findings include palpable purpura, petechiae, fever, arthralgias, and lymphadenopathy that usually begin within 10 days of the initial drug exposure**
- The sedimentation rate may be elevated; complement levels may be low
- Discontinuation of the drug should lead to resolution of symptoms within weeks; systemic corticosteroids may be necessary in severe cases

LICHEN PLANUS

See Figure 66-24 for an example of lichen planus.
- **Can be drug-induced, related to liver disease (e.g., hepatitis C), or idiopathic**
- Implicated drugs include β-blockers, methyldopa, penicillamine, quinidine and quinine, NSAIDs, angiotensin-converting enzyme inhibitors, sulfonylurea agents, carbamazepine, gold, and lithium
- Most lesions occur on the skin or mucous membranes
  - Skin lesions
    - Pruritic, violaceous, polygonal, flat-topped papules with white lacy lines (Wickham's striae)
    - Most common site is the flexor aspect of the wrists
  - Mucous membranes
    - Most common presentation
    - Milky-white papules with white lacework on the buccal mucosa
    - Patients with chronic disease may have an increased risk of oral SCC
- Withdrawal of the medication should lead to resolution of the lesions
- In cases that are not drug-induced, topical corticosteroids are first-line therapy

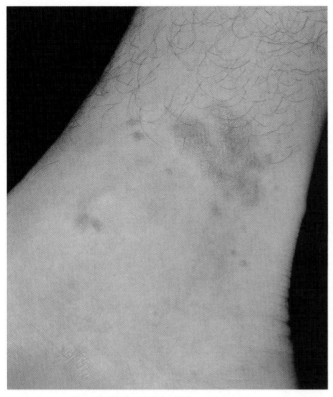

FIGURE 66-24 Lichen planus.

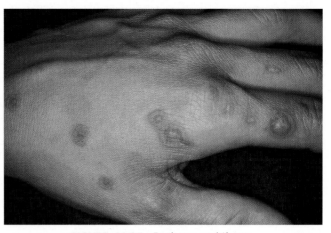

FIGURE 66-25 Erythema multiforme.

- Resistant disease can be treated with systemic corticosteroids, retinoid therapy, or phototherapy

ERYTHEMA MULTIFORME

See Figure 66-25 for an example of erythema multiforme (EM).
- Cell-mediated cytotoxic skin reaction triggered by infection (usually HSV or *Mycoplasma*) or drugs (e.g., sulfonamides, anticonvulsants, penicillins, or NSAIDs)
- Two basic forms of disease
  - EM major
    - Affects more than one mucosal surface (usually conjunctiva and oral mucosa)
    - Typical or raised atypical target lesions
    - Epidermal detachment involving less than 10% of body surface
    - Lesions usually located on the extremities or face
    - Usually associated with drugs
  - EM minor
    - Most are preceded by an HSV infection (a small percentage associated with *Mycoplasma pneumoniae*)
    - Limited or no mucous membrane involvement
    - Bullae and systemic symptoms are seen in some cases
    - Target lesions favor hands, feet, arms, and legs
    - Chronic suppressive acyclovir therapy prevents HSV and EM recurrences

STEVENS-JOHNSON SYNDROME AND TOXIC EPIDERMAL NECROLYSIS

- A spectrum of disease characterized by epidermal necrosis and mucous membrane involvement

- **Stevens-Johnson syndrome (SJS) involves less than 10% of the epidermis, whereas toxic epidermal necrolysis (TEN) involves over 30% of the epidermis. Involvement of 10% to 30% is considered SJS-TEN overlap.**
- Most commonly implicated drugs are sulfonamides, anticonvulsants, allopurinol, penicillins, and NSAIDs
- Lesions usually appear within a few days after the initiation of drug therapy; a prodrome of fever, malaise, and arthralgias can be present
- Skin lesions
  - Begin as tender erythematous macules, followed by formation of blisters that become confluent; the epidermis then begins to slough, leaving areas that resemble burns
  - Nikolsky's sign (separation of the outer layer of the epidermis from the basal layer with minimal pressure applied to the skin) may be present
- Mucous membranes
  - At least two mucosal surfaces are involved
- Erythema and sloughing of the lips, buccal mucosa, conjunctiva, or anogenital area can occur
- Complications of the disease include acute renal failure, fluid and electrolyte imbalances, GI hemorrhage, and sepsis
- **Treatment of TEN involves discontinuation of the offending agent, transfer to a burn unit, possible IV immunoglobulin, not corticosteroids**
- Death occurs in 40% of patients with TEN
- Patients with Stevens-Johnson syndrome may benefit from oral corticosteroids

HYPERSENSITIVITY SYNDROME

- Fever, rash, and lymphadenopathy occurring 2 to 6 weeks after initiation of drug therapy
- **Phenytoin, carbamazepine, phenobarbital, and sulfonamides are most commonly implicated**
- Erythematous papules and pustules or bullae are the typical skin manifestations
- Hepatitis and eosinophilia can also be seen
- Prompt withdrawal of the medication usually results in full recovery

66

TABLE 66-4 | *Autoimmune Blistering Diseases*

Disease	Basic Information	Clinical Presentation	Diagnosis	Treatment
Subepidermal blistering diseases				
Bullous pemphigoid (BP) (Fig. 66-26)	Most common type Typically affects older adults Usually chronic and recurrent Most cases are idiopathic related to drugs (e.g., diuretics, neuroleptics)	Starts as urticarial eruptions and evolves into crops of tense blisters with urticarial bases The edges of the blister do not extend with gentle manual pressure Often involve the axillae, groin, medial aspects of the thighs, lower legs, and flexor aspects of the forearm Cicatricial pemphigoid is a variant that involves the oral cavity, nasopharynx, or conjunctiva	Skin biopsy showing subepidermal blister with inflammatory cells (including eosinophils) Direct immunofluorescence (DIF) shows linear deposition of IgG and C3 in the epidermal-dermal junction (basement membrane zone)	Disease in some patients is self-limited Corticosteroids (topical or oral) can significantly improve symptoms High risk of complications because of systemic steroid therapy Immunosuppressives may be used
Epidermolysis bullosa acquisita	May be associated with inflammatory bowel disease, rheumatoid arthritis, and SLE	Blisters and erosions induced by minor trauma on the hands and feet Mucosal lesions can be present	Histology is similar to BP DIF shows IgG at the basement membrane zone NaCl-split skin technique applied to biopsy specimen shows IgG on the dermal side (as opposed to the epidermal side in BP)	Supportive therapy Does not usually respond to immunosuppressives
Dermatitis herpetiformis (Fig. 66-27)	Usually occurs between ages 20 and 50 yr Almost all patients have some degree of gluten-sensitive enteropathy (similar to celiac disease) Also associated with a number of other autoimmune disorders Linear IgA dermatosis is a variant associated with medications (e.g., NSAIDs, vancomycin) and not gluten-sensitive enteropathy	Clusters of pruritic, grouped vesicles on the elbows, knees, buttocks, or scalp Mucous membranes usually spared except in cases of linear IgA dermatosis Small-bowel lymphoma in a small number of patients	Histology reveals a subepidermal vesicle with neutrophils and eosinophils in the dermal papillae DIF shows granular IgA deposits at the basement membrane zone	Steroids not helpful Improvement seen with gluten-free diet Dapsone is the treatment of choice
Intraepidermal blistering diseases				
Pemphigus vulgaris (PV)	Usually occurs between the ages of 30 and 60 yr Has been associated with myasthenia gravis and thymoma	Begins with painful, nonhealing ulceration of the oral cavity Bullous lesions on the skin usually present months later Bullae are flaccid and rupture easily Pressure placed on the bulla leads to lateral extension of the blister (unlike BP) Nikolsky's sign* is positive when done on normal-appearing skin	Histologically there is intraepithelial acantholysis (separation of keratinocytes) Basement membrane is intact DIF reveals deposition of IgG and C3 at the epidermal cell surface Serum antidesmoglein antibodies	Fatal if not treated High-dose systemic corticosteroids initially Long-term steroid use may be needed Adjuvant immunosuppressives can help decrease steroid dose
Drug-induced pemphigus	Associated with pen-icillamine and captopril	Same as PV or PF	Same as PV or PF	Discontinuation of the drug
Mixed subepidermal and intraepidermal blistering disease				
Paraneoplastic pemphigus	Associated with lymphomas	Large, tense, bullous lesions on skin Oral and conjunctival involvement can be severe	DIF shows IgG in the intraepidermal layer and C3 involvement of the subepidermal layer	Difficult Steroids are attempted

*Nikolsky's sign, separation of the outer layer of the epidermis from the basal layer with application of minimal pressure to the skin.
Ig, immunoglobulin; SLE, systemic lupus erythematosus.

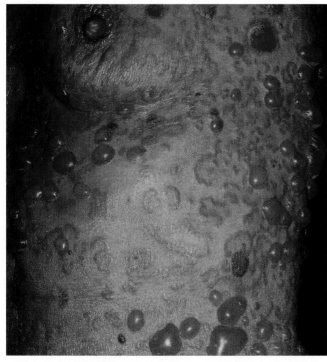

FIGURE 66-26 Bullous pemphigoid.

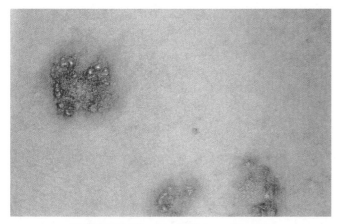

FIGURE 66-27 Dermatitis herpetiformis.

Autoimmune Blistering Disorders

Basic Information

- Blisters are fluid-filled skin lesions; small (<0.5 cm) blisters are called vesicles, whereas larger ones are referred to as bullae
- Most acquired forms of disease are autoimmune
- The unifying pathologic abnormality resulting in fluid-filled cavity formation is separation of skin at some level
- One method of classifying these diseases is by their level of tissue disadhesion; some diseases separate within the level of the epidermis, whereas others separate below the epidermis (Table 66-4)

Clinical Presentation, Diagnosis, and Treatment

See Table 66-4.

Cutaneous Manifestations of Internal Disease

CARDIOVASCULAR DISEASE

- LEOPARD syndrome: Generalized **l**entigines (brown macules), **e**lectrocardiogram abnormalities, **o**cular hypertelorism, **p**ulmonic stenosis, **a**bnormal genitalia, **r**etardation of growth (dwarfism), and **d**eafness
- LAMB syndrome: Generalized **l**entigines, **a**trial myxoma, **m**ucocutaneous myxomas, **b**lue nevi
- Pseudoxanthoma elasticum
  - Peau d'orange pattern of clusters of yellow papules found on the neck, axillae, or other body folds
  - Associated with peripheral vascular disease, stroke, myocardial infarctions, retinal hemorrhages, and GI hemorrhage
- Ehlers-Danlos syndrome
  - Defects in collagen biosynthesis result in hypermobility of joints and hyperelasticity of the skin
  - Associated with abdominal aortic aneurysm and GI hemorrhage

PULMONARY DISEASE

- Sarcoidosis (Fig. 66-28; see also Chapter 21)
  - **Lupus pernio: Violaceous plaques on the nose, cheeks, and ears**
    - Pathology reveals noncaseating granulomas
    - Course is chronic and requires treatment with intralesional steroids, antimalarials, or methotrexate
  - A number of other cutaneous diseases are seen with sarocoidosis, including EN (see preceding discussion)
- Yellow nail syndrome: Yellow nails, lymphedema, pleural effusions

ENDOCRINE DISEASE

- Diabetes mellitus (DM)
  - Acanthosis nigricans (Fig. 66-29)
    - Hyperpigmented velvety patches seen predominantly in skin folds such as the axillae, neck, and groin
  - Associated with insulin resistance (type 2 DM)
  - **Also associated with other endocrinopathies (e.g., acromegaly, Cushing's syndrome, polycystic ovary, thyroid disease) and GI malignancies**
  - Necrobiosis lipoidica diabeticorum (Fig. 66-30)
    - Multicolored plaques with atrophic centers found on the anterior and lateral aspects of the legs
  - Granuloma annulare
    - Skin-colored or erythematous fine papules that exhibit an annular arrangement
    - Seen on the hands, feet, arms, or legs
    - Diffuse form of granuloma annulare can be associated with diabetes
  - Stiff hand syndrome
    - Seen in type 1 diabetes
    - Scleroderma-like tightening of the skin over the hands with limited joint mobility
    - Associated with nephropathy and retinopathy
  - Scleredema
    - Induration of the skin of the posterior neck and back
    - Usually seen in men with poorly controlled type 2 diabetes

66

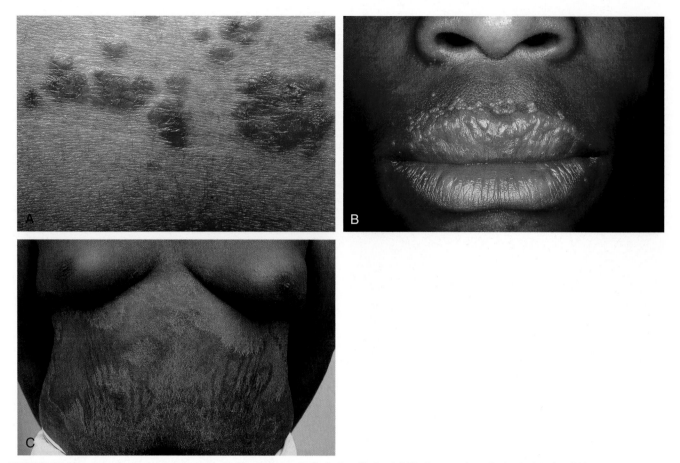

FIGURE 66-28 **A** to **C,** Cutaneous sarcoidosis. (From Bolognia JL, Jorizzo JL, Rapini RP: *Dermatology,* St. Louis, Mosby, 2003, p 1457.)

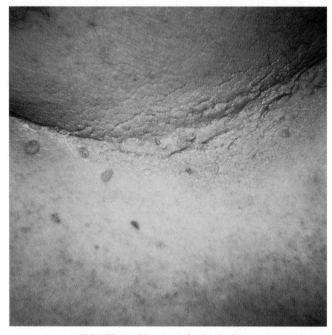

FIGURE 66-29   Acanthosis nigricans.

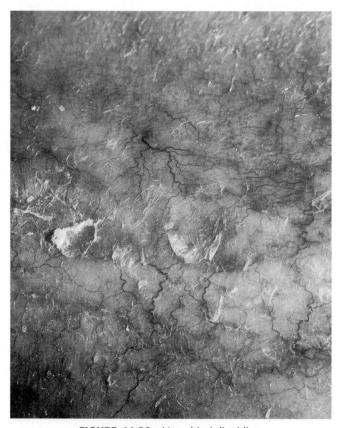

FIGURE 66-30   Necrobiosis lipoidica.

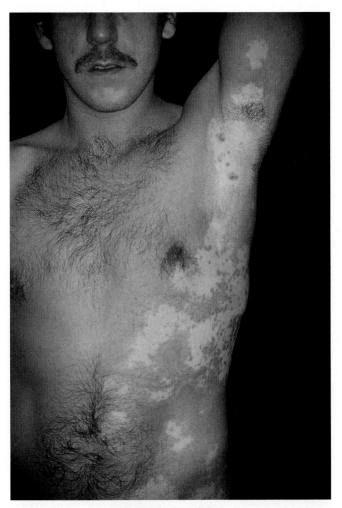

FIGURE 66-31 Vitiligo.

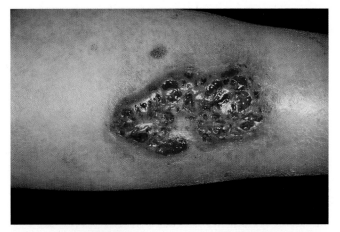

FIGURE 66-32 Pyoderma gangrenosum.

- Pyoderma gangrenosum (Fig. 66-32)
  - Rapidly progressing blue-red ulcers with irregular borders and purulent drainage
  - Can occur at sites of trauma (pathergy)
  - Also seen with inflammatory bowel disease, myeloproliferative disorders, rheumatoid arthritis, and chronic hepatitis; 50% of cases are idiopathic
- EN (see preceding discussion)
- Cutaneous Crohn's disease
  - Skin lesions with noncaseating granulomas on histology
  - Can take many forms
- Sweet's syndrome
  - Multiple erythematous nodules, most commonly on the head, neck, and upper extremities but can occur anywhere
  - May be associated with fever, arthritis, arthralgias, myalgias, ocular symptoms, neutrophilic pulmonary alveolitis, sterile osteomyelitis, acute renal failure, transient involvement of the kidney, liver, and pancreas, and aseptic meningitis
  - Also may be associated with infections, malignancy, autoimmune disorders, and pregnancy
- Celiac disease (gluten-sensitive enteropathy)
  - Aphthous stomatitis
  - Dermatitis herpetiformis (see Table 66-4 and Fig. 66-27)
- Hepatitis C infection
  - Porphyria cutanea tarda (Fig. 66-33)
    - Patients may present with fragile skin, vesicles, or bullae (usually on the dorsum of the hands) after minor trauma or sun exposure
    - Hypertrichosis, scleroderma-like induration, hyperpigmentation, and hypopigmentation can all occur as well
    - Also associated with alcohol and drugs (e.g., estrogens)
    - Diagnosis is made by showing elevated uroporphyrin levels
    - Patients who have been diagnosed should be screened for hepatitis C
  - Cryoglobulinemia (see Chapter 45)
  - Lichen planus
  - Pruritus

- Diabetic dermopathy
  - Hyperpigmented atrophic macules on anterior shins, from trauma
- Bulla diabeticorum
  - Bullae on anterior shins
- Hyperthyroidism
  - Thinning of hair
  - Onycholysis—separation of the nail from the nail bed
  - Pretibial myxedema (if Graves' disease)—edematous plaques primarily on anterior shins, can also get periorbital myxedema
  - Vitiligo (Fig. 66-31)
    - Depigmentation of skin, with white macules covering small or large amounts of the body surface
    - Can affect the hair and mucous membranes
    - **May be associated with autoimmune disorders (e.g., thyroid disease, type 1 diabetes, pernicious anemia, and adrenal insufficiency)**
- Hypothyroidism
  - Dull coarse hair with slow growth
  - Loss of lateral third of eyebrows
  - Dry skin, brittle nails

GASTROINTESTINAL AND LIVER DISEASE

- Inflammatory bowel disease
  - Aphthous stomatitis

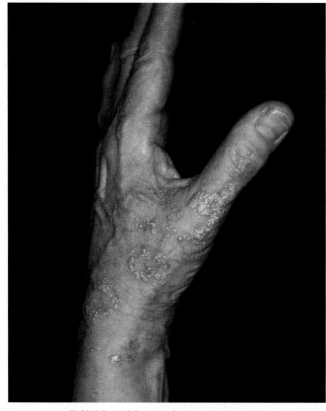

FIGURE 66-33　Porphyria cutanea tarda.

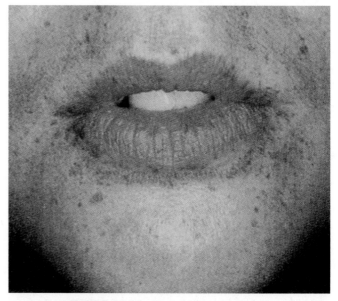

FIGURE 66-34　Peutz-Jeghers syndrome.

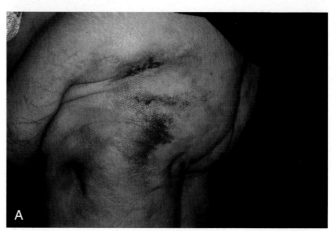

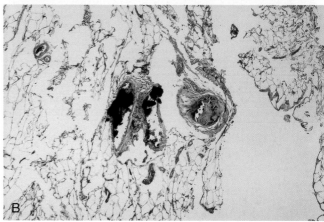

FIGURE 66-35　Calciphylaxis. (From Bolognia JL, Jorizzo JL, Rapini RP: *Dermatology,* St. Louis, Mosby, 2003, p 694.)

- Peutz-Jeghers syndrome (Fig. 66-34)
  - **Pigmented macules (freckles) on the lips, oral mucosa, palms, soles, fingers, and toes**
  - Associated with small-bowel hamartomas
- Hereditary hemorrhagic telangiectasia (Osler-Weber-Rendu disease)
  - Characterized by telangiectasias on the skin, lungs, GI tract, and CNS
  - Can cause life-threatening bleeding from noncutaneous sites

HEMATOLOGIC DISEASE

- Mastocytosis
  - Cutaneous and visceral infiltration of mast cells
  - **Urticaria pigmentosa: Reddish brown macules and papules that can urticate on stroking (Darier's sign)**
  - Can cause pruritus, flushing, diarrhea, abdominal pain, and wheezing
  - Diagnosis is made by demonstration of mast cell infiltration on skin biopsy specimen

RENAL DISEASE

- Fabry's disease
  - X-linked disorder resulting in deposition of glycosphingolipids in body tissues
  - Causes angiokeratomas (purple papules) on the trunk, extremities, palms, soles, and mucous membranes
  - Also results in paresthesias, renal failure, and cardiovascular disease
- Calciphylaxis (Fig. 66-35)
  - Localized areas of skin necrosis caused by vascular calcification
  - Seen in patients with end-stage renal disease
  - Parathyroidectomy may result in healing

- Nephrogenic systemic fibrosis
  - Thickening and hardening of the skin overlying extremities and trunk due to fibrosis of the dermis
  - Fibrosis can also affect deeper structures, including muscle, fascia, lungs, and heart
  - Seen exclusively in patients with kidney disease
  - **Associated with administration of gadolinium contrast medium for MRI**
    - Risk is thought to be about 5% after gadolinium exposure in a patient with end-stage renal disease
    - Disease is usually chronic and unremitting
    - No effective treatment at this time

NEUROLOGIC DISEASE

- Neurofibromatosis (Fig. 66-36)
  - Autosomal dominant disease characterized by soft, tan-colored nodules that arise from peripheral nerves
    - Cutaneous lesions develop before puberty and increase with age
    - Predominantly involves the trunk
    - Can be associated with severe pruritus

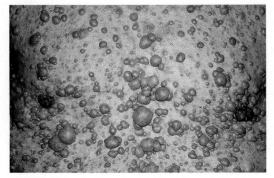

FIGURE 66-36 Neurofibromatosis. (From Bolognia JL, Jorizzo JL, Rapini RP: *Dermatology,* St. Louis, Mosby, 2003, p 855.)

- **Café-au-lait spots (pigmented patches), axillary freckling, and Lisch's nodules (pigmented iris hamartomas) are also seen in most patients**
- Tuberous sclerosis
  - Autosomal dominant disease characterized by skin lesions, mental retardation, seizures, and angiomyolipomas of the kidneys
  - Skin lesions include "adenoma sebaceum" (skin-colored facial papules that are angiofibromas), ash-leaf macules (hypopigmented macules), shagreen patch (connective tissue nevus), and periungual and subungual fibromas

ONCOLOGIC DISEASE

See Table 66-5 for a summary of the dermatologic manifestations of oncologic disease.

RHEUMATOLOGIC DISEASE

- Vasculitis
  - Livedo reticularis (Fig. 66-37)
    - Mottled, blue-purple discoloration in a netlike pattern usually on legs or arms
    - **Can be idiopathic or associated with vasculitis, syphilis, tuberculosis, atheroemboli, or drugs (e.g., amantadine, quinine)**
  - Purpura
    - Caused by extravasation of blood cells into the dermis
    - Nonpalpable purpura and petechiae
      - Primarily caused by thrombocytopenia, disorders of hyperglobulinemia, or disorders of capillary fragility (e.g., amyloidosis, Ehlers-Danlos syndrome, scurvy)
    - Palpable purpura (Fig. 66-38)
      - Seen in vasculitic disorders, embolic disorders (e.g., cholesterol emboli, atrial myxoma, endocarditis), and coagulopathies (e.g., antiphospholipid syndrome)

66

TABLE 66-5   *Dermatologic Manifestations of Oncologic Disease (Paraneoplastic Syndromes)*

Skin Disorder	Oncologic Disease(s)	Description
Acanthosis nigricans	Gastric cancer Colon cancer	Velvety hyperpigmentation in axillae, groin, neck Also associated with endocrinopathies (see text)
Acquired ichthyosis	Hodgkin's lymphoma Breast, lung, bladder carcinoma	Generalized scaling of the skin including palms and soles
Bazex's syndrome	Squamous cell carcinoma of the pharynx and esophagus Hodgkin's lymphoma	Psoriasiform lesions on the hands, feet, ears, and nose
Necrolytic migratory erythema	Glucagonoma	Weeping, eczematous lesions around the mouth, intertriginous areas, flexures, and perigenital area Weight loss, diarrhea, and glossitis also present
Paget's disease	Breast: Intraductal carcinoma Extramammary: Adnexal cancers, genitourinary cancers, gastrointestinal cancers	Breast: Erythematous eczematous, and scaly lesions around the nipple Extramammary: Erythematous plaques around the vulva, scrotum, or perianal area
Sweet's syndrome	Acute myelogenous leukemia	Acute onset of violaceous/erythematous papules or plaques usually on the face, neck, and upper extremities Fever, arthritis, leukocytosis may be present
Tylosis	Esophageal carcinoma	Inherited disorder presenting with yellow, smooth thickening of the palms and soles (palmar-plantar hyperkeratosis)
Tripe palm	Gastric cancer Bronchogenic carcinoma	Velvety thickening of the palms that leads to accentuation of palmar creases

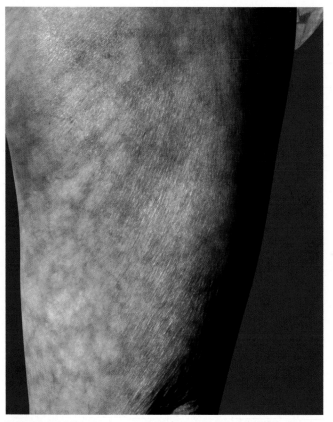

FIGURE 66-37 Livedo reticularis. (From Bolognia JL, Jorizzo JL, Rapini RP: *Dermatology,* St. Louis, Mosby, 2003, p 1652.)

ITCHING (PRURITUS) IN THE ABSENCE OF A RASH

- Commonly caused by xerosis or xerotic dermatitis ("winter itch")
- Many skin disorders have pruritus as a major finding (atopic dermatitis, infestations such as scabies)
  - Localized pruritus without evidence if a rash—nostalgia paresthetica (usually located on the upper back)
- May be a sign of systemic disease (generalized, chronic and progressive)
  - Biliary/hepatic disease (primary biliary cirrhosis, hepatitis)
  - Renal disease (end-stage renal disease)
  - Lymphoma (Hodgkin's lymphoma)
  - Polycythemia vera, myelodysplasia, essential thrombocythemia
  - Thyroid disorder
  - Mastocytosis
  - Hypereosinophilic syndrome
  - Diabetes
  - HIV
- Psychogenic pruritus
- Pregnancy-related pruritus

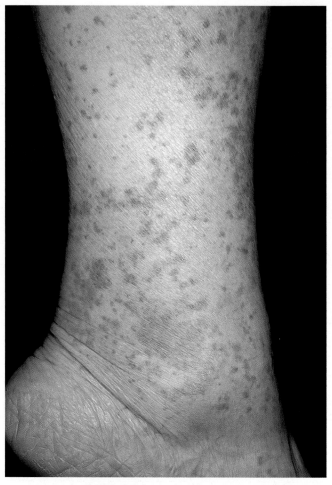

FIGURE 66-38 Palpable purpura.

REVIEW QUESTIONS

For review questions, please go to www.expertconsult.com.

SUGGESTED READINGS

Bachot N, Roujeau JC: Physiopathology and treatment of severe drug eruptions, *Curr Opin Allergy Clin Immunol* 1:293–298, 2001.

Bershad SV: In the clinic: acne, *Ann Intern Med* 1:149:ITC1-1-ITC1-16, 2008.

Bieber T: Atopic dermatitis, *N Engl J Med* 358:1483–1494, 2008.

Habif TB: *Clinical dermatology,* ed 4, St. Louis, Mosby, 2004.

Kazin RA, Lowitt NR, Lowitt MH: Update in dermatology, *Ann Intern Med* 135:124–132, 2001.

Nainani N, Panesar M: Nephrogenic systemic fibrosis, *Am J Nephrol* 29:1–9, 2009.

Whitmore SE: Atypical moles and common cancers of the skin. In Fiebach NH, Kern DE, Thomas PA, Ziegelstein RC, editors: *Principles of ambulatory medicine,* ed 7, Philadelphia, Lippincott Williams and Wilkins, 2007.

Ophthalmology for the Internist

JAMES P. DUNN, MD

Although most patients with underlying eye disorders are seen regularly by their ophthalmologists, it is imperative that internists recognize ophthalmologic emergencies, ocular manifestations of systemic diseases, and common causes of diminished visual acuity. Timely management and appropriate referral can serve to minimize potential visual loss and other ocular morbidity.

Review of Anatomy and Function

Figure 67-1 shows the cross-sectional anatomy of the eyelid and globe.

- Eyelids
  - Protect the eye
- Conjunctiva
  - Provides lubrication
  - Has immunologic functions (conjunctival-associated lymphoid tissue)
- Cornea
  - Most important refractile component of vision
- Anterior chamber and angle
  - Filtration of the aqueous humor through trabecular meshwork
- Lens
  - Responsible for accommodation (focusing for near tasks)
- Uvea (iris, ciliary body, choroid)
  - Produces aqueous humor (ciliary body)

- Nourishes outer retina
- Retina
  - Converts light to electrical impulses in first stage of visual processing
  - Macula (central retina) much more critical than peripheral retina; the fovea is the center of the macula and subserves central visual acuity
- Optic nerve
  - Connects retinal nerve fibers (~1 million per eye) to brain
  - The optic disc is nasal to the fovea and is the only visible part of the optic nerve
- Orbit
  - Contains extraocular muscles, adipose tissue, nerves, blood vessels, part of optic nerve

Common Causes of Visual Loss

REFRACTIVE ERROR

- Myopia (nearsightedness): Distance vision is blurred because light rays are focused anterior to the fovea
- Hyperopia (farsightedness): Near vision is blurred because light rays are focused posterior to the fovea
  - In children, accommodation of the ciliary body can overcome mild hyperopia but can induce accommodative esotropia ("crossed eyes")

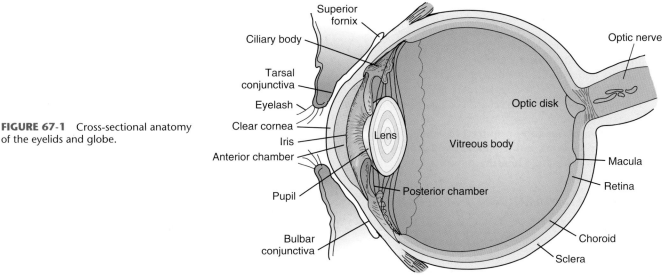

FIGURE 67-1 Cross-sectional anatomy of the eyelids and globe.

Superior fornix · Ciliary body · Tarsal conjunctiva · Eyelash · Clear cornea · Iris · Anterior chamber · Pupil · Bulbar conjunctiva · Lens · Posterior chamber · Vitreous body · Optic nerve · Optic disk · Macula · Retina · Choroid · Sclera

- In moderate and severe hyperopia, distance vision is also blurred
- Astigmatism
  - Refraction unequal in different parts of eyeball
  - Cylindrical (toric) lens needed to correct vision
- Presbyopia
  - Age-related diminution in near vision
  - Onset usually noticed around ages 40 to 45 years
- Laser in situ keratomileusis (LASIK) and photorefractive keratectomy (PRK) are used to alter the corneal surface and correct for some refractive errors

CATARACT

Basic Information

- Opacification of the lens of the eye
- Most cataracts are age-related (senescent)
- Other causes include uveitis, steroid use, trauma, diabetes, family history, radiation, poor overall nutrition, Wilson's disease (sunflower cataract)
- Usually bilateral with slow progression

Clinical Presentation and Diagnosis

- Symptoms include blurred vision, glare (especially at night), and difficulty with driving
- **No pain or redness**
- On examination, visual acuity is impaired; clouding of the lens can often be appreciated with an ophthalmoscope if slit lamp is unavailable (impairment of normal red reflex or difficulty visualizing optic disc and retina)

Treatment

- If refraction does not improve vision, surgery is the only effective treatment
- **Indications for surgery revolve around functional impairment and difficulty with activities of daily living; Snellen acuity (i.e., vision on eye chart) alone is a poor predictor of visual function (or dysfunction)**
- Standard treatment is phacoemulsification with posterior chamber (within capsular bag behind the iris) lens implant
- Cataract surgery nearly always performed as outpatient surgery
  - Anesthesia may be general (in children or uncooperative or extremely anxious adults), local (e.g., retrobulbar or peribulbar), or topical or intraocular (increasingly used)
  - Surgery performed through peripheral clear cornea using topical or intraocular (intracameral) anesthesia allows patients to remain on anticoagulants (e.g., warfarin) through cataract surgery
  - **IV sedation is usually required for surgery (e.g., midazolam), but preoperative laboratory testing in otherwise healthy patients is usually unnecessary**

AGE-RELATED MACULAR DEGENERATION

Basic Information

- Leading cause of legal blindness in patients aged 55 years and older in the United States

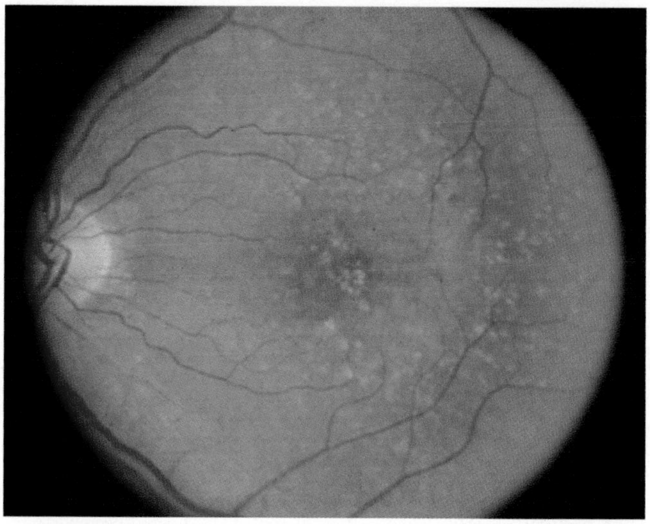

FIGURE 67-2　Drusen in non-neovascular age-related macular degeneration.

- 10% of population older than 43 years and 30% of population aged 75 years and older affected to some degree by age-related macular degeneration (AMD)
- 2% of those older than 65 years have vision of 20/200 or less in at least one eye because of AMD
- By 2020, nearly 3 million Americans will have advanced AMD
- Risk factors include increasing age, family history, cigarette smoking, light iris color
- Likely that different genetic and environmental factors influence different forms of AMD
- Two forms of disease
  - Non-neovascular ("dry," atrophic, nonexudative): 90% of cases
    - **"Drusen" are deposits of material in the macula that probably represent the accumulation of by-products of photoreceptor metabolism. On ophthalmoscopy they appear as small, bright yellow objects (Fig. 67-2).**
    - "Geographic atrophy" is well-circumscribed area of retinal pigment epithelium or choriocapillaris
  - Neovascular ("wet," exudative): Less common, more rapidly progressive
    - Choroidal neovascularization causes pigment epithelial detachment and photoreceptor damage
    - Hypertension is a risk factor for progression of dry to wet AMD

Clinical Presentation and Diagnosis

- Blurred central vision caused by loss of foveal function
- Distortion of straight lines may be an early presenting complaint
  - Amsler grid has been used to assess progression of disease (Fig. 67-3)
    - The patient covers one eye and focuses the other eye on the center dot of a hand-held copy of the grid; any new distortion in the lines (metamorphopsia) or scotoma (blind spots) suggests progression of disease
- No pain or redness
- Peripheral vision remains intact

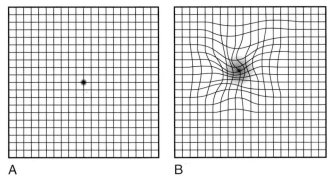

FIGURE 67-3 Amsler grid for monitoring age-related macular degeneration (AMD). **A,** How it would appear normally. **B,** How it might appear to someone with AMD.

Treatment

- Non-neovascular AMD
  - Antioxidants, zinc supplements, and carotenoids (e.g., lutein) often used, but value not proven for all types of AMD
  - A combination of zinc, vitamins C and E, and β-carotene may reduce the risk of progression from moderate to severe AMD, but has not been shown to reduce the risk of progression of mild to moderate AMD (and has no effect on development or worsening of cataracts)
- Neovascular AMD
  - Argon laser photocoagulation in some cases, but vision loss still severe
  - Less destructive laser treatments (photodynamic therapy), intravitreous corticosteroids, and especially intravitreous vascular endothelial growth factor antagonists (anti-VEGF) now routinely used
  - Anti-VEGF agents (bevacizumab, ranubizumab) injected intraocularly
  - Surgery to remove membrane or "translocate" the macula rarely effective
  - Referral to low vision specialist is highly recommended

Prevention

- Sunglasses or hats to block ultraviolet light possibly helpful
- Control of blood pressure to reduce risk of wet AMD may also be useful

Screening

- Comprehensive examination by ophthalmologist recommended every 2 to 4 years for patients ages 40 to 64 years and every 1 to 2 years for patients ages 65 years and older

PRIMARY OPEN-ANGLE GLAUCOMA

Basic Information

- Most common type of glaucoma
- Second-leading cause of legal blindness in United States (and leading cause of legal blindness among African Americans)
  - Incidence
    - Estimated 44.7 million people worldwide and 2.79 million Americans affected in 2010

- Primary open-angle glaucoma (POAG) undiagnosed in 50% of whites and 75% of African Americans
- Definition
  - Lowly progressive optic neuropathy characterized by optic disc cupping
  - Trabecular meshwork is blocked by excess glycosaminoglycan production, decreasing aqueous outflow
  - **Elevated intraocular pressure (IOP) and elevated cup-to-disc ratios are risk factors, but not diagnostic of POAG by themselves**
  - Other risk factors include increasing age, African-American or Latino heritage (10.3% cumulative probability for African Americans versus 4.2% for whites), family history, thinner corneas

Clinical Presentation and Diagnosis

- Asymptomatic until late stages, so measurement of visual acuity is not an adequate screening test
- Central visual loss occurs in end-stage disease
- **No eye pain or redness**
- Rarely causes headache unless IOP is extremely high
- Direct ophthalmoscopy may reveal an enlarged optic cup (cup-to-disk ratio of ≥0.5 is suggestive)
- Screening asymptomatic patients
  - Recommended every 2 to 4 years for patients ages 40 to 64 years, every 1 to 2 years for patients older than 65 years
  - Begin before age 40 years in African Americans

Treatment

- Medical
  - Prostaglandin analogues
  - Aqueous suppressants (topical β-blockers, topical or oral carbonic anhydrase inhibitors)
    - Side effects of oral carbonic anhydrase inhibitors render them poor long-term treatment options
  - Adrenergic agonists (brimonidine, epinephrine derivatives)
  - Cholinergic agonists (e.g., pilocarpine) now used infrequently because of side effects
  - Need to be aware of potential systemic effects of medications (Table 67-1)
- Laser therapy (argon laser trabeculoplasty, selective laser trabeculoplasty)
  - Easy to perform with low risk
  - Effect may only be temporary
- Surgical therapy
  - Trabeculectomy
  - Tube shunt surgery

NARROW-ANGLE GLAUCOMA

Basic Information

- One tenth as common as open-angle glaucoma in United States
- Seen in Asians more commonly than whites or African Americans

Clinical Presentation

- **Manifests with pain, redness, halos, and decreased visual acuity because of rapid elevation in eye pressure**

67

TABLE 67-1	Side Effects of Common Ocular Medications
Drug	**Effects**
β-Adrenergic blocking agents	Bronchospasm Bradycardia Hypotension Fatigue, depression Erectile dysfunction
Corticosteroids	Glaucoma Cataracts Corneal infection
Anesthetics	Poor epithelial healing Corneal melting (with chronic use)
Aminoglycosides α-Agonists	Toxic or allergic keratoconjunctivitis Hypotension Dry mouth Dizziness
Oral carbonic anhydrase inhibitors	Fatigue, depression Hypokalemia Acidosis Nausea Aplastic anemia (rare)

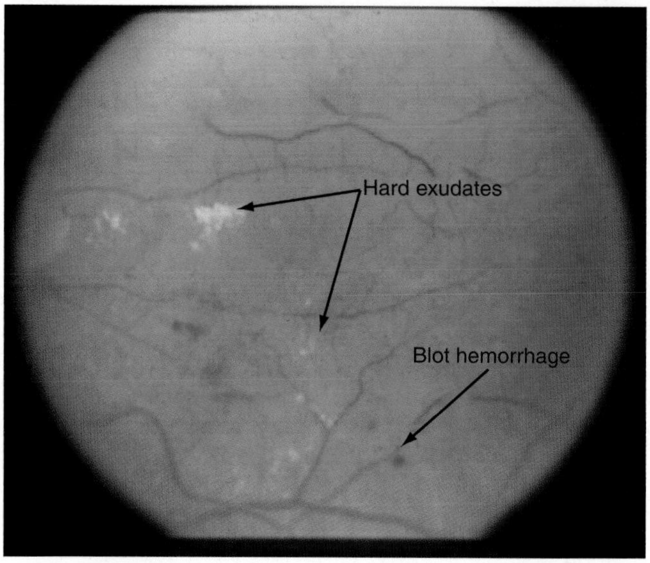

FIGURE 67-4 Nonproliferative diabetic retinopathy.

- Headache, nausea, and vomiting are commonly present
- Attack may be precipitated by mydriatic, sympathomimetic, and hypnotic medications

Treatment

- Requires urgent referral to ophthalmologist for laser iridotomy (and prophylactic laser in opposite eye)

DIABETIC RETINOPATHY

Basic Information

- Leading cause of blindness in patients ages 20 to 60 years in United States
- 4.1 million adults older than 40 years of age have diabetic retinopathy
- After 20 years of diabetes, more than 60% of patients with type 2 disease and nearly all patients with type 1 disease have some degree of retinopathy
- Among diabetics older than 40 years of age, prevalence rates for diabetic retinopathy and sight-threatening retinopathy are 40.3% and 8.2%, respectively
- **Risk of retinopathy directly related to duration of diabetes in both type 1 and type 2 patients**
- Level of glycemic control very important
  - Once retinopathy is present, degree of glucose control is a better predictor of progression to more serious disease than is duration of disease
  - Intensive therapy reduces onset and slows progression of retinopathy
  - Gestational diabetes is not associated with development of retinopathy, but pregnancy may exacerbate preexisting retinopathy

Clinical Presentation and Diagnosis

- Screening recommendations
  - Yearly dilated funduscopic examination for all diabetics
  - More frequent examinations if retinopathy is present
- Nonproliferative ("background," "preproliferative") retinopathy

  - Cotton-wool spots, microaneurysms, intraretinal hemorrhages, lipid ("hard") exudates, retinal edema, venous beading, and intraretinal microvascular abnormalities can be seen (Fig. 67-4)
  - 30% of patients blind after 5 years because of ischemia or macular edema
- Proliferative
  - Retinal vascularization caused by elaboration of angiogenic factors
  - 30% of patients blind after 5 years because of vitreous hemorrhage, retinal detachment, or neovascular glaucoma (angle closed by neovascularization)

Treatment

- Optimal control of diabetes, hypertension, and hyperlipidemia is crucial
- Laser photocoagulation effective for leaking vessels causing macular edema and for proliferative retinopathy
  - Most effective when patient has just reached high-risk proliferative diabetic retinopathy or before vision decreases due to macular edema
  - Laser may stabilize vision loss but often does not restore vision
  - Five-year risk of severe visual loss (<5/200) reduced to less than 5% if patients undergo appropriate panretinal photocoagulation for proliferative retinopathy
  - Risk of moderate visual loss (doubling of visual angle) reduced to less than 12% if patients undergo appropriate focal laser therapy for clinically significant macular edema
- Surgical treatment (often combined with laser photocoagulation) necessary to remove vitreous hemorrhage and repair retinal detachments
- Increasing role for anti-VEGF agents and other antiangiogenic agents likely

CAUSES OF SUDDEN VISUAL LOSS

- Usually monocular
- Can result from a number of different conditions (Box 67-1)

Causes of Sudden Visual Loss

Transient (Amaurosis Fugax)

Emboli (cholesterol or calcific plaques, cardiac myxoma, platelet-fibrin thrombi)

Vasospasm (migraine, subarachnoid hemorrhage, hypertensive crisis)

Sustained

Optic neuritis (MS, lupus, sarcoidosis)

Anterior ischemic optic neuropathy

   Arteritic—associated with giant-cell arteritis

   Nonarteritic—associated with advancing age, hypertension

Hemorrhage (neovascular AMD, vitreous hemorrhage in diabetes)

Occipital infarct

AMD, age-related macular degeneration; MS, multiple sclerosis.

Red Eye

See Table 67-2.

Eye Infections

HERPES SIMPLEX VIRUS

Basic Information and Clinical Presentation

- Major cause of blindness because of keratitis (infection of cornea)
- Usually caused by herpes simplex virus type 1 (HSV-1)
- **Unilateral redness, with a dendritic pattern on fluorescein staining is pathognomonic (Fig. 67-5)**
- May recur

Treatment

- Trifluoridine eyedrops
- Avoid topical corticosteroids (can cause exacerbation of HSV infection)
- Suppressive oral antiviral therapy (acyclovir 400 mg bid or equivalent) may help reduce recurrences

HERPES ZOSTER VIRUS

Basic Information

- Eye can be involved if there is vesicular eruption along any branch of the trigeminal nerve (VI most common)
- Can cause keratitis, uveitis, scleritis, and retinitis

Treatment

- Treat with acyclovir or similar antiviral therapy
  - Most effective if given within 72 hours of outbreak of vesicles

OCULAR COMPLICATIONS OF HIV INFECTION

Basic Information and Clinical Presentation

- Noninfectious retinopathy ("background HIV retinopathy")
  - Occurs in 50% to 100% of patients with CD4 counts less than 200 cells/mm³

- Clinical features: Cotton-wool spots, intraretinal hemorrhages
- Symptoms: None
- Clinical marker of advanced immunosuppression
- Need to rule out other causes of retinopathy (e.g., diabetes, hypertension, cytomeglaovirus [CMV])
- CMV retinitis
  - **Most common ocular opportunistic infection in AIDS**
  - CD4 count usually less than 50 cells/mm³
  - Floaters, flashing lights, blind spots (no pain, discharge, or redness) common
    - 15% to 50% of patients are asymptomatic
    - No external signs of inflammation
  - Retinal examination reveals white, fluffy lesions associated with hemorrhage (Fig. 67-6)
  - Screen at-risk patients every 4 to 6 months

Treatment

- Systemic
  - IV ganciclovir (less commonly, foscarnet or cidofovir) or oral valganciclovir
  - Reduces morbidity (extraocular disease), mortality, and second-eye involvement
- Local
  - Ganciclovir implant (with oral valganciclovir for previously listed reasons)
  - Intravitreous ganciclovir or foscarnet injections
- Effect of highly active antiretroviral therapy (HAART)
  - Reduces risk of ocular complications
  - CMV retinitis in less than 5% of patients versus more than 30% in pre-HAART era
  - In patients responsive and adherent to HAART (CD4⁺ count consistently > 100 cells/mm³), chronic anti-CMV therapy usually not necessary
  - "Immune recovery uveitis" (IRU) occurs in minority of eyes with CMV retinitis in patients responsive to HAART
    - Syndrome of uveitis, vitreitis, macular edema, and epiretinal membrane formation
    - Risk factors for IRU unclear

BACTERIAL AND VIRAL CONJUNCTIVITIS

See Table 67-2.

Disease of the Eyelid

BLEPHARITIS

Basic Information and Clinical Presentation

- Noninfectious lid margin inflammation (bacterial superinfection can occur)
- Symptoms: Crusting, irritation, chronic redness
- Common in patients with seborrhea, eczema, and rosacea

Treatment

- Warm compresses, lid scrubs; antibiotic ointment (erythromycin, bacitracin) if superinfection suggested

HORDEOLUM

Basic Information and Clinical Presentation

- Internal hordeolum: Infection of meibomian gland on the conjunctival side of the eyelid

67

TABLE 67-2   *Differential Diagnosis of the Red Eye*

	Allergic Conjunctivitis	Bacterial Conjunctivitis	Viral Conjunctivitis	Corneal Ulcer	Anterior Uveitis	Acute Glaucoma	Anterior Scleritis
Symptoms/findings	Bilateral, itchy eyes	No itching or adenopathy	Itching, preauricular adenopathy	Irregular corneal light reflex	Photophobia with ciliary flush	Headache, nausea, vomiting	Pain can be worse at night
Vision	Usually normal	Usually normal	May be impaired	Impaired	Slightly blurred	Decreased	Normal
Discharge	Watery	Mucopurulent	Watery	None	Tearing	Tearing	None
Pain	None	Minimal	Minimal	Present	Photophobia	Severe	Severe
Pupil size/shape	Normal	Normal	Normal	Normal	Miotic or irregular	Mid-dilated	Normal
Pupillary responses	Normal	Normal	Normal	Normal	May be nonreactive	Nonreactive	Normal
Redness	Diffuse	Diffuse	Segmental or diffuse	Localized or diffuse	Ciliary flush*	Diffuse with ciliary flush	Local or diffuse
Management/comments	Eliminate allergen Topical antihistamines or mast cell stabilizers	Topical antibiotics to cover S. aureus, S. pneumoniae, H. influenzae	Supportive Avoid close contact with other people for 7–14 days	Associated with trauma, contact lenses, topical steroid use	Topical corticosteroids† and cycloplegics Systemic workup usually necessary to assess for rheumatologic disease or sarcoid	Aqueous suppressants Laser Surgical iridectomy	Systemic corticosteroids or NSAIDs Systemic workup usually necessary to assess for rheumatologic disease or sarcoid

*Ring of injection around the limbus.

†Topical corticosteroids should never be used to treat a red eye without a specific diagnosis because they may cause glaucoma, cataract, or recurrent herpetic keratitis.

H. influenzae, Haemophilus influenzae; S. pneumoniae, Streptococcus pneumoniae; S. aureus, Staphylococcus aureus.

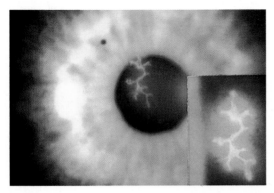

FIGURE 67-5 Dendritic pattern of herpes virus keratitis after fluorescein staining. *Inset* shows pattern after passing through cobalt blue filter. (From Goldman L, Bennett JC, Ausiello D: *Cecil textbook of medicine,* ed 22, Philadelphia, WB Saunders, 2004, figure 465-10.)

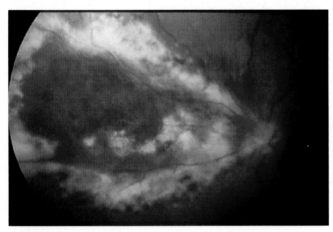

FIGURE 67-6 Cytomegalovirus retinitis in AIDS (note mixed hemorrhage and necrosis with optic nerve infiltration.)

- External hordeolum (stye): Infection of gland and eyelash follicle on skin side of the lid
- *Staphylococcus aureus* is the organism most commonly responsible for infection
- Symptoms: Pain, focal lid erythema; globe unaffected; patients often also have blepharitis

Treatment

- Warm compresses, topical antibiotics (e.g., erythromycin)

CHALAZION

Basic Information and Clinical Presentation

- Focal, noninfectious blockage of meibomian gland
- Symptoms: Nontender swelling of lid (unless superinfected)
- Upper lid more commonly affected
- Commonly associated with acne rosacea

Treatment

- Warm compresses; incision and drainage if chronic and bothersome

BASAL CELL CARCINOMA

Basic Information and Clinical Presentation

- Most common eyelid tumor
- Usually occurs on lower lid or medial canthus

Treatment

- Surgical excision preferred to radiation or cryoablation

Eye in Rheumatologic Disease

See Table 67-3. See Figure 67-7 for an example of anterior uveitis.

TABLE 67-3	*Ocular Manifestations of Rheumatologic Disease*	
Condition	**Description**	**Associated Diseases**

Keratoconjunctivitis sicca	Reduced or absent tear production
	Burning sensation in eye
	Photophobia may be present
	Eye(s) may be red
	Symptoms of dry mouth may also be present and are suggestive of Sjögren's syndrome
		Primary Sjögren's syndrome
		Secondary Sjögren's syndrome
		  Rheumatoid arthritis
		  Systemic lupus erythematosus
		  Polyarteritis nodosa
		  Scleroderma

Episcleritis and scleritis	Episcleritis
	  Redness of eye usually limited
	  Painless
	Scleritis
	  Redness more diffuse
	  Painful
		Rheumatoid arthritis
		Systemic lupus erythematosus
		Wegener's granulomatosus
		Polyarteritis nodosa
		Relapsing polychondritis
		Seronegative spondyloarthropathies
		Inflammatory bowel disease

Uveitis (see Fig. 67-7)	Pain Redness Photophobia Ciliary flush—ring of injection around limbus	Sarcoidosis (bilateral) Seronegative spondyloarthropathies (unilateral) Behçet's disease Lyme (bilateral)
Keratitis	Inflammation of the cornea May lead to ulceration Vision affected	Systemic lupus erythematosus Wegener's granulomatosus Polyarteritis nodosa
Anterior ischemic optic neuropathy	Sudden loss of vision	Giant-cell arteritis

67

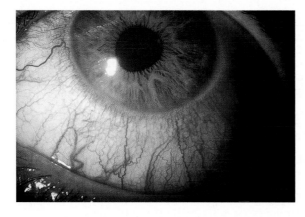

FIGURE 67-7 Anterior uveitis with ciliary flush. (From Henry MM, Thompson JN: *Clinical surgery,* ed 2, Philadelphia, WB Saunders, 2005, figure 36.14.)

REVIEW QUESTIONS

For review questions, please go to www.expertconsult.com.

SUGGESTED READINGS

Age-Related Eye Disease Study Group: A randomized, placebo-controlled, clinical trial of high-dose supplementation with vitamins C and E and beta-carotene for age-related cataract and vision loss, AREDS report no. 9, *Arch Ophthalmol* 119:1439–1452, 2001.

The Diabetes Control and Complications Trial/Epidemiology of Diabetes Interventions and Complications Research Group: Retinopathy and nephropathy in patients with type 1 diabetes 4 years after a trial of intensive therapy, *N Engl J Med* 342:381–389, 2000.

Pokhrel PK, Loftus SA: Ocular emergencies, *Am Fam Physician* 76:829–836, 2007.

Schein OD, Katz J, Bass EB, et al: The value of routine preoperative medical testing before cataract surgery: study of medical testing for cataract surgery, *N Engl J Med* 342:168–175, 2000.

Vogel R, Strahlman E, Rittenhouse KD: Adverse events associated with commonly used glaucoma drugs, *Int Ophthalmol Clin* 39:107–124, 1999.

Psychiatry for the Internist

THOMAS W. KOENIG, MD

Psychological and social problems are pervasive in our society. **An estimated 25% of adults experience some form of mental illness at some time in their lives.** This chapter provides the basic framework for diagnosing and treating a number of common conditions, including disorders of mood, anxiety, somatization, and body image. Additionally, issues involving the care of victims of domestic violence will be addressed.

Mood Disorders

DEPRESSION

Basic Information

- Everyone experiences periods in life when he or she feels "depressed"
- Depression is a symptom, not a diagnosis
- "Pathologic depression" refers to a condition that results in limitations to a person's functioning (i.e., social, occupational, or physical)
- **Major depression is seen in up to 15% of all outpatients and inpatients**
- Risk factors for major depressive disorders
  - History of a major depressive disorder in the past
  - Female gender: Major depressive episodes occur in women twice as often as in men
  - Family history of a depressive illness in a first-degree relative
- A number of medical conditions have been associated with depression, including coronary artery disease, stroke, diabetes, HIV, cancer, fibromyalgia, chronic fatigue syndrome, dementia, and other neurodegenerative disorders such as Parkinson's disease, and hypothyroidism (including subclinical disease)
  - Treatment of the underlying medical disorder may lead to improvement in the depressive symptoms in many cases
- A number of medications (e.g., β-blockers, reserpine, glucocorticoids, interferon) and illicit substances have also been associated with depression

Clinical Presentation and Diagnosis

- Symptoms vary from patient to patient
- Can coexist with other mental disorders (e.g., anxiety, somatization)
- The evaluation begins with an assessment of functional impairment and inquiry into the presence of a number of symptoms (Box 68-1)
- **Before making the diagnosis of a primary depressive disorder, inquiry should be made into**

BOX 68-1	*Symptoms and Classification of Depression*

Symptoms of a Depressive Episode
Depressed mood
Markedly diminished interest or pleasure (anhedonia)
Significant weight loss or weight gain
Insomnia or hypersomnia
Mental and physical agitation or slowing
Fatigue or loss of energy
Feelings of worthlessness or guilt
Poor concentration or indecisiveness
Recurrent thoughts of death or suicidal ideation

Major Depressive Disorder
Depressed mood or anhedonia must be present
At least five of the nine symptoms should be present
Symptoms persist for most of the day, every day, > 2 wk
Seasonal affective disorder is a subclassification used when patients present with recurrent depressive episodes at characteristic times of the year

Dysthymic Disorder
Depressed mood > 2 yr
Symptoms less severe than with major depression
Anhedonia, low self-esteem, and low energy are commonly present

Atypical Depression*
Most common mood disorder
Symptoms persist for most of the day, every day, > 2 wk
Less than five of the nine symptoms are seen

*Includes the subcategory minor depression.
Adapted from Task Force on DSM-IV: *The diagnostic and statistical manual of mental disorders,* ed 4, Washington, DC, American Psychiatric Association, 1994.

substance abuse, underlying medical disorders, and medication use
- The *Diagnostic and Statistical Manual of Mental Disorders-IV* (DSM-IV) divides depression into three subgroups: Major depression, dysthymia, and atypical depression (see Box 68-1)
  - Grief reactions are normal responses that are not considered depressive disorders, but they may progress to major depressive episodes (Box 68-2)
- **If the diagnosis of major depression is suggested, screening for the possibility of bipolar disorder (see following discussion) is recommended**

| BOX 68-2 | *Grief and Bereavement Reactions* |

Are considered normal responses to loss of someone of close relationship (usually a spouse)

Usually resolves within a few months of the death

Complicated grief reactions are the persistence of symptoms (e.g., preoccupation with thoughts of the deceased, auditory or visual hallucinations of the deceased, difficulty accepting the death)

The risk of major depression is very high (≤35%) within the first year of the loss of a loved one

Consider the diagnosis of depression in anyone whose grieving persists for longer than 2–3 mo

- Suicidal or homicidal risk should also be assessed
  - **Up to 15% of patients with untreated depression commit suicide**
  - Epidemiologic studies reveal increased suicide risk in the following populations:
    - Previous history of suicide attempt
    - Coexisting anxiety or panic disorder
    - Substance abuse
    - Older individuals (age > 65 years)
    - Whites or Native Americans
    - Patients living alone (e.g., single, divorced)
    - Patients with a recent stressful life event
    - Family history of completed suicide
  - If suicidal or homicidal ideation is present, an assessment of the patient's plan for such action should be obtained
  - **Patients with an imminent risk of suicide should be immediately referred for psychiatric services and evaluation**

Treatment

- The first step is an open discussion of and education about depression with the patient in an effort to minimize reluctance to accepting therapy
  - Emphasizing that clinical depression is a medical illness that affects numerous individuals should assist in such discussions
- Psychotherapy
  - Many different types of therapy (e.g., cognitive, behavioral, interpersonal, and group)
  - Effective as the sole mode of therapy for milder presentations of major depression
  - For more severe presentations, medications should be combined with psychotherapy
- Medications
  - A number of antidepressant medications are currently available with roughly equivalent efficacy rates (Table 68-1)
  - A number of factors should be considered when choosing a specific antidepressant, including
    - Patient's previous success with a specific medication
    - Coexisting medical conditions
    - Potential drug interactions
    - Cost
    - Anticipated side effects
    - History of response of a family member to a particular agent

- A response is usually seen within 6 to 8 weeks after a therapeutic dose of antidepressant is attained
  - Initially patients may not report any improvement in mood or anhedonia, but questioning may reveal improvement in other symptoms such as energy level, sleep, appetite, anxiety, or ability to concentrate
  - If there has been a partial response to therapy, the medication dosage can be increased, the medication can be changed, psychotherapy can be added, or augmentation therapy can be added (see following discussion)
  - If there is absolutely no response to therapy within 8 weeks, another medication should be chosen
- **The duration of therapy is usually 6 to 12 months. Patients with a history of recurrent major depressive episodes should be considered for maintenance therapy.**
  - Tapering of medications is usually necessary to prevent or observe for the return of depressive symptoms and withdrawal effect
- Electroconvulsive therapy (ECT)
  - Typically used for severe depression or cases refractory to other therapies
  - Requires general anesthesia
  - Typically requires 6 to 12 treatments over the course of 2 to 4 weeks
  - Patients usually require antidepressant treatment following a course of ECT to prevent relapse
  - Some patients benefit from "maintenance ECT" when medication trials have failed
- Augmentation therapy
  - Considered when there is a partial response to antidepressant therapy
  - A number of medications have been shown to be useful in conjunction with standard antidepressants (e.g., lithium, triiodothyronine, pindolol, and methylphenidate)

BIPOLAR AFFECTIVE DISORDER

Basic Information

- Refers to the occurrence (and recurrence) of manic or hypomanic episodes usually alternating with episodes of depression
- Affects 1% of the population
- First episode usually occurs in the second and third decades of life, and depression is most common as the index episode

Clinical Presentation and Diagnosis

- Mania consists of a persistently elevated, expansive, or irritable mood and three of the following lasting at least 1 week
  - Inflated self-esteem
  - Decreased need for sleep
  - Flight of ideas or racing thoughts
  - Hypertalkativeness, pressured speech
  - Distractability
  - Psychomotor agitation, hyperactivity, or increased activity
  - Excessive involvement in pleasurable activities (e.g., sexual indiscretions, spending money)

TABLE 68-1	*Antidepressant Medications*		
Drug Class	**Examples**	**Side Effects**	**Comments**
Selective serotonin reuptake inhibitors (SSRIs)	Citalopram Fluoxetine Paroxetine Sertraline Luvoxamine	Nausea, vomiting, diarrhea Sweating Headache Sedation or agitation Sexual dysfunction Serotonin syndrome*	Widely used because of tolerability and ease of use Also effective for cases of anxiety and panic disorder Can raise levels of many drugs including anticonvulsants, digoxin, warfarin, antiarrhythmics, β-blockers
Serotonin/norepinephrine reuptake inhibitor	Venlafaxine Duloxetine	Nausea, vomiting, diarrhea Headache Insomnia Hypertension	Activating rather than sedating so good for "understimulated" patients
Norepinephrine and dopamine reuptake inhibitor	Bupropion	Dry mouth Constipation Dizziness Weight loss Seizures (at high doses)	Also used for smoking cessation Low incidence of sexual dysfunction Activating rather than sedating Avoid in patients with eating or seizure disorders
Norepinephrine and serotonin antagonist	Mirtazapine	Sedation Weight gain Orthostatic hypotension	Low incidence of sexual dysfunction
Serotonin antagonist and reuptake inhibitor	Trazodone	Sedation Orthostatic hypotension Dry mouth Liver damage or failure (nefazodone) Priapism (trazodone)	Low incidence of sexual dysfunction
Norepinephrine/serotonin reuptake inhibitors (tricyclic antidepressants)	Amitriptyline Imipramine Desipramine Nortriptyline	Orthostatic hypotension Dry mouth Blurry vision Constipation Sedation Weight gain Urinary retention Sexual dysfunction QT prolongation and arrhythmias	Need to titrate dose and follow blood levels Should avoid in patients with cardiac disease Can be useful in patients with coexisting illnesses such as insomnia, migraine, panic disorder, neuropathic pain disorders
Monoamine oxidase inhibitor	Phenelzine Tranylcypromine	Orthostatic hypotension Dry mouth Constipation Sedation Urinary retention Sexual dysfunction Hypertensive crisis with intake of tyramine-rich foods, meperidine, decongestants, SSRIs	Useful for "atypical depression" (hypersomnia, overeating, worsening depression in the evenings, prominent anxiety) Can treat hypertensive crisis with phentolamine

*Serotonin syndrome is a change in mental status, diaphoresis, rigors, hyper-reflexia, and tachycardia because of hyperstimulation of brainstem serotonin receptors caused by coadministration of an SSRI and another agent that increases serotonin level.

68

- May be delusional or experience hallucinations
- Hypomania is considered an abnormal elevation of mood but not to the extent that it seriously impairs functioning
  - Delusions and hallucinations do not occur in hypomania
- Classification of bipolar disorder
  - Type I: Positive history of at least one manic episode, with or without past major depressive episodes
  - Type II: Positive history of at least one episode of major depression and at least one hypomanic episode
- Need to evaluate patient for medical conditions and drug use that may mimic bipolar disorder (e.g., substance abuse, personality disorders, thyrotoxicosis, steroid-induced mania)

Treatment

- Lithium carbonate
  - Most studied mood stabilizer
  - Also has antidepressant effects
  - Side effects include GI distress (nausea, vomiting, diarrhea), sedation, weight gain, acne, bradycardia, diabetes insipidus (polyuria, polydipsia, hypernatremia), hypothyroidism, renal insufficiency, and benign leukocytosis
  - **A creatinine level, thyroid function tests, electrocardiogram, and pregnancy test (if appropriate) should be obtained before beginning therapy**
  - Drug levels must be monitored

- Anticonvulsants (e.g., carbamazepine, valproic acid) can also be effective; lamotrigine shows promise as treatment for bipolar depression
- Antipsychotics (e.g., olanzapine, quetiapine) can be used
- Antidepressants for bipolar depression should be used cautiously as they can precipitate a manic or "mixed" state
- ECT can be helpful during an acute manic episode as well
- Psychotherapy should be employed in addition to pharmacotherapy in virtually all patients

Anxiety Disorders

GENERALIZED ANXIETY DISORDER

Basic Information

- Characterized by excessive anxiety and worry that result in some degree of functional impairment
- Affects women more than men
- Commonly coexists with substance abuse and other psychiatric disorders (e.g., depression, obsessive-compulsive disorder)

Clinical Presentation and Diagnosis

- Excessive, extreme anxiety and worry for more days than not, for at least 6 months
- The patient's worry is difficult or impossible to manage or control and out of proportion to the likelihood of negative events
- Three or more of the following must also occur:
  - Restlessness
  - Easy fatigability
  - Poor concentration
  - Muscle tension
  - Sleep difficulties
  - Irritability or edginess

Treatment

- Antidepressant medications (e.g., selective serotonin reuptake inhibitors [SSRIs], tricyclic antidepressants, and dual reuptake inhibitors) can all be effective
- Benzodiazepines can be useful for short-term therapy until antidepressants have taken effect
  - Avoid short-acting agents (e.g., alprazolam) because of the high incidence of dependence
- Buspirone
- Counseling or psychotherapy can be effective as sole therapy or in conjunction with medications

PANIC DISORDER

Basic Information

- Common problem seen in primary care
- Affects 4% to 6% of the population
- **Most patients present with unexplained somatic complaints (e.g., chest pain, abdominal pain, dizziness, fatigue) rather than the complaint of fear or anxiety**
  - Results in high use of health care resources from doctor visits, laboratory testing, hospitalization, and specialty referrals
- Seen more commonly in patients with mitral valve prolapse, asthma, and migraine headaches

Clinical Presentation and Diagnosis

- Presents with the abrupt onset of intense fear that may manifest with the sudden onset of somatic or cognitive symptoms
- The DSM-IV criteria for diagnosing a panic attack (Box 68-3)
- Attacks commonly occur after a significant life stress
- Often coexists with other psychiatric conditions (e.g., agoraphobia, major depression, personality disorders, post-traumatic stress disorder, and somatization disorders)
- Need to consider the presence of an underlying medical disorder that may mimic panic disorder (e.g., angina, arrhythmias, pheochromocytoma, thyroid disorders, and temporal lobe epilepsy)

Treatment

- **For mild cases that are infrequent and related to stressors, supportive psychotherapy and relaxation techniques may be the only necessary interventions**
- For more severe cases, with or without phobic tendencies, cognitive behavioral therapy or medications are useful
  - Cognitive behavioral therapy designed to modify maladaptive behavior is equivalent or superior to therapy with medications
  - Effective medications include SSRIs, tricyclic antidepressants, and monoamine oxidase (MAO) inhibitors
- Treatment should be continued for at least 12 months
  - Tapering of medications can be tried thereafter
  - There is a high rate of recurrence after discontinuation of therapy
- For acute treatment of panic attacks, benzodiazepines (e.g., lorazepam) are useful in the short term but carry the risk of dependence used long term

---

BOX 68-3	*Criteria for the Diagnosis of Panic Disorder*

A discrete period of intense fear or discomfort during which four or more of the following occur, reaching a peak within 10 min:
Palpitations
Diaphoresis
Shakiness or trembling
Shortness of breath
Sensation of choking
Chest pain or discomfort
Nausea or abdominal distress
Dizziness or lightheadedness
Depersonalization (being detached from oneself) or derealization (feelings of unreality)
Fear of losing control
Fear of dying
Paresthesias
Hot flashes

Adapted from Task Force on DSM-IV: *The diagnostic and statistical manual of mental disorders,* ed 4., Washington, DC, American Psychiatric Association, 1994.

OBSESSIVE COMPULSIVE DISORDER

- Occurs in 3% of the population
- Diagnosed in patients with either obsessions or compulsions
  - Obsessions: Recurrent thoughts, images, or impulses that cause marked anxiety and are perceived as being senseless or intrusive
    - Examples include the fear of contamination or fear of harm
  - Compulsions: Ritualistic behaviors or mental acts that are done in response to an obsession to decrease anxiety or avoid a feared consequence
    - Examples include excessive hand washing, skin-picking, or hair-pulling (trichotillomania)
- Has a significant negative effect on activities of daily living, social functioning, occupational functioning, and overall quality of life
- Treatment is psychotherapy with or without medications
  - Effective medications include SSRIs (e.g., paroxetine, fluvoxamine, fluoxetine, sertraline) or clomipramine

PHOBIAS

- One of the most common psychiatric conditions
- Divided into three basic categories
  - Specific phobia
    - Fear of objects (e.g., insects, snakes) or situations (e.g., heights, flying, drawing of blood)
    - Usually responds to behavior therapy (systematic desensitization)
    - Benzodiazepines or β-blockers can be used in some cases
  - Social phobia
    - Fear of social situations (e.g., public speaking)
    - Treated with psychotherapy and medications
    - SSRIs are considered first-line therapy
    - Benzodiazepines and MAO inhibitors are also effective
    - β-Blockers may be particularly useful in cases of performance anxiety where somatic sensations (e.g., palpitations) can be troubling
  - Agoraphobia
    - Fear or anxiety over being in a place or situation from which escape might be difficult (e.g., being alone when away from home, being in crowds)
    - Often results from panic disorder
    - Treatment is similar to that of panic disorder (see preceding discussion)

POST-TRAUMATIC STRESS DISORDER

- Severe response to a traumatic event that involved the risk of serious injury or death to the patient or someone close to the patient
- Characterized by intrusive recollections of the traumatic event, avoidance of any situations or activities associated with the event, increased arousal, and emotional detachment
- Results in significant functional impairment
- Because of the complexity of the disorder, most patients should be referred to a psychiatrist

- Treatment is with psychotherapy and medications (SSRIs)
- Recovery is expected within 1 year in one third of patients and within 10 years in two thirds of patients

SOMATOFORM DISORDERS

Basic Information

- Refers to the manifestation of psychological distress as unexplained physical symptoms
- Patients may be aware or unaware of this tendency
- **Leads to high use of medical resources through unnecessary testing, referrals, and procedures**
- Commonly coexists with other psychiatric disorders (e.g., anxiety, depression)
- Somatoform disorders are subdivided into a number of categories by the DSM-IV (Table 68-2)

Clinical Presentation

See Table 68-2.

Diagnosis

- Based largely on clinical presentation
- A thorough history and physical examination should be done to help establish a rapport with the patient and to identify coexisting psychiatric disorders and potentially overlooked medical conditions
- A review of previous patient records is invaluable in avoiding repeat testing and overuse of resources

Treatment

- No specific therapy is uniformly effective
- Should be treated as a chronic illness
  - Regular office visits should be scheduled, rather than urgent visits for new complaints
- Recognizing the disorder as a medical problem rather than a condition that is "all in your head" is imperative in developing a trusting relationship
- Avoid extensive medical testing and complicated medical regimens

EATING DISORDERS

Basic Information

- Affects over 2 million people in the United States with an overwhelming female predominance
- Usually manifests in late childhood, adolescence, or early adulthood
- Associated with a number of potential medical complications (Box 68-4)

Clinical Presentation and Diagnosis

- Two major disorders are described by the DSM-IV
  - Anorexia nervosa
    - Refusal to maintain weight within a normal range for height and age
    - Intense fear of weight gain and becoming fat
    - Disturbance in body image or denial of seriousness of current body weight
    - Absence of at least three consecutive menstrual cycles
  - Bulimia nervosa

68

TABLE 68-2   *Somatoform Disorders*

Disorder	Description
Somatization disorder	History of seeking treatment for multiple physical complaints before age 30 yr, resulting in significant functional impairment More common in women Symptoms cannot be explained by an underlying medical condition At some point during the disorder, should have complained of pain at four different sites: two gastrointestinal symptoms, one sexual symptom, one neurologic symptom
Undifferentiated somatoform disorder	One or more unexplained physical complaints lasting ≥6 mo Results in significant functional impairment Not caused by another mental disorder
Conversion disorder	One or more unexplained symptoms suggesting deficits in normal neurologic function Presentation follows the patient's view of the disease rather than neurophysiology Examples include amnesia, aphonia, blindness, paralysis, paresthesias, seizures
Hypochondriasis	Misinterpretation of bodily symptoms as a serious underlying disease Preoccupation exists despite appropriate medical evaluation and reassurance Disturbance lasts for >6 mo Usually presents in the third decade of life
Pain disorder	Unexplained or amplified complaints of pain Presents in fourth or fifth decade of life Specific psychological factors can often be related to the onset of the pain
Body dysmorphic disorder	Preoccupation with an imagined or exaggerated defect in appearance Onset is usually in the second or third decade of life
Factitious disorder	Intentional feigning or induction of physical signs or symptoms to assume the sick role Can lead to multiple hospitalizations (chronic factitious disorder or Munchausen's syndrome) Secondary gain not evident
Malingering	Intentional feigning or induction of physical signs or symptoms for secondary gain (e.g., compensation for injuries)

BOX 68-4   *Medical Complications of Eating Disorders*

Dental erosions (Fig. 68-1)

Enlarged parotid glands

Hair loss and brittle nails

Calluses over the knuckles (Mallory-Weiss tears) caused by induction of vomiting

Neurologic disease—seizures, myopathy, neuropathy, cognitive difficulties

Cardiac disease—bradycardia, arrhythmias, congestive heart failure, ECG abnormalities

Gastrointestinal disease—dysmotility, esophagitis, gallstones, Mallory-Weiss tears, superior mesenteric artery syndrome

Endocrinologic disease—amenorrhea, osteoporosis, sick euthyroid syndrome, growth retardation, infertility

Hematologic—anemia, leukopenia, thrombocytopenia

Electrolyte abnormalities—hypokalemia, metabolic alkalosis (in patients who purge), hyponatremia

- Episodes of out-of-control binge eating with compensatory purging (vomiting, laxative abuse) or nonpurging (excessive exercise, strict dieting or fasting) behavior to prevent weight gain
- Binging and compensatory behavior occurs at least twice per week for 3 months
- Self-evaluation is unduly influenced by body weight and shape

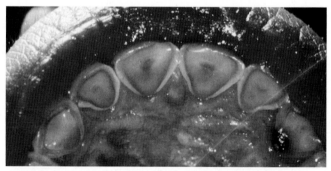

FIGURE 68-1   Advanced perimolysis of the maxillary incisors in which the pulp chambers of the teeth are visible due to acid erosion from chronic vomiting. (From Stefanac S, Nesbit S: *Treatment planning for dentistry,* ed 2, St. Louis, Mosby, 2007, figure 15-9.)

Treatment

- Requires a multidisciplinary approach with a mental health specialist, medical provider (to help treat potential complications), and dietician
- Goal is for weight gain of 0.5 to 1 pound per week in outpatients
- Refeeding syndrome
  - Seen in patients with severe anorexia nervosa within 2 to 3 weeks of refeeding
  - **Manifests as cardiac abnormalities and delirium primarily caused by hypophosphatemia and other electrolyte abnormalities; significant third-spacing of fluid**

- Psychotherapy is the treatment of choice
  - The addition of SSRIs (fluoxetine) or other antidepressants is effective for bulimia nervosa
  - Antidepressants may be helpful in patients with anorexia nervosa to prevent recurrences of illness or to treat comorbid depressive illness but do not significantly contribute to acute disease management

DOMESTIC VIOLENCE

Basic Information

- Defined as an ongoing physical, psychological, or sexual abuse in the home, associated with isolation, limited personal freedom, and limited access to resources (e.g., economic resources)
- An estimated 2 million people (usually women) are victims of abuse each year, resulting in over 2000 deaths
- Found in patients of all races, socioeconomic backgrounds, and ages
- Elder abuse
  - Refers to a subset of patients older than age 65 years who are subject to physical abuse, sexual abuse, neglect, or financial abuse
  - Associated with increased mortality
- Children who are victimized by sexual or physical abuse are more prone to be victims of domestic violence in adulthood

Clinical Presentation and Diagnosis

- A number of signs and symptoms are suggestive of domestic violence (Box 68-5)
- Injuries and bruising typically occur on the abdomen, genitalia, around the neck (from attempted strangulation), or around the breasts
- **The abuser may refuse to leave the examining room during the history and physical examination and may try to speak on behalf of the victim**

Diagnosis

- Most cases go unrecognized by physicians
- The key to identification is inquiry
  - Direct questions such as, "Has your partner ever punched or kicked you?" or "Are you afraid of your partner?" are more effective than general ones such as "Do you feel you are being abused?"
  - Questions about sexual and emotional abuse should also be included

Treatment

- Physicians need to identify local resources for dealing with domestic violence
  - Hospital social workers and local domestic violence hotlines can assist in this process

BOX 68-5	*Historical Clues Suggestive of Domestic Violence*

Chronic abdominal or pelvic pain
Chronic headaches
Chronic fatigue
Depression and anxiety
Frequent emergency room visits
Frequent physician visits with vague somatic complaints
History of sexually transmitted diseases
Recurrent, inconsistently explained injuries
Substance abuse

  - The National Domestic Violence Hotline (1-800-799-SAFE) can also assist in providing information about local resources
- If there is an imminent threat to life, immediate referral should be strongly encouraged
- Documentation should be specific and thorough with photographs or sketches of injuries (if present)
- Reporting
  - Only a few states require mandatory reporting of abuse against legally competent adult women
  - Abuse involving children, including children witnessing their parent being abused, should be reported to the local Department of Social Services
  - Elder abuse should be reported to the local elder abuse hotline or adult protective services

REVIEW QUESTIONS

For review questions, please go to www.expertconsult.com.

SUGGESTED READINGS

Gale C, Davidson O: Generalised anxiety disorder, *BMJ* 334:579–581, 2007.
McHugh PR, Slavney PR: *The perspectives of psychiatry*, ed 2, Baltimore, Johns Hopkins University Press, 1998.
Task Force on DSM-IV: *Diagnostic and statistical manual of mental disorders*, ed 4, Washington, DC, American Psychiatric Association, 1994.
Toohey JS: Domestic violence and rape, *Med Clin North Am* 92:1239–1252, 2008.
Yager J, Andersen AE: Clinical practice: anorexia nervosa, *N Engl J Med* 353:1481–1488, 2005.

Acknowledgment

This chapter is adapted from a chapter written by Todd S. Cox, MD, and Bimal Ashar, MD, MBA, for the first edition of *The Johns Hopkins Internal Medicine Board Review*.

68

Allergy and Immunology for the Internist

TAO ZHENG, MD, and SARBJIT S. SAINI, MD

The immune system is normally balanced to protect against foreign proteins and other allergens. However, reaction to extrinsic or intrinsic antigens can result in a cascade of events with clinical symptoms ranging from mild (pruritis, rhinorrhea) to severe (respiratory distress, vascular collapse, death).

Basic Information

- Allergens: Proteins of appropriate size that, after inhalation, injection (e.g., drug, venom), or ingestion, provoke an immunoglobulin E (IgE) antibody response and clinical symptoms in sensitive individuals. **Common aeroallergens include trees, grasses, and molds, as well as animals (e.g., domesticated pets, rodents), dust mites, and cockroaches.**
- **Acute-phase reaction:** Allergic response that begins within minutes of allergen exposure; **symptoms include pruritis and hives (skin), wheezing (lungs), rhinorrhea and sneezing (nose), erythema, and tearing of eyes**
  - Allergen cross-links specific IgE bound to the surface of mast cells and basophils
  - After surface IgE is cross-linked, mast cells and basophils release mediators such as histamine (stored in cytoplasmic granules) and leukotrienes/prostaglandins (rapidly synthesized from arachidonic acid)
- **Late-phase reaction:** Occurs 4 to 12 hours after acute phase and initial allergen exposure; **symptoms are similar to acute-phase reaction and mirror the inflammation seen in asthma and chronic rhinitis**
  - Pathogenesis includes leukocyte (eosinophil, T-helper type 2 cell [Th2 cell]) infiltration into tissues, which release Th2 cytokines (interleukin-4, -5, and -13 [IL-4, IL-5, and IL-13]) and chemokines (chemoattractant cytokines)
  - Histamine levels also increase

Clinical Presentation of Allergic Reactions

- **Anaphylaxis:** An IgE-related response after exposure to antigen, resulting in the rapid onset of systemic symptoms, including pallor, pruritis, dyspnea, wheezing, weakness, urticaria, erythema, flushing, cyanosis, angioedema, diarrhea, nausea, vomiting, abdominal cramping, and hypotension; some present with a biphasic illness, beginning with early abdominal symptoms before respiratory symptoms or vascular collapse set in; **may**

be fatal because of upper airway obstruction or cardiovascular collapse
  - Mechanism: Mast cell and basophil mediators released by allergen binding IgE; **mediators released include elevated serum β-tryptase level, histamine, platelet activating factor, prostaglandin D2, leukotrienes, and cytokines (e.g., tumor necrosis factor-α and IL-1); non-IgE-mediated factors include C3a and C5a**
  - Causes of anaphylaxis
    - Foods (especially nuts, shellfish, eggs, and milk)
    - Exercise (generally in people with an allergic background)
    - Medications (see following discussion)
    - Insect bites (for which immunotherapy > 97% protective)
    - Latex
  - **Idiopathic anaphylaxis: 30% to 40% of all recurrent anaphylaxis** (a diagnosis of exclusion)
  - Diagnosis of anaphylaxis is supported by the measurement of elevated serum tryptase (usually peaks in the first 2 hours)
  - **Cornerstone of treatment is avoidance of allergens;** treatment of an episode of anaphylaxis includes immediate treatment with epinephrine, followed by oxygen, antihistamines, corticosteroids, and β-agonists (as needed) for support; **patients with a history of anaphylaxis should be prescribed and carry an autoinjectable form of epinephrine**
- **Anaphylactoid reaction: A non–IgE-triggered process that clinically resembles anaphylaxis; may be caused by aspirin and NSAIDs, radiocontrast agents, and, rarely, opiate drugs**
  - Symptoms from aspirin and NSAIDs include rhinoconjunctivitis, urticaria, bronchospasm, angioedema, and laryngeal edema; treatment is avoidance or aspirin desensitization
  - Symptoms from radiocontrast agents include the spectrum of symptoms seen with anaphylaxis
    - **Despite common belief, there is no relationship of radiocontrast allergy with allergy to fish, shellfish, or iodine**
  - Pretreatment regimen includes prednisone (50 mg, administered at 13 hours, 7 hours, and 1 hour before procedure) and diphenhydramine (IM or PO) 1 hour before procedure

- Urticaria and angioedema
  - **Urticaria (Fig. 69-1) is characterized by well-circumscribed wheals from involvement of the upper layer of the dermis;** wheals are erythematous, with blanched centers, are pruritic, and may occur anywhere on the body; usually result from a type 1 hypersensitivity reaction
    - Lifetime risk of a single episode of acute urticaria is very high (i.e., one in four adults)
    - Urticaria lasting more than 6 weeks is labeled *chronic* urticaria; most are idiopathic
      - Biopsy of persistent lesions (>72 hours) should be done to exclude vasculitis
  - **Angioedema (Fig. 69-2) is characterized by the acute development of swelling and edema of submucosa or subcutaneous tissue in the skin, mucous membrane, and GI tract;** symptoms are based on tissue involved; typically nonpruritic

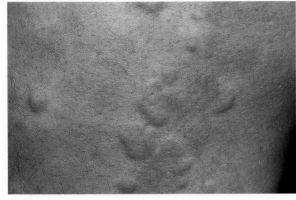

FIGURE 69-1 Urticaria with characteristic wheals surrounded by an erythematous flare. (From Forbes CD, Jackson WF: *Color atlas and text of clinical medicine,* ed 3, St. Louis, Mosby, 2003, figure 2.39.)

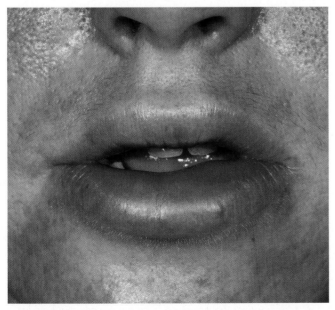

FIGURE 69-2 Angioedema commonly involves the lip. (From Habif TP: *Clinical dermatology: a color guide to diagnosis and therapy,* ed 4, Philadelphia, Mosby, 2004, figure 6-6.)

- Occurs with urticaria in approximately 50% of chronic cases
- 10% of chronic cases have angioedema alone and 40% urticaria alone
- Hereditary angioedema also occurs without urticaria (Table 69-1)
- **Differential causes of urticaria or angioedema**
  - Drugs (e.g., angiotensin-converting enzyme [ACE] inhibitors)
  - Thyroid disorders
  - Autoimmune disorders (e.g., vasculitis)
  - Infections (e.g., viral, including hepatitis, and parasitic)
  - Food
  - Malignancy
  - Cryoglobulins
  - Physical triggers of urticaria may also exist, including cold, heat, pressure, and exercise
  - Mechanism unknown; may involve chronic mast cell degranulation; a subset of patients will have antibodies against IgE or the IgE receptor
  - **Cornerstone of treatment is antihistamines;** may add histamine-2 (H_2) blocker or tricyclic antidepressant (e.g., doxepin) for severe cases; short-term oral corticosteroids are also used for severe eruptions

Clinical Presentation of Allergic and Immune-Related Diseases

- **Allergic rhinitis:** Allergen-induced inflammation of the lining of the nose characterized by nasal congestion, rhinorrhea, sneezing, itch, and postnasal drainage; **the most common adult allergic disease (15% of U. S. population)**
  - Overlap of symptoms with viral upper respiratory tract infection, nasal polyposis, nonallergic rhinitis with eosinophilia, and hormonally related nasal congestion (pregnancy, oral contraceptives, hypothyroidism)
  - Medications may also cause symptoms confused with allergic rhinitis (e.g., cocaine and β-blockers)
    - **Rhinitis medicamentosa: Overuse of over-the-counter topical nasal decongestants**
  - Other causes of symptoms that overlap with allergic rhinitis include vasomotor rhinitis (nasal congestion brought on by irritants such as cigarette smoke and cold air) and anatomic abnormalities (e.g., cerebrospinal fluid leak, deviated septum)
- Drug allergy: **Most adverse drug reactions (ADRs) do not have an immunologic basis** (<10% of all ADRs are immunologically based); the mechanism of many drug reactions is unknown
  - Most drugs are small molecules that cannot act as an antigen unless modified
  - Drugs may act as a hapten, in which the drug or its metabolite combine with a larger carrier protein and can thereby become immunogenic
    - Prior exposure is needed to generate an IgE antibody response
  - Time of onset from drug initiation assists in identifying allergic-type reactions

69

TABLE 69-1 *Allergic Skin Diseases*

Disease	Clinical Presentation	Pathogenesis	Diagnosis	Treatment
Hereditary angioedema	Autosomal dominant Recurrent swelling of face, airway, GI tract, extremities Bowel edema may result in severe abdominal pain that resolves spontaneously Trauma may trigger symptoms Urticaria uncommon	Absence of C1 esterase inhibitor (85%) Dysfunctional C1 esterase inhibitor (15%)	Clinical presentation Absence of C1 esterase inhibitor plus low C4 levels (caused by chronic complement consumption) C4 levels low even if symptoms absent	Synthetic androgens (e.g., danazol, stanazol) induce inhibitor synthesis Purified C1 esterase inhibitor concentrate also available Kallikrein inhibitors
Acquired angioedema	Same as above, with onset later in life	Autoantibodies develop to C1 esterase inhibitor Suggests underlying malignancy (leukemia, lymphoma)	C4 levels low Low C1q levels distinguish this from hereditary form	Treat underlying disease
Allergic contact dermatitis	Vesicular eruption with well-demarcated borders on exposed skin area Common causes include poison ivy, nickel, carrier substances in topical medications (e.g., thimerosal)	T cells activated, release γ interferon Macrophages then activated	Patch testing of suspected substance	Avoid offending agent Topical steroids Oral steroid taper
Atopic dermatitis	Dry, scaling skin with pruritis Commonly involves head and face Antecubital and popliteal fossae, as well as nape of neck commonly involved in adults	Unclear, but commonly an inherited pattern of elevated IgE, eosinophilia, and evidence of IgE sensitization to antigens	Patients often have positive family history Associated with asthma and allergic rhinitis Associated with dry skin Serum IgE often elevated	Topical corticosteroids to involved area Antihistamines Topical FK506 being used for more severe reactions Antistaphylococcal antibiotics
Chronic idiopathic urticaria	Recurrent urticaria or angiodema for >6 wk	Unknown May be related autoantibodies to IgE receptor	Exclusion of drugs or other diseases	$H_1 \pm H_2$ blockers Leukotriene receptor antagonists Steroids

IgE, immunoglobulin E.

- Immediate (<1 hour): Pruritis, urticaria, rhinitis, wheezing, anaphylaxis
- Accelerated (1–72 hours): Urticaria
- Late (>72 hours): Maculopapular eruption (Fig. 69-3), drug fever, hemolytic anemia, serum sickness, nephritis, leukopenia, exfoliative dermatitis, Stevens-Johnson syndrome (Fig. 69-4)
- **Penicillins and cephalosporins are the most common causes of immunologically based ADRs,** typically acting as haptens; cross-reactivity with cephalosporins is 6% to 30% (second- and third-generation cephalosporins are less likely to cross-react); carbepenems (i.e., imipenem) cross-react with minor determinants of penicillin [PCN], whereas monobactams (i.e., aztreonam) can be safely administered to PCN-allergic patients
  - Other ADRs from PCN include antibody-mediated hemolytic anemia and thrombocytopenia; immune complex disease (characterized by fever, rash, glomerulonephritis, and lymphadenopathy); cell-mediated contact dermatitis (with topical preparations); maculopapular rash seen in 5% to 13% of patients administered amoxicillin (incidence is increased with coincident Epstein-Barr virus and cytomegalovirus)
    - Basis of rash with amoxicillin is unknown; can often treat through the rash with close monitoring
- **Sulfonamides are the second most common antibiotic class to cause drug reactions,** usually via a T cell–mediated reaction; seen commonly in patients with HIV
- Allergic skin diseases: Include hereditary and acquired angioedema, allergic contact dermatitis (Fig. 69-5), and atopic dermatitis (Fig. 69-6; see Table 69-1)
- Immunodeficiency syndromes: Include immunoglobulin deficiencies, T-cell and B-cell deficiencies, as well as neutrophil and complement disorders
- Eosinophilia syndromes
  - Churg-Strauss vasculitis: A granulomatous vasculitis involving multiple organ systems, predominantly the lungs
    - Patients present with severe asthma in the setting of systemic illness (fevers, malaise, weight loss), accompanied by pronounced eosinophilia
    - Fleeting pulmonary infiltrates commonly seen on chest radiography
    - Skin rash may also be seen; sinus involvement also has been described
  - Hypereosinophilic syndrome
    - Systemic disorder characterized by dysfunction of several organs in the setting of persistent eosinophilia (>1500 cells/mL for at least 6 months)
    - Diagnosis involves exclusion of other causes of eosinophilia
    - Cardiac involvement is major cause of mortality
    - Recently identified genetic mutation (platelet-derived growth factor receptor alfa [FIP1L1-PDGFRA]) in some cases

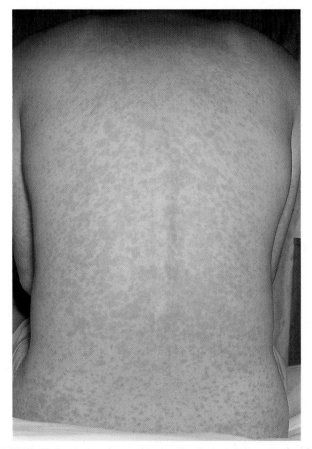

FIGURE 69-3 A maculopapular eruption in a patient treated with co-trimoxazole. (From Forbes CD, Jackson WF: *Color atlas and text of clinical medicine,* ed 3, St. Louis, Mosby, 2003, figure 2.147.)

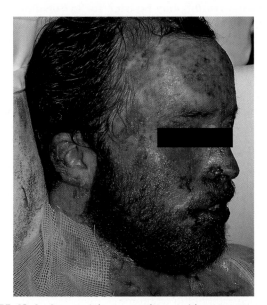

FIGURE 69-4 Stevens-Johnson syndrome with mucocutaneous facial lesions. (From Forbes CD, Jackson WF: *Color atlas and text of clinical medicine,* ed 3, St. Louis, Mosby, 2003, figure 2.49.)

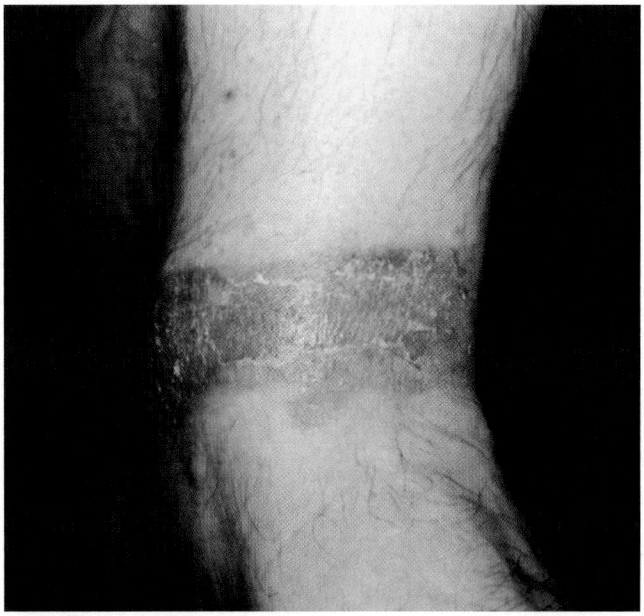

Diagnosis

- Diagnosis of allergic rhinitis
  - **Clinical presentation and historical features are often sufficient for treatment**

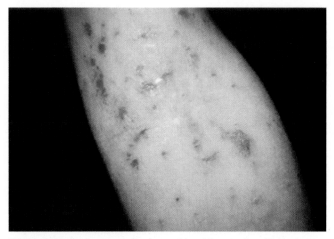

FIGURE 69-5 Allergic contact dermatitis caused by an ankle bracelet. (From Adkinson NF, Yunginger JW, Busse WW, et al: *Middleton's allergy: principles and practice,* ed 6, St. Louis, Mosby, 2003, plate 25.)

FIGURE 69-6 Acute atopic dermatitis with excoriated lesions. (From Adkinson NF, Junginger JW, Busse WW, et al: *Middleton's allergy: principles and practice,* ed 6, St. Louis, Mosby, 2003, plate 19.)

- Skin testing: Search for specific IgE to allergens; antihistamines must be avoided before skin testing
- **RAST (radioallergosorbent) test:** Detects the presence of allergen-specific IgE in a subject's serum by in vitro assay
  - **An alternative to skin testing if patient must continue antihistamines but less sensitive than puncture skin tests**
- Diagnosis of penicillin and related β-lactam antibiotic allergy
  - Skin test is performed with major and minor determinants to detect the presence of specific IgE; **skin test does not predict non–IgE-dependent reactions**
  - 80% to 90% of PCN "allergic" patients are not truly allergic because they lack specific IgE

69

TABLE 69-2	*Selected Immunodeficiency Syndromes*		
Disease	**Clinical Presentation**	**Diagnosis**	**Treatment**
Common variable immunodeficiency	Recurrent sinopulmonary infections Parasitic GI infections seen (esp. *Giardia*) Autoimmune diseases and malignancy risk increased	Quantitative immuno-globulin levels Plasma cells are absent Poor humoral response to immunizations	Antibiotics IV immunoglobulins every 3–4 wk
Selective IgA deficiency	The most common primary immunodeficiency (1:600) Recurrent sinopulmonary infections Asthma and atopic dermatitis more common, as are rheumatoid arthritis and lupus Anaphylaxis to blood or blood product transfusion	Low to absent IgA levels IgG and IgM levels normal	Antibiotics Avoid transfusion of blood or blood products unless donor is also IgA deficient
Adult T-cell deficiencies	Opportunistic infections (similar to HIV)	Exclude HIV Wiskott-Aldrich syndrome, a subtype, is associated with thrombocytopenia, small platelets, and eczema	Antimicrobials Wiskott-Aldrich syndrome is treated by bone marrow transplantation
Complement disorders	Early complement component deficiencies: Autoimmune disease C5–C8 deficiencies: Recurrent meningococcal or gonococcal infections	Assay of complement levels	Antibiotic

IgA, immunoglobulin A; IgG, immunoglobulin G; IgM, immunoglobulin M.

- Because most PCN or β-lactam allergic patients do not have an IgE-dependent reaction, and skin testing only tests for IgE-dependent reactions, a negative skin test does not exclude a reaction to penicillin or β-lactam antibiotic
- Stevens-Johnson syndrome and exfoliative dermatitis are contraindications for PCN use
- **Diagnosis of allergic skin diseases is often done based on the clinical presentation;** confirmation may be done with serum markers or skin testing (see Table 69-1)
- Diagnosis of immunodeficiency syndromes requires quantitative immunoglobulin levels or other serologic markers (Table 69-2)
- Diagnosis of eosinophilia syndromes
  - Churg-Strauss vasculitis is diagnosed by biopsy demonstrating granulomatous vasculitis with extravascular eosinophilic infiltration in the patient with a compatible clinical presentation
  - Hypereosinophilic syndrome is diagnosed by organ biopsy demonstrating eosinophils and tissue damage in the patient with persistent eosinophilia (>1500 eosinophils/μL for at least 6 months) when other causes of eosinophilia have been excluded

Treatment

- **Allergic rhinitis**
  - **Treatment should follow a three-tiered approach**
    - Avoidance or reduction of identified allergen triggers
    - Medications (Table 69-3)
      - Topical ocular agents may be used for coexisting allergic conjunctivitis
      - Leukotriene receptor antagonists are also approved in allergic rhinitis
    - Allergen-specific immunotherapy: Used in patients with severe allergic rhinitis who are intolerant to or refractory to medications

- Mechanism of action unknown, appears to involve shift to Th1 response to allergen
- Treatment risks anaphylaxis; 20 to 30 minutes of observation required after injection
- Maintenance dosing may be continued for 3 to 5 years
- **Drug allergy**
  - Treat with unrelated drug class if possible
  - **If no alternative antibiotic is available, desensitization may be tried for IgE-mediated hypersensitivity**
    - Can be administered either orally or intravenously with increasing doses of drug
    - Theory is that it prevents anaphylaxis by favoring univalent haptens that do not cross-link IgE and hence do not activate mast cells
    - **Duration of effect is limited to single treatment episode; must maintain uninterrupted treatment for duration of therapy**
    - **Future drug courses will require repeating the entire process**
- Allergic skin diseases: Treatment varies based on the underlying disorder (see Table 69-1)
- Immunodeficiency syndromes: Treatment includes antibiotics for infection, with other treatment based on the underlying disorder
- Eosinophilia syndromes
  - Churg-Strauss: High-dose steroids and cyclophosphamide
  - Hypereosinophilic syndrome
    - Corticosteroids
    - Hydroxyurea
    - Alfa-interferon
    - Potentially monoclonal anti-IL-5
    - Imatinib mesylate (Gleevec) used in cases with FIP-1-like mutation

TABLE 69-3	*Pharmacotherapy for Allergic Rhinitis*			
Class	**Example**	**Action**	**Symptoms Treated**	**Comments**
First-generation antihistamines	Diphenhydramine	Blocks H_1 receptor	Sneezing Rhinorrhea Pruritis	Sedation major side effect; limits use
Second-/third-generation antihistamines	Fexofenadine, cetirizine	Blocks H_1 receptor	Sneezing Rhinorrhea Pruritis	Do not cross blood-brain barrier, thus less sedating
Topical or oral decongestants	Pseudoephedrine	Stimulates α-adrenergic receptors to result in vasoconstriction	Congestion	CNS stimulation most common side effect Elevates blood pressure Phenylpropanolamine discontinued because it increases risk of CVA
Intranasal mast cell stabilizers	Cromolyn	Stabilizes mast cell membranes, preventing release of histamine, slow-reacting substance of anaphylaxis (SRS-A)	Sneezing Rhinorrhea Congestion	Best used before exposure to allergen Requires frequent dosing
Intranasal corticosteroids	Fluticasone	Reduces mast cell numbers in local tissues; inhibits cytokine synthesis	Sneezing Rhinorrhea Congestion Pruritis	Requires 1 wk of use before clinical response

CVA, cerebrovascular; H_1, histamine 1; H_2, histamine 2.

REVIEW QUESTIONS

For review questions, please go to www.expertconsult.com.

SUGGESTED READINGS

Joint Task Force on Practice Parameters; American Academy of Allergy, Asthma, and Immunology; American College of Allergy, Asthma, and Immunology; the Joint Council of Allergy, Asthma, and Immunology: The diagnosis and management of anaphylaxis, *J Allergy Clin Immunol* 101(Pt 2):S465–S528, 1998.

Middleton R, Reed S, Ellis B, et al: *Allergy principle and practice*, ed 6, St. Louis, Mosby, 2003.

Shearer WT, Li JT: Primer on allergic and immunologic diseases, *J Allergy Clin Immunol* 111:S441–S778, 2003.

69

Genetics for the Internist

HOWARD LEVY, MD, PhD

Although even the most common disorders attributable to mutation in a single gene are individually rare, when considered collectively, they constitute a major health burden. Genetic diseases affect people of all ages and ancestries and manifest symptoms in every organ system. With the completion of the human genome project and additional advances in complex disease genetics, there is growing recognition of genetic factors in common, everyday conditions encountered in internal medicine. Although cures for genetic disorders are rare, recognition and understanding of genetic factors in disease can improve detection and management of many conditions and prevent or reduce morbidity and mortality.

Basic Genetics Concepts

- Chromosomes
  - Each cell nucleus contains 46 chromosomes
    - 22 pairs of autosomes
    - 1 pair of sex chromosomes (X/Y)
  - In females, one of the two X chromosomes is permanently inactivated in each cell
    - X-inactivation is random and occurs early in embryonic development
    - Both of a woman's X chromosomes are expressed, but only one or the other in any single cell
    - Therefore, women may have some clinical manifestations of an X-linked disorder
- Genes are carried on chromosomes and thus occur in pairs
  - There are approximately 25,000 pairs of genes
  - Each member of a pair of genes is called an *allele*
  - 37 additional genes are carried on a small mitochondrial chromosome, whose inheritance and behavior are very different from that of the 46 nuclear chromosomes
- DNA variation
  - **Polymorphism: Alteration in DNA sequence that does not affect the function of the gene and typically has no clinical consequences**
  - **Mutation: Alteration in DNA sequence that changes gene function and potentially has clinical manifestations**
  - Alteration of a gene in a germ cell or zygote ultimately will be present in all cells of the resulting person, including his or her germline (the next generation of eggs or sperm), and thus can be inherited
  - Alteration of a gene in a somatic cell may result in clinical manifestations in all or part of an individual, but it will not be present in the germline and cannot be inherited

- Cancer cells accumulate multiple genetic changes that directly affect their behavior and response to therapy, but those changes are not transmitted to future generations
- One or both alleles of a gene may carry an alteration (mutation or polymorphism)
  - **Homozygosity: Both alleles are the same (either normal or altered)**
  - **Heterozygosity: One allele is normal and the other is altered**

Inheritance Patterns

- Multifactorial inheritance: Most of the common diseases and conditions seen by an internist are multifactorial, resulting from a complex interaction of genetic and environmental factors
  - **The relative contribution of genes and environment can vary, but both are important in virtually all medical conditions (Fig. 70-1)**
  - Examples
    - Mutation of a single gene may be the known cause, but environmental factors affect specific clinical outcome(s) (e.g., crises and other manifestations in sickle cell anemia)
    - An environmental exposure may be the known cause, but genetic factors affect the ultimate clinical outcome (e.g., resistance to HIV infection as a result of mutation of the CCR5 cell surface receptor)
    - Several genetic and environmental risk factors may be known to have major effects on a condition (e.g., thromboembolic disease; Fig. 70-2)
    - For most conditions, multiple genetic and environmental factors each contribute relatively small components of risk, and the complete spectrum of risk factors has yet to be fully elucidated
  - Characteristics of multifactorial inheritance
    - Males and females may be equally likely to be affected, or there may be skewing of the sex ratio
    - The condition may cluster in families with greater genetic and/or environmental risk, may appear to skip generations, and may seem to occur at random
    - No single gene inheritance pattern is obvious
    - **Estimation of risk to family members is largely empirical but increases with the number of affected relatives, closer degree of relation, and severity**
    - Box 70-1 lists red flags that should prompt consideration of increased genetic predisposition to a specific disease

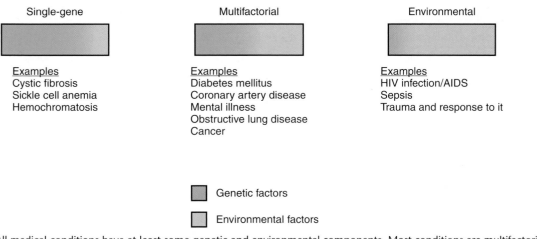

Single-gene

Examples
Cystic fibrosis
Sickle cell anemia
Hemochromatosis

Multifactorial

Examples
Diabetes mellitus
Coronary artery disease
Mental illness
Obstructive lung disease
Cancer

Environmental

Examples
HIV infection/AIDS
Sepsis
Trauma and response to it

Genetic factors

Environmental factors

FIGURE 70-1 All medical conditions have at least some genetic and environmental components. Most conditions are multifactorial, with varying mixes of both. Clinical expression of a single-gene disorder is subject to environmental effects. Response to infection or trauma depends in part on genetic susceptibility and capacity for recovery.

FIGURE 70-2 Thromboembolic disease as an example of a multifactorial condition. Several known genetic and environmental risk factors have been identified. Typically more than one risk factor is necessary to manifest the condition. Note that several risk factors are themselves multifactorial—both genetic and environmental factors contribute to cancer, inflammation, anticardiolipin antibody syndrome, hyperhomocysteinemia, and obesity.

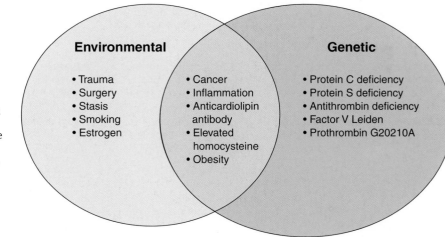

Environmental
• Trauma
• Surgery
• Stasis
• Smoking
• Estrogen

• Cancer
• Inflammation
• Anticardiolipin antibody
• Elevated homocysteine
• Obesity

Genetic
• Protein C deficiency
• Protein S deficiency
• Antithrombin deficiency
• Factor V Leiden
• Prothrombin G20210A

BOX 70-1 *Red Flags for Increased Genetic Risk for Multifactorial Condition*

Multiple affected relatives
Closely related affected relatives
Younger than expected age of onset
Occurrence in the less commonly affected sex
Multiple primary occurrences of the same or a related condition in an individual
Unusually severe manifestations
Other exceptions to usual epidemiology:
   Histopathology
   Anatomic location

- **Single gene (mendelian) inheritance: Applies when a trait or condition results from alteration of one or both alleles of a single gene**
  - One or the other of each pair of chromosomes (and thus genes) is passed along in each egg or sperm cell
  - An altered allele can be inherited from either parent (or both if they are both carriers)

- DNA polymorphisms and mutations do not have to be inherited from either parent; they can occur as new errors in an egg or sperm cell
- See Table 70-1 for characteristics of autosomal dominant, autosomal recessive, and X-linked inheritance patterns
- See Table 70-2 for examples of some mendelian disorders
- **Mitochondrial inheritance (see Table 70-1) applies when a trait or condition results from alteration of the mitochondrial DNA**
  - Each mitochondrion carries multiple copies of its chromosome, and each cell contains many mitochondria
  - **Heteroplasmy—the relative proportion of normal and abnormal mitochondria within individual cells, tissues, and organs—affects the severity and distribution of clinical manifestations**
    - Significant genetic variation exists within and between individual mitochondria in a single cell as well as between individual cells, tissues, and organs
    - Heteroplasmy can vary over time within a single person and even in different tissues within a single person

70

TABLE 70-1	*Inheritance Patterns*			
	Autosomal Dominant	**Autosomal Recessive**	**X-Linked Recessive**	**Mitochondrial**
Definition	Heterozygosity for mutation of a single gene is sufficient to cause the condition (unless the gene is on the X or mitochondrial chromosome)	Homozygosity for mutation of a single gene is necessary to cause the condition (unless the gene is on the X or mitochondrial chromosome) Carriers (heterozygotes) usually have no clinical manifestations	The condition results from mutation of a single gene located on the X chromosome Also called "sex-linked," because of characteristic inheritance patterns in men and women	Mutation of a gene contained on the mitochondrial chromosome causes the condition Most mitochondrial proteins are encoded on nuclear genes, and therefore follow autosomal or X-linked inheritance patterns
Distribution in the family	Multiple generations affected	One or more siblings affected, but only in one generation	Multiple generations affected May appear to skip generations when transmitted by a carrier female Affected males are related to each other through one or more carrier females	Multiple generations affected
Parents of an affected	Usually one or the other affected Sometimes neither affected	Usually both are carriers Usually neither affected	Mothers often carriers Fathers of affected sons are *never* affected	Mothers almost always affected Fathers never affected
Siblings of an affected	50% chance of being affected (unless neither parent affected)	25% chance of being affected 50% chance of being a carrier	Brothers have 50% chance of being affected Sisters have 50% chance of being a carrier	All are affected
Children of an affected	50% chance of being affected	All are carriers Can be affected only if the other parent is a carrier	Sons of affected fathers are *never* affected (always inherit father's Y and mother's X chromosomes) Daughters of affected fathers are *always* carriers (always inherit father's X chromosome) Sons of carrier mothers have 50% chance of being affected Daughters of carrier mothers have 50% chance of being a carrier	All children of affected mothers are affected No children of affected fathers are affected
Sex ratio	Males and females equally likely to be affected	Males and females equally likely to be affected	Almost all affected patients are male	Males and females equally likely to be affected
Other comments	Reduced penetrance and variable expression are common	Parental consanguinity is sometimes present Relatively high prevalence of some recessive conditions due to "heterozygote advantage," in which carriers have a survival advantage (e.g., carriers of sickle cell anemia are relatively resistant to malaria)	Male-to-male transmission does not occur Carrier females may have mild clinical manifestations	Heteroplasmy often results in variable expression, complicating recognition of some affected relatives

- **Mitochondria are inherited almost exclusively through the egg; sperm mitochondria only rarely are incorporated into a fertilized egg**
- Clinical manifestations vary but are primarily neuromuscular
  - Central nervous system: Encephalopathy, seizures, dementia, migraine, strokelike episodes, ataxia, spasticity
- Peripheral nervous system: Ptosis, external ophthalmoplegia, sensorineural deafness, optic atrophy, pigmentary retinopathy, peripheral neuropathy, autonomic neuropathy
- Skeletal muscle: Proximal myopathy, weakness, hypotonia
- Cardiomyopathy

TABLE 70-2	*Some Representative Single-Gene Disorders*
Condition	**Some Clinical Considerations**

Autosomal Dominant	
Marfan syndrome	Joint laxity; characteristic skeletal features; myopia and/or lens dislocation; aortic aneurysm/dissection
Neurofibromatosis type 1	Benign and occasionally malignant nerve sheath tumors; hypertension
Polycystic kidney disease	Renal, hepatic, and splenic cysts; renal failure; nephrolithiasis; hypertension; cerebral berry aneurysms occur in ~10% and correlate with specific mutations, so family history predicts risk of aneurysm
Hereditary breast and ovarian cancer	Breast and ovarian cancer; other associated cancers
Hereditary nonpolyposis colon cancer	Colon and other associated cancers
Familial adenomatous polyposis	Colon and other associated cancers; characteristic benign ocular manifestations; fully penetrant—100% chance of cancer
Multiple endocrine neoplasia syndromes	Benign and malignant endocrine tumors; benign tumors frequently hormonally active
Achondroplasia	Most common cause of dwarfism
Autosomal Recessive	
Hemochromatosis	Iron overload; cardiac, hepatic, endocrine, and joint complications; low clinical penetrance
Sickle cell anemia	Hemoglobinopathy; painful and degenerative ischemic complications; certain infections; more common in descendents of traditional malarial regions (especially Africa)
Cystic fibrosis	Defective ion transport; sinopulmonary, pancreatic, intestinal, and fertility complications; especially common in Northern Europeans; different specific mutations more common with different ancestry
α and β Thalassemia	Hemoglobinopathy; anemia; α more common in Chinese and Southeast Asians; β more common in Mediterranean peoples
Tay-Sachs disease	Neurodegenerative condition due to metabolic enzyme deficiency; common in Ashkenazi Jews and French Canadians, but disease itself is now rare in those populations due to effective screening programs
X-Linked	
Fragile X syndrome	Mental retardation; characteristic facial features; joint laxity
Hemophilia A	Classic hemophilia, due to factor VIII deficiency; bleeding diathesis; variable expression
Duchenne/Becker muscular dystrophy	Most common cause of muscular dystrophy; Becker less severe than Duchenne, but same gene

- Diabetes mellitus
- Susceptibility to aminoglycoside-induced ototoxicity
- **Chromosomal inheritance: Exists when all or part of a chromosome is duplicated or deleted**
  - **Numerical abnormalities: An extra or missing chromosome usually results from nondisjunction, or failure to properly divide one pair of chromosomes during meiosis; it is generally not inherited or passed along to future generations**
    - Monosomy of the X chromosome (45 chromosomes, only one X) is Turner's syndrome
      - 99% end in miscarriage
      - Always female
      - Short stature, characteristic physical features, but normal intelligence
      - Most are infertile
    - Monosomy of an autosome always results in miscarriage
    - Trisomy (three copies) of an autosome almost always results in miscarriage.
      - Trisomy 21 causes Down syndrome, characterized by mental retardation, short stature, cardiac defects, and other malformations
    - An extra copy of the X chromosome has milder manifestations, including tall stature and mild mental retardation
    - An extra copy of the Y chromosome usually has no clinical effect; contrary to older reports, this condition does not cause violent behavior or greater likelihood of incarceration
  - Structural abnormalities
    - Deletions or duplications of large segments of a chromosome
      - Clinical manifestations may include mental retardation, growth retardation, and malformations
      - May be inherited from a parent with a balanced rearrangement (see following discussion), but affected patients with large deletions or duplications usually do not reproduce
    - Microdeletions, or contiguous gene syndromes, involve loss of a short segment of a chromosome and affect only a few genes
      - Clinical manifestations may be similar to, or milder than, large deletions and duplications

70

- Many are compatible with a normal lifespan and fertility
- Can occur as a new genetic change or can be inherited in an autosomal dominant pattern
- Balanced rearrangements occur when segments are exchanged between two or more chromosomes, but no material is deleted or duplicated
  - May have no clinical manifestations
  - May cause symptoms by disrupting a gene
  - May cause symptoms by creation of a new abnormal gene (e.g., the Philadelphia chromosome in chronic myelogenous leukemia is a translocation that joins portions of two genes, producing a hybrid that contributes to unregulated growth)

Complications of Inheritance Patterns

- **Variable expression: Any feature of a condition may vary greatly from one patient to the next, including age of onset, severity and frequency of manifestations, and organ and tissue distribution of manifestations**
  - Variation occurs not only between unrelated individuals but also among members of the same family who all carry the same mutation
  - Environmental factors and small effects from other genetic changes contribute to variable expression
  - Distinguished from multifactorial inheritance because the condition is clearly caused by mutation in one or both alleles of a single gene
  - **An individual may carry and transmit a disease-causing mutation, even if the expression is so mild that it goes unrecognized**
  - Sex-limited expression is a subset of variable expression because of the physiologic differences between the sexes
    - Sex-limited expression is distinct from X-linked inheritance because the likelihood of inheriting or transmitting a mutation is independent of sex or degree of clinical expression
    - Daughters of a man carrying an autosomal dominant mutation predisposing to breast cancer are at increased risk for breast cancer, even though their father is unlikely to manifest breast cancer himself
  - See Box 70-2 for examples of variable and sex-limited expression
- **Reduced penetrance: Some genetic conditions fail to manifest any clinical features in a portion of people carrying the mutant allele(s)**
  - May occur in any type of inheritance
  - Distinguished from variable expression by the complete absence of any clinical manifestations
  - Likelihood of inheriting or transmitting a mutation depends only on the mode of inheritance (dominant, recessive, etc.), regardless of whether the individual manifests any clinical features
    - Daughters of a woman carrying an autosomal dominant mutation predisposing to breast cancer are at increased risk for breast cancer, even if their mother never develops breast cancer herself

---

BOX 70-2 *Examples of Variable and Sex-limited Expression*

Frequency and severity of crises are different in every patient with sickle cell anemia

Presence or absence of berry aneurysms in polycystic kidney disease tends to be consistent within a family, but age of onset and severity of hypertension and/or renal failure are quite variable

Severity, age of onset, and progression of skeletal, ocular, cardiovascular, and other complications in Marfan syndrome are highly variable, both within and between families

Some variation in pulmonary, gastrointestinal, pancreatic, and other manifestations in cystic fibrosis may be attributed to the specific mutation (thus consistent within families), but most of the variation is independent of the specific mutation

Prostate cancer cannot occur in a female

Ovarian cancer cannot occur in a male

Breast cancer is much less likely to occur, but not impossible, in a male

Females with hereditary hemochromatosis tend to have milder and later onset of symptoms than males because of menstrual blood loss

---

- **Anticipation: Some genetic conditions become more severe or onset at an earlier age in successive generations**
  - The most common mutational mechanism is expansion of trinucleotide (or triplet) repeats within a gene, which can increase in successive generations as a result of errors in DNA replication
    - Expansion beyond a threshold results in altered gene function and clinical manifestations
    - Severity increases and age of onset decreases in proportion to the length of the repeat
  - Most diseases in this category are adult- or late childhood-onset conditions that primarily affect the nervous system
    - Huntington's disease: Adult-onset chorea, dysarthria, dysphagia, cognitive dysfunction, and psychosis
    - Fragile X syndrome: Childhood-onset mental retardation, characteristic facial features and joint laxity, but shorter trinucleotide expansions result in adult-onset ataxia, tremor, and cognitive dysfunction
- **Imprinting: Some parts of the genome are chemically tagged (imprinted) to mark whether they were inherited through the egg or sperm; an imprinted gene is expressed only from the maternal or paternal allele**
  - Inheritance of a mutation follows the traditional 50-50 pattern, but clinical expression depends on the parent of origin
    - Mutations in the silenced (inactive) parental allele have no clinical effect
    - Mutations in the active parental allele will be clinically expressed
  - **The sex of the parent who passes along the mutation is the critical factor, not the sex of the child who inherits the mutation**

Genetic Testing

- **Although "genetic testing" is usually thought of as DNA testing, family history and virtually any test or procedure may yield a result with direct or indirect genetic implications**
- Risk assessment and full discussion of the potential risks and benefits (i.e., genetic counseling) should precede DNA testing and many other forms of genetic testing
  - Consultation with a genetic counselor or medical geneticist is often appropriate
  - With adequate experience and training, an internist or subspecialist can perform pretest counseling
- **Benefits of DNA testing**
  - Can help to confirm a clinical diagnosis
  - Can establish a specific genetic cause for a disorder
  - Can help predict natural history and guide management
  - Can facilitate presymptomatic or predictive testing in relatives, subject to variation in actual clinical expression and penetrance
  - DNA test results are generally independent of environmental factors and do not change over the lifespan; therefore no need to repeat unless laboratory error is suspected
- **Limitations of DNA testing**
  - **False negatives: A negative (or normal) DNA test usually does not completely rule out disease**
    - Most DNA tests have less than 100% sensitivity (i.e., not all potential mutations in a gene can be detected by most tests)
    - Multiple different genes may cause or contribute to a condition; thus the wrong gene may have been tested
    - The individual family member who underwent testing may coincidentally have a sporadic, nongenetic cause of the disease in the family; another relative might have a detectable mutation; this is of greatest concern for common diseases, such as breast cancer
  - **False positives: A positive (or abnormal) DNA test does not always rule in disease**
    - **Polymorphisms: Some DNA variations cause no clinical manifestations**
    - Reduced penetrance and variable expression complicate prediction of clinical manifestations based solely on DNA test results
- Determining who should undergo DNA testing
  - When trying to establish, confirm, or further elucidate a genetic diagnosis, a clinically affected person is appropriate to undergo testing
  - **For predictive, presymptomatic, or carrier testing in an unaffected person, the closest or most severely affected relative should be tested first to establish what genetic mutation(s) is(are) present in that specific family and to facilitate appropriately selected DNA testing in at-risk relatives**
  - For predictive, presymptomatic, or carrier testing in an unaffected person if the specific mutation(s) within the family is(are) unknown
    - A positive test in a clinically unaffected individual may be a false positive and not accurately predict disease (e.g., the DNA change may represent a meaningless polymorphism, unrelated to the affected relative's disease)
    - A negative test in a clinically unaffected individual may be a false negative and not accurately predict protection from disease (e.g., the actual disease-causing mutation may be in a gene other than the one tested)
  - If an affected relative has been tested and the specific mutation(s) in the family is(are) known
    - A negative DNA test in an unaffected relative means he or she did not inherit the known genetic mutation and is at average risk for the disease based on his or her other risk factors (high negative predictive value)
    - A positive DNA test in an unaffected relative means he or she did inherit the known genetic mutation and is at increased risk for the disease, but the positive predictive value for actual clinical manifestations depends on the variability and penetrance of the disease
  - If an affected relative is unavailable or has negative test results, predictive or carrier testing in an unaffected person can still be performed, but positive predictive value and negative predictive value will be reduced
- Ethical and social considerations regarding genetic testing and diagnoses
  - Potential issues for an affected individual
    - Stigmatization and isolation from the family or society
    - Anxiety
    - Guilt related to potentially transmitting a disease or risk to his or her offspring
    - Employment and/or insurance (both life and health) discrimination; some legal protections exist, and abuses are relatively rare, but this is a significant potential concern
    - Privacy; others gaining access to genetic diagnoses and test results
    - Results may reveal that biologic relationships are not the same as social relationships (most commonly that one's father is not who it was thought to be)
  - Additional potential issues for relatives of an affected individual
    - Right to know that they are at increased risk for a genetic condition
    - Right to not know that they are at increased risk for a genetic condition
      - Example: An adult at risk for Huntington's disease who elects not to undergo predictive genetic testing; if his or her child has a positive predictive genetic test, then he or she almost certainly carries the same genetic mutation
    - Duty to warn: In some cases, the physician or patient may have a duty to warn relatives of an affected patient of their risk for certain diseases, even if the relatives are not patients of that physician
    - Survivor guilt related to learning that one does not have the same genetic disease or risk as a sibling, parent, or child
  - Predictive or presymptomatic testing of children or adolescents for adult-onset conditions is almost always inappropriate because obtaining such knowledge is irreversible
    - It is preferable to wait until adulthood when the risks and benefits of testing can be evaluated by the individual at risk

70

- If the disease onsets in childhood, or effective childhood interventions to reduce or prevent disease are available, then such testing may be appropriate
- Diagnostic genetic testing of a symptomatic child is not subject to this concern, but still raises all of the other issues listed in this section

Select Clinical Examples

HEREDITARY BREAST AND OVARIAN CANCER

Basic Information

- Most breast cancer is multifactorial
- Approximately 5% to 10% of all breast cancer is hereditary
- Most (60–80%) of hereditary breast cancer is due to mutations in the *BRCA1* and *BRCA2* genes, accounting for approximately 3% of all breast cancer
  - Inheritance is autosomal dominant with reduced penetrance and variable expression
- Other known genetic causes include
  - Cowden syndrome: Associated with thyroid, skin, and GI hamartomas and cancers
  - Li-Fraumeni syndrome: Associated with sarcomas
- Male breast cancer is suspicious for hereditary breast cancer
- Men are equally as likely as women to transmit a hereditary breast cancer mutation to their children, even if they do not manifest breast cancer themselves; a paternal family history of breast and/or ovarian cancer is as significant as a maternal family history

Clinical Presentation of *BRCA1* and *BRCA2* Mutations

- Breast cancer can occur as young as 30 years old
- Lifetime risk of breast cancer for women is 40% to 85%
- Lifetime risk of ovarian cancer is 16% to 60%
- Other associated cancers include peritoneal, prostate, pancreas, and possibly colon

Diagnosis and Evaluation

- Genetic testing should be preceded by genetic risk assessment and counseling, usually available through a genetics, oncology, or cancer genetics consultation
- Clinical testing of the *BRCA1* and *BRCA2* genes is available, but sensitivity is less than 100%
- If a *BRCA1* or *BRCA2* mutation is identified in a family, relatives at risk need only be tested for that specific mutation
- Testing for some other genetic causes of hereditary breast cancer is also available and is best managed by a specialist
- Negative DNA testing in an unaffected person with strong family history has low negative predictive value if the specific genetic etiology in the family has not been identified

Treatment

- All first-degree relatives should be informed of their increased risk and offered genetic counseling

- Therapeutic response of identified cancer is similar to sporadic breast or ovarian cancer
- Bilateral mastectomy at the time of initial breast cancer diagnosis may be appropriate in patients with hereditary breast cancer

Prevention

- Breast cancer screening (breast self-examination, clinical breast examination, and radiologic imaging) should begin 10 years earlier than standard population screening or 10 years earlier than the earliest age of onset in an affected relative, whichever is younger
- Bilateral prophylactic mastectomy reduces (but does not eliminate) the risk of breast cancer
- Annual or semiannual ovarian cancer screening with pelvic examination, transvaginal ultrasound, and serum cancer antigen 125 (CA-125) beginning at age 25 to 35 years may improve detection and survival
- Bilateral prophylactic oophorectomy reduces (but does not eliminate) the risk of breast and ovarian cancer in patients with known or suspected *BRCA1* or *BRCA2* mutation, but it does not reduce the risk of peritoneal carcinoma
- For men with known or suspected *BRCA1* or *BRCA2* mutation, consider beginning prostate cancer screening 10 years earlier than standard population screening

HEREDITARY COLON CANCER

- Approximately 10% of all colon cancer is attributable to single-gene syndromes
- Hereditary nonpolyposis colon cancer (HNPCC) and familial adenomatous polyposis (FAP) are the most common causes; see individual sections that follow
- An additional 30% of all colon cancer occurs in individuals with a family history of colon cancer, consistent with multifactorial inheritance
- Patients with family history of hereditary multifactorial colon cancer should begin colon cancer screening 10 years earlier than the youngest age of onset in the family or at age 40 years, whichever is younger; colonoscopy should be repeated every 3 to 5 years

HEREDITARY NONPOLYPOSIS COLON CANCER SYNDROME

Basic Information

- HNPCC accounts for approximately 3% of all colon cancer
- Also known as Lynch syndrome
- Due to mutation in one of several DNA mismatch repair genes
- Autosomal dominant predisposition to multiple cancers with variable expression and reduced penetrance

Clinical Presentation

- **Average age of cancer onset (colon or other) is mid-40s**
- Often poorly differentiated and more aggressive than sporadic colon adenocarcinoma
- **Most colon cancers (two thirds) occur in proximal (ascending) colon, in contrast to sporadic colon cancer predominantly occurring more distally**
- Lifetime risk of colon cancer is approximately 80%
- Lifetime risk of endometrial cancer is 20% to 60%
- Other associated tumors include stomach or small bowel adenocarcinoma, transitional cell carcinoma of the

proximal ureter, sebaceous skin neoplasms, glioblastoma multiforme, and hepatobiliary and ovarian cancer

Diagnosis and Evaluation

- See Box 70-3 for clinical diagnostic criteria that suggest HNPCC
- When clinically suspected, test tumor tissue for microsatellite instability (MSI)
  - Microsatellites are regions of highly repetitive DNA
  - In tumor tissue with faulty DNA mismatch repair (i.e., in HNPCC), these regions demonstrate variable length (instability)
  - MSI within tumor tissue is highly predictive of HNPCC
- If MSI positive, proceed to DNA testing of mismatch repair genes
  - Genetic testing should be preceded by genetic risk assessment and counseling, usually available through a genetics, oncology, or cancer genetics consultation
  - Sensitivity of DNA testing is less than 100%
- **HNPCC is confirmed by positive Amsterdam II criteria or positive DNA testing**
  - Negative DNA testing does not rule out HNPCC, especially if Amsterdam II criteria are met

Treatment

- All first-degree relatives should be informed of their increased risk and offered genetic counseling
- HNPCC-associated colon cancer prognosis may be better than for sporadic colon cancer
- Total colectomy is preferred over partial colectomy in HNPCC patients with colon cancer

BOX 70-3	*Clinical Criteria to Suspect Hereditary Nonpolyposis Colorectal Cancer (HNPCC)*

Amsterdam II Criteria

All of (mnemonic "3-2-1")

    3 or more family members with HNPCC-associated cancer, each a first-degree relative of at least one other affected relative

    2 successive generations affected

    1 or more cancer(s) onset before age 50 yr

Sensitivity ~75–80%

Specificity ~50–60%

Bethesda Criteria

Any one of

    Positive Amsterdam II criteria

    Two independent HNPCC-related cancers

    Colon or endometrial cancer onset before age 50 yr

    Colonic adenoma onset before age 40 yr

    Colon cancer at any age, plus a first-degree relative with either an HNPCC-related cancer onset before age 50 yr or colonic adenoma before age 40 yr

    Poorly differentiated proximal colon cancer onset before age 50 yr

    Signet-ring cell type colon cancer onset before age 50 yr

Sensitivity ~95%

Specificity ~25%

Prevention

- Colonoscopy every 1 to 2 years beginning at age 20 to 25 years, or 10 years earlier than the earliest age of colon cancer diagnosis in the family, whichever is earlier
- Consider annual transvaginal ultrasound, endometrial biopsy, and serum CA-125 measurement, beginning at age 25 to 30 years
- **Prophylactic colectomy is not recommended because colon cancer screening is effective**
- Prophylactic hysterectomy and oophorectomy is an option

FAMILIAL ADENOMATOUS POLYPOSIS

Figure 70-3 shows an example of FAP.

Basic Information

- FAP accounts for approximately 1% of all colon cancer
- Due to mutation in *APC*, a tumor suppressor gene
- Autosomal dominant predisposition to colonic adenomas, which evolve into cancer
- **Expression is variable, but penetrance is complete (100%) for colonic adenomas and cancer**

Clinical Presentation

- Hundreds to thousands of colonic adenomas
- Average age of polyp onset is 16 years
- Average age of colon cancer is 39 years
- Other manifestations include gastric and small bowel polyps (~5–10% malignant), osteomas (never malignant), papillary thyroid cancer, hepatoblastoma, benign skin lesions (epidermoid cysts, fibromas, desmoid tumors), and extra or missing teeth
- **Congenital hypertrophy of the retinal pigment epithelium (CHRPE) occurs in 70% to 80%**
  - **Benign pigmented retinal hamartomas**
  - **When bilateral, highly suggestive of FAP, and thus a useful clinical diagnostic tool**
- Attenuated FAP (aFAP) is a milder presentation resulting from mutations in the same gene
  - Usually fewer than 100 adenomas, average is about 30
  - Average age of cancer onset is mid 50s
  - Other manifestations of FAP also occur at reduced frequency

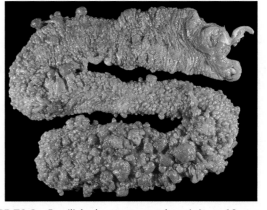

FIGURE 70-3 Familial adenomatous polyposis in an 18-year-old woman. The mucosal surface is carpeted by innumerable polypoid adenomas. (From Kumar V, Fausto N, Abbas A: *Robbins and Cotran pathologic basis of disease,* ed 7, Philadelphia, WB Saunders, 2004, figure 17.59.)

70

Diagnosis and Evaluation

- Genetic testing should be preceded by genetic risk assessment and counseling, usually available through a genetics, oncology, or cancer genetics consultation
- Among patients with typical clinical manifestations, *APC* gene analysis has a mutation detection rate of 80% to 90%

Treatment and Prevention

- First-degree relatives should be informed of their increased risk and offered genetic counseling
- Annual lower endoscopy beginning at age 10 to 12 years
- **Colectomy when there are 20 to 30 adenomas or when polyp histology is advanced; this is usually adolescence or very early adulthood**
- Postcolectomy lower endoscopic surveillance is still necessary
- NSAIDs and cyclooxygenase-2 (COX-2) inhibitors reduce the rate of adenoma formation and may help to delay colectomy from adolescence to young adulthood
- Endoscopic and radiologic visualization of the stomach and small bowel every 1 to 3 years beginning when colonic polyps are found
- Annual thyroid palpation (± annual thyroid ultrasound)

HEREDITARY HEMOCHROMATOSIS DUE TO *HFE1* MUTATIONS

Basic Information

- Homozygous mutation of the *HFE1* gene is the most common cause of iron overload in white patients
- Other genetic and environmental causes of hemochromatosis and iron overload exist
- ***HFE1* hemochromatosis is the most common autosomal recessive single-gene disorder among adults**
  - 1:200 to 1:400 white individuals has two mutant alleles (genetically affected)
  - 1:10 (10%) white individuals have one mutant allele (unaffected carrier)
- **The high carrier frequency results in pseudodominant inheritance**
  - 100% chance that a genetically affected person passes along a mutant allele to the offspring
  - 10% chance that a white spouse is a carrier
  - 50% chance that a carrier spouse passes along a mutant allele to the offspring
  - **1:20 (100% × 10% × 50% = 5%) chance that a child of a genetically affected person with a white partner will also be genetically affected**
- Only two specific mutations are clearly associated with clinical disease: *C282Y* and *H63D*
  - Homozygosity for the *C282Y* mutation accounts for approximately 90% of clinically manifest cases of hereditary hemochromatosis
  - Compound heterozygosity, with one *C282Y* allele and one *H63D* allele, accounts for most of the rest
  - Homozygosity for the *H63D* mutation almost never causes clinical symptoms
  - Other variations of *HFE1* are common, but likely represent benign polymorphisms

Clinical Presentation

- Manifestations are due to increased GI iron absorption and storage in multiple organs, especially liver, skin, pancreas, joints, heart, testes, and pituitary
  - Nonspecific symptoms include abdominal pain, weakness, fatigue, lethargy, and weight loss
  - Transaminase elevation and/or hepatomegaly may or may not occur
  - Cirrhosis, portal hypertension, and liver failure may occur late in the disease
  - Hepatocellular carcinoma occurs only in the setting of cirrhosis
  - Arthralgia is common, especially in the hands, but other joints may be involved
  - Hypogonadism may be central (pituitary) or peripheral (testicular)
  - Bronze-colored hyperpigmentation, insulin-resistant or insulin-dependent diabetes mellitus, cardiomyopathy, and arrhythmia are late manifestations
- Variable and sex-limited expression
  - *C282Y* homozygotes are more severely affected than compound heterozygotes
  - Men generally have earlier onset (in their 40s and 50s) and more severe disease than women (perimenopausal onset)
- Reduced penetrance
  - Estimates vary widely (<1% to >70%), depending on genotype, method of patient ascertainment, and how clinical disease is defined
  - Even with elevated iron levels, there may be no clinical signs or symptoms

Diagnosis and Evaluation

See Figure 70-4 for an evaluation algorithm for suspected hemochromatosis.

- Increased transferrin saturation on two independent assays is the most sensitive and specific blood test for iron overload but does not establish the specific cause
  - Traditional thresholds are 60% for men and 50% for women
  - A lower threshold of 45% has higher sensitivity but lower specificity
- Increased serum ferritin is common but is not specific for iron overload
- **DNA testing is used only to confirm the diagnosis in affected individuals and to facilitate evaluation of at-risk relatives**
  - The presence of only one mutant allele establishes carrier status but is insufficient to confirm a diagnosis of hereditary hemochromatosis
  - False-positive or false-negative analysis for *C282Y* and *H63D* is unlikely
- Quantitative phlebotomy and liver biopsy can help establish the diagnosis in equivocal situations but are rarely needed
  - Older affected patients usually can tolerate removal of 4 g or more of iron via phlebotomy (8 L of blood over 16 treatments) without developing anemia
  - Younger affected patients with smaller total iron stores may become iron depleted earlier

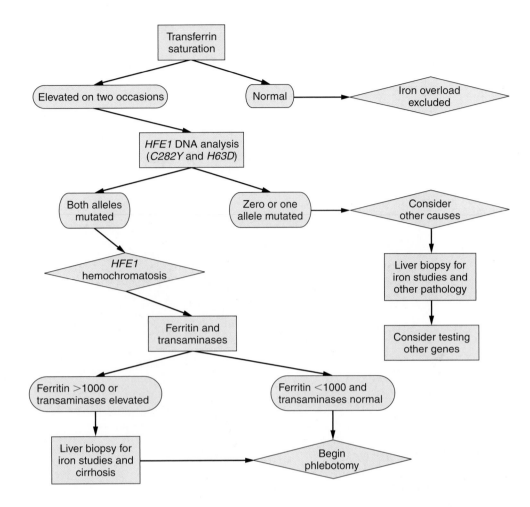

FIGURE 70-4 Algorithm for evaluation of suspected hemochromatosis.

Treatment

- **Iron-depletion therapy is appropriate only in patients with documented iron overload**
  - **Weekly phlebotomy until serum ferritin is less than 50 ng/mL**
  - If anemia occurs, decrease frequency of phlebotomy (and potentially reconsider the diagnosis)
  - **Maintenance phlebotomy about two to six times per year to keep ferritin level less than 50 ng/mL and transferrin saturation less than 50%**
  - Untreated patients with *HFE1* mutations and normal iron studies should have transferrin saturation and serum ferritin checked every 1 to 5 years
- Dietary restrictions: Avoid iron supplements, vitamin C, alcohol, and uncooked seafood
- If cirrhosis is present, screen for hepatocellular carcinoma every 6 to 12 months
- Prognosis
  - **Phlebotomy improves liver disease and may partially reverse cirrhosis but does not reduce the risk of hepatocellular carcinoma once cirrhosis has occurred**
  - Phlebotomy usually reverses cardiac complications and nonspecific symptoms (abdominal pain, weakness, fatigue, lethargy, and weight loss)
  - **Endocrine deficiencies and arthralgia usually do not improve with phlebotomy**

Prevention

- All first-degree relatives of an affected patient should be offered DNA testing
  - Siblings have a 25% chance of being affected and a 50% chance of being carriers
  - Both parents are likely to at least be carriers but may be affected
  - All children must at least be carriers but may be affected if the other parent is a carrier

NEUROFIBROMATOSIS TYPE 1

Basic Information

- **Autosomal dominant syndrome resulting in focal overgrowth of multiple tissues, especially (but not exclusively) those derived from the neural crest**
- One of the most common dominant single-gene disorders, affecting approximately 1 in 3000 people worldwide
- Results from mutation of the neurofibromatosis type 1 (*NF1*) gene, whose protein product, neurofibromin, functions as a tumor suppressor and regulator of cellular growth and differentiation

Clinical Presentation

- **Penetrance is complete (100%), but clinical expression is quite variable**

70

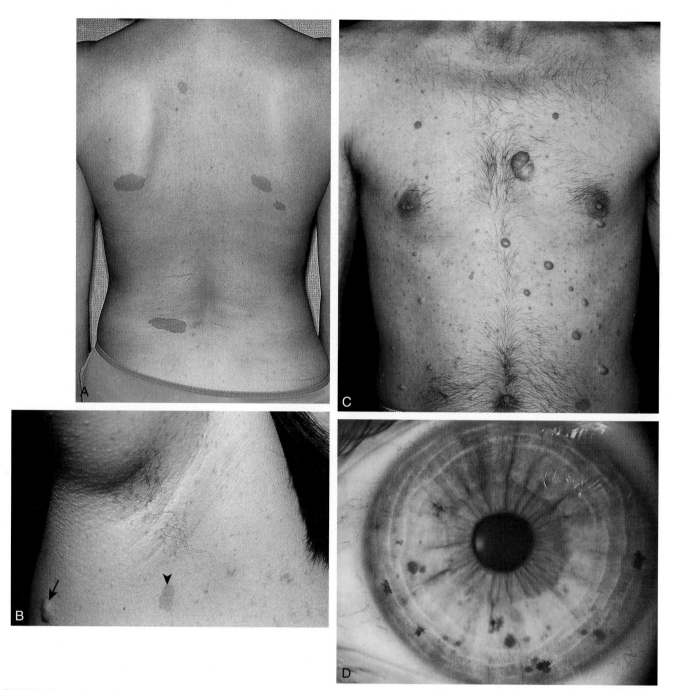

FIGURE 70-5   Some clinical features of neurofibromatosis type 1. **A,** Café-au-lait macules. **B,** Axillary freckling. There is also a small café-au-lait macule *(arrowhead)* and a dermal neurofibroma *(arrow)*. **C,** Dermal neurofibromas. **D,** Lisch nodules. (From Habif TP: *Clinical dermatology: a color guide to diagnosis and therapy,* ed 4, Philadelphia, Mosby, 2004, figures 26-11A, 26-11B, 26-12, and 26-13A.)

- Skin (Fig. 70-5A to C)
  - Café-au-lait macules occur in first year of life and increase in size and number throughout childhood
  - Axillary or inguinal freckling
  - Benign dermal neurofibromas (soft, fleshy nerve or nerve sheath–associated tumors) gradually increase in number and size throughout life but especially rapidly during puberty and pregnancy
- Plexiform neurofibromas (diffuse amorphous nerve sheath tumors) occur in up to 50% of patients, enlarge over time, and may cause significant morbidity

- Ocular
  - Lisch nodules are benign iris hamartomas present in nearly all patients by adulthood (see Fig. 70-5D)
  - Optic gliomas occur in approximately 15% of patients, but only half cause clinical manifestations (proptosis, strabismus, optic nerve pallor, reduced visual acuity, or vision loss)
- Skeletal manifestations include scoliosis, sphenoid dysplasia, and rarely long bone cortical thinning or bowing

- Pathologic fracture of thinned distal tibia is common and heals poorly, if at all, resulting in pseudarthrosis (creation of a "pseudo-joint")
- Hypertension is more frequent than in the general population
  - Occurs at any age, including childhood
  - Usually essential hypertension
  - Sometimes due to NF1 vasculopathy: Renal artery stenosis, aortic coarctation, narrowing of any other artery
- Malignancy
  - Malignant peripheral nerve sheath tumor develops from a plexiform neurofibroma in about 10% of patients
  - Pheochromocytoma, rhabdomyoma, neuroblastoma, and childhood leukemia may occur
- Unidentified bright objects are T2 hyperintensities on cerebral MRI imaging that occur anywhere in the brain in about 60% of patients and are of no apparent clinical consequence; they often regress or disappear by adulthood
- Premature death is primarily associated with malignancy and vasculopathy; average life span is about 15 years shorter than the general population

Diagnosis and Evaluation

- See Box 70-4 for clinical diagnostic criteria
- Genetic testing can detect *NF1* mutations in about 95% of affected patients but is almost never needed clinically
  - Can be used to establish the diagnosis in young children not yet meeting clinical diagnostic criteria
  - Useful for prenatal diagnosis if the affected parent's specific mutation is known
- Evaluation and monitoring
  - Annual physical examination seeking typical manifestations
  - Blood pressure measurement at every visit
  - Ophthalmologic examination annually in children, less frequently in adults (seeking Lisch nodules and optic glioma)

| **BOX 70-4** | *Neurofibromatosis Type 1 (NF-1) Clinical Criteria* |

Two or more of the following are required to establish a diagnosis of NF1

6 or more café-au-lait macules (each >5 mm in children or >15 mm after puberty)

2 or more neurofibromas of any type or one plexiform neurofibroma

Axillary or inguinal freckling

Optic glioma

2 or more Lisch nodules (iris hamartomas)

Characteristic osseous lesion (sphenoid dysplasia or thinning of long bone cortex with or without pseudarthrosis)

An affected first-degree relative as defined by these diagnostic criteria

---

- Routine cerebral MRI is not recommended because optic nerve or intracranial lesions that require monitoring or intervention will cause clinical manifestations

Treatment

- Secondary causes of hypertension should be considered at any age, especially renovascular hypertension, pheochromocytoma, and aortic coarctation
- NF1 vasculopathy should be considered in any ischemic condition, including acute coronary and cerebrovascular syndromes
- Plastic surgery or neurosurgery intervention for problematic dermal or plexiform neurofibromas
- Sudden rapid growth or pain in a previously stable plexiform neurofibroma is suspicious for malignant transformation
- Optic gliomas and other intracerebral tumors tend to be slow growing and occasionally regress spontaneously; serial assessment of tumor size and clinical manifestations before therapeutic intervention is appropriate

Prevention

- All first-degree relatives of an affected patient should be evaluated, including slit-lamp examination for Lisch nodules
  - One or the other parent is affected (or at least mosaic—some of the cells in the body are mutated) around 50% of the time; the remaining 50% represent new mutation, with neither parent affected
  - If neither parent is affected, the patient's siblings have a very low chance of being affected (there is a small chance that a parent has germline mosaicism—some of the eggs or sperm carry the mutation without any somatic features of neurofibromatosis)
  - If a parent is affected, each of the patient's siblings has a 50% chance of being affected
  - Each child of an affected person has a 50% chance of being affected

REVIEW QUESTIONS

For review questions, please go to www.expertconsult.com.

SUGGESTED READINGS

Adams PC: Hemochromatosis, *Clin Liver Dis* 8:735–753, 2004.
Beutler E: Hemochromatosis: genetics and pathophysiology, *Annu Rev Med* 57:331–347, 2006.
Galiatsatos P, Foulkes WD: Familial adenomatous polyposis, *Am J Gastroenterol* 101:385–398, 2006.
GeneTests: Medical genetics information resource, Seattle, University of Washington, 1993–2006, Available at: www.genetests.org.
Korf BR: Principles of genetics: overview of the paradigm of genetic contribution to health and disease. In Goldman L, Bennett JC, Ausiello D, editors: *Cecil textbook of medicine*, ed 22, Philadelphia, WB Saunders, 2004.
Mecklin J-P, Järvinen HJ: Surveillance in Lynch syndrome, *Fam Cancer* 4:267–271, 2005.
Vasen HFA: Clinical description of the Lynch syndrome (hereditary nonpolyposis colorectal cancer [HNPCC]), *Fam Cancer* 4:219–225, 2005.
Viskochil D: Neurofibromatosis type 1. In Cassidy SB, Allanson JE, editors: *Management of genetic syndromes*, ed 2, Hoboken, NJ, John Wiley, 2005.

70

Complementary and Alternative Medicine

BIMAL H. ASHAR, MD, MBA

Over the past two decades, the use of healing modalities outside the realm of Western allopathic medicine has increased dramatically. This movement has been a patient-driven phenomenon that has incited the need for physicians to expand their knowledge base beyond principles and concepts taught in medical school to solidify physician–patient relationships and protect patients from potential harm. This chapter provides a basic overview of the field of complementary and alternative medicine (CAM) and describes a few specific popular modalities.

Overview

Definitions

- Alternative medicine: Approaches not routinely used by conventional practitioners
- **Complementary medicine: Use of unconventional modalities as adjuncts to established Western medicine**
- Integrative medicine: Combination of conventional and complementary methods for preventing and treating disease

Classification

- There is no one universally accepted classification system for all of CAM
- **Most modalities are used to enhance the body's natural defenses in preventing and treating disease**
- The National Institutes of Health/National Center for Complementary and Alternative Medicine has developed a classification system designed primarily to facilitate research efforts (Fig. 71-1)

Alternative Medical Systems

ACUPUNCTURE

Background

- One modality used in traditional Chinese medicine
- Many different types (e.g., auricular, five elements, hand, traditional Chinese)
- Involves the insertion of fine needles into the skin to restore the balance of life energy, or qi (pronounced "chee")

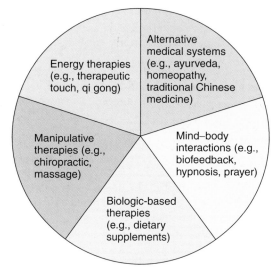

FIGURE 71-1 National Institutes of Health/National Center for Complementary and Alternative Medicine Classification of Complementary and Alternative Medicine Practices.

- **A block in the flow of qi can lead to an imbalance of flow of energy through channels in the body (meridians) and lead to disease**
- Accurate needle placement along these meridians corrects the imbalance and treats the disorder
- Heating of the needles with mugwort (moxibustion), electrical stimulation, or manual twisting of the needles may be used to achieve the desired response

Mechanism of Action

- No unifying mechanism currently exists
- Acupuncture needling has been shown to effect the release of endorphins and neurohormones and alter blood flow

Efficacy

- Data for most conditions are inconclusive
- Studies support the use of acupuncture for the following
  - Postoperative and chemotherapy-induced nausea and vomiting
  - Chronic low back pain: Equivalent to but not superior to other therapies
  - Lateral epicondylitis
  - Osteoarthritis of the knee
  - Tension headaches and migraine prophylaxis

71

- Strong data exist against its use for smoking cessation and tinnitus

Safety

- **Overall considered safe with the use of sterile needles by trained practitioners**
- Most common side effects include pain at the insertion site, localized bleeding, tiredness, and vasovagal syncope
- Rare case reports of pneumothorax, organ puncture, and hepatitis B

HOMEOPATHY

Background

- Homeopathy is based around two concepts
  - "Law of similars" suggests that substances that cause symptoms in healthy subjects can cure those symptoms in patients who are sick (e.g., digoxin is used to treat some arrhythmias that it is capable of causing)
  - "Principle of serial dilutions" suggests that medications can have a biologic effect even if diluted to levels at which the original substance is undetectable (a so-called homeopathic dose)
- Focuses on subjective symptoms rather than disease diagnoses
- Most commonly used to treat allergy, hypertension, otitis media, arthritis, and headache
- Most homeopathic remedies are sold over the counter

Mechanism of Action

- No clear mechanism identified
- Scientific implausibility of the homeopathic dose makes acceptance into mainstream medicine difficult

Efficacy

- Few good studies available
- Systematic reviews have suggested that homeopathy is superior to placebo, but data supporting the use for any particular condition are limited

Safety

- Serious adverse reactions are rare because there is little to no active ingredient in the preparation
- "Aggravation reactions" are worsening of symptoms shortly after a remedy is started and are not considered side effects by homeopaths
- Risk of adulteration exists because there is no requirement for finished product testing
- Potential for harm exists when homeopathic physicians recommend against conventional medications and/or immunizations

Manipulative Therapies

CHIROPRACTIC

Background

- Used by up to 20% of the U.S. adult population
- Most commonly used for low back pain, neck pain, and various musculoskeletal conditions
- Basic principles

- Spinal cord and nervous system are at the center of general well-being
- Malalignments of vertebrae (subluxations) cause and perpetuate disease
- Correction of the subluxations (usually via spinal manipulation) restores physiologic balance and allows the body to restore health
- Many chiropractors use massage, heat, and trigger-point injections as adjuncts to therapy

Mechanism of Action

- The mechanism of action is unknown

Efficacy

- **More effective than sham therapy for acute and chronic low back pain—equivalent to other modalities (e.g., physical therapy, analgesics, back exercises)**
- Data on efficacy for neck pain, headaches, and other conditions are quite limited
- Patient satisfaction seems to be high with this manual approach to treatment

Safety

- Low back manipulation is considered safe, although there are rare reports of cauda equina syndrome after therapy
- Most common side effects include tiredness, headache, and localized pain that are self-limited
- Reports of carotid artery dissection, vertebrobasilar vascular accidents, vertebral fracture, and tracheal rupture with cervical manipulation do exist
- **Contraindications to chiropractic therapy include coagulopathy, osteoporosis, spinal tumors or infection, and spinal instability. It should also be avoided in patients with rheumatoid arthritis.**

MASSAGE THERAPY

Background

- Involves manipulation of soft tissues
- Many different types (e.g., Swedish, deep-tissue, shiatsu)
- Goal is to effect the flow of energy through the body and restore balance and health
- Primarily used for relaxation and stress relief but also used for treatment of back or neck pain, fibromyalgia, headaches, etc.

Efficacy and Safety

- Useful for stress reduction, although duration and intensity of response are variable
- **Recent data suggest that it is a useful, cost-effective measure in the treatment of chronic low back pain**
- No clear data to support its use for other specific conditions
- Generally considered safe, although caution should be used in patients with coagulopathies, especially with deep-tissue techniques

Dietary Supplements

Overview

- Most widely used CAM modality
- Regulation in the United States

- Before 1994, regulated as foods with required premarket testing for safety and efficacy
- In 1994, the Dietary Supplement Health and Education Act (DSHEA) was enacted. It served to do the following:
  - Expand the definition of dietary supplements to include vitamins, amino acids, herbs, and other botanicals
  - Eliminate the need for companies to prove safety or efficacy before marketing their products
  - Place the burden of proof on the Food and Drug Administration (FDA) to show that a particular product is unsafe to keep it from the marketplace (e.g., ephedra ban took 7 years of data gathering)
  - Allow companies to make claims of "structure or function" (e.g., "for prostate health"), but not allow them to claim that their product was "intended to diagnose, treat, cure, or prevent any specific disease" (e.g., "for the prevention of prostate cancer")
- General issues surrounding dietary supplement safety
  - No product standardization exists (e.g., not all gingko biloba has the same active ingredients)
  - Active ingredient is often unknown, making standardization impossible
  - Potential for misidentification of herbs
  - Potential for adulteration of products with drugs or heavy metals
  - Little published data exist on the efficacy, safety, and potential for drug interactions with most dietary supplements
  - The FDA passed the Dietary Supplement Current Good Manufacturing Practices rule in 1997, which
    - Was designed to give consumers greater confidence that the dietary supplement they use has been manufactured to ensure its identity, purity, strength, and composition
    - Should apply to all companies by June 2010

Supplement Use for Selected Conditions

- Anxiety, insomnia
  - Kava kava
    - Used by natives of the South Pacific for many years
    - Superior to placebo for short-term treatment of anxiety but no data on long-term use
    - Side effects include GI upset and rash
    - Reports of idiosyncratic fulminant hepatic failure have led to its ban in Europe and Canada but it is still available in the United States
    - Avoid with other anxiolytics or alcohol
  - Valerian
    - Primarily used for insomnia
    - Very limited short-term data to support its use
    - Avoid with other anxiolytics
- Depression
  - SAMe (S-adenosylmethionine)
    - A metabolic intermediary thought vital for cellular functioning
    - Small studies suggest utility for treating depression, but most of these were done with parenteral formulations
    - **Oral bioavailability is poor**

- Considered safe but there is concern for interactions with tricyclic antidepressants
- St. John's wort (*Hypericum perforatum*)
  - Most commonly prescribed antidepressant in Germany
  - Data suggest that it is superior to placebo for treatment of major depression and may be equivalent to many standard antidepressants
  - Generally well tolerated
  - Great concern over drug–herb interactions (Table 71-1) because of its effect on the cytochrome P450 system
- Dementia
  - Ginkgo biloba
    - Thought to have a number of biologic effects, including increasing blood flow, inhibiting platelet activating factor, altering neuronal metabolism, and working as an antioxidant
    - No clear evidence to support its use for cognitive impairment or dementia
    - No evidence that it is effective for the prevention of memory loss or dementia
    - Side effects are usually rare and mild and include headaches and gastrointestinal discomfort
    - Case reports of spontaneous bleeding and seizures exist
    - Because of its potential antiplatelet effects, it should be avoided in patients taking warfarin
- Hypercholesterolemia
  - Fish oil
    - A source of omega-3 fatty acids (i.e., eicosapentaenoic acid, docosahexaenoic acid)
    - **Lowers triglycerides in a dose-dependent manner (30% reduction at doses of 2–4 g/day)**
    - Can raise low-density lipoprotein (LDL) levels by 5% to 10% at high doses

TABLE 71-1	*Potential Drug Interactions with St. John's Wort*	
Drug	**Effect**	**Potential Clinical Complication**
Cyclosporine	Decreased drug levels	Transplant graft rejection
Digoxin	Decreased drug levels	Improper rate control or CHF exacerbation
Oral contraceptives	Decreased drug effectiveness	Unplanned pregnancies
Protease inhibitors	Decreased drug levels	Increase in HIV viral load
Theophylline	Decreased drug levels	Asthma/COPD exacerbation
Selective serotonin reuptake inhibitors	Serotonin excess	Serotonin syndrome— confusion, agitation, diaphoresis, tremor, rhabdomyolysis
Warfarin	Decreased drug effectiveness	Reduced international normalized ratio value

CHF, congestive heart failure; COPD, chronic obstructive pulmonary disease.

- Little effect on high-density lipoprotein (HDL) levels
- Data have shown decrease in cardiovascular mortality in patients with coronary disease
- No current randomized controlled trials have shown reduced mortality in primary prevention
- American Heart Association has recommended the consumption of 2 to 4 g per day of fish oil capsules for patients who need to lower triglycerides
- An FDA-approved fish oil capsule (Lovaza) is now available by prescription
- Side effects include fishy aftertaste and GI upset
- Theoretical risk of bleeding at high doses due to antiplatelet effects
- Garlic (*Allium sativum*)
  - True active ingredient is unknown
  - May decrease total cholesterol and LDL in the short term
  - No data on impact on cardiovascular mortality
  - Side effects include bad breath, body odor, and GI upset
  - Case reports of bleeding and interactions with warfarin exist
  - Has been shown to decrease saquinivir (protease inhibitor) levels
- Menopausal symptoms (Table 71-2)
- Osteoarthritis
  - Glucosamine sulfate and chondroitin sulfate
    - Theoretically support cartilage and connective tissue formation
    - May also have anti-inflammatory properties
    - Conflicting data exist on their use for symptomatic and functional benefits for patients with osteoarthritis of the knees or hips. Studies are also conflicting regarding their ability to slow the progression of joint-space narrowing.
    - Treatment effect may not be seen for up to 12 weeks
    - Generally well tolerated
    - No known drug interactions
- Prostatic hyperplasia
  - Saw palmetto (*Serenoa repens*)
    - Mechanism of action unknown
    - Conflicting data on its efficacy for improving urologic symptoms and urinary flow measures; most larger recent trials have been negative
    - No data to suggest that it prevents the complications of prostatic hyperplasia (i.e., acute urinary retention) or the development of prostate cancer
    - Generally well tolerated
    - No effect on prostate specific antigen levels
- Probiotics
  - Microorganisms that have properties beneficial to the host
    - Examples include *Lactobacillus*, *Bifidobacterium*, *Streptococcus salivarius*, and *Saccharomyces boulardii*
    - Thought to work by preventing invasion by pathogenic bacteria and improving intestinal barrier function; may also play a role in perception of pain

		TABLE 71-2	*Popular Dietary Supplements Used for the Treatment of Menopausal Symptoms*

Supplement	Potential Toxicity	Potential Drug Interactions	Comments
Black cohosh (*Cimicifuga racemosa*)	Gastrointestinal discomfort Case reports of liver failure	None known	May be effective for short-term use (<6 mo)
Dong quai (*Angelica sinensis*)	Rash	Increased international normalized ratio (INR) in patients taking warfarin	No clinical evidence of efficacy
Red clover (*Trifolium pretense*)	Generally well tolerated	Theoretical risk of interaction with warfarin and tamoxifen	Is a source of isoflavones No clear efficacy in data
Soy isoflavones	Constipation, bloating, nausea, rash	Potential decreased INR in patients on warfarin; theoretical risk of competition with tamoxifen	Most studies have not shown a benefit

- **Data are limited, but some studies suggest that probiotics may be useful in the care of patients with inflammatory bowel disease, irritable bowel syndrome, antibiotic-associated diarrhea, chronic liver disease, and allergic disorders**
- Avoid in seriously ill or immunocompromised patients

REVIEW QUESTIONS

For review questions, please go to www.expertconsult.com.

SUGGESTED READINGS

Ashar BH: Complementary and alternative medicine. In Dale DC, Federman DG, editors: *ACP medicine*, New York, WebMD, 2007.

Ashar BH, Rowland-Seymour A: Advising patients who use dietary supplements, *Am J Med* 121:91–97, 2008.

Ernst E: Acupuncture—a critical analysis, *J Intern Med* 259:125–137, 2006.

Fugh-Berman A: Herb-drug interactions, *Lancet* 355:134–138, 2000.

Furlan AD, Imamura M, Dryden T, Irvin E: Massage for low-back pain, *Cochrane Database Syst Rev* 4:CD001929, 2008.

Jonas W, Levin JS: *Essentials of complementary and alternative medicine*, Philadelphia, Lippincott, Williams & Wilkins, 1999.

Linde K, Berner M, Kriston L: St John's wort for major depression, *Cochrane Database Syst Rev* 4:CD000448, 2008.

Substance Abuse

AMINA A. CHAUDHRY, MD, MPH

Substance abuse is a worldwide public health problem that is associated with significant personal morbidity and mortality, numerous adverse societal consequences, and high costs. Societal economic costs from lost productivity, medical expenses, motor-vehicle accidents, domestic violence, and drug-related crime have been estimated at more than $180 billion for alcohol abuse and more than $180 billion for drug abuse per year. The problem of substance abuse spans all racial and socioeconomic strata and continues to grow. *The Diagnostic and Statistical Manual of Mental Disorders* outlines accepted criteria for a spectrum of substance-related disorders based on the substances used and the severity of the disorder. Substances can be a drug of abuse, a medication, or a toxin.

Basic Information

- **Definitions: Two groups of disorders exist: Substance use disorders and substance-induced disorders**
  - Key features of substance use disorders are listed in Box 72-1
    - **Substance abuse is characterized by continued use of a substance despite evidence of harm, either physically, legally, socially, or in employment**
    - **Substance dependence also includes the manifestations of tolerance, withdrawal, and typically extreme behavioral changes in response to compulsive cravings for the substance**
      - Patients with substance dependence have often tried unsuccessfully to cut down or abstain
    - **Tolerance is defined as either an individual requiring an increasing amount of a substance to achieve a desired effect or the same amount of a substance producing a decreased specific effect**
      - The development of tolerance and withdrawal, by themselves, do not indicate the presence of substance dependence
      - The psychological dependence on a substance must also be present for this diagnosis to apply
  - The substance-induced disorders range from substance intoxication to substance withdrawal, substance-induced delirium, dementia, psychosis, mood or anxiety disorders, sexual dysfunction, and sleep disorder
    - **The hallmarks of substance intoxication are reversible, clinically significant behavioral or psychological changes that develop during or shortly after the ingestion of a substance**

BOX 72-1	*Key Features of Substance Use Disorders*

Substance use disorders include substance abuse and the more severe substance dependence

Although tolerance and withdrawal may be present, the key feature of substance dependence is the psychological dependence on a particular substance

- **Substance withdrawal involves characteristic physiologic and cognitive impairments as a result of the cessation of, or significant decrease in, the amount of a substance typically used continuously over a prolonged period**
  - Once withdrawal develops, most individuals will want to ingest the substance again to relieve the withdrawal symptoms
  - Substances with a recognized withdrawal state include alcohol, amphetamines, cocaine, nicotine, opioids, sedatives, hypnotics, and anxiolytics
- Common drugs of abuse
  - Marijuana: Peripheral and CNS depressant through the cannabinoid receptor system
  - Benzodiazepines: CNS depressants that have anxiolytic and hypnotic effects
  - Opioids: Potent analgesics such as heroin and prescription opioids
  - Alcohol: CNS depressant that rapidly equilibrates between blood and tissues
    - **Hazardous drinking is defined as more than seven drinks per week or more than three drinks in one sitting for healthy women and healthy men over age 65 and more than 14 drinks per week or more than four drinks in one sitting for healthy men up to age 65**
    - One standard drink equals 12 oz regular beer, or 5 oz wine, or 1.5 oz distilled spirits
    - Hazardous drinkers are at risk for injury, social and legal problems, and illness
  - Nicotine: Peripheral and central cholinergic agonist that paradoxically produces both stimulatory and relaxing effects
  - Cocaine: Peripheral and central stimulant with anesthetic and potent vasoconstrictive activity and duration of action of 20 to 30 minutes
  - Methamphetamine: Stimulant similar to cocaine in mechanism of action but with duration of action of 8 to 24 hours and a half-life of 12 hours
  - Club drugs: Numerous drugs, mostly serotoninergic agonists

- LSD (lysergic acid diethylamide)
- "Ecstasy" or MDMA (methylene-dioxymethamphetamine)
- "Love drug" or MDA (methylene-dioxyphenylaminopropane)
- GHB (γ-hydroxybutyrate): A short-acting, GABA-like aqueous solution with CNS sedating effects
- Anabolic steroids: Performance-enhancing, tissue-building compounds with concomitant androgenic effects
- Inhalants: Include volatile solvents (e.g., adhesives, aerosols, solvents, propellant gases) nitrites, and anesthetics; highly lipophilic
- Epidemiology
  - Prevalence and incidence of substance use disorders
    - In the United States, alcohol and nicotine are the most commonly abused substances across all age groups
      - More than 18 million people age 12 or older meet the criteria for an alcohol use disorder every year
    - The prevalence of cigarette smoking and nicotine dependence among adults has declined in the 21st century
      - The Centers for Disease Control estimates that 19.8% of adults in the United States, or 44.5 million people, currently smoke
      - Cigarette smoking in the United States results in an estimated 443,000 premature deaths and $193 billion in direct health-care expenditures and productivity losses each year
    - Marijuana is the most commonly used illegal substance among Americans, with more than 14 million people age 12 or older reporting past month use in 2007
    - Abuse of prescription drugs has risen dramatically over the past decade
    - The prevalence of alcohol and drug use disorders is highest among young adults age 18 to 25
    - **Alcohol- and drug-related disorders are more common among men than women**
    - The rates of substance use disorders vary by race and ethnicity; data from 2007 indicate that:
      - At less than 5%, Asians and Asian Americans have the lowest rates of both alcohol- and drug-use disorders
      - Native American and Alaskan Native persons have the highest rates of these conditions (13%)
      - African Americans and Hispanic Americans are less likely to consume alcohol than whites, but they are more likely to have persistent alcohol dependence if the disorder does develop
  - Risk factors for the development of substance use disorders (Fig. 72-1)
    - **Genetics may explain approximately 50% of the propensity to develop a substance use disorder**
    - **Other host factors, such as premorbid depression, anxiety disorders, and borderline and antisocial personality disorders**
      - Alcohol dependence is most likely an antecedent to the development of depression rather than a result of self-medication of a mood disorder
    - **Marital stability seems to have a protective effect**
    - Educational level
      - Youths who drop out of high school are at higher risk for developing alcohol and drug dependence later in life

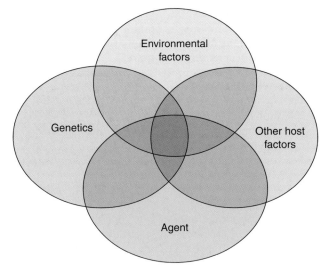

FIGURE 72-1 Risk factors for the development of substance use disorders.

- Drug use during adolescence and young adulthood is also a predictor for not completing high school
- Environmental factors
  - More frequent in populations in which drug use is more socially acceptable
  - Associated with community and family disorganization
  - Peer influence impacts the initiation and ongoing use of alcohol and drugs, particularly among adolescents and young adults
  - **The absence of employment and particular jobs or work settings (bartenders, anesthesiologists) may also carry risk**
- Agent factors
  - **Agents that quickly reach the brain, such as lipophilic substances that are injected intravenously, have a higher addictive potential**
  - Substances that are effective for self-medication, such as heroin or opiods for pain, may help explain addiction to certain drugs
  - Easily accessible substances obtained at low cost tend to have a higher abuse potential
- Common physiologic mechanisms of action
  - **Drugs of abuse and alcohol share a common final pathway: The dopamine reward pathway**
  - **In the early stages of drug use, reward pathway activation causes euphoria and intense pleasure**
  - **With repeated use, reward pathway activation results in diminished responses and the development of long-lasting memories linked to drug-using experiences**
  - These changes are responsible for the development of tolerance, psychological dependence, and the relapse that can happen after years of abstinence

Clinical Presentation

- Warning signs in the office setting
  - **Sudden change in behavior (e.g., sudden job loss, financial difficulty, or family problem)**
  - **History of two or more non–sports-related traumas in an adult**

- **Sexual dysfunction**
- **Intoxicated behavior secondary to active use (inebriated, agitated, extremely lethargic)**
- **Family concerns about patient**
- **History of "driving under the influence" (DUI) or other substance-related arrest**
- Overdose complications
  - Alcohol
    - Symptoms consist of somnolence, bradycardia, coma, and eventual death
    - Symptoms vary with blood alcohol concentration (BAC)
      - Cognitive and behavioral changes occur at BAC of 20 to 30 mg/dL
      - Legal intoxication is at BAC of 80 to 100 mg/dL
      - Death can occur at BAC of 300 to 400 mg/dL
    - Treatment is supportive with close monitoring of electrolytes and for evidence of alcohol withdrawal as the BAC decreases
  - Stimulants such as cocaine and methamphetamine
    - Overdose may result in seizures, arrhythmias, and death
    - Treatment is supportive and management of any medical complications that arise
  - Opioids
    - Symptoms include respiratory depression with shallow respirations, miosis, bradycardia, decreased levels of consciousness, coma, and eventual death
    - Treatment is with IV naloxone 0.2 to 2 mg immediately
      - May require frequent additional doses of naloxone over the first 24 hours because this medication may clear before the effects of the opioids have diminished sufficiently
- **Withdrawal syndromes**
  - **Alcohol withdrawal, which may be life-threatening, typically occurs in three stages (Table 72-1)**
  - Withdrawal from stimulants including cocaine and methamphetamine
    - Symptoms typically are mild and include depression, anxiety, hypersomnolence, anhedonia, difficulty concentrating, increased appetite, and increased drug cravings
    - Acute hospitalization is almost never warranted solely for cocaine withdrawal
  - **Opioid withdrawal typically occurs in two phases**
  - **Acute physiologic withdrawal: Generally not life-threatening, but may be fatal in people with**

underlying cardiac conditions or other medical illness
- **Protracted withdrawal phase**
  - **May involve insomnia, decreased blood pressure and heart rate, and persistent drug cravings**
  - **May last up to 6 to 12 months**
- Secondary medical complications
  - Complications from substance use in general
    - Trauma
    - Infectious diseases such as HIV/AIDS, sexually transmitted infections, hepatitis B and C
    - Renal complications such as acute tubular necrosis from rhabdomyolysis
    - Altered mental status with delirium
    - Malnutrition in general or specific vitamin B complex deficiency
    - Poor adherence to medical appointments and recommended treatments
  - Complications from injection drug use
    - Endocarditis, often with septic emboli
    - Cellulitis and deep tissue infections
    - Thrombophlebitis
    - Foreign-body granulomatosis, often called "talc lung" from talc or other fillers used in drug tablets
    - Secondary amyloidosis
    - Emphysema and bullous lung disease
    - Pulmonary hypertension
  - Complications from alcohol
    - Cardiovascular: Arrhythmias with atrial fibrillation or "holiday heart" being the most common, hypertension, dilated cardiomyopathy
    - GI: Esophagitis, esophageal varices, gastritis, pancreatitis, alcoholic hepatitis, cirrhosis, GI bleeding
    - Endocrine: Testicular atrophy, amenorrhea
    - Hematologic: Macrocytic anemia, thrombocytopenia, leukopenia
    - Neurologic: Peripheral neuropathy, alcoholic myopathy
      - **Wernicke's encephalopathy, a medical emergency, is a confusional state of abrupt onset caused by thiamine deficiency**
        Characterized by a triad of confusion, ataxia, and oculomotor dysfunction (usually cranial nerve VI palsy leading to ophthalmoplegia)
        The diagnosis is made clinically, although necrosis and atrophy of mamillary bodies are visible on brain MRI in 80% of cases
        Treatment is immediate administration of IV thiamine, admission for observation and

TABLE 72-1	*Stages of Alcohol Withdrawal*				
	Autonomic Dysfunction	→	**Withdrawal Seizures**	→	**Delirium Tremens**
Symptoms	Tremors Mild elevations in blood pressure and heart rate		Generalized motor seizures singly or in episodic bursts		Severe autonomic dysregulation Confusion Auditory, visual, or tactile hallucinations
Time course	Begins within 5–10 hr		Begins within 8–24 hr		Begins within 72–96 hr
Treatment	Frequent assessments Symptom-driven doses of benzodiazepines		Treat seizure with parenteral benzodiazepines followed by slow taper with oral benzodiazepine Other antiepileptics minimally effective		Frequent parenteral doses of benzodiazepines or continuous drip Close monitoring

continued IV thiamine therapy, and long-term oral supplementation on an outpatient basis

Symptoms may be precipitated or worsened by administration of glucose before thiamine

Patients usually improve over hours to days

- **Korsakoff's amnestic syndrome refers to profound memory impairment for ongoing events with a marked inability to retain new information**
  - Occurs often late in the course of chronic alcohol dependence
  - Usually seen after an episode of Wernicke's encephalopathy
  - **Both anterograde and retrograde memory are affected, although long-term memory is usually preserved**
  - **Patients often appear apathetic, unconcerned, or unaware of their illness and may confabulate**
  - Treatment with thiamine is usually ineffective, and recovery of memory is often poor
- **Alcoholic cerebellar degeneration is a syndrome characterized by gait abnormalities, including complaints of weakness, unsteadiness, or incoordination, with wide-based ataxic gait and abnormal heel-knee-shin test**
  - Occasionally patients may also have tremors or incoordination of the upper extremities, dysarthria, or blurred vision
  - Onset of symptoms can be progressive over weeks to months, but acute worsening of mild symptoms may occur
  - Head MRI may show evidence of cerebellar atrophy
  - Treatment consists of abstinence from alcohol and nutritional supplementation, but gait abnormalities may persist
- Complications from stimulants (cocaine and methamphetamine)
  - Cardiovascular: Arrhythmias and sudden death; severe, sometimes malignant, hypertension; myocarditis; cardiomyopathy
    - Myocardial infarction that is usually caused by vasospasm; cocaine may also accelerate atherosclerosis
    - Treatment consists of aspirin, benzodiazepines to reduce blood pressure and heart rate, and nitrates or calcium channel blockers to decrease vasospasm and prevent arrhythmias
    - **Avoid β-blockers because they enhance cocaine-induced vasoconstriction, allow unopposed α-activity, and may decrease survival**
  - Neurologic: Seizure, cerebrovascular accidents, intracranial hemorrhage, migraine headache, vasculitis, acute lead poisoning from methamphetamine use
  - Psychiatric: Psychosis, auditory hallucinations, paranoia, extreme violent behavior from methamphetamine use
  - Renal: Rhabdomyolysis

- Gastrointestinal: Bowel ischemia leading to infarction and perforation
- Pulmonary: Alveolar hemorrhage and infarction; pulmonary edema
- Complications from heroin
  - Renal: Focal, segmental glomerulosclerosis that may progress to renal failure
  - Pulmonary: Pulmonary edema
  - Endocrine: Amenorrhea, hypogonadism and erectile dysfunction, euthyroid increase in thyroxine-binding globulin concentration

Diagnosis and Evaluation

- Screening for problematic substance use and substance use disorders
  - History should include family history of alcohol or drug use disorders, presence of co-occurring psychiatric disorders, employment and family status, history of experimenting with or using illicit drugs
  - Screening instruments
    - AUDIT: The Alcohol Use Disorders Identification Test
      - A 10-item questionnaire developed by the World Health Organization specifically for identifying disorders of alcohol use in primary care
      - Has been extensively validated in many populations and languages
    - AUDIT-C: An abbreviated version of the AUDIT using only the first three questions; also performs well when the longer version is not feasible (Box 72-2)
    - **CAGE Questionnaire: Can be used to identify problematic alcohol use (Box 72-3)**
      - Has been adapted to include drug use as well
      - The more affirmative answers, the more likely the person is alcohol or drug dependent
- Assessment of severity of substance use and substance use disorders should be comprehensive and thorough (Box 72-4)
- Physical findings
  - Alcohol dependence: Secondary medical complications caused by use of the substance
    - Abdominal discomfort and/or hemoccult positive stool
    - Findings consistent with liver disease such as jaundice, palmar erythema, caput medusa, ascites, bruising, encephalopathy
    - Peripheral neuropathy

BOX 72-2	*AUDIT-C Questionnaire*

Question 1: How often did you have a drink containing alcohol in the past year?

Question 2: How many drinks did you have on a typical day when you were drinking in the past year?

Question 3: How often did you have six or more drinks on one occasion in the past year?

Each question is worth from 0–4 points, depending on the answer, for a total possible score of 12. In men, a total score of 4 or more is considered positive. In women, a total score of 3 or more is considered positive.

BOX 72-3	CAGE Questions to Screen for Substance Abuse

C: Have you ever tried to **cut down** on your alcohol or drug use?

A: Do you get **annoyed** when people comment about your drinking or drug use?

G: Do you feel **guilty** about things you have done while drinking or using drugs?

E: Do you need an **eye-opener** to get started in the morning?

BOX 72-4	Assessment Questions to Identify Severity of Substance Use Disorder

Duration of use or age at first use

Route of administration

Measurement of frequency and quantity of use

Timing of last use

Past history of blackouts, delirium tremens, withdrawal seizures, and/or hospitalizations for alcohol or drug withdrawal

Past legal problems because of use

Past treatment history and treatment impact on use

Duration of longest, continuous time clean and how achieved

Review of systems for physiologic consequences of substance use

- Smoked or snorted cocaine: Atrophy or perforation of nasal septum; acute respiratory wheezing; digit burns; nervous picking at skin (formication); and agitation
- Methamphetamine
  - Acute: Hyperthermia, hyperventilation, delusions, and paranoia
  - Chronic users: Poor dentition from bruxism, decreased saliva production, inadequate dental hygiene, skin findings such as burns or excoriations caused by formication
  - Intranasal or oral opioid use: Shallow breathing; lethargy, "pinpoint pupils" or miosis, and acute respiratory wheezing
  - Injection drug use: New and old needle track marks, healed and new abscesses
- Laboratory testing
  - **Toxicology screens**
    - **Alcohol: With acute alcohol intoxication, blood alcohol concentration should be measured**
    - **Cocaine: Urine tests for cocaine and metabolites**
      - **Positive for cocaine for less than 48 hours**
      - **The major metabolite of cocaine, benzoylecgonine, is detectable in urine for 5 to 10 days**
      - **Substances used to "cut" the drugs (quinine and quinidine) may be positive for up to 10 days**
    - **Opioids: Heroin is metabolized to morphine and will result in a morphine-positive urine test result**

- **Typical opiate assays do not cross-react with oxycodone or hydrocodone, so these must be tested for separately**
- **Poppy seeds and certain fluoroquinolone antibiotics may cause false-positive results**
- Hematology testing
  - Elevated mean corpuscular volume may be seen in chronic alcohol exposure
  - Acute alcohol consumption may cause pancytopenia, particularly thrombocytopenia
- Liver function tests
  - Alcohol has direct toxic effects on the liver, resulting in abnormalities in several liver enzymes
    - γ-Glutamyl transpeptidase (GGT) levels may be elevated, often greater than 1000 U/L
    - Aspartate transaminotransferase (AST) is typically elevated to a greater degree than alanine transaminotransferase (ALT), but neither increase to levels above 500 U/L
    - Serum bilirubin levels and prothrombin time may be abnormal in acute alcoholic hepatitis
- Chemistries
  - Abrupt cessation of alcohol consumption may result in an anion gap ketoacidosis secondary to poor nutrition and alcohol-induced increased lipolysis with decreased gluconeogenesis
  - Hypomagnesemia is common with chronic alcohol use and often is accompanied by hypokalemia and hypophosphatemia
- **Treatment of acute withdrawal and detoxification**
  - **Alcohol: Mainstay is benzodiazepines to prevent alcohol withdrawal seizures and delirium tremens (DTs)**
    - **In patients with liver disease, lorazepam and oxazepam are the benzodiazepines of choice because a higher proportion of patients will be renally cleared compared with other agents**
    - Dosing should be symptom-driven with frequent assessments for worsening or improvement of symptoms
    - Patients should also receive thiamine and folate, followed by dextrose-containing fluids
  - **Cocaine: Treatment is mostly supportive and typically does not require acute inpatient care; be alert, however, for other substance use and severe depression, which may necessitate hospitalization**
  - **Opioids: Symptoms are most effectively relieved with administration of either a long-acting full opioid agonist such as methadone or a partial opioid agonist such as buprenorphine**
    - Clonidine may decrease the autonomic dysfunction associated with opioid withdrawal but will not treat many of the other symptoms
    - Dicyclomine may relieve abdominal cramping, and ibuprofen treats the generalized myalgias and joint pains
    - Methocarbamol can ease muscle spasms
- **Assessment of motivation and interest in long-term treatment**
  - **Assess stage of readiness for change**
    - **Precontemplative: Patient has not yet considered stopping substance use; may not think substance use is a problem**

- **Contemplative: Patient is thinking about cessation**
- **Determination: Patient has decided to stop substance use but is not yet taking action to quit**
- **Action: Patient is actively goal-setting, problem-solving, and trying to quit**
- **Maintenance: Patient has successfully quit and is working on relapse prevention**
- **Relapse: Can occur at any point through this process; goal is then to get back to action stage**
- Nonpharmacologic interventions
  - A brief intervention by a physician in an office takes about 5 to 10 minutes to complete and takes advantage of the unique role in the doctor–patient relationship to effect change
    - Consists of assessment, feedback to the patient, and referrals or recommendations
    - Studies demonstrate that it reduces levels of hazardous drinking
  - **The FRAMES algorithm is useful in a primary care office (Box 72-5)**
  - Specialized substance abuse treatment programs are able to perform more comprehensive assessments and evaluation
    - Provide more intensive substance abuse treatment
    - Both group and individual addiction counseling
    - These programs usually do not offer psychiatric or medical care
  - Community support programs and self-help groups are common
    - Many, such as Alcoholics Anonymous and Narcotics Anonymous, are based on 12-step approach
    - "Rational Recovery" uses a cognitive-behavioral approach and may be an alternative for patients who are uncomfortable with the spiritual approach
- Pharmacologic therapies
  - All pharmacologic therapies for substance use disorders are most effective in combination with counseling or active self-help group participation
  - Alcohol
    - **Disulfiram acts as a deterrent to continued alcohol intake**
      - **Usual daily doses range from 250 to 500 mg**
      - **Patients develop severe flushing, shortness of breath, dizziness, nausea, vomiting, and abdominal pain, often with significant volume depletion if alcohol is consumed concomitantly**
      - Should be avoided in pregnant women and in patients with severe liver disease
      - Advise patients to avoid foods and beauty products that contain alcohol

- **Acamprosate is thought to affect GABA and excitatory glutamate neurotransmission in the CNS to decrease alcohol cravings**
  - Results from numerous clinical trials demonstrate modest reductions in number of drinking days compared with placebo
- **Naltrexone, an opioid antagonist, is modestly effective in preventing relapse to heavy drinking by diminishing cravings for alcohol**
  - Thought to act by decreasing some of the reinforcing effects of alcohol that may occur through opioid neurotransmission
  - Avoid the medication in patients with severe liver disease, pregnant patients, and those on chronic opioids
- Opioids
- **Methadone is a full opioid agonist at the μ-opioid receptor with a duration of action for opioid dependence treatment of 24 hours**
  - Available for opioid dependence maintenance; treatment occurs in tightly regulated, specialized treatment centers where patients are observed taking the medication unless they have earned privileges to take home individual doses
  - In combination with counseling, methadone reduces illicit drug use by 50% to 70%; keeps patients in treatment; reduces crime, unemployment, family disorganization, HIV and hepatitis C seroconversion; and improves health-related quality of life for patients
  - About 50% of patients relapse to heroin use within 1 year of stopping methadone treatment
  - Therapeutic doses range between 70 and 100 mg, but individualized dosing is key
- **Buprenorphine is a partial opioid agonist at the μ-opioid receptor with a higher affinity and a much slower dissociation rate compared with full opioid agonists**
  - **Dosed once daily or every other day**
  - Because of its partial agonist properties, buprenorphine has a ceiling beyond which increasing the dose will not result in any further opioid effects
  - Available in a parenteral formulation and sublingual formulations (buprenorphine and buprenorphine/naloxone); only the sublingual form is Food and Drug Administration (FDA) approved for treatment of opioid dependence
  - **Office-based physicians can prescribe sublingual buprenorphine to treat opioid-dependent patients**
  - The combination tablet (buprenorphine/naloxone) contains naloxone, which decreases the abuse and diversion potential of the medication because IV administration of crushed tablets may cause withdrawal
  - Buprenorphine may precipitate withdrawal in patients who have recently taken full-agonist opioids
- Naltrexone, an opioid antagonist, is used as a deterrent because patients attempting to use opioids in the presence of naltrexone develop precipitated withdrawal

---

BOX 72-5   *FRAMES Intervention Components*

F: Give **feedback** on personal risks and existing impairments

R: Put emphasis on personal **responsibility** for change

A: Give clear **advice** and recommendations

M: Offer a **menu** of options and alternatives

E: Interact with patient in an **empathic** way

S: Focus on **self-efficacy** to promote optimism and empowerment

72

BOX 72-6	*Key Steps in Relapse Prevention*

Establish a supportive patient-physician relationship

Schedule regular follow-up

Mobilize family support

Facilitate involvement in self-help and community groups

Help patients recognize and cope with relapse triggers and cravings

Facilitate positive lifestyle changes

Manage depression, anxiety, pain, and other comorbid conditions

Consider pharmacotherapy

Collaborate with addiction treatment specialists, if available

- Cocaine: Currently no effective pharmacologic agents exist for treatment of cocaine abuse or dependence
- Relapse prevention (Box 72-6)
  - Relapse is a common part of recovery
    - 50% to 80% of patients return to drug use within their first year of recovery
    - Most of these patients relapse within the first 3 months after stopping alcohol or drug use
    - As a chronic, relapsing condition, preventing relapse is a key component of long-term management of substance use disorders

Disclaimer

This chapter was updated and edited by Dr. Amina Chaudhry in her private capacity. No official support or endorsement by the Substance Abuse and Mental Health Administration, Department of Health and Human Services, is intended or should be inferred.

REVIEW QUESTIONS

For review questions, please go to www.expertconsult.com.

SUGGESTED READINGS

American Psychiatric Association: *Diagnostic and statistical manual of mental disorders*, ed 4, Arlington, VA, American Psychiatric Association, 2000.

Buchsbaum DG, Buchanan RG, Centor RM, et al: Screening for alcohol abuse using CAGE scores and likelihood ratios, *Ann Intern Med* 115:774–777, 1991.

Fiellin DA, O'Connor PG: Clinical practice: office-based treatment of opioid dependent patients, *N Engl J Med* 347:827–823, 2002.

Garbutt JC, West SL, Carey TS, et al: Pharmacological treatment of alcohol dependence: a review of the evidence, *JAMA* 281:1318–1325, 1999.

O'Connor PG, Fiellin DA: Pharmacologic treatment of heroin-dependent patients, *Ann Intern Med* 133:40–54, 2000.

Ries R, Fiellin D, Miller S, et al, editors: *Principles of addiction medicine*, ed 4, Chevy Chase, MD, American Society of Addiction Medicine, 2009.

Substance Abuse and Mental Health Services Administration: Office of Applied Studies: *Results from the 2007 National Survey on Drug Use and Health: national findings*. NSDUH Series H-34, DHHS Publication No. SMA. 08-4343. Rockville, MD, 2008.

Wilk AI, Jensen NM, Havighurst TC: Meta-analysis of randomized control trials addressing brief interventions in heavy alcohol drinkers, *J Gen Intern Med* 12:274–283, 1997.

World Health Organization (WHO): *The Alcohol Use Disorders Identification Test: guidelines for use in primary care*. WHO/MSD/MSB/01.6a. Geneva, 2001, WHO. Available at: http://whqlibdoc.who.int/hq/2001/WHO_MSD_MSB_01.6a.pdf.

Preoperative Evaluation

STEPHEN D. SISSON, MD

Preoperative evaluation is a common task for the internist. The primary objective of the preoperative evaluation is **to assess the patient's medical readiness for surgery.** Every operative procedure carries some level of risk; clinical judgment, accompanied by appropriate testing, is needed to define risk. The preoperative evaluation **includes three steps: clinical risk assessment, functional assessment, and surgery-specific risk assessment**. These assessments determine whether or not to proceed with surgery or to obtain cardiac testing before proceeding with surgery. Mounting evidence has demonstrated **the beneficial impact of β-blockers on cardiovascular outcomes** in some, but not all, patients undergoing noncardiac surgery.

Clinical Risk Assessment

- Clinical risk assessment is the first step in the preoperative evaluation; in this assessment, clinical predictors of increased risk are identified. The presence of certain conditions, termed *active cardiac conditions* (Table 73-1), should lead to the postponement of elective surgery until they are resolved.
  - Cardiovascular disease is commonly associated with increased operative risk
    - **The five areas of potential cardiovascular risk include ischemic cardiovascular disease, congestive heart failure (CHF), valvular heart disease, hypertension, and arrhythmia**
    - Operative risk associated with preexisting ischemic cardiovascular disease is the best studied; prior **history of myocardial infarction (MI)**, especially within the **past month,** is associated **with increased operative risk;** acute MI is an "active cardiac condition" that should delay elective surgery for at least 1 month
  - Stable angina that is mild (i.e., class I or II angina) is not a contraindication to surgery. Unstable angina and class III or IV angina are considered "active cardiac conditions" that should delay surgery until they are resolved.
  - In the absence of MI, surgery should also be postponed following percutaneous coronary intervention as follows
    - Balloon angioplasty: Delay surgery 2 to 4 weeks following angioplasty; ideally complete surgery before 8 weeks following angioplasty
    - Bare-metal intracoronary stent: delay surgery 4 to 6 weeks following stent placement
    - Drug-eluting intracoronary stent: Delay surgery 1 year following stent placement
    - In all cases, aspirin should be continued perioperatively, if possible
  - **Cardiac catheterization does not have a role in perioperative risk assessment;** performing

TABLE 73-1	*Clinical Risk and Elective Surgery*
Active Cardiac Conditions (should postpone or cancel surgery until resolved)	**Clinical Risk Factors (should be included in preoperative risk assessment)**

Unstable coronary syndromes:
  Unstable angina
  Class III or IV angina
  Recent (i.e., ≤30 days) MI
Decompensated heart failure
Significant arrhythmia
  Supraventricular tachyarrhythmias with heart rate > 100 bpm
  High-grade atrioventricular block
  Mobitz II atrioventricular block
  Symptomatic ventricular arrhythmias
  Symptomatic bradycardia
Severe valvular disease
  Severe aortic stenosis (i.e., mean pressure gradient > 40 mm Hg or aortic valve area < 1 cm, or symptomatic)
  Symptomatic mitral stenosis (i.e., progressive dyspnea on exertion, exertional syncope, or heart failure)
	History of heart disease
	History of compensated or prior heart failure
	History of cerebrovascular disease
	Diabetes mellitus (or specifically, anyone treated with insulin)
	Renal insufficiency (defined as serum creatinine > 2 mg/dL)

cardiac catheterization solely to evaluate a person for elective surgery should not be done

- **Similarly, performing cardiac revascularization procedures specifically to prepare a patient with known coronary artery disease (CAD) for elective surgery has not been shown to be of benefit and should not be done**
- CHF is associated with increased perioperative risk, especially if uncontrolled. **Decompensated CHF is another active cardiac condition that is a contraindication to elective surgery.**
- Valvular heart disease is poorly tolerated during surgery because of fluid shifts; severe **aortic stenosis** (defined as aortic valve area < 1 cm or mean pressure gradient > 40 mm Hg) is another active cardiac condition that should delay elective surgery until addressed
  - Similarly, symptomatic **mitral stenosis** is an active cardiac condition
  - Patients with prosthetic heart valves, prior infective endocarditis, intracardiac shunts, and/or prosthetic patches, as well as cardiac transplant patients with cardiac valvulopathy, should receive endocarditis prophylaxis when undergoing certain dental procedures or respiratory tract procedures
- Hypertension has not been demonstrated to affect surgery, but general consensus has been to control hypertension so that diastolic pressure is maintained at less than 110 mm Hg
  - **β-Blockers are the drug of choice for perioperative hypertension**
- Arrhythmias may be poorly tolerated with surgery
  - **Supraventricular arrhythmias** should be **rate-controlled** before surgery
  - Ventricular arrhythmias should prompt evaluation by a cardiologist to recommend perioperative management
- First-degree and Mobitz I heart block are well tolerated during surgery. **Mobitz II and third-degree heart block require intraoperative pacing.**
- Pulmonary disease is also associated with perioperative risk. **Pulmonary complications** (e.g., atelectasis, pneumonia) are the **leading cause of perioperative morbidity.**
  - Patients with chronic pulmonary disease should have local or epidural anesthesia whenever possible
  - Preoperative pulmonary testing is controversial; the American College of Physicians recommends against preoperative spirometry or chest radiography, except in patients with chronic obstructive pulmonary disease (COPD) or asthma
    - Serum albumin less than 3.5 g/dL is a marker for increased pulmonary complications
    - **Forced expiratory volume in 1 second (FEV$_1$) less than 1.5 L** is associated with **increased** risk of **pulmonary complications**
    - An **FEV$_1$ less than 1 L** is associated with **prolonged intubation** and should prompt consultation of a pulmonologist
- Other **diseases that are associated with increased operative risk** include cerebrovascular disease,

TABLE 73-2	*METs and Physical Activity*	
1 MET	**≥4 METs**	**>10 METs**
Take care of self Eat, dress, use toilet Walk indoors around house Walk 1–2 blocks on level ground at 2–3 mph Dusting/washing dishes (some classify this as 1–4 METs)	Climb 1 flight stairs or walk up a hill Walk on level ground at 4 mph Run a short distance Scrubbing floors, moving heavy furniture Golf, bowl, dance, doubles tennis, throw baseball or football	Participate in strenuous sports including: singles tennis, football, basketball, skiing

METs, metabolic equivalents.

diabetes mellitus, and **renal insufficiency** (defined as creatinine > 2 mg/dL) (see Table 73-1)
- **Patients should delay surgery in the presence of active infection**
- If **corticosteroids** have been administered for at least **2 weeks** in the year preceding surgery, **stress-dose corticosteroids should be administered perioperatively**

Functional Assessment

- Surgery creates a stress on the cardiovascular system, which may unmask subclinical cardiovascular disease, especially in someone who is physically deconditioned
- Functional status assessment is a means of quantifying the physical conditioning of a patient who is about to undergo surgery
  - Functional status is standardized into units of metabolic equivalents, referred to as METs
  - METs can be correlated with routine daily activities, allowing the physician to perform a functional status assessment by inquiring about those activities a patient is able to perform without developing limiting dyspnea or chest pain
  - The **inability** to perform at least **4 METs** of activity without symptoms is consistent with **poor functional status** and is associated with **increased operative risk**
  - If the patient **is unable to perform physical activity** (e.g., a patient who cannot walk because of severe degenerative arthritis), **assume that patient cannot perform 4 METs** and has poor functional status
- The amount of METs associated with common physical activities is summarized in Table 73-2

Surgery-Specific Risk Assessment

- Overall risks
  - For all surgeries, perioperative mortality is 0.3%
    - Most perioperative deaths (55%) occur in **the first 48 hours postoperatively**
    - Of perioperative deaths, 35% occur in the operating room, and 10% of deaths occur during anesthesia induction

TABLE 73-3	*Surgery-Specific Risk*		
Low Risk (<1%)	**Intermediate Risk (<5%)**	**High-Risk Vascular (>5%)**	
Endoscopic procedures	Carotid endarterectomy	Peripheral vascular surgery	
Superficial procedures	Endovascular abdominal aortic aneurysm repair	Aortic/major vascular surgery	
Cataract surgery	Head and neck surgery		
Breast surgery	Intraperitoneal surgery		
Ambulatory surgery	Intrathoracic surgery		
	Orthopedic surgery		
	Prostate surgery		

- ▪ **Pulmonary complications are the most common perioperative complications**
- ▪ **Cardiac complications are the most common cause of perioperative death**
- ▪ Perioperative MIs usually occur by postoperative day 3
- ▪ Of perioperative MIs, 50% are fatal
- Procedure-associated risk
  - ▪ Surgery-specific risk is determined by the operative procedure planned
    - ▪ **Low-risk** procedures are associated with a less than **1%** risk of death
    - ▪ Intermediate-risk procedures are associated with a 1% to 5% risk of death
    - ▪ **High-risk** procedures are associated with a **greater than 5%** risk of death
    - ▪ Emergency surgery is considered very high risk
- A summary of surgery-specific risks is provided in Table 73-3

Summarizing Preoperative Risk

- Preoperative risk is summarized by **combining clinical risk, functional status, and surgery-specific risk**
  - ▪ Patients with an active cardiac condition should not undergo elective surgery until the active cardiac condition has been treated
  - ▪ Patients with no clinical risk factors can proceed to surgery without noninvasive cardiac testing
  - ▪ Patients with good functional status can proceed to surgery without noninvasive cardiac testing
  - ▪ Patients undergoing low-risk surgical procedures can proceed to surgery without noninvasive cardiac testing
  - ▪ Patients with one or two clinical risk factors undergoing intermediate or vascular surgery or with poor or unknown functional status should be treated with perioperative β-blockers or consider noninvasive cardiac testing
  - ▪ Patients with three or more clinical risk factors should be managed similarly, unless undergoing vascular surgery, in which case they should undergo non-invasive cardiac testing

Instructions to the Patient

- Medication adjustments
  - ▪ **Check serum levels of all medications** that are monitored with serum levels preoperatively and adjust doses accordingly

- ▪ **Antihypertensives are continued** on the morning of surgery **with the exception** of diuretics and angiotensin-converting enzyme (ACE) inhibitors, which are held the morning of surgery
- ▪ Diabetes medications are adjusted as follows
  - ▪ **Oral hypoglycemics are held on the day of surgery**
    - ▪ **Metformin**, with its risk of lactic acidosis, is **held two days preoperatively**
  - ▪ **Regular insulin and rapid-acting insulins are held on the day of surgery**
  - ▪ **Glargine** insulin and **NPH** insulin doses are reduced by one half to one third
- ▪ **HMG CoA reductase inhibitors are continued** on the day of surgery and may reduce risk of a cardiac event
- ▪ Sedatives, hypnotics, and other CNS-active medications are held on the day of surgery
- ▪ **Aspirin is held 1 week before surgery;** although the effect on platelets of other NSAIDs is less pronounced than aspirin, they are typically held 1 week before surgery.
- ▪ Other idiosyncratic reactions include the following
  - ▪ **Lithium:** May cause myocardial suppression and is **held the day of surgery**
  - ▪ **Tetracycline:** May cause renal failure if administered with methoxyflurane (anesthetic) and is **held the day of surgery**
  - ▪ Neuroleptics may enhance neuromuscular blocking agents; if given, anesthesia may need to adjust neuromuscular blockade during surgery
  - ▪ All herbal remedies should be discontinued prior to surgery (e.g., St. John's wort and ginkgo biloba)
- ▪ New symptom monitoring
  - ▪ Patients should be reminded to contact the internist or surgeon if a febrile illness, chest pain, or new medical symptoms develop between the preoperative assessment and surgery
- Preoperative testing
  - ▪ Although routine preoperative testing is often performed, there are few data to support its use. Surgeons typically will make specific requests based on the type of surgical procedure.
  - ▪ The following preoperative testing is commonplace
    - ▪ For patients 65 years and older: Electrolytes, glucose, creatinine, and CBC
    - ▪ Electrocardiography: For men older than 40 years, women older than 50 years
    - ▪ Chest radiography: Consider in patients with chest complaints or greater than 10 pack-years of tobacco use
    - ▪ CBC: Consider in menstruating women
    - ▪ Glucose: Consider in younger African-American patients
    - ▪ Prothrombin time (PT)/(partial thromboplastin time [PTT]): Consider in patients with liver disease, malignancy, patients receiving anticoagulants, or patients having neurosurgery
    - ▪ Urinalysis: For prosthetic joint placement
- Role of β-blockers
  - ▪ The role of **perioperative β-blocker administration** in a selected population has demonstrated **a reduced risk of perioperative MI and death.** The benefit persists for at least 2 years postoperatively.

73

TABLE 73-4	*Recommendations for Perioperative β-Blockers*
Strength of Recommendation	**Recommendation**
Strongest	β-Blockers should be continued in patients undergoing surgery who are receiving β-blockers for other indications β-Blockers should be given to patients undergoing vascular surgery who have ischemia on preoperative testing
Intermediate	β-Blockers probably recommended for patients undergoing vascular surgery in whom preoperative assessment identifies CAD, or in patients with high cardiac risk, as defined by the presence of >1 clinical risk factor (i.e., known cardiac disease, diabetes, renal insufficiency, cerebrovascular disease, prior CHF) β-Blockers are probably recommended for patients in whom preoperative assessment identifies CHD or high cardiac risk as defined by >1 clinical risk factor and who are undergoing intermediate-risk or vascular surgery
Low	β-Blockers may be considered for patients who are undergoing intermediate or high-risk procedures in whom preoperative assessment identifies intermediate cardiac risk as defined by the presence of a single clinical risk factor β-Blockers may be considered in patients undergoing vascular surgery with low cardiac risk who are not currently on β-blockers

CAD, coronary artery disease; CHD, congenital heart disease; CHF, congestive heart failure.

- Studies have demonstrated that perioperative β-blockers (specifically **cardioselective β-blockers** such as atenolol, metoprolol, or bisoprolol) were well tolerated, including in those with COPD
- **Mortality may be reduced by 50%** in patients treated appropriately with **perioperative β-blockers**, but mortality may also increase when perioperative β-blockers are used inappropriately
  - American College of Cardiology/American Heart Association recommendations on use of perioperative β-blockers are listed in Table 73-4

REVIEW QUESTIONS

For review questions, please go to www.expertconsult.com.

SUGGESTED READINGS

Fleisher LA, Beckman JA, Brown KA, et al: ACC/AHA 2007 guidelines on perioperative cardiovascular evaluation and care for noncardiac surgery, *Circulation* 116:418–499, 2007.
Fleisher LA, Beckman JA, Brown KA, et al: ACC/AHA 2006 guideline update on perioperative cardiovascular evaluation for noncardiac surgery: focused update on perioperative beta-blocker therapy, *J Am Coll Cardiol* 47:2343–2355, 2006.
Wilson W, Taubert KA, Gewitz M, et al: Prevention of infective endocarditis: guidelines from the American Heart Association, *Circulation* 116:1736–1754, 2007.

Immunization and Prevention

BIMAL H. ASHAR, MD, MBA

Immunizations and screening for designated pathologic conditions are the cornerstones of preventative medicine. Several major medical societies have published guidelines for these practices, and these vary in several of their recommendations. The following is an overview of the necessary immunizations and side-effect profiles as well as other health maintenance screening guidelines.

Immunization

- General concepts
  - Active versus passive
    - Active immunization involves administration of antigen to induce an antibody response
    - Passive immunization involves administration of an exogenous antibody (temporary protection against a disease)
      - Usually done by infusion of human immunoglobulin (e.g., hepatitis A, tetanus)
  - Types of active immunization (i.e., vaccination)
    - Live attenuated
      - Usually confers lifelong immunity
      - **Should not be given to immunocompromised patients**
      - Examples: Measles, mumps, rubella (MMR); varicella-zoster (chickenpox); shingles, influenza (intranasal)
    - Inactivated (killed) whole pathogen
      - Examples: Influenza (flu shot), hepatitis A, rabies
    - Fractional protein-based
      - Examples: Hepatitis B, tetanus
    - Polysaccharide
      - Examples: *Pneumococcus, Meningococcus, Haemophilus influenzae*
  - Principles of administration
    - All vaccines can be given together (except yellow fever + cholera)
    - Live vaccines should either be given together or at least 4 weeks apart
    - **It is not necessary to restart an interrupted vaccine series (except oral typhoid)**
    - Live vaccines should not be given with immunoglobulin or blood products
  - Common patient misconceptions about vaccination
    - **Many vaccines cause a local reaction and fever that lasts 24 to 48 hours. This does not contraindicate using the vaccine again and should not be considered an allergic response.**
    - Mild acute illness (or recent illness) or the current use of antibiotics does not contraindicate the use of vaccines
    - Family history of adverse reaction to a vaccine does not contraindicate the use of vaccines
- Individual vaccines (see also Fig. 74-1)
  - Influenza
    - Vaccine characteristics
      - New formulation created each year for different strain
      - Ideally given in October or November, but can be given as late as January
      - Needs to be given annually
      - **60% to 80% effective in preventing disease, but 95% effective in preventing complications**
      - Two types: Live attenuated influenza vaccine (LAIV) can be used in healthy individuals aged 2 to 49 years; trivalent inactivated influenza vaccine (TIV) should be used for all others
    - Indications
      - Age 50 years or older
      - Pregnancy
      - Chronic disease
      - Immunocompromised (including HIV)
      - Contacts of chronically ill (e.g., health care workers)
      - Institutionalized patients (and employees there)
      - Any individuals who want to decrease their risk of contracting and disseminating influenza
      - Data show improved economic outcomes for inoculating healthy working young adults
    - Adverse reactions (TIV)
      - Local reaction 15% to 20%; soreness at the sight
      - Low-grade fever
      - Myalgias
    - Adverse reactions (LAIV)
      - Runny nose, sore throat
      - Headache
      - Cough
    - Contraindications
      - Egg allergy
      - History of severe postvaccine reaction or Guillain-Barré syndrome (GBS)
  - *Pneumococcus*
    - Vaccine characteristics
      - Polysaccharide vaccine made from 23 strains (90% of strains causing the morbidity of *Pneumococcus*)
    - Indications
      - Age 65 years or older

Recommended adult immunization schedule by vaccine and age group—United States, 2009

VACCINE ▼ AGE GROUP ▶	19–26 years	27–49 years	50–59 years	60–64 years	≥65 years
Tetanus, diphtheria, pertussis (Td/Tdap)*	Substitute 1-time dose of Tdap for Td booster; then boost with Td every 10 yr				Td booster every 10 yr
Human papillomavirus (HPV)*	3 doses (females)				
Varicella*	2 doses				
Zoster				1 dose	
Measles, mumps, rubella (MMR)*	1 or 2 doses		1 dose		
Influenza*	1 dose annually				
Pneumococcal (polysaccharide)	1 or 2 doses				1 dose
Hepatitis A*	2 doses				
Hepatitis B*	3 doses				
Meningococcal*	1 or more doses				

*Covered by the Vaccine Injury Compensation Program

☐ For all persons in this category who meet the age requirements and who lack evidence of immunity (e.g., lack documentation of vaccination or have no evidence of prior infection)

☐ Recommended if some other risk factor is present (e.g., as the basis of medical, occupational, lifestyle, or other indications)

☐ No recommendation

FIGURE 74-1 Recommended adult vaccination schedule. (From the Centers for Disease Control Advisory Committee on Immunization Practices. Available at: www.cdc.gov/mmwr/preview/mmwrhtml/mm5753a6.htm?s_cid=mm5753a6_e.)

- Chronic disease (e.g., diabetes, end-stage renal disease, congestive heart failure, liver disease, alcoholism, chronic obstructive pulmonary disease, asthma)
- Immunocompromised patients
- Asplenia
- Chronic cerebrospinal fluid leak
- Revaccination
  - Healthy patients do not need revaccination if first shot given at 65 years or older
  - If first shot given younger than 65 years, revaccinate after 5 years
  - Chronic disease or asplenia: Revaccinate once after 5 years
  - If patient is unsure if he or she has received the pneumococcal vaccine before, it is okay to revaccinate regardless of the time interval
  - **It is currently not recommended to vaccinate any individual more than twice**
- Tetanus (dT)
  - Vaccine characteristics
    - Fractional protein-based toxoid
    - Primary adult series if no history of vaccination: three-shot series at 0, 1, and then 6 to 12 months
    - Recommended every 10 years
    - Important to revaccinate elderly patients because the elderly and children are the at-risk populations for the illness
    - **Substitute Tdap (tetanus, diphtheria, pertussis) for dT once in adults younger than 65 years**
  - Treatment of exposure (i.e., dirty wound)

- Administer dT vaccine if last shot was 5 or more years before, or begin primary series if never given
- Administer tetanus immune globulin if dT never given (okay to give with first dT vaccine)
- Hepatitis A
  - Vaccine characteristics
    - Inactivated whole-virus vaccine (killed)
    - Given as two-shot series at least 6 months apart
    - First dose should be given at least a month before anticipated exposure
    - Unknown if booster doses are required; immune response appears to last at least 10 years
    - Hepatitis A immune globulin used for postexposure prophylaxis, although some data suggest that immunization in the acute setting may be equally protective
  - Indications
    - Men who have sex with men
    - IV drug users
    - Patients with chronic liver disease
    - Travelers to endemic areas
    - People who work with the virus or with primates
    - Recipients of clotting factors
    - Note that heterosexual promiscuity and health care workers are not indications
- Hepatitis B
  - Vaccine characteristics
    - Recombinant subunit (protein-based) vaccine
    - Three-shot series at 0, 1, and 6 months
    - Test for HBsAb 6 months after third shot

- **Nonresponders after three doses should be revaccinated**
- High risk of nonresponder in dialysis patients, elderly, obese, smokers, and males
- Use high dose (40 μg versus 10 μg standard) for dialysis patients and nonresponders after three standard doses
- A fall in titer does not mean loss of immunity; once titer is present, do not need to revaccinate
- Indications
  - Men who have sex with men
  - Multiple sex partners
  - IV drug users
  - Patients with chronic liver disease
  - Patients with HIV
  - Travelers to endemic areas
  - Contacts of patients with hepatitis B
  - Health care workers
  - Institutionalized developmentally disabled patients
  - Hemodialysis patients
  - Regular recipients of blood products (e.g., hemophiliacs)
  - Alaska and Pacific Islander natives
  - Now recommended for all adolescents
- Human papillomavirus (HPV) vaccine
  - Vaccine characteristics
    - Recombinant protein-based vaccine
    - Three-shot series at 0, 2, and 6 months
    - Efficacious in preventing infection from HPV types 6, 11, 16, and 18
    - About 70% of cervical cancers are caused by HPV 16 and 18
  - Indications
    - Currently approved for use in girls/women aged 9 to 26 years
    - Vaccine should ideally be given before the onset of sexual activity so current targeted group is girls aged 11 to 12 years
    - Recommended for sexually active women younger than age 27 years, but may be less efficacious in preventing disease
    - Need to continue screening Pap smears even in women who received the vaccine
  - Contraindications
    - Hypersensitivity to yeast
    - Patients with a moderate to severe acute illness
- Measles, mumps, and rubella (MMR)
  - Vaccine characteristics
    - Live attenuated vaccine
    - Given in two doses: typically at 0 and at 1 to 2 months
    - **Do not give to patients who are pregnant or trying to get pregnant**
    - May suppress a tuberculosis test (purified protein derivative [PPD]) response for 4 to 6 weeks
  - Indications
    - Patients vaccinated between 1957 and 1968 received a killed vaccine that is not effective, so they are not immune; if in an at-risk group, they need revaccination
    - Patients born before 1957 are considered immune

- Women of childbearing age (if rubella titer is negative)
- College students (if measles titer is negative)
- Travelers (if measles titer is negative)
- Health care workers (if measles titer is negative)
- Varicella-zoster (chickenpox)
  - Vaccine characteristics
    - Live attenuated vaccine
    - Given in two doses: one each at 0 and 1 month
    - **Diffuse varicella-like rash can occur in up to 5% of patients; transmission from a patient with the vaccine rash to immunocompromised children has been reported; patients should be advised not to have contact with immunosuppressed patients until rash is gone**
  - Indications
    - All adults without evidence of immunity (i.e., never had chickenpox or no serologic evidence of immunity)
    - Health care workers
    - Teachers and daycare workers
    - Contacts of chronically ill patients
    - Nonpregnant women of childbearing age
    - Military or institutional housing
  - Contraindications
    - HIV+ and immunocompromised controversial, Advisory Committee on Immunization Practices (ACIP) recommends for mild HIV in children and adults (CD4$^+$ count > 200 cells/mm^3)
    - Pregnancy (woman should avoid pregnancy for 1 month after vaccination)
    - Varicella-zoster immune globulin (VZIG) can be given postexposure in patients who cannot receive the varicella-zoster vaccine (may be effective when given up to 4 days postexposure)
- Herpes zoster (shingles) vaccine
  - Vaccine characteristics
    - Live attenuated vaccine
    - About 50% to 60% effective in preventing shingles
    - About 60% to 70% effective in preventing postherpetic neuralgia
    - Given as a single shot; no revaccination currently recommended
  - Indications
    - ACIP recommends for all patients older than 60 years
    - **Not necessary to ask about history of chickenpox or to conduct serologic testing for varicella-zoster immunity**
    - Patients who have a history of a shingles episode in the past can be vaccinated unless contraindications exist
  - Contraindications
    - History of anaphylaxis to vaccine components (e.g., gelatin, neomycin)
    - Anyone with acquired, primary, or medication-induced immunodeficiency
- Meningococcal vaccine
  - Vaccine characteristics
    - Polysaccharide-based vaccine
    - Active against groups A, C, Y, and W-135

74

- Does not protect against group B, the most common one in United States
- Indications
  - Terminal complement component deficiency
  - Travelers to endemic area (e.g., sub-Saharan Africa)
  - Asplenia
  - Military recruits
  - College freshman living in dormitories
  - ACIP recommends vaccinating all adolescents at age 11 to 12 years
- Rabies vaccine (pre-exposure)
  - Vaccine characteristics/background
    - Bats, skunks, raccoons, dogs, and cats can transmit disease
    - If given as pre-exposure prophylaxis, three doses given
    - If given after bite, five doses of vaccine plus rabies immune globulin should be given
  - Indications
    - Veterinarians, animal handlers
    - Travelers who will likely come in contact with animals in parts of the world where rabies is common
- Polio vaccine
  - Oral polio vaccine (OPV) no longer recommended
  - Unvaccinated adults should get the enhanced inactivated polio vaccine (eIPV) in three doses at 0,

1 to 2, and 6 to 12 months, particularly if they may be traveling to endemic areas (South Asia, sub-Saharan Africa)
- *Haemophilus influenzae* type B vaccine
  - Indications
    - Usually given in childhood
    - Patients should be revaccinated after bone marrow transplant and given the first dose before splenectomy (if possible)
- Other vaccines
  - Yellow fever vaccine for travelers to endemic areas only
  - Pertussis vaccine (Tdap) recommended for adults younger than age 65 years as a one-time substitute for dT
- Special populations (Fig. 74-2)
  - HIV
    - Only live attenuated vaccines are contraindicated
    - Flu vaccine had been thought to raise HIV viral load, but recent data show safety; it should be given annually to HIV patients
    - Should receive flu and pneumococcal vaccines; consider hepatitis A and B
  - Multiple sclerosis
    - No evidence of a risk from vaccination in multiple sclerosis patients despite concerns in 1990s; they should be vaccinated without reservation

Vaccines that might be indicated for adults based on medical and other indications—United States, 2009

INDICATION ▶ / VACCINE ▼	Pregnancy	Immuno-compromising conditions (excluding HIV)	HIV infection CD4+ T lymphocyte count <200 cells/μL	HIV infection CD4+ T lymphocyte count ≥200 cells/μL	Diabetes, heart disease, chronic lung disease, chronic alcoholism	Asplenia (including elective splenectomy and terminal complement component deficiencies)	Chronic liver disease	Kidney failure, end-stage renal disease, receipt of hemodialysis	Health-care personnel
Tetanus, diphtheria, pertussis (Td/Tdap)*	Td	Substitute 1-time dose of Tdap for Td booster; then boost with Td every 10 yr							
Human papillomavirus (HPV)*		3 doses for females through age 26 yr							
Varicella*	Contraindicated	Contraindicated		2 doses					
Zoster	Contraindicated	Contraindicated		1 dose					
Measles, mumps, rubella (MMR)*	Contraindicated	Contraindicated		1 or 2 doses					
Influenza*	1 dose TIV annually								1 dose TIV or LAIV annually
Pneumococcal (polysaccharide)	1 or 2 doses								
Hepatitis A*	2 doses								
Hepatitis B*	3 doses								
Meningococcal*	1 or more doses								

*Covered by the Vaccine Injury Compensation Program

☐ For all persons in this category who meet the age requirements and who lack evidence of immunity (e.g., lack documentation of vaccination or have no evidence of prior infection)

☐ Recommended if some other risk factor is present (e.g., as the basis of medical, occupational, lifestyle, or other indications)

☐ No recommendation

FIGURE 74-2 Immunization schedule for special adult populations. LAIV, live attenuated influenza vaccine; TIV, inactivated influenza vaccine. (From the Centers for Disease Control Advisory Committee on Immunization Practices. Available at: www.cdc.gov/mmwr/preview/mmwrhtml/mm5753a6.htm?s_cid=mm5753a6_e.)

- Bone marrow transplant
  - Need to be reimmunized with primary series
  - Killed vaccines should be given 12 to 24 months post-transplant
  - Live vaccines should be given 24 months post-transplant assuming no graft-versus-host disease or immunosuppressant drugs

Screening

- General principles
  - Recommendations for screening vary widely
    - United States Preventive Services Task Force (USPSTF)
      - Government-sponsored group whose mission is to make recommendations on which preventive services should be part of routine primary care
      - Cost-effectiveness does play a role in recommendations made
      - The USPSTF has a grading system for its recommendations (Table 74-1)
    - Specialty societies (e.g., the American Cancer Society [ACS], American Urologic Association [AUA], American Thyroid Association, and American College of Physicians [ACP])
      - Often make recommendations and develop independent guidelines for screening
      - Cost-effectiveness may or may not play a role in guidelines
  - Screening tests are generally a form of secondary prevention
    - **Primary prevention: Intervention designed to avert disease before it develops** (e.g., nutritional counseling)
    - **Secondary prevention: Intervention aimed at early detection of disease** (e.g., mammography)
    - **Tertiary prevention: Preventing complications of a symptomatic disease** (e.g., hepatitis B vaccine in hepatitis C patients)
  - An ideal screening test is one that does the following:
    - Screens for a disease that has high morbidity and mortality
    - Is sensitive with a confirmatory test available, inexpensive, and noninvasive
    - Screens for a disease that has a long premorbid phase during which intervention can affect outcome

TABLE 74-1	United States Preventive Services Task Force Grading System	
Grade	**Description**
A	Service recommended. Net benefit is thought to be substantial
B	Service recommended. Net benefit is thought to be moderate to substantial
C	Not routinely recommended. There may be some individuals for which service is appropriate
D	Not recommended. Data show no benefit or potential for harm
I	Current evidence insufficient to make a recommendation for or against the service

Cancer Screening

BREAST CANCER

- Mammography
  - Screen every 1 to 2 years for patients older than age 40 years
  - USPSTF states as long as comorbid disease does not decrease life expectancy one can continue mammograms beyond age 70 years
- Clinical breast examination
  - Screen yearly ages 50 years and older in conjunction with mammogram
  - **Has not been shown to reduce mortality either alone or in combination with mammography**
- Genetic testing
  - Indicated for women whose family history is associated with an increased risk of *BRCA1* or *BRCA2* mutation
  - Patients should be referred for genetic counseling and testing
- Chemoprevention
  - Should discuss use of tamoxifen or raloxifene in women at high risk for breast cancer
  - Can estimate risk with the use of online tools (e.g., the National Cancer Institute's Breast Cancer Risk Assessment Tool, http://cancer.gov/bcrisktool/)
  - Need to weigh risks of medications (i.e., venous thrombosis, uterine cancer) against benefits of prevention

COLORECTAL CANCER

- Screening options (by the USPSTF)
  - High-sensitivity fecal occult blood testing (FOBT) annually
  - Flexible sigmoidoscopy every 5 years plus high-sensitivity FOBT every 3 years
  - Colonoscopy every 10 years
  - CT colonography and fecal DNA may be useful tools in the near future but currently not recommended
- Timing
  - Start screening at age 50 years in individuals at average risk
  - Net benefit of screening between the ages of 76 to 85 years is small
  - Absolutely stop screening in adults older than 85 years (harm outweighs benefits)
- High-risk patients may need colonoscopy earlier than age 50 years or more frequently than every 10 years
  - Familial polyposis
  - Strong family history (first-degree relative aged younger than 60 years)
  - History of adenomatous polyps
  - History of inflammatory bowel disease

PROSTATE CANCER

- Prostate-specific antigen (PSA)
  - Insufficient evidence to recommend routine screening per the USPSTF
  - ACP just recommends discussion of pros and cons between physician and patient
  - Some groups (e.g., ACS and AUA) recommend annual screening starting at age 50 years (if life expectancy is greater than 10 years) and at age 40 years in high-risk

74

individuals (e.g., African Americans, those with family history)
- **USPSTF recommends against screening men older than age 75 years since harms outweigh benefits**
- Digital rectal examination
  - Insufficient evidence to recommend routine screening per USPSTF
  - ACS and AUA recommend same guidelines as for PSA

CERVICAL CANCER

- Papanicolaou test (Pap smear)
  - Perform on all sexually active women older than 21 years with a cervix (or within 3 years of onset of sexual activity)
  - If no risk factors (e.g., HIV, recurrent STDs, multiple partners, abnormal Pap in past), can perform every 3 years (per both USPSTF and ACP)
  - ACS agrees but recommends three annual negative Pap smears before doing 3-year intervals
  - If no history of abnormal Pap and no risk factors, can stop after age 65 years
  - If no or distant history of last Pap smear, the test should be performed regardless of age
  - USPSTF recommends against Pap smears in women who underwent hysterectomy for benign disease (e.g., fibroids)
- HPV testing
  - USPSTF found insufficient evidence for or against testing for HPV
  - The American College of Obstetrics and Gynecology suggests HPV testing in addition to Pap smear as an option for women older than 30 years; if both are negative, no need to repeat the Pap for at least 3 more years

OVARIAN CANCER

- **Screening not recommended for individuals at average risk; tests (cancer antigen 125 and ultrasound) are inaccurate with very low positive predictive value**
- Routine pelvic examinations done for ovarian cancer screening are not recommended (except by the ACS)

LUNG CANCER

- Currently, chest radiograph, sputum cytology, or low-dose CT are not recommended for early detection in smokers
- Low-dose CT scans are being studied as screening tool in high-risk patients and may prove beneficial, but mortality benefit has not yet been proven

Screening for Infectious Diseases

- HIV
  - USPSTF strongly recommends screening patients at increased risk
    - Recent history of STD
    - Men who have sex with men
    - Past or present IV drug users
    - Women or men whose sex partners have been HIV-positive, IV drug users, bisexuals, or those who have multiple partners without protection

- History of receiving blood products between 1978 and 1985
- USPSTF also recommends screening all pregnant women
- CDC recommends screening all individuals between the ages of 13 and 64 years
- All patients should be counseled on how to prevent HIV transmission
- STDs (USPSTF recommendations)
  - Hepatitis B: Routine screening not recommended except in high-risk individuals or pregnant women
  - Syphilis: Rapid plasma reagin for all pregnant women and high-risk patients (e.g., history of STD or HIV, multiple sex partners)
  - Gonorrhea: Routine screening not recommended but asymptomatic high-risk patients should be screened
  - ***Chlamydia*: Recommends screening all asymptomatic adolescent sexually active women (25 years or younger) and high-risk adult women; does not recommend routine screening of men or adult women at low risk**
  - Herpes simplex virus: Routine screening is not recommended
- Rubella immunity
  - USPSTF recommends all women of childbearing age be screened for rubella immunity; if nonimmune, they should receive the MMR
- PPD screening
  - Routine screening not necessary
  - USPSTF recommends screening in high-risk patients such as the following:
    - Chronic disease (e.g., diabetes, renal failure, HIV)
    - Recent emigrants from Africa, Asia, and Latin America
    - Health care workers and anyone with close contact of a patient with known tuberculosis
    - Medically underserved populations
    - Residents of long-term facilities (e.g., jails, nursing homes)
    - Immunosuppressed
    - Alcoholics and IV drug users
  - Frequency of screening is a matter of clinical discretion
  - Bacille Calmette-Guérin vaccine history is not an acceptable explanation for a positive PPD
  - Criteria for positive test are as follows:
    - Low-risk patients: 15-mm diameter or greater
    - High-risk patients (any of the previous indications for screening makes a patient at least high risk): 10-mm diameter or greater
    - Very high risk patients (HIV infection, abnormal chest film, recent contact of known infected patients): 5-mm diameter or greater

Screening for Cardiovascular Disease

- Hypertension
  - USPSTF suggests screening for all adults older than age 18, but they do not specify frequency
  - The seventh report of the Joint National Committee on Prevention, Detection, Evaluation, and Treatment of High Blood Pressure (JNC 7) recommends yearly

evaluations in everyone with a blood pressure over 120/80 mm Hg and every 2 years in those with pressures lower than 120/80 mm Hg
- Hypercholesterolemia
  - USPSTF recommends screening all men 35 years or older and men and women 20 years and older if they have another risk factor for coronary heart disease
  - USPSTF makes no recommendation for screening women without risk factors
  - National Cholesterol Education Panel (NCEP) screening all adults over age 20 years with a lipid profile
  - Ideal frequency of screening has not been established but NCEP recommends every 5 years if profile is normal
- Coronary heart disease
  - USPSTF recommends against resting electrocardiography, exercise treadmill testing, or electron-beam computed tomography (EBCT) for the prediction of coronary disease in low-risk patients
  - USPSTF reports that there is insufficient evidence for or against use of these modalities in adults at increased risk of CAD
- Abdominal aortic aneurysm (AAA)
  - USPSTF recommends one-time screening for AAA by ultrasound in men aged 65 to 75 years who have ever smoked
  - USPSTF recommends against screening in women
- Aspirin use
  - Recommended for physicians to discuss risk and benefits of aspirin use with patients at increased risk for CAD
  - Ideal dose is unclear since beneficial effects are shown for doses ranging from 75 mg to 325 mg

Other Disease Screening

See Table 74-2.

Psychosocial and Behavioral Screening

- The USPSTF does not make recommendations for or against routine screening for a number of behavioral and situational disorders (other than depression and smoking cessation). However, they do state that clinicians should be aware of them and address these issues when appropriate.
- The following areas of concern may need to be addressed in an individual patient
  - Depression
  - Eating disorders
  - Contraception and safe sex practices
  - Domestic violence
  - Nutrition
  - Exercise
  - Tobacco cessation
  - Alcohol and drug abuse
  - Injury prevention (e.g., seat belts, firearms, smoke detectors)
  - Advanced directives

Periodic Health Examination

- There is significant controversy as to the value of the periodic health examination
  - Evidence suggests increased receipt of preventive services including Pap smear, cholesterol testing, and FOBT
  - There is no definitive evidence on the long-term benefits and effect on morbidity and mortality
  - Significant variability in what services should be included in a periodic health examination and how frequently those services should be repeated

TABLE 74-2	USPSTF Screening Guidelines for Common Disorders	
Disorder	**USPSTF Guideline**	**Comments**
Obesity	Screen all patients for obesity by calculating body mass index	
Type II diabetes	Screen for diabetes in patients with blood pressures > 135/80 mm Hg	American Diabetes Association suggests screening everyone older than age 45 yr with a fasting glucose every 3 yr. Hemoglobin A$_{1C}$ may be the preferred screening method in the future
Thyroid disease	Insufficient evidence for or against screening	American Thyroid Association recommends screening all adults beginning at age 35 yr every 5 yr
Osteoporosis	Screen women > 65 yr with a DEXA scan. Start at 60 yr if risk factors exist	National Osteoporosis Foundation has much broader recommendations, including screening all men older than 70 yr
Alcohol abuse	Screen all adults for alcohol misuse and begin counseling	Screening tools are available at the National Institute on Alcohol Abuse and Alcoholism Web site: www.niaaa.nih.gov/Publications/AlcoholResearch/
Depression	Screen all adults	Many different short screening tools available
Smoking	Screen all adults and provide cessation interventions	
Chronic obstructive pulmonary disease	Screening with spirometry not recommended	American Thoracic Society recommends spirometry for all persons with tobacco exposure

DEXA, dual-energy X-ray absorptiometry; USPSTF, United States Preventive Services Task Force.

REVIEW QUESTIONS

For review questions, please go to www.expertconsult.com.

SUGGESTED READINGS

Advisory Committee on Immunization Practices: Recommended adult immunization schedule: United States, 2009, *Ann Intern Med* 150:40–44, 2009.

Boulware LE, Marinopoulos S, Phillips KA, et al: Systematic review: the value of the periodic health evaluation, *Ann Intern Med* 146(4): 289–300, 2007.

The guide to clinical preventive services, AHRQ Publication No. 08-05122, 2008. Also available online at: www.ahrq.gov/clinic/pocketgd.htm

Petitti DB, Teutsch SM, Barton MB, et al: U.S. Preventive Services Task Force. Update on the methods of the U.S. Preventive Services Task Force: insufficient evidence, *Ann Intern Med* 150(3):199–205, 2009.

Acknowledgement

This chapter was adapted from a chapter written by Jeffrey Magaziner, MD, for the second edition of the *Johns Hopkins Internal Medicine Board Review*.

CHAPTER 75

Clinical Epidemiology

L. EBONY BOULWARE, MD, MPH

Common Terms and Concepts in Research

- Many common terms and concepts derive from the 2 × 2 table (Fig. 75-1)
- Most research questions can be reduced to a 2 × 2 table
- **Prevalence:** The number of **existing cases** of a disease at any given time divided by the total population at that time (see Fig. 75-1)
- **Incidence:** The number of **new cases** of a disease that develop over a specific time divided by the population at risk for developing the disease
  - Prevalence and incidence are related to each other via the duration of disease: **Prevalence = incidence × duration of disease** (P = ID)
  - Example: Before 1972, the prevalence of end-stage renal disease (ESRD) patients was very low (the duration of disease was very short because ESRD patients died at a very high rate without dialysis). After the Medicare dialysis program, the prevalence of ESRD soared (the duration of disease was extended, so prevalence increased)

Validity and Reliability of Diagnostic and Screening Tests

- Sensitivity and specificity: Characteristics of the test that reflect the test's ability to correctly identify disease in any population (see Fig. 75-1)
  - **Sensitivity: The ability of the test to correctly identify persons who have the disease of interest**
    - Example: If a test is able to correctly identify 80 persons (among 100) who have diabetes as having diabetes, the sensitivity of the test is 80/100 (80%)
  - **Specificity: The ability of the test to correctly identify persons who do not have the disease of interest**
    - Example: If a test is able to correctly identify 95 persons (among 100) who do not have diabetes as not having diabetes, the specificity of the test is 95/100 (95%)
- Positive and negative predictive values: The **test result's** likelihood of reflecting disease presence or absence in a specific population (affected by both disease prevalence and specificity of test) (see Fig. 75-1)
  - **Positive predictive value:** The probability that a **positive test in a patient reflects disease**
    - Example: If 200 people test positive for diabetes, but only 80 of those people have diabetes, the positive

predictive value of a positive test is 80/200 = 40%. Note that positive predictive value increases as prevalence increases; of the preceding group of people, if 100 of the 200 had diabetes, positive predictive value would be 100/200 = 50%.
  - **Negative predictive value:** The probability that a **negative test in a patient reflects health (no disease)**
    - Example: If 200 persons test negative for diabetes, but only 40 do not have diabetes, the negative predictive value of the negative test is 40/200 = 20%. Note that negative predictive value increases as prevalence decreases. If 100 of the 200 preceding patients did not have diabetes, negative predictive value would be 100/200 = 50%.

Sources of Error in Measurement, Interpretation, or Analysis

- **Precision:** On repeated measurement of the same sample, **how closely do the results *cluster*?**
  - Precision does not consider how close a result is to truth
  - Precision depends on random error (greater random error results in lower precision; increasing sample size decreases effect of random error)
- **Accuracy: How close to the truth is the result?**
- **Bias: Systematic error,** resulting in decreased accuracy (Table 75-1)
  - Bias is reduced by careful study design
  - Randomization and blinding are powerful tools used in clinical trials to reduce selection and information bias
- Confounding (Fig. 75-2)
  - Confounding describes a relationship between an exposure and an outcome of interest that is distorted by a second exposure that is related to both the outcome and the exposure of interest
    - Simply termed, confounding is guilt by association
    - Confounding is a particular problem in observational studies
- Internal and external validity
  - **Internal validity in a study refers to whether the results accurately reflect the connection between exposure and disease within the population being studied**
    - Randomized clinical trials maximize internal validity through randomization, blinding, and placebo-control
  - **External validity** (i.e., generalizability)
    - Ability of a study to produce **results that can be applied to a target population (beyond the study participants)**

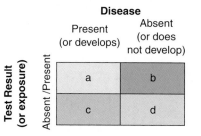

Sensitivity: Of those with disease, what percent test positive? ("sensitivity is positive in disease, or PID")

$$\text{Sensitivity} = a/(a + c)$$

Specificity: Of those without disease, what percent test negative? ("specificity is negative in health, or NIH")

$$\text{Specificity} = d/(b + d)$$

Prevalence: The percentage of a population that has a disease

$$\text{Prevalence} = (a + c)/(a + b + c + d)$$

Positive predictive value: If the test is positive, what percent will have disease? Markedly increases with increasing prevalence

$$\text{PPV} = a/(a + b)$$

Negative predictive value: If the test is negative, what percent will not have the disease? Markedly increases with decreasing prevalence

$$\text{NPV} = d/(c + d)$$

Relative risk: Risk of developing disease in those exposed, divided by the risk of developing disease in those not exposed

$$\text{RR} = \text{Risk(exp)}/\text{Risk(unexp)} = (a/[a + b])/(c/[c + d])$$

Attributable risk (AR): The absolute increase in risk of developing disease in those exposed compared to those not exposed. Absolute risk reduction (ARR) is the absolute decrease in risk among those taking a medication compared to those not taking it

$$\text{AR} = \text{Risk(exp)} - \text{Risk(unexp)} = a/(a + b) - c/(c + d)$$
$$\text{ARR} = \text{Risk(not taking)} - \text{Risk(taking)} = c/(c + d) - a/(a + b)$$

Number needed to treat: How many individuals will need to be treated to prevent a single event?

$$\text{NNT} = 1/\text{ARR}$$

Odds ratio: In individuals with disease, what are the odds of having been exposed compared to those who were exposed who do not have disease?

$$\text{OR} = \text{Odds (exposure in those with disease)}/\text{Odds}$$
$$\text{(exposure in those without disease)}$$
$$\text{OR} = (a/c)/(b/d)$$

FIGURE 75-1 The 2 × 2 table.

- To be externally valid, a study must also be internally valid. A study with restrictive inclusion criteria enhances internal validity at the expense of external validity.
- Analyzing "crossovers" in clinical trials: Intention to treat
  - **Intention to treat is a conservative approach to the analysis of a clinical trial, in which analysis is based on the original assignment of a participant regardless of what assignment the participant actually received in the study**
  - Example: Randomized clinical trial of medical versus surgical treatment of mild carotid stenosis; if some in the medical arm cross over into the surgical arm, why not analyze them in the surgical group? Suppose most of those who crossed over had transient ischemic attacks (TIAs): If they are counted in

TABLE 75-1	*Types of Bias*
Type of Bias	**Example**
Selection bias: When those chosen for a study (or those leaving a study) systematically differ from those not chosen (or those not leaving) with respect to characteristics important to the study question	In a case-control study of pancreatic cancer, controls are chosen from a GI clinic. If the controls from the GI clinic are avoiding coffee because of GI side effects, this will tend to create a false association between coffee drinking and pancreatic cancer, resulting simply from the control group that was chosen.
Information bias: Occurs when individuals of a particular exposure or outcome are systematically erroneously classified as having a different exposure or outcome. For instance, recall bias: When individuals with a particular outcome retrospectively recall an exposure, their memory may be influenced by the event itself	Mothers of infants with a birth defect are more likely to remember taking a medication than other mothers. This will tend to create a false association between the medication use and birth defects.
Lead-time bias: Seen in studies of screening tests, in which identification of disease at an earlier stage will "lengthen" apparent survival, even if prognosis is not improved	A new test for detecting pancreatic cancer is associated with a doubling of survival time. However, the test merely detected the cancer at an earlier, untreatable stage.
Length bias: Seen in studies of screening tests when screening a population will detect those with the longest survival (i.e., less severe disease) more than those with shorter survival (i.e., more severe disease), thus creating the illusion that the screening test prolongs survival when in fact it does not	A new screening test for renal cell cancer is performed every 5 yr. Survival rates in the screened group are 7 yr, as compared with 4 yr in an unscreened group. Those with more aggressive disease die before the screening interval, so that those screened have less aggressive disease.

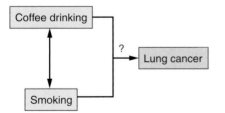

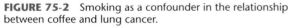

FIGURE 75-2 Smoking as a confounder in the relationship between coffee and lung cancer.

the surgical group, they will enrich (i.e., bias) the surgical arm with those who are more likely to have strokes (i.e., it will make surgery look worse than it really is).

- When performing analyses using "intention to treat," the preceding crossover will bias the relative risk

toward the null (result demonstrating less difference between study groups) but will never bias the association away from the null (result demonstrating more difference between study groups)
- "As-treated" analysis has potential to bias away from the null

Study Design

- **Observational studies: No intervention performed;** observations made between exposures and outcomes (Table 75-2)
  - Strengths
    - Only way possible to study a number of important research questions (e.g., prognostic effect of disease)
    - More likely to reflect real-world situations (external generalizability)
    - Less expensive and generally faster to perform than randomized controlled trials
  - Limitations
    - Lower validity
    - More subject to bias and confounding of results
- Experimental studies: The randomized clinical trial (RCT)
  - **RCTs are a true experiment, the purpose of which is to test interventions**
    - Example: Does treating hypertensive patients with antihypertensive therapy reduce cardiovascular events?
  - Strengths
    - The gold standard study design to evaluate therapeutic interventions without bias or confounding
    - Stronger internal validity than cohort studies
  - Limitations
    - Limited to questions of clinical equipoise and clinical benefit
    - The study is run under ideal conditions and therefore most often measures efficacy, not effectiveness: **Efficacy refers to how the intervention performs under ideal conditions. Effectiveness refers to how the intervention performs in the real world.**
    - Generalizability often can be questioned
- Data synthesis studies
  - Qualitative review article: No explicit methods; must trust author's judgment
  - Practice guidelines: Consensus statements; quality varies
  - Decision analysis
    - Create a decision analysis tree, assign probabilities and utilities
    - Calculate the expected value of various decisions
  - Systematic review and meta-analysis
    - Explicit methods to review and possibly pool or combine (meta-analysis) data from multiple studies
    - **Beware of meta-analysis of observational studies** (pooled results may reflect bias or confounding in individual studies)
    - Publication bias: Positive studies are published more than negative studies and are most often included in systematic reviews, meta-analyses

75

TABLE 75-2	*Types of Observational Studies*		
Name	**Design/Example**	**Strengths**	**Weaknesses**
Case report/series	Observations from clinical practice. *Example:* Case report of seizure associated with cat-scratch disease	Useful for generating hypotheses	Limited use in clinical decision making; no control group; selection bias
Ecologic study	Compare average exposure with average outcome between populations. *Example:* Comparison of mean salt intake and mean BP in United States and Japan	Useful for generating hypotheses; can be used to compare prevalence of disease or exposures in various populations	No individual data; not useful for demonstrating causation
Cross-sectional study	Determine exposure and disease status simultaneously in a representative sample of a population. *Example:* Prevalence of *Chlamydia* antibodies in patients with coronary artery disease	Good initial step in evaluating associations; useful for public health surveys	Causation cannot be determined; temporal relationship not defined; cannot evaluate prognosis
Case-control study (retrospective study)	Identify cases (with disease) and select controls (without disease). Determine exposure status retrospectively in both groups. *Example:* Is history of head trauma greater in Alzheimer's patients than in controls?	Lower cost than cohort studies; useful for studying uncommon diseases	Susceptible to recall bias and selection bias; cannot evaluate prevalence, incidence, prognosis; can only determine odds ratio
Cohort study (prospective study)	Prospective study of subgroup in a population that share a particular characteristic; determine exposure at beginning and ascertain outcomes with follow-up over time. *Example:* Incidence of mesothelioma in steel mill workers who smoke	Studies incidence and prognosis; establishes temporal relationships; strong external validity	Long and costly; limited in studying treatment effects

Measures of Risk Reduction

See also Figure 75-1

- Example: Results of a recently performed RCT demonstrating patients' 5-year risk of death from breast cancer on treatment A versus treatment B are 50% versus 40%, respectively
- **Absolute risk reduction** (absolute improvement provided by treatment B versus treatment A) is 50% − 40% = 10%
- **Relative risk reduction** (improvement provided by treatment B relative to treatment A) is 50% − 40%/50% = 20%
- **Number needed to treat** (NNT) (number of patients needed to treat with treatment B to prevent one

additional death over 5 years compared with what would happen with treatment A [NNT = 1/Absolute risk reduction]) is 1/0.1 = 10

REVIEW QUESTIONS

For review questions, please go to www.expertconsult.com.

SUGGESTED READINGS

Gordis L: Epidemiology, Philadelphia, WB Saunders, 1996.
Last JM: A dictionary of epidemiology, New York, Oxford Press, 1995.
Sackett DL, Haynes RB, Guyatt GH, et al: Clinical epidemiology: a basic science for clinical medicine, Boston, Little Brown, 1991.

Medical Ethics

MARK T. HUGHES, MD, MA

Ethics is the systematic study of human actions with respect to good and bad, right and wrong, what should and should not be done, and the character of the individuals involved in the actions. The field of bioethics had its birth about 30 years ago, but medical ethics can be traced back millennia to professional codes and standards of conduct, including the Hippocratic Oath. Clinical bioethics deals with the interface between moral philosophy and health care.

General Principles

- **Respect for autonomy: Self-rule, self-determination**
  - Respect for autonomy is the cornerstone principle for informed consent (allowing the patient to make an informed decision about his medical care) and confidentiality (respecting the individual's privacy)
  - Respect for persons acknowledges the patient as an individual and also as a member of various groups. The physician should pay attention to the individual and cultural identification of the patient when determining a treatment plan.
- **Beneficence: Acting in the best interests of the individual**
  - An inherent duty in medicine, in which a vulnerable patient seeks the help from one who professes to be a healer
- **Nonmaleficence: Enjoins the physician not to pursue interventions that are harmful to the patient, especially if the possibility of medical good cannot be achieved (primum, non nocere, or "first, do no harm")**
- **Justice: Fairness, similars should be treated similarly**
  - In health care ethics, one generally considers justice in terms of distributive justice—that is, how scarce resources are distributed
- **Professionalism: The elements of professionalism include expertise and competence, self-regulation, subjugation of self-interest, and an ongoing dialogue with society**
  - In medicine, professionalism is best exemplified in the Hippocratic tradition, in which one takes an oath to uphold certain values with respect to patients and colleagues on entering the profession
  - Codes of ethics propagate the standards of the profession. Professional organizations such as the American Medical Association (AMA) codify what it means to be a responsible physician attentive to the needs of the patient and society.

- Issues in professionalism include commitment to lifelong learning, the power differential between physician and patient, the societal role of physicians to prescribe medications and determine disability, truth-telling, communication skills in breaking bad news and engaging in difficult encounters, response to medical errors, physician impairment, reimbursement for services, competition, conflicts of interest, and conflicts of obligation

Selected Issues

- Medical economics: Response to the perceived scarcity of health care resources, the escalating costs of health care, the increasing number of uninsured and underinsured patients, and the fiduciary responsibilities of the physician caring for patients in the medical marketplace
  - Issues in medical economics include triage of patients for limited ICU beds, drug formularies, denial of services dictated by managed care organizations, gaming the system, pay-for-performance reimbursement standards, physicians as employees, and physicians as stockholders
- Confidentiality: Protection of information shared in confidence between physician and patient, extending also to information systems that need safeguards to ensure privacy
  - Confidentiality is felt to be important to adequately treat the patient (i.e., the patient must feel comfortable disclosing personal information, so that a complete picture of his condition can be made)
  - Confidentiality may be breached only if all of the following criteria are met
    - Identifiable third party at risk of harm
    - A high probability of serious harm exists
    - A likely benefit will result from breaking the confidence
    - All other avenues of disclosing the information are unavailable
- Informed consent: The patient should be an active participant in the decision-making process and has the right to accept or refuse medical treatment; involves the following
  - Disclosure of information: Providing sufficient information on condition, risks, benefits, and options; usual standard is what would be expected by a reasonable person to make a decision
  - Voluntariness: Ensuring that the patient's decision is made free of undue influence, such as coercion,

improper persuasion, or manipulation (framing effects when giving information)

- Comprehension: Confirming that the patient understands what has been disclosed about the proposed test or treatment, and the patient's questions have been answered
- Decision-making capacity (competency; Box 76-1)
  - Sliding scale notion of competency: Determination of capacity depends on the decision to be made, with complex or riskier decisions requiring a higher threshold in assessing capacity
- Surrogate decision making: **Situation in which a person is selected to make medical decisions on behalf of a patient who does not have the capacity to make her own decisions**
  - The surrogate can be preselected by the patient in an advance directive or selected by the medical team based on a hierarchy of relationships established by law (Box 76-2)
    - The morally appropriate surrogate for a particular patient might differ from the person selected by the legal hierarchy, as when a patient has been estranged from his family or has a close friend or significant other who knows his wishes and values more intimately. The physician in these circumstances should be guided by her conscience and legal advice as to whom to select as the surrogate.
  - Standards of surrogate decision making
    - Substituted judgment: Surrogate makes decision based on knowledge of the incompetent patient's previously expressed values and goals

- Best interests: Surrogate weighs risks and benefits of each option available in given situation for incompetent patient in order to make decision
- **Emergency situations: Physician can act without surrogate consent when an action to save life or prevent significant harm must be taken immediately and cannot wait for the time needed to contact next of kin**

End of Life Issues

- Patient Self-Determination Act of 1991: Federal law passed requiring health care organizations to inform patients that they have the right to make medical decisions and to execute advance directives
- Advance directives: Two types of documents completed by a competent patient in anticipation of one day being unable to speak for himself (Box 76-3)
  - Appointment of health care agent or proxy (i.e., the durable power of attorney for health care): Naming surrogate with or without explicit instructions about future care
  - Living will: Specifying wishes of medical care when the patient has a terminal medical condition, coma, or persistent vegetative state
- Advance care planning: Places an emphasis on finding out about the "authentic" preferences that reflect the values important to the patient
  - Includes traditional elements of advance directives such as health care agent appointment and scenario-based decisional preferences
  - Also covers such items as how to deal with medical uncertainty, patient wishes about comfort, how others should treat the patient at the end of life, what loved

---

BOX 76-1	*Decision-Making Capacity*

Decision-making capacity (competency): The ability to make health care decisions

Assessment of decision-making capacity involves the following:

Ability to communicate a choice and preference

Ability to understand medical condition

Ability to understand consequences of condition and treatment(s)

Judgment not impaired (e.g., through depression or substance abuse)

Consistency with previously expressed wishes or values

Ability to reason about medical situation, risks, and benefits

Making a decision (with some fixity in decision made)

BOX 76-2	*Legal Hierarchy of Surrogate Decision Makers*

1. Health care agent designated by patient
2. Court-appointed guardian
3. Spouse (or domestic partner in some states)
4. Adult child
5. Parent
6. Sibling
7. Other relative
8. Close friend

BOX 76-3	*Types of Advance Directives*

Durable Power of Attorney for Health Care (Health Care Agent)

Designated by the patient when competent

Takes effect once patient loses capacity

Applies even in nonterminal conditions

Most effective when prior discussion has occurred

When activated, designated health care agent can consent to or withhold or withdraw medical treatments

Some states make exceptions regarding decisions about artificial nutrition and hydration, involuntary psychiatric admission, psychosurgery, and sterilization

Living Will

Specifies patient's wishes in event of incapacitation

Applies in terminal condition, persistent vegetative state, coma

Typically advances comfort care approach when death is imminent

Wishes may be too general to provide guidance in particular situations

Must be witnessed by adults unrelated to patient, with no financial conflict of interest

ones should know about the patient, the patient's thoughts and feelings about death, options regarding organ donation, funeral arrangements and what the patient would want at a memorial service, and how the patient would want to be remembered by family and friends

- Do not (attempt to) resuscitate (DNR) orders: Applies only to resuscitation efforts (CPR, defibrillation, tracheal intubation) in the event of cardiac or pulmonary arrest
  - Other measures of concurrent care (monitoring in a critical care setting, vasopressors, chemical antiarrhythmics, electrical cardioversion, external pacemakers, mechanical ventilation for conditions short of pulmonary arrest, artificial nutrition and hydration) require separate consent procedure and are not included within a DNR order
  - "Do not intubate" orders are used by some health care facilities for patients who would opt against mechanical ventilation under any circumstances
  - Because DNR is a medical order written by a physician, a patient does not sign a DNR. Most states, however, require at least prior discussion with the patient or surrogate, if not a full informed-consent process, before the physician can institute a DNR order. The reasons for writing a DNR order should be documented in the medical record.
  - Generally, states have specific requirements for outpatient DNR orders and for transfer of DNR orders from a chronic nursing facility to a hospital. Typically, a separate form needs to be completed to specify that the DNR order endures after the hospitalization, and this documentation should be readily available to other health care providers, such as emergency medical technicians.
- Ordinary versus extraordinary care
  - Ordinary care: Benefits outweigh risks and burdens, such that care is to be pursued at the patient's or surrogate's discretion in an effort to preserve life
  - **Extraordinary care: Risks and burdens outweigh benefits.** If the means to preserve life are excessively burdensome and beyond that expected of a reasonable person, treatment is considered above and beyond the call of duty, and need not be pursued. Extraordinary care has nothing to do with how technologically advanced the treatment is, as even everyday treatments can be considered extraordinary if they are overly burdensome.
- **Futility: When treatment is medically ineffective or not able to achieve the desired goal as set forth by the treatment team, the patient, or the surrogate**
  - Quantitative futility (physiologic futility): Treatment cannot achieve the desired physiologic effect (e.g., restoration of heart rhythm)

- Most states have laws that recognize that physicians are not obligated to provide treatments that are ineffective or outside the bounds of good medical care
- Qualitative futility: Treatment is considered futile because certain goals with respect to the patient's quality of life cannot be met. For instance, a surrogate may judge mechanical ventilation to be qualitatively futile in a patient permanently comatose, even though it achieves the physiologic effect of maintaining respiration and ventilation.
  - The standards for determining qualitative futility ultimately reside with the patient or surrogate
  - The physician can help in discussing qualitative futility with the patient or surrogate but generally cannot unilaterally forego treatment on the basis of the physician's personal assessment of the patient's quality of life
- Conflict may arise when there is a dispute between the treatment team and the patient or surrogate regarding whether treatment constitutes futile care
  - Discussion regarding potentially futile treatment should focus on mutually agreed on goals of care
  - If dispute persists despite ongoing dialogue and involvement of ethics consultants, then transfer to another facility or physician should be pursued
  - State laws differ on whether and how physicians can unilaterally forego medical treatment without consent of surrogate
- Euthanasia and physician-assisted suicide
  - Euthanasia: Intentional act to cause the (immediate) death of another person, usually by administration of a lethal drug
    - Illegal in all states
  - Physician-assisted suicide: Physician prescribes medication to the patient with instructions on how to commit suicide
    - Legal only in Oregon
  - The physician should ensure proper palliative care so that patients do not view these as their only options

REVIEW QUESTIONS

For review questions, please go to www.expertconsult.com.

SUGGESTED READINGS

Beauchamp TL, Childress JF: *Principles of biomedical ethics*, ed 5, New York, Oxford University Press, 2001.
Fletcher JC, Hite CA, Lombardo PA, et al: *Introduction to clinical ethics*, Frederick, MD, University Publishing Group, 1995.
Junkerman CJ, Schiedermayer D: *Practical ethics for students, interns, and residents*, Frederick, MD, University Publishing Group, 1998.
Pellegrino ED, Thomasma DC: *A philosophical basis of medical practice*, New York, Oxford University Press, 1981.
Sugarman J: *Ethics in primary care*, New York, McGraw-Hill, 2000.

76

INDEX

Note: Page numbers followed by b refer to boxed material; those followed by f refer to figures; those followed by t refer to tables.

A

Abacavir, adverse effects of, 93t
Abatacept for rheumatoid arthritis, 349t
Abdominal aortic aneurysm, screening for, 593
Abscesses
  epidural, spinal, 494t
  hepatic, 236
Abuse, domestic, 553, 553b
Acamprosate for alcohol abuse, 581
Acanthocytes, 424f, 427t
Acanthosis nigricans
  in cancer, 537t
  in diabetes mellitus, 285, 287f, 533, 534f
Acarbose for diabetes mellitus, 288, 289t
Accuracy, definition of, 595
Acetaminophen, 346
  toxicity of, 183t
Achalasia, 202–203, 203f
Achilles tendinitis, 364
Achilles tendon rupture, 364
Acid-base disorders, 247f, 247–251. *See also specific disorders.*
Acidosis
  in chronic renal insufficiency, 273t
  metabolic. *See* Metabolic acidosis.
  renal tubular, 251–252, 251t
    type 1, 251, 252t
    type 2, 251–252, 251t
    type 4, 251t, 254
  respiratory, 247f, 250
Acne, adrenal androgen excess and, 337
Acne rosacea, 518, 518f
Acne vulgaris, 517–518, 517f
  clinical presentation and diagnosis of, 517
  differential diagnosis of, 518t
  treatment of, 517–518
Acquired immunodeficiency syndrome. *See* HIV infections.
Acromegaly, 329, 330, 330f
  paraneoplastic, 465
ACTH stimulation test in adrenal insufficiency, 339
Actinic keratosis, 529, 529f
Activated partial thromboplastin time, in bleeding disorders, 410
Activated protein C
  resistance to, 163, 412t
  for sepsis, 180
Acupuncture, 572–573
  for migraine prevention, 475
Acute coronary syndromes, 29–36. *See also* Angina, unstable; Myocardial infarction.
  care following myocardial infarction and, 35
  clinical presentation of, 30
  definitions of, 29, 31t
  diagnosis and evaluation of, 29–32, 31b, 31f, 32t
  differential diagnosis of, 31–32
  epidemiology of, 29
  pathophysiology of, 29, 30f
  secondary prevention of, 35
  treatment of, 32–34, 33f, 34f, 35t–36t
    pharmacologic, 32–34, 33f, 35t
    reperfusion therapy for, 33
Acute idiopathic demyelinating polyneuropathy, 496t
Acute-phase reactions, 554

Acute renal failure, 260–265, 261t
  intrarenal, 260, 260f, 262–264, 262t
    acute tubular necrosis and, 262f, 262t, 262–263
    contrast-induced nephropathy and, 262t, 263
    glomerulonephritis and, 262t
    interstitial nephritis and, 262t, 263, 263f
    pigment nephropathy and, 262t, 264
    renal artery embolic disease and, 262t, 263–264
  postrenal, 260, 260f, 264–265, 265f
    clinical presentation of, 265
    diagnosis of, 265, 265f
    treatment of, 265
  prerenal, 260–262, 260f
    clinical presentation of, 261
    diagnosis of, 261, 261t
    treatment of, 262
Acute respiratory distress syndrome, 178, 179f
Adalimumab for rheumatoid arthritis, 349t
Adenocarcinoma
  esophageal, 203–204
  of lung, 467
  pancreatic, 209
  prostatic, 44
  as unidentified tumor type, 461
  urothelial, 445
Adenomas. *See also* Familial adenomatous polyposis.
  adrenal, hypercortisolism due to, 330, 331f
  drug-induced, 227t
  hepatic, 236
  pituitary, 327, 327f
    hypercortisolism due to, 330
    hypopituitarism and, 331–332
Adhesive capsulitis, 360
Adrenal adenomas, hypercortisolism due to, 330, 331f
Adrenal disease, 335–340. *See also specific disorders.*
Adrenal gland, 335, 336t
Adrenal hormone excess states, 335–338
Adrenal hyperplasia, congenital, 320, 321b, 338f
Adrenal incidentalomas, 335
Adrenal insufficiency, 338–339
  clinical presentation of, 339
  diagnosis of, 339
  treatment of, 339, 340f
α-Adrenergic antagonists for hypertension, 13t
β-Adrenergic antagonists
  for acute coronary syndromes, 32, 34
  for coronary artery disease, 26–27
  for heart failure, 52
  for hypertension, 13t
  for portal hypertension, 238
  surgery and, 585–586, 586t
  for thyrotoxicosis, 298
  toxicity of, 182
Adrenocorticotropic hormone, 326, 328t
  deficiency of, 333
Adult T-cell deficiencies, 558t
Advance care planning, 600–601
Advance directives, 600–601, 600b
Age-related macular degeneration, 540–541, 540f
  clinical presentation and diagnosis of, 540, 541f
  treatment of, 541